Health Psychology

Applying Psychological Science to Health and Wellness

JEFFREY S. NEVID
St. John's University

SPENCER A. RATHUS
College of New Jersey

WILEY

Vice President: Amanda Miller
Senior Editorial Director: Justin Jeffryes
Executive Editor: Glenn Wilson
Senior Managing Editor: Judy Howarth
Senior Editorial Assistant: Kelly Gomez
Creative Product Design Lead: Nicholas Wehrkamp
Senior Creative Product Designer: Thomas Nery
Senior Manager, Content Enablement & Operations: Simon Eckley
Cover Photo: © PeopleImages/Getty Images

Published by John Wiley & Sons, Inc., Hoboken, New Jersey.
Published simultaneously in Canada.

Library of Congress Cataloging-in-Publication Data

Names: Nevid, Jeffrey S., author. | Rathus, Spencer A., author.
Title: Health psychology : applying psychological science to health and wellness / Jeffrey S. Nevid, Spencer A. Rathus.
Description: First edition. | [Hoboken, NJ] : Wiley, [2024] | Includes bibliographical references and index.
Identifiers: LCCN 2024018188 (print) | LCCN 2024018189 (ebook) | ISBN 9781394227631 (hardback) | ISBN 9781394227655 (adobe pdf) | ISBN 9781394227686 (ebook)
Subjects: LCSH: Clinical health psychology--Textbooks.
Classification: LCC R726.7 .N48 2024 (print) | LCC R726.7 (ebook) | DDC 613.01/9—dc23/eng/20240603
LC record available at https://lccn.loc.gov/2024018188
LC ebook record available at https://lccn.loc.gov/2024018189

SKY10097904_020625

DEDICATIONS

Jeff Nevid:
To my son Michael and daughter-in-law Ariel, who are healthcare professionals, to my daughter, Daniella, who is beginning her career as a healthcare professional, and to our grandson Asher, who is well on his way to living a healthy life.

Spence Rathus:
To Marchie, Eliot, and Theodora (Empress-in-training for the Byzantine Empire), Elio, and Wren—new delights, all.

Preface

Health Psychology: Applying Psychological Science to Health and Wellness

As we navigate our way in a post-pandemic world, one of the lessons we carry with us is the importance of practicing healthy behaviors to protect ourselves and others from infectious disease as well as fostering personal health and wellness throughout our lives. Psychological science is making major contributions to our understanding of factors determining health and longevity, and we are excited to bring these latest developments to students of health psychology.

Our overriding goal in writing this text was to bring research findings and applications in health psychology to students in a way that is accessible, engaging, and relevant to their lives. We adopt a pedagogical approach designed to help students succeed in the course and acquire an understanding of the many applications of health psychology in our daily lives.

This text takes a fresh, new look at health psychology through a lens that encompasses a broader perspective than many traditional texts. While we cover topics typically represented in a course in health psychology, we also explore important topics that may not have received as much attention, such as reproductive and sexual health (see Chapter 10) and psychological health (see Chapter 11). Health psychologists focus on the health and well-being of the whole person, and we believe that issues regarding reproductive, sexual, and psychological health should receive their proper emphasis.

We also approached the preparation of this text with several other important goals in mind:

- To provide students with an understanding of the body systems directly in the chapters in which they are relevant to the topic at hand to avoid such information becoming a jumble of unanchored biological facts; as examples, see the discussion of the immune system in Chapter 4, the digestive system in Chapter 7, the reproductive system in Chapter 10, and the cardiovascular system in Chapter 12.
- To present material in a fashion that engages students, using a more personal writing style that makes reading the text more appealing to students.
- To emphasize the applications of health psychology in our daily lives, as found in the ***Applying Health Psychology*** feature.
- To include features that pique curiosity and interest in reading further, such as the chapter-opening ***Did You Know That?*** feature, ***Self-Assessment***, ***Health Psychology in the Digital Age***, ***Health Psychology in Action***, and ***A Closer Look***.
- To incorporate a complete pedagogical package to help students understand and remember the subject matter by showing them where they are going (see the learning objectives at the start of each chapter)), and then showing them where they have been and what they have achieved (see the section reviews and the end-of-chapter reviews).
- To encourage critical and scientific thinking by outlining principles of critical thinking and providing the latest research findings in health psychology, with many hundreds of citations to research findings reported since 2020.

Designed to Expand Coverage in a Semester-Friendly Format

Health Psychology covers topics traditionally addressed in a mainstream health psychology course. However, it also provides more breadth and depth in many important health-related topics that might not be found in other texts, including dedicated chapters focusing on important topical areas relating to reproductive and sexual health (Chapter 10) and psychological health (Chapter 11).

With respect to reproductive health, we go beyond just identifying parts of the human reproductive system and noting some health-related concerns to encompass a more thorough exploration of reproductive health issues, including coverage of health-related topics such as managing menstrual discomfort, behavioral factors in coping with menopause, and postpartum psychological adjustment.

Similarly, issues relating to sexual health are more fully integrated in the text. Chapter 10 presents a health psychology perspective on issues relating to sexual behavior, including coverage of many sexually transmitted infections and their prevention (not just HIV/AIDS), decision making about reproductive options, sexual dysfunctions, and the health of sexual and gender minorities. *Health Psychology* takes the position that we should understand the specific health needs that affect sexual and gender minorities and the psychological and cultural barriers limiting access to health care for people from traditionally disadvantaged groups.

Other texts may briefly refer to issues of psychological health such as anxiety and depression. We believe, however, that psychological health is an important aspect of our overall health and well-being and that it should be examined more fully from the standpoint of the biopsychosocial model. Moreover, health psychology issues such as adherence to treatment and theories of health behavior apply to psychological health as well as they do to, for example, cardiovascular disorders and cancer.

The text is presented in a 15-chapter format designed to meet the contours of a typical semester course, so that instructors can schedule about one chapter a week during a standard semester. Here is a listing of the chapters:

1. Foundations of Health Psychology
2. Theories of Health Behavior: Adherence and Change
3. The Healthcare System
4. Stress and the Immune System
5. Resilience and Coping
6. Understanding and Managing Pain
7. Healthy Living: Nutrition, Weight-Management, and Physical Activity
8. Playing It Safe: Reducing Health Risks by Practicing Safety Behaviors
9. Substance Use and Abuse
10. Reproductive and Sexual Health
11. Psychological Health
12. Cardiovascular Health
13. Cancer
14. Chronic Diseases and End-of-Life Issues
15. New Directions in Health Psychology

Designed with Applications of Psychological Science in Mind

One of the cardinal themes in health psychology is the application of theory and research to fostering health and wellness. In the ***Health Psychology in Action*** feature, we explore how theory is applied to practice and focus on the many research contributions of health psychologists. Examples of the ***Health Psychology in Action*** features include the following:

- Field Studies Using the Health Belief Model
- A Health Psychologist Applies the CSM Model in the Hospital
- Lockdown! Building Resilience in Times of Crisis
- Knowing the Facts About Sugar and Health
- The Theory of Planned Behavior and Risky Subway Riding—Chinese Style
- Vape No More: The Use of Contingency Management in Quitting Vaping
- Role of Health Psychology in Prostate Cancer Prevention and Treatment
- Cognitive Behavior Therapy Goes Digital in Treating Illness Anxiety Disorder
- Should Salt Shakers Carry Tobacco-Style Health Warnings?
- Using the CSM Model to Change Intentions to Practice Sun Protective Behaviors
- A Day in the Life of a Cancer Care Psychologist
- Dia de los Muertos—Coping with Loss ... and with Discrimination

Designed to Engage Student Interest

The pedagogical features of *Health Psychology* are intended to stoke student interest as well as to inform. These features include ***Health Psychology in the Digital Age***, *Self-Assessment*, *Applying Health Psychology,* and *A Closer Look* sections.

Health Psychology in the Digital Age

No reader today will need convincing that professors and students alike have embraced the digital age. We shop online, find recipes online, conduct research online, share our lives through online social networks, and communicate online.

The ***Health Psychology in the Digital Age*** feature focuses on the role of digital devices in our health and well-being. These features highlight the dangers and pitfalls of the digital age but also emphasize ways in which mobile phones, tablets, laptops, and desktop computers can have positive impacts on our health and well-being. Here are some examples:

- Telemedicine for Pandemics—Virtually Perfect?
- "Calm"
- Texting Your Way to a Slimmer Figure
- Rape Prevention? There's an App for That (Actually, There Are Several)
- Internet Addiction
- Symptoms of Menopause There's an App for That—Actually, There Are Several
- Apps That Predict Safe Periods for Sex
- Little Miss Muffet Confronts a Spider—Virtually
- Is Social Media a Risk to Psychological Health?
- Texting to Manage Diabetes

Self-Assessment

Self-scoring questionnaires stimulate student interest and expand self-awareness of health-related attitudes and behaviors and underscore the relevance of course content to the daily lives of our students. These features also enhance the relevance of the text to students' lives.
Examples include:

- Locus of Control Scale
- What Would You Say? Beliefs Associated with Nonadherence to Medical Treatment
- Are You an Active or a Passive Healthcare Consumer?
- How Much Stress Have You Experienced?
- Are You an Optimist or a Pessimist?

- The Brief COPE
- The Short-Form McGill Pain Questionnaire
- Are You Getting Your Zs?
- Is Drinking Becoming a Problem for You?
- Are You Depressed?
- Assessing Personal Risk Factors for Cancer

Applying Health Psychology

Application sections highlight knowledge that students can apply in their daily lives to help them adopt healthier behaviors. We advise readers when we believe they might profit from visiting a health professional, but we also point out what readers can do for themselves. Examples of ***Applying Health Psychology*** features include the following:

- Thinking Critically When Surfing Online
- Preventing Burnout
- Eating Right on Campus
- Developing Healthy Habits for Getting to Sleep and Staying Asleep
- Managing Menstrual Discomfort
- Preventing Repetitive Stress Injuries
- Coping with Depression
- Putting Cancer-Preventive Behaviors into Practice
- Suicide Prevention

A Closer Look

A Closer Look provides in-depth discussions of high interest or current topics. Examples include:

- Colorectal Screening: Celebrate Life for Years to Come
- Stress in America
- Active Versus Passive Coping
- The Opioid Epidemic
- A Snapshot of College Drinking
- Women and Coronary Heart Disease
- Why Are More Women Depressed Than Men?

Did You Know That?

Did You Know That? chapter openers stimulate student interest by whetting their appetite to learn more about the material covered in the chapter. Here is a small sample:

Did you know that . . .

- More than a million deaths each year are preventable?
- Thinking that the flu is just a bad cold can make you less likely to obtain a flu shot?
- Subtle cues, such as the background color of a printed health message, affected students' intentions to use sunscreen to prevent skin cancer?
- People may commit microaggressions against other people even when they are unaware they are doing so?
- The neighborhood in which you live can be hazardous to your health?
- Fear can give you indigestion?
- You are more likely to contract the common cold when you are under stress?
- A person may rationalize not wearing face masks during a pandemic by saying, "I don't see other people wearing them"?
- Optimistic people tend to live longer?
- The brain produces its own pain-killing chemicals that are similar in chemical structure to narcotics?
- People with chronic pain are likely to do better by taking on more physical activity and household responsibilities than by doing less?
- Health psychologists find that people tend to eat more when food is served on larger plates?
- Exercise helps combat feelings of anxiety and depression?
- There's no place like home—for accidents, that is?
- More people in the United States die each year from smoking-related illnesses than from motor vehicle accidents, alcohol and drug abuse, suicide, homicide, and HIV/AIDS combined?
- Many of the risk factors for cardiovascular disease involve health behaviors that we can control?
- Persistent anger and hostility can be dangerous for your heart?
- Cancer is not one disease but many?
- Cancer of the lung and bronchus takes the lives of more women than breast cancer?
- Fewer than 2% of health claims made by eHealth apps have been validated in scientific studies?
- Only about one in three college students in a national survey fit a healthy profile in terms of health risk behaviors?

Designed to Help Students Learn

The pedagogical model we adopt in the text is adapted from the SQ4R study method originated by educational psychologist Francis Robinson. The SQ4R method enhances learning by encouraging students to adopt a more active role in the learning process. It is designed to help students develop more effective study habits and to absorb and apply the information in the text. The acronym SQ4R stands for the steps:

- Survey
- Question
- Read
- Recite
- Reflect
- Review

Survey

The learning objectives at the start of each chapter serve as advance organizers, guiding students to identify the major learning goals in the chapter. Learning objectives are framed in terms of active learning verbs that emphasize active learning—to Define, Describe, Discuss, Evaluate, and List.

Question

Many students find it helpful to read and complete assignments when they have a clear purpose in mind—in this case, to answer questions that challenge them to retrieve and recite knowledge they have acquired. As noted, the "Did you know that ..." questions that begin each chapter are explained in the body of the text. These questions highlight key issues and points that are addressed in the chapter. Students can be encouraged to test themselves after they have read the chapter to see whether they can explain why each of these items is true. Also, the "Think About It" questions in the section reviews are posed in question format to encourage students to reflect more deeply about material they encounter in the text.

Read

Surveying the material in each chapter by flipping through the pages and picking out key terms helps students prepare for their reading of the text. Key terms are defined directly in the margins of the text so as not to break the flow of reading when students encounter new terms. Students may also find it helpful to survey the chapter summaries before they read through the chapter itself. We made every effort to stimulate student engagement by using inviting chapter-opening features, personal stories and vignettes, and adopting an accessible writing style. We hope this will prompt engagement and further reading.

Recite

Students can be encouraged to consider converting section headings into questions they can pose to themselves as they read through the text. We help guide them through reciting what they have learned by posing questions in the Recite—An Active Summary sections at the end of each chapter. Answering these questions "in their heads" or aloud helps make their learning a more active process and connects learning with parts of the brain used in speech.

Reflect

Students learn more effectively when they reflect on what they are learning. Psychologists who study learning and memory refer to reflection as elaborative rehearsal. One way of reflecting on subject matter is to relate it to information one already knows about, whether it be related material or events or experiences in one's own life. Reflection makes material meaningful and easier to remember. It also makes it more likely that students will be able to apply the information to their own lives.

Think About It items in section reviews in each chapter are designed to help students reflect more deeply about information in the text and apply it to their own lives. Not only does reflection strengthen new learning, but it also encourages deeper processing and helps students relate course material to their own lives. Instructors can use these writing prompts for writing assignments or extra credit assignments. Examples of ***Think About It*** items include the following:

- How would you apply the concepts of predisposing factors, enabling factors, and reinforcing factors to help someone else, or help yourself, make healthy behavior changes?
- How do you respond to the first signs of illness? How might the common-sense model predict your illness behaviors?
- What challenges do you face in your life? Do you view the challenges as insurmountable obstacles or as opportunities to grow as a person? How does your answer relate to your sense of your psychological hardiness?
- Do you or someone close to you live with chronic pain? What steps can you take to help yourself or another person with chronic pain? What techniques discussed in the text might you find helpful?
- Do you or someone close to you suffer from a diagnosable psychological disorder? Have you or they sought professional help? Why or why not?
- What are your personal risk factors for CVD? Which of these factors can you change? How would you go about changing them?
- Do you or does someone you know have diabetes? What steps can you or they make to manage the disease more effectively? What can you do to reduce your risk factors for diabetes?
- Do you use health apps? Why or why not? What factors would determine whether you would choose to use a health app? What questions should you ask before using a health app?

Review

Each section of each chapter is followed by a ***Review*** section. The ***Review*** contains sentence completion items, which encourage students to retrieve from memory what they have learned in a more active way.

Each chapter also ends with a review section, called ***Recite: An Active Summary***, that revisits the ***Learning Objectives*** posed at the beginning of the chapter. We encourage students to provide their own responses to the learning objectives and then compare their responses with sample responses provided in the text. We also find it useful to encourage our students to apply the principle of distributed practice by reviewing text material on a regularly scheduled basis rather than cramming before exams.

Acknowledgments

We are especially grateful to the many scholars, teachers, and researchers whose contributions to the field of health psychology are represented in this text. We are also grateful to our professional colleagues who provided feedback, encouragement, and advice in helping us prepare and strengthen this manuscript. We would also like to acknowledge Jason S. Spiegelman, associate professor of psychology at the Community College of Baltimore County for creating the Instructor's Manual and Test Bank to accompany this text.

We are also indebted to many fine professionals at John Wiley & Sons who supported our work, showed incredible patience with the constant back and forth as we fine-tuned and updated our material, and who guided the process of bringing this effort to fruition. In particular, we wish to thank Senior Editor Glenn Wilson, who spearheaded the development of the text, kept us on track, and helped us sharpen our focus, and the fabulous team of production professionals who brought it all to life, especially Senior Managing Editor Judy Howarth, and Senior Project Manager Rajeev Kumar. We thank you all and appreciate all your efforts!

Finally, we would like to acknowledge our appreciation to our students and colleagues who continue to inspire us to find new ways of sharing and disseminating knowledge from psychology and the health sciences to help us all live longer and healthier lives.

Jeffrey S. Nevid
Spencer A. Rathus

About the Authors

JEFFREY S. NEVID is a professor of psychology at St. John's University in New York, where he has taught for many years at both the undergraduate and graduate levels, as well as directing the doctoral program in clinical psychology. He received his doctorate from the University at Albany and was awarded a NIMH Post-Doctoral Fellowship in evaluation research at Northwestern University.

Jeff is a fellow of the American Psychological Association and was awarded a diplomate in clinical psychology by the American Board of Professional Psychology. He has accrued more than 200 research publications and professional presentations and has conducted research in various areas in health psychology, including smoking cessation, hypertension, cancer, HIV/AIDS, and substance use disorders. His research on smoking cessation with Hispanic smokers was supported by the National Heart, Lung, and Blood Institute of the National Institutes of Health.

Jeff served as editorial consultant for the journals *Health Psychology* and *Teaching of Psychology* and as associate editor of the *Journal of Consulting and Clinical Psychology*. His research publications have appeared in such journals as *Health Psychology*, *American Journal of Health Promotion*, *Journal of Youth and Adolescence*, *Journal of Occupational Medicine*, *Journal of Consulting and Clinical Psychology*, *Professional Psychology: Research and Practice*, *Rehabilitation Psychology*, *Journal of Social Distress and the Homeless*, *Psychology and Health*, *AIDS Education and Prevention*, *Annals of Behavioral Medicine*, *Teaching of Psychology*, *Scholarship of Teaching and Learning in Psychology*, *Computers in Human Behavior*, *Behavior Therapy*, *Cultural Diversity and Ethnic Minority Psychology*, *Psychology of Addictive Behaviors*, *Journal of Substance Abuse Treatment*, and *Journal of Personality Assessment*. Along with his coauthored textbooks with Spencer Rathus, Jeff is author of the textbook *Essentials of Psychology: Concepts and Applications* (Cengage Learning), as well as the books *A Student's Guide to AIDS and Other Sexually Transmitted Diseases*, and *Choices: Sex in the Age of STDs* (Allyn & Bacon).

Jeff also conducts an ongoing program of pedagogical research designed to help students become more effective learners and has published findings from his research lab in several scientific journals and at many teaching conferences. In recognition of his many contributions to the teaching of psychology, he was honored as the 2022 recipient of the Charles L. Brewer Award for Distinguished Teaching of Psychology from the American Psychological Foundation, the highest national teaching award in psychology.

SPENCER A. RATHUS received his Ph.D. from the University at Albany and is on the faculty of the College of New Jersey. His research interests include treatment of obesity and eating disorders, smoking cessation, human growth and development, methods of therapy, assertive behavior, and sexual dysfunctions. He is the author of the Rathus Assertiveness Schedule and has published articles in the *Journal of Clinical Psychology*, the *Journal of Counseling Psychology, Behavior Therapy*, *Behaviour Research and Therapy*, and *Journal of Behavior Therapy and Experimental Psychiatry*. He has also written several college textbooks, including *PSYCH* (Cengage Learning), *HDEV* (Cengage Learning), *AIDS: What Every Student Needs to Know* (Cengage Learning), *Childhood and Adolescence: Voyages in Development* (Cengage Learning), and *The Lifespan* (Cengage Learning). His co-authored textbooks with Jeff Nevid include *Human Sexuality in a Changing World* (Pearson Education), *Abnormal Psychology in a Changing World* (Pearson Education), and *Adjustment and Growth: Psychology and the Challenges of Life* (Wiley).

Brief Contents

Contents

14 Chronic Diseases and End-of-Life Issues 413

15 New Directions in Health Psychology 436

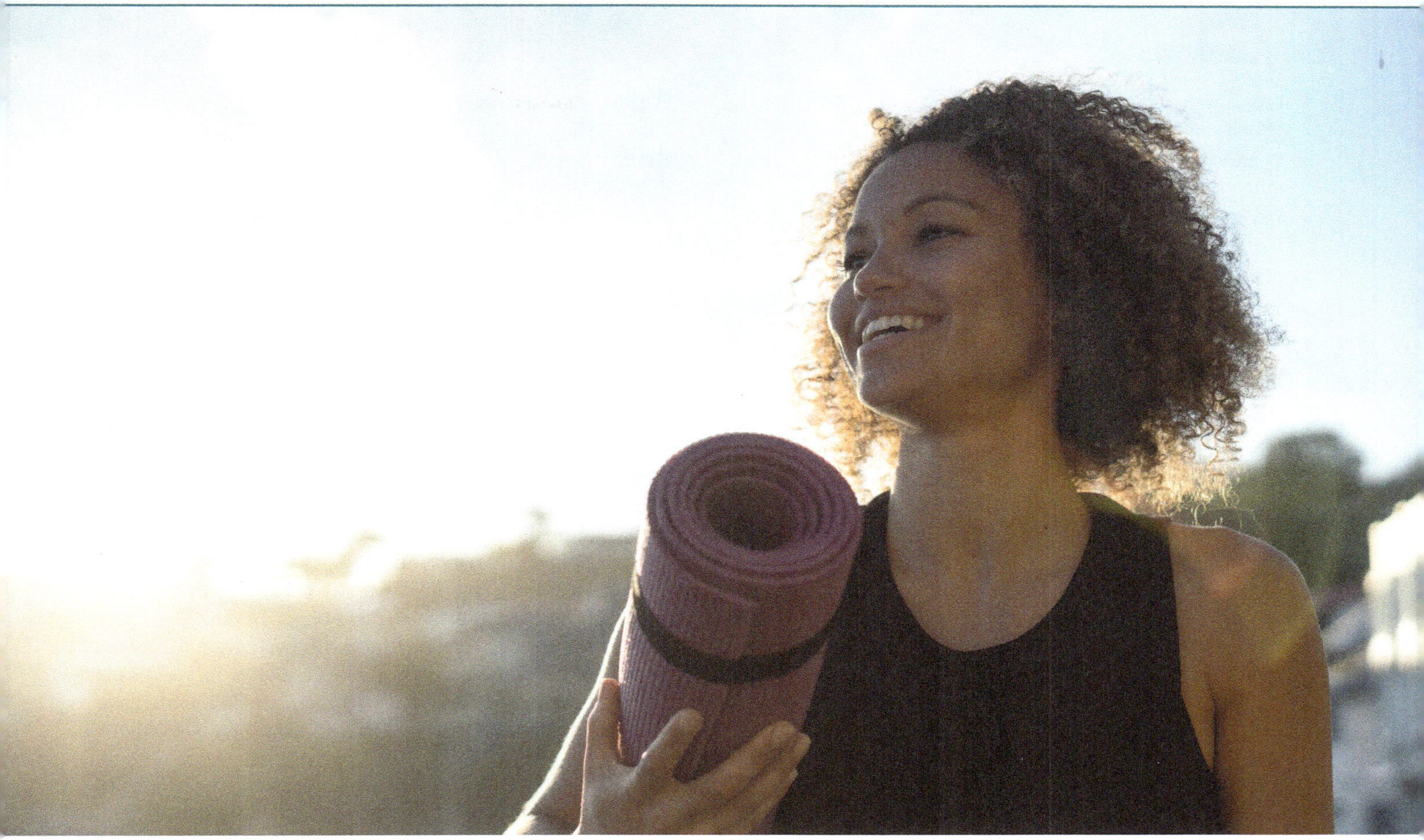

andresr/Getty Images

Foundations of Health Psychology

LEARNING OBJECTIVES

After studying this chapter, you will be able to ...

1. **Describe** the development of the field of health psychology.
2. **Describe** the biopsychosocial model of health.
3. **Describe** the relationships between health and human diversity.
4. **List** and **describe** the major research methods in health psychology.
5. **Describe** the major features of critical thinking about health-related information.

Did you know that ...

- People were more likely to use a hand sanitizer in a hospital setting when a citrus scent was diffused in the air?
- Depression is a causal factor in heart disease, asthma, and gastrointestinal disorders?
- Having more social connections and higher-quality social ties is linked to a lower risk of cardiovascular disease and cancer?
- More than a million deaths each year are preventable?
- Smoking cigarettes takes 10 years off the average person's life?
- Happier words are tweeted more often during the early morning hours?
- Health psychologists created an app designed to reduce fatigue in airline pilots?
- No experiments have been done with humans to show that smoking causes cancer?
- Researchers have found that placebos (pills with no medicine) work to reduce pain even when the people taking them know that they are phony?

Until the COVID-19 pandemic in 2020, most people paid little if any attention to hand-gel sanitizers. Placed in many public areas, including office buildings, schools, and hospitals, they went largely unused by passersby, even in hospital settings where their use could help curb the risk of infections. Although a hand sanitizer is not as effective as a thorough handwashing, it can reduce the risk of getting sick or spreading disease to others (CDC, 2019j).

Young people tend to be less compliant in using hand sanitizers, so health psychologists performed a field experiment in which they posted signs in university residence halls next to sanitizer dispensers with messages encouraging students to use them (Capps et al., 2022). The investigators found that sanitizer use was 36% greater for sanitizers with posted signs than for those without signs. Yet just simply posting reminder signs may not be enough to increase sanitizer use in sensitive settings, such as hospital units, so hospital staff members in an intensive care unit (ICU) in a teaching hospital in Miami went a step further (King et al., 2016). Let's have a closer look at what they did.

Years before the COVID-19 pandemic, staff members in the Miami hospital recognized they had a problem with hand hygiene of visitors to the unit. They wanted to encourage visitors to use a hand-gel dispenser placed outside the entrance to the unit but realized that simply posting a sign to remind people to use the sanitizer didn't work well enough, as many visitors simply just ignored it. Having a staff member stationed at the door to monitor whether people complied with proper hand hygiene would be too cumbersome and expensive. So they decided to try a behavioral experiment, enlisting the help of health psychologists.

priming Exposure to a stimulus, called a prime, that increases the likelihood of another response.

The health psychologists drew upon the psychological principle of **priming**, which is the use of a stimulus (called a *prime*) that increases the likelihood of a response to another stimulus, which in this case was a hand-gel dispenser posted just outside the entrance to the ICU. They tested the effects of two types of primes: one, a clean-smelling citrus scent infused in the hospital corridor by an aroma dispenser, and the second, a pair of observing female or male eyes placed strategically near the dispenser. Observers were discreetly placed so that they could monitor whether visitors used the hand-gel dispenser without making themselves obvious. Some days were designated as control days with no primes present, while on other days the clean-smelling citrus scent was infused in the air or the pair of observing eyes (male eyes on some occasions, female eyes on others) was posted just outside the unit.

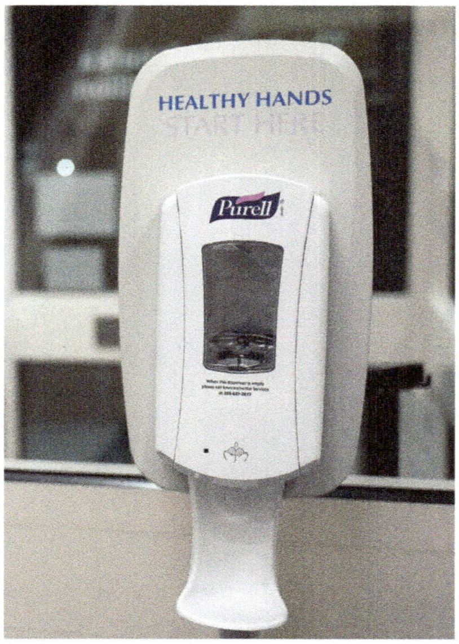

Erin Deleon/Shutterstock.com

Will You Use Me? It's there, it's free, and it helps prevent disease, but will passersby in hospital corridors and elsewhere stop to use it?

What results would you predict? Would a slight nudge—infusing the air with a clean-smelling scent or posting a set of observing eyes—make a difference in inducing people to use the sanitizer?

The results showed that 47% of people exposed to the citrus scent before entering the unit used the hand-gel sanitizer as compared to only 15% of controls—that is, visitors not exposed to priming. The experimenters argued that exposure to clean smells might bring associations with cleanliness to mind, inducing people to be more conscientious about sanitizing their hands. Moreover, significantly more participants (33%) exposed to the male watchful eyes used the gel as compared to visitors (controls) not exposed to any primes. Interestingly, only 10% of those exposed to the female eyes prime used the sanitizer, a result that was not significantly different than the (no-prime) control. Exposure to harsher male eyes turned out to be a more effective nudge than softer female eyes.

health psychology The scientific study of relationships between psychology and physical health and illness.

This hospital study introduces the field of **health psychology**, the branch of psychology that focuses on relationships between behavior and physical health. Health psychologists examine how psychological factors can affect a person's health and well-being. This work by a team of health psychologists may encourage other public institutions, such as schools, municipal buildings, and clinics, to use similar visual or olfactory primes to encourage people to practice hand hygiene in public places. It shows the role that psychological factors—in this case, primes—can play in promoting healthy behaviors.

Health psychologists also study relationships between psychological factors and physical illness. For example, they examine the role of psychological factors in disease, such as stress, lifestyles, behaviors, and attitudes. Examining these relationships enables psychologists to better explain the nature and mechanisms of disease and leads to the development of health-promotion and disease-prevention programs. Health psychologists also work directly with medical patients to improve their quality of life and help them cope with the challenges of living with health problems such as heart disease, cancer, chronic pain, and HIV/AIDS.

Research in health psychology informs our understanding of the psychological factors relating not only to health but to longevity. Consider, for example, a recent study that probed these links based on a large national survey, the Health and Retirement Study, which polled more than 21,000 older adults over the age of 50 several times over a 14-year period, a length of time long enough to track mortality (death) rates (Boylan, Tompkins, & Krueger, 2022). The survey measured various aspects of that psychological health or well-being, including positive affect (emotions), life satisfaction, purpose in life, social support, and optimism. Suffice it to say these factors predicted lower mortality rates, meaning that people with higher levels of psychological well-being tended to live longer. Our emotional and mental well-being bears a primary role in determining how long we are likely to live and how healthy we are likely to be.

We will see that health psychologists perform various roles. Some, like the psychologists in the Miami hospital study, conduct research in hospital settings in which they apply psychological theories, principles, and techniques to promote healthy behaviors. Others design or implement health-promotion programs in worksites, universities, or clinics or work directly with individuals to help them develop healthy behaviors and lifestyles. The work of health psychologists touches virtually every aspect of our lives, from our diets, exercise, and sleep habits, to how we cope with stress and manage illness.

A History of Health Psychology

The ancient Greeks and Romans believed that we should cultivate both our mental (or spiritual) well-being and our physical bodies. The need to take care of both mind and body was perhaps best summed up by Juvenal, a Roman poet of the late 1st and early 2nd century CE, who offered a simple prescription, *Pray for a sound mind in a sound body.*

But how do the body and the mind relate to one other? The ancient Greek physician Hippocrates (ca. 460–377 BCE) lived at a time when many people subscribed to spiritual explanations of physical illness, believing that the gods afflicted humans with ill health. Hippocrates was among the first to offer naturalistic explanations of disease. He also believed there is a two-way street between mind and body, that bodily processes affect the mind and the mind affects the body. For example, he argued that our emotional well-being was dependent on a balance of four vital bodily fluids he called *humors*: phlegm, black bile, blood, and yellow bile. Depression, he believed, was caused by a buildup in the body of a substance he called black bile, whereas lethargy or sluggishness was due to an excess amount of phlegm, from which we derive the

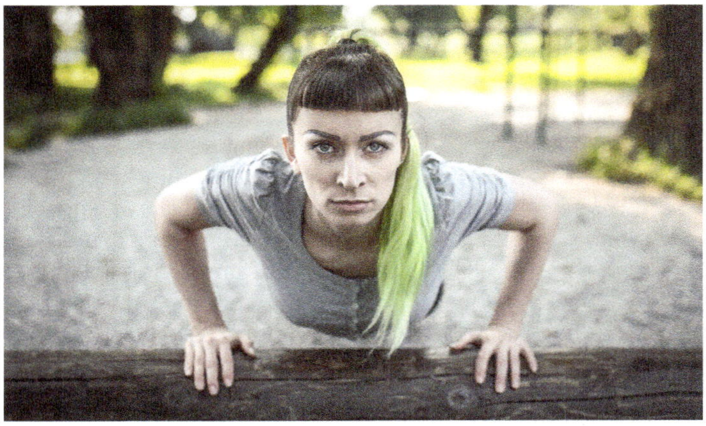

AzmanJaka/Getty Images

Just What Is Going On Here? The first answer that might pop into "mind" would be "pushups." Dualists might say we have an immaterial spirit animating a physical body. The scientific answer, of course, is that billions of neurons along with muscle fibers are involved in the decision to go outdoors and exercise, to show awareness of the environment, including the photographer's camera, to command the muscles to adopt a prone position and lift the body with the arms, and to experience the result through sensory awareness.

word "phlegmatic." Those with an excess of blood had a cheerful or sanguine disposition and were confident and optimistic. But an excess of another substance, yellow bile, or so Hippocrates claimed, would make you choleric or quick-tempered. Although we no longer subscribe to this theory of humors, we continue to honor the contributions of Hippocrates in the development of naturalistic explanations of disease by having medical school graduates take an oath named in his honor: the Hippocratic oath.

dualism A philosophical belief that mind and body are fundamentally separate entities.

Centuries later, the 17th-century French philosopher René Descartes (1596–1650) proposed the principle of **dualism**—the belief that mind and body are fundamentally different entities. Descartes recognized that the mind does indeed affect the body, as, after all, we intend to raise our arm and our arm complies by rising. However, he argued that mind and body operate according to different organizing principles. Like other animals, Descartes argued, humans possess a body of several parts that is controlled by mechanical forces, such as digestion and muscle contractions. But unlike other animals, humans alone possess an immaterial mind, a spiritual entity that houses the soul and that is not divisible into separate parts like the body. Today scientists recognize that the mind is a function of the brain, involving communication among billions of cells called **neurons**.

neurons Cells in the nervous system that receive and transmit messages involved in sensory awareness, consciousness, thinking, voluntary movements, and automatic function, such as the heart rate, blood pressure, and digestion.

Since the time of Descartes, philosophers have argued about the so-called *mind–body problem*, that is, the nature of the relationship between the mind and body—whether they are fundamentally different substances as Descartes believed or the same underlying substance. Scientists today have largely moved beyond the mind–body problem. The field of health psychology takes as its starting point this interaction of mind and body by focusing on how our mental or psychological functioning—our thoughts, beliefs, behaviors, lifestyles, attitudes—affect our physical health.

The Development of Psychosomatic Medicine

psychosomatic medicine A branch of medical science that focuses on understanding mind–body interactions in disease.

More formal scientific approaches to understanding mind–body interactions began in the 19th century with the development of a field of medicine called **psychosomatic medicine**. The term "psychosomatic" derives from Greek roots for *psyche* (mind or soul) and *soma* (body). The first use of the term "psychosomatic" is attributed to a German physician, Johann Christian Heinroth, in 1818. Interest in how psychological or mental processes can lead to diseases of the body arose at time of rapid scientific advances in the 19th century. Psychosomatic medicine emerged in the interface between behavioral and medical science, becoming a bridge that connected *psyche* to *soma* (Martin, 1978).

By the early 20th century, physicians were drawn to the teachings of psychological theorists such as Sigmund Freud, whose theory of the mind focused of how underlying psychological conflicts can lead to physical symptoms (Deter et al., 2018). Freud's early case studies featured individuals who complained of various neurological problems, such as numbness in parts of the body or paralysis of a limb, that could not be explained based on known medical causes. The cases generally carried a diagnosis of **hysteria** or *hysterical neurosis*. Freud's first book, coauthored in 1895 with colleague Josef Breuer and called *Studies in Hysteria*, featured case studies of these patients. Freud believed that problems of hysteria could be traced to psychological conflicts in early childhood involving socially unacceptable sexual and aggressive impulses. He argued that the mind converted these conflicts into physical symptoms to protect the self from having to come to terms with threatening or upsetting impulses, desires, and wishes. The impulses themselves remained hidden in an area of the mind he called the **unconscious**. In effect, hysterical symptoms shielded the conscious self from awareness of unacceptable unconscious impulses. The individual would only be aware of the physical defects or symptoms, not the underlying psychological issues that gave rise to them. Although Freud's theories have been mired in controversy, he was instrumental in paving the way for a broader recognition of psychological factors in physical health.

hysteria A psychological disorder characterized by physical symptoms that cannot be explained medically.

unconscious In Freud's view, the part of the mind that operates outside the range of ordinary consciousness.

Throughout the early and mid-20th century, physicians in the psychosomatic tradition became increasingly interested in the effects of many psychological factors, especially emotions, in the development and course of physical disease (Lipsitt, 2006). Early theorists largely followed in the Freudian tradition, especially the Hungarian American physician Franz Alexander (1891–1964), who studied the psychological bases of medical conditions. Alexander believed that certain diseases—*psychosomatic diseases* such as ulcers and hypertension—are strongly influenced by psychological factors. By 1939 the first journal devoted to this area of medicine appeared under the title *Psychosomatic Medicine*. By 1942 the American Psychosomatic Society was established to represent physicians, psychologists, and other health professionals who were interested in connections between the mind and diseases of the body.

The American physician Helen Flanders Dunbar (1902–1959) founded the American Psychosomatic Society. To Dunbar, there wasn't any special class of psychosomatic diseases. Rather, many physical disorders are influenced by psychological and social factors to some degree (Lipsitt, 2006). Even in cases with clear biological causes, as in certain genetic diseases, Dunbar believed that an individual's thoughts, feelings, and behaviors influence the person's coping with illness and its symptoms. Understanding how psychological factors influence somatic diseases is the core concept underlying the field of psychosomatic medicine and, later, the development of health psychology.

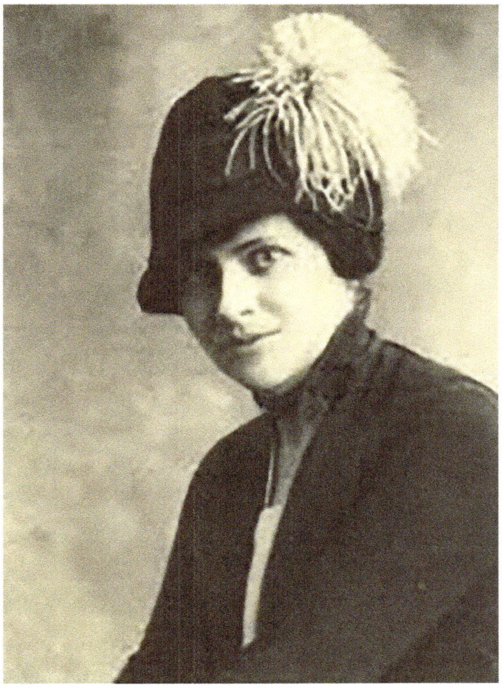

Helen Flanders Dunbar An early pioneer in the scientific study of the mind–body connection, Dunbar was an American physician who established the American Psychosomatic Society in 1942.

Although the early threads of the psychosomatic movement in medicine featured the theories of Freud and his followers, by the 1950s a broader view began to take hold that emphasized a multifactorial framework that takes into account biological, psychological, and sociocultural factors in physical disease, especially the role of stress.

Psychosomatic medicine today is an interdisciplinary field that brings together the work of physicians, psychologists, sociologists, and other scientists in exploring the relationships between psychological, behavioral, and social factors in health and illness (Jacob et al., 2015). The field of psychosomatic medicine embraces a holistic view of health and well-being by considering the whole person in physical health, not just the roles of microbes, genetics, and diseased organs. This holistic approach explores the roles of emotions, coping resources, and life stress in physical health.

Within contemporary medical practice, psychosomatic medicine is recognized as a subspecialty in the field of psychiatry called *consultation-liaison (C-L) psychiatry*. C-L psychiatry connects psychiatry to other medical specialists. **Psychiatrists** are medical doctors who specialize in the diagnosis and treatment of mental disorders. Psychiatrists who further specialize in C-L psychiatry are involved in developing new knowledge and providing consultation to other healthcare providers on relationships between mental and physical illness.

psychiatrists Physicians who specialize in the diagnosis and treatment of mental disorders.

The Emergence of Health Psychology

Early contributors to the developing science of psychology in the late 19th century and early 20th centuries were also concerned about understanding relationships between mind and body. Several of the early figures in psychology were trained as medical doctors, including Wilhelm Wundt (1832–1920), recognized as the founder of scientific psychology; William James (1842–1910), widely credited as the father of American psychology; and Walter Cannon (1871–1945), a Harvard physician and physiologist who conducted research on emotions.

Wundt established the first experimental psychology laboratory in Leipzig, Germany, in 1879. There he conducted studies of mental processes and mind–body interactions. Another early luminary figure in psychology was the Russian physiologist Ivan Pavlov (1849–1936), who focused on a form of learning called **classical conditioning**, or learning by association. Pavlov showed in his laboratory studies that dogs learned to salivate to the sound of a tone or bell by pairing the tone or bell with another stimulus, namely food, that naturally elicits salivation. From these not-so-humble beginnings, other psychologists, such as B. F. Skinner, went on to develop **operant conditioning**, which is central to the psychology of self-control and behavior therapy, one of the pillars of cognitive behavioral therapy. Psychologists also showed that it is possible to condition rats to increase or decrease their heart rates—learning to modify behaviors that are normally beyond conscious control (Fehr & Stern, 1965). Research with the rats led to the development of biofeedback training, in which individuals can control their heart rates, the generation of brain waves, and so on to obtain desired results, such as relaxation or sleep.

classical conditioning A form of learning by association in which a response is elicited by a previously neutral stimulus that has been paired or associated with a stimulus that originally elicited the response.

operant conditioning A form of learning in which an organism modifies its behavior because of the consequence of that behavior.

Both James and Cannon were interested in how the mind and body interact in the case of emotional responses, especially fear, and whether the experience of fear occurs at the same time

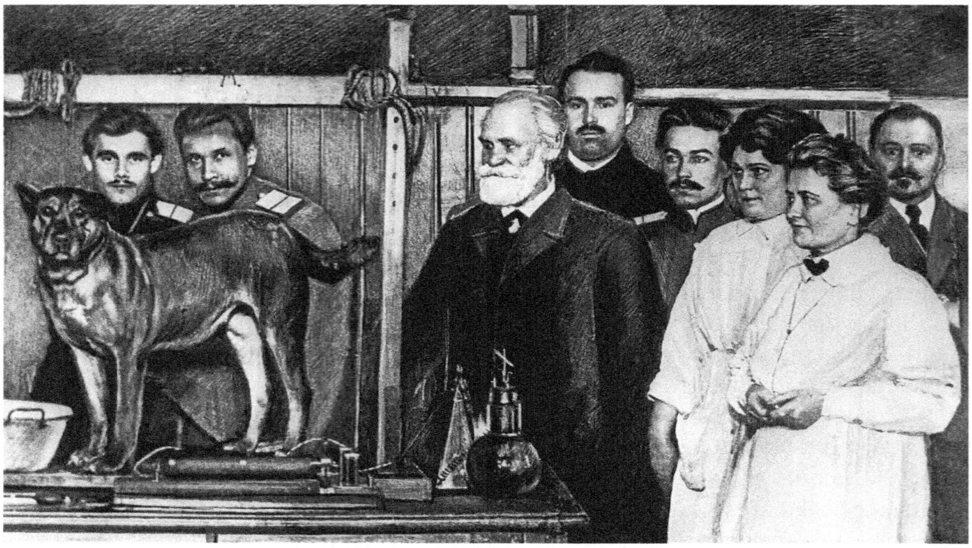

SPUTNIK/Alamy Stock Photo

Ivan Pavlov and his colleagues at the Military Medical Academy in Petrograd, Russia, in 1914.

as the bodily response. Consider a thought experiment proposed by James. Imagine that you are walking in the woods and suddenly encounter a bear. Do you first see the bear, then feel fear, and then run for your life? Or does your body first react, either by freezing or hightailing it out of there, and only then do you experience fear? James believed the bodily reaction occurs first. In other words, you see the bear, you run, and then you feel fear. He believed the felt experience of fear is based on sensing our bodily reactions—our heart beating faster and our muscles propelling our legs to run away as fast as we can, allowing us to live to tell the tale another day.

Cannon and his student Philip Bard (1898–1977) proposed that the emotion of fear and the body's emotional reactions to a threatening stimulus occur simultaneously, not sequentially. In other words, you see the bear, then experience fear and flee at the same time. In the 1960s, Stanley Schachter and Jerome Singer proposed a two-factor theory of emotion: We respond physiologically to a stimulus and then engage in cognitive appraisal of the situation, leading us to label the emotion and act accordingly. Psychologists still endorse the importance of cognitive appraisal in response to stressful situations, as we will see in Chapter 5. But these earlier theories highlighted the intersection of mind and body, which became a foundational principle in the development of health psychology.

The field of health psychology emerged during the 1960s and 1970s to meet the needs for research, education, and practice focused on the role of psychological factors in physical health. Before that time, psychologists were primarily concerned with problems of mental health, not physical health (Wallston, 1997). But psychologists began applying knowledge of behavioral science and behavior change techniques to help people develop healthier habits and cope with the many challenges of adjusting to serious or chronic illness. In the late 1960s and early 1970s, papers emerged in psychological journals focused on the role of psychologists in the healthcare system. It was at that time that groups of psychologists began to organize around their common interest in the interface of psychology and health. In 1978 the American Psychological Association established a new division, the Society for Health Psychology (Division 38), to advance the contributions of psychology to health and illness through research, education, and service (Wallston, 1997).

Today, health psychologists are involved in research, teaching, and practice on the connections between psychology and physical health, including issues such as these:

- How does stress impact the immune system? Does stress increase the risk of cancer?
- How can we help people adopt healthier behaviors and lifestyles?
- How are behavioral patterns, such as unhealthy diets and physical inactivity, related to negative health outcomes?
- How can we best assist people cope with chronic diseases?
- How does psychological theory inform efforts to help people adhere to medical advice, take their medications more reliably, and follow up with medical visits?

The Profession of Health Psychology

VIDEO CONTENT

Understanding Health Psychology

Health psychology is a specialty area or subfield in the broader field of psychology. Pursuing a professional career in health psychology generally requires completion of a doctoral program in health psychology or a related field. There are four general areas of practice in health psychology: clinical health psychology, occupational health psychology, community-based health psychology, and public services health psychology:

- **Clinical health psychology** focuses on helping individuals lead healthier lives and cope with chronic illness. Clinical health psychologists work with individuals to help them develop healthier behaviors and adopt healthier lifestyles. Other clinical psychologists treat mental health issues such as anxiety and depression, whereas clinical health psychologists focus on issues of physical health and well-being, using techniques like stress management and biofeedback training.
- **Community health psychology** focuses on improving the health of members of communities. Community health psychologists investigate factors accounting for differences between communities in the prevalence of certain diseases. They may focus their research on problems such as overcrowding, discrimination, pollution, and limited access to health services.
- **Occupational health psychology** focuses on improving the health and well-being of employees. Occupational health psychologists might be involved in developing worksite health and wellness programs, providing counseling services to employees, and consulting with companies to change workplace policies to improve the health and well-being of employees.
- **Public health psychology** seeks to improve the health and well-being of the general population by focusing on policies and programs of governmental agencies and public health services. Public health psychologists might gather evidence to assist lawmakers in drafting healthcare policies or assisting government officials in developing public health awareness campaigns.

clinical health psychology A branch of health psychology focusing on helping individuals live healthier lives and cope with chronic illness.

community health psychology A branch of health psychology focusing on improving the health of members of communities.

occupational health psychology A branch of health psychology focusing on improving health and well-being of employees.

public health psychology A branch of health psychology focusing on improving health and well-being of the general population.

Training in health psychology typically involves completion of a doctoral degree (either a Ph.D. or Doctor of Philosophy degree, or a PsyD or Doctor of Psychology degree). The American Psychological Association (APA) oversees the accreditation process for doctoral training programs in health psychology and other applied areas of psychology, such as clinical, counseling, and school psychology.

The typical Ph.D. program in health psychology involves 3 to 4 years of coursework and related training in health psychology settings, along with completion of a doctoral dissertation, a formal research project in which the student works closely with a faculty mentor to complete an original research project designed to make a contribution to the literature in the field. Students seeking to learn more about careers in psychology may access career-related materials made available by the APA. You can visit their website, www.apa.org, to access these materials.

The Biopsychosocial Model

Many health psychologists are guided by a conceptual framework called the **biopsychosocial model**, which recognizes that health and illness are best understood by examining the roles of biological, psychological, and social factors, and the interactions among these factors in the development, treatment, and prevention of physical illness (see **Figure 1.1**).

biopsychosocial model A conceptual framework in health psychology that incorporates biological, psychological, and social factors in understanding and treating physical disease and promoting health and well-being.

The biopsychosocial model has largely replaced the earlier **biomedical model** that understood disease in terms of defects in biological processes, exposure to pathogenic organisms such as bacteria and viruses, and genetic factors. The biopsychosocial model expands upon the biomedical model by also considering psychological factors (behaviors, attitudes, and emotions) and social factors (social relationships, ethnicity and gender, employment and marital status, immigrant status, **socioeconomic status (SES)**, and discrimination). The biopsychosocial model recognizes the importance of healthy behaviors in determining health outcomes and longevity.

biomedical model A traditional conception of disease as explained by disease processes.

socioeconomic status (SES) The social standing or class of an individual or group, often measured in terms of education, income, and occupation.

Biological factors such as genetics and exposure to disease-causing pathogens such as harmful bacteria and viruses play an important role in determining our risk of serious illness.

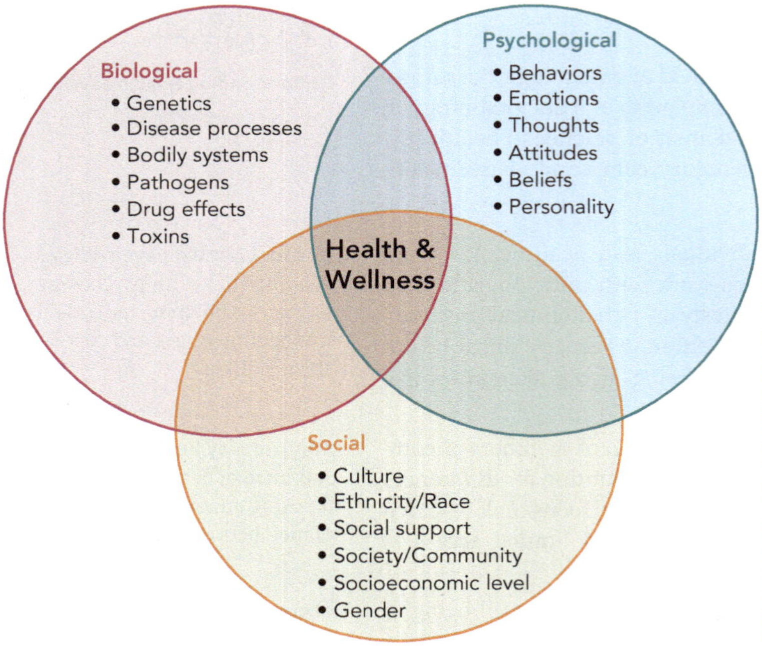

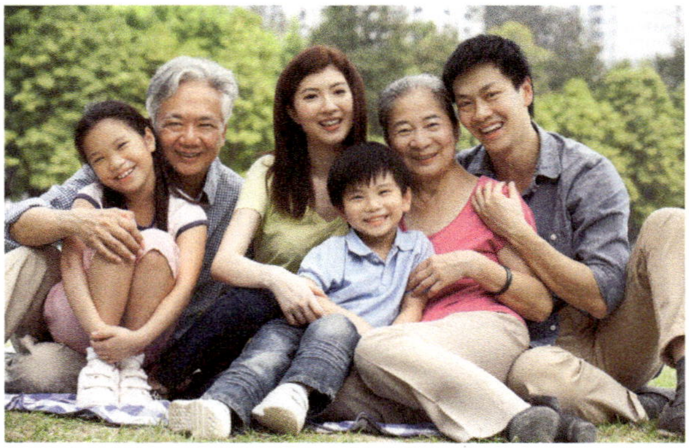

monkeybusinessimages/Getty Images

FIGURE 1.1 **The Biopsychosocial Model of Health** The biopsychosocial model posits that health and wellness are determined by biological, psychological, and social factors and their interactions. Which of these factors can we control? Which are beyond our ability to control?

But biology is not destiny. The likelihood of living a long and healthy life also depends on behavioral factors we can control, such as diet and exercise and avoidance of harmful substances such as tobacco.

immune system The body's system of defense against disease.

We have also learned that psychological states such as anxiety and depression can impair the functioning of the **immune system**, the body's system of defense against disease-causing organisms, leaving us more vulnerable to physical disorders. Recent research points to causal links between depression and diseases including coronary heart disease, asthma, and gastrointestinal disorders (Mulugeta et al., 2019). Identifying and treating emotional problems might not only improve one's mental health but also reduce the risks and chronicity of physical illness later in life.

Social factors can be associated with either positive or negative health outcomes. On the positive side, social support can help people cope with health problems and stress. Showing warmth and caring can be a soothing and consoling form of "medication" (Knoll et al., 2019). Having a shoulder to lean on can help people cope with health crises. Evidence shows that having more social connections and higher-quality social ties is a significant predictor of a wide range of positive health outcomes, including lower rates of cardiovascular disease and cancer and lower mortality (death) rates overall (Farrell & Sarah, 2019; Holt-Lunstad, 2018). On the other hand, negative social interactions, such as a troubled marriage, can be a stressful burden, making it more difficult to cope with health problems.

Social factors early in life can have telling implications for health outcomes later on. A study in the United Kingdom showed that socially isolated children were at greater than average risk during midlife of developing Type 2 diabetes and having blood markers of inflammation associated with coronary heart disease (Lacey et al., 2014).

The biopsychosocial model holds that body affects mind and mind affects body, that there are reciprocal relationships between psychological, biological, and sociocultural factors that bear upon our health and well-being, In Chapter 7, we will learn how regular exercise is good for both the body and the mind. Many psychotherapists today prescribe exercise programs for their patients to help them deal with their emotional problems (e.g., Tomasi, Gates, & Reyns, 2019). In Chapter 11, we examine the roles of biological factors, such as genes and neurotransmitter functioning in the brain, as contributing factors in the development of psychological disorders, such as depression and schizophrenia.

Sociocultural factors—SES, ethnicity, and discrimination—are also connected with health outcomes. One of the most robust findings in the health literature is that people from higher socioeconomic levels tend to live longer and healthier lives than people at lower income levels (Chetty et al., 2016; Glanz et al., 2015). The gap between the richest and poorest U.S. residents is nearly 15 years for men and about 10 years for women (Chetty et al., 2016). Wealthier people typically have greater access to high-quality health care. They tend to have greater awareness and knowledge about the health risks associated with unhealthy behavior patterns and to make healthier choices about their diets, perhaps because they can better afford them. Smoking, the major cause of preventable diseases, is concentrated among less well educated and affluent people in our society.

Consider some of the questions posed by health psychologists:

- Why are some people more prone to serious illness than others?
- What determines a person's risk of cancer? Or heart disease?
- How can I preserve my mental functioning as I age?
- Why do some people come down with whatever "bug" is going around while others remain resistant?
- Why are some people better able to maintain their health in their later years than others?

There are no simple answers to these questions. The biopsychosocial model leads us to take a broader view of these issues. We need to consider the role of biological influences, such as genetics, exposure to infectious organisms, and the workings of the immune system. Genetic (inherited) influences are fundamental in the transmission of physical traits, such as height, hair texture, and eye color. Genetics also appears to play a role in personality traits such as impulsivity, sociability, shyness, anxiety, empathy, and even interest in arts and crafts (Gustavson et al., 2019; Keum & Shin, 2019; Savage et al., 2018; Wasielewska & Bethke, 2019). Genetic factors are also involved in many health conditions, such as cardiovascular disorders, cancer, and substance use and abuse (Dunn et al., 2020; Forsyth & Asarnow, 2020; Walsh et al., 2020; Zhang et al., 2019). We will return to the role of genetics in understanding both psychological and physical health throughout this text. Biological factors such as genetics and exposure to disease-causing pathogens such as harmful bacteria and viruses play important roles in determining our risk of serious illness. However, biology is not destiny. From a psychological perspective we need to consider behavioral factors such as the adoption of a healthy lifestyle and use of coping responses to handle daily stress, as well as cognitive factors (attitudes, expectancies, and beliefs) and personality traits (conscientiousness, extraversion, hostility). The likelihood of contracting an illness—be it the flu or cancer—can reflect the interaction of many factors, including genetics and lifestyle factors.

Health psychologists examine relationships between unhealthy behavior patterns and many forms of physical illness. How long we are likely to live and how healthy we are likely to be is often determined by behavioral factors that lie within our control, such as whether we adopt healthy dietary and exercise habits, avoid harmful substances such as tobacco, have regular medical care visits, adhere to medical advice, control our alcohol intake, and take steps to prevent accidents, such as by wearing seat belts. The good news is that healthy behaviors save lives.

Health psychologists also place health and illness within a broader sociocultural context. We will examine throughout our exploration of health psychology the importance of sociocultural factors such as gender, ethnicity, socioeconomic status, and exposure to social ills, such as poverty, discrimination, and racism.

The nearby Self-Assessment on locus of control provides insight as to whether you believe that you are in charge of your own life or you are subject to the whims of external forces.

Healthy Behaviors Save Lives

The COVID-19 pandemic focused public attention on the importance of adopting healthy behaviors, such as handwashing, wearing a facial mask or facial cloth covering, and keeping a safe distance from other people. COVID-19 represented the most significant health threat to the nation and the world at large since the influenza pandemic of 1918, which claimed an

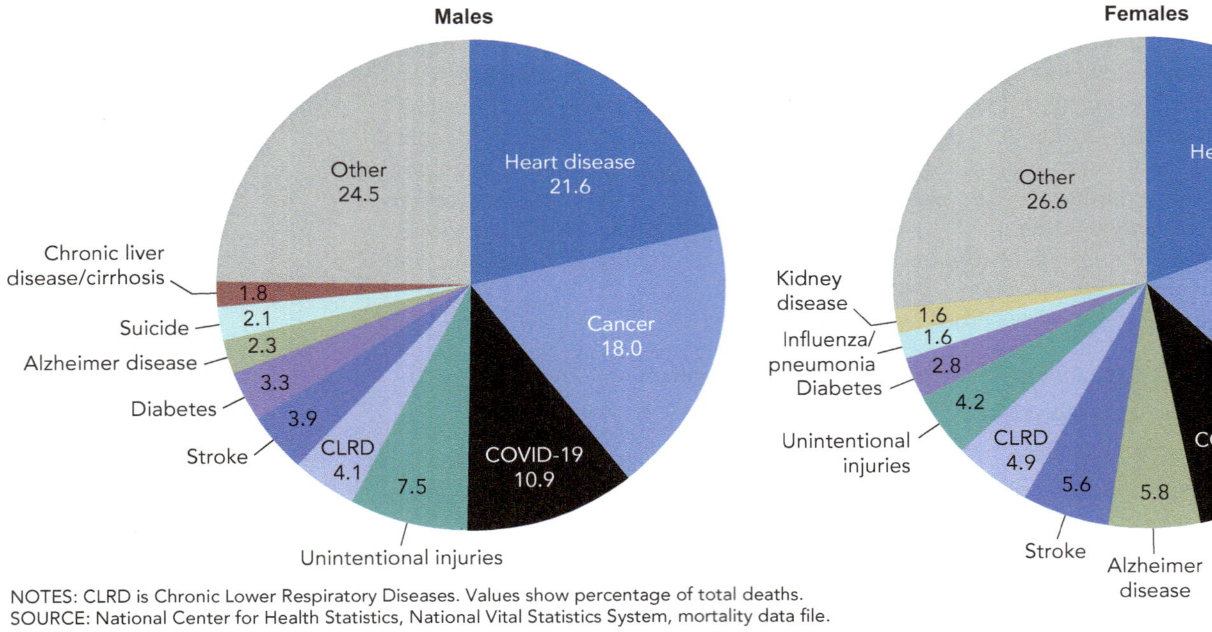

FIGURE 1.2 Leading Causes of Death, United States Unhealthy behaviors contribute to the most common causes of death in the United States, including the number 1 killer, heart disease. Does your behavior increase or decrease your risk of death from heart disease or another leading cause of death?

Source: Curtin et al. 2023 / U.S. Department of Health & Human Services/ Public Domain

estimated 50 million lives worldwide and about 675,000 in the United States (CDC, 2023r). COVID-19 joined the nation's leading causes of death in 2020.

Despite the enormity of the health threats posed by COVID-19 and other infectious diseases, the perennial leading causes of death in the United States have not involved pathological agents such as bacteria and viruses. They are noncommunicable (noninfectious) chronic diseases, including the nation's leading cause of death, heart disease, and the second leading killer, cancer (see **Figure 1.2**). All together, these 10 causes of death account for about three quarters of all deaths in the United States (Heron, 2019; Xu et al., 2020a).

Preventable Causes of Death

Approximately one death in three is preventable, a result of unhealthy behaviors (Holman, 2016; Taksler et al., 2018). Smoking is the leading preventable cause of death in the United States, accounting for nearly one in every five deaths, especially including deaths from heart disease, cancer, and respiratory problems (CDC, 2023g). Unhealthy dietary patterns including overeating, eating saturated fats, and ingesting large amounts of sodium (in salt) play roles in preventable causes of death. Excessive drinking of alcohol contributes to many health problems, including liver disease, and is associated with risky behaviors, such as driving under the influence and risky sexual behavior. Failure to use seat belts and obey traffic laws also increases the risk of fatal accidents. **Figure 1.3** shows the estimated number of deaths attributable to individual risk factors. Eliminating these risk factors could save more than a million lives each year in the United States.

These risk factors are all controllable by practicing healthier lifestyles and going for regular medical and dental checkups. We can avoid tobacco use and adopt healthier diets and exercise regularly to manage our weight. Regular medical care can help us to control diabetes, hypertension, and high levels of blood cholesterol, which are risk factors for heart disease. Medical care, healthy diets, and exercise can prevent hundreds of thousands of deaths due to heart disease and diabetes each year (Hagger et al., 2020; Naar, Czajkowski, & Spring, 2018). Control of underage and excess drinking of alcohol can prevent tens of thousands of deaths from motor vehicle accidents, falls, drowning, and risky sex. Ensuring that we and our children are immunized against infectious agents saves thousands of lives. We can avoid more needless deaths by improving worker training and safety. We can go for screening for various kinds of cancer.

Self-Assessment

INTERACTIVE SELF-ASSESSMENTS

Locus of Control Scale

It is, or can be, within our control to fend off preventable illnesses and to enhance our well-being. Do you believe that your health and well-being lie within your control? Or do you believe that what happens to you in life depends on the whims and fancies of others or just blind luck? To find out, answer the following questions by selecting "Yes" or "No." Then check the answer key at the end of the chapter.

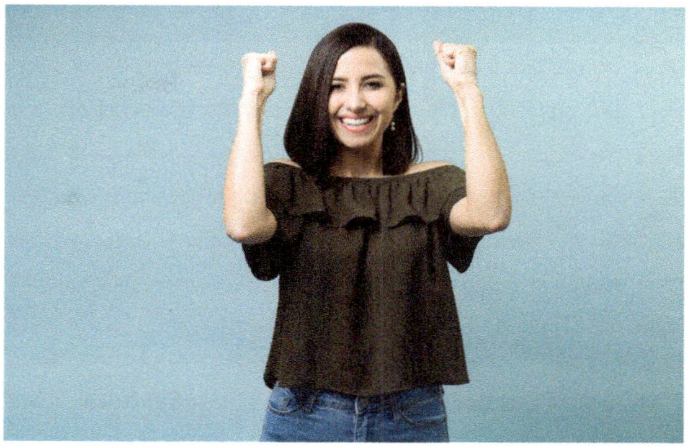

Antonio_Diaz/Getty Images

		YES	NO
1.	Do you believe that most problems will solve themselves if you just do not fool with them?	___	___
2.	Do you believe that you can stop yourself from catching a cold?	___	___
3.	Are some people just born lucky?	___	___
4.	Most of the time, do you feel that getting good grades means a great deal to you?	___	___
5.	Are you often blamed for things that just aren't your fault?	___	___
6.	Do you believe that if somebody studies hard enough, he or she can pass any subject?	___	___
7.	Do you feel that most of the time, it doesn't pay to try hard because things never turn out right anyway?	___	___
8.	Do you feel that if things start out well in the morning, it's going to be a good day, no matter what you do?	___	___
9.	Do you feel that most of the time parents listen to what their children have to say?	___	___
10.	Do you believe that wishing can make good things happen?	___	___
11.	When you get punished, does it usually seem to be for no good reason at all?	___	___
12.	Most of the time, do you find it hard to change a friend's opinion?	___	___
13.	Do you think cheering more than luck helps a team win?	___	___
14.	Do you feel that it is nearly impossible to change your parents' minds about anything?	___	___
15.	Do you believe that parents should allow children to make most of their own decisions?	___	___
16.	Do you feel that when you do something wrong, there's very little you can do to make it right?	___	___
17.	Do you believe that most people are just born good at sports?	___	___
18.	Are most other people your age stronger than you are?	___	___
19.	Do you feel that one of the best ways to handle most problems is just not to think about them?	___	___
20.	Do you feel that you have a lot of choice in deciding who your friends are?	___	___
21.	If you find a four-leaf clover, do you believe that it might bring you good luck?	___	___
22.	Do you often feel that whether or not you do your homework has much to do with what kind of grades you get?	___	___
23.	Do you feel that when a person your age is angry with you, there's little you can do to stop him or her?	___	___
24.	Have you ever had a good-luck charm?	___	___
25.	Do you believe that whether or not people like you depends on how you act?	___	___
26.	Do your parents usually help you if you ask them to?	___	___
27.	Do you ever feel that when people are angry with you, it is usually for no reason at all?	___	___
28.	Most of the time, do you feel that you can change what might happen tomorrow by what you do today?	___	___
29.	Do you believe that when bad things are going to happen, they are just going to happen, no matter what you try to do to stop them?	___	___
30.	Do you think that people can get their own way if they just keep trying?	___	___
31.	Most of the time, do you find it useless to try to get your own way at home?	___	___

		YES	NO
32.	Do you feel that when good things happen, they happen because of hard work?	___	___
33.	Do you feel that when somebody your age wants to be your enemy, there's little you can do to change matters?	___	___
34.	Do you feel that it's easy to get friends to do what you want them to do?	___	___
35.	Do you usually feel that you have little to say about what you get to eat at home?	___	___
36.	Do you feel that when someone doesn't like you, there's little you can do about it?	___	___
37.	Did you usually feel it was almost useless to try in school, because most other children were just plain smarter than you were?	___	___
38.	Are you the kind of person who believes that planning ahead makes things turn out better?	___	___
39.	Most of the time, do you feel that you have little to say about what your family decides to do?	___	___
40.	Do you think it's better to be smart than to be lucky?	___	___

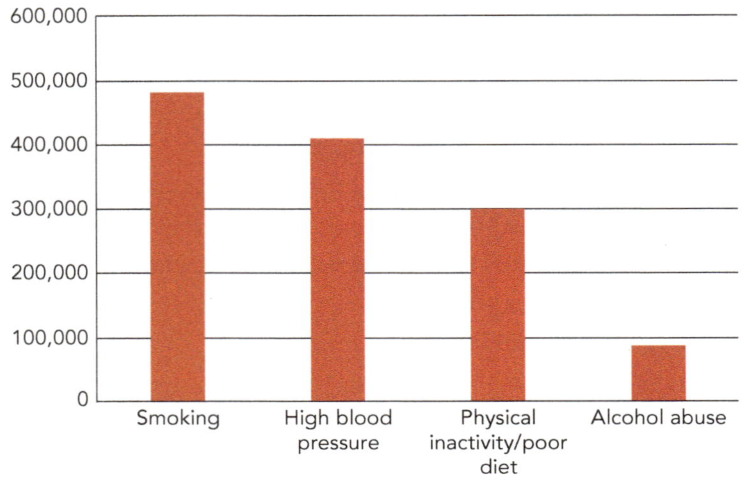

FIGURE 1.3 Estimated Annual Deaths Attributable to Individual Risk Factors Unhealthy behaviors and lack of appropriate medical care for chronic health conditions such as high blood pressure and high blood cholesterol are responsible for more than a million premature deaths in the United States each year.

Sources: CDC (2017d, 2019b), Danaei et al. (2011), NIAAA (2020), and Taksler et al. (2018).

The story of health psychology is largely about the efforts of behavioral scientists to identify unhealthy behavior patterns and apply psychological science to develop behavior change programs to help people live longer and healthier lives.

Historically, the leading cause of preventable deaths has been tobacco use. Despite progress in reducing the prevalence of cigarette smoking (see Chapter 9), we still lose some 480,000 people in the United States annually due to smoking-related causes. Cigarette smoking reduces a person's life span by about 10 years on average (United Health Foundation, 2019). Obesity is also a major contributor to preventable deaths, along with high blood pressure and high levels of cholesterol (Elmaleh-Sachs et al., 2023; Mangione et al., 2022). The math shows that every kilogram (2.2 pounds) of excess body weight takes more than 2 months off the average person's life span, although there are obviously individual differences (Joshi et al., 2017).

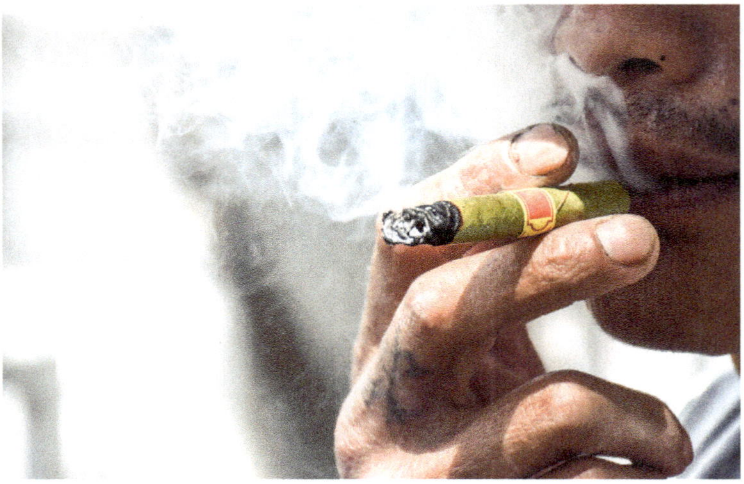

Aknarin Thika/EyeEm/Getty Images

What's the payoff in health and longevity of adopting a healthier lifestyle? Harvard University researchers conducted a long-term study that followed more than 100,000 people at age 50 through the next several decades of their lives (Li et al., 2020). They measured lifestyle factors repeatedly and tracked the development of serious diseases and deaths. A healthy lifestyle was defined as not smoking, maintaining a healthy body weight, regularly engaging in moderately vigorous physical activity, and following a healthy diet. The question was: How many additional years of living free of cancer, cardiovascular disease, and diabetes could people expect if they met all of these health objectives—a few months? A few years? The answer is an average of 7.6 years for men and 10.7 years for women.

Other preventable causes of death lie in the realm of medical errors (Rodziewicz & Hipskind, 2020). There are two types of errors:

- Errors of omission, resulting from actions not taken, such as failing to strap a person into a wheelchair, failing to use proper diagnostic techniques, or failing to provide a needed medicine or surgical procedure.
- Errors of commission, resulting from erroneous actions that are taken, such as administering a medicine to a person with a documented allergy to the medicine, incorrectly naming the person who has provided a laboratory specimen, or surgical mistakes. (It is reassuring that most surgeons routinely check that they will be operating on the correct leg by marking it.)

We do not have precise figures on the deaths that result from medical errors. However, we can note that some investigators consider them to be a leading cause of death. Fear of punishment obviously makes many healthcare professionals reluctant to report errors. When errors do come to light, they tarnish the reputations of hospitals and professionals. In later chapters we outline factors to consider when selecting healthcare professionals. Health psychologists note that it is crucial that we become knowledgeable consumers of health care. Physicians and other healthcare professionals are authority figures in our society, and sometimes it is necessary to question authority.

Health and Wellness

Health can be defined in different ways. The classic view of health, as understood within the biomedical model of disease, is that health is simply the absence of disease. If you are fortunate to be free of disease or injury, you are, by this definition, healthy. Health researchers who conceive of health in terms of the biopsychosocial model take a broader view of health, defining it not simply as the absence of disease but also as a state of physical, psychological, and social well-being.

health The state of physical, psychological, and social well-being.

The concept of health differs in a subtle but important way from that of **wellness**, which is a state of *optimal* physical, psychological, and social well-being. Wellness involves adoption of a healthy lifestyle. You may be healthy and free of disease, but you may still lack wellness if you are not attempting to optimize your well-being, as by making physical activity a routine part of your lifestyle.

wellness An optimal state of physical, psychological, and social well-being.

Health psychologists are concerned with helping people adjust to the challenges posed by serious or chronic illness. But that's only part of the story. They are also involved in developing health promotion programs that focus on wellness. The pursuit of wellness involves keeping physically fit, obtaining regular medical checkups, adhering to medical advice, developing healthier relationships, avoiding use of harmful substances, and seeking personal meaning to create a sense of purpose and self-fulfillment. It basically comes down to taking an active role in making the personal choices that lead to a healthier and more fulfilling life.

Many health psychologists work with businesses to help them develop wellness programs in the workplace. About four of five large companies in the United States provide wellness programs to their workers (Kaiser Family Foundation, 2018). Typically, these programs offer a range of services and resources, including comprehensive health assessments and education and coaching to help workers make healthy

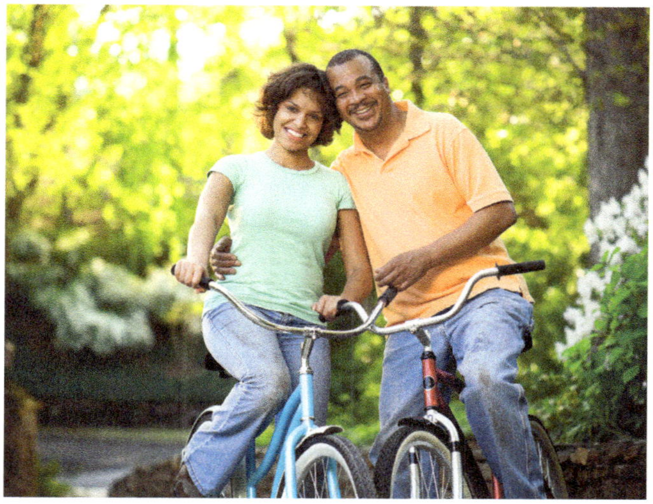

stevecoleimages/Getty Images

Health and Wellness Health and wellness are not defined by the absence of disease but by one's overall state of physical, psychological, and social well-being. How we live our lives plays a major role in our health and wellness.

behavioral changes, such as help quitting smoking, becoming more physically active, reducing stress, and managing weight (Abraham, 2019).

But do wellness programs have a positive health impact? Some psychologists have found that physical activity in workplace wellness programs not only improves physical health but also decreases absenteeism (Losina et al., 2017). Other researchers report mixed findings, some positive, some negative (Abraham, 2019; Raymond et al., 2019). Workplace wellness programs may boost some health-related behaviors, as by increasing regular exercise and promoting weight management, but they may not reduce healthcare costs (Song & Baicker, 2019).

One nagging problem in studying wellness programs is the variability in employee participation. If these programs are to boost healthy outcomes, they need to ensure a high level of participation (Raymond et al., 2019). Health psychologists are involved in designing programs that workers will use more consistently.

Psychological Science Applied to Health and Wellness

Health psychologists apply psychological science to many of the health problems we face in life. In the pages of this text, you will encounter the work of a great many health psychologists and other health researchers who apply psychological principles and theory in scientific studies across a wide range of health-related issues. They use scientific methods to better understand health-related behavior and evaluate health promotion and disease-prevention efforts. Among the many health-related issues they address, and that are discussed in this text, are the following:

- How do health behavior theories help us better understand the factors involved in the decision to get vaccinated for the flu, tuberculosis, or COVID-19, or to use condoms to protect oneself and one's partners from sexually transmitted diseases?
- How might we apply principles of reinforcement to reduce sugar consumption, help people lose excess weight and keep it off, and increase tooth-brushing behavior in children?
- What are the stages of change that determine whether a person is ready to make healthier behavior changes?
- How does our mental health affect our physical health and well-being?
- How do the workings of the body affect our health and well-being?
- What is the role of regular exercise in determining health outcomes and why is prolonged sitting a potential health risk?
- How do psychological principles like priming lead to ways of increasing the use of hand sanitizers in healthcare settings?

Review 1.1

INTERACTIVE SELF-SCORING QUIZZES

Sentence Completion

1. The subfield of psychology that explores relationships between behavior and physical health is called _______.
2. Dualism is the belief that mind and _______ are fundamentally different entities.
3. The scientific study of mind–body interactions began in the 19th century with the emergence of the field of _______ medicine.
4. The American physician who founded the American Psychosomatic Society was Helen Flanders _______.
5. _______ health psychologists focus on helping individuals lead healthier lives.
6. _______ health psychologists focus on improving the health of members of communities.
7. The biomedical model of disease defines health as the _______ of disease or injury.
8. A broader conception of health defines it not simply by the absence of disease but also as a state of physical, psychological, and social _______.
9. The leading conceptual model in health psychology is a multidimensional framework called the _______ model.
10. Anxiety and depression can impair the _______ system, making us more vulnerable to physical disorders.

Think About It

If you worked for a company that offered a wellness program, would you use it? What features of the wellness program would you be most likely to use? Which would you be least likely to use, and why?

Health Psychology in the Global Context

Promoting health and combating disease are global challenges, ever more so today because the world is so closely interconnected. As the COVID-19 pandemic illustrated, a person with an infectious disease can board an international flight and within hours arrive anywhere in the world, infecting people in these locales who in turn infect still others in a spreading web of disease that does not respect national borders. On a positive note, advances in medical research can also have far-reaching consequences, improving the health and well-being of people in distant countries and remote villages.

Global health is the field of study, research, and practice that focuses on improvement of health of people worldwide. Health psychology is also a global endeavor, as health psychologists seek to understand behavioral factors contributing to global health challenges, the spread of infectious diseases such as COVID-19 and HIV/AIDS, and the devastating effects of smoking and the use of other harmful substances. They develop initiatives designed to promote healthier behaviors. For example, health psychologists implemented a health promotion program with university students in South Africa, finding that students who received the intervention were more likely to meet physical activity guidelines and show lower levels of self-reported consumption of fried foods (Heeren et al., 2018).

Health psychologists recognize the need to take cross-cultural differences in health into account. Consider, for example, that mortality (death) rates from cancer are higher in the Netherlands, Denmark, England, Canada, and—yes—the United States. Although many factors—including genetic and environmental factors—may contribute to an increased risk of cancer, a common denominator in these countries is a relatively high intake of fat, especially the saturated fat found in meat and dairy products. Death rates from cancer are much lower in Thailand, the Philippines, and Japan, where the daily fat intake is lower. Do not assume that the difference is racial because Thailand, the Philippines, and Japan are Asian nations. The diets of Japanese Americans are similar in fat content to those of other Americans—and their death rates from cancer are also higher.

Health psychologists also study how folk beliefs may affect the provision of health care. For example, African researchers conducted interviews with people living with diabetes in a poor urban area of Ghana (de-Graft Aikins, Awuah, & Pera, 2015). They found that attributing symptoms of diabetes to supernatural causes, such as sorcery or witchcraft, was associated with a lack of disclosure of their illness to others for fear that revealing symptoms would put them at risk of the listener's using sorcery against them.

One of the challenges of global health is the wide disparity in access to health resources worldwide. People in poorer countries have limited access to medicinal drugs and medical care that people in more affluent countries may take for granted. Diseases that have been effectively eliminated in affluent countries, such as malaria, continue to spread misery and death in less developed nations. Yet there has been substantial progress in improving health and longevity worldwide. For example, infant mortality has declined by more than 50% worldwide since 1990, and maternal mortality (death of women during pregnancy) has fallen 43% (Filippi et al., 2016; World Bank, 2023; World Health Organization, 2018). But we will see that health disparities are a national as well as an international concern.

In some respects, global health concerns mirror those seen in the United States. Noncommunicable diseases (NCDs) such as heart disease, stroke, chronic lung diseases, and cancer are the leading causes of disease worldwide, as they are in the United States. Worldwide, NCDs account for about seven of 10 deaths overall and more than one in three premature deaths (Alcántara et al., 2020). Health psychologists are involved in developing health initiatives by assisting people here and abroad to make changes that can lower their risk of developing these chronic diseases.

Among the leading chronic health conditions globally is high blood pressure (hypertension), which is a major risk factor for cardiovascular diseases such as heart disease and stroke (see Chapter 12). Achieving control over blood pressure is especially problematic in developing countries that lack health resources that are available to people in more technologically developed countries.

Recently, health researchers adapted methods used in more developed countries to improve health outcomes of people with hypertension from rural communities in several South Asian countries (Bangladesh, Pakistan, and Sri Lanka) (Jafar et al., 2020; Poulter, 2020).

People with hypertension in the study received either a low-cost (<$11 per person annually) multicomponent intervention or usual care. Those receiving the multicomponent intervention had regular home visits in which trained government health workers measured their blood pressure and provided health education and counseling focused on adopting healthier diets and lifestyles. Health care was also coordinated with local physicians who followed a structured treatment protocol for prescribing medications. At a 2-year follow-up, people receiving multicomponent treatment showed greater reductions in blood pressure than the control group receiving usual care. This type of program offers an affordable strategy for improving blood pressure control in many areas of the world in which healthcare resources are scarce.

We should also note that infectious or communicable diseases pose a much greater threat to health and survival in other parts of the world than they do in the United States. Communicable diseases such as diarrheal diseases are among the 10 leading causes of death worldwide, though they are largely controlled in the United States and other developed countries. Other communicable or infectious diseases, such as malaria, are grim threats faced by many of the world's poorest, which have less developed public health care and sanitation systems. The threats posed by communicable diseases globally require greater resources directed toward infection control procedures (WHO, 2018).

Health and Diversity in the United States: Nations Within the Nation

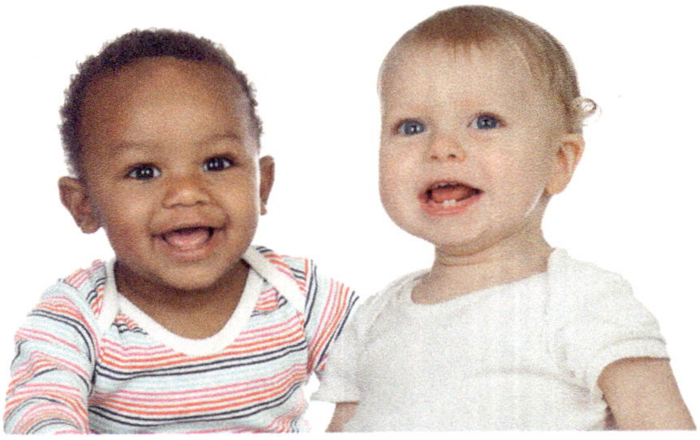
Gelpi/Shutterstock.com

Which of These Babies Is Likely to Live Longer? Non-Hispanic White baby boys, on average, can expect to live about 5 years longer than African American baby boys. For girls, the difference in longevity is nearly 3 years in favor of non-Hispanic Whites. To what extent does access to health care play a role in these discrepancies?

From the perspective of health and health care, we are many nations, not just one. Various factors, including ethnicity and gender, have a bearing on how long we are likely to live and how healthy we are likely to be.

Life Expectancy in Relation to Race, Ethnicity, and Socioeconomic Status Life expectancy in the United States had been rising steadily for many decades but began to decline in 2014, first as a result of a spike in drug overdoses in the wake of the nation's opioid epidemic (see Chapter 9) as well as increased rates of suicide, and then in the early 2020s as the result of the COVID-19 pandemic (Xu et al., 2020a). The good news is that life expectancy at birth, based on the latest available statistics, turned upward again in 2022, rising to 77.5 years overall, 74.8 years for males, and 80.2 years for females (Arias et al., 2023).

Average life expectancy can be a misleading statistic because it does not take gender or ethnicity into account (see **Figure 1.4**) (Arias & Xu, 2019; Carnethon, Kershaw, & Kandula, 2020). Notice that, on average, the life span of non-Hispanic Black Americans is nearly 5 years less than that of non-Hispanic White Americans. The life expectancy of (non-Hispanic) Asian Americans is the longest.

How might we account for these racial and ethnic differences? An important factor is SES. Non-Hispanic Blacks are disproportionately represented among the lower income levels in our society, and people on the lower rungs of the socioeconomic ladder—especially Black men—have lower life expectancies (Johnson et al., 2022; Khan et al., 2022). Social or economic disadvantage in the form of poverty and unemployment is associated with a significant increase in the risk of death (Alcántara et al., 2020). Not only are wealthier people likely to live longer, but they also more likely to remain healthy and free of age-related disabilities for about 9 years longer than the least affluent people (Picheta, 2020).

We also need to consider other factors, including greater proneness among Black Americans to risk factors for cardiovascular disease, such as hypertension, obesity, and diabetes. But other factors may also contribute, including differences in diet, physical activity, and access to health care. A different story emerges when we look at life expectancies of Latino/Hispanic Americans, who live about 3 years longer, on average, than non-Hispanic White Americans.

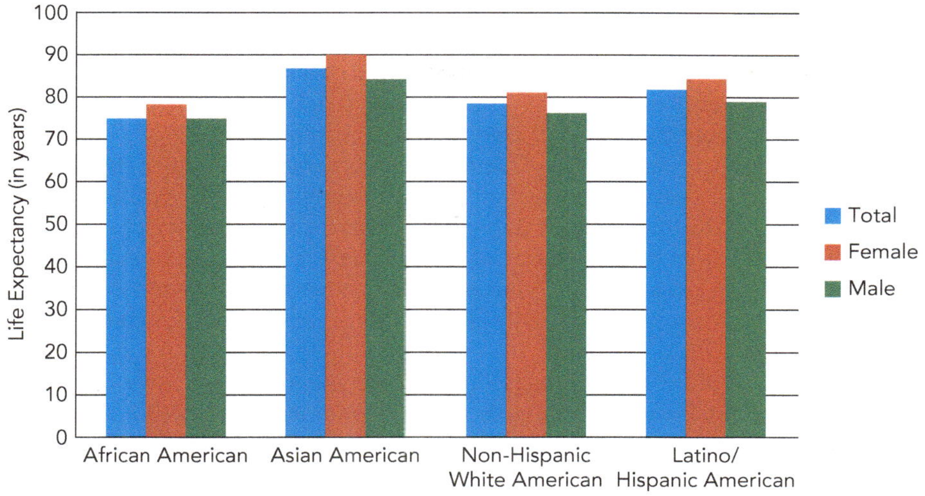

FIGURE 1.4 **Life Expectancy by Sex and Race/Ethnicity, United States**
Source: Arias & Xu, 2019 / Centers for Disease Control and Prevention / Public Domain.

Latino/Hispanic Americans have a lower death rate from several killer diseases as compared with Whites, including heart disease and cancer (Arias et al., 2015).

Longevity is but one marker of living a full and healthy life. We need to look at other health indices as well. For example, Spanish-speaking Latino/Hispanic Americans are less likely to be screened than non-Hispanic White Americans or English-speaking Latinos/Hispanics for colorectal cancer, a leading cancer killer (NCI, 2019). Latino/Hispanic Americans are also at greater risk than non-Hispanic White Americans of developing HIV/AIDS and adult-onset diabetes.

Genetic factors also play a role in racial/ethnic group differences in health. For example, the incidence of sickle-cell anemia is highest among Black Americans and Latino/Hispanic Americans. The incidence of Tay-Sachs disease is greatest among Jews of Eastern European origin.

Other risk factors differentially affecting (non-Hispanic) Blacks are overweight and hypertension (high blood pressure), which are two of the major risk factors for heart disease and stroke (Lee, 2019). Cardiovascular illness and deaths are higher among Blacks than Whites (Bauer & Thompson, 2018; Cunningham et al., 2017). Black people also tend to have more risk factors linked to complications and death from COVID-19, such as heart disease and diabetes (Egede & Walker, 2020; Yancy, 2020).

Although there may be a genetic component in these risk factors, lifestyle factors such as diet and physical activity play significant roles. Interestingly, Black Americans are more likely to suffer from hypertension than are Black Africans, suggesting that environmental factors affecting many Black Americans—such as stress, diet, and smoking, may contribute to their increased risk of hypertension. Black Americans may also face life stressors that can have a negative impact on health and longevity, such as insecure housing, poverty, crime, and exposure to discrimination.

Another factor contributing to racial/ethnic differences in health outcomes is quality of treatment. Non-Hispanic Black Americans tend to receive different levels of treatment by medical practitioners. They are less likely than (non-Hispanic) White Americans to receive hip and knee replacements, kidney transplants, mammograms, and flu shots (Ghomrawi et al., 2018; Quinn, 2018; Yeary et al., 2018). Black women are 42% more likely to die from breast cancer than White women in the United States, even though they are less likely than White women to develop breast cancer. This discrepancy is partly explained by the fact that Black women tend to develop breast cancer at an earlier age but to be diagnosed at a later age than White women. The later diagnosis may be a result of less access to healthcare services, especially cancer care. However, genetic factors are also apparently involved, making breast cancer generally more aggressive in Black women (Centers for Disease Control and Prevention, 2017b).

The United States and Canada have the resources to provide the most advanced health care in the world. But not all of us have access to these advantages. People of color tend to have less access to quality health care than do White people (Dickman et al., 2022; Hamed et al., 2022; Shuman & Malani, 2018). Why do these discrepancies exist? Various explanations have been offered, including cultural differences, cost and lack of access to specialized medical services at the neighborhood level, cultural mistrust of the healthcare system among people of color, lack of awareness or knowledge about health risks, and racism.

Early diagnosis and treatment might help reduce racial gaps in life expectancy. However, evidence bears out that people of color may not receive the same quality of medical services as their (non-Hispanic) White American counterparts. For example, Black adults in the United States with heart disease patients are less likely than their White counterparts to receive aggressive treatments, such as bypass surgery, even when it appears that they would benefit equally from the procedure (Stolberg, 2001). Black Americans and other ethnic minorities tend to have less access to cardiovascular and other healthcare services than White Americans—services that might potentially identify health conditions before they reach more serious stages (NCHS, 2023).

Underutilization of health services is a pressing problem among Latinos/Hispanics, as they tend to engage in fewer medical visits than Black Americans and White Americans. A number of factors are involved in accounting for lower use of medical services among Latinos/Hispanics, such as lack of health insurance; financial difficulties to manage medical fees, even copays; linguistic difficulties communicating with English-speaking healthcare providers; fewer neighborhood healthcare providers; and concerns about immigration status and fear of deportation for undocumented people. Latino/Hispanic preschoolers are also less likely than their Black or White counterparts to be immunized against childhood diseases.

One major factor contributing to racial or ethnic disparities in utilization of medical services is the fact that greater percentages of Black Americans and Latino/Hispanic Americans and other ethnic minorities, such as American Indian and Alaska Native peoples, are uninsured as compared to Whites (Cohen et al., 2019)—a topic we explore further in Chapter 3.

Socioeconomic Disparities in Health Outcomes

Racial or ethnic differences in markers of health and longevity may mask differences in SES, which encompasses income and educational level. African Americans are disproportionately represented among the lower income levels in our society, and people on the lower rungs of the socioeconomic ladder have lower life expectancies and more risk factors for life-threatening diseases, such as heart attack and stroke (Mariotto et al., 2018; Murphy et al., 2017; Rehm & Probst, 2018).

We need to consider social determinants of health inequalities. Evidence shows that social factors such as housing instability and food insecurity disproportionally affect minoritized groups and represent sources of life stress that adversely affect the physical and mental health of these groups (Alegria & Cheng, 2023).

We also need to consider that people on the lower rungs of the socioeconomic ladder tend to be medically underserved, often because of a lack of affordable health insurance. They also tend to have more risk factors for heart disease and cancer, such as smoking, inactivity, and obesity (He et al., 2021; NCHS, 2023). Unhealthy lifestyles can take a toll on health outcomes and longevity.

Black Americans have higher death rates from many (though not all) forms of cancer (NCI, 2019) (see Chapter 13). Again, lower SES may help explain these differences, as people in the lower rungs of SES tend to smoke more frequently, exercise less regularly, and consume a diet richer in unhealthy fats, all of which are factors implicated in various forms of cancer.

Wealthier, better-educated people tend to take better care of themselves, in large part because they have greater financial resources that allow them to join a gym or participate in exercise programs and obtain more regular health care. They are less likely to smoke and have the resources to shop for healthier (and often more expensive) foods. By contrast, people living in poorer neighborhoods face a type of environmental racism, with a proliferation of nearby fast food restaurants and grocery stores that offer limited healthier food choices. The stressful burden imposed by financial strains may also lead people in poorer neighborhoods to rely on junk food or overeating as a way of coping with stress.

Health promotion efforts designed to help people change unhealthy habits have been less successful in reaching people of lower socioeconomic standing. The problem is compounded by the fact that people of low SES are also less likely to receive health education messages about the importance of regular health checkups and early medical intervention when symptoms arise. They also tend to have poorer access to healthcare services (AHRQ, 2019). As we noted, factors such as costs of health care and lack of health insurance or underinsurance are major contributors to healthcare disparities.

Stress places people at greater risk of physical illness, ranging from gastrointestinal disorders to heart attacks. People at lower SES levels are more likely to suffer the effects of stress for two reasons. First, people from economically-distressed neighborhoods are more likely to encounter more significant life stressors, such as financial hardship, insecure housing, and crime. Second, poorer people are less likely to have the resources to cope with stress, such as access to healthcare professionals.

All in all, health psychologists and other health researchers are aware of the complex matrix of factors that underlie racial and ethnic disparities in health outcomes and longevity and of the need to find ways of providing prevention and treatment services to all members of the population.

Life Expectancy and Gender

Being male shaves about 5 years off the average person's life expectancy. On average, women live about 5 years longer than men (life expectancies are about 75 years for men and about 80 years for women) (Arias et al., 2023; Mueller, 2023; Yan et al., 2023).

A major factor explaining this gender discrepancy is that men typically engage in riskier behaviors. They are more likely to smoke, to consume larger amounts of alcohol (contributing to cirrhosis of the liver and other serious medical problems), and to die from acts of violence, accidents, and suicide (de Visser, 2019). They also tend to pay less attention to their health and to follow their doctors' recommendations.

Surveys of physicians and of the general population find that women are generally more willing than men to seek health care (Mursa, Patterson, & Halcomb, 2022; Ramos-Vera et al., 2022). Women are also more likely to perform regular self-exams, such as checking their breasts for lumps, than men are to examine themselves for possible early signs of cancer, such as checking for lumps in their testicles or elsewhere. Perhaps because of the lingering gender stereotype that men are expected to be self-sufficient and shouldn't rely on help from others, men may just let symptoms go until a problem that might have been prevented or readily treatable becomes serious or life-threatening.

Many men seem to have a *bulletproof mentality*, believing they are too strong to need a doctor, or too busy. Health psychologists study attitudes and beliefs people hold about seeking healthcare services and following through with treatment, recognizing that negative beliefs are a major impediment not only to obtaining help but also to adhering to medical treatment.

Review 1.2

INTERACTIVE SELF-SCORING QUIZZES

Sentence Completion

1. Mortality or death rates from cancer are (higher or lower) than in Asia in the Netherlands, Denmark, England, Canada, and the United States.

2. Diseases that have been effectively eliminated in more affluent countries, such as ________, continue to spread misery worldwide.

3. Life expectancy in the United States is (higher or lower) overall for men as compared to women in recent years.

4. Non-Hispanic Black American males live nearly 5 years (less or more), on average, than non-Hispanic White American males.

5. Black people with heart disease are (less likely or more likely) than their White counterparts to receive aggressive treatment.

6. Survey research indicates that women are (more willing or less willing) to seek health care than men.

7. Many men seem to have a ________ mentality when it comes to seeking health care.

Think About It

What factors contribute to socioeconomic differences in health outcomes? What do you think can be done to reduce these disparities?

Research Methods in Health Psychology

Is there a link between diet and risk of cancer? Is light to moderate use of alcohol a health risk or a health benefit? Do health apps work? These are some of the research questions we will pose in later chapters. But here, let us focus on the scientific method and the research methods health psychologists use to address these and other questions about our health and well-being.

The Scientific Method

The scientific method is an organized way that scientists use to test ideas and expand and refine their knowledge based on careful observation and experimentation (see **Figure 1.5**). It is not a recipe that psychologists and other scientists follow but rather a set of general principles that guides their research. Psychologists usually begin by formulating a research question. Research questions can have many sources. Our daily experiences, psychological theory, even folklore and intuition all help generate questions for research. A research question may be studied as a question or reworded as a hypothesis—a specific prediction about behavior or mental processes that is tested through research. Let us consider the various research methods used by health psychologists.

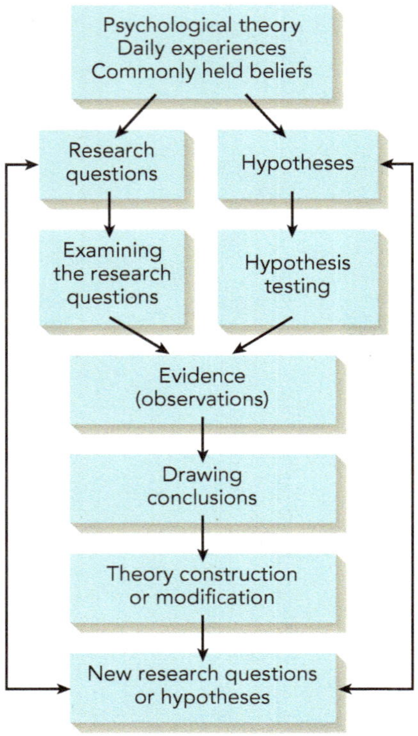

FIGURE 1.5 The Scientific Method The scientific method provides a systematic way of organizing and expanding scientific knowledge.

VIDEO CONTENT
The Scientific Method

VIDEO CONTENT
Psychological Research

The Case Study Method

The **case study method** is an intensive and detailed study of an individual or a few individuals with particular health conditions. Sigmund Freud relied on the case study method, studying his clients in depth in an attempt to understand factors that lead to abnormal behavior patterns, such as troubling psychological problems.

That said, researchers recognize the limitations of the case study method. There are bound to be gaps in memory when people are questioned. People may also distort their pasts because of a **social desirability bias**. Interviewers may also have certain expectations and may subtly encourage subjects to fill in gaps in ways that are consistent with their theoretical perspectives. All in all, case studies may provide useful or revealing information, but they lack the rigorous controls found in experimental methods.

The case study method represents a type of **qualitative research**, a method of research that relies on gathering nonnumerical or nonquantitative data from interviews, observations in natural setting, personal narratives, and textual analysis of written records, in order to learn about people's behaviors, beliefs, and attitudes (Pathak, Jena, & Kalra, 2013). We will see examples of qualitative research in this text, including a study in Chapter 14 that cataloged responses of terminally ill people to questions about wisdom and the meaning of life. Evidence from qualitative studies can be combined with quantitative measures to provide a richer understanding of health-related issues.

case study method
A method of research based on a carefully drawn biography obtained through interviews, questionnaires, or psychological tests.

social desirability bias
The tendency of people to respond in socially desirable ways.

qualitative research
A non-numerical method of research based on collecting and analyzing information drawn from interviews, observations, personal narratives, and written materials.

The Correlational Method

Health psychologists use the **correlational method** to study links between behavioral risk factors and health outcomes. These links are expressed in the form of a statistical association, or **correlation**, between variables under study. Through this method, we learn about relationships between diet and cancer (discussed in Chapter 13) and exercise and heart disease (discussed in Chapter 8), among many others.

A correlation is an association between two variables, which is expressed in the form of a correlation coefficient that can vary in size from −1.00 to +1.00. A positive sign means there is a positive relationship between the two variables, so that as one of the variables increases, the other tends to increase as well. A negative sign points to an inverse relationship such that as one variable increases, the other tends to decrease. For example, and hardly surprisingly, ice cream sales tend to be positively correlated with ambient temperature, as people tend to buy more ice cream as temperatures rise during the summer. As for an inverse or negative relationship, we shouldn't be surprised to find that as hours of sleep decrease, the number of errors on test performance tends to increase.

correlational method
A method of research examining relationships among variables.

correlation A statistical association or relationship between two variables, expressed in the form of a correlation coefficient.

Notice the use of the words "tend" and "tends." Unless there is a perfect +1.00 or −1.00 correlation coefficient, changes in one variable do not perfectly correspond to changes in the other. It's like trying to predict the path of a hurricane based on a set of meteorological factors. Our predictions may be better than chance, but lacking a perfect correlation between the variables of interest, we cannot make predictions with absolute certainty. The size or magnitude of the correlation coefficient indicates the strength of the relationship between the two variables. The larger the magnitude, the more reliably we can use changes in one variable to predict changes in the other.

Consider relationships between stress and the likelihood of a common cold. Let's assume there is a positive correlation such that increases in stress tend to be associated with increased vulnerability to the common cold. Based on this evidence, we could make a better-than-chance prediction that people under high levels of stress are more likely to develop a cold (upper respiratory infection). That being said, while correlational relationships may *suggest* a cause-and-effect relationship, they are not *sufficient* to establish a causal relationship between two variables.

It may be the case that stress is a causal factor determining vulnerability to the common cold. One possibility is that stress negatively affects the body's immune system, the body's line of defense against disease-causing organisms, such as bacteria and viruses (see Chapter 4). However, it is also possible that people under stress take poorer care of their health (not exercising as regularly, getting less sleep, etc.) and that these factors, not stress per se, account for poorer immune system functioning. The possibility that other factors account for the variables in a study represents the so-called *third variable problem*, namely that some alternative factor, say insufficient sleep, may account for a relationship between two other factors (stress and the common cold). Another possibility is that the causal links are actually reversed, such that people in poorer health may encounter higher levels of stress.

Observational studies use the correlational method to observe relationships between variables that are not directly controlled or manipulated by the experimenter. Consider evidence of linkages between negative thinking and depression. As we'll see in Chapter 11, depressed people tend to show more negative thinking than nondepressed people, such as exaggerating disappointments or failures, focusing only on the negatives, and heaping blame on themselves for negative outcomes. While thinking negatively in the face of disappointing life events may lead to depression, we need to consider alternative possibilities, such as depression leading to negative thinking.

Chinese investigators used the observational method to examine the relationships between tea consumption and cardiovascular disease (Wang et al., 2020). The researchers didn't control whether people drank tea or how much tea they drank. They merely analyzed the frequency of cardiovascular incidents (heart attacks, strokes, and other problems) between people at higher and lower levels of tea consumption. Tea, especially green tea, is rich in certain plant chemicals called *flavonoids* that may have healthy effects on the heart and circulatory system (Bakalar, 2020). The investigators analyzed health records from more than 100,000 Chinese adults and compared these data to self-reports of tea consumption. Correlational analysis showed a relationship between tea consumption and cardiovascular incidents over a period of 7 years, which when broken down further revealed that individuals who drank more than three cups of tea weekly had a 20% lower risk of cardiovascular incidents and also lower risks for cardiovascular death and premature death from any cause.

Can we say from this data that drinking tea is actually good for the heart and circulatory system? Perhaps it is, but finding a correlation between two variables, in this case between tea consumption and cardiovascular incidents, doesn't suffice to establish a causal link. We need to await experimental data in which tea consumption over a period of years is directly controlled by experimenters to see if tea actually has beneficial effects on cardiovascular health.

The bottom line is that while correlational research may suggest possible causal relationships, we need experimental methods to pinpoint cause-and-effect relationships. Although correlation is not causation, there are at least three ways in which correlational studies provide importance sources of evidence in health psychology and other fields:

1. *They help us predict future outcomes or behaviors.* When we find that two variables are correlated, we can use one to predict the other. For example, evidence shows that teenagers who hold more positive expectancies about the use of alcohol, such as expecting that

drinking alcohol will make them more confident or sociable, are more likely to develop problems with alcohol use and abuse than those with less favorable expectancies. Consequently, knowing factors that predict future problems with some degree of confidence can help us direct preventive efforts toward high-risk groups, such as adolescents with positive alcohol expectancies. We might even be able to change their attitudes about alcohol before problems develop.

2. *They offer clues to causal influences.* We may not be able to determine causal relationships based on correlational data alone, but correlational relationships can point us toward identifying possible underlying causes. For example, knowing there is a correlation between exposure to lead paint in the home and academic performance of schoolchildren can lead to studies that determine the causal role of lead exposure on cognitive abilities.
3. *They help us better understand relationships among variables.* We can use correlational methods to better understand relationships between health behaviors and health outcomes. Correlational studies allow us to address questions we pose in later chapters, such as: Does regular physical exercise predict longevity? Do personality factors relate to health and longevity? Is the risk of cancer linked to stress?

Health Psychology in the Digital Age

Health Research in the Smartphone Era

Health researchers and healthcare providers are turning to smartphone apps to help them collect data from patients and research participants. Using these apps, physicians can monitor patients' symptoms and adherence to medication. Researchers can directly cull data from daily experiences of participants in their studies. Researchers are also equipping people with wearable devices, such as smart watches and activity trackers, to help people keep track of their levels of physical activity, levels of pain, and other physical symptoms in real time (Chau et al., 2019; Eccleston et al., 2018; Ranby, 2019). People with chronic pain have been outfitted with wearable devices they can use to report their levels of pain during the day, providing data that health professionals can use to see how pain fluctuates in relation to time of day, activities (sitting, walking, etc.), and states of mind (bored, feeling down, anxious, etc.). In another example, people with epilepsy wore sensor-infused bands that transmitted alerts to their healthcare providers when a seizure was about to happen (Poh et al., 2012).

Researchers are also using Web-based survey tools to conduct online surveys rather than using traditional questionnaires administered in person or by (snail) mail. Investigators realize that samples drawn from the internet may be biased in certain ways, as people who respond to online surveys may not be representative of the target audience. However, online surveys offer opportunities to expand research samples to a worldwide laboratory of potential participants who are but a few keystrokes away.

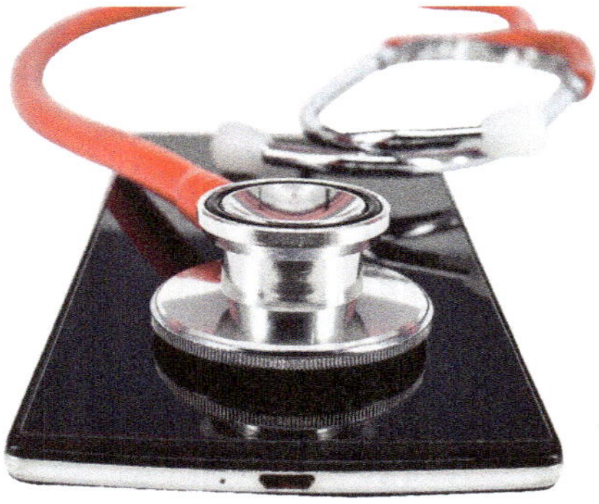

Hilalabdullah Hilal/EyeEm/Getty Images

Researchers are also mining social media sites to detect relationships between online behavior and health outcomes (Gosling & Mason, 2015; Kosinski et al., 2016). Cornell University researchers turned their attention to the content of Twitter messages at various times of day. By analyzing more than a half billion messages, the researchers noticed some interesting patterns. It turned out that happier words associated with more positive mood states were tweeted more often during the early morning hours (Weaver, 2012). But as the day dragged on, tweets became more negative in tone. As one of these researchers, Michael Macy, pointed out, "We found people are happiest around breakfast time in the morning and then it's all downhill from there." Consider you own daily fluctuations in mood. Do you feel chipper early in the day and grumpier as the day grinds on? Do the demands of daily life affect your mood in predictable ways?

Occupational health psychologists created an app designed to reduce fatigue in airline pilots (van Drongelen et al., 2016). The app provided information on optimal light exposure, sleep, nutrition, and physical activity and was tailored to the pilot's personal characteristics and work assignments (short haul vs. longer flights). More than 80% of pilots who received the app said they had used the advice and a majority (65%) said that the app met its purpose of helping them prevent fatigue and improving health outcomes (van Drongelen et al., 2016).

Many people today are using mobile health apps. But are they using them consistently? In one recent study, researchers found that people who had intentions to lose weight and exercise more often were more likely to own a mobile health app (Tuman & Moyer, 2019). But owning an app is one thing and using it consistently is quite another. Questions remain about how consistently smartphone apps are used and whether they lead to measurable changes in health-related behaviors, or whether they sit docked on the user's phone. Where things now stand, researchers say, is that while smartphone apps and other digital health tools are widely available, only a few of them have been scientifically evaluated in clinical trials (Kwasnicka et al., 2022).

A cross-cultural study examined relationships between family factors and health status of a sample of 53 Native American, 132 Black American, and 155 Latino/Hispanic families with an adolescent living at home (Bradley, 2019). Investigators made home visits to these families, administering measures of family connectedness and evaluating the health status of the adolescent family member. Correlational analysis showed that adolescents in families with higher levels of family connectedness tended to have fewer health problems. Might it be that spending more productive time with family members helps protects adolescents from health problems? *Possibly*, but we simply can't say based on correlational analysis alone. But the fact that these factors are related suggests it may be worthwhile to test whether programs aimed at promoting better engagement between parents and their adolescent children may be helpful. After all, building these family connections at a time when teens tend to pull away from their families and are prone toward engaging in risky behaviors, such as drug use, may help keep them safe and healthy.

The Case-Control Method

In the **case-control method**, investigators identify individuals with known health conditions and compare them to healthier people. The individuals with known health conditions are called index cases or **probands**, while the healthy participants are classified as control cases. Investigators match probands and controls on as many characteristics as possible, such as gender, age, ethnicity or race, educational levels, and so on, and then look for distinguishing factors that might explain differences between the groups. This type of research uses correlational methods, but it can point to possible causes, such as in early studies comparing smokers and nonsmokers in the attempt to determine whether smoking causes cancer.

case-control method A method of comparing cases of individuals with a particular disease with control cases who are free of the disease in order to find differences that might explain the development of the disease.

probands Index cases of individuals identified as having a particular disease or physical condition.

You're probably aware that the federal government requires all cigarette packs to carry a warning label that smoking causes cancer (and other diseases). A classic example of a case-control study first raised awareness that smoking may cause cancer. This 1939 study in Germany identified 86 cases of people with lung cancer and a similar number of control cases of people without cancer. The investigators found much higher rates of smoking among the people with lung cancer, suggesting a possible causal link (cited in Proctor, 2012). Later case-control studies in the United Kingdom and the United States confirmed a much greater frequency of smoking in people with lung cancer as compared to control cases. But as we'll see later in this chapter, nailing down the causal connections between smoking and cancer required follow-up studies using the experimental method.

The Epidemiological Method

In using the **epidemiological method**, investigators examine community- or population-wide variations in the rates of various disorders and socioeconomic differences in health and longevity. They then try to identify factors that account for these variations, in effect acting as public health detectives in trying to account for why some population groups are more vulnerable than others.

epidemiological method A method of research in which researchers conduct surveys, examine databases, and perform field studies to identify communities and subgroups of individuals at higher risk of developing particular disorders.

In an epidemiological study mentioned earlier in this chapter that mined one of the largest databases to date, researchers culled income data from 1.4 billion tax records for the U.S. population between 1999 and 2014 (Chetty et al., 2016). The names of individual taxpayers were shielded. The investigators examined mortality data in relation to life expectancy while statistically adjusting for race and ethnicity. The most prominent finding was that higher income was associated with greater longevity. The gap in longevity between the richest 1% of the population and the poorest 1% was nearly 15 years for men and about 10 years for women. One of the running themes in our study of health psychology is that more advantaged groups are typically healthier and live longer than less advantaged groups. We'll see that factors such as access to quality healthcare services and adoption of healthier behaviors (e.g., smoking less, exercising more regularly) play an important role in accounting for differences between groups of different income levels.

incidence The number of new cases of a disorder occurring within a specific period of time.

prevalence The number of existing cases of a disorder within a given population.

To determine rates of specific disorders, we need to distinguish between **incidence**, which is the number of new cases occurring during a specific period of time, and **prevalence**, which is the overall number of cases of a given disorder within a population for a particular period of time. Prevalence rates are necessarily higher than incidence rates, as they include both new cases and existing cases.

Researchers can use epidemiological methods to determine whether particular diseases or disorders cluster in certain groups or locations. They then seek to determine what characteristics put these clusters at higher risk. One limitation of the epidemiological method, like that of the case-control method, is that it cannot determine causal influences. In other words, epidemiological research may identify characteristics that may account for the increased risk of particular diseases in certain groups, but it cannot determine causal factors. For determining causal relationships, we need to turn to experimental studies, as we'll soon see.

survey A method of information gathering by which large numbers of individuals are interviewed or asked to complete questionnaires in order to learn about their attitudes or behaviors.

population A complete group of organisms or events.

sample A portion of a population selected for research.

random selection A process of randomly selecting research participants from a population of interest.

random sample A sample drawn such that every member of a population has an equal chance of being selected.

random assignment A procedure for assigning subjects to experimental or control groups by chance so that experimenters can have confidence that differences between groups are due to the independent (treatment) variable and not the types of participants making up the groups.

selection bias A type of bias in which differences between experimental and control groups are due to the differences in the types of participants in the groups rather than the variable(s) of interest.

The Survey Method

A **survey** is a method of correlational research involving the use of questionnaires and structured interviews to measure opinions, behaviors, values, and other attributes of members of particular groups. Epidemiological researchers often rely on surveys to measure health-related behaviors and health conditions of residents in particular communities or members of particular groups. The survey method allows investigators to determine whether various groups are more likely to be affected by different types of health conditions, such as heart disease, diabetes, and cancer. They can also collect data to determine relationships between rates of particular disorders and factors such as race, ethnicity, gender, and social class.

In the best of all possible worlds, researchers would survey every member of a **population** of interest. Health researchers who are interested in examining links between binge drinking and academic grades on a particular college campus might survey the drinking habits of every matriculated student. However, surveying every member of the student body is unrealistic, or at least unlikely. Therefore, imagine the problems in trying to survey every college student in the country in order to generalize the findings across campuses. Consequently, most surveys are conducted on samples of participants.

A **sample** is a subset of a population. Instead of surveying drinking habits of every student on campus (the population of interest), an investigator might obtain a sample of perhaps 10% of students on campus. In order to generalize results based on a sample to the population of interest, the researcher needs to ensure that the sample represents the target population.

The best way of ensuring a representative sample is by using **random selection**, which is a procedure in which way each member of the population has an equal probability of participating in the sample. When properly constituted, a **random sample** may represent but sliver of the population, but it is robust enough that its results can be generalized to the larger population. A proper random sample of but a few hundred voters, for example, may be sufficient to represent the voting preferences of the entire population.

Random selection should not be confused with random assignment. Random selection means choosing members of a population at random to participate in a research study or complete a survey instrument. Use of random selection enables a researcher to generalize results based on a sample of individuals to the population from which it was drawn. **Random assignment** refers to randomizing the placement of research participants into experimental or control groups in order to balance the individual characteristics of the participants across the groups. In this way, experimenters can control for a potential **selection bias**, in which the types of people who make up the experimental and control groups, rather than the experimental variables, explain the different research outcomes.

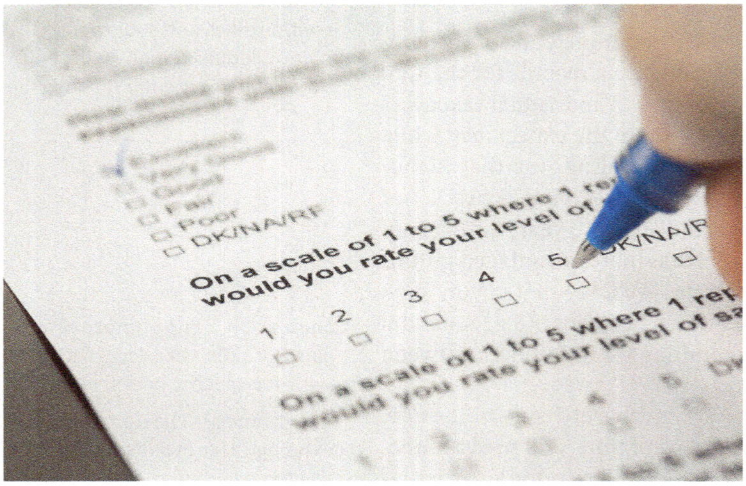

enis izgi/E+/Getty Images

The Experimental Method

Does smoking cause cancer? You say, "Of course it does," but how do you know that it does? Early case-control studies pointed the way, but later experimental studies were needed to confirm the causal role of smoking in cancer.

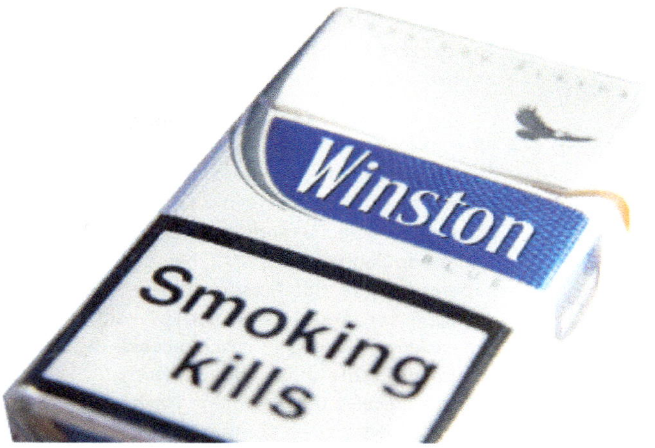

LWH/Alamy Stock Photo

Can we be certain that smoking is a cause of cancer in humans when no experiments have been conducted with humans to confirm the matter? What are our sources of evidence?

But there was a problem in applying the **experimental method** to determining whether smoking causes cancer. Conducting experimental research with humans was neither feasible nor ethically responsible, as it would require participants to be assigned randomly to smoke or not to smoke over a lengthy period of time and then to assess whether differences emerged in rates of cancer between the comparison groups. Researchers could only observe the effects of **natural experiments** by following the health of people who chose to smoke and people who did not. The lack of random assignment in natural experiments is often associated with selection bias; that is, the same factors that lead people to smoke may be responsible for their health problems, rather than the smoking itself. Packs of cigarettes in the United States carry warning messages such as "Cigarettes cause cancer." What kinds of psychological and behavioral factors might we find among people who see such messages yet choose to smoke? Could some of these factors contribute to the health problems of people who choose to smoke?

Because of the limitations of correlational studies and natural experiments, researchers turned to animal studies to examine whether tobacco was a **carcinogen**. In classic laboratory research, laboratory mice were held in cages in which tobacco smoke was infused into the air they breathed (IARC Working Group, 2004). When compared to control groups of mice who were not exposed to tobacco smoke in their cages, those held in smoking cages showed significantly greater incidence of cancerous tumors in the lungs. Of course, mice differ from humans in many ways, but their lung tissue is similar, so this evidence can be construed as confirming that smoking causes lung cancer.

Researchers use experimental methods with humans and other species to explore cause-and-effect relationships. In the experimental method, researchers test hypotheses through experiments in which they directly control the variable or variables of interest, called the **independent variable** or variables, and measure their effects on an outcome measure or measures, called the **dependent variable** or variables, while holding constant other variables that might affect the results (see **Figure 1.6**). Using the experimental method, experimenters test the effects of new medications or psychological interventions, surgical procedures, even the effects of texting while driving (as shown in Figure 1.6). They manipulate or control the independent variable or variables by determining which participants receive the experimental treatment.

Participants who receive the experimental treatment, say medication treatment or psychotherapy, constitute the **experimental group**, and those who do not receive the treatment constitute the **control group**. The control group may be placed in a *waiting-list condition* during the active treatment of the experimental group. Differences in outcomes between the experimental and control groups are then analyzed to determine whether there was a causal effect of the independent variable(s) on the dependent variable(s) of interest. Researchers perform statistical tests on these differences to determine whether they reach **statistical significance**, which is a level at which it is highly unlikely (generally set at a level of less than a 5% probability) that the differences between the groups are a result of chance fluctuation. Controlled research trials using the experimental method provide the best evidence of the effectiveness of medical and psychological methods of helping. Through experimental research, health researchers address many of the research questions we pose in this text, such as whether physical activity helps lower high blood pressure (see Chapter 8) or whether cognitive behavioral therapy helps lift people out of depression (see Chapter 11).

experimental method A method of research that seeks to confirm or discover cause-and-effect relationships by introducing independent variables and observing their effects on dependent variables.

natural experiments A study in which the participants are not randomly assigned to experimental or control groups but have determined on their own the group to which they belong.

carcinogen A cancer-causing chemical or substance.

independent variable A condition or factor in a scientific study that is manipulated so that its effects can be measured.

dependent variable Measures of the effects of an independent variable.

experimental group A group of research participants who receive a treatment in an experiment.

control group A group of research participants in an experiment whose members do not obtain the treatment, while other conditions are held constant.

statistical significance A level at which differences between groups are deemed large enough to make it very unlikely that the differences are a result of chance fluctuation.

Step 1 The experimenter begins by identifying the hypothesis.

Step 2 Next, the experimenter solicits volunteers for the experiment. In order to avoid sample bias, the experimenter first attempts to select a random sample of the entire population of interest. Then the experimenter randomly assigns these participants to two different groups—either the experimental group, which receives the treatment, or the control group, which does not receive the treatment. Having two groups allows a direct comparison of responses between the two groups.

Step 3 Both the experimental and the control groups are assigned to a driving simulator. The experimental group then texts while driving, whereas the control group does not text. Texting or not texting are the two levels of the independent variable (IV).

Step 4 The experimenter counts the number of simulated traffic accidents for each group and then analyzes the data. The number of simulated traffic accidents is the dependent variable (DV). (Note that the DV is called "dependent" because the behavior [or outcome] exhibited by the participants is assumed to *depend* on manipulations of the IV.)

Step 5 The experimenter interprets the results and writes them up for publication. The experimenter discusses the utility of the study, its limitations, and possible future directions for further research.

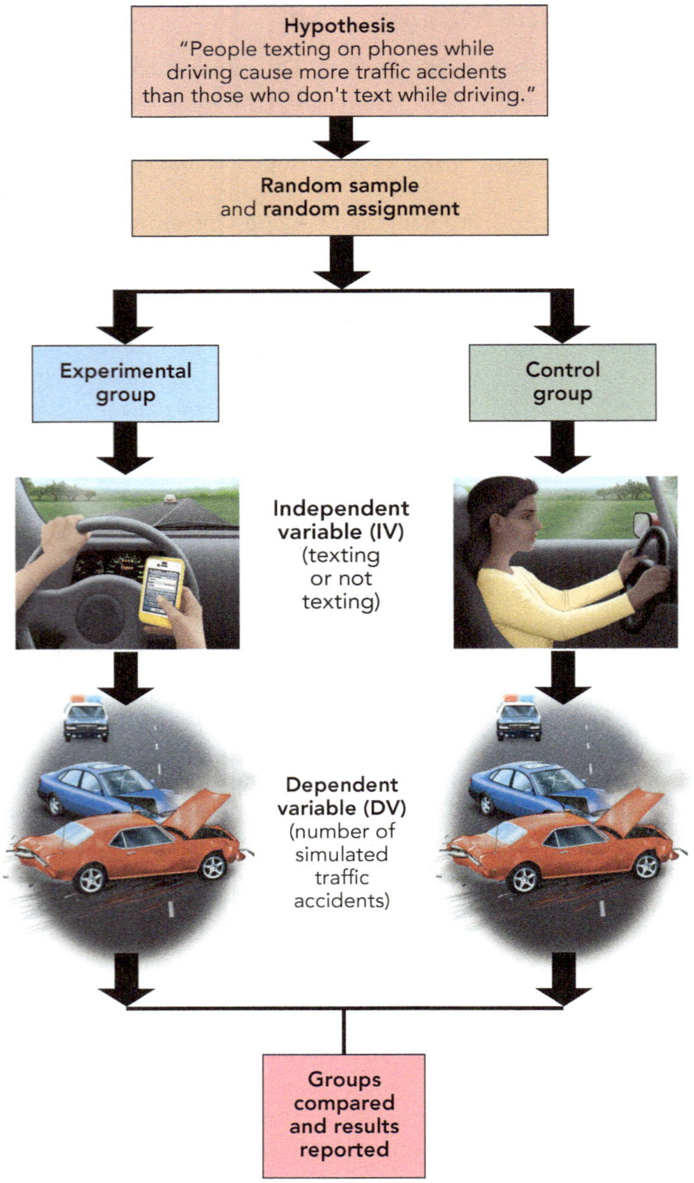

FIGURE 1.6 Experimental and Control Groups in Experimental Design

expectancy effects A set of expectations that research participants may have that may affect the outcomes of an experiment.

placebo A bogus treatment that has the appearance of being genuine.

placebo effects Beneficial effects of positive expectancies on the outcome of an experiment or treatment.

single-blind placebo control design An experimental method in which research participants are kept unaware of whether they are placed in an experimental (active medication) or placebo (inert medication) group.

The *randomized clinical trial* (RCT) is considered the standard for determining the efficacy of treatments or interventions in psychology and medical research. An RCT is a controlled experiment in which participants in a clinical trial are assigned randomly to experimental and control conditions (Finkelstein, 2020). Random assignment balances groups on individual characteristics of participants, so that experimenters can be confident that differences between groups are due to the independent (experimental) variable and not a selection factor or bias. However, one limitation of the experimental method is that random assignment is not always feasible or ethically responsible. For example, ethical experimenters would not randomly assign children to be exposed to abuse or neglect to assess the effects of these experiences on their development. They may rely on correlational methods to examine these relationships, even though correlation alone does not determine cause and effect. Health investigators use randomized controlled trials to evaluate the outcomes of health behavior interventions, such as programs designed to help people improve their nutritional quality, increase physical activity, or avoid harmful substances like tobacco (Freedland, 2022).

Placebo and Nocebo Effects An early study on the effects of alcohol on aggression reported that men at parties where beer and liquor were served acted more aggressively than men at parties where only soft drinks were served (Boyatzis, 1974). But subjects in the experimental group knew they had drunk alcohol, and those in the control group knew they had not. Aggression that appeared to result from alcohol might not have reflected the influence of alcohol per se. Instead, it may have reflected the subjects' expectations about the effects of alcohol.

People tend to act in stereotypical ways when they believe they have been drinking alcohol. For instance, men tend to become less anxious in social situations, more aggressive, and more sexually aroused. You may have experienced this *power of suggestion* yourself. Perhaps you've had the experience of taking antibiotics and beginning to feel better shortly after downing the first pill, even though you later learn that the medication doesn't actually take effect for perhaps 12 to 24 hours.

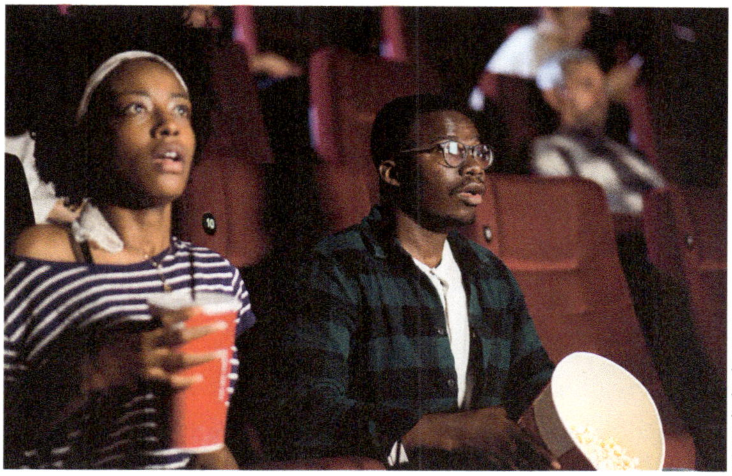

Placebo Effects at the Movies The power of suggestion may lead you to experience fear while watching a scary movie, which we can liken to a type of placebo effect since there is no actual physical threat.

Experimental studies may control for **expectancy effects**. Experimenters control for expectancies by keeping participants "blind," or unaware their assigned experimental condition—whether they receive an active medication or a **placebo**. A placebo is a chemically inactive substance that is made to look like a real drug. They are used as a basis of comparison with an active drug to evaluate whether treatment effects might be explained by a patient's hopeful expectancies about the effects of the drug rather than the chemical properties of the drug itself (Liu, 2021; Liu et al., 2022). The effects of positive expectancies on the outcomes of an experiment or a treatment are called **placebo effects**. You may have experienced a type of placebo effect while watching a scary movie and experiencing physiological sensations of fear, such as a rapid heartbeat. The fear might feel very real, even though you knew the action on the screen was fake and you were never in any real danger (Benedetti, 2021).

double-blind placebo control design An experimental method in which neither the research participants nor the researchers themselves know which participants receive the experimental (active medication) treatment and which receive a placebo.

Blinds

Experimental blinds are intended to prevent the biasing of results by the expectations of the participants and the researchers (see **Figure 1.7**).

A **single-blind placebo control design** keeps participants unaware of their group assignments in order to control for expectancies that participants may have that might affect the results. A **double-blind placebo control design** keeps both investigators and participants in the dark about assignments to the medication or placebo to control for the expectancies of both participants and investigators. In both types of placebo control designs, experimenters randomize assignments to the medication or placebo conditions and then evaluate differences in outcomes between these conditions. If active medication participants show significantly better results than placebo or untreated participants, experimenters can be reasonably confident that the medication effects are due to the medication itself and are not a placebo or suggestion effect.

Placebo control designs may also be used in evaluating psychological treatments. In these cases, the placebo group is an alternate psychological treatment that has the look and feel of the experimental treatment but without the specific techniques of the active treatment. The U.S. health watchdog agency, the Food and Drug Administration (FDA), requires double-blind studies before it allows the marketing of new medications. After the final measurements have been made, a neutral panel (a group of people who have no personal stake in the

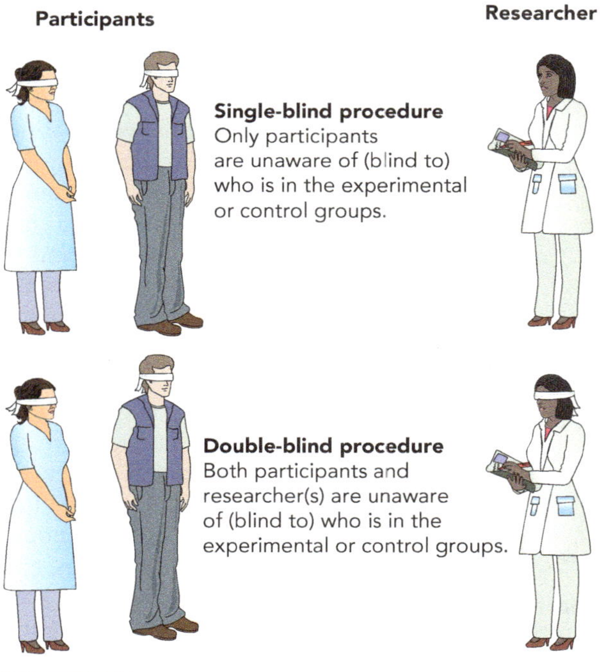

FIGURE 1.7 Single- and Double-Blind Experimental Designs To validly evaluate the effectiveness of something such as a new medication, the researchers administering the medication and the participants taking it need to be unaware of (or "blind to") who is receiving the medication and who is receiving a placebo (a fake pill). Blinds are necessary because participants' beliefs and expectations can affect their responses; this is the so-called placebo effect. Similarly, researchers' beliefs about the effectiveness of the drug could alter the experimental outcome.

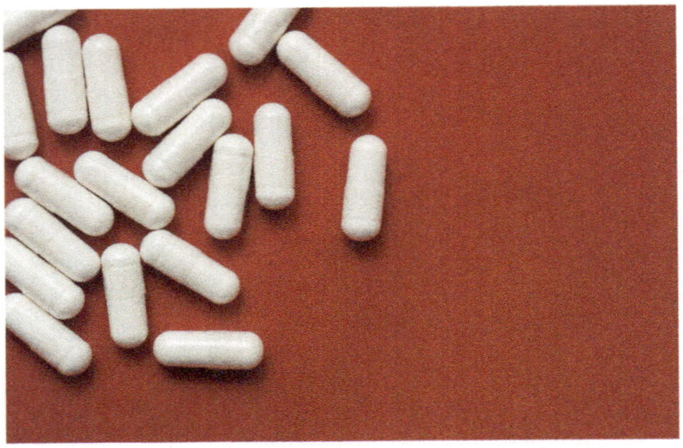

Yana Kho/Shutterstock.com

The Power of Placebos Are they the real thing or are they placebos? Placebos can have powerful effects on health outcomes, including effects on the brain's processing of pain signals. Placebos may even produce beneficial effects when people know the "drug" they receive is in fact a placebo. But nocebo effects are harmful or dangerous.

outcome of the study) judges whether the effects of the medication differed from those of the placebo.

Double-blind controlled studies are not perfect, however. Prescribing physicians as well as many of their patients can often tell whether a medication is a placebo or the real thing based on telltale side effects (Schulz et al., 2010). Thus, double-blind designs may sometimes resemble Venetian blinds with the slats slightly open. Despite their limitations, they remain the most important means of determining effectiveness of new medications—essentially the gold standard in testing new medications (Perlis et al., 2010).

Placebos can actually have powerful effects on health outcomes. Placebos can work on reducing pain even when participants know they are receiving a placebo and not an active medication (Kam-Hansen et al., 2014; Schafer et al., 2015). Research shows that placebos have measurable effects on parts of the brain involved in processing pain signals (Koban et al., 2017; Zunhammer et al., 2021).

Placebos may also block pain signals from reaching the brain, perhaps by triggering the release of the brain's own pain-killing chemicals, called *endorphins* (Colloca & Barsky, 2020; Merchant, 2016). However, we should point out that placebos tend to have stronger effects on subjective measures, such as self-reports of pain, than they do on objectively measured outcomes, such as blood pressure (Meyer et al., 2015).

Investigators also focus on the opposite side of the placebo coin. Placebo effects involve positive or hopeful expectancies that can lead to beneficial outcomes. But people sometimes have negative expectancies that can lead to negative outcomes. These effects, called **nocebo effects**, can lead to harmful or even dangerous outcomes (Colloca & Barsky, 2020). For example, people with negative expectancies about the outcomes or adverse side effects of medications may stop using them, which can have adverse effects on their health. Negative expectancies may arise from misinformation about medication effects, which is sometimes spread on social media, as well as from general pessimistic attitudes, negative experiences with prior treatment, and other factors. Like placebo effects, nocebo effects can directly affect brain functioning. For instance, brain imaging studies link nocebo effects to increased transmission of pain signaling from the spinal cord to the brain (Geuter & Büchel, 2013; Tinnermann et al., 2017).

nocebo effects Negative effects of an experiment or treatment that may result from negative expectancies.

Placebo and nocebo effects offer us a perspective on the importance of psychological factors in health care. Expectancies—whether positive or negative—are psychological factors that can affect how people respond to medication or other treatments (Colloca & Barsky, 2020). Investigators use placebo control designs to control for both placebo and nocebo effects in experimental research. But what about clinical practice? People bring their expectancies with them to medical visits with healthcare providers. Physicians can take a proactive approach to counter nocebo effects by directly asking patients about any negative expectancies, as in posing questions such as: "Have you had negative experiences in the past with this type of medication? What concerns do you have about side effects? Are you worried about how you might respond to these medications?" Positive expectancies, or placebo effects, can have beneficial effects on outcomes. But responsible treatment providers need to set patients straight on how quickly the medication is likely to work, the side effects that might occur, and how effective the medication is likely to be.

ANIMATION CONTENT

Important Components of an Experiment

Becoming a Critical Thinker About Health-Related Information

Critical thinking is a form of thinking in which you adopt a questioning attitude and carefully weigh the evidence when judging claims or arguments of others (Rozenkrantz et al., 2022). Critical thinkers do not accept claims at face value. They question what people say on the internet, on TV, or in passing conversations and hold the claims they make up to the light of evidence.

critical thinking An approach to thinking characterized by skepticism and thoughtful analysis of statements and arguments—for example, probing the premises of arguments and the definitions of terms.

Health Psychology in Action

Placebos and the Power of Suggestion

In a remarkable demonstration of the power of suggestion, researchers conducted a randomized clinical trial to test the effects of an open-label placebo on severity of symptoms in patients with irritable bowel syndrome, a type of gastrointestinal disorder characterized by recurring abdominal pain and changes in bowel movements (Lembo et al., 2021).

As the term suggests, an *open-label placebo* is a pill that is clearly marked on its container that it is really a placebo, a chemically inactive substance made to resemble the active drug. In effect, patients in the IBS study knew they were taking a placebo, not a real drug. And yet the results showed that patients assigned to the open-placebo condition reported significantly greater symptom reduction than control patients who received no drug at all. Not only that, but patients receiving the openly labeled placebo pills showed similar benefits as those who had been assigned to a double-blind placebo condition who weren't told whether they were taking a placebo or an active drug. The reduction in symptom severity of patients in the open-placebo condition represented clinically meaningful symptom reduction. The patients felt better overall and reported less severe IBS symptoms after taking pills—now get this—that were clearly marked as placebos.

Other researchers report that pain patients given placebos report lower levels of pain, even when they knew they were given a placebo (e.g., Flowers et al., 2021; Guevarra et al., 2020; Liu, 2021). We have a growing body of evidence showing that placebos can produce some degree of relief even when patients know that the pills they are taking are fakes. These findings lead researchers to wonder whether offering open-label placebos may actually play a role in managing symptoms in patients with IBS or other medical conditions (Lembo et al., 2021).

Relatedly, we have evidence of the power of belief in how people experience COVID symptoms. A recent study in France showed that reports of persistent symptoms of COVID-19 were more strongly related to a person's beliefs about having been infected with the virus than with actual laboratory evidence of a confirmed infection (Matta et al., 2022).

Critical thinkers challenge conventional wisdom and knowledge that many people tend to take for granted, such as claims that vitamin C helps ward off the common cold. Critical thinkers suspend judgment until scientific evidence is gathered, sifted through, and analyzed. Rather than relying on gut feelings or taking the word of others, even the word of respected authorities, critical thinkers assume a skeptical attitude toward what they hear, see, and read, even what they read in the pages of a college textbook. Critical thinkers accept nothing as true until they have had the chance to examine the evidence supporting the claim.

Features of Critical Thinking

Developing critical thinking skills can help you succeed in your college years and beyond. Here are some of the key features of critical thinking about health claims:

1. *Maintain a healthy skepticism.* Advertisers try to persuade you to purchase products they claim will keep you healthy or help you treat health problems.
2. *Examine definitions of terms.* Some statements are true when a term is defined in one way but not when it is defined in another way. Consider the label on a container of "low-fat" ice cream: "97% Fat-Free!" One day at the supermarket we were impressed with an ice cream package's claims that the product was 97% fat-free. Yet when we read the label closely, we found that a 4-ounce serving had 160 calories, 27 of which were contributed by fat. Fat, then, accounted for 27/160ths, or about 17%, of the ice cream's calorie content. But fat accounted for only 3% of the ice cream's weight—most of which was calorie-free water weight. The packagers of the ice cream knew that labeling the ice cream as "97% fat-free" would make it sound healthier than "Only 17% of calories from fat." Read carefully. Think critically.

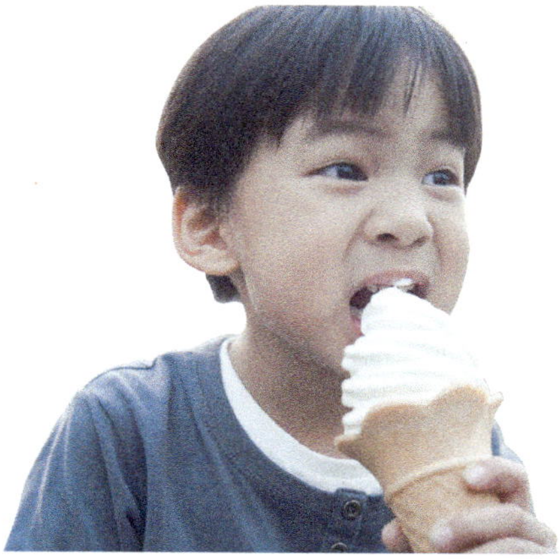
Clover No.7 Photography/Getty Images

It's 97% Fat-Free! Is that good enough? How can you determine whether or not it is?

3. *Examine the assumptions or premises of arguments.* If you hear a health claim that a weight loss product in combination with following a healthy low-calorie diet plan will help you lose excess weight, question the premises on which the claim is based. Is the advertiser assuming that the weight loss product will help users reduce excess weight without changing their diet? Or that the weight loss product will increase weight loss above that which would be achieved by following a low-calorie diet plan alone?
4. *Examine the sources of evidence.* Self-help books often rely on testimonials to tout their claims. They may point to the cases of a few individuals who achieved positive health

outcomes, such as losing excess weight, stopping smoking, or reducing stress by following the methods described in the books. But how do you know if these testimonial endorsements mean that people in general, or you in particular, would achieve the same results?

A celebrity might report losing 20, 30, or more pounds following the latest diet plan in a TV commercial or described in a self-help book. Perhaps you say to yourself if this famous person could do it, then why not me? What you may not realize is the celebrity is paid handsomely for the endorsement and is thus motivated financially to lose excess weight, and that the weight loss product may have little if anything to do with the positive results. Or think of those people (actors really) who appear deeply depressed at the start of a commercial for an antidepressant but suddenly spring back to life by the end of the commercial, presumably because they started using the medication. Is the evidence presented persuasive, based on claims drawn from carefully conducted scientific trials, or are the images manipulated by an advertising company seeking to promote their products? Are the claims supported by studies reported in respected scientific journals or from questionable sources?

5. *Consider alternative interpretations of research evidence.* Ask yourself whether there are other ways of explaining a given set of facts or findings, especially evidence that seems to show cause-and-effect relationships. Consider this research question: "Does alcohol cause aggression?" That is, many people who commit violent crimes have been drinking alcohol. But is the connection causal? Could other factors, such as gender, age, willingness to take risks, or social expectations, account for links between drinking alcohol and the aggressive behavior?
6. *Do not oversimplify.* Consider the statement "Alcoholism is inherited." Genetic factors may create a predisposition to alcoholism, but the origins of alcoholism and many other health problems involve a complex interplay of biological and environmental factors. People may inherit a predisposition to heart disease but never develop it if they watch their diet, exercise regularly, and learn to manage stress. On the other hand, people may develop heart problems if they overeat, smoke, and fail to exercise, even when there is no family history of the disease.
7. *Do not overgeneralize.* We shouldn't assume that health-promotion efforts that work in some settings with some types of people would work as well in other settings or with other groups of people. We may find that the effectiveness of these programs varies across settings and populations.
8. *Do not confuse correlation with causation.* People may assume that because two variables are linked, for example, alcohol use and poor grades, that one (alcohol use) causes the other (poor grades). Alcohol use may indeed be a cause of slipping grades, but we can't assume this is the case based only a correlational link between the two. It's conceivable that the two variables are linked because both are associated with a third variable, such as problems with self-control. Or students who are depressed or anxious may obtain poorer grades and also become dependent on alcohol because they turn to alcohol as self-medication for emotional problems.

Thinking Critically About Health Claims

Every now and then, we hear claims touting some miracle drug, vitamin, hormone, or alternative therapy that promises to enhance health and vitality, cure or prevent disease, or even reverse the effects of aging. Some of these claims are outright hoaxes. Others take promising scientific leads and exaggerate or distort the evidence. Although the federal watchdog agency, the FDA, regulates health claims for drugs and medications, many of the substances found in your health food store or neighborhood supermarket purporting to have disease-preventive or anti-aging effects are classified as foods and are not regulated as drugs. It's basically a matter of "buyer beware" (see **Table 1.1**).

Critical thinkers do not take health claims at face value. They recognize that alternative therapies and healthcare products may not work as promised and could even be harmful. Another concern is that people advocating particular therapies may have a vested interest in getting consumers to try their services or use their products and may play fast and loose with the truth.

TABLE 1.1 Thinking Critically About Health Claims

What They Claim About Their Product	What They Might Actually Mean
Designed to enhance vitality and well-being	"We may have designed our product to enhance vitality and well-being, but we do not have scientific evidence that it actually does."
Promotes muscle growth	"Yes, we put amino acids the body uses to build muscle into our product, but many other foods you can buy also contain amino acids, such as meat and dairy products."
Recommended by leading physicians	"We found a few physicians who have respectable credentials who were willing to say they would recommend our product to their patients, and they were well paid for their endorsements."
Backed by advanced research	"What we mean by 'backed' is that we have some research that tested our product. We're not saying what the research showed, or how well it was carried out, or whether it was conducted by impartial investigators. What we mean by 'advanced' is that, well, the research methods went beyond just asking people if they liked our product."
It can supercharge your metabolism!	"We do not really know what this means, but it sure sounded good in the advertising copy."
Our ice cream is 97% fat-free!	"We know our ice cream is 3% fat and to be honest, that 3% is saturated. We also know you wouldn't buy milk labeled 3% saturated fat, so why should we advertise that our product is 3% saturated fat?"
Clinically tested formula!	"Yes, we tested it clinically. We asked a few patients what they thought of our product and they all liked it."
Laboratory tested	"We paid some guys who have this clinical lab and they tested it. We're not sure what they tested, but they said it went well."

Source: Adapted from Nevid (2022).

Use your critical thinking skills to read between the lines in evaluating health claims. What do you think the following claims for products found in your neighborhood health store might actually mean?

Applying Health Psychology

Thinking Critically When Surfing Online

The internet is the digital version of the old Wild West, a place where just about anything goes and where just about anything can get posted, whether true or not. Nothing much gets vetted on the internet for its validity or the trustworthiness of the source. People with significant health problems may find emotional and social support from peers on Facebook, but they need to be aware that information from users is highly variable in quality and often inaccurate, especially where health issues are concerned (Yardley et al., 2019). You'll find all kinds of claims about health-related products and services. Anyone with a mouse and keyboard can post just about anything, so the expression *Caveat emptor*—buyer beware—has special salience when you go online. So whom and what can you trust?

Critical thinkers bring a skeptical attitude to what they read and see on the internet. They check out the credentials of the source by asking themselves questions like "What is the source of the claim? Who's posting it? Do they have a vested interest in selling a health-related product? The person in the ad may claim to be a 'doctor,' but what kind of doctor? Where did the person get their degree? Might the person or people posting the information have an axe to grind with the medical or scientific establishment? Is the source a respected scientific or medical organization, respected university, or government agency or institute?" Postings are especially sketchy if the source is not clearly identified.

To be sure, there is some trustworthy online information, but you need to sift through the clutter. These trustworthy sources, which your authors rely on as well, are scientific journals, government agencies such as the National Institutes of Health (NIH) and the FDA, and major professional organizations like the American Psychological Association (APA) and the Association for Psychological Science. You can find health-related information that has been carefully scrutinized by scholars in the field in articles published in the APA journal, *Health Psychology*, the *Journal of the American Medical Association*, *The New England Journal of Medicine*, and from the various institutes of the NIH.

When viewing material posted online, bring to bear the same skeptical attitude that you would when watching a TV commercial. Take health claims with a proverbial grain of salt and keep a tight grip on your wallet, especially if vendors make claims that rely on testimonials. Read the fine (electronic) print. Understand that an offer of a "guaranty" doesn't mean the product will work as advertised, only that you'll get your money back if the product fails, but with such tight strings attached to make it very unlikely you'll ever see your money again. And you'll never recoup those shipping and handling costs.

Though we need to think critically about online information, we should also recognize that the internet can be an extremely valuable channel for distributing health-related information that may not be as readily accessible through other sources.

Review 1.3

INTERACTIVE SELF-SCORING QUIZZES

Sentence Completion

1. A correlation coefficient is a statistical measure of association between two variables that can vary from −1.00 to + _______.

2. The size or magnitude of the correlation coefficient indicates the _______ of the relationship between the two variables.

3. Correlational research is helpful in _______ future outcomes or behaviors.

4. Researchers find that _______ words are tweeted more often during the early morning hours.

5. The _______ of a disease is the number of new cases occurring during a specific period of time.

6. The _______ of a disease is the overall number of cases of a disorder within a given population.

7. A _______ is a subset of a population.

8. Random _______ is a procedure in which way each member of the population has an equal probability of participating in the sample.

9. Researchers randomize research participants to experimental or _______ groups to balance the individual characteristics of the participants in these groups.

10. A _______ is an inert pill that looks like the genuine medication.

11. A _______blind placebo control design keeps both the participants and the experimenters themselves in the dark about which participants are assigned to which experimental conditions.

Think About It

Cigarette smoking has been on decline in the United States. The main reasons for the decline might be widespread knowledge that smokers are more likely to develop serious health problems such as lung cancer than people who do not smoke. We noted that packs of cigarettes in the United States carry messages such as "Smoking causes cancer." What kinds of cognitive and behavioral factors might we find among people who are aware of such warnings yet choose to smoke? How might these factors be related to their other health behaviors? How might some of these factors contribute to their health problems?

Recite: An Active Summary

INTERACTIVE SELF-SCORING QUIZZES

Chapter 1 Practice Quiz

1. Describe the development of the field of health psychology.

Health psychology is the scientific study of the relationships between psychology and physical health. It has a long history, dating back to ancient times, when it was recognized that mind and body influence each other. With the emergence of medical science in the 19th century, the medical subfield of psychosomatic medicine was established to study connections between psyche (mind) and soma (body). Health psychology emerged as a subfield in psychology during the 1960s and 1970s to meet the needs for research, education, and practice focused on the role of psychological factors in physical health.

2. Describe the biopsychosocial model of health.

The biopsychosocial model represents a broadly based conceptualization of health that takes into account biological (genes, disease processes, etc.), psychological (personality, behaviors, attitudes), and social (socioeconomic level, social support, ethnic or racial background) in health and well-being. It has largely replaced the earlier biomedical model of disease that was limited to biologically based disease processes. Wellness is a state of optimum health with respect to the quality of our lives. It takes into account physical, psychological, and social functioning and addresses whether our lifestyles, habits, and behaviors are helping us achieve a healthy and fulfilling life.

3. Describe the relationships between health and human diversity.

Cross-cultural differences affect health, as in dietary differences and the prevalence of various forms of cancer. Health psychologists attempt to encourage people from different backgrounds to obtain available health care, even when scientific methods are in conflict with local traditions. In the United States, people from higher socioeconomic backgrounds lead longer, healthier lives, in part due to access to high-quality health care.

4. List and describe the major research methods in health psychology.

Research methods in health psychology include the case study method, the correlational method, the case-control method, the epidemiological method, the survey method, and the experimental method. Some of these methods—the case study, correlational, case control, and epidemiological methods—are descriptive or observational. They allow us to examine relationships among variables and suggest possible cause-and-effect relationships, but they cannot pinpoint causal factors. The experimental method, which allows investigators to directly manipulate possible causal factors and measure their effects, provides investigators with the means of determining causal factors in health outcomes.

5. Describe the major features of critical thinking about health-related information.

Thinking critically about health-related information involves maintaining a healthy skepticism about health claims, examining definitions of terms, examining assumptions and premises of health claims or arguments, examining the sources of evidence supporting health claims, taking into account alternative interpretations of research evidence, avoiding oversimplification and overgeneralization of findings, and distinguishing between correlation and causation.

Answers to Review Sections

1.1

1. health psychology
2. body
3. "psychosomatic" medicine
4. Dunbar
5. Clinical
6. Community
7. absence
8. well-being
9. biopsychosocial
10. immune

1.2

1. higher
2. malaria
3. lower
4. less
5. more willing
6. less likely
7. bulletproof

1.3

1. 1.00
2. strength
3. predicting
4. happier
5. incidence
6. prevalence
7. sample
8. selection
9. control
10. placebo
11. double-

Scoring Key for the Locus of Control Scale

(Place a checkmark for each response that matches the answer in the scoring key and then sum the checkmarks to compute your total score.)

1. Yes ___
2. No ___
3. Yes ___
4. No ___
5. Yes ___
6. No ___
7. Yes ___
8. Yes ___
9. No ___
10. Yes ___
11. Yes ___
12. Yes ___
13. No ___
14. Yes ___
15. No ___
16. Yes ___
17. Yes ___
18. Yes ___
19. Yes ___
20. No ___
21. Yes ___
22. No ___
23. Yes ___
24. Yes ___
25. No ___
26. No ___
27. Yes ___
28. No ___
29. Yes ___
30. No ___
31. Yes ___
32. No ___
33. Yes ___
34. No ___
35. Yes ___
36. Yes ___
37. Yes ___
38. No ___
39. Yes ___
40. No ___

Total Score _____

Interpreting Your Score

Low scorers (0–8): About one person in three earns a score of from 0 to 8. These people typically have an internal locus of control. They see themselves as responsible for their fate and for the success or failure they experience in life.

Average scorers (9–16): Most respondents earn from 9 to 16 points. Average scorers may see themselves as partially in control of their lives. Perhaps they see themselves as in control at work but not in their social lives—or vice versa.

High scorers (17–40): About 15% of respondents attain scores of 17 or above. High scorers largely tend to see life as a game of chance, and success as a matter of luck or the generosity of others.

CHAPTER 2

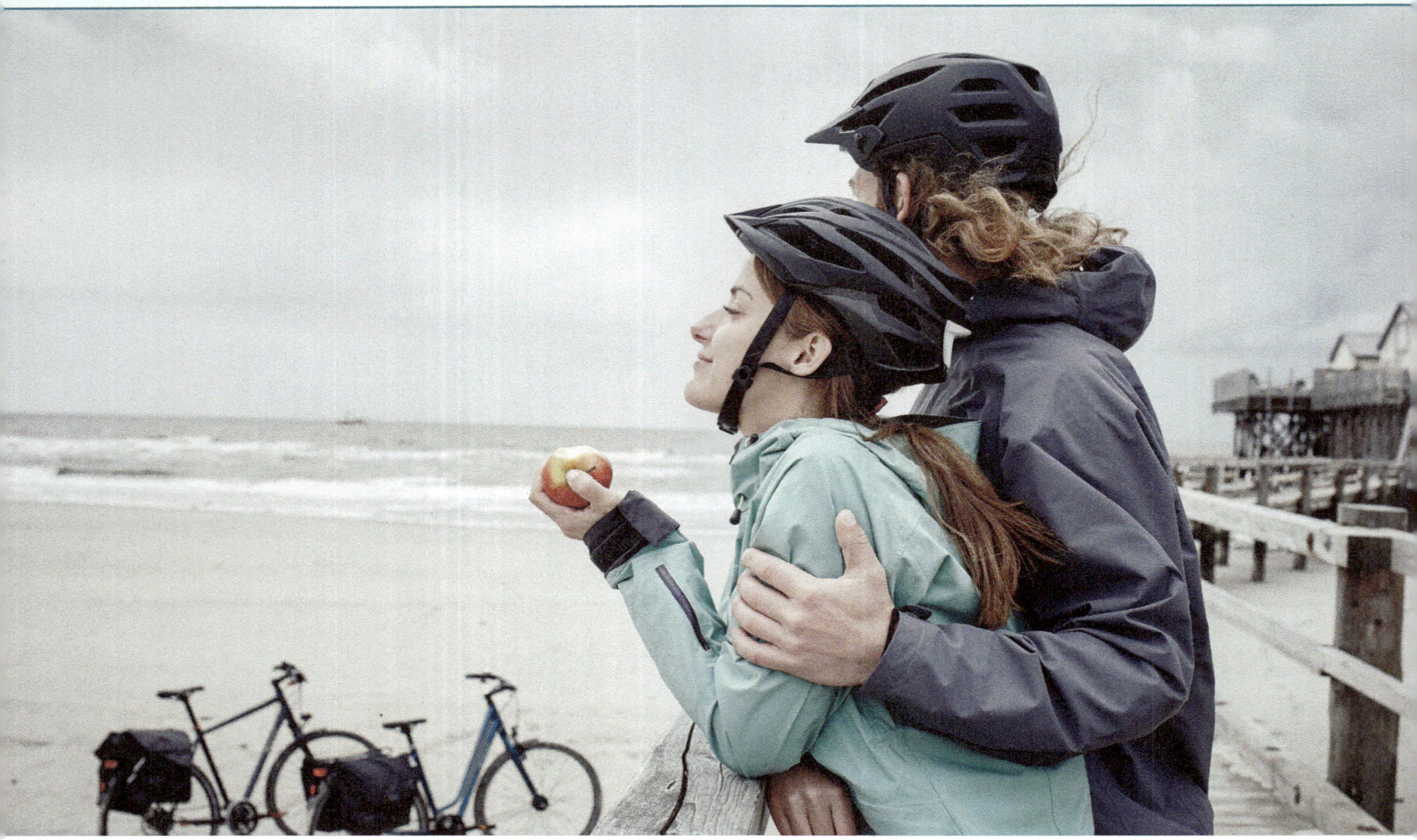

Westend61/Getty Images

Theories of Health Behavior: Adherence and Change

LEARNING OBJECTIVES

After studying this chapter, you will be able to ...

1. **Describe** the factors involved in changing health behaviors.
2. **Describe** the factors involved in adherence to medical treatment.
3. **Describe** the Health Belief Model of behavior change.
4. **Describe** the role of social cognitive theory in explaining health behavior.
5. **Describe** how the Theory of Reasoned Action, the Theory of Planned Behavior, and the Transtheoretical Model help us understand health behavior change.

Did You Know That ...

- About half of patients with chronic diseases do not take their medicine as prescribed?
- Thinking that the flu is just a bad cold can make you less likely to obtain a flu shot?
- Whether people make healthy behavior changes is best predicted by how they evaluate the benefits and costs of making these changes?
- One of the major risk factors of cardiovascular disease is a silent health problem—one that you cannot see or feel?
- Showing an educational video to HIV patients while they are waiting to be seen in a clinic was associated with higher rates of starting HIV medication and lower HIV viral loads?
- Subtle cues, such as the background color of a printed health message, affected students' intentions to use sunscreen to prevent skin cancer?
- The intention to make a healthy change in behavior may be necessary, but it is not a sufficient condition for making the change?
- Adolescents who believe their peers eat more fruits and vegetables than they do boost their intake of fruits and vegetables?

- Lose 10 pounds
- Watch the salt
- Exercise 30 minutes, 3–5 times per week
- Stop smoking—now!
- Reduce the carbs
- Increase your fiber intake
- Reduce consumption of red meat and saturated fat
- Schedule a colonoscopy
- Eat more fruits and vegetables

Countless numbers of people receive advice like this from their physicians and other healthcare providers. They may be advised of the benefits of making healthier food choices, engaging in regular physical activity, taking medication as prescribed, avoiding smoking, and controlling other forms of substance use. But medical advice only works if it is applied consistently. Although most people want to live longer and healthier lives, many do not adopt the lifestyles needed to foster good health and longevity. In this chapter, we seek to understand the behavioral factors that promote healthy living and the obstacles that may hinder them.

Healthcare providers are often frustrated, wondering why patients do not follow sound medical advice. Physicians themselves are not immune; they too often fail to follow their own advice. To one extent or another, we all struggle with following medical advice or adopting healthier lifestyles. Sometimes we don't know what's healthy. We wonder if we should cut back on salt, or adopt a vegetarian or vegan diet, or start tracking our steps. We may know that many of the leading causes of death are linked to behavioral choices, but we may still make unhealthy choices. Knowledge of the behavioral risk factors in disease is a good starting point, but knowledge alone is often insufficient to induce healthy changes in behavior. Health psychologists understand that other factors are involved.

We approach the problem of health behavior change by drawing upon the biopsychosocial model. We will also draw upon several leading theories in our exploration of health behavior change. Theories weave together interrelated concepts, propositions, and research findings to explain and predict outcomes and phenomena, such as health outcomes and longevity. Physicists may theorize about the workings of the visible universe and of the invisible universe within the nucleus of each cell. Psychologists develop theories that help explain mental processes and behavior, including health-related behavior.

Theories must be tested in the light of evidence to judge how well they allow us to understand and predict behavior. We also need to gauge their usefulness in designing disease prevention and health-promotion programs to help people live healthier lives.

Health behavior is too complex to be explained by any single theory, so we consider several of the key theories in play today: the Health Belief Model, social cognitive theory, the Theory of Reasoned Action, the Theory of Planned Behavior, and the Transtheoretical Model. Each of them contributes to our understanding of health behavior.

Factors in Health Behavior

Imagine you are on a hunt for a treasure box. You are given a map to follow and certain tasks to accomplish along the way. The treasure box may be worth more than a king's ransom because it holds a gift that may lead to living a longer and healthier life.

The tasks you need to accomplish to obtain the treasure box are all within your reach. Unlike the Greek myth of Jason and the Argonauts who set out on their quest for the Golden Fleece, you won't need to slay dragons or confront a giant Cyclops. All you need to do is adopt a healthy lifestyle. You need to watch what you eat, obtain regular medical checkups, follow the advice of your healthcare providers, become physically active, avoid harmful substances, get vaccinated against infectious diseases, get sufficient sleep, and engage in stimulating mental activities. And, yes, you need to make these behaviors a staple of daily life.

Are you willing to set out on this adventure? What obstacles might you encounter along the way? How would you overcome them? Let's begin with a roadmap of sorts, a set of guidelines to help you get started making healthy changes in your behavior.

Changing Unhealthy Habits

When asked about quitting smoking, the famed writer Mark Twain quipped that it was easy—he had done it many (many!) times. Changing unhealthy behaviors may not be easy, but it can be done. As did Twain, people who "succeed" in making changes often revert to their former unhealthy habits. Making changes in your health behavior, and maintaining these changes, depends on three sets of factors:

- Predisposing factors,
- Enabling factors, and
- Reinforcing factors.

Predisposing Factors

Predisposing factors can either promote or hinder healthy changes in behavior. These factors include beliefs, attitudes, knowledge, expectancies, and values. For example, believing that smoking is dangerous only to people with a family history of lung cancer can hinder people without a family history of the disease from making a commitment to changing their behavior. Similarly, young people who think that vaping or smoking cigarettes is "cool" or glamorous are more likely to engage in these behaviors than peers who hold a negative view.

Knowledge can lead to change. Millions of Americans quit smoking after the Surgeon General in 1964 first reported on the dangers of smoking. Knowledge about the risk factors in conditions such as heart disease and cancer can lead people to make changes that reduce their risks of developing these diseases. But, as noted, knowledge alone is often insufficient to induce lasting behavior change. Virtually all smokers today know of the dangers of smoking but continue to smoke. Most sexually active people know about the dangers of unprotected sex, but many surrender to impulse.

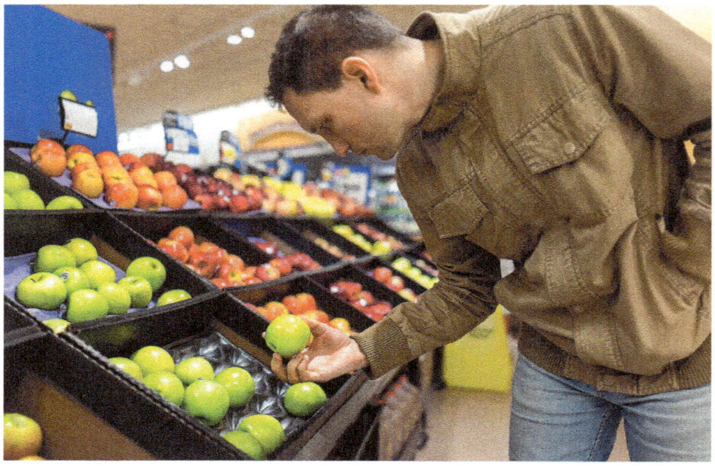
Kristina Blokhin/Alamy Stock Photo

Making Healthy Choices What factors contribute to making and maintaining healthy changes in behavior?

Psychologists also recognize that expectations play an important role in change. Young people who expect that drinking alcohol will make them popular, sexier, or more outgoing are more likely to drink than their peers who don't have these expectations.

Values are yet another determinant of change. Young people who value their popularity over their future health are more likely to succumb to peer pressures to smoke than those who place a greater value on long-term health.

Enabling Factors Factors that enable change include skills or abilities, physical and mental capabilities, and the availability and accessibility of resources. You are more likely to begin an exercise program, or stick with one, if

- There's a gym in your building or around the corner rather than a half-hour drive away,
- You have developed the skills to accomplish the task (you can follow the steps in an aerobics dance class or serve a tennis ball), and
- You possess the physical and mental capabilities required to perform the behavior (e.g., the strength, coordination, endurance, and concentration).

Accessibility to services is another enabling factor. People who lack health insurance or access to facilities may not receive the care they need.

Reinforcing Factors Reinforcing factors for healthy behavior changes include praise and support—including self-praise. If you shrug off the changes you make (e.g., starting a beginner's exercise class) by saying to yourself, "It's no big deal," you are less likely to stick with it than if you credit yourself for getting started. You're more likely to continue making healthy changes if the important people in your life make reinforcing comments ("Good job!") than if your efforts go unnoticed. However, it's best if reinforcement becomes internalized. Whether it is about losing weight, quitting smoking, or maintaining an exercise routine, you need to feel that what you are doing will ultimately lead you to feel better about yourself and to live a healthier life.

Increasing Adherence to Medical Treatment

Failure to adhere to medical advice and treatment is widespread. For example, about half of people treated for chronic diseases do not take their medications as prescribed (Dawson, 2019; Moon et al., 2019). Factors such as cost, access to pharmacies, literacy, and availability of health insurance all play a role in adherence to taking prescribed medication as directed (Choudhry et al., 2022). Therefore, health psychologists work with healthcare providers to help them boost compliance with treatment.

Guided by research on factors in adherence, healthcare providers can take a proactive role to help improve people's adherence to treatment, as seen in **Table 2.1**. Adherence to medical treatment depends on processes involving *self-regulation*, or ability to regulate our own behavior, as in taking medication as prescribed, obtaining regular medical and dental check-ups, and monitoring our daily behavior to ensure we are following medical guidance. Research evidence supports the value of efforts to improve adherence to medication for chronic health conditions, as by targeting people's self-monitoring of medication use, providing personalized feedback to people about their adherence to treatment, and helping them become better able to manage their medication (Wilson et al., 2020).

The problem of nonadherence is complex and involves many factors, as we see represented in **Figure 2.1** (Zullig & Bosworth, 2017). Some of these are *patient-related factors*, such as forgetfulness about taking medication, negative expectations or beliefs about medication, or difficulties understanding medication labels. A medication label might read, "Take one pill twice a day," but does that mean taking one pill at breakfast and another at lunch? Clearer labeling may help avoid dosing errors, as in specifying "Take one pill every 12 hours." Other patient-related factors leading to problem with adherence are

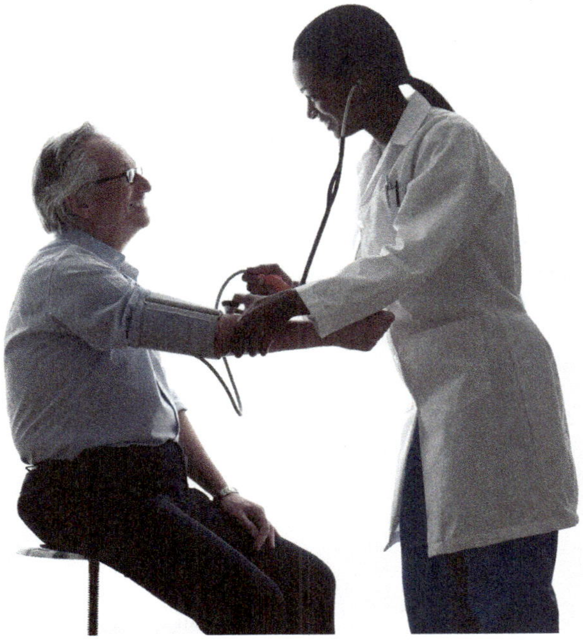

Image Source/Getty Images

Fostering Adherence About 50% of patients do not take medicine as prescribed. This man is reluctant to take his blood pressure medication "forever" because he doesn't experience the problem and doesn't like the idea of chemicals in his body. What can his physician say?

TABLE 2.1 Tackling Nonadherence: What Healthcare Providers Can Say and Do

INTERACTIVE FIGURES, CHARTS, & TABLES

Clinician Responses to Nonadherence	Examples
Explain	... the need for treatment and address how the treatment relates to the person's goals and interests. ... the importance of adherence at the time treatment is initiated, addressing the negative consequence of nonadherence, and then asking about adherence at each medical visit.
Address	... individual barriers to adherence. ... people's concerns about stigma associated with some types of medical treatment, such as taking psychiatric medications. ... any concerns patients may have about treatment.
Seek	... opportunities for group programs for weight management and fitness programs in which people may benefit from mutual support from others. Evidence shows that people seeking to increasing their physical activity achieved better results when they participated in group-led programs than when they were individually outfitted with pedometers (Norton et al., 2015). ... ways of providing medications at subsidized costs.
Provide	... the time needed to answer any questions from people. ... educational programs to modify health-related beliefs patients may hold about the need for treatment. ... individualized medical information that is tailored to the needs of the particular person. ... people with choices and control over their treatment alternatives.
Integrate	... behavioral changes within the person's lifestyle. For example, to increase physical activity, suggest walking around the living room during TV commercials, playing with a child or pet, taking the stairs rather than an elevator or escalator, or parking a little further away than usual in a parking lot. ... use of memory aids such as linking doses to daily events (e.g., dinnertime) or using a pill trigger alarm as a reminder to take a scheduled dose.
Simplify	... the medication plan whenever possible by reducing the number of medications and frequency of doses and making sure to carefully explain the importance of the dosing schedule.
Help	... people achieve attainable goals in a stepwise fashion to increase self-efficacy. Evidence points to better results in adopting healthy diet and physical activity programs when treatment providers work to increase people's self-efficacy through a series of healthy behavior changes (Schneider et al., 2016). ... people deal with emotional factors involving medical treatments and screening procedures, such as feelings of uncertainty, guilt, and fear (Hunleth et al., 2016).
Enhance	... outcome expectations. A recent major review highlighted the importance in survivors of cancer of building positive outcome expectations, such as by having participants imagine attainable desirable outcomes of physical activity (Sheeran et al., 2019).

Sources: Al-Noumani et al. (2019), Horne et al. (2019), Nigg and Harmon (2018), Sublette et al. (2018), WHO (2003), and Wilson et al. (2019), among others.

psychological problems, such as depression and the stigma associated with taking certain medications, such as those used to treat mental health problems.

Treatment-related factors include problems posed by complex dosing regimens and taking multiple medications, especially when they carry different dosing schedules or different sets of instructions. One medication label might specify, "Take only with food" whereas another might state, "Take on an empty stomach." *Complex indeed.*

Health-related factors affecting adherence include high copayments (copay), restricted formularies (limited choices of affordable medications), and lack of access to services or providers.

The following Self-Assessment encourages you to put yourself in the shoes of a healthcare provider who is attempting to field people's objections to adhering to advice or treatment. Do you know people who have raised some of these objections?

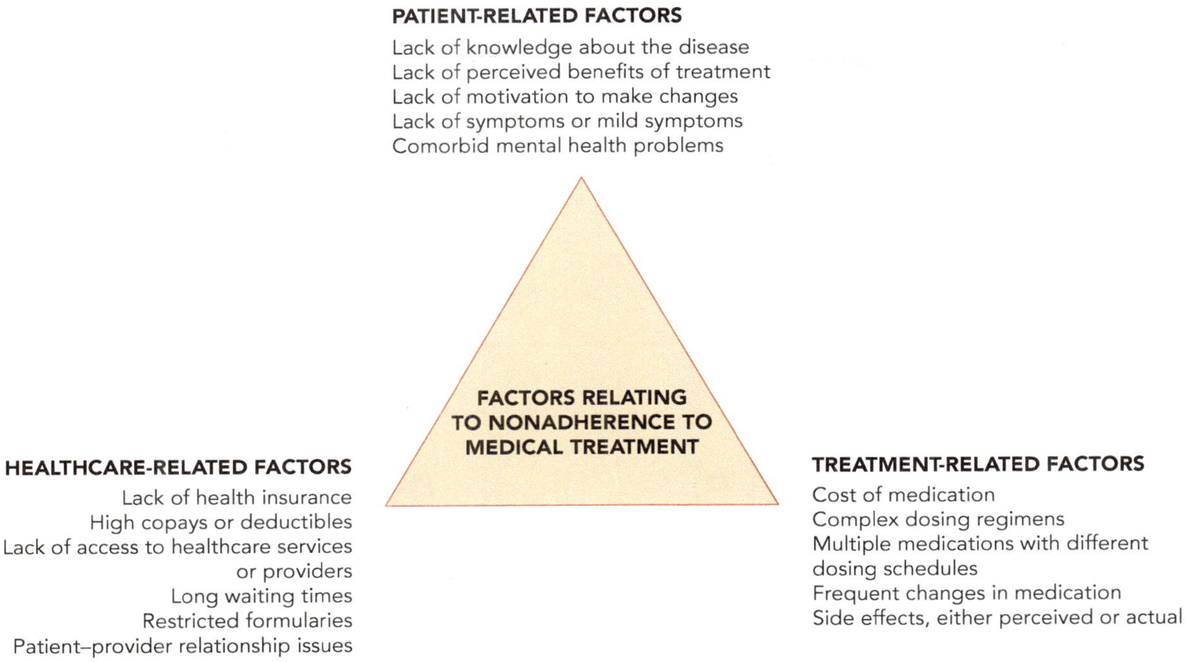

FIGURE 2.1 **Factors Relating to Nonadherence to Medical Treatment** We can conceptualize problems with adherence to medical treatment in terms of three sets of factors: patient-related factors, treatment-related factors, and healthcare-related factors.

INTERACTIVE FIGURES, CHARTS, & TABLES

Self-Assessment

INTERACTIVE SELF-ASSESSMENTS

What Would You Say? Beliefs Associated with Nonadherence to Medical Treatment

Imagine that you are a healthcare provider advising a person about the need to follow through with a course of medical treatment. Consider the responses in the left-hand column. Now consider what you would say to encourage the person adhere to treatment. You can compare your responses to sample clinician responses at the end of the chapter.

Patient's Response	What Would You Say?
"This medical issue is no big deal and so it doesn't warrant much effort from me."	
"I know the doctor says that I need to take the medications and exercise to stay healthy, but I feel good, so I'm not worried."	
"I am a healthy person overall, so I don't need to take medications. I'm not sick."	
"I'll wait until I'm not feeling good."	
"I don't like chemicals in my body, so I avoid taking any medications."	
"I'm worried about side effects of the medication."	
"My uncle had this medical issue, never saw a doctor, took medication, or had any treatment, and he did OK."	
"I don't want to do this."	
"It takes too much time."	

Source: Labbott (2018). Reprinted with permission of the American Psychological Association.

Review 2.1

INTERACTIVE SELF-SCORING QUIZZES

Sentence Completion

1. __________ factors either promote or hinder healthy changes in behavior.
2. Factors that enable change are called __________ factors.
3. __________ factors for healthy changes include praise and support.
4. __________-related factors in adherence include forgetfulness about taking medication.
5. __________-related factors in adherence include dosing regimens.
6. __________-related factors in adherence include high copays.

Think About It

How would you apply the concepts of predisposing factors, enabling factors, and reinforcing factors to help someone else, or help yourself, make healthy behavior changes?

The Health Belief Model (HBM)

Health Belief Model (HBM) A conceptual framework for predicting health behavior changes based on a person's beliefs about the perceived threat and severity of harm posed by an illness or health condition and the perceived benefits and costs of making behavioral changes.

tuberculosis A respiratory illness caused by a bacterium and characterized by coughing and pain in the chest.

The **Health Belief Model (HBM)** was developed to deal with a specific problem facing health officials back in the 1950s: Why were so few people seeking screening for tuberculosis when it became widely available? (Skinner et al., 2015).

Tuberculosis (TB) is a bacterial infection that is typically spread through the air when an infected person coughs, sneezes, or talks. The bacterium attacks the lungs and other organs and, if left untreated, can lead to severe respiratory and other problems, and possibly to death. Symptoms of TB include coughing, chest pain, and coughing up blood, but the bacterium may remain alive in the body in a latent state that does not cause any symptoms until it becomes activated at some later time. The only way to know for certain if a person is infected is through a screening test called the *tuberculin skin test* that detects the presence of the TB bacterium in the blood. A chest X-ray may also be used for screening purposes but is not sufficient to make the diagnosis. If TB is detected, doctors can successfully rid the body of the bacterium before it does extensive damage, through an extended course of antibiotic treatment.

In the early 20th century, tuberculosis was a leading cause of death in the United States, but today it can be cured in most cases with a 6- to 9-month course of antibiotics. The number of new TB cases in the U.S. has been dropping steadily since the early 1990s, and now account for fewer than 9,000 new cases annually and fewer than 625 deaths (CDC, 2024). These welcome changes are largely the result of widespread screening and greater availability of treatment. Worldwide, however, TB remains among the top causes of death, accounting for more than 1.6 million deaths per year (WHO, 2023). The contrast between the national and international figures underscores the lack of health resources in many of the world's poorest countries.

Widespread screening for TB in the United States was introduced in the 1950s, including the use of mobile X-ray vans that brought screening equipment directly into neighborhoods. However, relatively few people in the United States took advantage of screening at the time (Gehlert & Browne, 2019). The HBM was developed to better understand and predict health behaviors needed to detect, prevent, and control illnesses such as TB (Skinner et al., 2015). An earlier study had shown the importance of health-related beliefs in TB screening (Hochbaum, 1958). People who believed themselves to be more susceptible to TB and who also believed that early detection would be beneficial were nearly four times more likely to have at least one chest X-ray screening than those who did not see themselves as susceptible or perceive benefits in screening.

The HBM seeks to explain factors involved in making a health behavior change, such as getting screened for TB, getting a flu shot, attempting to lose weight, or trying to stop smoking, or getting vaccinated for COVID-19. The model recognizes that the decision to act is often based on a *cue to action*, such as the appearance of a symptom or a public health campaign raising awareness about the importance of getting an annual flu vaccine. But whether the change is put into effect depends on a process of weighing the pros and cons of making a change (Barley & Lawson, 2016).

The HBM predicts that people make healthy changes when they believe these changes will reduce a serious health threat they are either facing or likely to face. It emphasizes two major components in making a health-related behavior change: (1) perceived threat and (2) perceived benefits and costs.

1. **Perceived threat:** People judge a health threat based on the likelihood of the threat to their own personal health and the severity of harm the threat poses to themselves. The perceived threat involves two principal factors:
   a. *Perceived susceptibility*. Perceived susceptibility refers to the person's belief in the likelihood of contracting a disease or developing a medical condition. A person discounting their own risk of getting the flu is unlikely to obtain a flu shot.
   b. *Perceived severity*. Perceived severity refers to the person's belief about the seriousness of the disease or condition if it is contracted or untreated. If you think the flu is just a bad cold, you are probably less likely to go ahead and have a flu shot than if you believed the flu poses a serious risk to your health or your life. Perceived severity is not simply about the illness or condition itself, but also about how it will affect the person's daily life, ability to work, and family relationships ("I do not want to become a burden to my family").
2. **Perceived benefits and costs:** According to the HBM, people weigh the pros and cons, or perceived benefits of carrying out a course of action and the perceived costs, as in barriers or obstacles they are likely to face in making changes. Should I join a gym or sign up for an exercise program? Should I reduce my carbs or go "keto"? Should I wear a mask to help prevent transmission of an airborne infection? Taking action hinges on whether the person believes the outcomes will be beneficial and that barriers to taking action can be overcome. People are likely to join a gym or start an exercise program if they believe it will lead to tangible benefits, such as losing weight, increasing physical fitness, and reducing the risk of illness.

Perceived benefits include both positive health outcomes, such as controlling or preventing a disease or negative health condition, and non-health-related outcomes, such as saving money by not needing to purchase cigarettes or pleasing a family member (Skinner et al., 2015). Factored into a decision to take action are judgments the person makes about the costs and inconvenience of enacting health behavior changes, such as making regular exercise a routine part of their lifestyle (Gehlert & Ward, 2019).

The HBM offers insight into the role of maladaptive beliefs in accounting for nonadherence to treatment (failure to take medication as prescribed or to follow other medical recommendations). People's beliefs about the seriousness of their illness, the need for medication or other medical treatments, the potential of adverse side effects, the costs of treatment and expected outcomes or benefits all figure prominently in determining compliance with medical treatment. The HBM predicts that a person is likely to engage in a health-related behavior when the following conditions are met (Skinner et al., 2015):

1. *Perceived susceptibility to an illness or health condition* (e.g., "I'm at high risk of a stroke"). Recent evidence shows that smokers who have negative attitudes toward smoking but nonetheless continue to smoke tend to minimize the risks they face or believe any likely risk lies far off in the future (Alashoor & Han, 2021).
2. *Belief that the illness or condition can have serious consequences* (e.g., "A stroke could kill me or leave me paralyzed or unable to speak").
3. *Belief that engaging in a specific behavior or course of action can have beneficial consequences in reducing the risk of suffering from the illness or condition or lessening its severity* (e.g., "If I quit smoking, it will significantly lower my risk of a stroke").

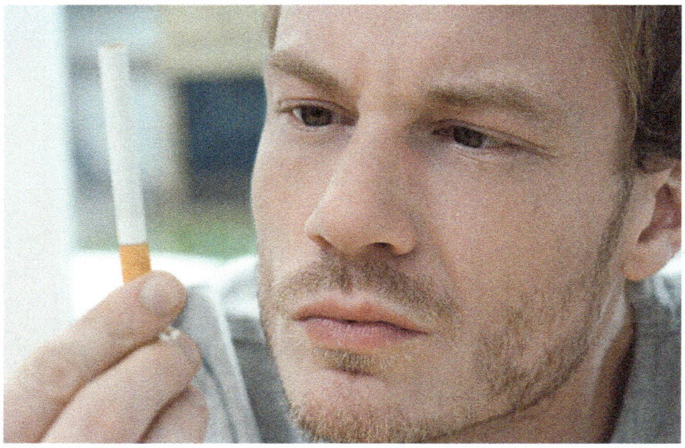

Image Source/Getty images

"Will I or Won't I?" The Health Belief Model looks at the question in terms of the perceived threat of smoking and the perceived benefits and costs of turning away the cigarette. Waking up with a cough or learning of a relative developing lung cancer could be cues to action.

4. *Belief that the costs of engaging in the behavior change are outweighed by the potential benefits* ("I may have unpleasant withdrawal effects if I quit smoking, but in the end it will be worth it").
5. *A cue for action.* A cue for action serves as a trigger for following through on a health recommendation. These cues can be internal, such as having chest pains, or external, such as receiving health advice or reminders from family members.

hypertension High blood pressure, a known risk factor of cardiovascular disease in which blood pressure exceeds healthy limits.

Consider an example of two people with **hypertension**, Avi and Maya, whose healthcare providers prescribe the same daily dose of a blood pressure medication and encourage both of them to make certain lifestyle changes to help lower blood pressure, such as curbing salt intake and losing excess weight. Avi questions whether he needs to take the medication and believes that changing his diet would require too great a sacrifice. He says, "I'm feeling fine, so why do I need to take these pills? They only make me need to go to the bathroom more often. And giving up the food I love? I'd rather just enjoy my life and not worry about a health problem that might never happen or could be 20 or 30 years down the road."

Maya focuses on the perceived benefits of treatment and recognizes that barriers to making health-related changes can be overcome. She says, "Getting my blood pressure under control will reduce my risk of heart disease and likely add years to my life. Sure, it's inconvenient to remember to take my pills, and it will be a pain to keep my weight in check and watch my salt intake, but taking care of my health is worth it."

Health psychologists help people like Avi and Maya adjust to living with a serious or chronic illness. They are aware that people's beliefs may sometimes impede the treatment process, and thus they encourage people to rethink their beliefs and consider treatment alternatives, as shown in the sample clinician responses at the end of the chapter.

Figure 2.2 presents an example of the HBM in predicting compliance with taking medication for hypertension. Notice how the perceived threat (perceived susceptibility and severity) and outcome expectations (perceived benefits and costs) influence the likelihood of engaging in behavior (taking the medication reliably).

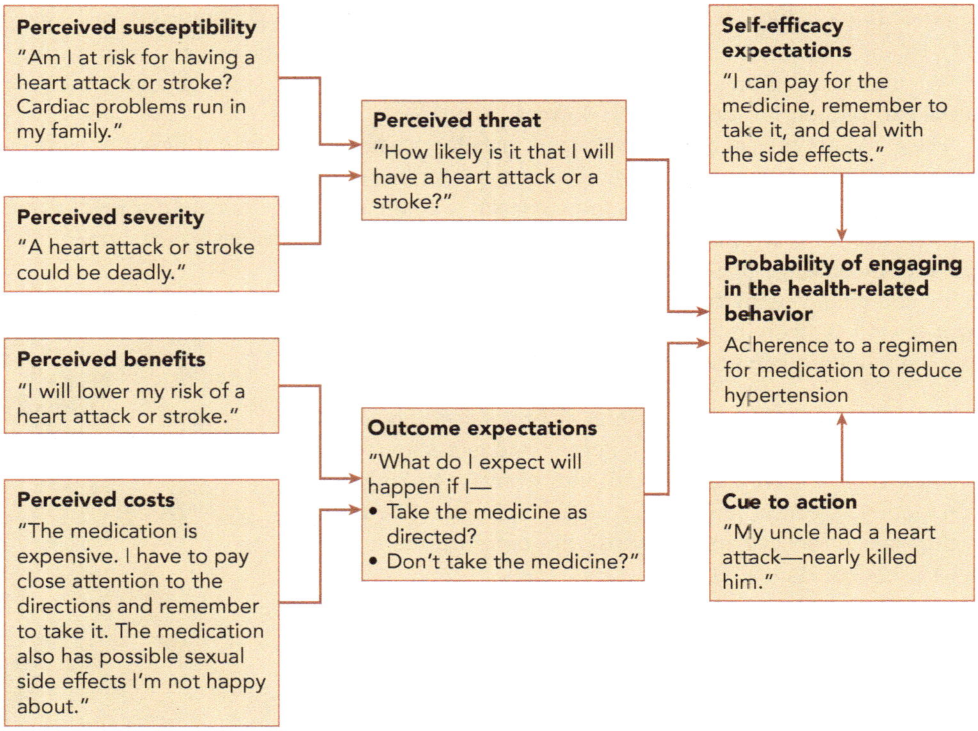

INTERACTIVE FIGURES, CHARTS, & TABLES

FIGURE 2.2 Application of Health Belief Model (HBM) to Adherence to Medication for Hypertension Perceived susceptibility and perceived severity contribute to the perceived threat posed by hypertension. Weighing the perceived benefits and costs leads to outcome expectations. The perceived threat, outcome expectations, self-efficacy expectations, and cues to action all feed into the probability the individual will adhere to a medication plan to reduce hypertension.

The scientific literature shows many examples of the use of the HBM in predicting a wide range of health behaviors, including increasing adherence to taking medications, following a healthy diet, obtaining needed vaccinations, undertaking cancer screenings, and making other healthy lifestyle changes.

The HBM sheds light on reasons that people do not follow through with medical treatment. Although concerns about side effects of medication may be understandable, they need to be weighed against the benefits of taking a medication. At the same time, healthcare providers need to hear people's concerns and consider treatment alternatives that may carry fewer side effects.

But how do health beliefs translate into improved medical outcomes? One possible pathway is that positive health beliefs lead to greater adherence to medical recommendations and greater adherence in turn leads to better outcomes. People who hold positive beliefs and attitudes about their doctors and other healthcare providers tend to comply more consistently with treatment recommendations, and their greater adherence results in better physical and mental health outcomes.

fibromyalgia A pain syndrome involving pain in muscles and soft tissues throughout the body.

Health Psychology in Action

Field Studies Using the Health Belief Model

Consider some recent studies applying the HBM to adherence to medical treatment for various diseases and health conditions:

- *Fibromyalgia:* Researchers applied the HBM to a study of people with **fibromyalgia**, a chronic physical condition that leads to pain and fatigue (Rowe et al., 2019). Consistent with the model, the researchers found that patients with fibromyalgia who held more positive or adaptive health beliefs tended to follow medical advice more closely and to report a better quality of life.
- *Breast cancer:* Prediction of medication adherence based on the HBM was tested in a study that tracked 345 patients with breast cancer in the United Kingdom who were prescribed the cancer medication tamoxifen during their first year of treatment (Moon et al., 2019). The women completed follow-up questionnaires throughout the year. The most prominent factors associated with failure to take the medication as directed were negative beliefs about the benefits of the medication and lack of confidence in their own ability to take the medication as prescribed. These results support the validity of the HBM and identify potentially modifiable factors—negative beliefs and lack of confidence (lack of self-efficacy, as we will see later) as a barrier in following a plan—that can become a focus of behavioral interventions aimed at improving adherence.
- *High blood cholesterol:* Other researchers examined factors predicting adherence to taking statin medications, which are a class of medications widely used to lower blood cholesterol levels. High blood cholesterol is linked to cardiovascular disease and stroke. The problem of nonadherence to statin medications is well recognized by treatment providers, with estimates suggesting that at least 40%, but perhaps as many as 80%, of people don't fully comply with their prescribed treatment (Hope et al., 2019). Consistent with the HBM, people who perceive more barriers to taking these medications, such as concerns about side effects, have lower rates of adherence than those perceiving fewer barriers. Concerns about side effects figure prominently in lack of adherence to many medications (Ismail et al., 2017; Rottman et al., 2017; Yeam et al., 2018).
- *Hypertension:* The role of perceived barriers to taking medication also comes into play with people with hypertension. Hypertension (high blood pressure) is a major risk factor for cardiovascular disease, increasing the risk of heart attacks and stroke. Hypertension is considered a silent killer because it typically does not produce any noticeable symptoms, so people are often unaware that they have it. Fortunately, following proper medical guidelines and making healthy changes in lifestyle behaviors, such as reducing excess weight and exercising regularly, as well as taking medication for hypertension as prescribed, can help manage hypertension and reduce the risk of complications.

  About half of people with hypertension discontinue their blood pressure medications within a year, even though they know about the risks posed by uncontrolled hypertension (Thirumurthy et al., 2019). Why don't these people take their meds? Applying the HBM, researchers find that high on the list of barriers to taking medication, as in the case of statins, are health beliefs and concerns about side effects (Al-Nouman et al., 2019; Jarab et al., 2018).
- *Flu vaccine*: European researchers tested the HBM with community residents who were eligible for free flu immunizations because of chronic diseases (Arsenović et al., 2022). Consistent with the HBM model, people who perceived influenza as more serious, or reported more cues to action (e.g., telephone reminder calls), or perceived fewer barriers to getting the shot were more likely than others to get a flu vaccine.
- *COVID-19 vaccine:* The HBM predicts that people make healthy changes when they believe these changes will reduce a serious health threat they are facing or likely to face. Consider the public health challenge of getting people vaccinated during the COVID-19 pandemic. Health officials recognized that vaccine hesitancy was a major impediment to the success of COVID-19 immunization programs. Researchers found the HBM to be useful in predicting COVID-19 vaccine hesitancy (Limbu, Gautam, & Pham, 2022). The HBM factors most strongly associated with lower vaccine hesitancy and hence greater willingness to get vaccinated were the following: (1) perceived benefits of the vaccine, (2) perceived susceptibility to COVID, (3) perceived severity of the illness, (4) presence of cues to action (prompts from others or news reports), and (5) self-efficacy (belief in one's ability to get vaccinated). Armed with this information, health promotion programs need to overcome these obstacles to vaccination by providing people with accurate information about the benefits of vaccination and the risks they face by remaining unvaccinated.

Health psychologists are working on ways of increasing adherence to treatment, as we see in a study of people with HIV (Neumann et al., 2018). For example, treatment of HIV infection involves the use of antiretroviral medications to keep the infection at bay. People who maintain a lower viral load are unlikely to transmit HIV. But at the time the study was conducted, achieving a good clinical outcome depended on people following complex dosing schedules. The researchers used an educational intervention in the form of a video that depicted barriers people might face in following their prescribed regimen and also keeping regular medical appointments.

The investigators showed the video to more than 2,000 people with HIV as they waited to be seen for medical appointments. People who saw the video showed 10% higher rates of initiating antiretroviral medication, and 6% lower viral loads, than people in the same clinic a year before the video was used. This pilot study showed that a relatively low-cost intervention can have a positive impact on treatment engagement and suppression of HIV.

Today, as researchers continue to use components of the HBM to predict the likelihood of health behavior change, they have expanded the model by considering roles for other factors, and also have incorporated other theoretical constructs, including self-efficacy.

Other Factors in Adherence The HBM focuses on how people's beliefs affect their likelihood of adhering to medical treatment. But other factors also play important roles in adherence. Taking medication involves more than just taking a pill as prescribed. It requires closely following dosing regimens, which sometimes can be quite complicated, and also adhering to the timing of intervals between doses (Ismail et al., 2017; Rottman et al., 2018; Yeam et al., 2018).

Scientific reviews highlight other factors involved in poor medical adherence, such as low income level and lack of social support, underscoring the need for treatments that people can afford and the importance of involving family members as supportive partners in the treatment effort (Gast & Mathes, 2019). The HBM assumes that demographic factors such as age and educational level affect a person's belief system, but the model does not specify how these types of factors interact with the other components of the model (Skinner et al., 2015). Lack of trust in health professionals, especially among people of color who feel neglected or mistreated by healthcare institutions, also contributes to nonadherence to medical treatment (Cuevas & O'Brien, 2019).

Knowledge is yet another critical factor in adherence. Managing the care of people with cardiac problems depends largely on their following medical advice, such as taking medication as prescribed, getting regular exercise, limiting salt intake, exercising regularly, and so on. Evidence shows that failure to adhere to medical recommendations in people with heart disease contributes to increased need for hospitalization, poorer health outcomes, and increased risk of death (Seid et al., 2019). Researchers who studied people with heart failure showed that those with a good level of knowledge about heart failure were more likely to adhere to treatment recommendations than were people who were less well informed (Seid et al., 2019).

Lack of adherence is not simply about failure to take medications as prescribed. Among the factors that reduce compliance with cancer screenings are low income and poor accessibility to medical clinics. As our nation grapples with disparities in health care, let us note that people with lower income levels and those who have less access to services, especially those who are underinsured or uninsured, are less likely to obtain regular cancer screenings (Hunleth et al., 2016; Kiviniemi et al., 2018).

A person's emotional reactions also need to be considered. Many health decisions are made in an emotionally laden context (Ferrer & Klein, 2015; Ferrer & Mendes, 2019). For example, receiving a cancer diagnosis may elicit fears not only about death, but also about the adverse consequences of treatments (surgery, chemotherapy, radiation) and their side effects. People may need help managing fear in order to carefully weigh treatment alternatives and follow through with medical tests and procedures. Fear of being proven cancer positive may prevent people from undergoing recommended screening procedures that would detect cancer in its early, more manageable stages. An important role for health psychologists in cancer care is to provide psychological assistance to people in managing fear so that it does not prevent them from making necessary treatment decisions or following health directives.

Fear may also motivate disease-preventive efforts. In a recent study conducted during the COVID-19 pandemic, health researchers showed that perceived risk was associated with more COVID-19 preventive behaviors, such as wearing masks (Serpas & Ignacio, 2022). The link in the chain that explained how perceived risk predicted preventive behavior was fear. Increased risk was associated with higher levels of fear, which in turn led to more preventive behaviors. In other words, the greater the risk people perceived COVID-19 to be, the more fearful they became, and the more fearful they became, the more likely they were to take measures to prevent infection.

What about positive emotions? Do they also help promote healthier behaviors? The color red, for example, is more strongly linked to avoidance behaviors (think "stop sign" or a teacher's red pen) whereas bluish colors are associated with more peaceful imagery that evokes approach tendencies (the calming image of a blue sky or sea). Investigators in one study (Voss et al., 2018) therefore reasoned that different colors evoke different emotional associations. But would the use of color affect the effectiveness of health-persuasion messages? To answer the question, the investigators prepared a pamphlet promoting sunscreen protection. They distributed two versions of the pamphlet, one with "cooler" colors (blue/purple) in the background and another in "warmer" colors (red/orange). The message was the same (promoting the use of sunscreen). The only difference was the background color framing the message.

It turned out that a health message framed by cooler colors (blue and purple) was a more effective persuader, as measured by student expression of intentions to use sunscreen. The health message with warmer colors in the background (orange and red) did not increase persuasion. Therefore, if you want to encourage people to use a health-related product or adopt healthier behavior, think blue, not red.

Also note that intentions do not necessarily translate into actions (Michie et al., 2019). Intentions may only have weak relationships with behavior, so weak in fact that they may not be very useful in making predictions of behavior (Rhodes & Dickau, 2012). People may have the best of intentions to engage in healthy behaviors—to exercise regularly or make healthier foods choices, for instance. However, when it comes to working out or eating right, people often do not follow through. Therefore, we also need to consider factors beyond intentions in determining whether people are likely to follow through on making healthy changes in their behaviors—factors such as motivation and self-efficacy. These considerations bring us to other models that help us predict health behavior change—social cognitive theory, the Theory of Reasoned Action (TRA) and Theory of Planned Behavior (TPB), and the Transtheoretical Model (TTM).

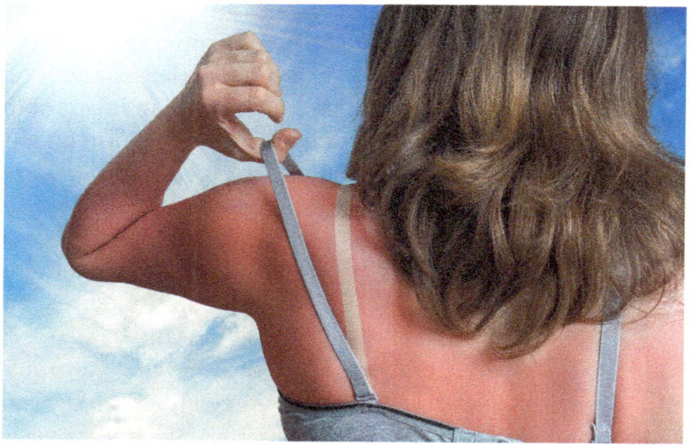

vchal/Shutterstock.com

Protection Needed! The persuasiveness of health messages may depend in part on subtle cues, even the background color framing the message.

Review 2.2

INTERACTIVE SELF-SCORING QUIZZES

Sentence Completion

1. The __________ model was developed to explain why so few people were seeking screening for tuberculosis.

2. The Health Belief Model emphasizes two major components, (1) perceived __________ and (2) perceived __________ and __________.

3. Perceived __________ refers to a person's belief in the likelihood of contracting a disease or developing a medical condition.

4. Perceived __________ refers to a person's belief about the seriousness of the disease or condition and of letting it go untreated.

5. Enacting healthy behaviors hinges on whether a person believes the results will be beneficial and that __________ to taking action can be overcome.

6. __________ health beliefs lead to greater adherence to medical recommendations.

7. People with fibromyalgia who held more positive or adaptive health beliefs reported having a (better or worse) quality of life.

Think About It

How might the HBM apply to making changes in your health behavior? How might the model help you predict the likelihood of carrying out a health behavior change? What factors would make the behavior change more likely or less likely to occur?

Social Cognitive Theory

social cognitive theory A conceptual model that expands upon traditional learning theory by incorporating roles for cognitive factors and learning through observing others in the social environment.

Social cognitive theory (formerly called *social learning theory*) emerged in the 1960s and 1970s as psychologists sought to expand traditional learning theory to include roles for cognitive factors and learning by observing others in the social environment.

Classic Learning Theory

Classic learning theory is based on principles of classical conditioning and operant conditioning first formulated through laboratory research by the Russian physiologist Ivan Pavlov (1849–1936) and the American behaviorist B. F. Skinner (1904–1990), respectively, in the early and middle 20th century.

classical conditioning A form of learning by association in which a response is elicited by a previously neutral stimulus that has been paired or associated with a stimulus that originally elicited the response.

VIDEO CONTENT

Classical Conditioning

Classical conditioning is a form of learning based on the association or pairing of stimuli. Pavlov showed that dogs learned to salivate to the sound of a bell when this stimulus was repeatedly paired with food powder. To a person with cancer undergoing chemotherapy, the lessons learned in Pavlov's laboratory have special significance. Chemotherapy often produces intense nausea that becomes associated with stimulus cues in the treatment center. People may become nauseous upon entering the treatment facility or even on the way to the clinic. Health psychologists help people with cancer manage unpleasant side effects treatments by teaching them relaxation skills to combat conditioned nausea and using attention distraction techniques to divert their attention as they are awaiting chemotherapy.

A case example illustrates the role of classical conditioning with respect to another health-related problem, drug cravings. A construction worker in New York City battled heroin addiction and underwent a detoxification program that cleared his body of the drug. Upon his release, and looking to put his life back together, he got a job working on a construction site in lower Manhattan. Taking the subway on his first day of work, he suddenly experienced intense cravings for heroin when the subway car doors opened at a particular stop in Queens. When the doors closed, the symptoms disappeared and he went on to work, but they would return whenever the subway doors opened at this location. What was the connection between his cravings and that particular subway stop? You might well have guessed it was the same station where he had scored drugs when he was using. His cravings were a conditioned response to conditioned stimuli (cues) associated with that particular subway station.

In a similar way, people who are primarily "stimulus smokers" reach for a cigarette whenever they are exposed to smoking-related stimuli, such as observing someone else puffing a cigarette or when they get a whiff of tobacco smoke. Smoking can become a conditioned habit when it is linked to situational cues in the environment, such as watching TV, driving in the car, or relaxing after dinner.

Classical conditioning also comes into play in other health-related behaviors, such as dietary control. External food cues, such as passing by a favorite bakery or watching a food commercial on TV, can induce cravings for treats, resulting in cued overeating (Kirsten, Seib-Pfeifer, & Gibbons, 2022).

operant conditioning A form of learning in which the consequences of a response determine the probability that the response will be repeated or become stronger.

VIDEO CONTENT

Operant Conditioning

Operant conditioning is a form of learning in which the consequences of responses, such as rewards and punishments, influence the strength of the behaviors they follow, including health-related behaviors. B. F. Skinner referred to rewards as *reinforcers*, or stimulus events that strengthen behaviors they follow. For example, use of alcohol, tobacco, or other drugs may be reinforced by the pleasurable effects of the drugs themselves, which strengthens their continued use. Drug-using behavior may also be strengthened by another form of reinforcement, social reinforcement, as in the form of social approval from drug-using friends (see Chapter 9).

Skinner identified two types of reinforcement, *positive reinforcement*, in which a rewarding stimulus is presented after a response occurs, and *negative reinforcement*, in which a response leads to the removal of an unpleasant or aversive stimulus. In drug use, positive reinforcement may involve the pleasurable effects of taking a drug or social approval from others. But negative reinforcement may also come into play, as when people use a drug to reduce withdrawal symptoms or to self-medicate; that is, to attempt to soothe negative feeling states, such as anxiety or depression by using a drug like alcohol (see Chapter 9).

Punishment is the flip side of reinforcement. Punishments are unpleasant or undesirable consequences that decrease or suppress the likelihood of the behavior they follow. Examples include the case of a parent scolding a child for slamming a door or a driver receiving a ticket for speeding. The punishment might decrease the likelihood of an undesirable behavior and have undesirable consequences, especially when it is applied frequently to children or is harsh or severe. It can leave emotional scars and may only result in suppressing the undesirable behavior for a time rather than teaching an alternative, more desirable form of behavior.

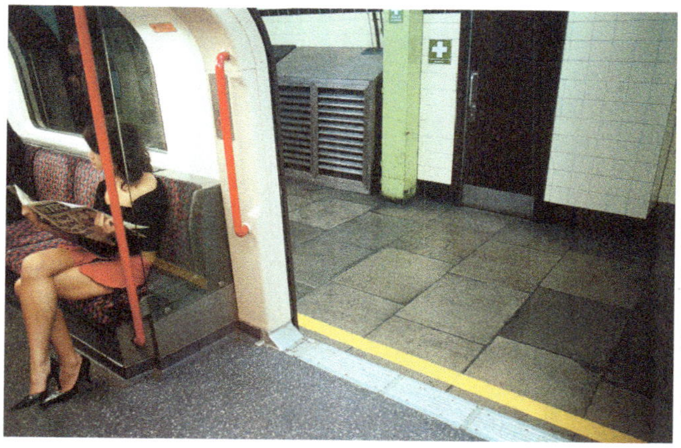

agefotostock/Alamy Stock Photo

A Conditioned Craving? When the doors on a subway car opened at a particular stop, a passenger recovering from heroin addiction suddenly experienced intense cravings for heroin. The question is: Why?

Albert Bandura and Social Cognitive Theory

Social cognitive theorists such as psychologist Albert Bandura (1925–2021) recognize the importance of classical and operant conditioning, but believe that behavior is best understood by adding to the mix cognitive factors and how we learn new behaviors by observing others in the social environment. Cognitive factors include expectancies, goals, and personal values. Bandura emphasized the importance of two types of expectancies as determinants of behavior, **self-efficacy expectations** and **outcome expectations**. He also famously demonstrated the role of modeling (also called observational learning) by showing that children imitated aggressive behaviors they had observed in adults who modeled these behaviors.

A key element in Bandura's social cognitive theory is **reciprocal determinism**, the belief that cognitions, environmental or situational factors, and behavior all mutually influence each other (see Figure 2.3). Let's say you are considering quitting smoking. Whether you are likely to begin taking steps to quit smoking, such as discarding leftover cigarettes, ashtrays, and the like, depends on cognitive factors, including self-efficacy (belief in your ability to quit) and the perceived value you place on quitting, as well as situational factors, such as exposure to cues associated with smoking or praise from loved ones from attempting to quit. Each factor influences the other. For example, on the first day you go without smoking, you pass someone in the street who is puffing away (a situational factor) and the whiff of tobacco smoke triggers cravings that lead you to resume smoking (a behavior). This then reduces your self-efficacy (belief in your ability to succeed in quitting), which in turn further increases your likelihood of smoking. In order to make meaningful changes in behavior, we need to consider each of these components—behaviors, environment, and cognitions—as part of system of interlinking parts.

The main components of social cognitive theory as outlined by Bandura and other theorists include:

1. *Reciprocal determinism:* The belief that cognitions, behaviors, and the environment all influence one another.
2. *Behavioral competencies:* If we possess competencies needed to perform skilled actions, we are more likely to perform these actions.
3. *Outcome expectations:* The more strongly we believe that making a health-related change in our behavior, such as exercising regularly, will have a tangible payoff, the more likely we are to engage in that behavior.
4. *Self-efficacy expectations:* The stronger our belief in our ability to accomplish the tasks we set out for ourselves and to overcome barriers in our way, the more likely we will be to make healthy behavior changes.
5. *Observational learning (modeling):* When we observe others in our social environment modeling healthy behaviors, we are more likely to engage in those behaviors ourselves.

VIDEO CONTENT

Insight, Latent, and Observational Learning

self-efficacy expectations
Beliefs people hold about their ability to accomplish certain tasks or achieve certain outcomes or goals.

outcome expectations
Predictions people make about the outcomes of their behavior.

reciprocal determinism
Bandura's social cognitive model in which cognitions, behaviors, and environmental factors mutually influence each other.

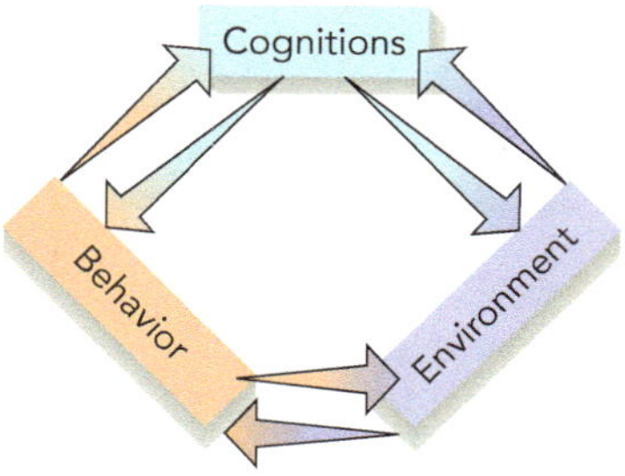

FIGURE 2.3 Albert Bandura's Model of Reciprocal Determinism Bandura proposed that cognitions, behaviors, and environmental factors interact with one another to determine behavior.

Source: Adapted from Bandura (1986).

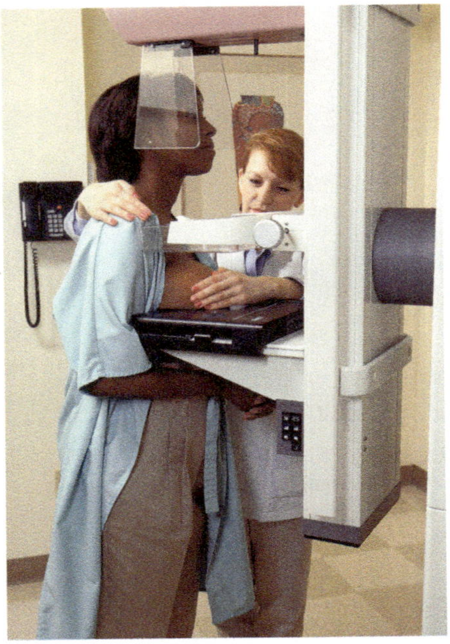

A Technician Assisting a Woman Having a Mammogram Health psychologists find that self-efficacy predicts greater likelihood of engaging in screening for cancer.

6. *Reinforcement:* The stronger the reinforcement or reward for making healthy behavior changes, the greater the likelihood the behavior will recur. If you start a weight loss program and are reinforced by losing a few pounds, you are more likely to continue the program than if your weight refused to budge.

Social cognitive theory has been applied to a wide range of health behaviors, from improvement of dietary behaviors, to participation in cancer screening, to contraceptive use, smoking cessation, reduction of alcohol use, and adoption of healthy sexual behaviors (Gehlert & Ward, 2019; Glanz & Bishop, 2010).

Self-Efficacy: "Yes, I Can"

Self-efficacy expectations are an important element in social cognitive theory. Health psychologists recognize that people are more likely to make healthy changes in their behavior, such as choosing healthier foods and exercising regularly, when they have confidence in their abilities to put these changes into practice—that is, when they have high levels of self-efficacy.

As an example, health psychologists find that higher self-confidence in taking prescribed breast cancer medication (tamoxifen) in breast cancer survivors was associated with a greater likelihood of adherence to taking the medication (Moon et al., 2019). Other researchers tie higher self-efficacy to increased physical activity in cancer survivors (Hirschey et al., 2020).

A study cited earlier that looked at adherence to medication among people with heart problems on statin medications reported that self-efficacy, a factor that was not included in the original HBM, played an important role in determining which people reliably followed the treatment regimen (Hope et al., 2019). Because nothing quite succeeds like success, getting started making healthy changes in behavior can help boost self-efficacy, which in turn can lead to yet healthier behavior changes, becoming a positive loop, or *virtuous cycle,* in which success breeds success (Schneider et al., 2016).

Before we move on, let us note that theories make a difference in designing health promotion efforts. A recent systematic review showed that interventions designed to promote oral health in teens were more effective in reducing plaque when they were grounded in theory, especially social cognitive theory, than when they were based on simply disseminating health-related information (Xiang et al., 2021). Among the social cognitive factors that can be incorporated in oral health interventions is social influence, such as by using peer-led social networking to get oral hygiene messages across to teens, and also building their self-efficacy or confidence in their ability to consistently practice better oral hygiene.

Review 2.3

INTERACTIVE SELF-SCORING QUIZZES

Sentence Completion

1. Social cognitive theory expanded upon traditional __________ theory.
2. Social cognitive theorists emphasize the role of cognitive factors, such as expectancies, goals, and personal __________.
3. In social cognitive theory, stimulus cues and rewards and punishments represent __________ or environmental factors.
4. Reciprocal __________ is the belief that cognitions, behaviors, and the environment all influence other.
5. __________ expectations are beliefs we hold about whether behavioral changes will have a tangible payoff.
6. Self-__________ is the belief you hold in your ability to enact behavior changes or succeed in tasks you attempt to accomplish.
7. A health message was (more or less) persuasive when it was framed by blue rather than red.

Think About It

Do you believe in your ability to succeed in tasks you set out to accomplish? Are there some areas of life in which you are higher in self-efficacy than others—academics, sports, social relationships? Do you have the confidence in yourself to follow through in making healthy changes in your behavior? Why or why not? And if not, what can you do to boost your level of health-related self-efficacy?

Health Psychology in Action

Applying Operant Conditioning in the Snack Aisle in the Supermarket

Sugar consumption is a leading contributor to many types of health problems including diabetes, obesity, and tooth decay. In order to reduce the purchase and consumption of sugary drinks, governments have applied the principle of *response cost* by imposing an added sales tax on these products. A response cost is simply that: a monetary consequence or penalty for performing an undesirable response, such as buying sugary drinks. States have long imposed additional sales taxes as response costs for other consumer products linked to negative health outcomes, such as cigarettes and alcohol.

The effects of taxing specific products may be limited because they are typically levied on distributors and passed along to consumers who may be unaware they are paying an added tax. But what if the added tax was more salient, say by stating it plainly on the product sales tag? Behavioral scientists in San Francisco conducted a field experiment in a university store in which they affixed the phrase "includes sugary drink tax" on the sales tag of sugary drinks (Donnelly et al., 2021). They found that purchases of sugary drinks dropped by about 10% from the pretax period. These reductions were largely offset by increased purchases of water and diet soda.

Further research is needed to determine whether reducing purchases of sugary products improves health outcomes, such as reducing excess weight. Do you think that seeing a product carrying a "sugar tax added" label might influence your purchasing decisions, perhaps prompting you to make healthier choices? More broadly, do you think it's fair for the government to impose additional taxes on certain products because their use may be associated with negative health outcomes?

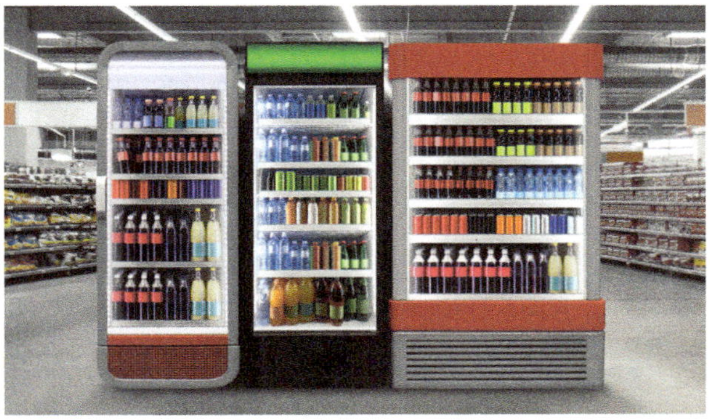

Hitra/Shutterstock.com

The Theories of Reasoned Action and Planned Behavior

According to the Health Belief Model (HBM), a person's beliefs about making healthy changes in behavior—the balance between the pros and cons of taking action—are key determinants of behavior change. The **Theory of Reasoned Action (TRA)** expands upon the HBM to consider the larger social context in which intentions to act translate into actions (Fishbein & Ajzen, 1975). The theory has evolved into a broader model, called the **Theory of Planned Behavior (TPB)**, that incorporates a role for perceived control over behavior. Let's take a closer look.

Theory of Reasoned Action (TRA) A conceptual framework used to predict intentions to act, which is based on a person's attitudes toward the behavior and perceptions of subjective norms.

Theory of Planned Behavior (TPB) An expanded TRA model that includes the additional factor of perceived control over behavior.

The Theory of Reasoned Action

The TRA emphasizes the importance of intentions to act (Hennessy et al., 2018; Lezin, 2019). Consider an intention as a plan to engage in a particular behavior, such as starting an exercise program. Intentions precede actions, but there is no guarantee that an intention will translate into action. For example, a person may intend to see a specialist but not follow through.

The TRA posits that the following factors affect whether intentions lead to actions:

1. the person's attitudes toward a behavior, and
2. the person's perception of the **subjective norms** of people and groups the person deems to be important.

subjective norms The perceived social pressures to perform or not perform a certain behavior.

First, expecting that an intended behavior will lead to a valuable outcome will likely result in a positive attitude toward the behavior (e.g., "If I join a gym, I'll lose weight and firm up my body"). However, expecting a negative outcome will likely lead to development of a negative attitude toward the behavior (e.g., "I'm just kidding myself that I'll lose weight or change how I look").

normative beliefs A person's beliefs about how others are likely to judge a particular behavior.

Subjective norms derive from a person's **normative beliefs** about how others will judge the behavior. If I believe my friends and family will approve of the intended behavior and support my efforts to make a change, I am more likely to follow through (e.g., "My partner will be very pleased if I started going to the gym"). Normative beliefs that underlie perceived social norms may be correct or incorrect, because other people may not act as expected. Yet for a person contemplating a behavior change, perception carries weight and guides behavior.

In sum, to predict whether a person who intends to get off the couch and start an exercise program actually follows through, we need to evaluate the person's attitudes about the behavior in question (beliefs about the expected results or outcomes of the behavior) and the person's perceptions of subjective norms—what the person believes others think about the behavior.

Let's see how researchers applied the Theory of Reasoned Action to vaccine resistance during the COVID-19 pandemic (Akther & Nur, 2022). Health researchers in Bangladesh recruited 351 university students between the ages of 19 and 30 years. They found that a person's belief in conspiracy theories about the vaccine negatively impacted both their attitudes toward the vaccine and their perception of subjective norms (beliefs about what other people think about the vaccine). To promote vaccine acceptance and likelihood of getting the vaccine, the researchers encourage health officials to focus health campaigns on reducing misinformation about COVID-19 vaccination.

injunctive norms Expectations of other people's approval or disapproval of particular behaviors or actions.

prescriptive norms Perceptions of what one believes other people do, think, or feel.

Revisions to the model divide subjective norms into two subtypes, **injunctive norms** (what you believe other people expect you to do) and **prescriptive norms** (what you believe other people actually do) (Conner, 2015). In considering factors that determine whether intentions carry over into actions, we need to account for the person's expectations about what others think and what others do.

The TRA is based on the concept of reasoned action. But we shouldn't confuse "reasoned" with "reasonable." The TRA doesn't assume people act reasonably or correctly but rather that their intentions to act are based on their reasons or motives for engaging in the behavior and their beliefs about what other people will think about it (Lezin, 2019). It may be, or perhaps not be, reasonable to quit smoking cold turkey, but the person who reasons that success is likely and desirable, and that the effort will be supported by friends and family, is more likely to form the intention to do it and quit all at once.

The Theory of Planned Behavior

The Theory of Planned Behavior (TPB) expands upon the TRA by incorporating another factor, perceived control over one's behavior (Ajzen, 1991, 2005).

The TPB is based on the belief that the ability to predict whether a person is likely to carry out an intended action depends in part on the person's perception of control over the behavior. Perceptions of control are shaped by past experiences. You may intend to join a gym but fail to follow through if your past experience with gyms has been unsuccessful, creating the perception that your effort will be disappointing ("What's the point? I've tried before and never followed through"). The basic components of the TPB are shown in **Figure 2.4**.

Perceived behavioral control has two components, (1) *self-efficacy* (the belief that one is capable of carrying out the intended action successfully even in the face of obstacles or barriers); and (2) *controllability* (the belief that the behavior is under the person's control and that the person has the resources and opportunity needed to perform the action) (Ajzen, 2002). That is, perceived behavioral control has *perceived confidence* (self-efficacy) and *perceived control* (controllability) (Conner & Sparks, 2005).

Return to the gym example. Luna plans to exercise three times a week for 30 minutes each time in a nearby gym. Luna may believe in her ability to carry out the behavior ("I am confident that once I get to the gym I can use the cardio equipment for a 30-minute workout") but lack perceived control over the behavior ("With my work schedule, I just don't see how I can fit it in").

The TPB predicts that despite strong intentions, lack of perceived control over the behavior will likely lead to inaction. So the combined TPB model, as shown in Figure 2.4, predicts that when the intended behavior is more strongly aligned with favorable attitudes and subjective norms, and with perceptions of control over the behavior, the stronger the intentions to act are likely to be and the more likely the person will follow through.

Are you ready to make a healthy change in behavior in your own life? **Table 2.2** can help you assess your readiness, based on the TPB.

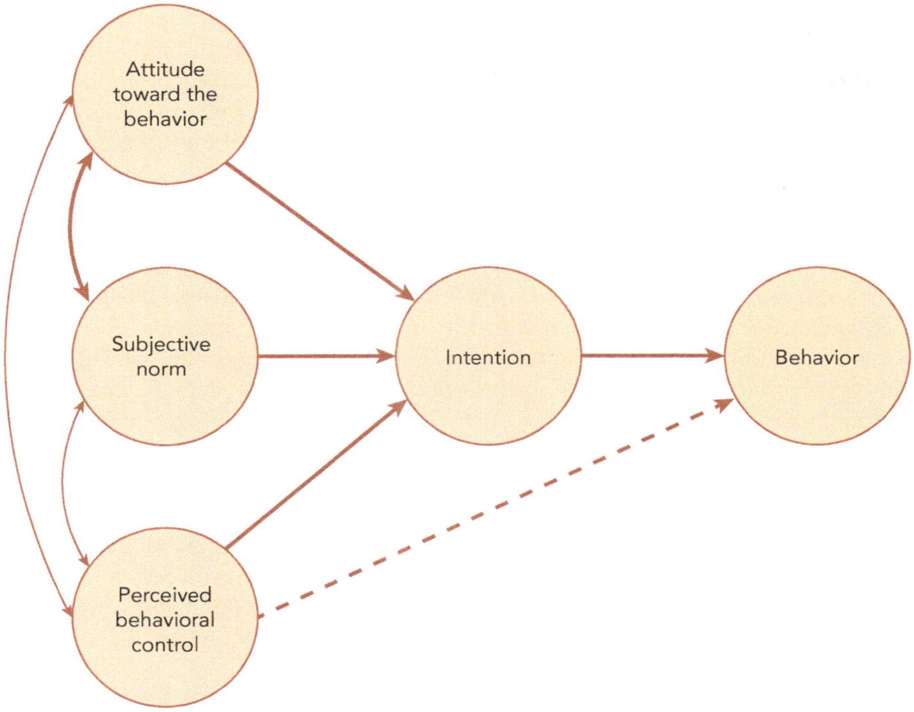

FIGURE 2.4 Components of the Theory of Planned Behavior (TPB) The TPB proposes three factors that contribute to intentions to make behavioral changes. Perceptions of behavioral control influence both intentions and the behavior itself.

Applying the TRA/TPB Model to Health-Related Behaviors

Research supports the value of the TPB and combined TRA/TPB models in predicting changes in health-related behaviors (Gehlert & Browne, 2019; Lo et al., 2019; Michie et al., 2019). A study in Northern Ireland put the TPB into practice in predicting children's intentions to regularly brush their teeth (Davison et al., 2019). Poor dental health can negatively impact both physical and emotional health. The investigators measured children's intentions by means of a questionnaire that asked them to rate how strongly they intended to brush their teeth. Each of the major concepts in the TPB model—attitudes, subjective norms, and perceived control—predicted tooth-brushing intentions.

TPB concepts may not contribute equally in predicting intentions to make healthy changes in behavior. In the tooth-brushing study, the strongest predictor of intentions was self-efficacy, which is a facet of perceived control ("I know how to brush my teeth and can do it regularly"). This finding underscores the importance of building self-confidence for performing healthier behaviors.

A Taiwanese study of smokers attending a smoking cessation clinic showed that the strongest predictors of intention to quit were perceived control over quitting and belief that one was susceptible to the health threats posed by smoking (Tseng et al., 2018). In this particular study, subjective norms failed to predict intentions. It seems that the predictive utility of the TPB may vary with the type of behavior under study and the population of interest, among other factors.

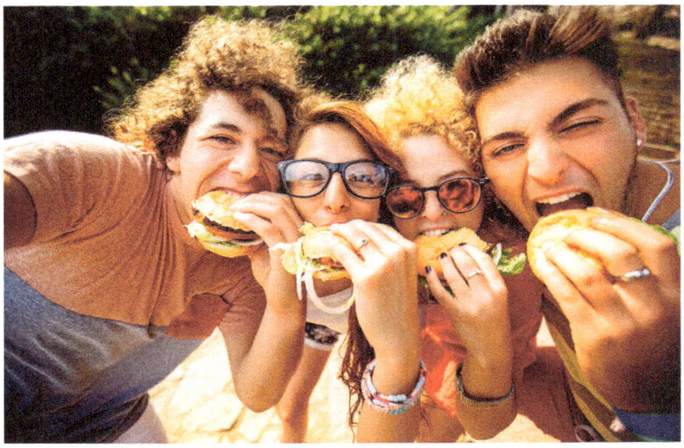

wundervisuals/Getty Images

All Together Now? Adolescents often follow the crowd—eating as the crowd eats, exercising if and when the crowd exercises. These adolescents apparently perceive their peers to be voracious consumers of junk food.

We noted that intentions do not necessarily translate into behavior. That is, behavior change depends on having an intention to act, but intention alone is not sufficient to determine whether an action occurs. Even if children intend to brush their teeth regularly, parents may still need to monitor their compliance with oral hygiene practices. An Australian study of oral hygiene in children focused on the role of parents not only as conveyors of information ("Darius, you need to brush your teeth so that you don't get cavities") but also as monitors of their children's tooth-brushing behaviors (Hamilton et al., 2018). Applying the TPB, the investigators found that predicting parental monitoring of children's tooth brushing improved when they considered factors such as parental intentions ("I intend to make sure my children brush their teeth"), self-efficacy ("I'm confident I can get them to brush their teeth"), and planning ("I established a regular schedule for brushing their teeth"). Predicting health-related behaviors apparently depends on a combination of factors, as the TPB model teaches.

A review of research evidence supports the value of perceived behavior control (PBC) in determining whether intentions to perform healthier behaviors are actually carried out (Hagger et al., 2022). This suggests that the degree to which you believe in your ability to perform a certain healthy behavior (self-efficacy) and expect that performing the behavior is under your control (controllability) influences whether your healthful intentions will translate into healthier actions.

The role of prescriptive norms was featured in a study of handwashing among university students in the United Kingdom. Prescriptive handwashing norms (beliefs about how often peers washed their hands) were associated with students' own handwashing (Dickie et al., 2018). If you want people to wash their hands more frequently, induce their friends to wash up.

Researchers also find that perceptions of peer norms may be linked to healthy as well as unhealthy behaviors (Rice & Klein, 2019). In this study involving 1,859 adolescents of 12–17 years of age, the individuals who perceived their peers as eating more fruits and vegetables and as being more physically active were more physically active themselves and ate more fruits and vegetables. However, those perceiving their friends as not exercising regularly and as frequent consumers of junk food and sugary drinks showed similar unhealthy behaviors.

Review 2.4

INTERACTIVE SELF-SCORING QUIZZES

Sentence Completion

1. The Theory of Reasoned Action (TRA) emphasizes the importance of __________ to act.
2. The TRA emphasizes the roles of two factors, (1) the person's __________ toward the behavior and (2) the person's __________ of subjective norms.
3. Subjective norms fall into two subtypes, __________ norms (what you believe other people expect you to do) and __________ norms (what you believe other people actually do).
4. Perceived behavioral control has two components, self-efficacy and __________.
5. The Theory of Planned Behavior expanded the TRA to include the factor of perceived __________ over behavior.
6. Perceptions of control are shaped by past __________.
7. In a tooth-brushing study, the strongest predictor of intentions was __________, a facet of perceived control.
8. The role of __________ norms was featured in a recent study of handwashing behavior among university students in the United Kingdom.
9. In a recent study, teens who perceived their peers as eating more fruits and vegetables ate (more or less) fruits and vegetables.

Think About It

How do your attitudes, perceptions of social norms, and perceived control affect a health-related behavior you would like to change? How might an attitude adjustment help you move toward putting that change into practice?

The Transtheoretical Model

Transtheoretical Model (TTM) A conceptual framework for understanding the stages and processes involved in behavior change.

The **Transtheoretical Model (TTM)** views behavioral change as a process that unfolds in discrete stages. The model is transtheoretical in that it integrates and synthesizes elements of different theoretical models including the HBM, social cognitive theory, and the Theory of Planned Behavior.

The TTM adopts the view that change is an ongoing process rather than fixed at a point in time. It challenges professionals to meet the client "where the client is" with respect to readiness to change, rather than assuming that everyone is equally likely to benefit from a health behavior program such as an exercise or weight loss program (Gehlert & Ward, 2019). The model posits that behavior change occurs through six definable stages of change.

The Precontemplation Stage

People in the **precontemplation stage** are not intending to change their behavior in the near future (typically a 6-month period), nor are they thinking about making changes. People at this stage may be unaware of the consequences of their unhealthy behaviors such as smoking, excessive alcohol consumption, physical inactivity, or a high-fat diet. Or perhaps they tried unsuccessfully to make healthy changes in the past and now feel frustrated or demoralized about trying new behaviors. They may avoid reading or thinking about health-related behaviors or try to not think about their risky behaviors.

precontemplation stage The first stage in the TTM in which people are not thinking about, or intending to make, a behavior change in the near future.

The Contemplation Stage

In the **contemplation stage**, people are intending to make behavioral changes within the next 6 months. They have not yet begun change, but they are starting to think seriously about it. They may be weighing the pros and cons of making a change but can get stuck for months as they vacillate about whether they are ready to change. As long as they remain ambivalent about following through on a course of action, they are not ready for programs that require immediate actions, such as weight loss or smoking cessation programs.

contemplation stage The second stage in the TTM in which people are planning to make a behavior change within the next 6 months and have begun to take steps in that direction.

The Preparation Stage

People in the **preparation stage** plan to take action in the near term, typically within a month. They develop a plan of action and have taken steps to put the behavioral change into effect, perhaps speaking to their physician about it or researching weight loss programs in their community. People at this stage are ready and willing to get started and would likely benefit from participating in an action-oriented program. Self-efficacy—the belief a person holds about their ability to successfully carry out a planned course of action—is an important factor in change, especially during the preparation stage.

preparation stage The third stage in the TTM in which people are actively preparing to take action in the near future, typically within the next month.

The Action Stage

In the **action stage**, people have begun making changes in their behavior within the past 6 months. They may have started a weight loss program or been going to the gym several times a week. The question now becomes whether they will persevere.

action stage The fourth stage in the TTM in which people have begun making changes within the past 6 months.

The Maintenance Stage

The **maintenance stage** describes the period of time when changes in behavior are becoming solidly integrated within the person's lifestyle. This stage may stretch from 6 months to about 5 years. In this stage, people become increasingly more confident that their healthy behaviors will last but are aware that they need to make efforts to prevent relapse, such as by varying their gym schedule or weight loss efforts to keep themselves motivated and engaged. Even so, relapses may occur if the person resumes unhealthy patterns of behavior, such as by starting to smoke again after quitting or dropping out of an exercise program. Achieving long-term changes requires readiness to reinstate change efforts after a relapse, perhaps by seeking support from others to help them get back on track.

maintenance stage The fifth stage in the TTM in which changes in behavior are becoming solidly integrated within the person's lifestyle.

The Termination Stage

People reach the **termination stage** when they have complete confidence (high self-efficacy) in maintaining the behavior change and zero temptation to relapse. Now they are certain the changes they have made—quitting smoking, exercising regularly, taking antihypertensive medication daily, following a healthier diet—are a fixture of their daily routine. It's as if the new habits have become automatic and people don't need to work on their new habits for them to stick.

termination stage The sixth and final stage in the TTM in which behavior changes have fully integrated as a permanent feature of a person's lifestyle.

Processes of Change

Processes of change involve the means people use to move through the stages of change. These processes are associated with particular stages.

- *Consciousness raising* may take the form of a healthcare professional sharing information about a health concern, as in a physician raising people's awareness of the risks posed by their elevated blood pressure. This process is most helpful during the precontemplation change.
- *Self-reevaluation* involves taking stock of oneself and realizing that making healthy changes in behavior is part of who and what one wants to become. Self-reevaluation is critical during the stages of contemplation and preparation when a person seriously contemplates change.
- *Healthy relationships* involve efforts to find supportive relationships to help the person make healthy changes, as in the action stage where a person might seek a support group or join a group exercise or weight loss program.
- *Counterconditioning* is a process targeted to the action stage in which the person substitutes healthy forms of behavior for unhealthy behaviors, as in substituting mints or sunflower seeds for cigarettes when a craving for tobacco occurs.
- *Stimulus control* is another action stage process by which the person redesigns the environment to link cues with healthier behaviors and eliminate cues associated with undesirable behavior. For example, a smoker attempting to quit may remove all smoking paraphernalia from the home, including lighters and ashtrays; the person might also spend more time in nonsmoking environments, where the stimuli are healthy rather than unhealthy.
- *Contingency management* brings to bear principles of reinforcement to strengthen healthy behaviors during the action stage, as in rewarding oneself for meeting exercise or weight management goals.

Applications of the TTM

The TTM is a leading model for guiding the development of health behavior programs. It has been successfully applied across a wide range of health behaviors including smoking cessation (Robinson & Vail, 2012), self-care in people with heart disease (Paradis et al., 2010), substance abuse interventions (Velasquez et al., 2005), and weight loss and exercise programs (Han et al., 2017). A recent scientific review found that applying the TTM model improved medication adherence in chronically ill patients who had struggled to take their medications regularly (Imeri et al., 2022).

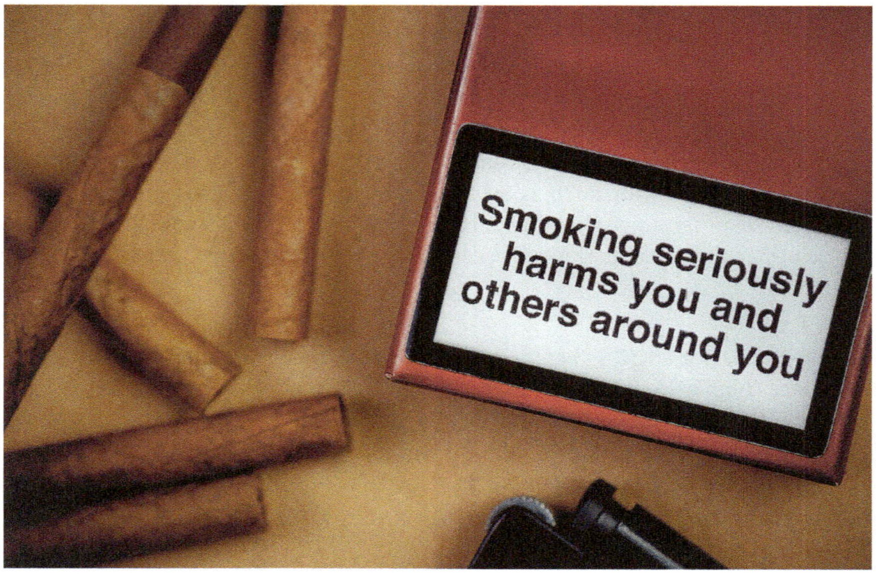

Igor Stevanovic/Alamy Stock Photo

Raising Public Awareness At which stage of the transtheoretical model is raising awareness of a health issue the most critical need?

A central theme of the TTM is that an intervention should match the person's stage of change (Weinberg, 2018). For people in the contemplation stage, for example, an intervention might focus on building motivation to change rather than on how to use specific change strategies or techniques. Similarly, precontemplators would likely benefit more from a health message that seeks to raise their awareness (consciousness raising) about the need to make a change, whether it is about undergoing a colonoscopy, quitting smoking, managing high blood pressure, or reducing intake of high fat and high cholesterol foods. Those in the preparation stage might engage in more active behavior, such as taking steps to enroll in a smoking cessation program.

The major unsettled issue with the TTM is whether matching individuals to interventions based on their current stage of change is more effective than nonmatched health promotion programs that recruit participants irrespective of their current stage of change. Although the staged or matched approach has broad appeal within the health research community, evidence about its effectiveness remains mixed, as some studies show that designing interventions targeted to people at particular stages works better while other studies fail to show a significant benefit of stage-based matching (Gehlert & Ward, 2019; Weinberg, 2018).

Applying Health Psychology

Using the TTM to Change Health Behavior

The TTM posits that making lasting changes in behavior does not happen all at once but progresses through a process that occurs in stages. Old habits, as the familiar expression goes, die hard. To get started making healthier behavior changes, we need to take stock of our current stage of change and then progress to the point at which healthy changes become a permanent fixture in our lives.

Assume that you are thinking about making a change in your health habits, having already progressed from precontemplation to contemplation. Here is a rundown of some processes of change you can begin to work through to make healthy habits a way of life (adapted from NIDDK, 2019):

Contemplation: "I'm Thinking About It"

In thinking about making healthier changes, it may be useful to lay out the pros and cons. Consider how much better your life would be if you made healthy changes in your behavior, such as losing excess weight, quitting smoking, or starting a regular exercise program. Consider the barriers you may face, such as coping with withdrawal symptoms from quitting smoking or the cost or inconvenience of starting an exercise program. None of the cons may be a deal breaker, but it is useful to think them through so that you are prepared for them.

Preparation: "I Have Made Up My Mind to Take Action"

You enter the preparation stage when you decide to make changes and are about to get started. Prep work maximizes your chances of success. Identify potential roadblocks and how you plan to overcome them. Table 2.2 provides common roadblocks (barriers or "cons" you have identified) and possible solutions. Consider these as you construct your plan.

The key steps in preparation are making a plan and setting goals. Do you want to increase your physical activity level? Start with small changes and make a realistic and attainable plan. For example, you might begin with a goal of a vigorous walk in your neighborhood or local park two or three times a week for 30 minutes each time. Plan your walks to fit into your schedule and post them to your calendar, treating them like any other important event. Think through any obstacles you might face, such as inclement weather

TABLE 2.2 Preparing to Take Action: Identifying Roadblocks, Finding Solutions

Roadblock	Possible Solutions
I don't have time	Make your new healthy habit a priority. Fit in physical activity whenever and wherever you can. Try taking the stairs or getting off the bus a stop early. Set aside one grocery shopping day a week and make healthy meals that you can freeze and eat later when you don't have time to cook.
Healthy habits cost too much	You can walk around the mall, a school track, or a local park for free. Eat properly on a budget by buying in bulk and when items are on sale.
I can't make this change alone	Recruit others to join you. Consider signing up for a fun fitness class like salsa dancing. Get your family or coworkers on the healthy eating bandwagon. Plan healthy meals with your family or start a healthy potluck dinner once a week at work.
I don't like physical activity	Forget the old notion that being physically active means lifting weights in a gym. You can be active in many ways, including dancing, walking, or gardening. Make your own list of appealing physical activities. Explore options you may never have considered and stick with those that you enjoy.
I don't like healthy foods	Try making your old favorite recipes in new, healthier ways. Trim visible fat from meats and reduce the amount of butter, sugar, and salt you use in your cooking. Use low-fat cheeses or milk rather than whole milk. Add a cup or two of broccoli, carrots, or spinach to casseroles or pasta.

and unexpected events. In the event of inclement weather, plan to substitute a stay-at-home exercise routine or find an indoor space, such as a local mall, to serve as your track. Have alternative times available in case other scheduling demands bump you from your usual exercise time.

Action: "I Have Started to Make Changes"

When you begin making changes, evaluate your progress. Are you meeting your goals, or are obstacles impeding your progress? Treat setbacks as challenges to be met, not as failures. Figure out how to overcome obstacles to get yourself back on track and reward yourself with a pat on the back or a small gift for making healthy changes. Track your progress on a regular basis, as by keeping weekly records of your physical activity. Jot down not only what you did but how you felt when you were doing it. Negative emotional states can get in the way of following through with behavior plans, so become mindful of your emotions and take steps to keep on course. For example, if you are bored while exercising, try listening to music or podcasts to divert your attention, but avoid activities that may become dangerously distracting, such as talking on the phone while crossing an intersection.

Maintenance: "I Have a New Routine"

Congratulate yourself for making a healthy behavior change a part of your new lifestyle, but recognize that adopting a healthier lifestyle involves a lifelong commitment. Add variety to your routine so you don't feel that you are in a rut. Modify your exercise program. Join a gym. Take an exercise class. Explore different locations for walking, biking, or running. Seek exercise buddies to help you maintain your commitment. The more varied your routine, the more likely it will remain part of your lifestyle. Build upon your success by expanding your goals in small steps. If you've cut back on saturated fat in your diet, as by avoiding greasy foods, begin limiting your intake of added sugars. Transition from a 20-minute exercise routine to a 30- or 40-minute program. But don't overdo, as the more you tax your body, the greater the risk of muscle strains and overtraining injuries. Know your limits and consult with your healthcare provider if you have questions about the type of exercise routine that is best suited to your needs.

Figure 2.5 provides a schematic representation of applying the TTM.

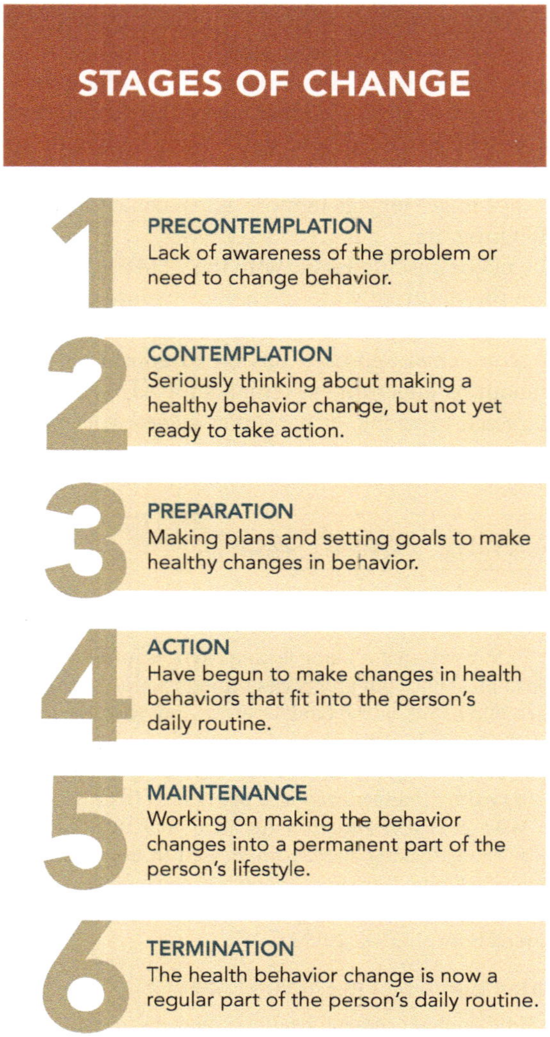

FIGURE 2.5 Stages of Change

Review 2.5

INTERACTIVE SELF-SCORING QUIZZES

Sentence Completion

1. The transtheoretical model (TTM) views changes in behavior as a process that unfolds in discrete __________.

2. People in the __________ stage do not intend to make any significant changes in their behavior in the near future.

3. People in the __________ stage intend to make changes in their health-related behavior in the next 6 months.

4. People in the __________ stage plan to take action in the near term, typically within the next month.

5. In the __________ stage, people have begun making changes in their health behavior within the past 6 months.

6. The __________ stage describes a time when changes in behavior are becoming solidly integrated in the person's lifestyle.

7. People reaching the __________ stage are certain they can stick with the behavior change.

8. Self-__________ is a process of appraising oneself and realizing that making healthy changes in behavior is part of who one wants to become.

9. A central theme of the TTM model is that an intervention should match the person's __________ of change.

Think About It

Are you thinking about making a change in health behavior, perhaps starting an exercise program, quitting smoking or vaping, losing excess weight, or establishing a regular sleep–wake schedule? What stage of change best describes your current status? What can you do to move through the stages of change?

Recite: An Active Summary

INTERACTIVE SELF-SCORING QUIZZES

Chapter 2 Practice Quiz

1. Describe factors involved in changing health behaviors.

Factors involved in changing health behaviors include predisposing factors, enabling factors, and reinforcing factors. Predisposing factors include beliefs, attitudes, knowledge, expectancies, and values that either promote or hinder healthy changes in behavior. Enabling factors include skills or abilities, physical and mental capabilities, and the availability and accessibility of resources that make it possible to change and sustain health-related behaviors. Reinforcing factors include praise and support that strengthen and maintain health-related behavior.

2. Describe the major factors involved in adherence to medication.

Patient-related factors include forgetfulness about taking medications, negative expectations or beliefs about medication, and difficulties understanding medication labels. Treatment-related factors include complex dosing regimens and use of multiple medications. Factors related to the healthcare system include high copays, restricted formularies, and lack of access to healthcare services or providers. Perceived stigma also affects adherence to treatment.

3. Describe the Health Belief Model (HBM) of behavior change.

The Health Belief Model focuses on the role of people's perceptions in determining health-related behavior change with respect to (1) perceived threat to oneself of the illness or disease and (2) perceived benefits and costs of making behavior changes. Perceptions of threat break down into perceptions of susceptibility to the disease and perceptions of the severity of the disease in terms of seriousness of the symptoms or the health threat it poses.

4. Describe the role of social cognitive theory in explaining health-related behavior.

Social cognitive theory posits roles for cognitive factors and observational learning in accounting for health-related behavior. Among the major concepts are reciprocal determinism, behavioral competencies, outcome expectations, self-efficacy, modeling or observational learning, and reinforcement.

5. Describe how the Theory of Reasoned Action, the Theory of Planned Behavior, and the Transtheoretical Model help us understand health behavior change.

The Theory of Reasoned Action (TRA) posits two major factors that underlie intentions to engage in behaviors involving health: (1) attitudes toward the behavior and (2) perceptions of subjective norms. The Theory of Planned Behavior (TPB) expanded the TRA to include perceived control over behavior. The Transtheoretical Model conceptualizes behavior change as progressing through a series of six stages: precontemplation, contemplation, preparation, action, maintenance, and termination stages. Processes of change are the means by which change happens.

Answers to Review Sections

2.1

1. Predisposing
2. enabling
3. Reinforcing
4. Patient
5. Treatment
6. Healthcare

2.2

1. health beliefs
2. threat/benefits/costs
3. susceptibility
4. severity
5. barriers
6. Positive
7. better

2.3

1. learning
2. values
3. situational
4. determinism
5. Outcome
6. efficacy
7. more

2.4

1. intentions
2. attitudes/perception
3. injunctive/prescriptive
4. controllability
5. control
6. experiences
7. self-efficacy
8. prescriptive
9. more

2.5

1. stages
2. precontemplation
3. contemplation
4. preparation
5. action
6. maintenance
7. termination
8. reevaluation
9. stage

Sample Clinician Responses to Patients' Responses

You may have arrived at excellent answers that differ from the ones offered in the following table. These are intended to be sample answers, not "right answers."

Suggested Clinician Responses
"What does your doctor say about the importance of doing this? Do you believe the doctor? Does your doctor have any reason to be dishonest with you?"
"It's great that you feel good, and this isn't about making you worry. I think the idea is that your doctor feels you won't continue to feel this good if you don't begin the regimen now. Do you see any benefits to doing this?"
"It's good to be healthy. Many healthy people have medical issues to deal with and take maintenance medications to stay healthy. Does taking medication, changing your diet, etc., mean you are sick?"
"Sometimes people do that, but by the time they decide to take action, the disease has progressed, so it is usually better to start now before it gets bad."
"Avoiding unnecessary medication is always a good idea, but it sounds like there are times when medications are necessary. When in the past have you taken medication; under what conditions would you consider doing so again? Does this situation meet those conditions?"
"What do you know about this medication? What side effects are expected—their frequency of occurrence? Severity? You need to weigh the possible side effects against the potential benefits."
"It is true that some people don't have treatment and seem OK, and back then we didn't have the options for treatment that we have now anyway. There was lots of data, though, that most people do better if they take the medication. I wonder if your uncle was just one of the lucky ones?"
"Why not? Why wouldn't you make some changes to keep yourself as healthy as possible? What would you say to your wife if she said she didn't feel like taking her medication?"
"Let's talk about ways to make this easier."

Source: Labbott (2018). Reprinted with permission of the American Psychological Association.

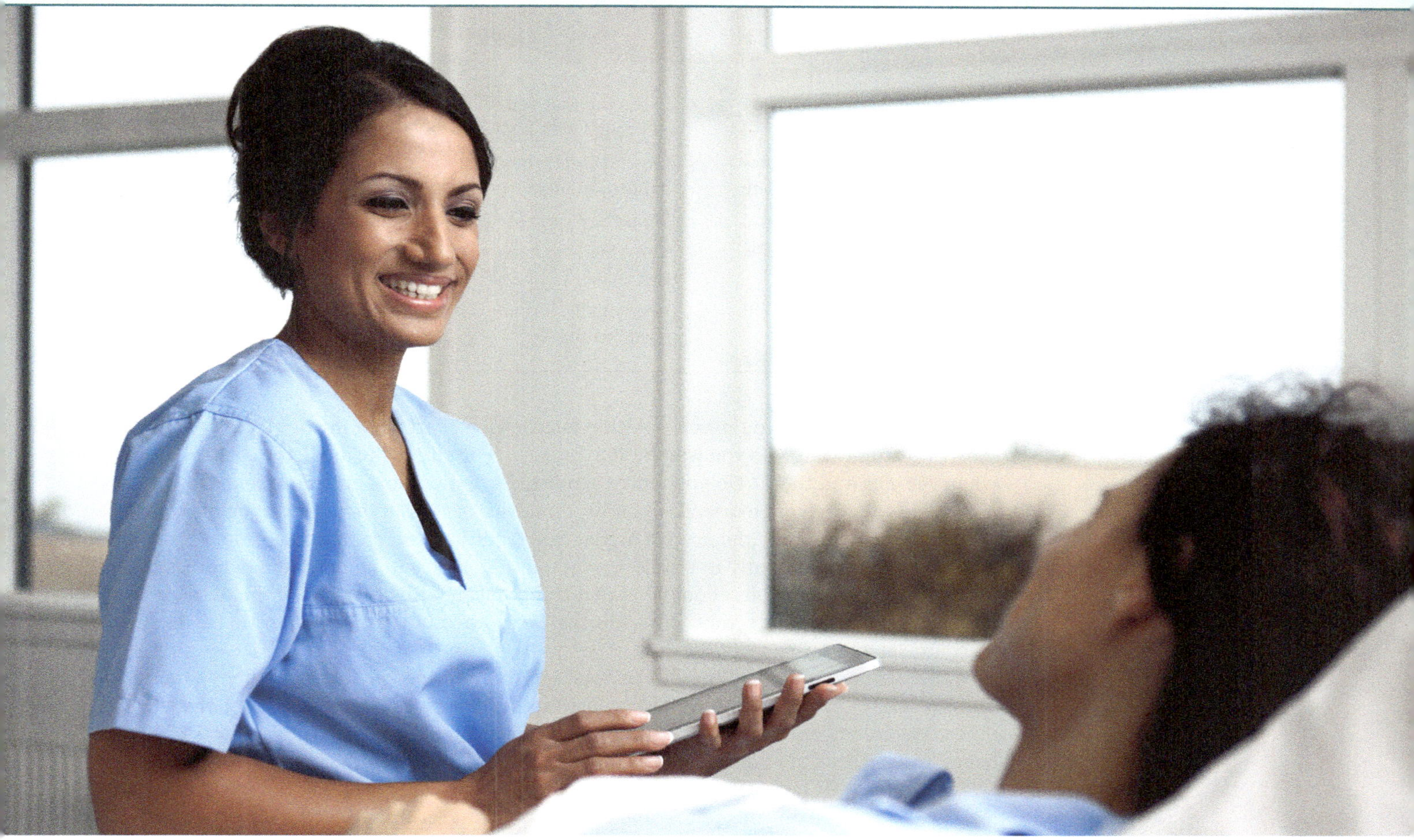

Cultura RM/Alamy Stock Photo

The Healthcare System

LEARNING OBJECTIVES

After studying this chapter, you will be able to …

1. **Define** the concept of illness behavior and identify some of the determinants of health-seeking behavior.
2. **Apply** the common-sense model of self-regulation to understand how people respond to physical illness.
3. **Describe** health disparities in relation to income level and race/ethnicity.
4. **Identify** and **describe** the major types of health insurance plans.
5. **Identify** and **describe** various methods of complementary and alternative medicine.

Did You Know That ...

- People with asthma who believe in their ability to control their symptoms show better control of asthma?
- The number of uninsured persons in the United States has dropped by about 40% since the passage of the Affordable Care Act (ACA)?
- People may commit microaggressions against other people even when they are unaware they are doing so?
- The neighborhood in which you live can be hazardous to your health?
- Expecting that you will be belittled because of your weight is associated with higher levels of the stress hormone cortisol?
- General Motors has been called a healthcare company that also happens to make cars?
- Managed care is perhaps better described as managed costs?
- The American healthcare system isn't really an organized system at all?
- Nearly half of Americans aged 40 and above report praying for good health?

What do you do when you have a splitting headache, a sharp pain in your side, or a burning sensation after eating? Do you wait for it to pass? Do you run to the medicine cabinet and take whatever you find there? Do you worry about the symptom and what it might mean? How much? Do you reach out to friends or family for advice or reassurance? Or do you immediately call the doctor or head to the nearest urgent care facility or emergency department?

People react differently to physical symptoms. Some try to ignore them, whereas others become worried or anxious about what they might mean. Still others go online to track down information about their symptoms—and they may encounter information that is rife with inaccuracies and misconceptions.

This chapter is about "illness behaviors"—the actions people take when they experience physical symptoms. Working from a biopsychosocial perspective, health psychologists and other researchers examine the biological, psychological, and sociocultural aspects of illness behaviors and seek to understand why and when people seek health care.

Consider your own use of the healthcare system. Do you list your doctor or local health facility as a favorite on your phone and reach out whenever a physical symptom appears? Or do you wait weeks or months before seeking assistance despite persistent symptoms?

Speaking of the "healthcare system," is it really a *system* at all? Actually, the U.S. healthcare system is not so much an organized network of healthcare providers as a patchwork of healthcare services that is often difficult to navigate—not just for the average healthcare consumer but also for healthcare professionals. People are often confused about their healthcare options, and understandably so, as even legislators in Congress don't seem to know the intricacies of the policies the government has enacted. The acronyms alone cause confusion, as when trying to decipher between a preferred provider organization (PPO), a point-of-service (POS) plan, or a health maintenance organization (HMO), or figuring out how Part D of Medicare works.

At the outset we need to recognize that the responsibility for managing our own healthcare needs does not lie with healthcare providers, government programs, or insurance carriers. It is our individual responsibility to become active, informed healthcare consumers to manage our own health care. To that end, we need to educate ourselves about different types of healthcare services that may be available to us, choose our healthcare providers (HCPs) carefully, and weigh treatment alternatives.

Health psychologists help people navigate a patchwork quilt of healthcare services. They assist people in becoming better-informed consumers of healthcare services and help them adopt a more active role in managing their own healthcare needs.

Illness Behavior

illness behavior A pattern of behavior in response to acute or chronic illness.

The term **illness behavior** refers to the ways in which people respond to symptoms and illness. It includes the experience of being ill as well as healthcare-seeking behavior.

Illness behavior begins with perception of a change in physical or mental functioning that the person interprets as a threat to health (Leventhal et al., 2015). Illness behavior has a protective function, in that it includes efforts aimed at restoring and maintaining health.

The concept of illness behavior was introduced by sociologists David Mechanic and Edmund Volkart (1960), who defined it in terms of the ways in which different people perceive, evaluate, and act upon (or do not act upon) the emergence of physical symptoms.

Illness behavior is influenced by psychological, social, and cultural factors as well as the symptoms. Note that we use the term "illness behavior" rather than "disease behavior." Although the terms "illness" and "disease" are often used interchangeably, they have different meanings and implications. We say we "feel ill" but that we "have a disease." This usage reflects our understanding that a disease is an affliction, but "illness" reflects the experience of being ill and the meanings we attribute to our condition. People may have a significant physical disease (such as heart disease) but not feel ill. Therefore, they may not attend to the disease until it progresses to a point at which it threatens their survival. Our focus is on the psychological experience of illness and how we cope with it.

Healthcare-Seeking Behavior

What determines when people see a doctor or other healthcare professional? Health psychologists recognize that our use of healthcare services depends on many factors, including our gender, age, type of illness, access to services, insurance coverage (or lack thereof), and ability to afford services even if we are insured (yes, deductibles and copayments often present barriers to accessing healthcare services). Some people immediately seek medical help when they experience troublesome symptoms, such as chest pain, whereas others may wait even in the case of a life-threatening disease for which prompt medical attention may spell the difference between life and death (Sirri et al., 2013).

Healthcare-seeking behavior concerns the ways in which we seek help when we are ill. People seek not only traditional healthcare services, such as medical services, but also informal channels, such as the internet; laypersons such as friends, family members, and colleagues; homespun or traditional remedies; or complementary and alternative medicine.

Consider a simple question: How do you know if you are ill? For many people, the answer starts with a symptom. A **symptom** is an alteration in our typical or normal physical or psychological functioning. Pain is a symptom. Loss of movement in a limb is another. Feelings of depression or anxiety are also symptoms—psychological symptoms. But some medical conditions and diseases, such as hypertension, may have no noticeable symptoms. The concept of illness behavior applies only when we experience ourselves as being ill—attributing a change in physical functioning to a symptom of an underlying disease or health condition.

symptom A physical or psychological feature that is regarded as indicating a condition of disease, particularly a feature that is apparent to the individual with the disease.

Health psychologists are concerned not only with how individuals respond to illness but also with the larger social context that determines accessibility and affordability of health care. Socioeconomic class is a major determinant of healthcare utilization and health outcomes. There are major disparities in health indices; people at lower socioeconomic levels tend to have poorer health outcomes (greater risks of chronic disease and increased mortality) and poorer access to healthcare services.

Styles of Coping with Illness

A serious illness is a stressful life event to which people tend to respond in different ways. When we try to understand the different ways in which people respond to illness, we must recognize that people have different styles of coping with stress demands and challenges. Some people face the challenge of illness head-on, while others avoid dealing with it or deny that they are ill.

Active Versus Passive Coping

Some people take an active role in coping with stressful life events, including physical illness. They actively engage in learning more about their illness, consulting health professionals, seeking help from others, and following a prescribed course of treatment. Others adopt a passive approach characterized by

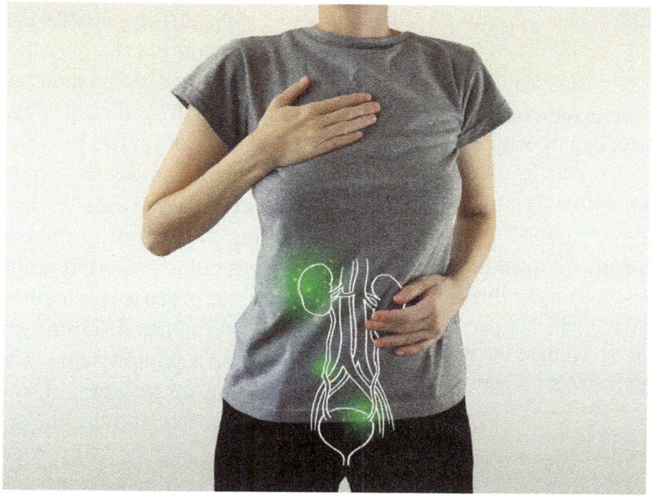

mi_viri/Alamy Stock Photo

A Simple Question How do you know when you are ill?

disengagement or withdrawal from the health threat, as by denying or ignoring it, by leaving it up to some external source of control such as the will of God, or by relying on others to manage their health needs. Active and passive coping represent *approach* and *avoidance* dimensions of coping, respectively (Choi et al., 2012).

Active coping is generally a more adaptive form of adjustment in which people seek information and engage in problem solving to deal directly with a health challenge. By contrast, passive coping involves avoidance of a stressor that typically results in maladaptive or ineffective ways of handling a health threat, such as ignoring it, refusing to consult a health professional, or avoiding diagnostic tests. Ignoring a serious health threat can lead to unfortunate, even life-threatening consequences. Avoidance is a form of denial in which people decide to act as if the threat doesn't exist, feel there is no need to change their behavior, or feel that the situation is so hopeless that changing their behavior is pointless (Sahler & Carr, 2009). Passive or avoidant coping can also take the form of defensive behaviors that can make matters worse, such as resorting to alcohol or drugs to blunt emotional reactions to a health problem.

Active coping is generally associated with better health outcomes; people who engage in active coping are likely to avail themselves of support, assistance, and appropriate medical care. People who use active coping adjust better to the challenges of living with a chronic disease or health condition (Helgeson & Zajdel, 2017). A study of 80 survivors of breast cancer found that those who used more active coping strategies were less emotionally distressed and had lower levels of stress hormones than did passive copers (Perez-Tejada et al., 2019).

A study in China focused on the role of active versus passive coping in determining quality of life of frontline healthcare workers (HCWs) during the COVID-19 pandemic (Li et al., 2021). Active coping was associated with higher quality of life whereas passive coping was linked to lower quality of life. The investigators point to a need to develop psychological interventions to improve the resilience and coping style of HCWs.

Problem-Focused Versus Emotion-Focused Coping Psychologists Richard Lazarus and Susan Folkman's (1984) theory of stress and coping incorporates a cognitive dimension to help us better understand how people cope with stressful life events, including physical illness (Folkman & Lazarus, 1985; Lazarus, 1999). The cognitive dimension involves appraising, or making judgments about, the threat posed by a stressor, such as a physical symptom. The theory proposes primary and secondary appraisal processes:

1. In *primary appraisal*, we evaluate the degree to which a stressful threat poses a risk to our health and well-being. Believing a symptom like stomach pain is a sign of indigestion leads to an appraisal of a less serious threat than attributing the symptoms to a more serious cause, such as ulcers or cancer.
2. In *secondary appraisal*, we evaluate what can be done to address the threat while taking into account the resources and coping strategies we have available or can readily access. People ask themselves, "What can I do about it? ... What options are available to me? ... Will they work? ... Will I be able to follow through?"

Appraising a stressor as threatening or harmful produces negative emotions, such as fear, which prompts the person to use coping responses either to directly address the stressor or to manage the distress associated with the stressor (Biggs et al., 2017). These two types of coping responses are called **problem-focused coping** and **emotion-focused coping**. In problem-focused coping, the person attempts to remove the stressor, whereas in emotion-focused coping, the person seeks to regulate their emotional responses to the stressor, as in trying to lessen anxiety or emotional distress associated with a health threat. (Examples of problem-focused coping and emotion-focused coping are shown in Table 3.1.) Afterward, the person weighs the outcomes of coping efforts, along with any new information that may change the situation; the process is one of *reappraisal*, which can lead to relief if coping efforts are succeeding or to trying out different strategies if the initial attempts proved unsuccessful.

problem-focused coping A style of coping with stressful life events in which a person takes steps to directly confront the stressor to reduce or remove it.

emotion-focused coping A style of coping with stressful life events in which a person takes steps to regulate the emotional response to a stressor.

For a person with stomach pains, for example, problem-focused coping might involve reaching for an antacid or calling for an appointment with a general physician or specialist. Emotion-focused coping may involve practicing a relaxation exercise or distracting oneself from the problem in order to lessen states of emotional arousal. Some forms of emotion-focused coping overlap with passive coping, as in denying or ignoring a threat to relieve anxiety. Other emotion-focused coping strategies involve more active coping strategies, as in practicing meditation or relaxation.

TABLE 3.1 Examples of Problem-Focused and Emotion-Focused Coping Strategies

INTERACTIVE FIGURES, CHARTS, & TABLES

Problem-Focused Coping Strategies	Emotion-Focused Coping Strategies
• Obtaining information about the medical condition or health threat • Seeking a consultation with a health professional • Making healthy changes in behavior • Talking to other people who have experienced similar health problems • Using prescription or over-the-counter medication to treat the problem	• Using distraction techniques to get your mind off of the problem, such as engaging in hobbies, watching videos or TV, or exercising • Calming oneself through relaxation, meditation, or prayer • Expressing feelings in a journal • Using alcohol or other drugs to blunt emotional responses, or using medication to relieve anxiety or depression • Using denial to avoid thinking about the problem

Emotion-focused coping may have benefits on health outcomes as well. For example, psychologist James Pennebaker (2018) finds that writing about traumatic experiences in a journal can improve the physical and emotional health of people who survive trauma. Meditation and relaxation can help relieve stress and lead to more healthful outcomes, as we explore further in Chapter 5. Though emotion-focused coping may yield a short-term benefit in relieving emotional discomfort, it can lead to negative outcomes when people rely on this form of coping for a prolonged period of time rather than taking a more direct, problem-solving approach to a health challenge.

The person's appraisal of a health threat is affected by factors other than the illness itself, such as their financial situation (Labbott, 2018). People who lack the financial resources to handle the healthcare needs that may arise may have more negative appraisals of serious illness or health concerns than people.

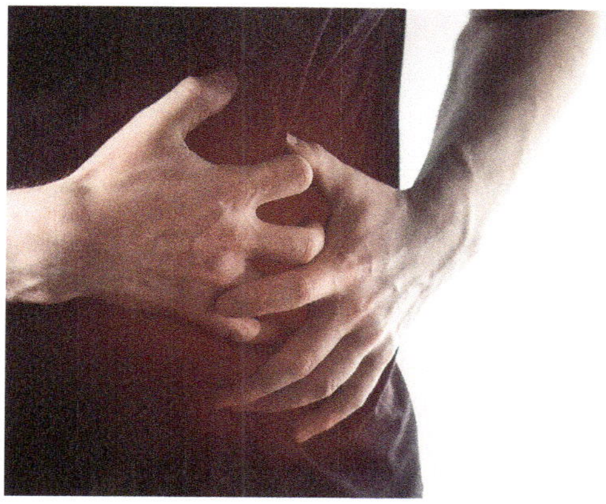

Sjstudio6/Shutterstock.com

Coping with Health Threats How do you cope with physical symptoms that may pose threats to your health? Do you ignore them and hope they disappear on their own? Do you reach out to others or to healthcare professionals? What psychological models help explain how people respond to health threats?

The Common-Sense Model of Self-Regulation

Another model designed to help us understand how people respond to threats to health and well-being is the **Common-Sense Model (CSM) of self-regulation**, developed by health psychologist Howard Leventhal and his colleagues (Benyamini & Leventhal, 2019; Diefenbach & Leventhal, 1996; Leventhal et al., 2016). The crux of the model is *self-regulation*, the process by which individuals manage their behaviors, emotions, and thoughts in pursuing their life goals and reacting to life events, including how they deal with the threat of physical illness. The model posits that people react to illness by forming two types of representations, cognitive representations and emotional representations. **Figure 3.1** shows how the model works.

Common-Sense Model (CSM) of self-regulation An understanding of how people react to threats to health and well-being by forming cognitive and emotional representations of illness that determine their coping behaviors and healthcare-seeking behaviors.

The model adopts a common-sense view of how people respond to illness in terms of how they make sense of a health threat (cognitive representations) and how they react to it (emotional representations). These representations determine how they cope and whether they seek healthcare services. The CSM breaks down the response to illness into two separate but interlinking processes (Hagger & Orbell, 2022).

- *Cognitive representations* are ways in which people think about their illness in relation to the following:
  - *Identity* (What is it?)
  - *Perceived cause or causes* (What caused it?)
  - *Degree of threat it poses* (How serious a threat is this?)
  - *Duration* (How long is this going to last and what course will it follow?)
  - *Impact on daily life* (How is this going to affect my life ... my relationships ... my job ... my finances?)
  - *Control* (Can it be cured or minimized? What can I or medical care providers do to control the illness or mitigate its consequences?)

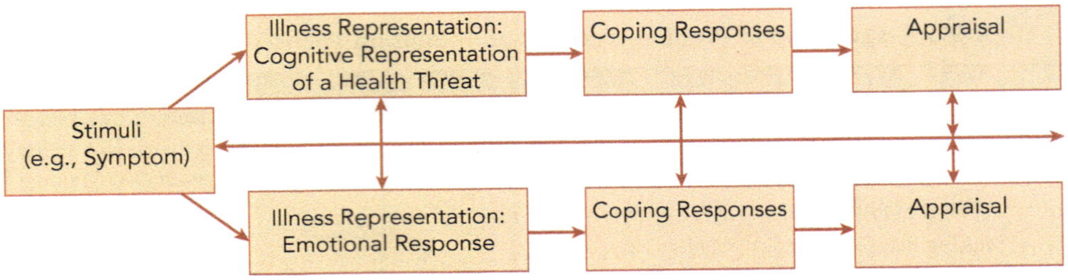

FIGURE 3.1 Main Elements of Common-Sense Model of Self-Regulation The CSM breaks down the process of responding to physical health threats into a cognitive track involving how people think about their illness and an emotional track involving how they emotionally respond to it.

Source: Adapted from Diefenbach and Leventhal (1996).

- *Emotional representations* of (or reactions to) illness run the gamut of negative emotions from fear (e.g., of dying or of long-term disability) to anger (at oneself for not taking better care of one's health or toward the medical establishment for failing to prevent the disease or not picking it up at an earlier and more treatable stage) to depression (which may be characterized by feelings of hopelessness and helplessness).

Applying the CSM, health researchers identified three types of illness representations that rely on the ability to adjust to a chronic illness: (1) *illness consequences*; (2) *illness identity*; and (3) *illness controllability* (Hagger & Orbell 2003; Helgeson & Zajdel, 2017). Individuals adjust more poorly to illness when they perceive more negative consequences ("I'm likely to die"), when they identify themselves more closely with the illness ("I am a cancer patient"), and when they perceive a lack of control over the illness ("There's little I can do about it"). Conversely, people who expect more positive outcomes ("I'll beat this"), who disconnect their identity from their illness ("Cancer is something I'm dealing with, but it does not define me or my life"), and who perceive more control over the illness ("I can handle this") tend to show better psychological and physical adjustment to chronic illness.

The CSM posits an interaction between cognitive and emotional processes. Consider a person who experiences chest pains. The person may form a cognitive representation that chest pain is a symptom of a serious underlying condition (heart disease), but one that can be controlled through changes in lifestyle (weight loss, regular exercise, etc.) and appropriate medical treatment (drugs or surgery). These cognitive representations might lead the person to engage in active coping responses, such as making healthful changes in behavior and obtaining appropriate medical care. These coping responses, in turn, may reduce emotional reactions such as the anxiety and fear that may attend the symptoms. Emotional reactions to illness can also lead to effective coping responses that involve healthful behavior changes, such as using relaxation or meditation to control anxiety or seeking the assistance of a therapist to correct worrisome or catastrophizing thoughts and beliefs.

The results of coping responses are evaluated time and again, leading to changes in cognitions (e.g., "Things are getting better" or "This doesn't seem to be working") and in emotional responses (either increased or decreased negative emotions). Changes in cognitions and emotions, in turn, lead to other coping responses and then further appraisals.

The CSM has been applied to a wide range of diseases, such as cancer, diabetes, and heart disease. Reviews of scientific findings generally support the value of the CSM in predicting health outcomes (Dempster et al., 2015; Hagger & Orbell, 2022). Both cognitive and emotional representations are predictive of healthier outcomes, but coping behavior (i.e., what people do in response to illness) is an even stronger predictor of healthier outcomes.

A study of people with asthma found that those with a better understanding of asthma and a stronger belief in their ability to control their symptoms showed better improvement (Achstetter et al., 2019). Those who believed that asthma had a large negative impact on their lives and who felt more distressed about it showed less improvement in asthma control. The investigators believe the CSM can help clinicians identify people at an early stage in treatment who are less likely to benefit and so may need interventions that focus directly on helping them change negative, dysfunctional thoughts.

Health Psychology in Action

A Health Psychologist Applies the CSM Model in the Hospital

The Common-Sense Model (CSM) examines how people respond to illness based on two types of representations, (1) how they make sense of a threat to their health and (2) how they respond emotionally to a threat. The CSM recognizes that negative emotions in response to a health threat can impede efforts to cope with serious illness. Health psychologists play important roles in helping patients manage their emotional responses to illness.

In some cases, health psychologists may apply the CSM to help hospital patients cope with their emotional responses to a health condition. In one example, health psychologist Susan Labbott (2018) described the case of a 70-year-old woman who had been recently diagnosed with breast cancer. The medical team reported that the woman felt overwhelmed and was not handling discussions of her treatment very well. A consultation was requested and the health psychologist was brought in to help the woman learn to manage her emotions, teaching her a technique called relaxation breathing (discussed in Chapter 5) she could use to calm herself before speaking with her doctors.

The psychologist also arranged to have the woman's daughter schedule visits just before the medical team made its rounds so that the woman and her daughter could prepare a list of questions for the doctors. If the medical team seemed about to leave before all her questions were answered, the daughter was tasked with asking the team to wait a minute to answer any additional questions. Afterward, the woman and her daughter discussed the information they received from the medical team.

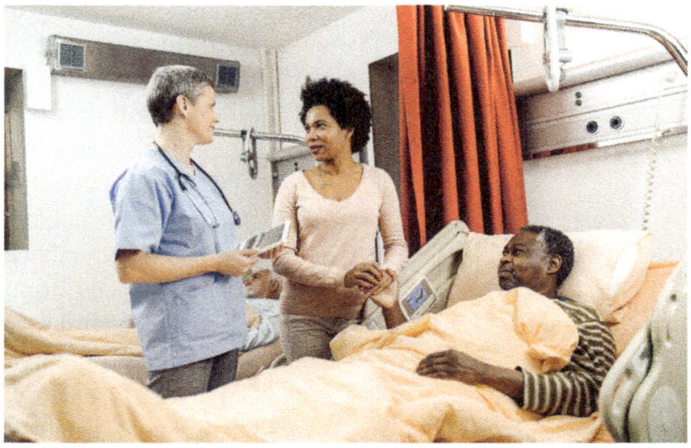

RgStudio/Getty Images

Determinants of Illness Behaviors

We noted how people vary in their response to illness. Let's take a look at the determinants of these responses through the lens of the biopsychosocial model, which incorporates biological, psychological, and sociocultural factors.

A useful way of representing these factors takes three sets of variables into account: *illness variables*, *patient-related variables*, and *healthcare-system variables* (Sirri et al., 2013). As we can see in **Figure 3.2**, these types of variables directly affect illness behaviors, and illness behaviors lead to different types of health outcomes, such as utilization of healthcare services, adherence to medical treatments, and preventive screenings.

Illness-Related Variables Illness-related variables are biological factors linked to disease processes, such as the type and severity of symptoms, the course of the disease, and disability and functional limitations associated with the disease. People with relatively mild symptoms, such as outbreaks of eczema or acne, may not contact healthcare professionals, preferring to manage them on their own. However, when symptoms become persistent or severe, or when they lead to negative psychological consequences, such as the social embarrassment associated with bumps and redness of the skin, people are more likely to seek medical attention and to adhere to treatment, as by using prescribed skin medication. Although illness-related variables may be grounded in disease processes, they interact with psychological factors in determining illness behaviors.

The severity of pain and disability are among the disease factors that determine whether a person seeks healthcare services. The greater the severity, frequency, and persistence of pain, or the greater the disability, the more likely it is a person will seek medical care and adhere to treatment. Among the other illness-related variables accounting for seeking medical care

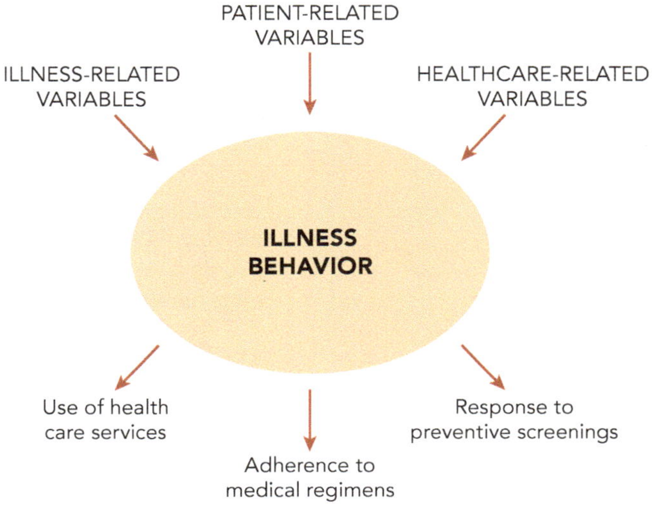

FIGURE 3.2 Determinants of Illness Behavior Variables related to the illness, the person, and the healthcare system all affect illness behavior, which in turn affects health outcomes.

Source: Adapted from Sirri et al. (2013).

services are rapid onset, sense of control, and uncertainty about the meaning of the symptoms (Sirri et al., 2013). A person who experiences sudden chest pain will likely seek medical attention sooner than a person whose chest pain develops gradually. People who believe they can control their symptoms on their own, such as controlling chest pain by stopping vigorous activity, tend to delay seeking help.

Patient-Related Variables Demographic factors, such as gender and age, also influence illness behaviors. Most research indicates that women are more likely than men to seek medical care (Koskela et al., 2010; Nabalamba & Millar, 2007). The traditional male stereotype in Western cultures associates masculinity with toughness and independence, which can lead men who adopt the stereotype to avoid asking for help. Unfortunately, men who "tough it out" may delay until a disease has progressed beyond its most treatable stages.

The ability to self-regulate one's health-related behavior—to marshal one's efforts to cope with the challenges of dealing with a health challenge—can lead to better outcomes. Health psychologists find that the use of behavior change techniques, such as setting goals, problem solving, and self-monitoring, can boost self-regulation (Hennessy et al., 2019; Miller et al., 2020; O'Carroll, 2020). For example, effective self-regulation of high blood pressure would likely include such behavior change techniques as self-monitoring (checking blood pressure regularly), setting goals (losing excess weight, curbing salt intake, exercising, taking medication as prescribed), and problem solving (arranging to put these techniques into practice).

Older people tend to utilize medical services more frequently than younger adults, in part because they face a greater risk of serious illnesses, such as cancer and heart disease (Cornally & McCarthy, 2011). People with disabilities are often deterred from seeking healthcare services because of limited mobility, especially those living in rural areas that lack accessible transportation (Dassah et al., 2018).

Another CSM patient characteristic that influences illness behavior is cognitive representation—how the person appraises the symptoms. Older people who attribute pain to aging are less likely to seek medical assistance than if they attribute it to a treatable condition (Sanders et al., 2004).

Misinterpretations of physical symptoms also affect healthcare-seeking behavior. A person who believes that low back pain is a sign of bone cancer is more likely to immediately seek medical attention than someone who attributes it to a minor muscle strain.

Personality factors also emerge as predictors of medical care utilization. For example, people who are more "emotionally unstable" (who score higher on the neuroticism scale of a personality test discussed in Chapter 11) tend to show lower levels of adherence to medical treatments (Sirri et al., 2013).

Patient-related factors in illness behaviors also include family interactions. Having social support and encouragement from others in the social or family environment prompts appropriate healthcare-seeking behavior and adherence to treatment (Sirri et al., 2013).

Family interactions also provide learning opportunities for illness behaviors. Both *observational learning* (learning by observing others) and *operant conditioning* (reinforcement-based learning) come into play. Family members may learn how to act when they are sick by observing how other family members respond to illness. Patients may also seek social reinforcement from family members in the form of attention, sympathy, and support for their complaints. Family members may similarly reinforce relatives for assuming the passive, dependent sick role by relieving them of responsibilities. Health psychologists who work with families of people with chronic pain or other chronic health conditions may try to change the reinforcement patterns in the family to encourage the ill person to adopt more active roles within the family structure.

Healthcare-Related Variables The patient–physician relationship is an important part of the helping process (Cifu et al., 2020). Having a trusting relationship with a physician or other healthcare provider plays a critical role in determining the use of healthcare services. Patients are more likely to seek services from providers whom they see as showing concern and empathy and who are able to communicate clearly (Sirri et al., 2013). Many patients complain that their doctors don't spend the time to listen to them; they feel that they are not being heard (Sanders et al., 2020). Physicians too are aware of the importance of establishing a relationship with their patients. Evidence shows that good doctor–patient communication is associated with higher levels of patient satisfaction, better adherence to medical advice, and better health outcomes (Labbott, 2018).

Researchers have identified several ways that physicians can forge a meaningful connection with patients (Labbott, 2018; Zulman et al., 2020):

- Taking a moment to prepare for greeting a patient
- Not talking too fast or using medical jargon the patient doesn't understand
- Listening carefully and fully, speaking clearly, sitting down with the patient, leaning forward, and avoiding interruptions
- Finding out what matters most to the patient
- Taking into account the patient's life story, including life circumstances affecting the patient's health, and acknowledging and validating the patient's efforts and successes in meeting health goals
- Recognizing and validating the patient's emotions

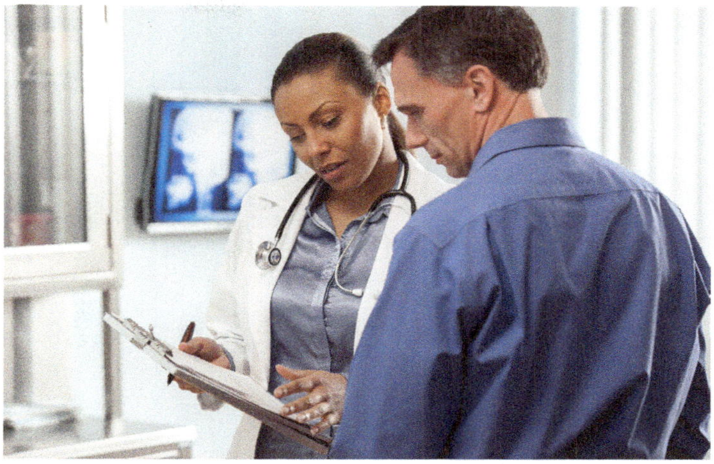

stevecoleimages/E+/Getty Images

Talking to Your Doctor Be seen and be heard when talking to your doctor. You are responsible for your own health care. Be certain that you take the time to communicate your health issues to your doctor. If you don't understand an explanation, say so. Ask the doctor to rephrase it in a way that you can understand. If you have a bad feeling about the doctor, or the diagnosis or the suggested course of treatment, get a second opinion.

Patients are more likely to follow medical advice when they perceive that the healthcare provider respects their ideas, provides accurate information, spends enough time with them, presents information in a way that is easily understood and addresses their concerns, and is willing to discuss the risks and benefits of proposed treatments.

Considering the broader social context, the question of whether ill people will seek healthcare services depends on factors including access to services as well as costs. With the introduction of the Affordable Care Act (ACA) (often called Obamacare after then-president Barack Obama who championed the effort), insurance coverage expanded to a larger number of Americans, making health services more affordable and accessible. From 2010, the year in which the ACA was enacted, the number of uninsured Americans fell by nearly 20 million people, from some 46.5 million in 2010 to about 27.5 million in 2021, a decline in the uninsured population of about 40% (Kaiser Family Foundation, 2022).

Health insurance saves lives; the odds of dying are greater among people who are uninsured (Woolhandler & Himmelstein, 2017). But Latino/Hispanics and Black Americans lag White and Asian Americans in the percentages of people who have health insurance (Cohen et al., 2019). Even people with health insurance may avoid or delay seeking health care because of concerns about deductibles and copays (Smith et al., 2018).

Cultural mistrust and discrimination play important roles in determining utilization of healthcare services among minority and disadvantaged groups. Black Americans often feel that the healthcare system does not care about them or treat them with the same level of concern and respect accorded to White Americans. They may feel that their symptoms or problems are overlooked or discredited, a sentiment expressed in the title of an article in a health psychology journal, "African American Experiences in Healthcare: 'I Always Feel Like I'm Getting Skipped Over'" (Cuevas et al., 2016). Medical mistrust may lead people of color to avoid seeking healthcare services or taking advantage of disease prevention efforts, such as cancer screenings. Feeling that their concerns are "skipped over" can lead people to wonder whether their healthcare providers are discriminating against them.

Because of healthcare disparities, might Black people fare better if they see Black doctors? One study found that Black men were more likely to obtain preventive care, such as flu vaccinations and screenings for blood pressure, cholesterol, and diabetes, if they were recommended and administered by Black male physicians (Alsan et al., 2018). The men also felt freer to open up about their health concerns.

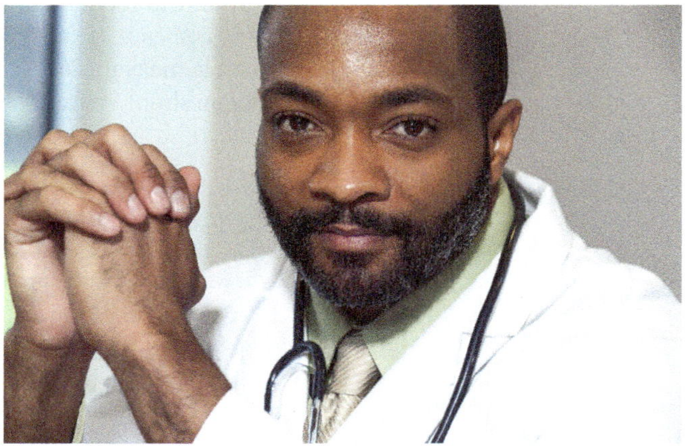

Spotmatik/Alamy Stock Photo

Do Black Men Fare Better with Black Male Doctors? Perhaps they do. A study found that Black men were more likely to undergo screenings for high blood pressure, cholesterol (a risk factor for heart disease), and diabetes when these preventive measures were recommended by a Black male physician.

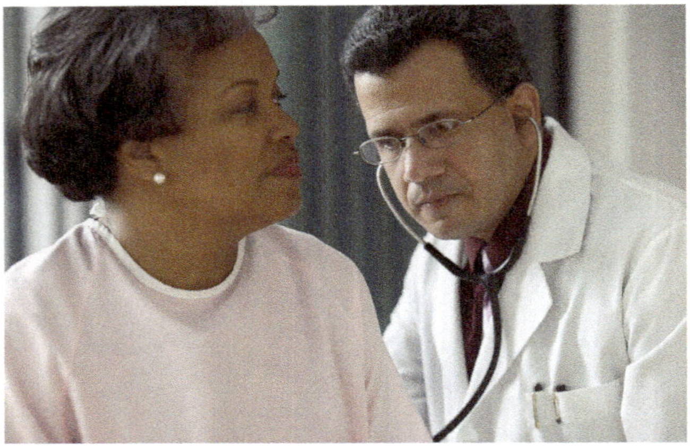

Jose Luis Pelaez Inc/Getty images

What Did He Just Say? Healthcare microaggressions are subtle expressions of bias by healthcare providers. Although they may be unintentional, they may discourage patients from seeking healthcare services or from following through with medical treatment.

Microaggressions People of color are also frequently subjected to **microaggressions** by healthcare providers that feed mistrust and resentment (Cruz et al., 2019). Microaggressions are subtle expressions of implicit bias or prejudice that often occur without conscious awareness (Fattoracci & King, 2023; Williams, 2020). Examples of microaggressions in the healthcare context include comments that serve to deny the distinctive cultural experiences of oppressed groups, as when a healthcare provider says "I don't see color" or "We are all the same." Other microaggressions convey negative stereotypes about people of color or show outright hostility toward them. **Table 3.2** shows items from a rating scale that measures patient perceptions of microaggressions by healthcare providers.

Eliminating implicit biases among healthcare providers is a daunting challenge, but one approach deserving of further study is development of culturally informed training that not only raises awareness among clinicians about their underlying biases but also provides opportunities for them to practice more culturally aware interactions with patients. Another direction toward reducing bias in healthcare providers involves promoting direct, high-quality contact with people of color. Investigators found that medical students of non-African descent who had more favorable interracial contacts with African American hospital staff, fellow students, faculty, and residents during medical school were less likely to show racial biases when they were tested 2 years later during their medical residency (Onyeador et al., 2020). Studies like this point to the need for more direct and favorable interactions between people of different racial or ethnic groups.

microaggressions Everyday slights, snubs, insults, or instances of discrimination that are usually directed against members of marginalized groups, such as racial, ethnic, and sexual minorities. Microaggressions may be purposeful or unintentional.

The Sick Role

sick role A social role that prescribes the expected rights and responsibilities of people who are sick.

American sociologist Talcott Parsons (1902–1979) described the **sick role** in terms of a set of rights and responsibilities of people who are sick. From this perspective, a sick person can expect to be relieved or freed from certain work or family responsibilities. If we come down with the flu, we can expect time off from work or school to allow us to rest at home; we also can expect that family members will pick up our share of household and childcare responsibilities.

A more severe illness or medical condition, such as a heart attack, would typically lead to a longer recuperative period during which we would be freed from normal work and social obligations. From the standpoint of medical sociology, assigning a person to a sick role removes the person from being a productive member of society and makes the person dependent upon the medical profession (Crossman, 2018; Gerhardt, 2022). But along with these "rights" comes a set of responsibilities. If we call in sick to work, we are expected to take reasonable measures to recover by arranging to see a physician and following medical advice. Our focus should be on getting better as soon as possible so that we can resume our usual

TABLE 3.2 The Microaggressions in Healthcare Scale

My Healthcare Provider:

1. Avoided discussing or addressing cultural issues
2. Sometimes was insensitive about my cultural group
3. Seemed to deny having any cultural biases or stereotypes
4. At times seemed to overidentify with my experiences related to my race or culture
5. At times seemed to have stereotypes about my cultural group, even if he or she did not express them directly
6. Sometimes minimized the importance of cultural issues

Source: Cruz et al. (2019)/ Elsevier/ CC BY 4.0.

Self-Assessment

INTERACTIVE SELF-ASSESSMENTS

Are You an Active or a Passive Healthcare Consumer?

Are you an active or passive healthcare consumer? For each of the following pairs of statements, place a check mark by the statement that best represents your beliefs and attitudes concerning your health care. Then consult the scoring key at the end of the chapter.

1. I put off thinking about my health care until a healthcare need arises.	*or*	I regularly consider my healthcare needs and plan ahead to meet them.
2. I don't know how to locate a personal physician and other healthcare providers (HCPs) in my area.	*or*	I have established a relationship with a primary HCP and other HCPs, such as a dentist and (if I'm female) a gynecologist.
3. I'm not aware of the major hospitals and clinics in my area or what services they provide.	*or*	I know the major healthcare facilities in my area, what services they offer, and how to get to them in case of emergency.
4. I don't have a list of phone numbers for hospitals and doctors I can call for help.	*or*	I keep handy a list of phone numbers and know whom to call for medical needs.
5. I have skipped regular medical exams because I didn't have the time or wasn't sure how to arrange them.	*or*	I have regular medical exams and have established a relationship with a primary HCP who knows my health history.
6. I cannot afford health care and have not made arrangements in case I need medical services.	*or*	I maintain healthcare coverage.
7. To be honest, I tend to ignore symptoms as long as possible in the hope that they will disappear.	*or*	I pay attention to any changes in my body and bring symptoms to the attention of my HCP in a timely manner.
8. I sometimes use emergency services, such as emergency departments or urgent care clinics, for minor problems.	*or*	I always try to work through my primary HCP when I am in need of care.
9. I really don't know what I would do or where I would go in case of a medical emergency.	*or*	I know how to handle a medical emergency—whom to call and where to go.
10. I sometimes or often fail to keep medical appointments or arrive late.	*or*	I keep appointments and arrive on time.
11. I sometimes or often fail to call to cancel appointments ahead of time.	*or*	I always call to cancel appointments when necessary.
12. I sometimes hold back information from my HCP or believe that doctors should be able to figure problems out by themselves.	*or*	I readily offer information to my HCP and describe my symptoms as clearly as possible.
13. I sometimes or often omit information on medical histories due to embarrassment, forgetfulness, or carelessness.	*or*	I give complete information and do not withhold, embellish, or distort information about my health.
14. I sometimes or often fail to pay attention to the doctor's instructions.	*or*	I listen carefully to instructions and ask for explanations of my condition and treatment.
15. I generally don't ask my physician to explain medical terms I don't understand.	*or*	I always ask my physician to explain technical terms I don't understand.
16. I generally accept what my doctor tells me without questioning.	*or*	I ask questions when I don't understand or agree with the diagnosis or treatment plan.
17. Sometimes I don't fill prescriptions or take medications according to schedule.	*or*	I follow instructions and call the doctor or pharmacist for clarification when necessary.
18. I sometimes fail to keep follow-up appointments or neglect to update my HCP on my condition.	*or*	I reliably keep follow-up appointments and make update calls when indicated.

19. I simply stop following a treatment that has troubling side effects or no apparent effects and don't inform my HCP.	*or*	If a treatment doesn't appear to be working or produces negative effects, I call my HCP before making changes in the treatment plan.
20. I don't examine medical bills carefully, especially those that are paid by my insurance company.	*or*	I carefully examine bills for any errors or duplication of services and bring discrepancies to the attention of my HCP.
21. I don't question charges for medical services, even if they seem excessive or inappropriate.	*or*	I question my HCPs about charges that seem excessive or inappropriate.
22. I generally neglect filling out insurance claim forms for as long as possible.	*or*	I promptly complete insurance forms and submit them.
23. I generally don't keep records of my medical treatments and insurance claims.	*or*	I generally keep records of my medical treatments and insurance claims.

Source: ©Jeffrey Nevid & Spencer Rathus.

social roles and obligations. The sick role is thus a temporary social arrangement, lasting only as long as necessary.

People adapt to the sick role in different ways. Some people abuse the rights accorded them by failing to fulfill their obligations to get well, as in refusing to see a doctor or to adhere to medical advice. Others exaggerate their illness behaviors by overusing medical services, over-reporting symptoms, or claiming excessive disability (Finkelstein et al., 2020; Hamilton et al., 2015).

Having a prescribed social role for people who become ill is well integrated in society. Companies typically offer paid sick days to employees, and schools make arrangements for students who miss school because of illness to make up any missing work or tests. It's generally understood that when you are running a fever, it's best to stay home for everyone's sake. We should, however, note a major limitation in applying the sick role model to illness behaviors: The model is better suited for illness behaviors associated with acute illnesses, like the flu, or recovery from injury or surgery than it is for long-term chronic diseases. In effect, a sick role is a temporary social designation, a time out from ordinary life responsibilities and not a lifestyle.

There is a disconnect between the expectations underlying the sick role and treatment approaches for people dealing with chronic health conditions. The sick role places the affected person in a passive and dependent role with respect to healthcare providers and supportive family members. But healthcare providers often encourage people faced with chronic health conditions like coronary heart disease and cancer to assume a more active role in their treatment, make healthful lifestyle changes, engage in reasonable physical activity, and assume as many household responsibilities as possible.

Conflict within the family may arise when a person with severe or prolonged illness remains dependent on others and is relieved of household chores or childcare responsibilities for a lengthy period. This disruption of family roles can lead to anger and resentment among other members of the family and to feelings of guilt in ill people for imposing additional burdens on the family.

Review 3.1

INTERACTIVE SELF-SCORING QUIZZES

Sentence Completion

1. __________ behavior refers to how people respond to acute or chronic illness.

2. Illness behaviors begin with a perceived change in physical or bodily functioning that the person interprets as a __________ to health.

3. There are major disparities in health indices, as people in (lower or higher) socioeconomic levels of our society tend to have poorer health outcomes.

4. The __________ Model (CSM) of self-regulation describes how people react to threats to their health and well-being by forming cognitive and emotional representations of illness.

5. The CSM is based on the process of __________ by which individuals manage their behaviors, emotions, and thoughts in pursuing their life goals and reacting to life events.

6. A review of the CSM found that __________ behavior was a stronger predictor of healthier outcomes than cognitive and emotional representations.

7. Determinants of illness behaviors can be broken down into three sets of variables, __________ variables, patient-related variables, and healthcare-system variables.

8. In the first several years following enactment of the ACA, the number of uninsured Americans (increased or decreased).

9. The sick role model is better suited to explaining illness behaviors in response to (acute illness or chronic) illness.

Think About It

How do you respond to the first signs of illness? How might the CSM predict your illness behaviors?

Health Disparities

Health disparities are differences in health outcomes or health status between groups based on race, ethnicity, or level of income. Health disparities reflect differences in rates of disease and mortality that involve factors such as wealth, neighborhood characteristics, and underlying health risks. Your income level and your racial or ethnic identity play important roles in determining how healthy you're likely to be and how long you are likely to live (Brady et al., 2023; Gordon, 2024). Even the neighborhood in which you live can be hazardous to your health, as people from poorer communities carry disproportionate health burdens. Consider what health researchers report about the health consequences of poverty:

health disparities Particular types of differences in health that are linked to socioeconomic and environmental advantages or disadvantages.

- People are likely to have poorer health outcomes if they lack resources needed to obtain good education, stable housing, safe environments, and health insurance coverage (Brady et al., 2023; Roesch et al., 2024).
- Disadvantaged groups are more likely to reside in neighborhoods lacking access to nutritious food, quality housing, good jobs, and properly funded schools (Stringhini et al., 2017).
- The reduction in life expectancy associated with low socioeconomic status is about the same as the reduction associated with physical inactivity (Stringhini et al., 2017). The life expectancy of a child born into the upper middle class, mostly White American neighborhood of Streeterville, Chicago, can expect to live to 90 years; whereas a child born into the poorer, mostly Black Chicago neighborhood of Englewood can expect to live fewer than 60 years (Soth, 2020).
- People with heart failure who live in poorer neighborhoods have poorer health outcomes than do those who live in wealthier neighborhoods (Bikdeli et al., 2014).
- All told, health disparities cost lives. A recent estimate put the number of lives lost among Black Americans at more 1.6 million excess deaths from 1999 to 2020 (Caraballo et al., 2023). More Black men, nearly a million, lost their lives prematurely as compared to Black women, who accounted for more than 600,000 excess deaths. The leading cause of these premature deaths in Black men and women, researchers say, was heart disease, which disproportionally affects Black Americans (see Chapter 12).

Health disparities in the United States came into sharper focus with the COVID-19 pandemic in 2020, in which people of color, especially Blacks and Latinos/Hispanics, were disproportionally affected, suffering higher rates of hospitalizations, serious complications, and deaths (Aubrey, 2020; Chowkwanyun & Reed, 2020; Van Dorn et al., 2020; Walsh, 2020). There are many reasons for these disparities, including greater prevalence in people of color of preexisting conditions that increase vulnerability to the effects of the virus, especially obesity, diabetes, and hypertension. Also adding to the increased risk were environmental factors such as the generally denser housing conditions in communities of color, which increased the risk of transmission of the virus, and the greater proportion of Blacks and Latino/Hispanic Americans working in essential services, such as retail grocery workers, public transit employees, and healthcare workers, which bring them into closer contact with the public, nursing homes, and hospitalized patients.

Not only inner-city neighborhoods were besieged by the coronavirus. The virus hit its deadly mark even in the remotest pockets of humanity in the United States, the vast stretches of New Mexico highlands desert that are home to the Navajo nation (Kovich, 2020; Romero, 2020). Here, where social distancing is a fact of life, but where families live tightly packed in traditional Navajo dwellings and where health services are sparse, the virus took its toll as it spread within families. Health disparities are not necessarily an urban or a rural problem but a problem of inequities involving poverty and access to health care.

Yet there is some good news. A federal watchdog agency, the NIH Agency for Healthcare Research and Quality (AHRQ), which tracks changes in health disparities, found that some disparities in health outcomes have shrunk since the year 2000 (AHRQ, 2019). That said, many disparities remain, and poorer and uninsured groups bear the brunt of them.

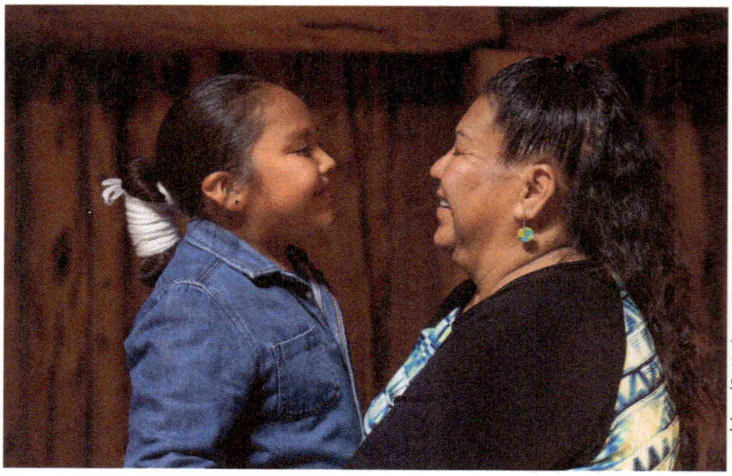
grandriver/Getty Images

Disparities in Health Insurance Coverage Many traditionally disadvantaged groups in the United States remain underinsured.

Serving the Underserved

One of the principal aims of the Affordable Care Act was to reduce health disparities by expanding insurance coverage to underserved communities. How well is it working? Pretty well, it happens. Insurance coverage increased substantially in the first few years after the introduction of the ACA across all major ethnic and racial groups, helping to close the insurance gap between rich and poor and among racial and ethnic groups (Artiga & Orgera, 2019; Chaudry et al., 2019; Griffith et al., 2017). However, Black Americans and Latino/Hispanic Americans still lag White Americans in insurance coverage (Office of Minority Health, 2022). Yet disparities continue, as we can see in **Figure 3.3**. Nearly 12% of Blacks remain uninsured, as compared to about 8% of Whites. Uninsured rates are even higher among Latinos/Hispanics and American Indian/Alaska Native Americans. The only ethnic/racial minority on par with White Americans in insurance coverage is Asian Americans. Although gaps in insurance coverage between racial/ethnic groups persist, they have narrowed in most states and may narrow still further

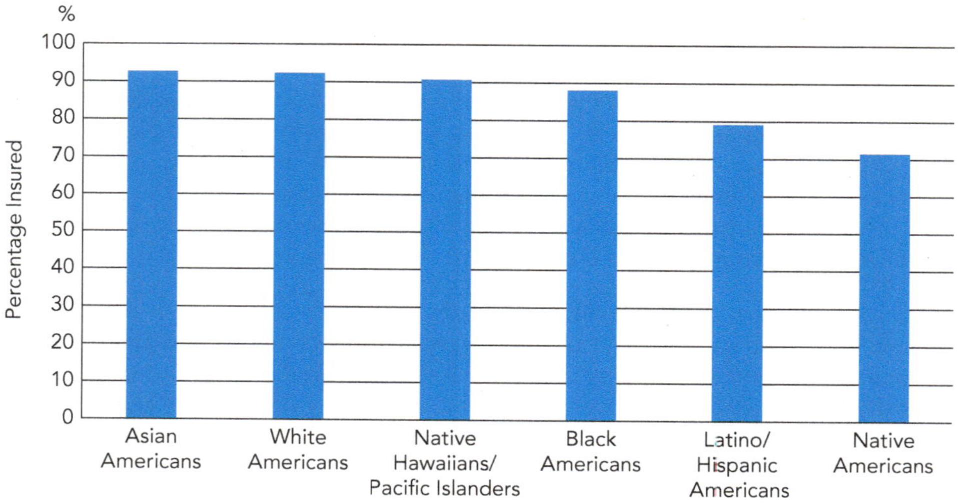

FIGURE 3.3 **Rates of Insured Groups, by Race/Ethnicity, United States** Despite gains in health insurance coverage since the passage of the Affordable Care Act, members of most racial/ethnic groups lag White Americans.

Source: National Health Interview Survey. 2020/ U.S. Department of Health & Human Services/ Public Domain if there is an additional expansion of Medicaid (Chaudry et al., 2019).

In the United States, in contrast to other developed countries, health insurance is generally tied to one's place of employment. Therefore, unemployment is a factor in lack of health insurance coverage. Blacks and Latinos/Hispanics have higher-than-average rates of unemployment, which can make it more difficult to acquire or afford health insurance. Another factor is that rates of uninsured persons are higher among groups who are over represented on the lower rungs of the socioeconomic ladder, including people of color.

Among the groups with the highest uninsured or underinsured rates are recent immigrants, migrant workers, and people working in small business concerns that do not provide healthcare coverage. American Indian/Alaska Native Americans are another underserved group. Though they are eligible for free health care through the Indian Health Service, many live in remote areas with few available healthcare providers (Adakai et al., 2018). Many cannot afford to travel to obtain medical services.

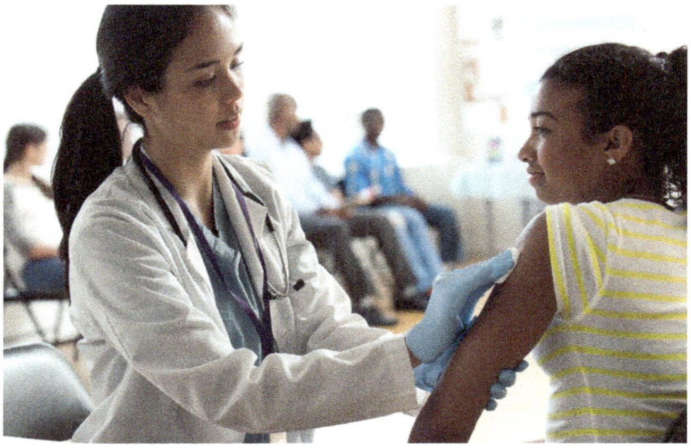

Jose Luis Pelaez Inc/Getty Images

Getting Vaccinated This patient is about to receive a vaccination, but with the exception of Asian Americans, members of racial and ethnic minorities are generally less likely to obtain the services—including preventive services—that they need.

It is not just the uninsured or underinsured who lack access to medical services. Most people who are underserved actually have some form of health insurance. But for many people with health insurance, cost remains a barrier, as deductibles, copayments, the need for time off from work, and transportation costs make it difficult to afford medical care, especially for people in poorer neighborhoods. About 1 in 7 people in the United States lives in a family that has trouble paying medical bills (Cha & Cohen, 2020).

Another problem for low-income families is that many healthcare providers are unwilling to accept Medicaid patients. Language incompatibility between patient and healthcare provider is yet another limiting factor. Long waiting times in clinics serving Medicaid recipients also contribute to lower levels of healthcare access. Moreover, economically disadvantaged people are often put in a position of juggling family needs for food, shelter, and education with the need for doctors' visits or prescription drugs. People living in remote rural areas are especially vulnerable; they may need to travel 50 miles to visit a doctor or farther for a specialist or hospitalization. Access to primary health services varies from state and state, with more rural areas of the United States having fewer primary health care providers available (Equity [Hope] Initiative et al., 2020).

Researchers find that race and ethnicity matter in determining access to health care regardless of socioeconomic standing (Williams et al., 2016). Even when health insurance or government programs like Medicare and Medicaid are available, members of ethnic minorities tend to receive lower-quality care than White Americans. Blacks are less likely than Whites to receive hip and knee replacements, kidney transplants, mammograms, and flu shots. Black people with heart disease are also less likely to receive aggressive medical treatment.

There are many reasons for these disparities, including cost of services, lack of nearby facilities—especially facilities that provide specialized services—and lack of knowledge about health risks and screening procedures, such as mammography. Cultural mistrust is another prominent factor limiting utilization of healthcare services among people of color, many of whom can recount experiences of indifferent or callous treatment by healthcare providers.

Exposure to discrimination is a source of stress that takes its toll over time on the physical and psychological health of minoritized groups (Benner et al., 2018; Comas-Diaz et al., 2019). Experiencing discrimination may lead to negative health outcomes by working through a pathway that leads to unhealthy behaviors, such as substance use or abuse and adoption of unhealthy diets and eating behaviors (Pascoe, Lattanner, & Richman, 2022). Facing unfair treatment day after day can become such a stressful burden that it leads to unhealthy behaviors, such as use of harmful substances and a diet rich in high-fat, high-calorie foods, which in turn can lead to adverse health outcomes.

Children are not immune to the pernicious effects of discrimination; evidence shows that exposure to discrimination in childhood can have negative health effects that endure into adulthood (Carter et al., 2019). Researchers find that maintaining close ties to one's traditional culture can help protect against the negative effects of discrimination by providing a sense of belonging, connection, and social support (Cobb et al., 2019; Seaton & Zeiders, 2021; Yip et al., 2019).

Consider the health effects of discrimination among the Sikh Asian Indian community. A study of a Sikh community in Queens, New York, found that Sikhs who wore traditional turbans and scarves reported higher levels of discrimination than those not wearing them (Nadimpalli et al., 2016). Furthermore, exposure to discrimination was associated with poorer mental and physical health. Sikh Asian Indians are an understudied but high-risk population group with respect to exposure to discrimination, and the researchers hope that their efforts will spur development of community-based programs to reduce discrimination or help buffer its effects.

Reducing Health Disparities

Despite the expansion of health insurance coverage under the ACA, barriers remain that limit access and availability to health care. The government's *Healthy People 2020* initiative identified several of them (see **Figure 3.4**):

- *Lack of availability:* Many people live in areas that lack sufficient numbers of healthcare providers. As noted, this is especially true in rural areas in which few physicians or health clinics are available or in which people need to travel considerable distances to access these services.
- *High cost:* Even when medical insurance is available, high premiums and costly copays deter many people from obtaining needed medical services, especially people at lower income levels who can least afford these out-of-pocket expenses.
- *Lack of insurance coverage:* Though the ACA has increased insurance coverage for Americans, there are still millions of people in the United States who remain uninsured or fail to qualify for government health programs like Medicaid.
- *Limited language access:* A major deterrent to effective health care is language incompatibility between patient and healthcare provider. We are a nation of many peoples who speak many languages. Finding a healthcare provider who can speak the same language as the patient can be difficult. The use of translation services in hospitals and medical centers can help bridge the language gap, but these services may be limited by cost and availability.

Barriers to accessing health services contribute to negative health outcomes in several ways. They lead to unmet health needs, as people fail to receive the treatment they need. They also lead to delays in receiving appropriate care, which can compromise health outcomes by failing to initiate care at a more treatable stage. By the same token, they can delay or prevent people from obtaining preventive services that can avert serious health threats.

What can be done to reduce or eliminate health disparities? While there may be no easy answers, health experts recognize that it will take a coordinated effort between legislators and public health officials to make health care more affordable and accessible to a broader range of people, especially people at the lower levels of the socioeconomic spectrum. Changes in social policies are needed to advance economic development in disadvantaged neighborhoods in order to attract healthcare providers and facilities. We also need to redouble public health efforts that focus on prevention and early detection of disease, from expanding vaccination programs to reducing sources of pollution in distressed neighborhoods. Our health and well-being is affected by many social determinants, such as social, economic, and political factors and the characteristics of the neighborhoods and communities in which we live (Alcantara et al., 2020; Swain, 2016).

Barriers →

- Lack of availability
- High cost
- Lack of insurance coverage
- Limited language access

Consequences

- Unmet health needs
- Delays in receiving care
- Inability to obtain preventive services
- Hospitalizations that could have been prevented

FIGURE 3.4 Barriers to Accessing Health Care and Consequences

Source: Adapted from Determinants of Health, Healthy People, 2020. https://www.healthypeople.gov/2020/about/foundation-health-measures/Determinants-of-Health.

Stigma and Health

Stigma is yet another barrier to utilization of healthcare services. Sociologist Erving Goffman (1963) described stigma as "as a mark of social disgrace" that carries with it the social perception of taint or untrustworthiness. The stigma attached to mental illness, for example, may prevent many people with psychological disorders from seeking help. Pejorative terms are often used to apply to people who are stigmatized, such as people with mental illness—terms like crazy, nuts, psycho, weirdo, or, as a particularly troublesome adjective for men—weak. Stigma may also be attached to physical illness, making people feel that seeking help is a sign of weakness or a mark of stain.

stigma A mark of disgrace associated with a person's mental or physical condition or behavior.

People may avoid or delay seeking help for conditions associated with stigma. For example, someone who has smoked for a long time may avoid medical care for a hacking cough out of concern for being the target of stigma associated with continued smoking. A person who is overweight or obese may avoid joining a gym for fear of fat-shaming.

The historical tradition in many cultures of avoiding and even forcibly separating people with certain types of communicable diseases, like leprosy, is an example of the stigmatization of physical illness. Even today, stigma is attached to some types of illness, such as sexually transmitted infections (e.g., herpes and HIV/AIDS), leading people who are affected by these diseases to feel tainted or ostracized, creating barriers to seeking health care. Stigma is often assigned to physical conditions that have observable physical marks, such as herpes or acne, leading others to devalue or discredit people with the conditions. In turn, the person who is stigmatized may feel shame or embarrassment and try to disguise or hide the marks, avoid social interactions and healthcare services. Evidence also shows that healthcare workers are less willing to help patients who have visual marks or characteristics they believe are the patients' own fault, such as patients with obesity, lung cancer, or addictions (Major et al., 2018).

Social identity is another basis for stigmatization and unfair treatment. Your social identity is about your identification with particular social groups, such as ethnic and racial groups; family, kinship, and religious groups; nations; or sports clubs or teams. Social identity speaks about the ways in which we categorize or classify people based on the groups to which they belong or identify with, or to which they are assigned by others. Because of lingering prejudices, people may stigmatize others from groups that are marginalized or disadvantaged.

Others may assign us to group memberships even when we see ourselves differently. For example, others may classify us in a binary gender category, as either male or female, even though we identify ourselves as transgender, intersexual, or something else. Members of minority or disadvantaged groups in our society are often stigmatized by those in more advantaged or powerful groups. They may be devalued in a number of ways, as others may view them as untrustworthy, deviant, and intellectually inferior.

Stigma can have harmful effects on health (Lucas et al., 2018). The experience of stigma is a source of stress that can lead to repeated activation of the body's stress response (as discussed in Chapter 4), which in turn can increase vulnerability to stress-related diseases (Major & Schmader, 2018). Even the mere expectation of being stigmatized by others based on one's body weight (weight stigma) is linked to greater levels of the stress hormone cortisol in a person's blood (Tomiyama, 2014).

Another way in which stigma can affect physical health is through exposure to discrimination. Members of racial and ethnic minority groups often face discrimination associated with racial and ethnic stereotypes. Being the target of discrimination can have negative health effects. Members of racial and ethnic minority groups who report more encounters with discrimination tend to have more physical health conditions (Richman et al., 2018).

Primary Prevention: "An Ounce of Prevention"

The American founding statesman Benjamin Franklin left a rich and enduring legacy, including quips that remain instructive today. Among these was his saying "An ounce of prevention is worth a pound of cure." One of the pillars on which efforts to reduce health disparities is based is **primary prevention**, that is, health-promotion programs designed to prevent the development of disease.

primary prevention Efforts aimed at preventing illness or disease.

Prevention programs seek to avert the suffering, pain, and costs associated with disease. Health psychologists find that markers of socioeconomic status, especially levels of income and education, contribute to the likelihood of engaging in preventive activities such as early detection screenings (Haught et al., 2015). For health psychologists, prevention efforts may be focused on helping young people control their weight and establish healthful dietary and exercise habits to keep them from developing heart disease and other chronic diseases. Health psychologists and other health professionals also aim to increase adherence to regular screenings for hypertension (to reduce the risk of heart disease and stroke) and colorectal cancer (colonoscopies to detect the cancer itself and to remove polyps that might develop into cancerous lesions).

Health psychologists also work with at-risk populations to assist them in screening programs targeting early detection of diseases at their most treatable stages. Major health organizations, such as the American Cancer Society and the American Heart Association, along with the government's National Institutes of Health, provide guidelines for health screenings, including screenings for the country's leading killers, heart disease and cancer. Health psychologists work with patients to educate them about the importance of early detection and helping them follow through with recommended health screenings at recommended intervals, such as those listed in Table 3.3.

TABLE 3.3 **Key Screening Tests**

INTERACTIVE FIGURES, CHARTS, & TABLES

Testing for	How It's Done	When Should You Be Tested
Blood pressure	Uses an inflatable cuff wrapped around the upper arm to gauge blood pressure.	Blood pressure should be checked during an annual physical exam. People with elevated blood pressure will likely need to have their blood pressure monitored more frequently.
Breast cancer (mammograms)	A mammogram is a specialized X-ray of the breast to deduct small lumps that may not be felt upon clinical examination.	The American Cancer Society recommends that women aged 40–44 years should have a choice of whether to start annual screening mammograms. Women aged 45–54 years should have an annual mammogram, and those aged 55 years or older should either have mammograms every 2 years or continue with annual screenings if they wish.
Cervical cancer	Typically a Pap test will be performed in which a sample of cells is gently scraped from the surface of the woman's cervix and analyzed for signs of cervical cancer.	Most physicians recommend annual Pap smears for women by age 21.
High cholesterol	A blood sample is analyzed to measure blood cholesterol levels in milligrams per deciliter, with desirable levels set at less than 200 mg/dl for total cholesterol, less than 100 mg/dl for LDL ("bad") cholesterol, and 40 mg/dL or higher in men and 50 mg/dL or higher in women for HDL ("good cholesterol").	Recommendations vary with some medical sources favoring early testing (beginning in the 20s) and others preferring to start testing when people are in their 40s. People presenting with a family history of heart disease, diabetes, or high cholesterol may need to have their blood cholesterol levels checked more frequently or start testing earlier.
HIV	Blood, saliva, and urine tests detect antibodies to HIV, the virus that causes AIDS. If antibodies are found, a follow-up test can confirm the presence of the virus itself.	People concerned about possible exposure to HIV through needle-sharing or unprotected sexual contact with partners of unknown HIV status can be tested at any time.
Low bone density, osteoporosis	A specialized X-ray may be used, called *dual X-ray absorptiometry*, or DXA, which detects bone loss.	Generally recommended for women aged 65 years and older or those at high risk of bone density loss associated with osteoporosis. Screening recommendations for men vary.
Prostate cancer	A physician may perform a digital (manual) rectal exam to detect abnormalities in the prostate that may indicate possible prostate cancer. A specialized blood test may be used to measure levels of prostate-specific antigen (PSA), which seeps out of the prostate when it is cancerous or enlarged. The PSA test may detect cancer cells before abnormalities can be felt by digital exam. However, only a follow-up biopsy can determine whether cancer is present.	The American Cancer Society recommends that men aged 50 who can expect to live at least another 10 years talk with their doctors about the potential risks and benefits of screening tests. Men in high-risk categories should start these conversations at an earlier age. The exam generally consists of a digital rectal exam and a PSA test.

(Continued)

TABLE 3.3 Key Screening Tests (*Continued*)

Testing for	How It's Done	When Should You Be Tested
Rectal and colon cancer	Several types of cancer screening tests may be used, including a *fecal occult blood test*, which analyzes a stool sample for the presence of blood, which may be a sign of cancer. A *colonoscopy* is a medical procedure for examining the colon for the presence of cancerous growth or polyps. In a *double-contrast barium enema*, a series of X-rays of the colon and rectum are taken after use of a special enema.	Screening generally begins at age 50 for most people and follows a schedule for colonoscopy and other tests based on a person's age, family history, and other medical conditions.
Skin cancer	A dermatologist (skin doctor) will perform a full head-to-toe examination for the presence of suspicious moles or growths. Any suspicious moles or growths may be removed and examined in a biopsy for the presence of cancerous cells.	Typically, a full skin exam is part of an annual medical checkup. More frequent screenings are recommended for people at higher risk of skin cancer.

Review 3.2

INTERACTIVE SELF-SCORING QUIZZES

Sentence Completion

1. __________ is associated with many negative health outcomes.

2. Some health disparities in health outcomes have become (smaller or larger) since the year 2000.

3. African Americans, Latino/Hispanics, and Native Americans are (less likely or more likely) than White Americans to have health insurance.

4. Most people who are unable to obtain the medical care they need (do or do not) have health insurance.

5. Ethnic minority groups tend to receive (lower-quality or higher-quality health care) than White Americans.

6. Stress resulting from ethnic or racial __________ can take a toll on both physical and psychological health.

7. A major deterrent to effective health care is __________ incompatibility between patient and healthcare provider.

Think About It

What changes need to be made to reduce or eliminate health disparities? To what extent do these changes involve individuals themselves or the larger society?

Health Care, USA

The healthcare system might be better described as a loosely coordinated network of healthcare providers, hospitals, clinics, and healthcare services than as an organized system for meeting the nation's healthcare needs. Navigating the "healthcare system" requires knowledge of its parts, how to access them, and how to pay for the services they provide. It's a complicated puzzle indeed, leaving many healthcare consumers confused about how they can obtain the services they need at a cost they can afford.

Three general types of healthcare programs provide access to healthcare services and help offset the costs:

1. *Private health insurance programs* directly enroll consumers either privately or through their places of employment. These programs include traditional fee-for-service plans and managed care plans, as discussed below.
2. *Government health insurance programs*, such as Medicare (for older people and people with disabilities) and Medicaid (for low-income people).
3. *Public health programs*, such as well-baby clinics and family planning clinics.

Cost is often the driving force in determining how healthcare services are delivered. Health care in the United States is big business, so big that it is the second only to retailing among the leading industries in the country. Determining how to provide and pay for health care is among the most important issues facing our country and is often the centerpiece of

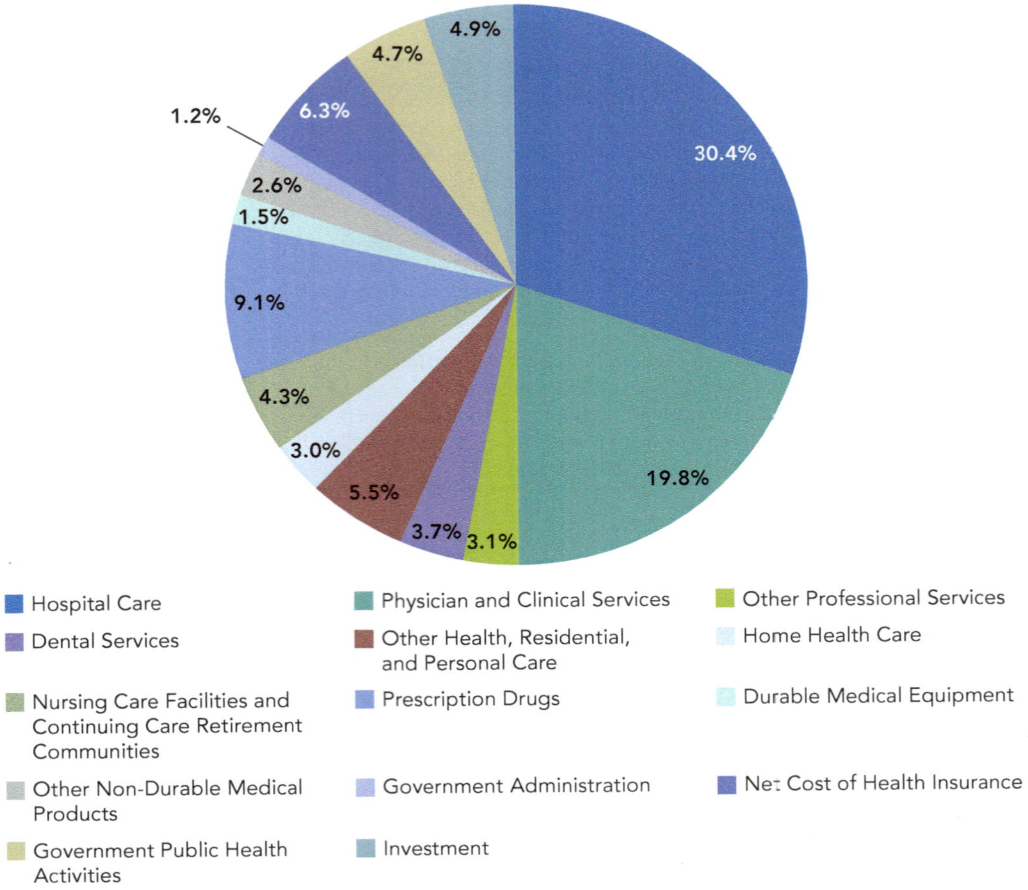

FIGURE 3.5 **Where We Spend Our Healthcare Dollars** We spend about 30% of our healthcare dollars on hospital care, followed by physician and clinical services and retail sales of medical products, mostly prescription drugs.

Source: Adapted from NHE Fact Sheet, December 2023

political debates. Although lack of availability of health care for people in need is a prominent concern, the United States actually spends more on health care (as a percentage of gross domestic product) than any other of the world's leading economically developed countries, far more than Canada, the United Kingdom, Germany, France, or Japan, and almost twice the average among the world's wealthiest nations. **Figure 3.5** shows where our health dollars are spent.

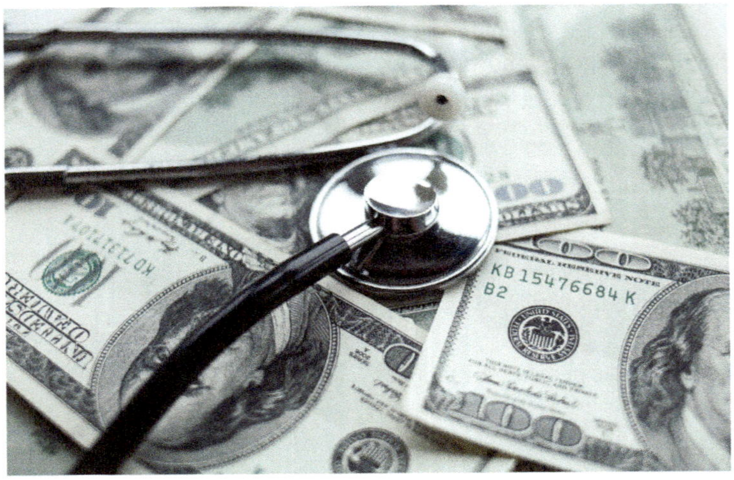

Foremniakowski/Getty Images

The Cost of Health Care The United States spends more than $10,000 per year on health care per capita, including every adult and child—more than any other developed nation spends. Although we spend more, our health outcomes are not generally any better.

Overall, the United States spends more than $10,000 per year on health care for every person, including every child, in the country, which is greater on a per capita basis than the expenditure made by any other developed nation (Peter G. Peterson Foundation [PGPF], 2019). Even with the expenditure of such large amounts of money, health outcomes in the United States are not generally better than those in other developed countries (PGPF, 2019). Simply put, we spend more, but we don't do better. Many factors account for the disconnect between spending and health outcomes, including the enormous administrative costs involved in managing U.S. healthcare services, as well as the cost of litigation for medical malpractice.

The healthcare system shields the consumer from many of the costs. Consumers with health insurance obtained through their places of employment do not directly bear the full brunt of healthcare costs, paying only part of the costs in the form of insurance premiums, deductibles, and copays. Most healthcare costs are borne by companies that subsidize health insurance programs for their workers and by government programs, such as Medicare and Medicaid, that provide health care, respectively, for older people, people with disabilities, and people without financial resources. Though tongue-in-cheek, there's a kernel of truth in the saying that General Motors is a healthcare company that also happens to make cars. Were it not for the availability of health insurance and government programs, only the wealthiest few would be able to afford quality health care. Even a regular visit to a doctor's office can cost hundreds of dollars when we consider the doctor's fees, lab fees, diagnostic tests—and office staff, rent (or mortgage and real estate tax costs if the physicians own the premises of their practice), and malpractice insurance. Costs for hospitalization and surgery can quickly spiral to five or six figures, although people who receive coverage for these services may pay only a nominal amount of the bill and sometimes nothing at all.

Types of Health Insurance Programs

There are two general types of health insurance plans, an **indemnity insurance plan** and a **managed care plan**. Let's look under the hood of these different plans.

indemnity insurance plan A traditional insurance plan in which covered individuals can choose to see any approved healthcare provider for a set fee (copay) or proportion of the costs (typically 80%), after any deductibles are met, or seek services from an out-of-network provider at higher cost to the individual.

managed care plan Generally, a system of health care for managing healthcare costs, typically in the form of prepaid health insurance plan in which a health benefits company or a group of doctors or hospitals provide healthcare services to groups of employees on a capitated basis.

Indemnity Insurance Plan (also called a Fee-for-Service Plan)

This is a traditional health insurance plan offered by large insurance companies and by carriers like Blue Cross/Blue Shield. Under this traditional insurance plan, covered individuals can see any licensed physician or other healthcare provider within a network of registered providers for a set fee (copay) or proportion of the costs (typically 80% are covered), after any deductibles are met, or seek services from an out-of-network provider, which typically incurs a higher fee or lower proportion of reimbursed expenses. These plans also provide coverage for approved hospital stays and surgical or other medical tests and procedures. As companies try to constrain healthcare costs, fewer workers, about 1 in 4 today, are covered by these types of traditional plans that provide flexibility in choice of doctors and medical care services. Most workers today are covered under company-sponsored managed care plans.

Managed Care Plan

In a managed care plan, also called a prepaid health insurance plan, a health benefits company or a group of doctors or hospitals agree to provide healthcare services to groups of employees on a "capitated" basis, meaning that they charge a set premium for each member or enrollee. Once enrolled, members can access medical services from a list of approved providers or clinics, paying a modest copay for each medical visit. Typically, few if any deductibles need to be met. Large employers may pay the annual premium as a benefit of employment or pass along some portion of the premium to employees. Members who decide to use a doctor who is not on the plan's list of approved healthcare providers can expect to pay more of the bill or the entire bill.

Managed care plans are based on the assumption that employers can reduce costs while still providing quality care by contracting to provide access to medical care on a capitated basis. It may be more accurate to describe these programs as managed cost plans than managed care plans, as they are focused more on managing the costs of health care than providing medical services. Ever focused on the financial bottom line, some managed care plans may reward doctors for limiting their use of outside specialists and expensive medical tests. The two most common types of managed care plans are PPOs and HMOs.

Preferred Provider Organization

In a **PPO**, a group of physicians or other healthcare providers (HCPs) who want to ensure a steady stream of referrals agrees to provide healthcare services to members of a managed care group at reduced rates, typically 15–20% lower than their customary rates. Members see HCPs in their regular offices as they would for a conventional fee-for-service plan, and the HCPs are free to see other patients who are not on the plan. The plan member only pays a modest co-payment and deductibles for approved medical services. Members are free to see a HCP outside the PPO, but will pay additional costs.

preferred provider organization (PPO) A group of healthcare providers who agree to provide health care to members of a managed care plan on a discounted basis.

health maintenance organization (HMO) A managed healthcare plan that provides members with a choice of providers within a network of affiliated physicians and hospitals or freestanding clinics, with costs based on a fixed amount for each enrolled member.

staff model A type of HMO offering comprehensive healthcare services to members of the plan within a freestanding clinic or health center that employs its own healthcare providers.

point-of-service (POS) plan A type of HMO offering members a choice of doctors within its network of approved providers or out-of-network physicians at a higher cost.

Health Maintenance Organizations More than half of employees today are members of an **HMO**, which is a prepaid medical service plan in which services are offered through a network of affiliated doctors and hospitals or freestanding clinics. There are two general types of HMOs, a *staff model* and a *point-of-service* model.

The traditional model of an HMO is based on a **staff model** in which a company-operated clinic or healthcare facility provides a range of medical and related services directly to members of the plan and their families. The HCPs on staff are limited to treating only members of the HMO. The major limitation of the traditional HMO is that it limits the ability of members to choose doctors who are not members of the HMO. To provide a wider range of choices of HCPs, a HMO may be structured as a **point-of-service (POS) plan**, in which members can choose either to use HCPs within the plan or to seek a provider who is outside the network for a higher per-visit charge.

Health psychologists and other health professionals help patients sort through the different types of insurance plans and government health programs for which they are eligible to ensure that they can find a program best suited to their healthcare needs. Informed healthcare consumers need to be aware of the potential pitfalls of managed care programs to avoid mismanaged care (see Table 3.4).

Medical professionals also need to be mindful of the rights of healthcare consumers, such as those listed in the American Medical Association's bill of rights for members of HMOs and other managed care plans (see Table 3.5). A qualifier is in order here, as the "bill of rights" lists the expectations that physicians are expected to meet, but it does not carry the force of law.

TABLE 3.4 Avoiding Mismanaged Care

Healthcare consumers need to take an active role in managing their healthcare needs and guarding against mismanaged care. To do so, they should:

- *Discuss coverage for hospital stays:* When planning a surgical procedure or expensive medical test, consumers should find out in advance what costs are involved and the extent to which the managed care company covers them.
- *Insist on seeing a specialist:* If a health condition requires a specialist but the person's healthcare plan requires that the person's regular HCP refer the person for a visit to a specialist, people can insist that their conditions be reviewed to justify the need.
- *Learn in advance what to do in case of emergencies:* When faced with a medical crisis or emergency, the person's first concern should be getting proper care, not haggling over costs with the managed care company. But before a need for emergency services arises, consumers can take the time to learn about their plan's coverage for emergency care.
- *Appeal refusal of coverage:* If coverage for services is denied, healthcare consumers have a right to file an appeal. (The appeal process is usually described in the plan's handbook.) Taking an active role in the process, the consumer should document the need for services and include supporting documents from physicians involved in their care regarding the need for the services. If an appeal is denied, the consumer may still have recourse to appeal to the employer's benefits manager. Failing that, a consumer can file a formal complaint with the department of insurance in the state in which the consumer resides. Sometimes a consumer may need to hire a lawyer specializing in these types of cases.

TABLE 3.5 A Healthcare Bill of Rights for Managed Care Patients

- The healthcare provider is required to place the patient's interests first.
- The healthcare provider is required to push for care that will benefit the patient's health.
- The healthcare provider is required to discuss all treatment options, even options not covered by the plan. The patient can then decide whether or not to appeal for coverage of an uncovered option or to go outside the plan.
- There should be established adequate means appealing disputes.
- Plans should disclose limitations or restrictions in coverage to prospective members deciding whether or not to join.
- Plans should not encourage or permit substandard care.
- Plans should disclose incentives to healthcare providers that limit care.
- Plans should limit the incentives healthcare providers receive for limiting care.

Source: Adapted from S. Rosenbaum (2003). Managed care and patients' rights. *Journal of the American Medical Association*, 289, 906–907.

Applying Health Psychology

Managing Your Own Health Care

You've learned about the concept of managed care. What you may not realize is that you are responsible for managing your own health care—wisely.

Some people are passive healthcare consumers. They wait until they get sick to seek health care or learn about healthcare options. They may carry an insurance card but know little about the services covered by their plan. Passive healthcare consumers typically do not get the best health care. They do not obtain regular physical examinations that might prevent the development of serious and costly medical conditions or reduce their severity.

Passive healthcare consumers may see the healthcare system as too complicated to understand. Their beliefs undercut their motivation to manage their own health care—beliefs such as "I prefer to leave medical matters in the hands of my doctor," "I do not really care what it costs, my insurance will cover it anyway," and "I assume that all healthcare providers are competent and have my best interests at heart."

In contrast, people who take an active role in managing their health care ask their healthcare providers questions—plenty of them—to ensure they get the best quality care. They see themselves, and not their HCPs or their insurance carriers, as ultimately responsible for managing their own health care. They take steps to protect themselves from mismanaged care.

What about you? Are you an active or a passive healthcare consumer? Evaluate whether you actively manage your own health care by completing the Self-Assessment on page 69. Then ask yourself what changes you can make in your attitudes and behavior to get the most out of your health care.

Deciding When to Seek Help

Being a rugged individual is fine—as long as you remain rugged. Part of responsible management of your health is knowing when not to go it alone. Here are some suggestions for when to seek help:

- If you experience sudden pain that doesn't fade quickly.
- If you have symptoms you don't understand that do not go away on their own, such as a persistent burning sensation when you urinate, a rash that does not fade, or any kind of unexplained pain.
- If you experience unexplained pain in the chest or in an arm or a shoulder, especially when accompanied by shortness of breath.
- If you have had an accident—or have been assaulted!—and you are experiencing loss of blood, sizable lacerations (cuts) of the skin, difficulty breathing, difficulty moving, loss of consciousness, or difficulty remaining awake and alert.
- If you are having persistent or recurrent diarrhea.
- If you are experiencing an unexplained loss of weight or unexplained changes in your sleeping habits.
- If your nail beds, lips, mouth, or skin take on a bluish color.
- If you are experiencing unexplained bleeding or a discharge from a body opening.
- If your temperature spikes or if you have a persistent or recurrent fever.
- If you feel a lump under your skin, or swelling, or a sore that grows or does not fade away.
- If you believe that you are pregnant, or if an over-the-counter test kit shows that you are pregnant.
- If a healthcare provider recommends a schedule for certain kinds of checkups and the time has come.
- If a healthcare provider recommends further workup of a symptom or a condition.

Early diagnosis and treatment of problems is most likely to lead to a cure or, depending on what is wrong, control of an unhealthful condition or a disease. Generally speaking, men in our society may be more reluctant than women to seek help. Men may see themselves as being "take charge" kinds of guys—but not necessarily when it comes to being active about their health care. Working to loosen the effects of traditional gender roles on health care empowers both men and women to become active healthcare consumers.

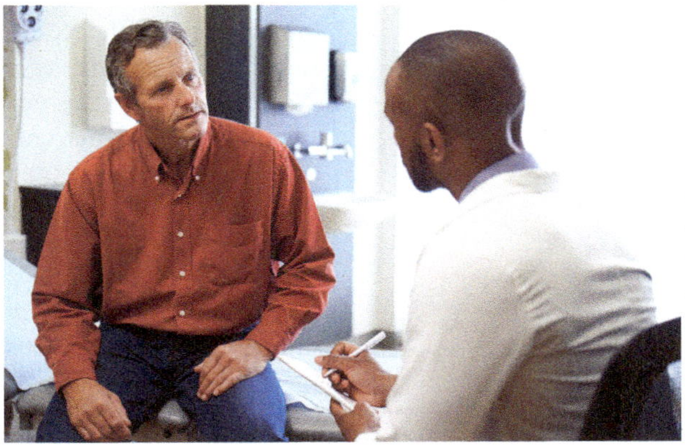

monkeybusinessimages/ Getty Images

Becoming an Active Healthcare Consumer Active healthcare consumers ask questions of the healthcare providers to help ensure they get the best quality care.

Review 3.3

INTERACTIVE SELF-SCORING QUIZZES

Sentence Completion

1. The healthcare system (is or is not) an organized system for meeting the nation's healthcare needs.

2. The three general types of healthcare programs providing access to healthcare services and helping to offset costs are: (1) private health insurance programs; (2) __________ health insurance programs; and (3) __________ health programs.

3. The United States spends (more or less) on health care (as a percentage of gross domestic product) than any other of the world's leading economically developed countries.

4. Annual Healthcare spending in the United States amounts to more than $__________ for every man, woman, and child.

5. An __________ insurance medical plan is also called a fee-for-service plan.

6. In a __________ care plan, which is also called a prepaid health insurance plan, a health benefits company or a group of doctors or hospitals agree to provide healthcare services to groups of employees on a capitated basis.

7. Managed care plans are based on the assumption that they can reduce __________ while still providing quality care.

8. The two most common types of managed care plans are __________ provider organizations and health maintenance organizations.

9. The traditional model of an HMO is based on a __________ model in which medical services are offered within a company-operated clinic or healthcare facility.

10. An HMO may be structured as a __________-service (POS) plan, in which members can choose either to use HCPs within the plan or to seek a provider who is outside the network on a higher per-visit charge.

Think About It

What type of health insurance plan best suits your healthcare needs? What do you like about your current health insurance plan (if you have one)? What don't you like?

Complementary and Alternative Medicine

Many people use alternative methods of treatment that lie outside conventional medicine. These methods are collectively called *complementary and alternative medicine* (CAM), and they range from homespun remedies and dietary supplements to prayer to healing methods practiced in various folk cultures across the world, especially in the Far East.

complementary medicine Alternative techniques used along with conventional medicine, such as dietary supplements.

alternative medicine Alternative ways of healing used in place of conventional medicine.

To clarify our terms, **complementary medicine** is the use of alternative methods of health alongside conventional medicine, as in the case of a cancer patient who undergoes chemotherapy and also turns to prayer or spiritual healing. **Alternative medicine** is practiced in place of conventional medicine, as when patients who have been diagnosed with cancer opt for radical changes in their diets rather than recommended surgery. Alternative medicine carries a significant risk, as patients may forgo conventional therapies in favor of alternative methods that might be unproven or—in the case of tackling cancer by dietary changes—lethal.

The government watchdog agency for CAM, the National Center for Complementary and Integrative Health (NCCIH), offers sound advice when it comes to use of complementary or alternative methods, as well as use of prescription or over-the-counter (OTC) medications (NCCIH, 2015). They encourage patients to speak directly with their healthcare providers about any treatments, conventional or otherwise, that they are using or considering to ensure that they are safe and are integrated with other aspects of their general healthcare plan.

integrative medicine Efforts to integrate conventional and alternative medicine in a coordinated fashion.

Americans spend billions of dollars annually on CAM, but is the money well spent? Some alternative forms of treatment are at least partially supported by scientific research, but others have scant, if any, evidence supporting their effectiveness. Researchers also raise concerns about the safety of alternative methods, especially those involving use of dietary supplements that are not subject to the same oversight as prescription medication.

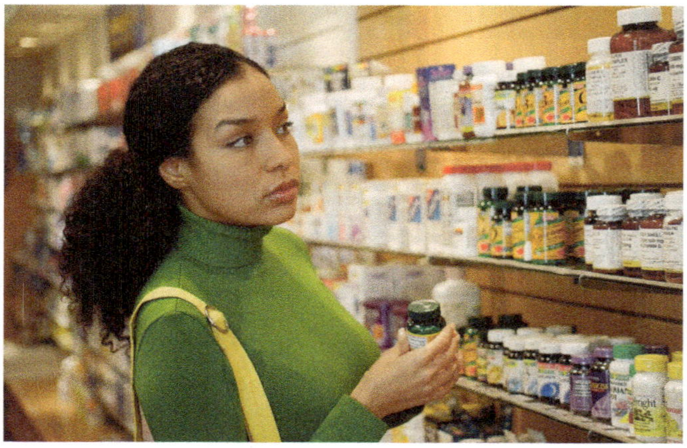

Hill Street Studios/Getty Images

Thinking about CAM? About 4 in 10 Americans use some form of CAM. Should you? What are the questions you should ask before using a complementary or alternative method of improving your health?

Integrative medicine combines conventional and complementary treatment methods in a coordinated fashion, as when a physician prescribes pain medications to a person with migraine headaches but also refers the person for biofeedback training for pain relief as an additional avenue of treatment. Integrative methods of health care tend to adopt a *holistic approach* that focuses on many aspects of the person's physical, mental, emotional, spiritual, social, and occupational functioning. The effort is placed on treating the whole person, not just a particular organ system or disease process.

As medical science continues to evolve, some of the alternative treatments of today may become established medical practice tomorrow. For example, healthcare providers are incorporating some forms of complementary treatment in their regular practice, such as exercise programs to treat depression, heart disease, and diabetes. Practitioners are also using meditation and hypnosis in treating stress-related

TABLE 3.6 Research Evidence Supporting Uses of CAM

- In a study of 60 women who survived breast cancer, women who used hypnosis reduced the number and severity of hot flashes and also reported improvements in mood and sleep.
- A study of 63 people with rheumatoid arthritis found that mindfulness-based stress reduction helped to improve quality of life and reduce psychological distress.
- A study of 298 college students found that transcendental meditation helped students reduce stress and improve coping strategies.
- In a study of 50 women, regular practice of yoga benefited mood and physiological response to stress.
- People with fibromyalgia may benefit from practicing tai chi, according to a study of 66 people. Study participants who practiced tai chi had a significantly greater decrease in total score on the Fibromyalgia Impact Questionnaire. In addition, the tai chi group demonstrated greater improvement in sleep quality, mood, and quality of life.
- Tai chi may also be a safe alternative to conventional exercise for maintaining bone mineral density in postmenopausal women, thus helping to prevent or slow osteoporosis, increase musculoskeletal strength, and improve balance.

Source: National Center for Complementary and Integrative Health. (2019). National Institutes of Health, *Mind–Body Medicine Practices in Complementary and Alternative Medicine.* http://nccam.nih.gov/Public Domain.

disorders and chronic pain (Schwenk, 2019). Table 3.6 lists examples of research evidence supporting particular forms of CAM.

Researchers have also looked at the health benefits of prayer and religion. A survey of some 5,100 Americans 40+ years of age showed that nearly half (47.2%) reported praying for health and 90% believed that prayer had a positive health effect (O'Connor et al., 2005). We should caution that these surveys tap perceptions, not direct evidence of health benefits of the "power of prayer." We do have evidence connecting attendance at religious services with more positive health outcomes (see Chen & VanderWeele, 2019; Suh et al., 2019). In one illustrative example, Blacks who attended religious services more than once a week outlived those who never attended church by 13–14 years (Marks et al., 2005). Other research also links religious attendance to healthier outcomes, including a longer life. But as critical thinkers, we need to examine the evidence more carefully. This correlational evidence cannot pinpoint cause and effect. It could be that the personality characteristics that lead people to attend church regularly are linked with healthier behavior patterns, such as adhering to medical advice, avoiding harmful habits such as smoking and excessive drinking, and maintaining social relationships.

Who Uses CAM?

Nearly 40% of adult Americans reported using some form of CAM during the previous 12 months (NCCIH, 2017). Women are more likely to use CAM, as are older adults. CAM is most popular among adults aged 50–69 years (NCCIH, 2015). Among people using CAM, most report they used these methods to prevent illness or for overall wellness (77%), to reduce pain or treat painful conditions (73%), to treat a specific health condition (59%), or to supplement conventional medicine (53%) (NCCIH, 2015).

What Types of CAM Do People Use Most Often?

Figure 3.6 shows the most commonly used forms of CAM. Use of herbal products or dietary supplements tops the list, followed by deep breathing, yoga and other East Asian practices, chiropractic manipulation, and meditation and massage. Types of CAM are listed in Table 3.7.

Should You Use CAM?

The National Center for Complementary and Integrative Health of the National Institutes of Health offers advice about using CAM. It reflects the issues health psychologists are likely to address with their clients—issues relating to obtaining trustworthy health information and thinking critically about health decisions:

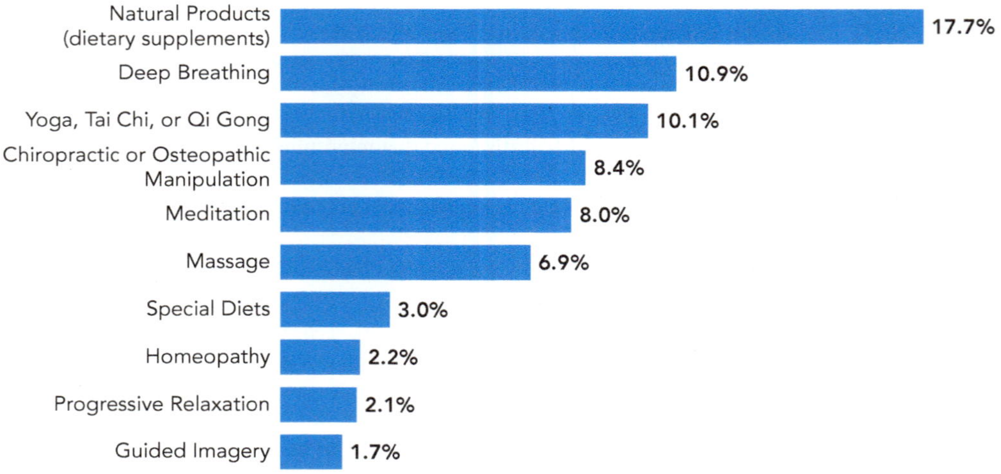

FIGURE 3.6 **10 Most Common Complementary Health Approaches Among Adults**

Source: National Center for Complementary and Integrative Health. (NCCIH) (2021). https://www.nccih.nih.gov/health/complementary-alternative-or-integrative-health-whats-in-a-name/Public Domain.

TABLE 3.7 **Types of Complementary and Alternative Medicine**

INTERACTIVE FIGURES, CHARTS, & TABLES

Type of CAM	About
Alternative medical systems	Alternative medical systems are complete systems of theory and practice that often developed earlier than conventional American medicine. Systems that developed in Western cultures include homeopathic medicine and naturopathic medicine. Systems that have developed in non-Western cultures include traditional Chinese methods, including acupuncture, and ayurveda.
Mind–body interventions	Mind–body techniques attempt to enhance the mind's ability to enhance bodily function and relieve symptoms. Some techniques that were once considered CAM, such as cognitive behavioral therapy and patient-support groups, have become part of the mainstream. Other mind–body techniques are still classified as CAM, such as meditation; mental healing; prayer; and art, music, or dance therapies.
Biologically based therapies	Biologically-based CAM therapies use natural substances, such as foods, herbs, and vitamins. Examples include dietary supplements, herbal products, and scientifically unproven methods, such as treating cancer with shark cartilage. But some dietary supplements are now mainstream, such as the use of folic acid to prevent certain birth defects or the use of vitamins and zinc to retard the development of the eye disease age-related macular degeneration.
Manipulative and body-based methods	Manipulative and body-based methods include chiropractic or osteopathic manipulation and massage.
Energy therapies	Energy therapies use energy fields. "Biofield therapies" aim to affect energy fields that are thought to surround and penetrate the body but whose existence remains unproven. Qi gong, Reiki, and therapeutic touch attempt to manipulate "biofields" by pressure on or manipulation of the body. Bioelectromagnetic-based methods are the unconventional use of electromagnetic fields, such as magnetic fields, pulsed fields, or alternating-current or direct-current fields.
Acupuncture	Developed in ancient China, the term "acupuncture" today describes procedures involving stimulation of anatomical points on the body. American acupuncture incorporates medical traditions from China, Japan, Korea, and other countries. The acupuncture technique that has been most studied scientifically involves penetrating the skin with thin, solid, metallic needles that are manipulated by the hands or by electrical stimulation. According to the National Center for Complementary and Integrative Health of NIH, acupuncture may help ease some types of chronic pain.
Aromatherapy	Use of oils (extracts or essences) from flowers, herbs, and trees to promote health and well-being.
Ayurveda	An alternative medical system that has been practiced primarily in the Indian subcontinent for 5,000 years. Ayurveda includes diet and herbal remedies and emphasizes the use of body, mind, and spirit in prevention and treatment of disease.

(Continued)

TABLE 3.7 Types of Complementary and Alternative Medicine (*Continued*)

Type of CAM	About
Biofeedback	Use of specialized equipment to provide people with information ("feedback") about their internal bodily states or activities, such as heart rate, muscle tension, and body temperature. Feedback may be provided in the form of tones that increase or decrease in pitch in relation to changes in internal bodily states. By learning to change the tone in the desired direction (making it rise or lower in pitch, e.g., as a measure of muscle tension), people may learn to induce states of relaxation by relaxing selected muscle groups or by increasing the frequency of certain brain wave patterns. Biofeedback is commonly used to treat hypertension, headaches, and stress.
Chiropractic	An alternative medical system that focuses on the relationship between bodily structure (primarily the spine) and function, and how that relationship can preserve and restore health. Chiropractors use manipulative therapy as a treatment tool.
Natural products (dietary supplements)	Products taken orally that contain a "dietary ingredient" intended to supplement the diet. Ingredients include vitamins, minerals, herbs or other botanicals, amino acids, enzymes, organ tissues, and metabolites. They come in many forms, including extracts, concentrates, tablets, capsules, gel caps, liquids, and powders. Under the Dietary Supplement Health and Education Act, dietary supplements are considered foods, not drugs, but they have special requirements for labeling.
Electromagnetic fields	Invisible lines of force that surround electrical devices or are produced by geological forces are sometimes used to reduce pain.
Homeopathic	An alternative medical system based on a belief that "like cures like," meaning that small, diluted quantities of medicinal substances can cure symptoms, when the same substances given at higher or more concentrated doses would cause the symptoms.
Massage	Manipulation of muscle and connective tissue to enhance function of those tissues and promote relaxation and well-being. 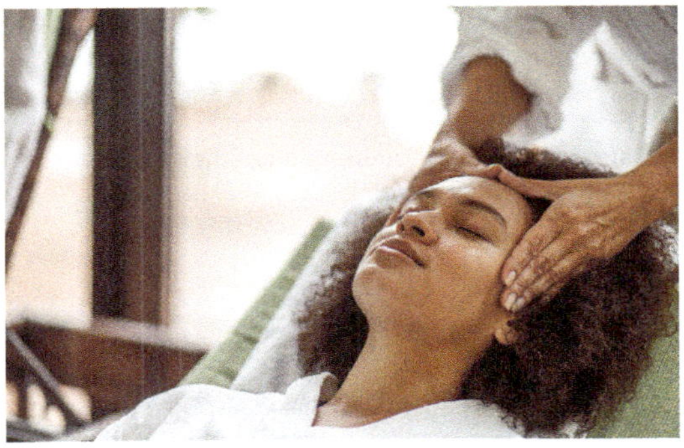 fotostorm/Getty Images
Meditation	Induction of relaxation by focusing attention on some activity, object, or image. In some cultures, meditation is believed to help people achieve spiritual or creative enlightenment. Traditional medicine has increasingly come to accept meditation to combat stress and high blood pressure.
Naturopathic medicine or naturopathy	An alternative medical system that proposes that there is a healing power in the body that establishes, maintains, and restores health. Practitioners work with people with a goal of supporting this power, through treatments such as nutrition and lifestyle counseling, dietary supplements, medicinal plants, exercise, homeopathy, and treatments from traditional Chinese medicine.
Osteopathic medicine	A form of conventional medicine emphasizing diseases arising in the musculoskeletal system. There is an underlying belief that the body's systems work together and disturbances in one system may affect others. Some osteopathic physicians practice osteopathic manipulation, a full-body system of hands-on techniques to alleviate pain, restore function, and promote health and well-being.
Prayer	The act of making a reverent petition to God or another object of worship (to prevent health problems or restore health).
Qi gong ("chee-GUNG")	A component of traditional Chinese medicine that combines movement, meditation, and regulation of breathing, which is believed to enhance the flow of qi (believed to be vital energy) in the body, improve circulation, and enhance immune function.
Reflexology	Manipulation of pressure points on the hands and feet to relieve stress and pain.

(*Continued*)

TABLE 3.7 Types of Complementary and Alternative Medicine (*Continued*)

Type of CAM	About
Reiki ("RAY-kee")	A traditional Japanese method based on the belief that when spiritual energy is channeled through a Reiki practitioner, a person's spirit is healed, which in turn heals the body.
Therapeutic touch	Also called laying-on of hands, a method based on the beliefs that (1) the healing force of the therapist affects a person's recovery; (2) healing is promoted when the body's energies are in balance; and (3) by passing their hands over someone, healers can identify energy imbalances.
Traditional Chinese medicine	An ancient system of health care based on a concept of balanced qi (pronounced "chee"), or vital energy, that is believed to flow throughout the body. Qi is proposed to regulate a person's spiritual, emotional, mental, and physical balance and to be influenced by the opposing forces of yin (negative energy) and yang (positive energy). Disease is proposed to result from disruption of the flow of qi and the imbalance of yin and yang. Methods include herbal and nutritional therapy, physical exercises, meditation, acupuncture, and massage.
Visualization	 Zenith Pictures/Shutterstock.com Use of mental imagery to alter bodily functions, such as heart rate and blood pressure. Like meditation, visualization (such as by mentally picturing oneself lying on a warm, tropical beach) can help people achieve a relaxed state, which can calm the nervous system and lower the heart and breathing rates. People in pain may use mental imagery to detach themselves from their pain.

Note: The listing of these complementary and alternative treatments is not an endorsement of their effectiveness or safety. As always, it is good advice to consult with a qualified health professional before beginning any nontraditional treatment.

Source: Adapted from NCCIH (2021).

- *Become an informed consumer:* Investigate the scientific literature to examine the results of scientific studies on the safety and effectiveness of CAM treatments before using them. You can search for scientific studies from reputable journals by using Google Scholar or by consulting your college or public librarian or course instructor.
- *Think critically about the source of information:* Ignore testimonials (anecdotes). Like online reviews of consumer products, testimonials may be planted or doctored. Even if genuine, they are impressionistic and don't measure up to scientific standards. One person's opinion is just that—an opinion—not scientific evidence. Also examine the source of the information. Was it vetted by a respected journal through a careful review process? Or does the information come from a manufacturer or marketing firm that stands to profit from people using the product or service?
- *Explore respected online sources for health-related information:* Trustworthy sources of information include professional organizations, such as the American Heart Association, the American Cancer Society, the American Diabetes Association, the various institutes of the National Institutes of Health, and leading universities or medical centers. Another helpful source of reliable information is the United States Food and Drug Administration (FDA), which provides health-related information about food products and dietary supplements (www.fda.gov). This is especially important for CAM products sold over the counter (without a prescription), such as dietary supplements. But be aware that the FDA does not require testing of dietary supplements prior to marketing. It can only remove items from the marketplace if they are shown to be dangerous.

- *Consult with your primary healthcare provider:* Your HCP is in the best position to evaluate your medical needs, history, and any conditions that might be impacted by use of CAM and to integrate any CAM methods within a comprehensive treatment plan.
- *If you decide to use a CAM practitioner, check out the person's credentials with care:* Check with your insurance carrier as to whether the services are covered. Check the person's credentials through your state or province's state licensing bureau or authority.

Review 3.4

INTERACTIVE SELF-SCORING QUIZZES

Sentence Completion

1. __________ medicine is the use of alternative methods of health alongside conventional medicine.

2. __________ medicine is practiced in place of conventional medicine.

3. __________ medicine combines conventional and complementary treatment methods in a coordinated fashion.

4. Integrative methods of health care often adopt a __________ approach.

5. In a large-scale survey, (30% or 90%) of respondents believed that prayer had a positive health effect.

6. In a study of women who survived breast cancer, hypnosis reduced the number and severity of __________ and improved mood and sleep.

7. Nearly (40% or 80%) of American adults report using some form of CAM during the previous 12 months.

8. The most commonly used form of CAM involves use of herbal products or dietary __________.

Think About It

Would you use CAM? Why or why not? If yes, what CAM would you be most likely to use? Is there evidence to support its effectiveness and safety?

Recite: An Active Summary

INTERACTIVE SELF-SCORING QUIZZES

Chapter 3 Practice Quiz

1. Define the concept of illness behavior and identify some of the determinants of health-seeking behavior.

The term "illness behavior" refers to how people respond to acute or chronic illness. It incorporates the experience of being ill as well as healthcare-seeking behavior. The determinants of illness behavior include psychological, social, and cultural factors as well as biological factors involved in disease processes. The determinants of health-seeking behavior include disease-related variables, patient-related variables, and healthcare system related variables.

2. Apply the common-sense model of self-regulation to understanding how people respond to physical illness.

Adopting a common-sense view of how people respond to illness, the CSM focuses on processes of self-regulation by which people manage their behaviors, emotions, and thoughts when they confront an acute or chronic illness. The model breaks down these responses in terms of two interlinking tracks, cognitive representations and emotional representations.

3. Describe health disparities in relation to income level and race or ethnicity.

People of lower socioeconomic status carry a disproportionate health burden with respect to increased rates of serious illness and higher mortality rates. Ethnic minority groups also carry a heavier health burden, which is partially explained by differences in income level across ethnic or racial groups but also by the stressful demands of discrimination, lack of access to health insurance, and unequal access to quality health care. Health disparities are narrowing but still persist.

4. Identify the major types of health insurance plans.

The major types of health insurance programs are (1) traditional indemnity insurance plans, which operate on a fee-for-service basis, and (2) managed care plans, which are prepaid health insurance plans organized as either a preferred provider organization (PPO) or a health maintenance organization (HMO). Fee structures and access to networks of providers vary across these types of insurance plans. The major types of healthcare programs are private health insurance programs, government health insurance programs (Medicare and Medicaid), and public health programs.

5. Distinguish between complementary and alternative medicine approaches to healing.

Complementary approaches to healing are alternative treatments that are used along with mainstream medical approaches, such as meditation and exercise programs. Alternative medicine is the use of healing practices in place of conventional medical approaches, which can incur risks as these treatments may be unproven or even harmful.

Answers to Review Sections

3.1

1. Illness
2. threat
3. lower
4. Common-Sense
5. self-regulation
6. coping
7. illness
8. decreased
9. acute illness

3.2

1. Poverty
2. smaller
3. less likely
4. do
5. lower-quality
6. discrimination
7. language

3.3

1. is not
2. government/public
3. more
4. 10,000
5. indemnity
6. managed
7. costs
8. preferred
9. staff
10. point-of

3.4

1. Complementary
2. Alternative
3. Integrative
4. holistic
5. 90%
6. hot flashes
7. 40%
8. supplements

Scoring Key for "Are You an Active or a Passive Healthcare Consumer?"

Statements in the left-hand column reflect a passive approach to managing your health care. Statements in the right-hand column represent an active approach. The more statements you circled in the right-hand column, the more active a role you take in managing your health care. For statements checked in the left-hand column, consider whether it is to your advantage to change your behavior to become an active rather than a passive healthcare consumer.

CHAPTER 4

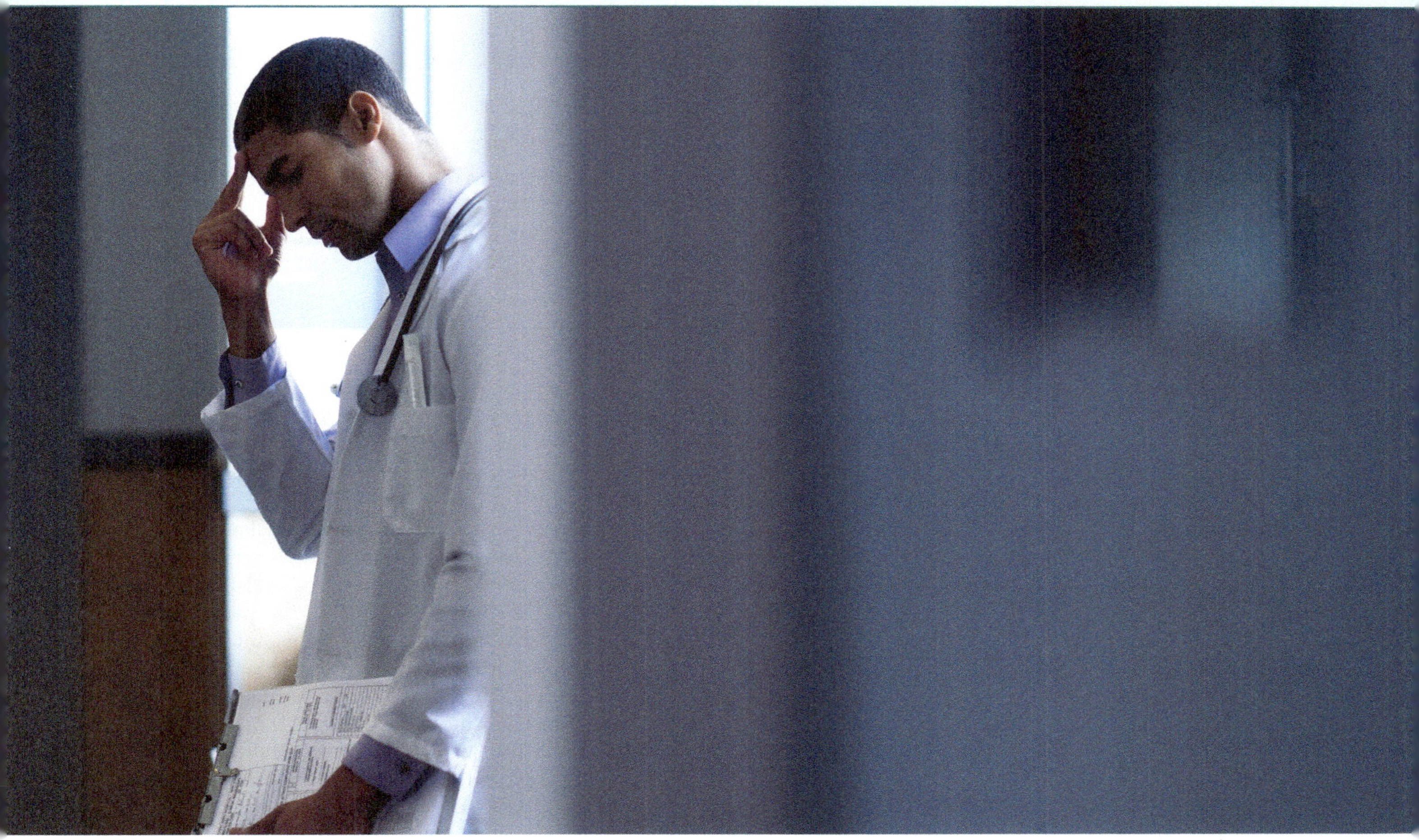

Tetra Images/Getty Images

Stress and the Immune System

LEARNING OBJECTIVES

After studying this chapter, you will be able to ...

1. **Define** *stress* and *eustress*.
2. **Discuss** stress as an event that requires adaptation.
3. **Discuss** other ways of thinking about stress—stress as a threat, as a situation in which demands exceed resources, and as an interruption of goals.
4. **Describe** the effects of stress on the body, focusing on the roles of the endocrine system and the autonomic nervous system.
5. **Discuss** the pathogens that serve as infectious agents.
6. **Describe** the functioning of the immune system.
7. **Discuss** the different types of immunity and the controversies surrounding vaccinations for measles and human papillomavirus.
8. **Discuss** immune system disorders.
9. **Discuss** common infectious diseases, referring to research concerning cortisol levels and vulnerability.

Did You Know That ...

- There may be *trillions* of species of viruses?
- We need some stress to keep ourselves alert and occupied?
- Generation Z is stressed out about mass shootings and global warming?
- Going on a first date and making new friends are sources of stress?
- Hot temperatures can make us hot under the collar—that is, trigger aggression?
- You can be literally wide-eyed with fear?
- Fear can give you indigestion?
- As you are reading this page, your body is engaged in search-and-destroy missions against foreign agents?
- You are more likely to contract the common cold when you are under stress?

There are nearly 7,000 named species of viruses, and there may be *trillions* of other species (Zimmer, 2020). (Yes—trillions of species.) Now and then a few cause widespread concern, as in the 1918 flu pandemic, Middle East respiratory syndrome, severe acute respiratory syndrome (SARS), and the seasonal flu.

COVID-19, another kind of SARS, proved to be at least 10 times as lethal as the seasonal flu. It is mainly characterized by fever, a cough, and shortness of breath. It arrived suddenly and overwhelmed the health systems of many countries throughout the world. People were told to wash their hands and to use hand sanitizers, but soon after the outbreak became known, there were shortages of hand sanitizers. There were shortages of test equipment, hospital beds, hospital gowns, protective masks, and ventilators, all contributing to the death toll. The world quickly learned the acronym PPE (personal protective equipment), which, as healthcare workers discovered, was in short supply. Ideal hospital conditions required isolation wards with separate rooms (Schwartz et al., 2020). These protective measures were not enough, and in some cases people with the virus simply walked into emergency departments, infecting hospital staff and causing them to quarantine themselves rather than be available to help others.

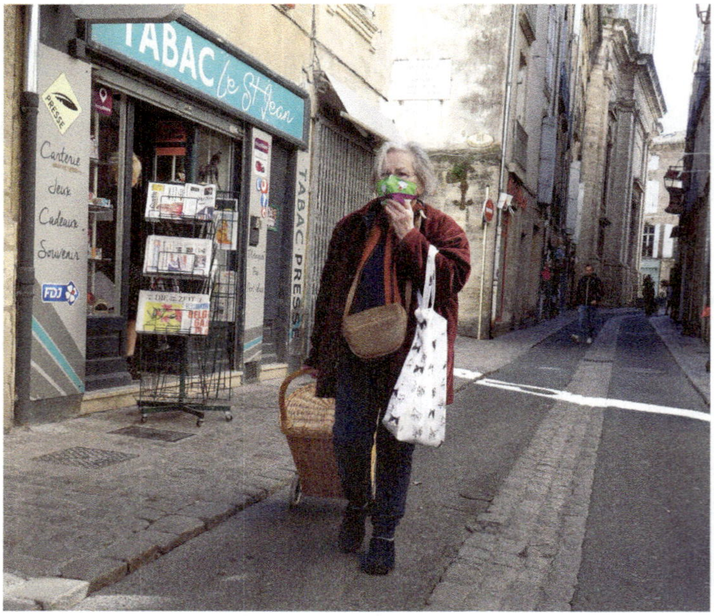

David Bagnall/Alamy Stock Photo

An older woman in France, wearing a protective face mask, does some essential food shopping on a nearly deserted street after the city was struck by COVID-19 progressed, rf.

State and local governments responded by closing schools, restaurants, bars, movie theaters, museums and other cultural venues, sports arenas, and cruise ships, while keeping grocery and drug stores open. The most open route for transmission of the virus was person to person, hand to hand, or by inhaling infected droplets shed by people exhaling. A new phrase became heard everywhere—social distancing. People stopped flying unless travel was necessary. At first people were advised to remain 3 feet apart, then 6 feet apart. Then people were told to work from home when they could and to avoid social gatherings. A great many sheltered in place in their homes, emerging masked, sometimes gloved, only to do necessary shopping—and to walk the dog.

pandemic A disease that is prevalent over a whole country or the world.

In Chapter 3, we learned about the Health Belief Model, which helps us understand health-related behavior changes during the **pandemic**. The HBM proposes that people are more likely to engage in healthful behavior when they feel they are in danger of contracting a disease, based on their beliefs about the severity of the disease and their own susceptibility. They evaluate the barriers to, and benefits from, their behavior, such as practicing social distancing. Cues to action and demographic factors also play key roles. Let's have a closer look at these factors.

COVID-19 poses a significant threat, especially to people who live in crowded urban conditions or college dormitories. Barriers to taking protective action involve factors such as the inconvenience of using gloves and masks and repeatedly washing one's hands. For many residential college students in the fall of 2020, a key barrier to avoid being infected was mingling with other students in dormitories, leading to surges of new cases on many campuses across the country (Watson et al., 2020).

Some of the obvious benefits of grappling with the inconveniences are remaining healthy and not infecting other people, including one's own family. Cues to action include statements by public health officials, politicians, and one's own healthcare providers. A major demographic factor is one's age; the younger one is, the more likely it is that one will survive if infected, and, consequently, the perceived personal risk may be seen as lower by younger people. During spring break of 2020, some young people cavorting on Miami Beach were interviewed. They said they didn't think they would get the disease and, if they got it, they'd be okay. But minimizing perceived risk can have unfortunate consequences to one's own health and the health of others.

Misconceptions such as these can be countered only by truthful, factual, scientific information from trusted communicators, including those from leading professional organizations, universities, and research institutes such as the National Institutes of Health. When the virus arrived in the United States, some politicians minimized its likely impact to avoid being blamed for it, whereas health professionals and other scientists were painting a very different and more serious picture (Fishel et al., 2020). To the credit of a majority of Americans, however, a poll taken in March 2020 found that 84% of Americans trusted statements by public health officials as compared with only 37% who believed what they heard from politicians (Montanaro, 2020).

COVID-19, like other epidemics and pandemics, places great stress upon healthcare workers, especially in hospital settings (American Medical Association, 2020; Huang et al., 2020). Not only do they fear being infected themselves, but they are also concerned about spreading the virus to their families and other people outside the hospital. The thought of possibly spreading the disease is also connected with feelings of guilt. The results of a study of nurses and nursing students found that women nurses self-reported more anxiety and fear than men did (Huang et al., 2020). Nurses who were not heavily impacted by anxiety tried to solve the problems they faced by using **problem-focused coping** (which we discuss in Chapter 5) to deal with their feelings.

problem-focused coping A method of dealing with stress that views stressors as problems to be solved rather than as insurmountable obstacles.

A Chinese hospital provided a model for how to handle stress among healthcare professionals and staff who were attempting to help people survive the pandemic (Chen et al., 2020). The hospital:

- Provided a place where staff could temporarily isolate themselves from their families and rest,
- Provided the quarantined staff with food and other living supplies,
- Helped the staff to make video records of their hospital activities and share them with their families to alleviate families' and staff members' concerns that their families were worried about them,
- Developed precise rules as to how to use protective measures,
- Provided leisure activities and training in how to use emotion-focused psychological methods of reducing stress,
- Provided psychological counseling for staff members, and
- Made security personnel available to help healthcare staff deal with uncooperative patients.

The Centers for Disease Control and Prevention (CDC, 2020b) offered some good health psychology advice to help us all deal with the stress of pandemics and other kinds of health crises:

- Take breaks from watching, reading, or listening to news stories about the problem, including social media. Endless exposure to such reports can be upsetting. Listen enough to become and remain informed, but don't let the problem become your entire life.

Health Psychology in the Digital Age

Telemedicine for Pandemics—Virtually Perfect?

Is telemedicine a key vehicle for helping health professionals tackle pandemics like the COVID-19 pandemic? Perhaps. Patients prioritize convenient and inexpensive care, and telemedicine might be just the ... tonic.

A major piece of the puzzle in responding to pandemics is "forward triage"; that is, sorting patients before they arrive en masse at emergency departments (Hollander & Carr, 2020). Telemedicine employs patients' smartphones or webcam-enabled computers to protect patients, clinicians, and the community at large from exposure. Telemedicine effectively screens patients away from sites in which they might infect others or in cases in which they were not infected but had symptoms, say, of the common cold, enabling them to keep their distance from sites in which they might themselves be infected with—in this case—COVID-19.

Using telemedicine, healthcare professionals can obtain detailed travel and exposure histories. Automated screening algorithms, in the form of apps, can also be part of an intake process. Such apps can also standardize screening patterns across providers.

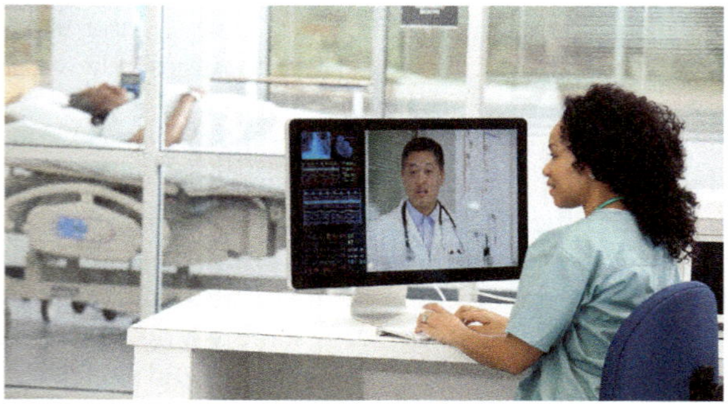
Ariel Skelley/Getty Images

A Nurse in a Telehealth Conference with a Physician.

Consider the scenario in which a patient arrives at a hospital screening center or an emergency department. Table computers, sanitized between patient use, can be used to isolate patients who appear to be infected in an exam room. Similar televisits enable patients to remain connected with family and friends at home, and social and emotional support are vital in the effort to promote recovery.

- Take care of your body. Take deep breaths, stretch, or meditate. Try to eat healthy, well-balanced meals, exercise regularly, get plenty of sleep, and avoid alcohol and drugs.
- Make time to unwind. Try to engage in some activities you enjoy, like watching an old movie.
- Social and emotional support is extremely valuable in a crisis. Connect with other people in your lives: Call them, text them, email them, and connect with them on social media or video calling. Share your concerns and your feelings with people you trust.

Pandemics are extreme sources of stress, but there are many other sources of stress, including run-of-the-mill stressors that may not be as threatening or taxing in the moment but accumulate over time to weigh on our lives and impair our ability to cope. Stress is a major topic in the study of health psychology. In this chapter we examine the sources of stress, how stress affects the body, and the role of stress in infection and immunity.

VIDEO CONTENT
Stress

stress The physical and psychological pressure experienced as a result of events that make demands on an organism to adapt.

Stress

Just what is **stress**? In physics, stress is the pressure or force exerted on a body or object. Tons of rock crushing the earth, one car smashing into another, a rubber band stretching—all are types of physical stress. Psychological forces, or stresses, also press, push, or pull. We may feel "crushed" by the weight of a big decision, "smashed" by adversity, or "stretched" to the point of snapping. We may encounter high levels of stress daily in the form of demands involved in juggling school, work, and family responsibilities; caring for infirm relatives; or coping with financial adversity or health problems. Let's consider various ways of looking at stress, as suggested by health psychology researcher Sheldon Cohen and his colleagues (2019).

Stress as a Demand That Requires Adaptation

Many sources of stress place demands on an organism to adapt, cope, or adjust. The implication is that stress is cumulative, so that the more changes in life circumstances that one experiences, the more stressful life they become. From this perspective, positive changes are also stressful. For example, graduating from college, obtaining a new job, dating a new person or deciding to live together with a partner, and even going on vacation are all life changes that require adaptation.

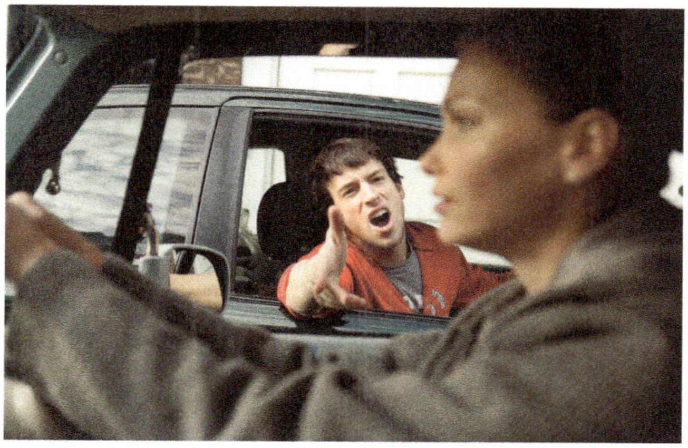
Dimitri Otis/Photodisc/Getty Images

Famed stress researcher Hans Selye (1956; Szabo et al., 2012) noted that some stress is necessary and healthful in that it keeps us alert, focused, and occupied. He referred to such positive stress as **eustress** (pronounced YOU-stress). Selye also hypothesized that intense or prolonged stress can overtax our physical and psychological resources, making us more vulnerable to stress-related disorders, such as digestive ailments, cardiovascular disorders, and depression. He referred to such disorders as "diseases of adaptation" (Selye, 1946).

eustress Healthful stress.

Extending the example of the advent of COVID-19, the virus required many adaptations in daily life, such as wearing protective masks and gloves, maintaining at least 6 feet of distance from others, sheltering in place (meaning not leaving home unless necessary), ordering in food or shopping very carefully and being mindful of others, working from home or adjusting to being laid off, and on and on.

It's not just adjusting to a pandemic that is stressful. Even the ordinary hassles of daily life and life changes that occur from time to time also require adaptation.

Daily Hassles

Which straw will break the camel's back? The last straw, according to the saying. Similarly, stresses can pile up until we can no longer cope with them. Some of these stresses, as listed by the American Psychological Association (APA, 2017), are **daily hassles**; that is, annoyances of daily life, such as traffic congestion and shopping, that we all face but which can add up to a point that it overtaxes our ability to cope. Evidence links hassles to health complaints among undergraduate students (Tran et al., 2021). Psychologist Richard Lazarus and his colleagues (1985) analyzed responses to a scale that measures daily hassles and their opposites—**uplifts**—and found that daily hassles could be grouped as follows:

daily hassles Routine, stressful sources of annoyance or aggravation.

uplifts Lazarus's term for regularly occurring enjoyable experiences.

1. Household hassles: preparing meals, shopping, and home maintenance
2. Health hassles: physical illness, concern about medical treatment, and side effects of medication
3. Time-pressure hassles: having too many things to do, too many responsibilities, and not enough time
4. Inner-concern hassles: being lonely and fearful of confrontations
5. Environmental hassles: crime, neighborhood deterioration, and traffic noise
6. Financial responsibility hassles: concern about owing money, such as mortgage payments and loan installments (reported by 62% in a Stress in America survey conducted by the APA)
7. Work hassles: job dissatisfaction, not liking one's duties at work, and problems with coworkers (61%)
8. Future security hassles: concerns about job security, taxes, property investments, stock market swings, and retirement

Life Changes

Another type of stress involves substantial changes in our life situation, whether positive or negative. The impact of life changes can make us wonder whether too much of a good thing can make us ill. You might think that marrying Mr. or Ms. Right, finding a prestigious job, and moving to a better neighborhood all in the same year would propel you into a state of bliss. They might. But the impact of these events, one on top of the other, can also lead to headaches, high blood pressure, and asthma. As pleasant as they may be, they all

life changes Notable changes in life circumstances, such as getting married, starting (or losing) a job, or losing a loved one.

involve **life changes**, and, as Hans Selye noted, change can be a source of stress. Life changes differ from daily hassles in two ways:

1. Many life changes are positive and desirable. Hassles, by definition, are negative.
2. Hassles occur regularly. Life changes occur at more irregular intervals.

Some life changes are more stressful than others. As you see in the Self-Assessment, negative changes, such as sexual assault or the death of a friend or family member, impose much greater burdens than positive changes, such as making new friends or attending a football game.

Investigators find that people who experience more life changes during a given period of time are more likely to develop physical conditions that are recognized as risk factors for the onset of cardiovascular disease (Steptoe & Kivimaki, 2013). Experiencing stressful life changes, especially enduring changes such as significant academic issues or problems in interpersonal relationships, also increase the likelihood of being infected by pathogens, such as viruses and bacteria (Cohen, 2016; Cohen et al., 2019).

The quality of the relationship with an intimate partner is another factor that may contribute to a person's stress level. Frequent criticism and bickering between intimate partners are sources of stress that can have negative effects on health. Researchers find that negative relationship quality, most notably in the form of criticism from one's spouse or partner, increases the risk of death among older adults (Bookwala & Gaugler, 2020).

Stress as Threat or Harm

Yet other stressors are events that are seen as harmful or threatening (Cohen et al., 2019). The imminence of the harm, its intensity, its duration, and the extent to which the threat is perceived to be beyond our control all contribute to the magnitude of the stress it entails. Again, COVID-19, of course, qualifies as a harmful threat, indeed a death threat. Assault and battery, wars, intimate partner violence—all are sources of stress resulting from harm. Threats to our self-esteem and negative social evaluation also make the list of stressors that are harmful.

Pain(!) Pain may be the clearest source of stress we can experience. Not only is pain discomforting on its own, but it also threatens worse things to come, for example, as a symptom of an illness. Most pain is transient, as when you are injured or have a toothache, but for 50 million American adults, chronic pain, especially headaches and backaches, can be unrelenting day after agonizing day (Dahlhamer et al., 2018). The rates of pain are higher among women, people who are older, and people who are obese. Additional sources of chronic pain include arthritis; back or joint pain; carpal tunnel syndrome; pain in tendons, nerves, muscles, and ligaments; and sore feet. About two of three people with chronic pain say their pain is constantly present, and about half say their pain is sometimes unbearable (Kennedy et al., 2014; Nashin, 2015). But it is estimated that more than 126 million American adults have had at least some pain in the last 3 months (Nashin, 2015).

We discuss pain in depth in Chapter 6.

Racism and Discrimination Exposure to racism and discrimination represent an important source of daily stress for immigrant and ethnic minority groups, which can impact their emotional and physical health and well-being (Anderson et al., 2020; Curci et al., 2023; Mekawi et al., 2021; Seaton & Zeiders, 2021). Researchers find that exposure to discrimination in the form of unfair treatment almost instantly triggers a burst of stress hormones released into the bloodstream (Ortega, 2021). Over time, the oversecretion of stress hormones can wear down the cardiovascular and immune systems, leading to the development of stress-related disorders.

Health psychologists find that maintaining strong family connections helps counter the negative emotional effects of frequent exposure to discrimination (Curci

Self-Assessment

INTERACTIVE SELF-ASSESSMENTS

How Much Stress Have You Experienced?

How stressful is your life? The College Life Stress Inventory provides a measure of stress associated with life changes or events that college students may encounter. Circle each of the events that you have experienced during the past 12 months, then sum the stress ratings for each of the circled responses to yield a total score. The scoring key at the end of the chapter can help you interpret your score.

	Life Change	(✓) Experienced During Past Year	Life Event Stress Rating
1.	Being raped		100
2.	Finding out that you are HIV-positive		100
3.	Being accused of rape		98
4.	Death of a close friend		97
5.	Death of a close family member		96
6.	Contracting a sexually transmitted infection (other than HIV/AIDS)		94
7.	Concerns about being pregnant		91
8.	Finals week		90
9.	Concerns about your partner being pregnant		90
10.	Oversleeping for an exam		89
11.	Flunking a class		89
12.	Having a boyfriend or girlfriend cheat on you		85
13.	Ending a steady dating relationship		85
14.	Serious illness in a close friend or family member		85
15.	Financial difficulties		84
16.	Writing a major term paper		83
17.	Being caught cheating on a test		83
18.	Drunk driving		82
19.	Sense of overload in school or work		82
20.	Two exams in one day		80
21.	Cheating on your boyfriend or girlfriend		77
22.	Getting married		76
23.	Negative consequences of drinking or drug use		75
24.	Depression or crisis in your best friend		73
25.	Difficulties with parents		73
26.	Talking in front of a class		72
27.	Lack of sleep		69
28.	Change in housing situation (hassles, moves)		69
29.	Competing or performing in public		69
30.	Getting in a physical fight		66
31.	Difficulties with a roommate		66
32.	Job changes (applying, new job, work hassles)		65
33.	Declaring a major or concerns about future plans		65

	Life Change	(✓) Experienced During Past Year	Life Event Stress Rating
34.	A class you hate		62
35.	Drinking or use of drugs		61
36.	Confrontations with professors		60
37.	Starting a new semester		58
38.	Going on a first date		57
39.	Registration		55
40.	Maintaining a steady dating relationship		55
41.	Commuting to campus or work, or both		54
42.	Peer pressures		53
43.	Being away from home for the first time		53
44.	Getting sick		52
45.	Concerns about your appearance		52
46.	Getting straight A's		51
47.	A difficult class that you love		48
48.	Making new friends; getting along with friends		47
49.	Fraternity or sorority rush		47
50.	Falling asleep in class		40
51.	Attending an athletic event (e.g., football game)		20

Source: Reproduced from M. J. Renner and R. S. Mackin (1998) / with permission of Sage Publications.

acculturative stress Pressures faced by immigrant people in adjusting to a host culture.

et al., 2023). Developing a strong sense of ethnic identity may help solidify feelings of belongingness and acceptance within immigrant and ethnic minority groups that can bolster social support and serve to buffer the stressful effects of racism and discrimination.

Exposure to discrimination can also have indirect effects on health by affecting the behavior of people from marginalized groups. Frequent exposure to unfair treatment may lead people to adopt unhealthy behaviors, such as alcohol or drug use, or make unhealthy food choices, which in turn may set the stage for development of significant health problems (Pascoe, Lattanner, & Richman, 2022).

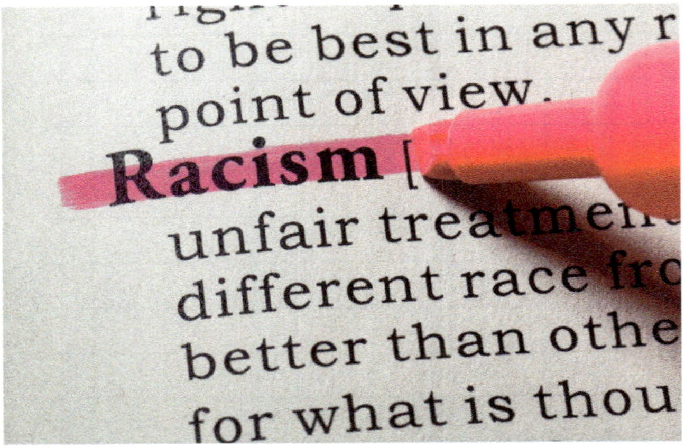

Devonyu/Getty Images

Discrimination as a Source of Stress Exposure to racism and discrimination is a source of stress affecting the emotional and physical well-being of targeted groups.

Acculturative Stress For immigrant groups, the adjustment to a new culture and way of life in the host country imposes demands that represent a significant source of stress. This type of stress, called **acculturative stress**, may be compounded by differences in language and the financial hardship that many immigrants face in making their way in a new country. There is also an additional source of stress in the form of pressure to acculturate—to adopt the values, language, customs, and even style of dress of the dominant or host culture. A recent study of Hispanic youth linked acculturative stress to higher levels of depression and anxiety (Wasserman et al., 2021).

A lack of acculturation can make it difficult for immigrant groups to achieve a foothold in their adopted culture, leading to financial difficulties and emotional consequences such as depression and anxiety. Yet acculturation can become a double-edge sword if it leads to erosion of family networks and traditional values and lifestyles. Evidence links greater acculturation to adoption of unhealthy behaviors commonly found in mainstream U.S. culture, such as substance abuse (Salas-Wright, Kagotho, & Vaughn, 2014; Zhang et al., 2013). Moreover, researchers find that erosion of traditional cultural identity and values in Latino teens is associated with increased prevalence of premarital intercourse (Adam et al., 2005). Forsaking traditional cultural values may come at a considerable cost. Overall, researchers find that better psychological adjustment in immigrant groups is generally associated with maintaining ties to traditional cultural values or heritage while also making efforts to participate more fully in the mainstream culture (Johnson et al., 2023; Serrano-Villar & Calzada, 2016; Thibeault, Stein, & Nelson-Gray, 2018).

Environmental Stressors: It Can Be Dangerous Out There

Some say the world will end in fire

Some say in ice.

—Robert Frost

In 2018, Hurricane Florence was supposed to slam into the coast of the Carolinas. It didn't. What was a category 3 or 4 hurricane out at sea meandered in as a category 1 hurricane, with winds at around 75 miles per hour. The winds did their damage—eroding beaches, felling trees, cutting power lines—but Florence lingered in the region for days, pouring up to 40inches of rain on parts of North Carolina that were already saturated from earlier rains. The rainwater had nowhere to go. Rivers overflowed their banks, and people died.

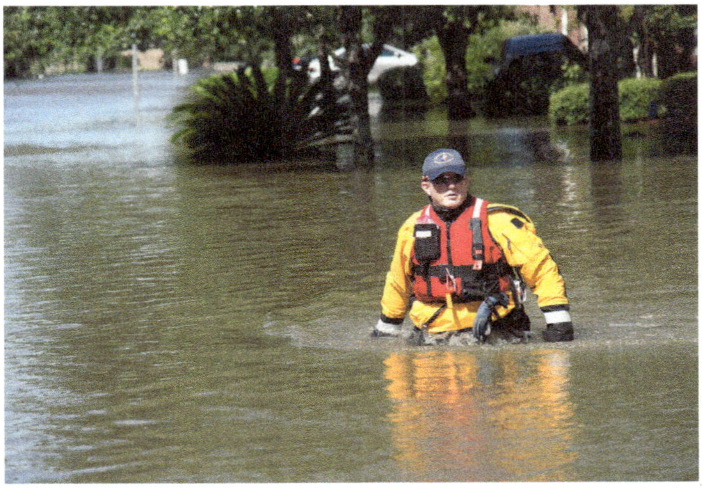

US Army Photo/Alamy Stock Photo

Some drowned. Others were exposed to submerged sharp objects, bacterial infections, mosquitoes bearing diseases, waste products from toilets and sinks, invisible storm drains, manure and agricultural runoff, and snakes. Houses developed mold and many would be beyond repair. People trapped by the rising water ran out of drinking water. Loss of electricity prevented people with diabetes from refrigerating their insulin. People in need of kidney dialysis could not get treatment. Some people were infected with bacteria from rodents and farm animals through cuts in the skin, or by way of their eyes or mouths. Storm drains and open manholes became death traps. If you were trudging along in 3 or 4 feet of water, you could not see the drains from the surface, but they sucked down hundreds of gallons of water every second, too strong a force to fight.

Florence, Harvey, Katrina, Maria, Sandy—a handful of names that represent some of the costliest disasters in recent history. Psychologist Jean Rhodes, who worked with survivors of Hurricane Katrina in New Orleans, said that people are traumatized first by the violence of the storm or the flooding, then by the loss of their homes, and also by the loss of family and friends and neighborhood—all of which give rise to spikes of anxiety and depression (Sun, 2018). Rhodes did not suspect one finding: Loss of a pet was a key predictor of feelings of depression. Disasters like hurricanes take an emotional toll as well as a physical toll (Bromet et al., 2017; Pennington et al., 2018). Most survivors in communities devastated by earthquakes, floods, hurricanes, terrorist attacks, and oil spills eventually adjust to their losses, their grief, and their memories. But many develop a lingering mental health problem called posttraumatic stress disorder (PTSD). Their sleep is killed by nightmares. Flashbacks, depression, and irritability darken their days (Bromet et al., 2017).

We face many environmental stressors, from routine stressors of blaring traffic noise on city streets to traumatic stressors, such as natural and technological disasters and acts of terrorism. There are hurricanes, earthquakes, blizzards, tornadoes, windstorms, ice storms, monsoons, floods, mudslides, avalanches, volcanic eruptions, and fires, such as the fires visited upon California in dry seasons. Natural disasters are hazardous in themselves and also cause life changes to pile on top of another by disrupting community and family life. Services that had been taken for granted, such as electricity and water, may be lost. Businesses and homes may be destroyed, and people must rebuild or relocate. Natural disasters reveal the thinness of the veneer of technology on which civilization depends. It is understandable that many survivors report stress-related problems, such as anxiety and depression, for months after the fact.

We owe our dominance over the natural environment to technological progress. Yet technology can also fail or backfire and cause disaster, such as in the case of airplane accidents, major fires, bridge collapses, leaks of poisonous gases or toxic chemicals, and blackouts. These are but a sample of the technological disasters that can befall us. When they do, we feel as though we have lost control of things and experience traumatic forms of stress.

Survivors of natural and technological disasters may experience psychological and physical effects of stress for years afterward. The stress of piecing together one's life or grieving for lost loved ones may be compounded by the additional burdens of filing claims and pursuing lawsuits against people and organizations identified as responsible for disasters of human origin.

Temperature: Getting Hot Under the Collar Adopting the biopsychosocial model, psychologists expand their study of social factors to include environmental conditions affecting behavior. Rising temperatures may also make some people hot under the collar. Evidence shows that higher temperatures are linked to increased aggressive behavior, including sexual assaults, violent confrontations, aggressive driving and road rage (Bushman et al., 2005; Groves & Anderson, 2018). Psychologist Brad Bushman puts it this way—"If someone cuts you off in traffic, you're much more likely to honk at them or flip them off if it's a hot day rather than a cool day" (Dahl, 2013). Even professional baseball pitchers are more likely to retaliate on hot days against an opposing team by hitting one of their players with a pitch during games in which one of their own players had been hit earlier (Larrick et al., 2011). Hot temperatures incite aggressive behavior by arousing angry or hostile thoughts and feelings, thereby increasing people's readiness to respond aggressively when provoked or frustrated. At very hot temperatures, however, aggressive behavior may begin to decline, as people become primarily motivated to escape the unbearable heat.

Air Pollution: Just Don't Breathe the Air? Psychologists and other health scientists investigate the effects of pollution and noxious odors on our health and adjustment. For example, ingesting lead dust or chips from decaying paint can impair children's intellectual functioning. High levels of air pollution are linked to heart disease and dementia (Bishop et al., 2018; Thurston & Newman, 2018). Unpleasant-smelling pollutants, like other forms of aversive stimulation, decrease feelings of attraction and heighten aggression (Branscombe & Baron, 2017; Xiang et al., 2017). And, of course, the air can carry droplets of diseases.

Crowding and Other Stresses of City Life Big-city dwellers are more likely to experience stimulus overload and to fear crime than suburbanites and rural folk (Lofland, 2017). Overwhelming crowd stimulation, bright lights, and multitudes of distracting shop windows may lead them to narrow their perceptions to a particular face, destination, or job. The pace of life increases. We even walk more quickly through city streets. Many people, of course seek out the stimulation, diversity, and cultural opportunities afforded by big cities. For them, much of the stress of city life is, using Selye's term, eustress.

personal space The physical space immediately surrounding a person, into which any encroachment feels threatening to or uncomfortable for the person.

Personal Space and Social Distancing One adverse effect of crowding is the invasion of one's **personal space**. Personal space is an invisible boundary, a sort of bubble surrounding you. You are likely to become anxious and perhaps angry when others invade your space. This may happen when someone sits down across from or next to you in an otherwise empty cafeteria or stands too close to you in an elevator. Personal space seems to serve both protective and communicative functions. People usually sit and stand closer to people who are similar to themselves in race, age, or socioeconomic status. Dating couples come closer together as the attraction between them increases.

Some interesting cross-cultural research on personal space has emerged. For example, North Americans and northern Europeans apparently maintain a greater distance between themselves and others than do southern Europeans, Asians, and Middle Easterners (Branscombe & Baron, 2017; Burgoon, 2016).

People in some cultures apparently learn to cope with high density and also share their ways of coping with others. Asians in crowded cities such as Tokyo and Hong Kong interact more harmoniously than North Americans and Europeans, who dwell in less dense cities. Chinese municipalities have designated women-only subway cars to protect women from being groped by men during rush hour. The Japanese are used to being packed sardine-like into subway cars by white-gloved pushers employed by the transit system. Imagine the rebellion that would occur if such treatment were attempted in American subways!

With the advent of COVID-19, Americans were advised to remain at least 6 feet apart from people out in the open, or when interacting with friends or family. They were asked not to visit others at home or in the hospital for fear of contaminating dwelling places or contracting the disease. Evidence from China suggests that social distancing, quarantining people who are infected, and isolating groups that were infected helped contain the spread of the pandemic (Anderson et al., 2020). Of course there was no control group, so one could argue that other factors might have brought about the slowing of the curve of infection, but one can also ask how likely a rival explanation would be. In the United States, there were several natural experiments in which some states mandated use of masks and social distancing, whereas others did not. The states that attacked the disease more aggressively saw fewer infections and deaths, and many states that originally did not require use of masks changed their policies over time (Goldstein, 2020).

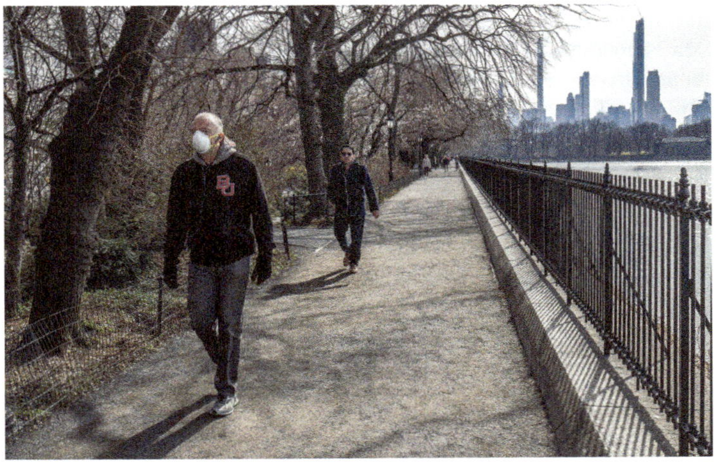

Enrique Shore/Alamy Stock Photo

Physical Distancing As COVID-19 spread across the United States, people were advised to remain at least 6 feet apart so as to try not to transmit the virus. Many wore masks in an effort not to inhale droplets (aerosols) shed by other people as they exhaled or coughed.

Health Psychology In Action

Framing the Message

One of the principal health measures designed to reduce the risk of infection during the COVID-19 pandemic was encouraging people to keep at least a six-foot distance from others. Though the use of the term "social distancing" may have been regrettable, as it implied that people should detach themselves from social interactions with others, the underlying principle of keeping a physical distance was sound. Health psychologists recognize the importance of maintaining social connections, albeit virtually or at a physical distance during a time of pandemic.

A team of health psychologists in Germany wondered whether the way in which a message is framed affects health-related behaviors, such as physical distancing. They framed a health message either in terms of potential gains of physical distancing ("to foster health") or potential loss of physical closeness ("it can be deadly") (Neumer et al., 2022). As part of a larger study, investigators posted signs with these health messages in the front of shopping carts in a supermarket. They also varied the message by directing it at the shoppers themselves ("do it for your own sake") or for the benefits of others ("do it for the sake of your fellow citizens"). The researchers then measured physical distancing behavior among customers who were exposed to these different messages.

Which way of framing the message do you think worked best? It turned out that framing the message in terms of loss was more effective in fostering physical distancing than framing the message in terms of gains. Also, independent of the message content, messages directed at the customers themselves were more effective in promoting physical distancing than messages targeting the effects on others ("fellow citizens"). The influence of framing effects, such as gain vs. loss or self vs. others, may depend on the targeted behavior, so it is possible that gain messages may work better in some contexts (healthy eating, for example) than in others. The uptake here is that in the face of a deadly virus like COVID-19, if you want to encourage people to practice healthier behaviors, such as keeping a physical distance, it might be best to highlight the risks they face and to make it personal.

A Closer Look

Stress in America

The APA (2017, 2018, 2019, 2020) commissions annual surveys of stress in America. Perennial stressors for the majority of Americans have been money (62%) and work (61%). Health is an enduring area of concern (46%), as are intimate relationships (58%). In 2017, for the first time, nearly two-thirds of Americans (63%) said that the future of the nation is a significant source of stress, citing social divisiveness (59%), health care (32%), trust in government (32%), and hate crimes (31%). And in 2018, a majority of members of Generation Z, aged 15–21, reported that they were stressed by mass shootings (75%), climate change and global warming (58%), and widespread reports of sexual harassment and assault (53%) (APA, 2018). There was no let-up of concerns in the 2019 survey (Bethune, 2020). More than half of American adults (56%) said the upcoming 2020 presidential election was a significant stressor. Mass shootings were identified as a significant source of stress by approximately 7 in 10 (71%), as was health care (69%). The majority (56%) of respondents were stressed by climate change. Almost half of Americans (48%) reported concern about immigration, and 25% were worried about discrimination. Nearly 2 of 3 LGBTQ adults (64%) said that discrimination had prevented them from leading a full and productive life.

And in the spring of 2020, the APA (2020) conducted an online Stress in America survey of 3,013 adults to learn about their sources of stress during the COVID-19 pandemic. Parents reported the following sources of stress:

- 74% reported worrying that a family member would get the virus.
- 74% expressed concern about the government response to the virus.
- 74% mentioned disrupted routines and adjusting to new routines.
- 73% were concerned about being infected with the virus.
- 73% reported stress as a result of managing distance/online learning for their children.
- 70% had concerns about meeting basic needs, as for food and housing.
- 67% reported self-isolation as a source of stressed.
- 66% mentioned being stressed about healthcare services.

In 2020, following the death of George Floyd when a police officer placed his knee on Floyd's neck, 83% of respondents to the Stress in America survey also said that the future of the nation is a significant source of stress (DeAngelis, 2020). Nearly 3 in 4 (72%) said that this era of racial protests and COVID-19 marked the lowest point in the country's history that they could personally remember. More than half of non-Hispanic Black Americans (55%) reported that discrimination was a significant source of stress.

Respondents to the 2019 survey reported physical and psychological signs of distress, such as feeling irritable or angry (45%). Two out of 5 (41%) survey respondents felt tired or worn out, and more than 1 in 3 (36%) said they had headaches. Respondents reported indigestion (26%) and tension (23%). About 1 in 3 said they felt depressed (34%) or could cry (30%). **Figure 4.1** shows warning signs of stress as compiled by the APA (2018).

- Headaches, muscle tension, neck or back pain
- Upset stomach
- Dry mouth
- Chest pains, rapid heartbeat
- Difficulty falling or staying asleep
- Fatigue
- Loss of appetite or overeating "comfort foods"
- Increased frequency of colds
- Lack of concentration or focus
- Memory problems or forgetfulness
- Jitters
- Irritability
- Short temper
- Anxiety

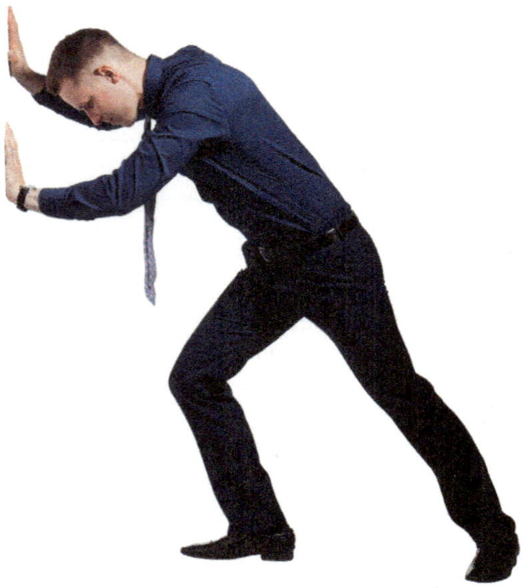

Vladimir Melnikov/Alamy Stock Photo

FIGURE 4.1 Sign of Stress How do you know that you are under stress? The APA (2018) has compiled these warning signs. We can try to remove, tamp down, or avoid sources of stress, or seek professional help.

Source: Adapted from APA (2018). Help Center. Listening to the warning signs of stress. http://www.apa.org/helpcenter/stress-signs.aspx.

TABLE 4.1 Percentages of Americans Reporting Stress-Related Symptoms in the Week Following the Terrorist Attacks of September 11, 2001

	Depression (%)	Difficulty concentrating (%)	Insomnia (%)
Men	62	44	26
Women	79	53	40

Source: Adapted from Pew Research Center (2002).

Terrorism: When Our Sense of Security Is Threatened Some of the social factors affecting our personal health involve geopolitical conflicts. On September 11, 2001, everything changed. Americans who had always felt secure and protected from acts of terrorism within the borders of their own country experienced the sense of vulnerability and fear that had become a part of daily life in many other countries. The effects of traumatic events like 9/11 affect most all of us in one way or another. As you can see from Table 4.1, a clear majority of Americans reported feeling depressed in the immediate aftermath of 9/11, and a sizable proportion had difficulty concentrating or suffered from insomnia.

Stress as Situations in Which the Demands Exceed Our Resources

Stressful demands at work and elsewhere can impact our psychological and physical health. One of the primary factors relating to stress in the workplace is job strain, which characterizes occupational settings in which workers are burdened by high responsibilities but do not have the power to make decisions or exercise control. The combination of high demands and little personal control places workers at higher risk of cardiovascular disease (Cohen et al., 2019; Karasek et al., 1981). As we see in Figure 4.2, restaurant servers are in the unenviable position of having repeated heavy demands placed on them yet having little control in the workplace.

frustration A state of feeling upset or annoyed, especially because of the thwarting of a goal or inability to change or achieve something.

The job–strain model can also apply to working women, who frequently work multiple shifts, one in the workplace and one at home (see Figure 4.3). Working mothers often bear the brunt of responsibility of childcare (Hass & Hwang, 2019). Mothers are the sole or primary breadwinners in approximately 40% of households with children (Cohn, 2016).

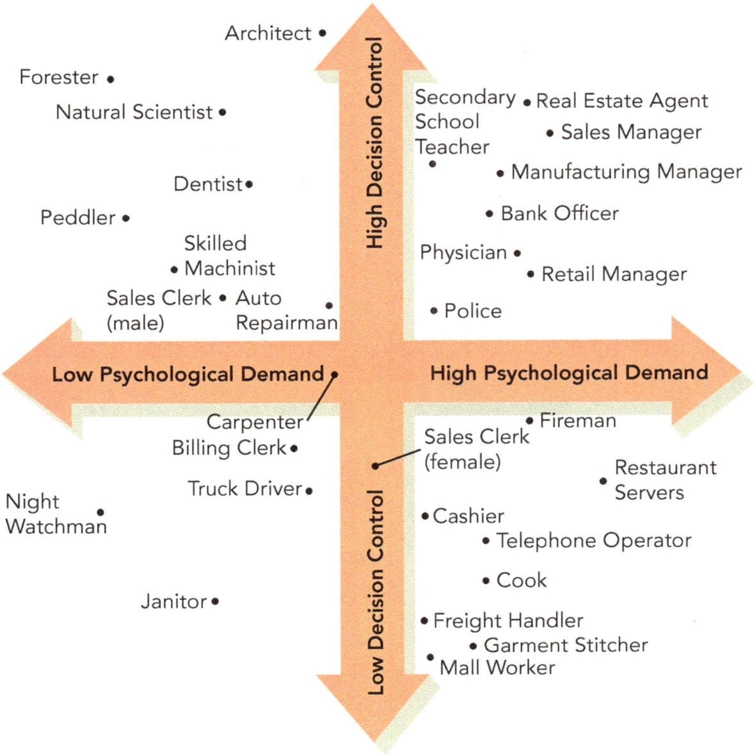

FIGURE 4.2 The Job-Strain Model This model highlights the demands of various occupations and the amount of personal (decision) control they allow. Occupations characterized by high demand and low personal control may place workers at risk of cardiovascular disease.

Stress as Interruption of Goals

You may want to be a point guard for your varsity basketball team but lose the ball every time you dribble. You may have been denied a job or an educational opportunity because of your ethnic background or favoritism. These situations give rise to **frustration**, the emotional state that occurs when a person's attempts to attain a goal are thwarted or blocked. Many sources of frustration are obvious. Adolescents are used to being told they are too young to wear makeup, drive, go out, engage in sexual activity, spend money, drink, or work. Age is the barrier that requires them to delay gratification. We may frustrate

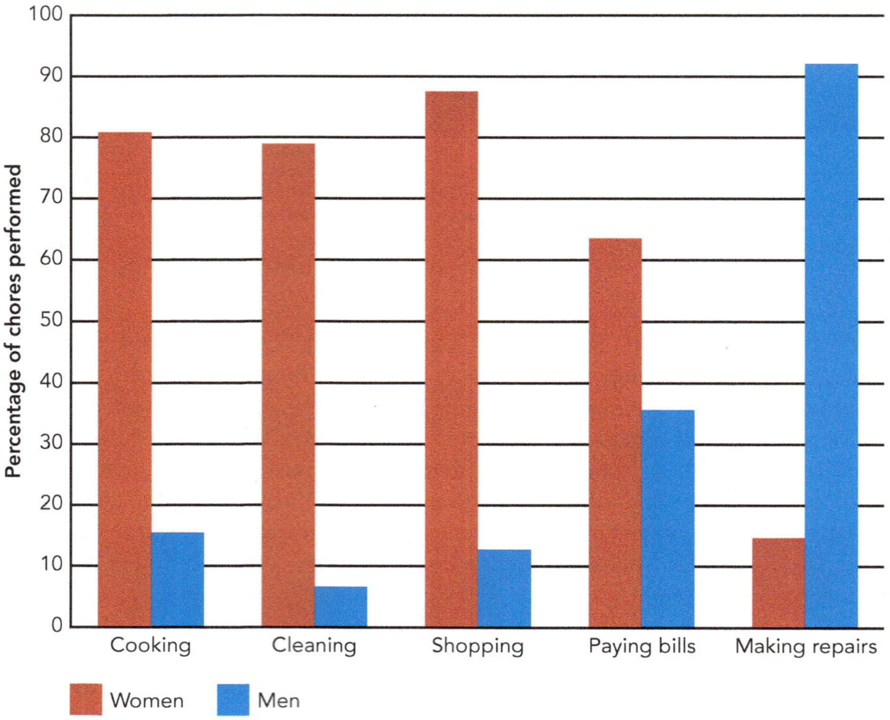

FIGURE 4.3 **When the Mother Is in the Workforce, Who Does the Cleaning, Cooking, and Shopping?** Good guess. Most American women put in a second shift when they get home from the workplace, handling most childcare and homemaking chores.

ourselves as adults if our goals are set too high or if our self-demands are irrational. If we try to earn other people's approval at all costs, or insist on performing perfectly in all of our undertakings, we doom ourselves to failure and frustration.

Commuting

One of the common frustrations of contemporary life is commuting. Distance, time, and driving conditions are some of the barriers that lie between us and our work or school. How many of us fight the freeways or crowd ourselves into train cars or buses for an hour or more before the workday begins? For most people, the stresses of commuting are mild but persistent. Still, lengthy commutes on crowded highways are linked to increases in heart rate, blood pressure, chest pain, and other signs of stress. Noise, humidity, and air pollution all contribute to the frustration involved in driving to work. If you commute by car, try to pick times and roads that provide lower volumes of traffic. It may be worth your while to take a longer, more scenic route that has less stop-and-go traffic.

Challenges for Women in the Workplace

Women with careers often find themselves stymied not only by sexism in promotions, the glass ceiling, a gender gap in earnings, and sexual harassment. They are also more likely than men to be the ones to stay home when the children are running a fever. Figure 4.4 shows that mothers are more likely than fathers to report career interruptions in order to care for children or other family members (Graf et al., 2019).

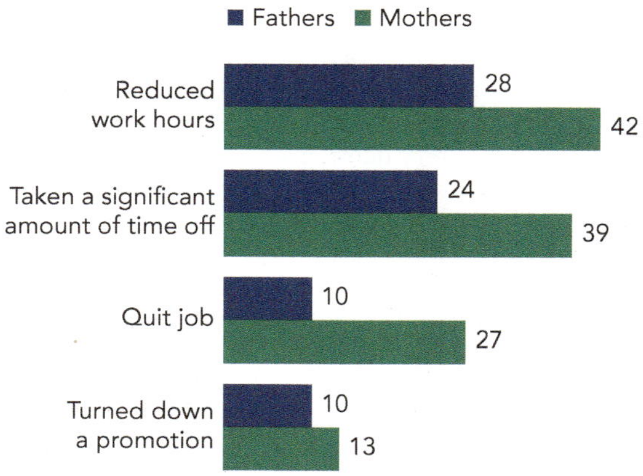

FIGURE 4.4 **Percentages of Fathers and Mothers Saying They Have Done Each of These to Care for a Child or Family Member**

Source: Graf et al. (2019). Reproduced with permission of Pew Research Center.

Psychological Barriers

Anxiety and fear may serve as emotional barriers that prevent us from acting effectively to meet our goals. A high school senior who wishes to attend an out-of-state college may be frustrated by the fear of leaving home. A young adult may not ask an attractive person out on a date because of fear of rejection. A woman may be frustrated in her desire to move up the corporate ladder, fearing that coworkers, friends, and family will view her assertiveness as compromising her femininity.

Frustration Tolerance Getting ahead is often a gradual process that requires us to live with some frustration and delay gratification. Yet our tolerance for frustration may fluctuate. Stress heaped upon stress can lower our tolerance. We may laugh off a flat tire on a good day. But if it is raining, the flat may seem like the last straw. People who have learned that it is possible to surmount barriers or find substitute goals are more tolerant of frustration than those who have not experienced it or who have experienced it in excess.

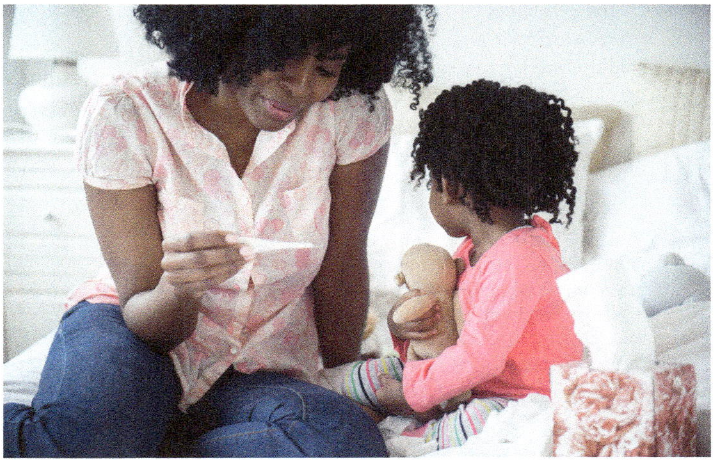

JGI/Jamie Grill/Getty Images

In Male–Female Partnerships, Which Parent Is More Likely to Stay Home with a Sick Child? Is this a trick question?

The Type A Behavior Pattern: Burning Out from Within?

The **Type A behavior pattern (TABP)** is another source of stress, one that arises from within. People with the TABP are highly driven, competitive, impatient, and aggressive. They feel rushed and under pressure all the time and keep one eye firmly glued to the clock (Matthews, 1982). They are not only prompt for appointments but often arrive early. They eat, walk, and talk rapidly and become restless when others work slowly. They attempt to dominate group discussions.

type A behavior pattern A pattern of stress-producing behavior, characterized by aggressiveness, perfectionism, unwillingness to relinquish control, and a sense of time urgency.

People with TABPs find it difficult to give up control or share power. They are often reluctant to delegate authority in the workplace, and as a result they increase their own workloads. They also find it difficult just to go out on the tennis court and bat the ball back and forth. They watch their form, perfect their strokes, and demand continual self-improvement. They hold to the irrational belief that they must be perfectly competent and achieve success in everything they undertake.

Review 4.1

INTERACTIVE SELF-SCORING QUIZZES

Sentence Completion

1. Daily __________ are regularly occurring annoyances or events that threaten our well-being.
2. Life __________, even pleasant ones, are stressful because they require adjustment.
3. The emotional state of __________ occurs when a person's attempts to accomplish a goal are thwarted.
4. __________ behavior is characterized by a sense of time urgency, competitiveness, and aggressiveness.
5. Disasters (increase or decrease) our sense of control over our lives.
6. High levels of heat tend to (increase or decrease) aggressiveness.

Think About It

What hassles do you encounter on a daily basis? Do you see them as impossible obstacles or as opportunities to solve problems and grow as a person?

The Body's Response to Stress

ANIMATION CONTENT

Physical Responses to Stress: The HPA Axis and the General Adaptation Syndrome

Stress is more than a psychological event; it is more than a feeling of being pushed and pulled. Stress also has clear effects on the body. A body under persistent stress can be likened to an alarm clock that does not shut off until its energy has been depleted. The field of health psychology studies the relationships between psychological factors, including stress, and physical health.

general adaptation syndrome (GAS) Hans Selye's term for a hypothesized three-stage bodily response to stress.

alarm stage The first stage of the GAS, which is triggered by stress and characterized by heightened activity of the sympathetic branch of the autonomic nervous system (see Figure 4.5).

The General Adaptation Syndrome

Hans Selye, who was playfully dubbed "Dr. Stress," observed in laboratory animals that the body shows a generalized response pattern to different kinds of stressors, such as pain, changes in temperature, perceived threats, or chronic noise. For this reason, he labeled the body's response to stress the **general adaptation syndrome (GAS)** (Selye, 1946). The GAS is a cluster of bodily changes that occur in three stages—an alarm stage, a resistance stage, and an exhaustion stage (see Figure 4.5).

fight-or-flight reaction Walter Cannon's term for a hypothesized instinctive response to the perception of danger.

The Alarm Stage

The **alarm stage** (also called the *alarm reaction*) is the body's initial response to a stressor. This reaction mobilizes or arouses the body in preparation to defend itself against a stressor. Early in the 20th century, physiologist Walter B. Cannon termed this alarm response the **fight-or-flight reaction** (Robinson, 2018). The mobilization prepares the body to fight or flee a threat.

The alarm reaction involves a number of bodily changes that are initiated by the brain and regulated by the endocrine system (**Figure 4.6**) and the nervous system (see

1 Alarm Stage
When faced with a threatening stressor, your body enters an alarm stage during which your sympathetic nervous system is activated (e.g., increased heart rate and blood pressure) and blood is diverted to your skeletal muscles to prepare you for the the fight-or-flight reaction response.

2 Resistance Stage
As the stress continues, your body attempts to resist or adapt to the stressor by summoning all your resources. Physiological arousal remains higher than normal, and there is an outpouring of stress hormones. During this resistance stage, people use a variety of coping methods. For example, if your job is threatened, you may work longer hours and give up your vacation days.

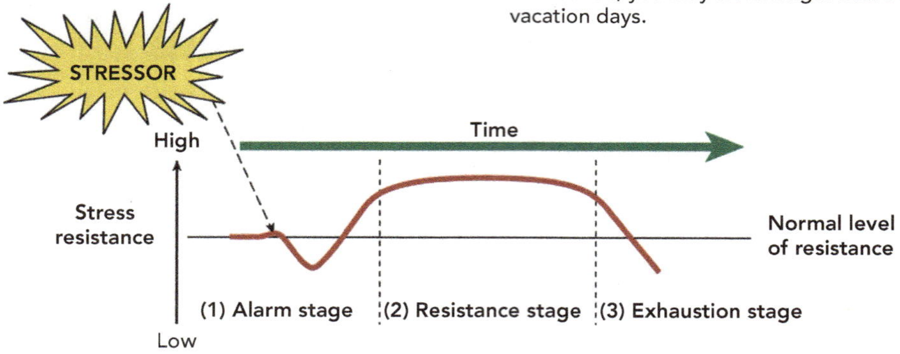

3 Exhaustion Stage
Unfortunately, your body's resistance to stress can last only so long before exhaustion sets in. During this final stage, your reserves are depleted and you become more susceptible to serious illness as well as potentially irreversible damage to your body. Selye maintained that one outcome of this exhaustion stage for some people is the development of *diseases of adaptation*, including asthma and high blood pressure. Unless a way of relieving stress is found, the eventual result may be complete collapse and death.

INTERACTIVE FIGURES, CHARTS, & TABLES

FIGURE 4.5 The Stages of the General Adaptation Syndrome

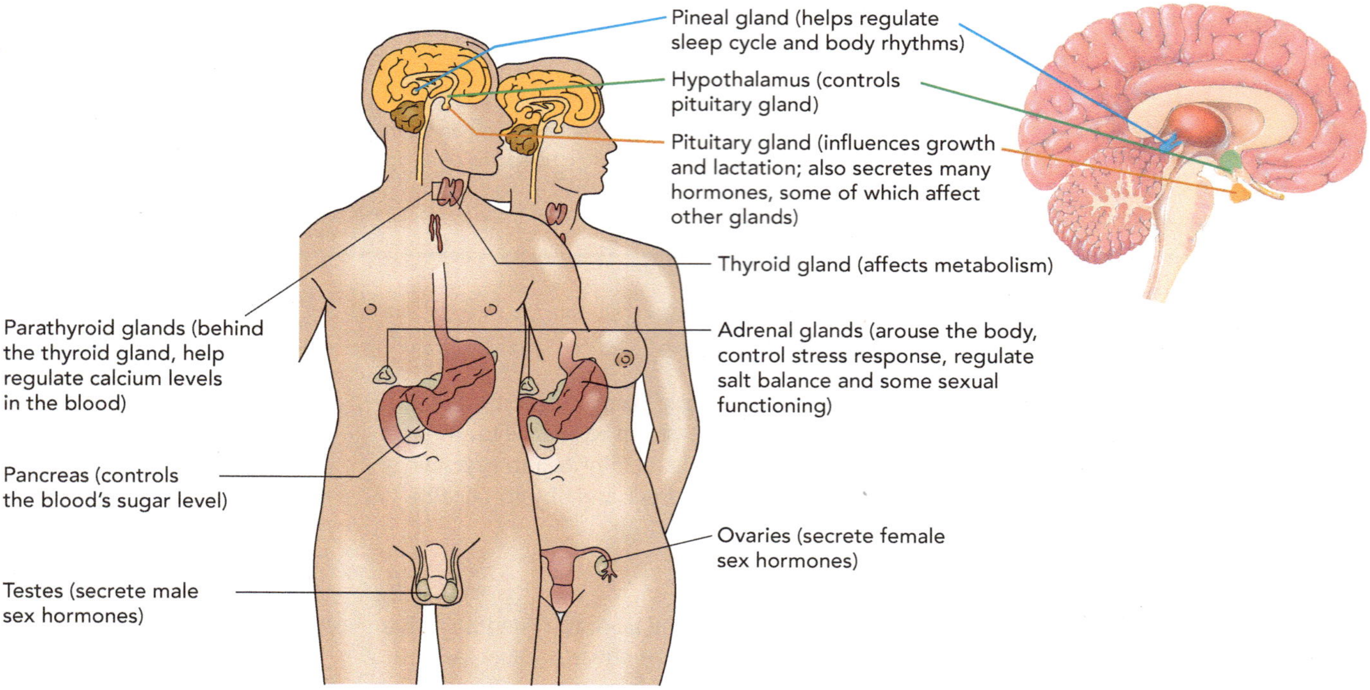

FIGURE 4.6 Glands of the Endocrine System The endocrine system consists of a network of glands located throughout the body that secrete hormones directly into the bloodstream. The endocrine system plays important roles in reproduction, growth, metabolism, and the body's response to stress.

INTERACTIVE FIGURES, CHARTS, & TABLES

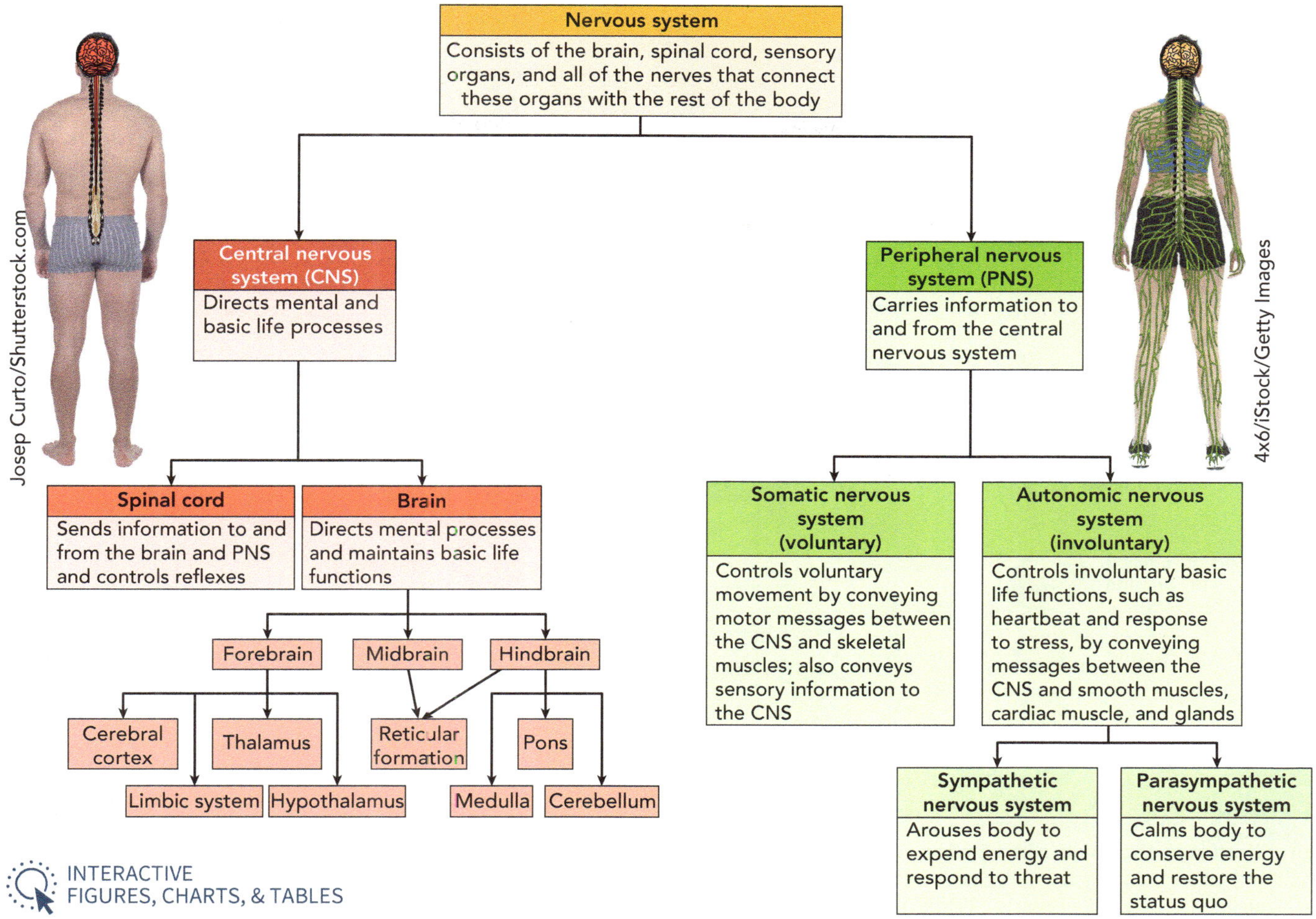

FIGURE 4.7 Divisions of the Nervous System The nervous system contains two main divisions—the central nervous system (CNS) and the peripheral nervous system. The CNS consists of the brain and the spinal cord. The peripheral nervous system contains the somatic and autonomic nervous systems. The somatic nervous system controls voluntary movement by conveying messages between the CNS and skeletal muscles; it also conveys sensory information to the CNS. The autonomic nervous system controls involuntary basic functions such as the heart beat and the responses to stress by conveying messages between the CNS and smooth muscles (e.g., the cardiac muscle) and the glands.

Figures 4.7 and **4.8**). The endocrine system is made up of the glands that pour their secretions, called hormones, directly into the bloodstream. The nervous system consists of the brain, the spinal cord, and the nerves linking them to the sensory organs, muscles, and endocrine system. As we see in **Figure 4.7**, the brain and the spinal cord make up the **central nervous system (CNS)**. The CNS is like the central processing unit in your computer that receives and processes information from other parts of the body and issues commands to control the body's "peripheral devices," as in deciding to look at something or lift your arm. The **peripheral nervous system (PNS)** receives and transmits information to and from the CNS, to various parts of the body, including the sensory organs, muscles, and glands.

The **autonomic nervous system (ANS)** (see **Figure 4.8**) is the part of the peripheral nervous system that automatically (autonomic means "automatic") controls involuntary bodily processes such as heartbeat and respiration. It consists of two parts or divisions—the **sympathetic nervous system** and the **parasympathetic nervous system**. The sympathetic division is most active during activities and emotional responses—such as anxiety and fear—that expend the body's reserves of energy. The parasympathetic division is most active during processes that restore the body's reserves of energy, such as digestion. These systems have largely opposing effects. The sympathetic nervous system accelerates bodily processes

central nervous system (CNS) The body's "command and control" system, comprising the brain and spinal cord.

peripheral nervous system (PNS) The part of the nervous system comprising nerve pathways that connect the central nervous system with the body's sensory organs, muscles, and glands.

autonomic nervous system (ANS) The part of the nervous system involved in controlling automatic bodily functions such as heart rate, respiration (breathing) rate, dilation of the pupils of the eyes, salivation, digestion, elimination, and sexual responses such as erection and vaginal lubrication.

sympathetic nervous system The division of the ANS that mobilizes bodily processes involved in expending the body's reserves of energy, which are needed to perform strenuous activities or respond to threatening stressors.

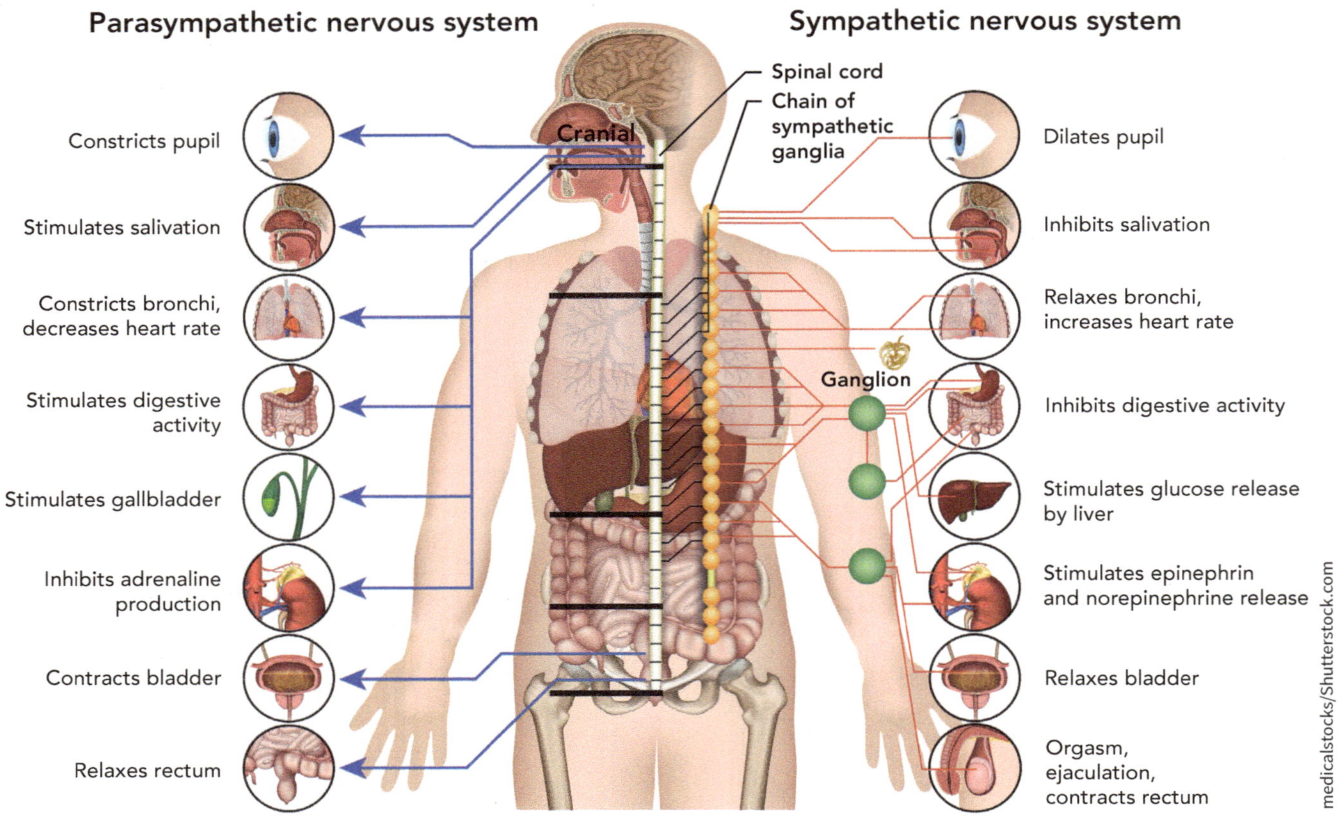

FIGURE 4.8 The Autonomic Nervous System The ANS helps regulate automatic bodily responses, such as heart rate, respiration, and digestion. The parasympathetic branch, or division, of the ANS is generally dominant during activities that replenish the body's store of energy, such as digestion and rest. The sympathetic branch is most active during activities in which the body expends energy, as in fighting or fleeing a threatening stressor, and when we experience strong emotions such as fear and anger.

ANIMATION CONTENT

Illustrating the Sympathetic and Parasympathetic Nervous Systems

such as heart rate and breathing and leads to the release of energy from stored reserves during times when the body needs additional oxygen and fuel to work harder or to defend itself from threats. The sympathetic division of the nervous system takes control during the alarm reaction. Because the sympathetic nervous system dilates the pupils of the eyes and is active when we feel fear, we can be literally wide-eyed with fear. The parasympathetic nervous system tones down states of bodily arousal and controls bodily processes that replenish resources, such as digestion. The saying that "fear gives you indigestion" is accurate because fear is connected with sympathetic nervous system activity that opposes digestion, which is a parasympathetic activity. Let us now consider the roles of the endocrine and autonomic nervous systems in the stress response.

Stress has a domino effect on a set of endocrine glands that are labeled the *hypothalamus–pituitary–adrenal* axis. This is how it works (see **Figure 4.9**):

1. A small gland in the brain called the **hypothalamus** secretes corticotropin-releasing hormone (CRH).
2. CRH causes another gland in the brain, called the **pituitary gland**, to secrete *adrenocorticotropic hormone* (ACTH).
3. ACTH then travels in the bloodstream to the adrenal glands and causes the outer layer, the *adrenal cortex*, to secrete **corticosteroids**.

Corticosteroids help the body resist stress by making nutrients that are stored in the body and available to meet the demands of coping with stressors. Although corticosteroids initially help the body cope with stress, continued secretion can harm the cardiovascular system, which is one reason that chronic stress can impair one's health. People who use steroids to build muscle mass may also develop cardiovascular problems.

parasympathetic nervous system The division of the ANS involved in regulating bodily processes that replenish the body's stores of energy.

hypothalamus A small endocrine gland in the brain that is involved in many bodily processes, including hunger, sleep, emotions, aggression, and body temperature.

pituitary gland A pea-sized endocrine gland in the brain that secretes various hormones, such as growth hormone, prolactin (which regulates maternal behavior in lower mammals), vasopressin (which inhibits production of urine when body fluids are at low levels), and oxytocin (which stimulates labor and is connected with nurturing behavior).

Health psychologists are particularly concerned about the role of *cortisol*, a key corticosteroid that is produced by the adrenal glands. One study observed changes in levels of cortisol in hair samples among 56 college (mean age, 19 years) undergraduates as an academic term progressed (Stetler & Guinn, 2020). The measures of cortisol were taken during the summer break and during an academic term. The students completed checklists of negative events weekly across a period of 10 weeks. Cortisol levels were 78% higher at the end of the semester. It was also found that stressful events in the form of increasing academic pressures and negative social peer evaluation were associated with increasing levels of cortisol. A recent study of LBGT young adults linked higher cortisol levels to daily stress associated with sexual minority status, such as unfair treatment or discrimination (Figueroa et al., 2021).

Two other hormones classified as *catecholamines* play a major role in the alarm stage and are secreted by the inner part of the adrenal glands, called the *adrenal medulla*. The sympathetic division of the ANS activates the adrenal medulla, causing it to release a mixture, or "cocktail," of the hormones *adrenaline* and *noradrenaline* (also called *epinephrine* and *norepinephrine,* respectively). These hormones are often referred to as stress hormones because they arouse the body during times of stress by accelerating the heart rate and stimulating the liver to release stored energy in the form of glucose (sugar).

The alarm reaction, or fight-or-flight mechanism, evolved during human prehistory when many stressors were life-threatening. At that time in our evolutionary history, the alarm reaction might have been triggered by the sight of a predator at the edge of a thicket or by a sudden rustling in the undergrowth. Today it may be aroused when you need to battle stop-and-go traffic on a daily basis or when you are confronted with an upsetting or challenging event, such as a major examination. Once the threat is removed, the parasympathetic nervous system takes control and returns the body to a lower state of arousal. Many of the bodily changes that occur during the alarm reaction are listed in Figure 4.10.

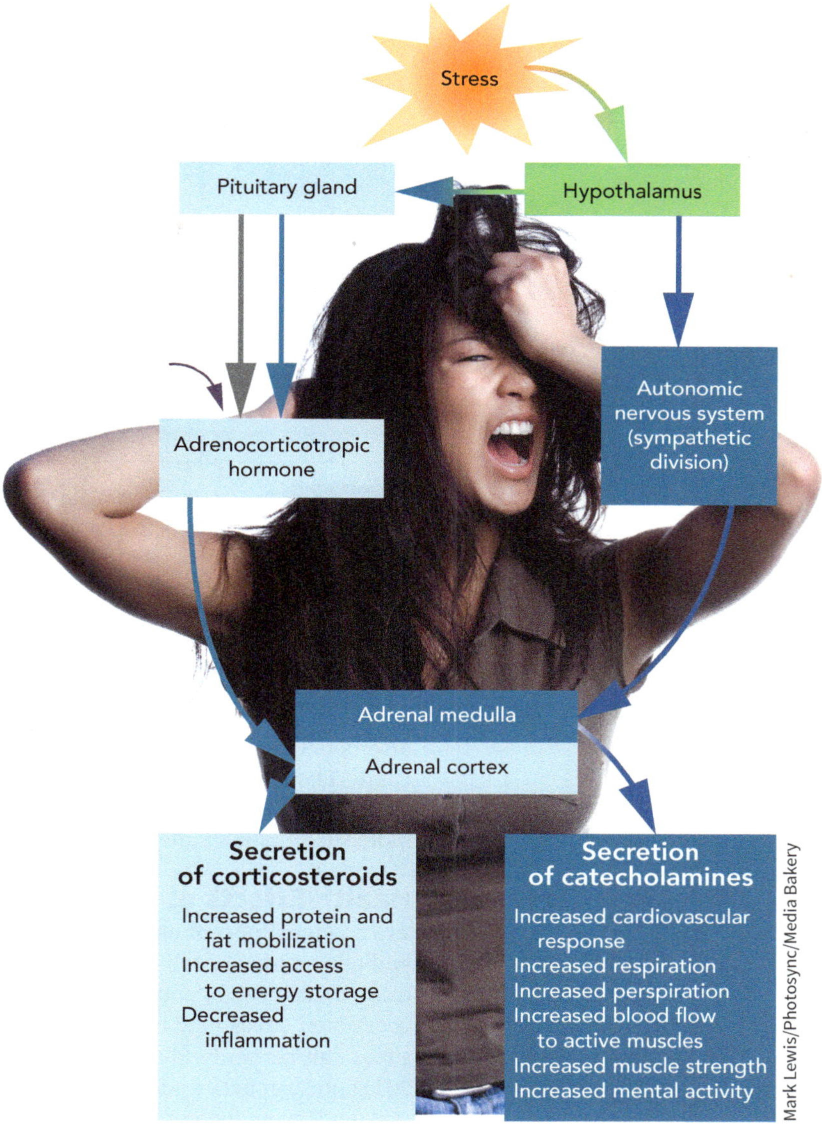

FIGURE 4.9 Stress, the Endocrine System, and the Autonomic Nervous System Under stress, the hypothalamus secretes a hormone that causes the pituitary gland to secrete ACTH, which in turn causes the adrenal cortex to secrete corticosteroids, which increase resistance to stress. The hypothalamus also causes the ANS to secrete catecholamines, which increase cardiovascular response and other responses that are associated with the alarm reaction.

The Resistance Stage

If the alarm reaction mobilizes the body and the stressor is not removed, we enter the **resistance** or adaptation stage of the GAS. Levels of endocrine and sympathetic nervous system activity are lower than in the alarm reaction but remain above normal. In this stage the body attempts to restore lost energy and repair bodily damage.

The Exhaustion Stage

If the stressor persists and is not dealt with adequately, we may enter the **exhaustion stage** of the GAS. Individual capacities for resisting stress vary, but when stress continues indefinitely, the body eventually becomes exhausted. The muscles become fatigued. The body is depleted of the resources required to combat stress. With exhaustion, the parasympathetic nervous system becomes dominant. As a result, our heartbeat, respiration rate, blood pressure, and bodily arousal decline. It might sound as if we would profit from the respite, but remember that we remain under stress—possibly an external threat. Continued stress in the exhaustion stage may lead to what Selye calls *diseases of adaptation*—medical

corticosteroids Hormones produced by the adrenal cortex that increase resistance to stress by fighting inflammation and stimulating the liver to release stores of sugar. Also referred to as steroidal hormones.

resistance stage The second stage of the GAS, characterized by a lowering of sympathetic nervous system activity and bodily processes involved in replenishing energy reserves and bodily repair.

exhaustion stage The third stage of the GAS, characterized by weakened resistance, increased vulnerability to stress-related disorders, and greater parasympathetic activity.

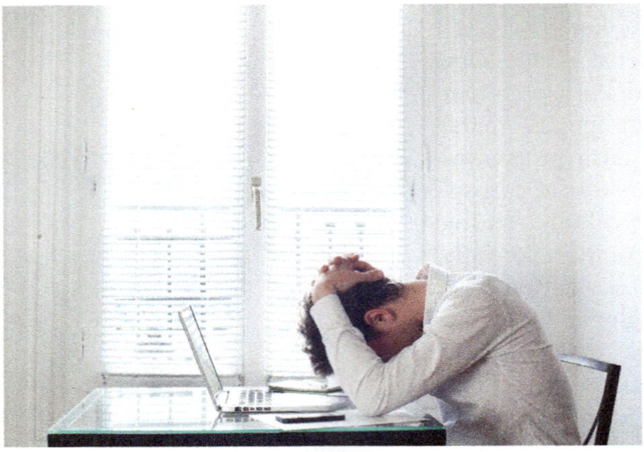

- Corticosteroids are secreted.
- Adrenaline is secreted.
- Noradrenaline is secreted.
- Respiration rate increases.
- Heart rate increases.
- Blood pressure increases.
- Muscles tense.
- Blood shifts from internal organs to muscles.
- Digestion is inhibited.
- The liver releases sugar.
- Blood coagulability increases.

Anna Berkut/Alamy Stock Photo

FIGURE 4.10 Components of the Alarm Reaction Under stress, we may also have difficulty thinking clearly or remaining focused on what we need to do. The high levels of bodily arousal produced by stress can impair memory functioning and problem-solving ability. During stressful examinations, for example, the anxiety that accompanies sympathetic nervous system activation might have prevented you from recalling material you were sure you had banked in memory. Afterward, you might have thought, "I just drew a blank." Our attention may also become so riveted on increased bodily tension and expectations of failure or doom that we cannot focus on the problems at hand.

disorders that can range from allergies to hives to coronary heart disease and, ultimately, to death. Though people differ in their ability to sustain stress, high levels of persistent or unrelieved stress eventually overtax the body's resources to the point where the person becomes more susceptible to infectious agents and stress-related disorders (Cohen et al., 2016, 2019).

Health Effects of Chronic Stress Stress can take the form of single events, such as a sudden illness or an accident, or a combination of life stressors of daily life that mount up and pile on top of each other, such as hassles, financial strain, working at two or more jobs to make ends meet, or coping with ongoing health problems or those of family members. While occasional stress may not have lasting effects on our physical or emotional health, chronic stress can certainly take its toll (Kiecolt-Glaser et al., 2020; O'Connor, Thayer, & Vedhara, 2021). Researchers find that chronic stress can impair the functioning of the body's immune system, leaving us more susceptible to various health problems, including infectious disease, cardiovascular problems, and digestive problems (Klopack et al., 2022; NIH, 2022).

A Closer Look

"Fight or Flight" or "Tend and Befriend"? Gender Differences in Response to Stress

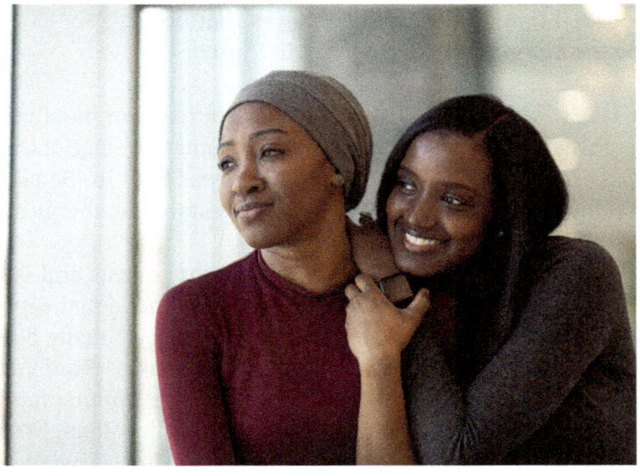

FatCamera/Getty Images

About a century ago, Harvard University physiologist Walter Cannon labeled the body's response to a threatening stressor the *fight-or-flight reaction*. He believed that the body was prewired to become mobilized or aroused in preparation for combat when faced with a predator or a competitor or, if the predator was threatening enough, that discretion—that is, a strategic retreat—would sometimes be the better part of valor. The fight-or-flight reaction includes the cascading sequence of bodily changes involved in the body's alarm reaction to stress—a sequence involving the autonomic nervous and endocrine systems, under the control of structures in the brain.

Emerging research examines stress-related responses through the lens of gender. Psychologist Shelley Taylor (2006, 2011) argues that at least half of us are more likely to seek or extend support to others in the face of stress than to fight or flee. Which half of us would that be? That would be the female half.

Taylor explains that her interest in the fight-or-flight reaction was prompted by an offhand remark of a student who had noticed that nearly all of the rats in studies of the effects of stress on animals were male. Taylor did an overview of the research on stress with humans and noted that before 1995, when federal agencies began requiring more equal representation of women if they were to fund research, only 17% of the subjects were female. That is quite a gender gap—and one that had allowed researchers to ignore the question of whether females responded to stress in the same way as males.

Taylor dug more deeply into the literature and found that men and women typically have different responses to stress (2006, 2011). She called the characteristic response to stress in women the "tend and befriend" response. It involves nurturing and seeking the support of others rather than fighting or fleeing in times of stress. Taylor and her colleagues reviewed studies showing that when women faced a threat, a disaster, or even an especially bad day at the office, they often responded by caring for their children and seeking contact and support from others, particularly other women. After a bad day at the office, men are more likely to withdraw from the family or become argumentative or hostile. This response may be prewired in female humans and in females of other mammalian species.

From the perspective of evolutionary theory, we might suggest that the tend-and-befriend response became imprinted in our genes because it promoted the survival of females who are tending to their offspring. (Females who choose to fight may die off or at least be separated from their offspring—no evolutionary brass ring here.)

Gender differences in behavior are frequently connected with gender differences in hormones and other biological factors. This one is no different. Taylor and her colleagues point to the effects of the pituitary hormone *oxytocin* in the woman's body. This hormone stimulates labor and causes the breasts to eject milk when women nurse. But oxytocin has also been dubbed the cuddle hormone because it is linked to social behaviors, such as the mother's attachment to her infant child and our development of empathy and sense of trust in other people (Jakubiak & Feeney, 2017; Piadeh Zavardehi et al., 2018).

But wait a minute! Men also release oxytocin when they are under stress. So why the gender difference? The answer may lie in the presence of other hormones, the sex hormones estrogen and testosterone. Females have more estrogen than males do, and estrogen seems to enhance the effects of oxytocin.

Males, in contrast, have more testosterone than females, and testosterone may mitigate the effects of oxytocin by prompting feelings of self-confidence (which may be exaggerated) and fostering aggression (Reed & Meggs, 2017; Turanovic et al., 2017). It is thus possible that males are more aggressive than females under stress because of biological differences in the hormone balance in their bodies, whereas females are more affiliative and nurturant.

Not all psychologists agree with an evolutionary or biological explanation. Psychologist Alice Eagly and her colleagues (2012) allow that gender differences in response to stress may be rooted in hormones but suggest we consider an alternative: that differences may reflect learning influences and cultural conditioning. Women, according to Eagly and her colleagues, may be somewhat more affiliative than men, but is the difference biologically hardwired or does it reflect the fact that women, historically, have been expected to assume family responsibilities? As in so many cases, the answer might lie in the interaction between nature (biology) and nurture (experience).

The accumulation of life changes and the stresses and strains of daily life contributes to the overall stress burden we carry. Biomedical researchers measure the overall stress burden by looking at various biomarkers of stress and evaluating the person's ability to function effectively. This stress burden is called **allostatic load**, and when it mounts up, it can result in wear and tear on the body that over time leads to negative health outcomes, including increased risk of infectious diseases (Guardino & Dunkel Schetter, 2022). In this chapter, we examine various types of infectious diseases and the contributions of health psychologists in efforts to help us protect ourselves from these types of health threats.

allostatic load A measure of the stress burden on physiological systems in the body.

Review 4.2

INTERACTIVE SELF-SCORING QUIZZES

Sentence Completion

1. Selye observed that the body's response to stress was similar regardless of the stressor and therefore labeled the body's response the __________ adaptation syndrome.

2. Physiologist Cannon labeled the alarm stage the __________-or-__________ reaction.

3. The __________ system pours stress hormones into the bloodstream.

4. The autonomic nervous system has sympathetic and __________ divisions.

5. Corticosteroids are secreted by the __________ glands.

6. The __________ secretes corticotrophin-releasing hormone.

7. Continued secretion of __________ can harm the cardiovascular system.

8. Psychologist Shelley Taylor argued that women show a __________ and __________ response to stress rather than a fight-or-flight reaction.

Think About It

What stressors trigger sympathetic arousal in you? What are the bodily changes you observe when you are experiencing sympathetic arousal? Do you find them to be uncomfortable? How so? What do you do to try to ameliorate sympathetic arousal? When confronted by a stressor, do your thought patterns tend to exacerbate or ameliorate your sympathetic arousal?

Infection and Immunity

Bubonic plague, the common cold, COVID-19, and HIV/AIDS are all infectious diseases—diseases caused by microorganisms. Because of worldwide air travel, someone who sneezes or coughs in Switzerland might infect a traveler who spreads the disease anywhere in the world in the space of a day.

The environment is a veritable soup of infectious organisms, so it is not surprising that colds, sore throats, flu, and sinus infections are among the health problems that affect college students and others who share classrooms, locker rooms, or stadium seats; those who sit next to you in a movie theater or at a play; those who are in the same airplane or on the same cruise ship; those who are in romantic relationships; those who attend a concert with you may all come down with the same diseases.

Infectious diseases are also called communicable diseases. They are caused by pathogens that multiply within the body. Pathogens include bacteria, viruses, fungi (yeast and molds), and parasites such as insects and worms (see **Figure 4.11**). Most pathogens are too small to be seen with the naked eye. They reproduce on or in a host—a plant or animal that provides a breeding ground. Pathogens enter the body through pores or sores in the skin or through the body's openings, such as the oral or nasal cavities. If unchecked they can establish beachheads in the body. They use the body's own resources to multiply and produce illness. Infectious organisms are transmitted by contact with infected people or animals, through insect bites, or by way of contaminated air, food, soil, or objects.

Some microorganisms are normally found in the body. When we use antibiotics to kill invading bacteria, we also kill healthful bacteria in our digestive system. This is why substances that promote the growth of bacterial colonies in the human gut, called *probiotics*—the opposite of antibiotics—might be recommended to restore the balance.

Infectious diseases may be localized, or restricted to a particular part of the body, as in some skin infections. Or they may be systemic—generalized, involving many organs and systems.

It may take minutes, hours, days, months, or years from the time a pathogen enters the body until symptoms occur. These latent or hidden infections may turn active when the individual's health in compromised by stress or other diseases.

It may take a decade or more for a person infected with HIV to show symptoms, although the virus is at war with their immune system for years. A person who engages in cunnilingus with a woman who is infected with human papillomavirus (HPV) may become infected themselves. However, the infected person may never develop symptoms or may develop oropharyngeal cancer 25 years or so later. Health psychologists are concerned about infectious diseases because of the health-related behaviors needed to prevent or mitigate their spread, as in the case of social distancing measures during the COVID-19 pandemic, and because of the need to facilitate access to medical services and promote adherence to medical advice and directives.

bacteria Single-celled organisms that have cell walls but lack a distinct cell nucleus. Some bacteria cause infections, whereas others are beneficial.

Bacteria (singular: bacterium) are microscopic, single-celled organisms that live in soil, air, plants, and animals, including humans. Bacteria thrive under warm, moist conditions, like those of the lining of the mucous membranes of the mouth, throat, and nasal passages. Yet some bacteria are so hardy they can survive in virtually any environment, from subarctic to desert conditions. Tuberculosis, some kinds of pneumonia, urinary tract infections, Lyme disease, dysentery, botulism (food poisoning), and periodontal (gum) disease are a few of the many diseases caused by bacteria.

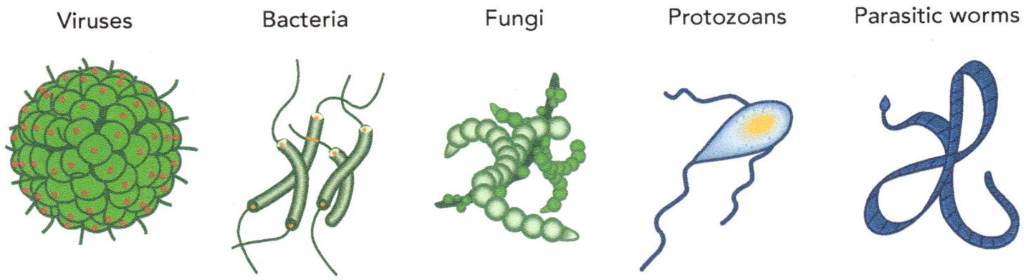

FIGURE 4.11 **Kinds of Pathogens**

Some bacteria are shaped like a sphere (*cocci*), others resemble a rod (*bacilli*), and still others have a spiral shape (*spirochetes*). Each bacterium reproduces itself using nutrients from the host organism. They reproduce by dividing into two identical cells; depending on the type of bacterium and environmental conditions, the rate of reproduction varies from slow to lightning fast.

Bacteria release poisonous chemical substances, or toxins, that can damage body cells, tissues, and organs. They can also invade body cells, destroying bodily tissue directly or reproducing so rapidly that they prevent body organs from functioning normally. Though some bacterial infections can be identified by the person's symptoms, a definitive diagnosis is made from laboratory tests. In some cases, a sample of blood can be analyzed under a microscope to identify bacteria. In other cases, the *culture method*, a throat swab, urine or blood sample, or another specimen of body fluid is placed in a plate with nutrients that allow bacteria to multiply. The presence of a particular strain is then identified by its shape and growth pattern. In still other cases, the *staining method* is used—stains made of colored dyes are mixed with bacteria-laden cells on a microscope slide. The stains bind to different bacteria in characteristic ways, allowing identification of particular bacteria.

Bacterial infections are typically treated with antibiotics. Some antibiotics, such as *penicillin*, destroy bacteria outright; others, such as *tetracycline*, slow their rate of reproduction. Some bacterial infections, such as diphtheria, whooping cough, and tetanus, can be prevented by vaccination.

Viruses are the smallest pathogens, perhaps 1/100th the size of bacteria. They consist of a core of genetic material (DNA or RNA) and a surrounding coat of protein. The only life activity they can perform is reproduction; they cannot metabolize food. They survive by taking over the machinery that makes the host's cell work. In effect, the virus hijacks the host to participate in its reproductive process. When a virus invades a cell, it injects its DNA or RNA into the cell. The virus provides the genetic code for replication, and the host cell provides the energy and raw materials to make new copies of the virus. The viral genes supplant the host cell's reproductive mechanisms and program them to make new viruses.

viruses A large group of infectious agents that consist of complex molecules containing genetic material and a protein coating; they are unable to reproduce except within a host.

Some viruses, such as HIV, remain dormant within host cells for long periods with no noticeable symptoms. Others reproduce quickly and burst out of cells with a vengeance, producing acute infections such as influenza—the flu. Some viruses have relatively mild effects, such as cold sores or warts; others, such as HIV, can produce lethal conditions. Virus families include *adenoviruses*, responsible for some respiratory and eye infections, and *retroviruses*, which cause HIV/AIDS and other health problems. The Epstein-Barr virus (EBV), a type of herpes virus, causes infectious mononucleosis, a disease primarily affecting children and young adults that is spread by close contact, including kissing. Coronaviruses are a large family of viruses that are common in people and many kinds of animals, including cattle, cats, and bats. COVID-19 is a coronavirus that may have spread from animals to humans (**Figure 4.12**).

The Immune System: Search and Destroy

When invading **pathogens** breach the body's external barriers, the immune system springs into action. Sometimes it conquers the invaders so quickly that we are not aware we have been infected. In other cases, the infection takes root and we become ill.

The immune system commands an army of billions of specialized *white blood cells* in the bloodstream and tissues of the body. These cells—known more technically as **lymphocytes**–circulate continuously throughout the body and are alert to foreign agents or **antigens** (literally *anti*body *gen*erators). An antigen is a substance that the immune cell recognizes as foreign to the body, such as a bacterium or virus, even a cancerous or worn-out body cell. Chemically, antigens are proteins on cell surfaces that stimulate an immune response.

The *immune response* is the sequence of events that takes place when lymphocytes detect antigens and attack them. Some lymphocytes directly attack and destroy antigens. Others produce **antibodies**. Antibodies are molecules of protein called *immunoglobulins*. A particular antibody fits an invading antigen like a key fitting a lock (**Figure 4.13**). By locking into an antigen, the antibody marks it for destruction by other immune cells.

pathogens Bacteria, viruses, or other organisms that can cause disease.

lymphocytes White blood cells that are responsible for immune system responses such as attacking cancerous body cells and invading bacteria and viruses.

antigens Foreign substances that induce an immune system response in the body, such as the production of antibodies.

antibodies Proteins produced by the immune system when it detects antigens. Antibodies combine with and neutralize invading viruses and bacteria.

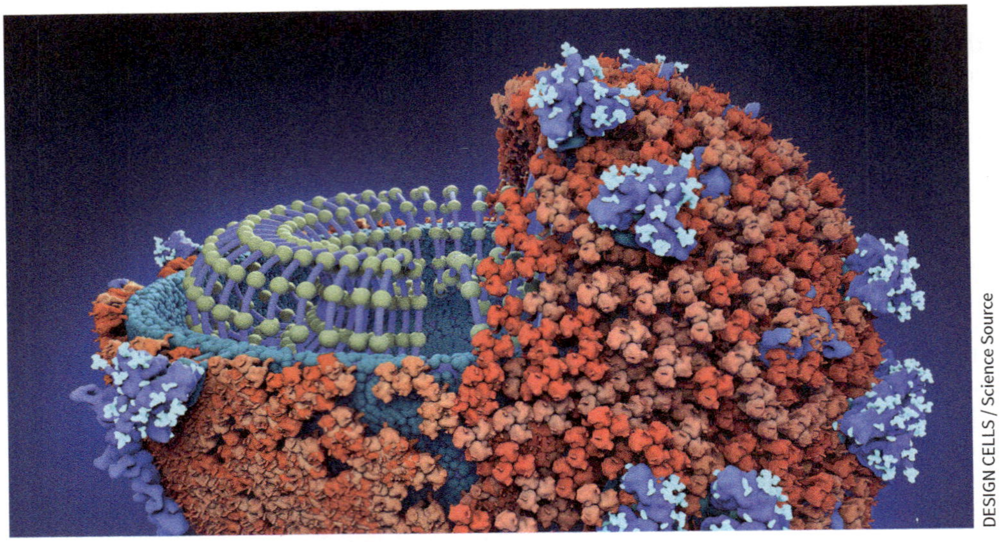

FIGURE 4.12 **Illustration of a Coronavirus Particle** The coronaviruses are composed of an RNA (ribonucleic acid) core surrounded by an envelope (depicted in light blue) containing surface proteins (shown in red and blue). Spike proteins (shown in dark blue) are used to attach and penetrate their host cells. Once inside the cells, the particles use the cells' machinery to make more copies of themselves. Different strains of coronavirus are responsible for various diseases, such as the common cold, gastroenteritis, and severe acute respiratory syndrome (SARS). The novel coronavirus called COVID-19 emerged in China in December 2019. The virus causes a respiratory illness that can develop into pneumonia and be fatal, especially among older people with compromised immune systems and preexisting conditions such as obesity.

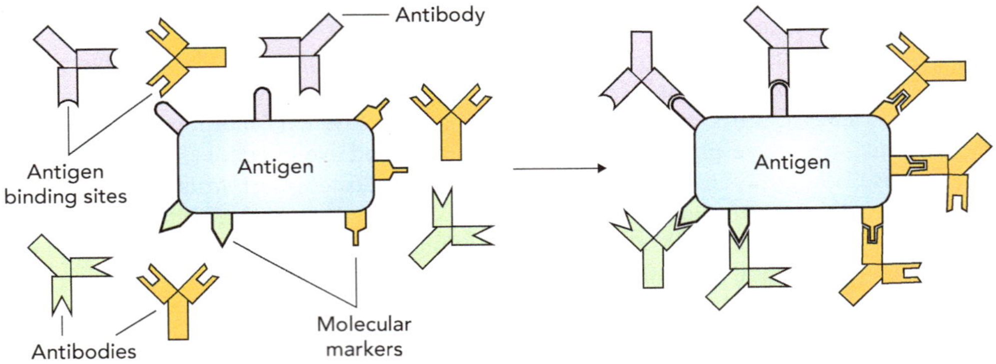

FIGURE 4.13 **Antigens and Antibodies** A particular antibody fits a particular antigen like a key in a lock. Once locked in, the antibody marks the antigen for destruction by other cells of the immune system.

Some research with different populations shows that as more of the stress hormone cortisol is secreted, levels of a type of immunoglobulin called immunoglobulin A decline, which has the effect of compromising the functioning of the immune system (**Figure 4.14**).

In one experiment, investigators looked at the effects of exercise on levels of cortisol and immunoglobulin A in people living with HIV/AIDS and people without HIV/AIDS (Melo et al., 2019). The treatment was a combination of aerobic exercise and weight training. The exercise program reduced the amount of cortisol in participants' saliva and increased their levels of immunoglobulin A. There were no significant differences in these levels between people living with HIV/AIDS and people who did not have HIV/AIDS. In sum, a healthful intervention, exercise, decreased levels of a stress hormone and improved the functioning of the immune system in both groups.

Let us take a closer look at several kinds of immune responses in the body's effort to rid itself of infectious organisms:

- **Cell-mediated immunity:** When immune cells directly attack and kill antigens without the aid of antibodies, the response is called *cell-mediated immunity*.
- **Antibody-mediated immunity:** When antibodies join the fray, the response is called *antibody-mediated immunity*.
- **Nonspecific immune response:** When the body is invaded by a pathogen, a nonspecific immune response is initiated. This first line of defense is carried out by *phagocytes* (large white blood cells called cell eaters) and natural killer (*NK*) cells.

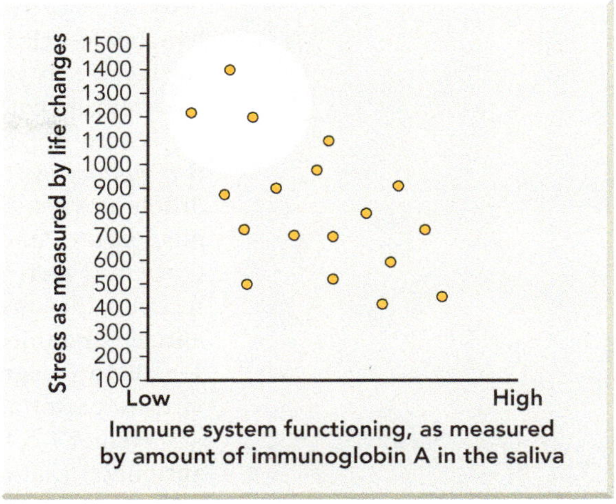

FIGURE 4.14 Negative Correlation between Stress as Measured by Life Changes and Levels of Immunoglobulin A in Saliva This figure shows that higher levels of stress are associated with poorer immune system response.

Phagocytes and NK cells are referred to as *scavenger cells* because they continuously roam the bloodstream and body tissues, hunting foreign microbes and cellular debris. When phagocytes encounter antigens, they swallow and digest them. NK cells also destroy antigens by filling them with a lethal burst of poisonous chemicals. The body defends itself by consuming its own diseased parts, and NK cells perform this function.

Phagocytes also play a key role in inflammation—the body's nonspecific defense reaction to tissue damage (such as cuts, burns, or splinters) caused by invading pathogens. When an area is infected, capillaries (small blood vessels) at the site enlarge to allow more white blood cells to flow to the injury. This activity causes the redness, swelling, warmth, and pain characteristic of inflammation. The pus that often accompanies inflammation contains the dead cells and fluids that participated in the fight between immune cells and antigens.

Tough as they are, some antigens are too powerful to be dealt a death blow by immune cells comprising the nonspecific response team alone. In such cases, phagocytes signal other lymphocytes to move into action, initiating a specific immune response. These other lymphocytes act in concert with phagocytes to disarm and destroy antigens. **Figure 4.15** shows the various parts and functions of the body's immune system.

Lymphocytes and the Lymphatic System

Lymphocytes are produced in the bone marrow and various organs of the *lymphatic system*, including the lymph nodes, spleen, and thymus. The lymphatic system is the body's other circulatory system. It carries the fluid *lymph*, which is collected from tissues throughout the

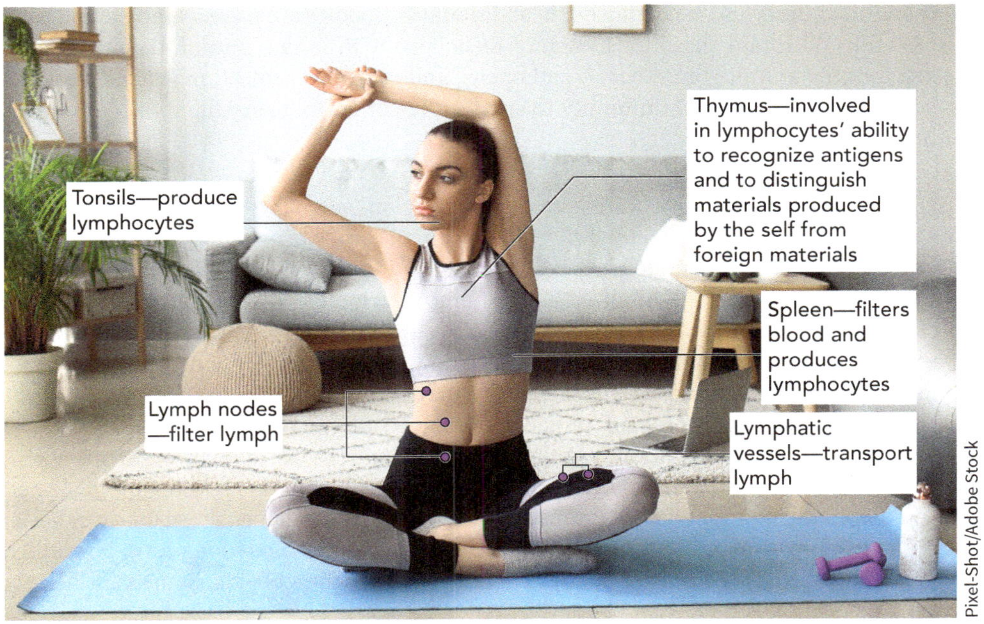

FIGURE 4.15 Structure of the Immune System The organs of the immune system are found throughout the body. They are home to white blood cells, or lymphocytes, that are key players in the immune system.

body, through its network of vessels. Lymph passes through the *lymph nodes*, or glands, where lymphocytes cleanse it of infectious agents and debris. This is why your lymph nodes become swollen when you come down with an infection. Lymphocytes are also released into the bloodstream, where they battle invaders.

There are two major types of lymphocytes—*T-lymphocytes* (simply, *T cells*) and *B-lymphocytes* (or B cells). Both T cells and B cells attack and disarm antigens, but in different ways. *Helper T cells* prowl the bloodstream for antigens, much like free-floating phagocytes. Once they find them, they secrete chemical messengers called *cytokines*. Cytokines alert *killer T cells* and phagocytes to swing into action. Killer T cells have a receptor that matches only one antigen. When it finds that antigen, it "locks" into the antigen and injects it with lethal chemicals. At birth, each of us is endowed with enough T cells to recognize at least 1 million different kinds of invading organisms, including viruses, bacteria, even dust mites.

Helper T cells also trigger production of B-lymphocytes—immune cells that produce antibodies that attack antigens. Antibodies do not kill antigens themselves. They act as "vises" that hold antigens in place so that T cells and other immune cells can destroy them. Each B cell makes only one kind of antibody that targets a particular antigen. Surrounded by phagocytes, T cells, and antibodies, most antigens don't stand much of a chance. But some overwhelm the body's immune system, causing serious illness and even death.

Memory cells are specialized B-lymphocytes that remain after the battle against a specific antigen is over, even for a lifetime. They are called *memory cells* because they produce antibodies that have a "memory" for the antigens to which they were exposed. This allows them to react swiftly when the same antigen invades the body again. Because of them, you will not come down with chicken pox twice. Memory cells specific to the chicken pox virus remain poised in your body, ready to rapidly disarm the virus should it reappear.

Suppressor T cells regulate the activities of B cells and other T cells. They prevent the immune response from damaging healthy cells in the vicinity of the infection. Suppressor T cells also signal the various T and B cells to cease activity when the infection has been eradicated.

Immunity and Immunization

The human body is capable of several kinds of immunity, or ways of protecting itself against disease. Let us begin as people begin, with innate immunity.

Innate Immunity Inborn or *innate immunity* results from transmission of the mother's antibodies to the fetus. Following birth, additional antibodies are passed along to the baby in breast milk. With rare exceptions, each of us is born with innate immunities. Babies are protected for only a limited number of pathogens, and even this protection is temporary. As we develop, we need acquired immunity to survive the continuous onslaught of many kinds of pathogens.

Acquired Immunity Acquired immunity develops after birth. Acquired immunity can be active or passive. *Active immunity* can develop naturally, as when we are infected by a pathogen and the immune system produces *antibodies* against it. It can develop artificially, as by vaccination. In naturally acquired active immunity, foreign agents cause an infection, which leads memory lymphocytes to develop antibodies that target the specific antigen. The antibodies protect us from reinfection. However, many viral and bacterial organisms mutate, or change their genetic structure. This is especially true of influenza, which is why a case of the flu during one flu season does not protect us when we are exposed to a different strain the following year. Artificially acquired active immunity involves the use of an immunizing agent, such as a vaccine. A vaccine—also called an immunization—contains a killed or weakened pathogen to stimulate production of antibodies. Many vaccines, such as those for diphtheria, measles, and mumps, are administered in early childhood and provide long-term immunity. Teenagers and adults may be given booster shots to enhance their effects. Some vaccines are injected. Others are taken orally.

Some infections—such as those produced by snakebite toxin—act so fast that they can prove lethal unless passive immunity is induced. *Passive immunity* is a short-lived form of protection against infections that can damage or kill before the immune system can produce antibodies. It is used in the treatment of snakebites, rabies (along with a vaccine), and other infections for which there are no vaccines.

Passive immunity can be transferred from one person to another through injecting antibody-rich blood serum *(antiserum)* called *gamma globulin* into the person needing protection. Once in the recipient's bloodstream, the antibodies attack antigens.

Immunization and Preventable Diseases

Health psychologists join the battle against infectious diseases by applying conceptual models, such as the health belief model (HBM), to better understand obstacles impeding participation in vaccination efforts and to design behavior change strategies designed to increase access and utilization of these public health programs (see nearby *Health Psychology in Action* feature). Vaccination is used to prevent many infectious diseases. Some vaccines are routinely recommended for children through the age of 6 years. The CDC also publishes, and frequently updates, recommended vaccinations for older children and adolescents, and for adults. For example, vaccines for HPV—Gardasil 9 and Cervarix—were originally prescribed for "tweens" and early adolescents. However, they are now recommended for older adolescents, young adults, and middle-aged adults through the age of 45 years. HPV infections have been linked to cervical, vaginal, and vulvar cancers in women, penile cancers in men, and anal cancers in both women and men (CDC, 2019g), so it is useful to know that one might still receive some benefit from the vaccines if they are obtained in adulthood.

Gardasil and Cervarix prevent people from being infected with several strains of HPV, and their advent was met with the open and often virulent opposition by some groups of people. The vaccines were originally given only to girls, tweens and early teenagers. Because they prevent the sexual transmission of HPV, some opponents argued that the vaccines signal young girls that "we expect you to be sexually active" (Dempsey & O'Leary, 2018). Some believe it would be better for girls to have the threat of HPV and eventual cervical cancer hanging over their heads. Some pediatricians also resisted vaccination, as in the case of one who said, "It may encourage risky sexual behavior in my adolescent patients." Another point of controversy was whether schools should require HPV vaccination as a condition of enrollment. In response to the controversy, the CDC began to include HPV vaccination in its recommended vaccination schedule for children and adolescents—and added boys and men to the list.

Immune System Disorders

Immune system disorders occur when the immune system overreacts to normally harmless antigens, when it misidentifies the body's own cells as foreign, or when it is unable to protect the body from common pathogens.

Allergies: An Overly Sensitive Alarm Allergies provide a good example of the interface between health-related behavior and physical health (see the next "Applying Health Psychology" feature). More than a quarter of American adults and children have allergies (CDC, 2023l). Twenty-one percent of U.S. college students report seeking professional help for an allergy within the past year (American College Health Association, 2018). An allergy is hypersensitivity to a normally harmless substance, such as dust, foods, mold, pollen, animal dander, and insect bites. An allergic reaction occurs when the immune system mounts too vigorous a response to substances that actually pose no threat. Substances that trigger allergic reactions are called *allergens.*

It remains unclear why some people are affected by allergies and others are not. Genetics presumably plays a role. The immune systems of people with allergies respond to allergens by releasing *histamine,* an inflammatory chemical that causes a runny nose and other symptoms typical of allergies. The particular symptoms depend in part on where histamine is released—for instance, in the nose, chest, skin, or intestine. Some of the most common allergic responses include sneezing, itchy skin, hives, eczema, diarrhea, nasal congestion, or constriction of the lungs such that one finds it difficult to breathe.

Health Psychology in Action

Changing Parents' Beliefs about Measles Vaccinations

Immunization represents one of the greatest public health achievements. Vaccines save lives, make communities more productive and strengthen health systems.

Salzburg Statement on Vaccine Acceptance (Ratzan et al., 2019)

One of the tragedies of these post-truth times is that the lies, conspiracy theories and illusions spread by social media and populist politicians can be downright dangerous. The denial of human responsibility for climate change is one example; another is opposition to vaccination.

Editorial Board, *The New York Times*, May 2, 2017

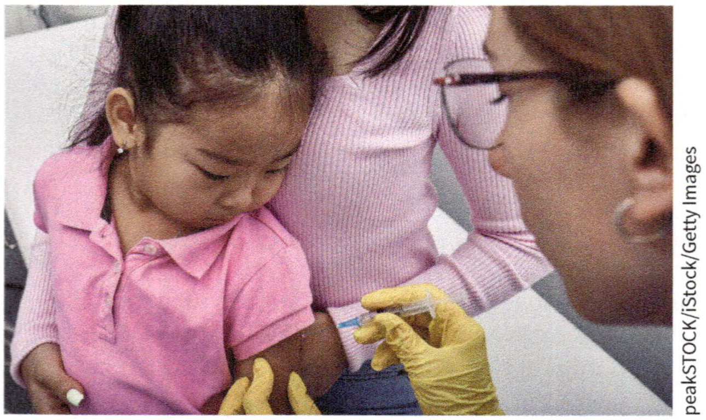

Getting Vaccinated How does the HBM help us understand the factors involved in making important health decisions, such as receiving vaccinations for measles and other serious illnesses?

Consider a remarkably successful public health campaign: the national effort to eradicate measles. By the year 2000, as a result of near-universal childhood vaccinations, measles was virtually eliminated from the United States (Gostin et al., 2019). This victory against measles literally saved hundreds of lives and needless suffering of millions of children annually in the United States. Measles is a highly contagious viral infection that can result in a severe flu-like illness and can lead to harmful, even life-threatening consequences and complications including pneumonia, encephalitis, and hearing loss. The measles vaccine is part of the combination MMR vaccine that is routinely administered to young children to protect them against measles, mumps, and rubella.

Before the introduction of a measles vaccine in the early 1960s, the disease accounted for upward of 500 deaths and 3–4 million cases annually in the United States. However, in recent years, false information about immunization, largely spread through social media, persuaded many parents to withhold vaccinations from their children for measles and other infectious diseases.

The anti-vaccination movement contributed to a dramatic rise in measles outbreaks, with the number of cases reported in 2019 reaching the highest level in the past 25 years. Thankfully, the number of reported cases dropped considerably in the early 2020s, falling to only 121 in 2022 (CDC, 2023k).

People identified as "anti-vaxxers" have perpetuated various myths about vaccines, including the false belief that the measles vaccine causes autism or that it can be deadly. Let's be clear: Drawing upon many scientific studies, the CDC unequivocally affirmed that vaccines do not cause autism (CDC, 2015, 2020e). However well-intentioned parents who refuse vaccinations for their children may be, the result is that measles has spread among unvaccinated children, especially among clusters of families claiming religious exemptions (this despite the appeals of many religious leaders in these communities who advocate childhood vaccinations). Not only does misinformation lead to needless suffering of unvaccinated children, but the spread of the virus can be harmful to vaccinated children with weakened immune systems (Gostin et al., 2019).

Looked at from the standpoint of the HBM, we need to examine the beliefs the parents hold about the perceived threat posed by measles and the perceived benefits and costs of having their children vaccinated. By changing their beliefs, the model posits, we can increase the likelihood that they will seek to have their children vaccinated.

- *Changing perceptions of threat:* Raising awareness about the threats posed by measles may involve bringing to the parent's attention information from the CDC and other reputable medical sources about the risks that measles poses. This educational intervention also needs to address tendencies to minimize the risk by thinking that the disease is like the common cold or that the chance of contracting or spreading the disease is remote.
- *Changing perceptions of benefits and costs:* Sharing health information about the effectiveness of the vaccine and debunking myths about harmful consequences can help parents change the decisional balance in favor of vaccination. It may also be helpful to appeal to religious and community leaders to speak with parents to counter tendencies for misinformation to spread within the community.

To combat the surge in measles cases, the CDC prepared a measles toolkit for healthcare providers, which is available at https://www.cdc.gov/measles/toolkit/healthcare-providers.html The toolkit provides fact sheets and immunization schedules healthcare providers can share with their patients, as well as suggestions about how to talk to parents about immunization. Examples of what healthcare providers can say to parents to help change their antivaccination beliefs include the following:

- "I strongly recommend your child get these vaccines today ..."
- "These shots are very important to protect them from serious diseases."
- "I believe in vaccines so strongly that I vaccinated my own children on schedule."
- "This office has given thousands of doses of vaccines and we have never seen a serious reaction."

On a broader societal level, health researchers have called upon the government to ensure that all children get vaccinated and have petitioned social media companies to step up and block misleading and false information from being spread on their networks.

Allergic rhinitis, commonly called *hay fever*, occurs when airborne allergens, such as pollen, dust, mold, and particles of dried dog or cat saliva, enter the nose and throat of a person with allergies. Common symptoms include puffy and itchy eyes, a runny or stopped-up nose (or both), and sneezing. People who are sensitive to pollens and ragweed suffer most during the pollination seasons of spring and fall.

Mold allergies involve reactions to seeds or spores of plants in the fungus family. Molds can survive anywhere there is moisture, including piles of fallen leaves and walls of damp basements. Dust allergies are caused by the tiny droppings (feces) of microscopic bugs called *dust mites,* which dwell in mattresses, carpeting, and upholstery.

Some people with allergies experience a severe allergic reaction called *anaphylaxis* or *anaphylactic shock* in response to insect bites, stings, and certain foods, such as peanuts. The throat may swell and shut down and fluid may begin to fill the lungs. Anaphylaxis can be life-threatening but can be treated with administration of adrenaline. Nut and peanut allergies are responsible for several hundred deaths a year from anaphylactic shock.

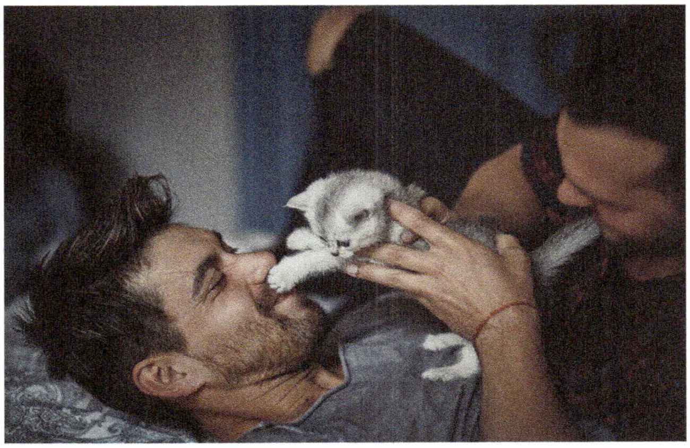

Oliver Rossi/Getty Images

Do We Really Want the Kitten On the Bed? It is doubtful that the animal will do any harm, but many people are allergic to animal dander.

Autoimmune Disorders

In autoimmune disorders, the immune system attacks healthy cells as though they were foreign. Two of the more prevalent autoimmune disorders are *rheumatoid arthritis*, a painful, potentially disabling condition involving chronic inflammation of the membranes that line the joints, and *lupus erythematosus*, a chronic inflammatory disorder of connective tissue. Both diseases strike women more often than men. These diseases are treated with varying degrees of success with medications that suppress the immune response. Psychological forms of treatment, such as cognitive-behavioral therapy, also shows beneficial effects with respect to enhancing immune system functioning in patients with immune-related disorders (Shields, Spahr, & Slavich, 2020).

Multiple sclerosis (MS) is a chronic and often crippling nervous system disorder in which *myelin*, the coating that insulates nerve cells in the brain and spinal cord, is damaged or destroyed. When myelin is damaged, communication between the brain and spinal cord breaks down, leading to symptoms that can impair speech, walking, or writing. MS strikes women about twice as often as men. MS may be an autoimmune disease in which white blood

Applying Health Psychology

Protecting Yourself from Allergies

Allergies can be diagnosed by a test in which a drop of the suspected allergen is injected just below the skin. Depending on the type of allergy, people can make behavioral changes to control it or reduce discomfort.

- *Environmental engineering:* Avoiding allergens is the most direct way of preventing an allergic response. People who are sensitive to pollens might benefit from checking the daily pollen count in their local newspaper or on the internet. On days when the pollen count is especially high, they might minimize outdoor activities. If you are sensitive to dust mites, keep your home and workplace as free of dust as possible. Venetian blinds, down-filled blankets, feather pillows, and wall-to-wall carpeting are natural dust collectors. Protect your bedding with allergen-proof covering and wash it regularly. You can dust furniture, but vacuuming may raise more dust than it removes. (There are low-emission vacuum cleaners.) You might use cleaning products containing *acaricides*, which kill dust mites.
- *Allergy medications:* Allergy medications help control the symptoms of allergies. Your primary healthcare provider or allergist can help identify the nature of the allergen(s) causing your symptoms and the appropriate course of treatment. *Antihistamines* counteract histamines and are useful in treating sneezing, runny nose, and itchy eyes and throat. Decongestants help unclog stuffy noses. Follow the instructions on the label. Steroid nasal sprays offer greater relief of nasal congestion than nasal decongestants do. Another type of nasal spray contains the anti-inflammatory drug *cromolyn sodium*.
- *Allergy injections:* Allergy shots contain tiny amounts of an offending allergen and gradually desensitize the individual. Though effective in most cases, they must be taken regularly for months or years. People who cannot control their exposure to particular an allergen are especially good candidates for allergy shots. They need to incorporate obtaining regular allergy shots as part of their routine lifestyle.

cells attack the body's nerve cells, causing inflammation that depletes myelin. A viral infection may trigger the autoimmune response, but no specific causal agent has been found.

Immune Deficiencies In rare instances, generally resulting from a genetic defect, children are born with immune systems that fail to protect them from common pathogens. They must live in a sterile environment to prevent exposure to pathogens that children with healthier immune systems can fight off. In the case of HIV/AIDS, a virus attacks the immune system, crippling it and leaving the person vulnerable to opportunistic infections. HIV is the acronym for *human immunodeficiency virus*. We will learn more about HIV/AIDS in Chapter 10. Immune system deficiencies have also been implicated in the development of cancer. Cancerous cells that would normally be eradicated may replicate out of control if the immune system is weakened by age or other factors.

Common Infectious Diseases

Now that we have considered the nature of pathogens and immunity, let's discuss several types of respiratory tract infections and other common infectious diseases. We discuss sexually transmitted infections (STIs) in Chapter 10.

Respiratory tract infections range from the common cold and milder cases of flu to more serious conditions like pneumonia and tuberculosis. Although bacteria and viruses are most often the pathogens involved, smoking and exposure to pollutants increase susceptibility to these infections.

The Common Cold The common cold is a contagious viral infection of the upper respiratory tract. Colds are the most common infectious illness. Most adults get two to four colds per year; children have about six to ten. About 200 different viruses cause the common cold, with *rhinoviruses* (from the Greek *rhino*, meaning "nose") causing 30–35% of them. Symptoms include nasal congestion, sore throat, fatigue, headache, and perhaps a low-grade fever. Colds typically last 1–2 weeks.

Colds may be transmitted by airborne exposure to viruses expelled by an infected person through sneezing, coughing, or just talking. They may also be contracted by touch, that is, by contact with a surface (e.g., a tissue, doorknob, or hand) that contains nasal secretions left by an infected a person with an infection. The best way to recover from a cold is to rest and drink plenty of fluids. No medications or vaccines prevent or cure the common cold, but many medications alleviate the symptoms.

Health psychologists have studied the relationships between stress and being infected with the common cold. In landmark research, Sheldon Cohen and his colleagues applied an experimental method in which healthy adults (with their permission, of course) were exposed to a virus that causes the common cold (Cohen, 2016; Cohen et al., 1998). The research participants were then quarantined and followed for 5 to 6 days to observe which ones developed a cold, as defined objectively by evidence of viral shedding, mucus production, and congestion. The results pointed directly to links between stress and the common cold. Participants with a greater occurrence of recent and especially chronic stressful life changes and events showed an increased risk of developing a cold after exposure to the challenge virus. Although this evidence does not demonstrate that stress is a direct causal factor in the common cold, the message is clear that people under high levels of stress are more susceptible to catching one.

Influenza (the Flu) Influenza or the flu is another infection of the respiratory tract—a highly contagious viral disease that affects the lungs and other parts of the body. It is transmitted like the common cold and caused by three families of influenza viruses—type A, type B, and type C. Type A influenza is most common and associated with the most severe outbreaks. Now and then new strains of influenza virus and other viruses, such as COVID-19, appear, which may lead to worldwide epidemics, or pandemics, because few people have antibodies against a newly emerging strain.

People infected with the flu generally experience a fever between 102°F and 104°F, chills, headache, general aches and pains, fatigue, weakness, and possibly a sore throat, dry cough, nausea, and burning eyes. The three major symptoms of COVID-19 are fever, a cough, and shortness of breath. Most healthy persons who are infected with the seasonal flu recover in about a week. In vulnerable groups, however, such as children, older people, and people with other health problems, the flu can lead to serious, possibly fatal complications. The best approach to the seasonal flu is prevention. The CDC advises people to obtain annual flu shots as early as the age of 6 months.

As with colds, the flu is best treated with rest, fluids, and pain and fever relievers. There is some evidence that antiviral drugs have some effect on the flu, but they tend to be of minimal value in severe cases.

Pneumonia Pneumonia is a serious lung infection in which invading pathogens cause the air sacs in the lungs—the alveoli—to fill with pus and other liquid, making it difficult for oxygen to reach the blood. Lack of oxygen may cause death. Prior to the COVID-19 pandemic, pneumonia claimed about 41,000 lives annually in the United States, although recent times have seen a large jump in COVID-19-related pneumonia. Most cases involve viral or bacterial infection, but pneumonia may also result from irritation to the lungs due to pollutants or, in hospitalized patients, from lung irritation caused by anesthesia or intravenous foods and

Applying Health Psychology

Wash Those Hands!

Hand washing is the simplest, easiest, and most effective way to prevent contracting or spreading infectious diseases, including the flu (CDC, 2020d). Amazingly, it is also one of the most overlooked prevention methods. People are taking heed, however, perhaps because of the raised awareness of risks posed by COVID-19 and other infectious agents. Women are more conscientious hand washers in public restrooms, washing their hands 93% of the time as opposed to 77% for men. However, a higher percentage (96%) of people reported in a separate telephone study that they always wash their hands, so it would seem that some people who say they wash their hands after using a public restroom actually don't.

Health professionals recommend scrubbing your hands vigorously for at least 20 seconds with soap and water, about as long as it takes to sing "Happy Birthday" two times. You will wash away cold viruses and staph and strep bacteria as well as many other disease-causing microbes. Hand washing also helps prevent transmitting the pathogens to others and to curb the spread of COVID-19. It is especially important to wash your hands:

- Before preparing or eating food
- After coughing or sneezing
- After changing a diaper
- After using the restroom

Health psychologists are involved in efforts to encourage people to practice good hand hygiene. Consider a research study in which self-designed poster interventions were installed in a college campus in the United Kingdom (Lawson & Vaganay-Miller, 2019). Rather than rely on self-reports, hand washing was indirectly observed for 2 months. Prior to the intervention, about 51% of the college population washed their hands with soap and dried them afterward. Nearly 8% (7.88%) washed their hands for 20 seconds. Following the intervention, the percentage of students who washed their hands with soap and dried them rose to about 55% (not a statistically significant difference), and washing for 20 seconds remained at nearly 8% (7.97%). Analysis of gender differences showed that the intervention had more of an effect on women than men. Prior to the intervention, about 49% of women washed their hands with soap; following intervention, the percentage rose to nearly 63%—a statistically significant difference. There was no such improvement for men. Women in the study were more compliant with the poster message than men were, perhaps because, as numerous studies find, women are relatively more concerned about health-related issues. Yet one-third of the women still did not wash their hands adequately, possibly suggesting that stronger messages are needed to change behavior.

A poster similar to this one was used in the British study.

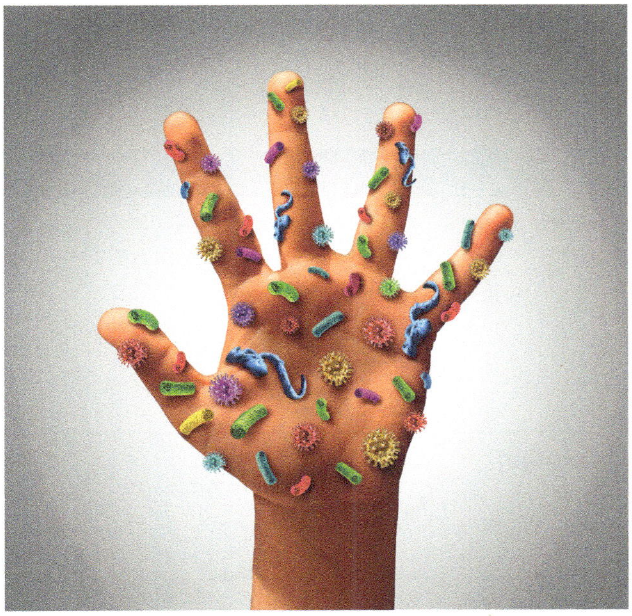

Brain light/Alamy Stock Photo

Germs Spread Easily! Wash Your Hands! The time it takes you to read this paragraph is the amount of time you should spend washing your hands. This helps prevent the spread of germs and illnesses like the cold and the flu that are easily transmitted from person to person by hands that are not washed and dried properly. Please help reduce the spread of germs and illnesses by washing your hands with soap and water for 20 seconds and drying them afterward for the same amount of time. Thank you.

A Closer Look

Is It a Cold, the Flu, or an Airborne Allergy?

Many of the symptoms of the common cold, flu, and airborne allergies are similar, and it is important to be able to tell the difference because these health problems require different types of responses. Here are some suggestions from the National Institutes of Health to help tell them apart.

Systoms	Cold	Flu	Airborne Allergy
Fever	Rare	Usual, high (100–102°F), sometimes higher, especially in young children); lasts 3–4 days	Never
Headache	Uncommon	Common	Uncommon
General Aches, Pains	Slight	Usual; often severe	Never
Fatigue, Weakness	Sometimes	Usual, can last up to 3 weeks	Sometimes
Extreme Exhaustion	Never	Usual, at the beginning of the illness	Never
Stuffy, Runny Nose	Common	Sometimes	Common
Sneezing	Usual	Sometimes	Usual
Sore Throat	Common	Sometimes	Sometimes
Cough	Common	Common, can become severe	Sometimes
Chest Discomfort	Mild to moderate	Common	Rare, except for people with allergic asthma

The National Institutes of Health also provides information about the treatment, prevention, and complications of each of these problems.

	Cold	Flu	Airborne Allergy
Treatment	Get plenty of rest. Stay hydrated. (Drink plenty of fluids.) Decongestants. Aspirin (ages 18 and up), acetaminophen, or ibuprofen for aches and pains	Get plenty of rest. Stay hydrated. Aspirin (ages 18 and up), acetaminophen, or ibuprofen for aches, pains, and fever Antiviral medicines (see your doctor)	Avoid allergens (things that you're allergic to). Antihistamines Nasal steroids Decongestants
Prevention	Wash your hands often. Avoid close contact with anyone who has a cold.	Get the flu vaccine each year. Wash your hands often. Avoid close contact with anyone who has the flu.	Avoid allergens, such as pollen, house dust mites, mold, pet dander, cockroaches.
Complications	Sinus infection Middle ear infection Asthma	Bronchitis, pneumonia; can be life threatening	Sinus infection Middle ear infection Asthma

Source: National Institutes of Health (2014) / Public Domain.

liquids. Symptoms usually include fever and chills; chest pain; a cough with rust, yellow, or greenish sputum (mucus-laden material coughed up from deep inside the lungs); and difficulty breathing. Pneumonia is especially dangerous in older people and the very young.

Bacterial pneumonia is treated with antibiotics. Though there are no effective drugs for viral pneumonia, most cases resolve on their own. Rest, fluids, proper diet, and avoidance of smoking are all helpful. A vaccine is available for *pneumococcal pneumonia*, a form of bacterial pneumonia.

Tuberculosis Tuberculosis (TB) was one of our most dreaded diseases until the 1940s and 1950s, when antibiotics were discovered. TB is a chronic infection caused by the bacterium *Mycobacterium tuberculosis,* which usually affects the lungs and sometimes other parts of the body, including the brain, kidneys, or spine. Symptoms include a racking cough, fever, night sweats, fatigue, hoarseness, chest pain, weight loss, and blood in the sputum.

The prevalence of TB is at a low ebb in the general population, but there is a high incidence of the disease among people who use intravenous drugs, people with HIV/AIDS, people who are homeless, and people in confined living quarters. TB is generally contracted through months of contact with people who are infected and is transmitted via sneezed or coughed-up airborne droplets. The bacteria multiply in the air sacs in the lungs, forming cheese-like clumps or lesions called *tubercles*. If left untreated, the entire lung can become scarred with these clumps, leading to respiratory failure and death.

The advent of screening tests for TB played a pivotal role in the development of the health belief model (HBM). The presence of the TB bacterium is detected by a tuberculin skin test (or *Mantoux* test), in which a small amount of fluid, called *tuberculin*, is injected under the skin of the forearm. If a red welt appears 48–72 hours later, TB may be present. Additional diagnostic tests determine whether an infected person has TB. Treatment for TB involves the prolonged use of antibiotics.

Infectious Mononucleosis Infectious mononucleosis (mono) is caused by the Epstein-Barr virus (EBV). Mono is often referred to as the kissing disease because the virus reproduces in salivary glands, making saliva especially contagious. Other means of transmission include sharing toothbrushes and eating utensils. Mono typically affects young adults in the 16- to 30-year age range, but almost everyone catches mono at some time. Underscoring the role of both behavior and stress in the transmission of disease, mono is common among college students because of deep kissing and the accumulation of academic stresses as a semester wears on (Choi et al., 2020). In cases in which health psychology ventured into space, investigators report that the stress of spaceflight puts astronauts at greater risk of dysregulation of the immune system (Crucian & Choukér, 2020) and is connected with reactivation of the symptoms of EBV (Stowe et al., 2020).

Symptoms of EBV begin to develop after an incubation period of perhaps 30–50 days and may include fever, sore throat, swollen glands, and fatigue, followed by high fever (101–105°F), sore throat (caused by enlarged, often pus-covered tonsils), and swollen lymph glands in the neck, arm, and groin. The clinical stage typically lasts 2–3 weeks, although some symptoms linger for months.

Numerous other studies have shown the connection between vulnerability to the EBV and stress. A classic study by health researcher Janice Kiecolt-Glaser and her colleagues (1984) examined blood samples from 42 medical students who were infected with EBV during three time periods—1 month before final exams, the first day of final exams (when stress was hypothesized to be at its highest), and during the first week after students returned from summer vacations. The students also completed the UCLA Loneliness Scale to gain insight into their levels of social and emotional support. As measured by levels of B lymphocytes, students' immune systems were most compromised during the hypothesized period of stress. The immune systems of students who had high levels of social and emotional support were significantly less compromised, it was found, suggesting that psychological factors can help mitigate the effects of stress.

Researcher Catherine Panter-Brick and her colleagues (2019) examined the relationships among adversity, biological markers of stress, and psychological outcomes among war-torn refugees and nonrefugees. All participants were 12–18 years old. The refugees were Syrian children living in Jordan, alongside Jordanian nonrefugees of similar socioeconomic status. The measures of adversity included poverty, exposure to trauma, and refugee status

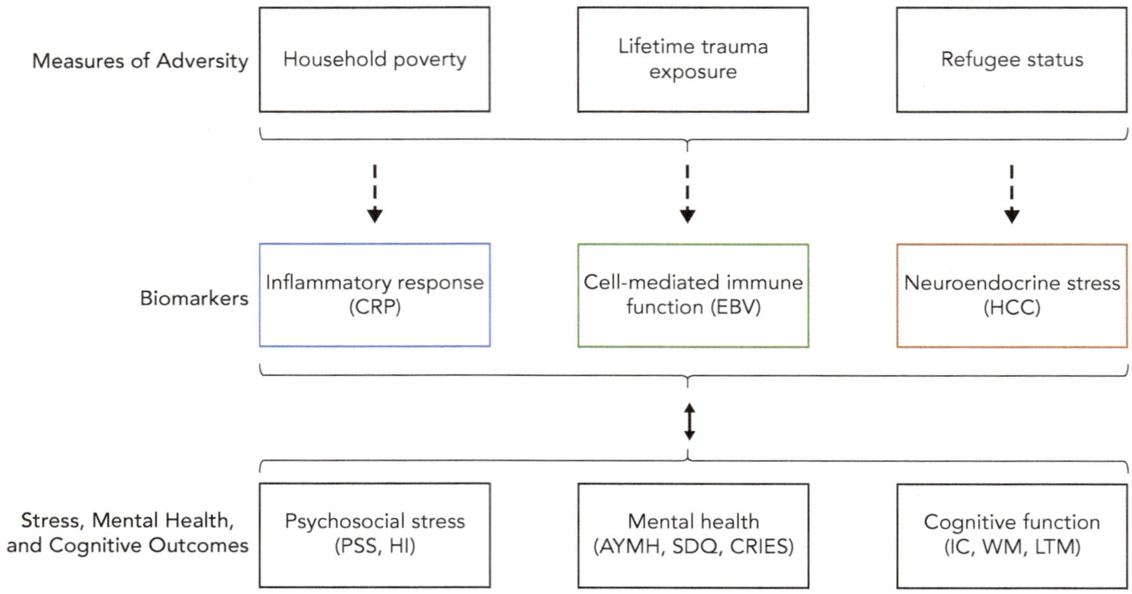

FIGURE 4.16 **Associations Between Adversity, Biomarkers, and Outcomes** Key: EBV = Epstein–Barr virus as identified by blood test; HCC = Concentration of cortisol in the hair; PSS = Perceived stress scale scores; HI = Human Insecurity Scale; AYMH = Arab Youth Mental Health scale; SDQ = Strengths and Difficulties Questionnaire; IC = Inhibitory control; WM = Working memory; LTM = Long-term memory.

(see **Figure 4.16**). The biological markers included presence of the EBV and stress, as measured by the concentration of cortisol found in the hair of the participants (HCC). The outcomes were perceived stress (PSS); feelings of insecurity as measured by the Human Insecurity Scale (HI); mental health as measured by a mental health scale tailored to Arab children; psychological strengths and weaknesses (SDQ); cognitive functioning, as measured by ability to conform one's behavior to the requirements of the social and educational setting (IC); and the functioning of working memory and long-term memory. The researchers also used a trial intervention to reduce the children's stress.

To some degree, the results were predictable. The prevalence of EBV was greater among refugee children than controls, and the refugees also showed higher inflammatory responses and hair concentrations of cortisol. Refugees were more insecure than controls. There were also positive correlations between insecurity, exposure to trauma, and stress scores. Hair cortisol concentrations were negatively associated with perceived stress, measures of mental health, and measures of cognitive functioning. The intervention had no effect, but to their credit, the researchers tried to help. Nevertheless, the study is of value for demonstrating solid connections among stress, the functioning of the immune system, and various health (EBV) and psychological outcomes.

Another study found similar results with a population thousands of miles away, in Appalachian Ohio, a relatively impoverished area in the United States (Brook et al., 2017). The participants were 185 Appalachian women aged 18 to 26 years. Of the 185 participants, blood tests showed positive for EBV in 169. The blood tests also enabled researchers to measure the level of EBV antibodies. There was a strong positive relationship between levels of perceived stress and levels of antibodies, suggesting that increased stress produces a stronger immune system response to EBV. Social support was linked with lower levels of antibodies in the women's serum, suggesting that having a helping hand (or two) made it easier for their bodies to fend off EBV. Perceived stress was also associated with the quality of sleep and with smoking behavior. This study showed that the greater the stress the women perceived, the less well they slept and the more they smoked.

No available medications or vaccines will cure or prevent mono. Rest, ample fluids, and a balanced diet are the best route to recovery. Pain relievers may be used for headaches and other discomfort. Sore throats may be treated with salt gargles.

It is apparent that stress is a major health problem in the United States—in fact, around the world. In the following chapter we explore psychological means of coping with stress and enabling people to lead healthier lives.

Review 4.3

INTERACTIVE SELF-SCORING QUIZZES

Sentence Completion

1. Bacteria, viruses, fungi, and yeast are examples of __________.

2. Bacteria thrive in the lining of the __________ membranes of the mouth, throat, and nasal passages.

3. __________ consist of a core of genetic material and a surrounding coat of protein.

4. The Epstein-__________ virus causes infectious mononucleosis.

5. The immune system contains billions of specialized __________ blood cells.

6. Antibodies are produced by __________.

7. There is a negative correlation between levels of immunoglobulin A and levels of __________.

8. Scavenger cells include NK cells and __________.

9. The bone marrow, lymph nodes, spleen, and thymus produce __________.

10. Acquired immunity can develop artificially, as by __________.

11. Some parents and commentators expressed concern that vaccination for __________ might disinhibit sexual restraint among teenage girls.

12. A(n) __________ reaction may occur when the immune system mounts too vigorous a response to substances that actually pose no threat.

13. __________ shock is a life-threatening response to an allergen in which airways narrow, threatening breathing.

14. HIV/AIDS is an example of an immune __________ disorder.

15. People are more vulnerable to the common cold when they have experienced __________ __________.

16. __________ __________ is the simplest and most effective way to prevent contracting or spreading infectious diseases, including the flu.

Think About It

How do people you know respond to the seasonal flu? How did they (and you) respond to the COVID-19 crisis? Did they wash their hands regularly and follow the other guidelines for protecting themselves and others from the deadly virus? Why or why not? How about you? Did you follow the guidelines; if not, why not?

Recite: An Active Summary

INTERACTIVE SELF-SCORING QUIZZES

Chapter 4 Practice Quiz

1. Define stress and eustress.

Stress refers to the pressures we experience when we face the demands in our daily lives that require adjustment. Eustress, however, is a positive form of stress in that it helps keep us alert and occupied.

2. Discuss stress as an event that requires adaptation.

One view looks upon stress as the demand made on an organism to adapt. Sources of stress that require adaptation include daily hassles and life changes (also called life events). There are household, health, time-pressure, inner-concern, environmental, financial, work, and future security hassles. Life changes differ from daily hassles in that they are intermittent, and some are positive—but they also require adaptation. Examples of highly stressful life changes include rape, finding out that one is seropositive for HIV, death of a friend or family member, concerns about pregnancy, and finals week.

3. Discuss other ways of thinking about stress—stress as a threat, as a situation in which demands exceed resources, and as an interruption of goals.

Viewing stress as threat or harm brings us into the realm of pain, environmental stressors (an overlap with daily hassles), and terrorism; stress as situations in which the demands exceed our resources, as in the examples of job strain and the demands on women in the workplace; and stress as interruption of goals, as with the stresses of commuting and those faced by who interrupt their careers to care for families. Yet another source of stress is the Type A behavior pattern. When under threat, Shelley Taylor argues that women may engage in a tend-and-befriend reaction rather than a fight-or-flight reaction.

4. Describe the effects of stress on the body, focusing on the roles of the endocrine system and the autonomic nervous system.

Hans Selye identified a three-stage biological response to stress, which he termed the general adaptation syndrome. The alarm stage is characterized by activity of the endocrine system, leading to the secretion of stress hormones—corticosteroids, adrenaline, and noradrenaline—by the adrenal glands. It also involves arousal of the sympathetic division of the autonomic nervous system, which stimulates rapid heartbeat and respiration rates, dilates the pupils of the eyes, causes sweating, and impairs digestion and sexual arousal. The resistance stage involves continued sympathetic activity but at a lower level, and the exhaustion stage may be associated with the deterioration of resistance and increased vulnerability to so-called diseases of adaptation.

5. Discuss the pathogens that serve as infectious agents.

Pathogens that serve as infectious agents include bacteria, viruses, fungi, protozoa, and parasitic worms. Some bacteria are beneficial, but others release toxins that harm the body. Bacterial infections are typically treated by antibiotics. Viruses consist of a core of genetic material and a surrounding coat of protein. They "hijack" the body's life processes to reproduce.

6. Describe the functioning of the immune system.

The immune system is armed with white blood cells, or lymphocytes. Lymphocytes detect antigens (antibody generators) and produce antibodies—immunoglobulins—that mark antigens for destruction. Phagocytes swallow and digest antigens. There is a negative correlation between life changes and levels of immunoglobulin A; in short, stress is associated with impaired functioning of the immune system.

7. Discuss the different types of immunity and the controversies surrounding vaccinations for measles and human papillomavirus.

Immunity may be innate (inborn) or acquired. Innate immunity in a newborn results from the mother's transmission of her antibodies to the baby. Acquired immunity may be obtained by successfully fighting a pathogen and developing antibodies to it or by vaccination (immunization). Anti-vaxxers have perpetuated the myth that the measles vaccine is associated with autism; this belief has no foundation in scientific evidence. The vaccine for HPV was met with suspicion by some people who feared that it would disinhibit sexual behavior in teenage girls.

8. Discuss immune system disorders.

Immune system disorders typically occur when the immune system overreacts to typically harmless antigens (such as pollen or nuts) or when it misperceives the body's own cells as foreign. Allergies reflect an overly sensitive immune system, now and then resulting in anaphylactic shock, which is symptomized by a possibly fatal narrowing of the respiratory passageways. In immune deficiencies, the immune system has a weakened ability to protect against disease. Immune deficiencies may be inborn or acquired, as in the case of an infection by the human immunodeficiency virus (HIV).

9. Discuss common infectious diseases, referring to research concerning cortisol levels and vulnerability.

Common infectious diseases include the common cold and the flu. Experimental research involving viral challenges have shown that experiencing recent and chronic life changes increases the risk that a person who has been exposed to the virus that causes a cold will develop a clinical illness. Seasonal flu is best prevented by annual flu shots. Research with people who have been infected with the Epstein-Barr virus, which causes mononucleosis (mono), shows a clear association between stressors and cortisol levels.

Answers to Review Sections

4.1

1. hassles
2. changes (events)
3. frustration
4. Type A
5. decrease
6. increase

4.2

1. general
2. fight, flight
3. endocrine
4. parasympathetic
5. adrenal
6. hypothalamus
7. corticosteroids (cortisol)
8. tend, befriend

4.3

1. pathogens
2. mucous
3. Viruses
4. Barr
5. white
6. lymphocytes
7. cortisol
8. phagocytes
9. lymphocytes
10. vaccination (immunization)
11. human papillomavirus (HPV)
12. allergic
13. Anaphylactic
14. deficiency
15. recent or severe chronic life changes or life events
16. Hand washing

Scoring Key for the "How Much Stress Have You Experienced?"

The developers of the College Life Stress Inventory administered their inventory to a sample of 257 students in introductory psychology. Though we can't say that their student sample was representative of undergraduate students in general, the scores they report provide a context for interpreting your own stress level. The average or mean score of the students was 1,247. About 2 of 3 students scored in the range of 806 to 1,688. Scores outside that range could be considered to reflect either low or high stress levels, respectively.

CHAPTER 5

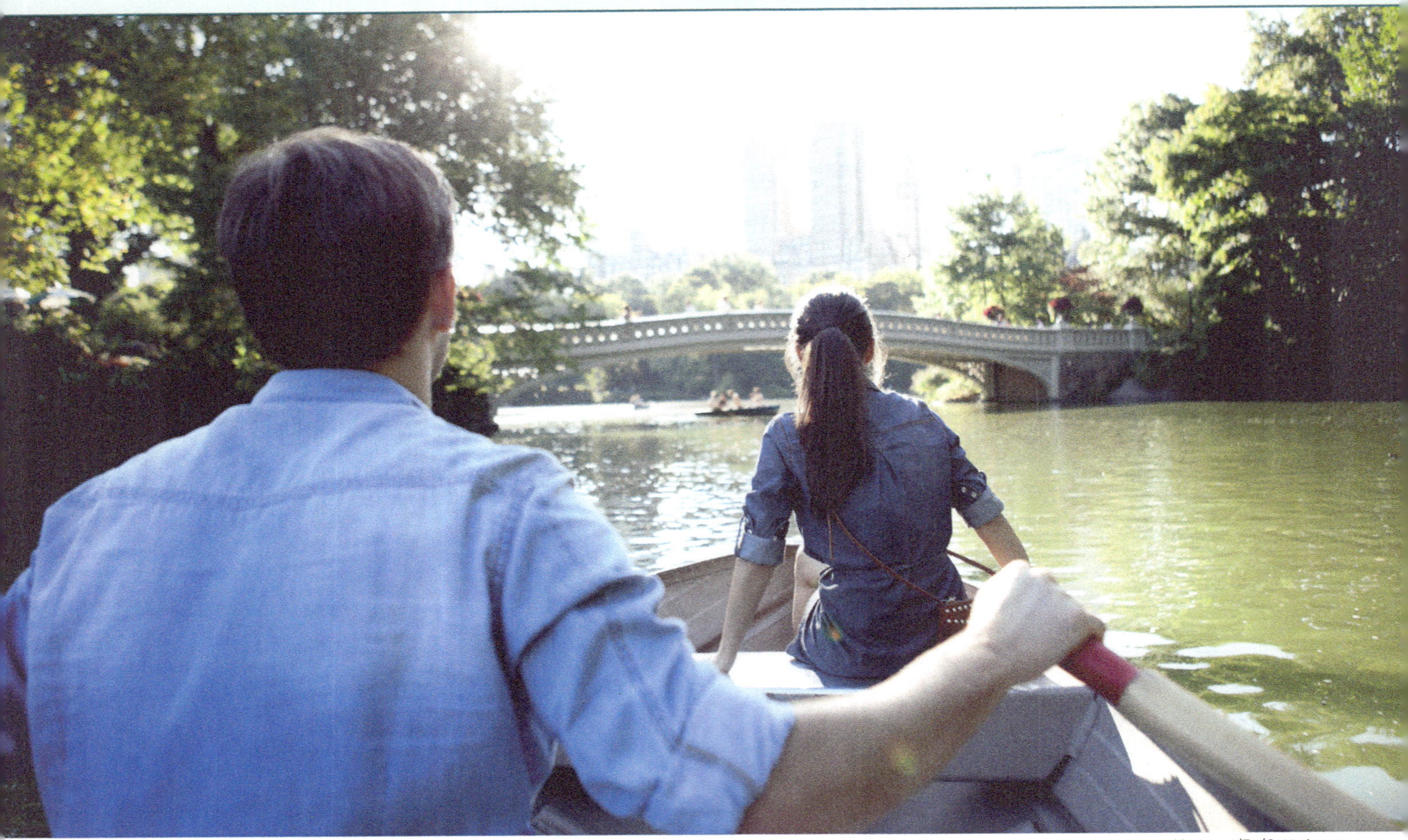

M_a_y_a/E+/Getty Images

Resilience and Coping

LEARNING OBJECTIVES

After studying this chapter, you will be able to …

1. **Identify** factors that foster resilience to stress.
2. **Explain** problematic ways of coping with stress.
3. **Explain** the role of cognitive appraisal in coping with stress.
4. **Describe** problem-focused methods of coping with stress.
5. **Describe** emotion-focused methods of coping with stress.

Did You Know That …

- Viewing stressors as challenges that make life more interesting helps us cope with them?
- Conscientious workers are the ones who are most likely to "burn out"?
- Laughing may strengthen your immune system?
- Loneliness is associated with elevated blood pressure and higher mortality rates?
- A person may rationalize not wearing face masks during a pandemic by saying, "I don't see other people wearing them"?
- Optimistic people tend to live longer?
- The belief that we must have the love and approval of almost everyone who is important to us is a recipe for heightening stress?
- Meditation may be good for your blood pressure?
- Stopping to smell the roses may really be good for your health (unless you're allergic to roses, of course)?
- To relax yourself, it may be helpful to tense up your muscles first?

> *People and groups differ in their sensitivity and vulnerability to certain types of events, as well as in their interpretations and reactions. Under comparable conditions, for example, one person responds with anger, another with depression, yet another with anxiety or guilt; and still others feel challenged rather than threatened. Likewise, one individual uses denial to cope with terminal illness whereas another anxiously ruminates about the problem or is depressed. One individual handles an insult by ignoring it and another grows angry and plans revenge.*
>
> **—Lazarus & Folkman, 1984, pp. 22–23.**

Resilience

As noted by Lazarus and Folkman (1984), some people are more resilient in the face of stress than others. Though we all have our limits, there is no one-to-one relationship between the amount of stress we experience and outcomes such as physical disorders or psychological distress. Biological factors account for some of the variability in our responses. For example, some people may inherit predispositions that increase their risk of developing certain physical and psychological disorders following stressful experiences. But psychological factors also influence our resilience to stress.

Psychological Hardiness: Tough Enough?

Health psychologists focus on psychological factors associated with resilience to stress. One such factor that helps people resist stress is a personality trait called **psychological hardiness**. Our understanding of this construct is derived largely from the pioneering work of Suzanne Kobasa and her colleagues (1994). They studied business executives who seemed to be able to resist illness despite stress. The psychologically hardy executives in Kobasa's research showed three key characteristics:

psychological hardiness A cluster of traits that buffer stress and are characterized by commitment, challenge, and control.

1. *Commitment:* They were strongly committed to their work and pursuit of their life goals.
2. *Challenge:* They felt challenged by new experiences and opportunities. They believed that change, rather than stability, is normal in life, not a threat to their security.
3. *Control:* They were high in perceived control over their lives. They felt and behaved as though they were effective, rather than helpless, in managing various demands placed on them and controlling the outcomes in their lives. Psychologically hardy people tend to have what psychologist Julian Rotter (1990) called an **internal locus of control**.

internal locus of control The place (locus) to which an individual attributes control over the receiving of reinforcers—in this case, the belief that one is in control of one's own life. Contrast with *external locus of control*.

Psychologically hardy people tend to interpret stress as a fact of life that makes life more interesting. They view themselves as choosing to lead challenging lives (Maddi, 2016). For example, they see a conference with a supervisor as an opportunity to persuade the supervisor rather than as a risk to their position. Researchers find that psychologically hardy people tend to get better grades, report fewer physical symptoms, cope better with stress, and experience less depression than their less hardy peers (e.g., Hystad et al., 2011; Sandvik et al., 2013; Taylor et al., 2013). Psychological hardiness also contributes to the success of federal law enforcement officials and military personnel, including candidates for Special Forces (Maddi, 2007; Soccorso et al., 2019; Stein & Bartone, 2020).

body mass index (BMI) A measure used for weight categories based on the relationship between height and body weight. A lower BMI means that one is slimmer, having less body fat; a higher BMI means that one is heavier (see Chapter 7).

high-density lipoprotein (HDL) The kind of cholesterol that absorbs cholesterol in the bloodstream and carries it to the liver, lessening the likelihood of the buildup of harmful plaque in the arteries. Contrast with LDL, low-density lipoprotein, the "bad" form of blood cholesterol that leads to a buildup of plaque in the arteries (see Chapter 12).

One study investigated links between psychological hardiness and immune system markers among Norwegian navy cadets (Sandvik et al., 2013). Measures of psychological hardiness were obtained 2 days before the cadets were exposed to a highly stressful field exercise. Blood serum levels were assessed halfway through the course and again toward the end, when levels of stress were at their highest. All participants were hardy according to the measures, but some were "unbalanced"; that is, they scored high only in commitment and control, but not in challenge. Cadets high in all three aspects of hardiness showed a more robust immune response.

Consider one of several studies connecting psychological hardiness with cardiovascular health (Bartone et al., 2016). The study assessed **body mass index (BMI)** and blood cholesterol levels in a sample of 338 adults. Greater hardiness was associated with higher levels of **high-density lipoprotein (HDL)**, also known as "good cholesterol") in the bloodstream and less body fat, both of which are predictors of better cardiovascular health.

Applying Health Psychology

Fostering Psychological Hardiness

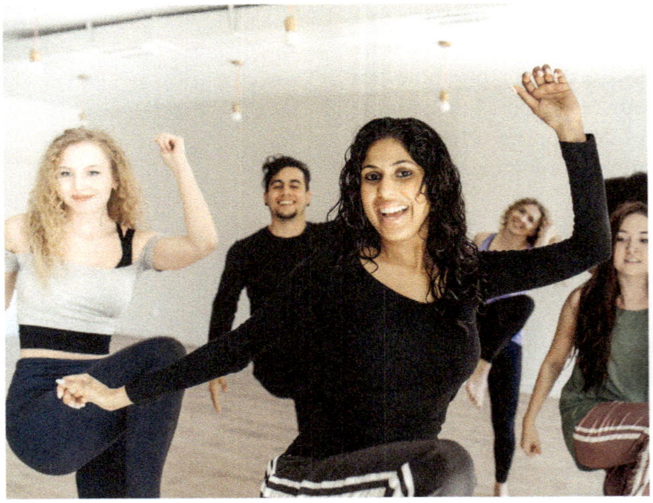

kate_sept2004/Getty Images

Why Not Aerobics? Yasmin became depressed when her girlfriend decided to end their relationship. Her psychologist suggested she take up aerobics as a form of compensatory self-improvement. It not only sculpted her body; it also boosted her self-esteem and her resilience.

Health psychologists examine factors that foster resilience by buffering the effects of stress. As proposed by psychologist Salvatore Maddi (2016), the psychological construct of psychological hardiness works as a mental shock absorber that makes stress more manageable. Psychologically hardy people feel that they are in control of the stressors that they encounter. They choose to attack problems and solve them rather than avoid them. Maddi offers three suggestions for enhancing psychological hardiness.

1. *Situation reconstruction:* Put stressful situations in perspective by imagining how situations could be worse and how they could be better. This approach helps prevent us from blowing things out of proportion. It also prompts us to use our problem-solving skills.
2. *Focusing on what is really bothering you:* Sometimes you're unhappy or stressed out, but you're not sure exactly why. In using focusing, you attend to all the body sensations that are disturbing you, such as tightness in the chest. Then you think back to previous times when you experienced the same sensations to better understand your feelings. Maddi offers the case study of a woman who felt churning in her stomach. She thought back and recognized that she had the same sensations when she had not completed her homework and feared that her teachers would reproach her. Her recognition that she feared being reproached raised her awareness that she was confronted with a concrete challenge, not a nameless fear. As a result the women felt that she gained control over the situation and that she could resolve the problem by developing more efficient study schedules.
3. *Compensatory self-improvement:* "If not love, then perhaps aerobics," Maddi writes. Let's add our own case study—Yasmin became depressed when her girlfriend decided their relationship was at an end. She spoke to a psychologist who said, "Why not aerobics?" Aerobics? Why not? Yasmin could undertake something healthy and seek to succeed at it, which might help boost her mood. She was clumsy at first in an aerobics class, but quickly caught on and began to excel. She enjoyed the exercise and appreciated the changes in her body—less fat, more muscle, more endurance—and she also made some new acquaintances. If you can't win doing one thing, it may be advisable to try another. It might boost both your self-esteem and your resilience.

Burnout: When Commitment Is Too Heavy a Burden **Burnout** is a state of mental and physical exhaustion brought on by excessive demands we face at work, or in caretaking roles, or in pursuing personal causes. People who experience burnout feel emotionally exhausted and lack motivation. They may also have a sense of detachment or depersonalization ("This doesn't feel real"; "I can't believe I'm here") (Lopes & Nihei, 2020). Burnout is associated with increased risk of depression and may actually be a type of depression (Bianchi et al., 2020; Frajerman et al., 2019). Burnout is not just emotionally exhausting; it can also lead to stress-related health problems, such as headaches, stomach distress, sleep problems, high blood pressure, and heart disease (Frajerman et al., 2019).

burnout A state of mental and physical exhaustion brought on by excessive demands at work or by other responsibilities.

Who is most likely to experience burnout? One vulnerable group of people consists of overly conscientious workers, frequently referred to as *workaholics*, who may set the stage for burnout by extending themselves too far. College students, too, can experience burnout, especially when they take on more work, family, and school responsibilities than they can reasonably handle.

A particularly troublesome component of burnout is low **self-efficacy**. From the perspective of social cognitive theory, people who burn out tend to have low self-efficacy expectations about their ability to cope with job strain or meet the many role demands they experience (Lloyd et al., 2017; Lopes & Nihei, 2020).

self-efficacy Self-efficacy is, according to psychologist Albert Bandura who originally proposed the concept, one's judgment as to how well one can execute the courses of action they set out to accomplish.

People who experience burnout may become so consumed by their work that they neglect other areas of life, such as social relationships and leisure activities. Typically, people who develop burnout are competent, efficient people who become overwhelmed by the demands of their jobs and by the recognition that they are unlikely to have the impact they had anticipated.

Teachers, healthcare workers, police officers, corrections officers, social workers, and criminal and divorce lawyers appear to be particularly prone to job burnout (Candeias et al., 2019; Frajerman et al., 2019; HaGani, Yagil, & Cohen, 2022). Many frontline healthcare workers experienced burnout during the COVID-19 pandemic, affecting not only their quality of life but also putting patients are greater risk because of the increased likelihood of medical errors (Parandeh et al., 2022). The demands of parenting may also place one at risk, especially when demands on the job are also extreme (Mikolajczak et al., 2020).

Burnout is also common among people who have high levels of role conflict, role overload, or role ambiguity. People in role conflict face competing demands for their time. They feel pulled in several directions at once. People with role overload find it hard to say "no." They take on more and more responsibilities until they burn out. People with role ambiguity are uncertain as to what other people expect of them. Thus they may work hard at trying to be all things to all people. It is not apathetic workers who are most likely to experience job burnout. Burnout tends to affect the most dedicated workers.

Behaviorally, highly stressed workers may become accident-prone, engage in excessive eating or smoking, turn to alcohol or other drugs, and experience temperamental outbursts. Perhaps the risk of injury is increased when stress impairs workers' ability to attend to potentially harmful situations, such as those involving machine tools.

The cognitive effects of excessive stress on the job include poor concentration and loss of ability to make sound decisions. Physiological effects include high blood pressure and other diseases of adaptation. The organizational effects of excessive stress include absenteeism, alienation from coworkers, decreased productivity, high turnover, and loss of commitment and loyalty to the organization.

Burnout develops gradually. The warning signs may develop over the years and may take these forms:

- Loss of energy and feelings of exhaustion, both physical and psychological
- Irritability and shortness of temper
- Stress-related problems, such as depression, headaches, backaches, or apathy
- Difficulty concentrating or feeling distanced from one's work
- Loss of motivation
- Lack of satisfaction or feelings of achievement at work
- Loss of concern about work in someone who was previously committed
- Feeling that one has nothing left to give

Applying Health Psychology

Preventing Burnout

All work and no play makes Jack a dull boy.
—**Traditional proverb**

All work and no play also makes Jack a burned-out boy. The same holds true for Jill, especially when she is working 40 hours a week, holds the major responsibility for the kids, and is also trying to manage the needs of her aging parents (Mikolajczak et al., 2020).

Health psychologists often use cognitive behavioral techniques to help people cope with, or reverse, the effects of burnout, such as the following (Lloyd et al., 2017):

- *Become aware of irrational or distorted thought patterns, as well as the effects that the thought patterns have on their work and their social relationships*: A study reported in the *Journal of Occupational Health Psychology* used mindfulness training as a means to help workers identify and replace the irrational thoughts and expectations that may underlie burnout, such as "If I don't get all my work done by the end of the day, I'll have failed" (Lloyd et al., 2017).
- *Establish priorities*: Make a list of the things that are truly important. If the list starts and ends with work, rethink your priorities. Ask yourself, "Am I making time for the relationships and activities that bring a sense of meaning, fulfillment, and satisfaction to life?"
- *Set reasonable goals*: People at risk of burnout drive themselves to extremes. Set realistic long-term and short-term goals and do not attempt to push yourself beyond your limits without fully examining the reasons.
- *Take things one day at a time*: Work gradually toward your goals. Burning the candle at both ends is likely to leave you burned (out).
- *Set limits*: People at risk of burnout often have difficulty saying "no." They are known as the ones who get things done. Yet the more responsibilities they assume, the greater their risk of burnout. Learn your limits and respect them. Share responsibilities with others. Delegate tasks. Cut back on your responsibilities before things pile up to the point where you have difficulty coping.
- *Share your feelings*: It is stressful to keep feelings under wraps, especially negative feelings like anger, frustration, and sadness. Share your feelings with people you trust.
- *Build supportive relationships*: Developing and maintaining relationships helps buffer us against the effects of stress. People headed toward burnout may become so invested in their work that they let supportive relationships fall to the wayside (J. Chen et al., 2020).
- *Do things you enjoy*: Balance work and recreation. Do something you enjoy every day. Breaks clear your mind and recharge your batteries.
- *Engage in physical activity*: Set aside time to do so. A study of 309 Swiss workers found that those who engaged in higher levels of physical activity experienced fewer symptoms of burnout under stress (Gerber et al., 2020).
- *Don't skip vacations*: People who are headed for burnout often find reasons to skip vacations, but vacations give you time off from the usual stresses.
- *Be attuned to your health*: Be aware of stress-related symptoms. These include physical symptoms, such as fatigue, headache or backache, and reduced resistance to colds and the flu. They also include psychological symptoms, such as anxiety, depression, irritability, or shortness of temper. Changes in health may represent the first signs of burnout. Take them as signals to examine the sources of stress in your life and do something about them. Consult health professionals about symptoms that concern you. Get regular checkups to help identify developing health problems.

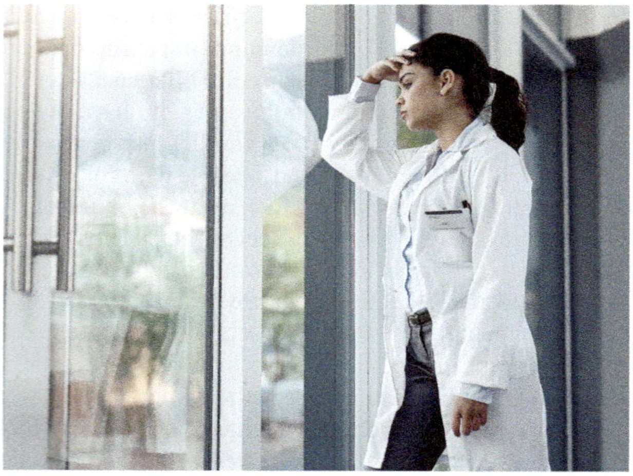
PeopleImages/Getty Images

Burnout Overly conscientious workers are those who are most likely to experience burnout. Burnout is a state of mental and physical exhaustion that is brought on by excessive demands.

Humor: "A Merry Heart Doeth Good Like a Medicine"?

Whenever I date a guy, I think, is this the man I want my children to spend their weekends with?
—**Rita Rudner**

My wife and I were considering a divorce, but after pricing lawyers we decided to buy a new car instead.
—**Henny Youngman**

Divorce is one of the most stressful events we can experience, yet finding something to laugh about may be helpful in handling the stress with greater equanimity.

Laughter may help buffer the effects of stress (Powell, 2023: Zander-Schellenberg et al., 2020). The idea that humor lightens the burdens of life and helps people cope with stress has been with us since biblical times. Consider the biblical maxim, "A merry heart doeth good like a medicine" (Proverbs 17:22). A dose of humor not only makes us laugh but also helps get our minds off the sources of stress in our lives, at least for a time. Think of humor as an antidote to stress, an elixir that provides at least a temporary reprieve from the stressful demands of life.

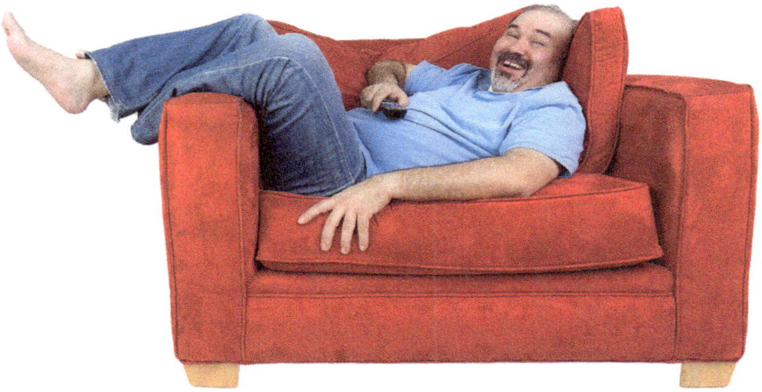

Ozgur Coskun/Alamy Stock Photo

"A Merry Heart Doeth Good Like a Medicine" (Proverbs 17:22) Humor can help lighten the stressful burdens we face in everyday life. Here is a painless prescription for you: Why not take in a comedy tonight?

A Norwegian study followed up 53,556 participants in the population-based Nord-Trondelag Health Study (Romundstad et al., 2016). The researchers measured the cognitive, social, and affective components of a sense of humor and their links to mortality caused by cardiovascular disease (CVD), infections, cancer, and chronic obstructive pulmonary disease. Among the findings was that high scores on the cognitive component of the sense of humor were significantly associated with lower mortality in women due to CVD and with lower mortality in both women and men due to infections.

Research also supports a role for laughter as a method of lessening the levels of cortisol in the body—a stress hormone that over time can impair the functioning of the immune system. One study assessed the effects of laughter on salivary cortisol levels among Taiwanese adolescents (Chang et al., 2013). An experimental group participated in a standardized laughing program during study halls for a period of 8 weeks. Control participants spent their time in study hall doing homework. Relative to controls, the mood states of experimental participants improved and their cortisol levels declined, which is suggestive that the laughing program lowered stress levels.

Another study was also designed to assess the effects of laughter therapy, tailored to "tickle the funny bones" of 48 fourth-year student nurses who were experiencing stress from final exams and job searches (Lee & Lee, 2020). The student nurses were randomly assigned to an experimental group and a wait-list control group. The intervention was administered weekly across a period of 4 weeks. It led to a one-third reduction in salivary cortisol compared to baseline measures and to concomitant self-reported reductions in psychological stress and increases in subjective happiness. Taking a cognitive perspective, the researchers suggest that the intervention helped the students replace negative thoughts with more optimistic thoughts. Laughter may not just "make merry" but may also induce changes in a person's mental outlook.

Predictability and Control

If I can stop the roller coaster, I don't want to get off.

—Suzanne M. Miller

The ability to predict a stressor may lessen its impact. Predictability allows us to brace ourselves for the inevitable and, in many cases, plan ways of coping with it. A sense of control is one of the keys to psychological hardiness. When we are at a concert, dance club, or sports event, we may encounter more crowding than we do in a ticket line that is moving at a frustratingly slow pace. But we may be having a wonderful time. Why? Because we have chosen to be at the concert and are focusing on our good time (unless a tall or noisy person is sitting in front of us). We feel that we are in control. Even in stressful situations, such as when riding in a crowded subway car or waiting in a frustratingly slow line, we can exercise control by distracting ourselves, such as by daydreaming, reading newspapers and books, or finding humor in the situation. Some people just catch a snooze and wake up before their stop.

Control—even the illusion of being in control—allows us to feel that we are not at the mercy of the fates (Brooks et al., 2017). There is also a relationship between the desire to assume control over one's situation and the usefulness of information about impending stressors (Lazarus & Folkman, 1984). People who want information about medical procedures and what they will experience cope better with pain when they undergo those procedures (Ludwick-Rosenthal & Neufeld, 1993).

Social and Emotional Support: On Being in It Together

We are social beings, so it is not surprising that social support acts as a kind of buffer against the effects of stress (Diaz & Bui, 2017; Wittig et al., 2016). There are many different sources of social support, including:

1. *Emotional concern,* such as by listening to people's problems and expressing feelings of sympathy, caring, understanding, reassurance—and hugs!
2. *Instrumental aid,* such as material support and services that facilitate adaptive behavior. For example, after a disaster, a government may arrange for low-interest loans to help survivors rebuild. Relief organizations may provide food, medicines, and temporary living quarters.
3. *Information,* such as providing guidance and advice that enhances people's ability to cope.
4. *Appraisal,* such as feedback from others about how one is doing. This kind of support helps people decide whether they are moving in the right direction or need to adjust their behavior or goals.
5. *Socializing,* such as through simple conversation, recreation, even going shopping with another person. Socializing has beneficial effects, even when it is not oriented specifically toward solving problems.

Research validates the value of social support (APA, 2015; see **Figure 5.1**). For one thing, people who report higher levels of social support tend to show lower levels of stress hormones, which indicates that their bodies are better able to fight off infections such as the common cold (Cohen et al., 2015; Wittig et al., 2016). Social support may be especially important to help members of immigrant groups, including international students, as well as people in racial/ethnic minorities, helping them cope with the stresses of adjusting to a new culture (Diaz & Bui, 2017; Lu et al., 2019; Sullivan & Kashubeck-West, 2015).

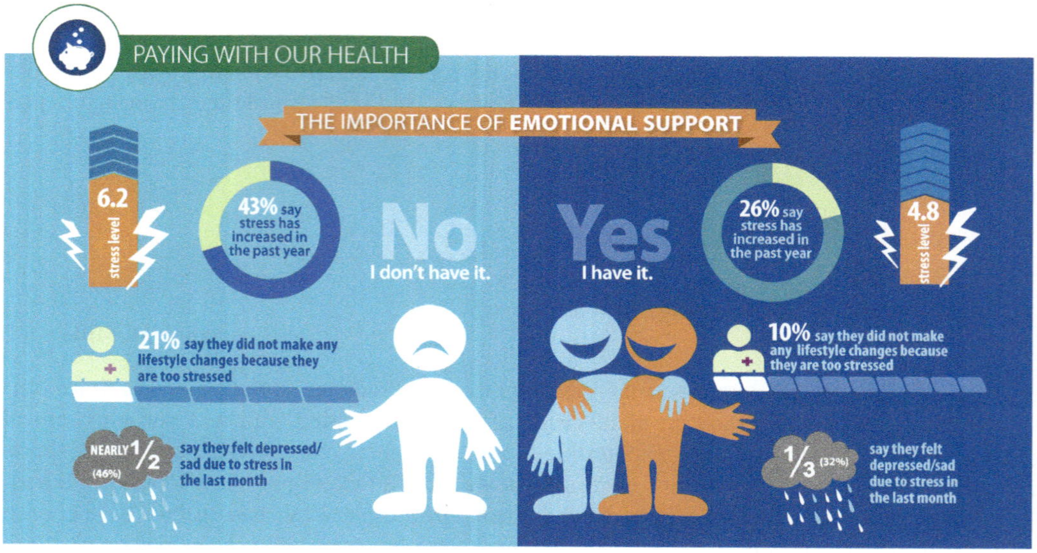

FIGURE 5.1 The American Psychological Association (2015) has found that people with social and emotional support fare better under stress than people who do not have it.

Source: APA (2015), Stress in America. Paying with our health. https://www.apa.org/news/press/releases/stress/2014/stress-report.pdf. © 2015, American Psychological Association.

Another aspect of social support is embedded in the concept of **familism**—also known as familialism—a behavior pattern that stresses the centrality of one's family in life. Research evidence suggests that familism may be protective against the elevated health risks faced by members of minority groups in the United States (Chiang et al., 2019). One study examined whether familism was related to different inflammatory processes among non-Hispanic White, non-Hispanic Black, and Latino/Hispanic youth. Participants included 257 youth drawn from the three groups. They completed measures of familism values. They were then exposed to a bacterial challenge, and blood samples were collected to determine whether there were differences in immune system responses. Black youth who placed greater value on familism showed lower cytokine responses to the bacterial challenge, suggesting that the challenge did not prompt dysregulation of their immune systems. But not all groups showed this healthy sign. The White and Latino/Hispanic youth did not show a strongly directional cytokine response to the bacterial challenge. The reasons for these ethnic group differences need to be further explored.

familism An ideology that places priority on the family, particularly the family of origin.

Loneliness: Moving from Day to Day in the Absence of Social Support Loneliness is a state of painful isolation, of feeling cut off from others. People who are lonely tend to spend a lot of time by themselves, eat alone, spend weekends alone, and participate in few social activities. Some people who are lonely report having friends, but a closer look suggests that these "friendships" are sometimes shallow. People who are lonely often feel that other people look past them or dismiss them.

Loneliness is common among older people, especially when they have been widowed or friends have passed on (Freedman & Nicolle, 2020). In our mobile society, family and friends are frequently on the move, and they often leave older relatives behind. One in six older adults reports feeling isolated from other people, even when others are nearby (Brady et al., 2020). Young adults also often feel lonely, even in college dormitories. Some of them have social anxiety and fear of rejection; they try to substitute social media for physical relationships, but virtual relationships may not offer the same level of social support that is found in real relationships (Singh et al., 2020). Use of social media to maintain contact with friends and family does, however, help some students make the transition from home to college life (Thomas et al., 2020).

Loneliness is connected with a host of problematic psychological and physical outcomes, including depression (Leigh-Hunt et al., 2017; Wang et al., 2018). Numerous studies and reviews of the literature find that loneliness is associated with high blood pressure and higher morbidity (sickness) and mortality rates (Xia & Li, 2018). Experiments with animals reared in social isolation find that they are more prone than animals raised in groups to developing plaque on artery walls (atherosclerosis) (Xia & Li, 2018). A study of 20,007 Swiss people aged 15–75+ found that people who are lonely were more likely to develop chronic diseases, such as diabetes, have high cholesterol levels, and show psychological distress (Richard et al., 2017). Moreover, loneliness was also associated with unhealthy lifestyle factors, such as drinking heavily and smoking cigarettes. A study with Latinas found similar results (Foti et al., 2020). Loneliness is also related to sleep disturbances (Griffin et al., 2020). The list goes on.

To better understand the links between loneliness and negative health outcomes, researchers administered a salmonella vaccination to healthy young adults to prompt an inflammatory response controlled by the body's immune system (Balter et al., 2020). Participants with higher scores on a widely used psychological measure of loneliness showed an elevated inflammatory response to this immune challenge. Thus it is possible that loneliness affects immune system functioning, which in turn may lead to health problems.

Health professionals have investigated many avenues for decreasing social isolation and feelings of loneliness, for example, exercise, psychological treatment, befriending

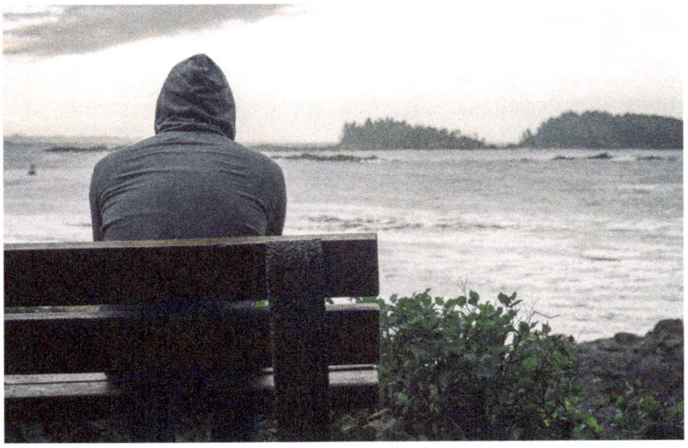

Marc Bruxelle/Alamy Stock Photo

Loneliness The vista is lovely, but the person has no one to share it with. Loneliness is a common problem among older people and even among young adults. It is associated with psychological and physical health problems, including dysregulation of the immune system. People who are lonely are also more likely to engage in unhealthy behaviors, such as heavy drinking and smoking cigarettes.

Health Psychology in Action

Lockdown! Building Resilience in Times of Crisis

Consider the title of an article in *New Scientist*—"World in Lockdown" (Hamzelou, 2020). Much of the world locked down in 2020 in an effort to combat the COVID-19 virus. Hubei Province in China, where the outbreak began, locked down to prevent the spread of the virus. So did hard-hit countries in Europe and parts of the United States. Italy first locked down its northern provinces and then the entire country. Spain followed, as did almost all of Europe. The United Kingdom announced that people should stay at home and leave their homes only for necessities, such as food and medicine, to meet their medical needs or those of others, or to exercise—once a day.

Lockdown in the United States was spotty because there was no general directive from the federal government. Decisions about lockdowns were left to the individual states, with some issuing stay-at-home orders and others resisting general lockdowns or reopening even while the virus continued to spread.

There were many other lockdowns and quarantines throughout history and in the 2000s: Taiwan, Hong Kong, China, and Canada quarantined people who had been in contact with people infected with the SARS[1] virus; South Korea quarantined people because of the MERS[2] virus; Senegal, Liberia, and Sweden (yes, Sweden) quarantined people because of Ebola[3] (Swedish healthcare workers had attempted to help Ebola patients in Africa); the United States and Canada quarantined people who lived in areas affected by H1N1.[4]

Health psychologists have studied the psychological effects of quarantines on people who are locked down. They find increased rates of psychological problems such as low moods and depression, irritability, insomnia, and exhaustion (Brooks et al., 2020). Anxiety, fear, frustration, and anger were common as well. Quarantined healthcare workers reported substantially more feelings of annoyance and anger, helplessness, loneliness, nervousness—even guilt—than non-healthcare workers under the same circumstances. Key stressors they reported included lengthy quarantines, fear of infection, frustration and boredom, lack of adequate supplies to see them through, and inadequate information about the outbreak in the community and possible changes in their status.

Health psychologists have been called upon to investigate factors that may help improve adherence to quarantine restrictions (Webster et al., 2020). Among the factors they identify are the following:

- *Demographic and employment characteristics of the people being quarantined:* Groups showing better adherence to quarantine measures include healthcare workers, parents who are able to supervise their children at home in contrast to parents who rely on third parties for childcare, and people with lower income levels. In Chapter 4, we noted that students on spring break in Florida swarmed the beaches and engaged in close contact despite media messages that doing so would place them and their families—when they returned home—at risk of infection with COVID-19. In such cases, the lure of short-term pleasures may outweigh fears of longer-term risks, especially among adolescents and young adults.
- *Knowledge about the disease and the quarantine procedures:* Adherence to quarantine was high in Taiwan due to well-communicated information about the disease and the nature of the outbreak. Ironically, in the case of Ebola in African villages, healthcare professionals did not adhere to the procedures as well as nonprofessionals did because they thought they knew everything there was to know and that the protocols were overly restrictive.
- *Sociocultural factors:* Canadians quarantined during a SARS outbreak showed high adherence rates largely because of social pressure from peers. Villagers in Senegal adhered to being quarantined during an Ebola outbreak when the head of the household set an example of compliance; it was expected that other members of the household would follow suit. Yet some villagers broke quarantine in order to care for the sick, because helping the ill was perceived as a higher-order cultural value.
- *Perceived benefits of the quarantine:* In accordance with the Health Belief Model (HBM), people who believed that adhering to the quarantine would protect them and those they cared about were more likely to comply. When African villagers saw that adherence slowed the spread of Ebola, their motivation to comply grew stronger. Canadians complied with quarantine due to SARS in large part because of the belief that doing so would protect others.
- *Perceived risk of the outbreak:* Also consistent with the HBM, greater fear of SARS as a health threat prompted high levels of adherence to quarantining in both Canada and Taiwan.
- *Competing concerns:* People who more strongly fear loss of income may choose to work outside the home despite lockdown or quarantine procedures.

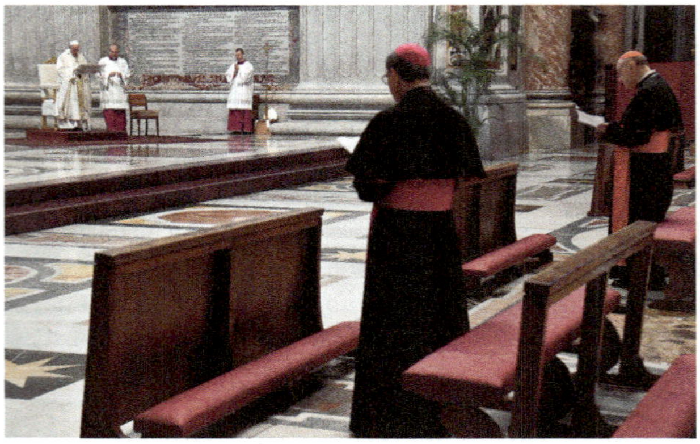
ALESSANDRO DI MEO/Getty Images

Commemoration of the Last Supper of Jesus In 2020, Pope Francis (left) celebrated the Mass of the Lord's Supper on Maundy Thursday behind closed doors at St. Peter's Basilica in the Vatican during the lockdown aimed at curbing the spread of COVID-19. The priests in attendance practiced social distancing.

[1]Severe acute respiratory syndrome, a contagious disease caused by a coronavirus that appeared in China in 2002.

[2]Middle East respiratory syndrome, another contagious disease caused by a coronavirus. It also is called camel flu, but it is derived from bats.

[3]A contagious viral disease spread through contact with other people's bodily fluids.

[4]A contagious strain of influenza that originated in pigs, also called swine flu.

- *Duration of the quarantine:* Not surprisingly, the longer the quarantine, the more likely people are to violate it, as seen in an outbreak of mumps at Harvard University in 2016 (Narayanan & Shimozaki, 2016).

Samantha Brooks and her colleagues (2020) reviewed the health psychology literature concerning ways in which health professionals and makers of public policy can help people cope with the stress of lockdowns and quarantines. They found that adequate information was the key. People who were expected to conform to procedures such as social distancing, staying at home, and quarantines needed to fully understand the specifics of the disease that was threatening them and their communities—that is, the risks they faced—and the procedures of the lockdown. Public officials in local, state, and federal governments must be consistent and "on the same page." Clearly, mixed messages do not relieve stress very well.

Supplies need to be adequate. It is difficult for people to be stressed about a disease and at the same time be stressed as to whether they will have food to eat and whether healthcare professionals will have the equipment they need to save lives.

Because involuntary restrictions on personal liberty are a major source of stress, it is better to enlist people's voluntary cooperation in maintaining social distancing, lockdowns, and quarantines than to impose the authority of the state. With voluntary compliance, people can then view themselves as adhering to restrictive measures because they choose to do so, not out of fear they will be deemed criminals and subjected to hefty penalties if they do not comply.

Above all, most people need accurate information. They need to know how a disease is progressing, why restrictive measures such as quarantines are needed, and whether efforts to manage the disease are proving to be beneficial.

people, animal therapy, prompting the development of social skills and hobbies to fill leisure time, and even social interactions in social media (Freedman & Nicolle, 2020).

From the perspective of the Health Belief Model (HBM), people who are lonely may see themselves as being susceptible to the threat of unhappiness resulting from social rejection. They may perceive the benefits of pushing themselves to engage in more social interactions, but barriers may include social anxiety, fear of rejection, and beliefs that they are unworthy and that other people will reject them. Some unfortunate experiences may have led them to believe that other people are only out for themselves and not worth their time. Will they attempt to fight through these barriers? Some social support in the form of encouragement might enable them to do just that.

Review 5.1

INTERACTIVE SELF-SCORING QUIZZES

Sentence Completion

1. Kobasa found that psychologically hardy executives are high in ______, challenge, and control.
2. People who (are or are not) committed to their work are most likely to burn out.
3. Being able to predict and control the onset of a stressor (increases or decreases) the impact of the stressor on us.
4. The kind of emotional and social support that we refer to as material support is also known as ______ aid.
5. Studies show that loneliness is associated with (high or low) blood pressure.
6. According to the Health Belief Model, people who are lonely may find fear of rejection to be a(n) __________ to engaging in more social interactions.
7. It is psychologically best to make quarantines (voluntary or involuntary).

Think About It

What challenges do you face in your life? Do you view the challenges as insurmountable obstacles or as opportunities to grow as a person? How does your answer relate to your sense of your psychological hardiness?

Problematic Ways of Coping with Stress

Stress is a part of life. At least some amount of stress is needed to help us remain active, alert, and motivated. Some people have good coping resources for handling stress, but others rely on less effective ways of coping with stress.

What do you do when the pressures of work or school begin to get to you? What do you do when you feel that your instructor or your supervisor doesn't appreciate your performance? When your partner begins showing less interest in you? When you're uptight before a test or irritated because you're stuck in traffic?

defensive coping A defensive reaction to stress characterized by avoidance, withdrawal, denial, self-deception, or inappropriate behaviors, such as substance abuse.

Many techniques for coping with stress are either ineffective or defensive. **Defensive coping** may reduce the immediate impact of the stressor, but at a cost. Costs include socially inappropriate behavior (as in alcoholism, aggression, or regression), avoidance of problems (as in withdrawal), or self-deception (as in rationalization or denial). Defensive coping may grant us time to marshal our resources, but it does not deal directly with the source of stress or enhance our effectiveness in responding to stressful challenges. In the long run, defensive methods can be ineffective or harmful if they lead us to forgo the chance to find better ways of coping. Next we note some examples of defensive coping.

Withdrawal

When you face a stressful situation you feel unable to control, your first tendency may be to withdraw from it. You might withdraw your interest or investment in what you were doing or withdraw physically by moving away, changing your lifestyle, or dropping out of college, the workforce, or a relationship. Temporary withdrawal may be helpful in some cases by providing you the chance to find better methods of coping or by giving you the opportunity to start over. But withdrawal from social involvement prevents people from getting on with their lives and finding other sources of support. In one case, a young man who had always dreamed of becoming a firefighter withdrew from the training academy after only 3 days because he found it too stressful. He later regretted his decision and fortunately was able to become reinstated. Given a second chance, he successfully completed the program and fulfilled his lifelong ambition.

Denial

Denial ain't just a river in Egypt.

—American humorist Mark Twain

People who rely on denial when facing the stress of coping with a serious illness refuse to acknowledge the seriousness of their health situation. They may think, "Oh, it's no big deal," misattribute their symptoms to benign causes ("It's probably just my arthritis acting up") or assume that symptoms will pass if left alone. But people who dismiss chest pains or suspicious lumps as "no big deal" may not avail themselves of the medical assistance they may require. Denial may minimize the effects of stress in the short run, but the eventual consequences of leaving a serious medical condition untreated can be tragic.

Sigmund Freud considered denial a type of defense mechanism that operates unconsciously to protect us from anxiety that might stem from recognition of unacceptable ideas and impulses. According to his psychodynamic theory, everyone uses defense mechanisms from time to time. However, defense mechanisms can become problems in adjustment when people come to rely on them to cope with stress rather than deal with stressful challenges more directly, or when they lead people to forgo seeking necessary medical treatment or making desirable life changes. **Table 5.1** provides a fuller list of Freud's defense mechanisms. Which ones do you use? Which ones are used by people you know?

Substance Abuse

Another common but problematic means of handling stressful situations is the use of alcohol or other drugs. The use of psychoactive substances may blunt awareness of sources of stress but fails to resolve the underlying problems. Moreover, drinking regularly or using other drugs to cope with stress can lead to problems with substance use and abuse, which only compounds the problems the person is facing. In Chapter 9 we explore the psychological and health-related problems posed by substance use and dependence.

Aggression

Some people lose their tempers when they feel stressed and become verbally or physically abusive to other people. Violence is often used to cope with social provocations and, sometimes, as a response to frustration. But lashing out at others verbally or physically is a source of stress in

TABLE 5.1 Defense Mechanisms in Freud's Psychodynamic Theory

INTERACTIVE FIGURES, CHARTS, & TABLES

Defense Mechanism	What It Is	Examples
Repression	The ejection of anxiety-evoking ideas from awareness	• A person forgets to keep an appointment for a blood test. • A client in therapy forgets an appointment when anxiety-evoking material is about to be brought up.
Regression	The return, under stress, to a form of behavior characteristic of an earlier stage of development	• An adolescent cries when forbidden to use the family car. • People become dependent again on their parents following the breakup of their marriage.
Rationalization	The use of self-deceiving justifications for unacceptable behavior	• "You can't blame me for smoking when _____ gets me upset." • A man justifies his failure to wear a mask and protective gloves during a pandemic by saying "I see other people not wearing masks and gloves either."
Displacement	The transfer of ideas and impulses from threatening or unsuitable objects to less threatening objects	• A worker picks a fight with their spouse after being criticized sharply by their supervisor.
Projection	The thrusting of one's own unacceptable impulses onto others so that others are assumed to harbor them	• A hostile person perceives the world as being a dangerous place. • A person who is sexually frustrated interprets innocent gestures of others as sexual advances.
Reaction formation	Assumption of behavior in opposition to one's genuine impulses in order to keep impulses repressed	• A person who is angry with a relative behaves in a sickly sweet manner toward that relative. • A sadistic individual becomes a physician.
Denial	Refusal to accept the true nature of a threat (e.g., according to the HBM, denying susceptibility to a health problem)	• A person believes that they will not contract cancer or heart disease although they smoke heavily. • "It can't happen to me"—an emerging adult parties with peers on a crowded beach during a pandemic.
Sublimation	The channeling of primitive sexual or aggressive impulses into positive, constructive efforts	• A person paints nudes for the sake of "beauty" and "art." • A hostile person becomes a football player.

itself and can damage relationships. It can have serious consequences, even lethal results in the case of physical assault. Physical violence is not only illegal but dangerous. Aggressive behavior also heightens interpersonal conflict by creating motives for retaliation.

In sum, defensive ways of coping can make matters worse. Let us consider healthier and more effective ways of managing stress. One method involves cognitive restructuring—rethinking our cognitive appraisal of events. When we come to believe that we can take charge of our situations, are optimistic about outcomes in life, and don't fall into the pattern of sabotaging ourselves by adopting distorted or irrational ways of thinking, we can more effectively manage stressful situations.

Another effective method is *problem-focused coping*—viewing stressors as problems to be solved rather than as insurmountable obstacles. We then apply problem-solving efforts to directly deal with problems to remove or control stressors. Sometimes stressors cannot be eliminated or controlled directly. In those situations we can profit from *emotion-based coping*—using research-driven methods to cushion their emotional impact.

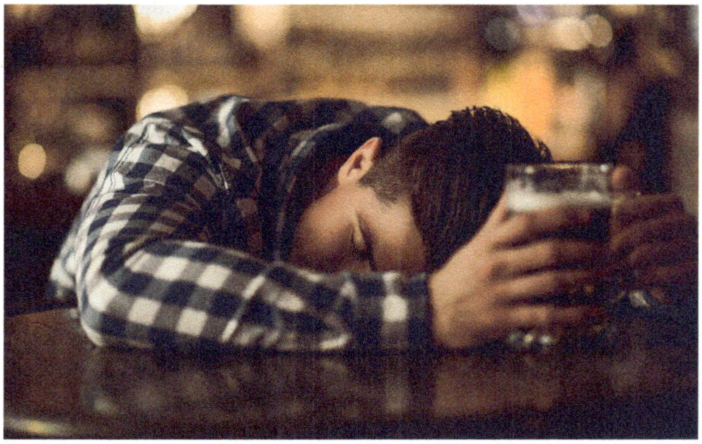

skynesher/E+/Getty Images

A Problematic Way of Coping with Stress Problematic ways of coping with stress—such as drinking, withdrawal, or use of defense mechanisms—can reduce the immediate impact of the stressor, but with costs—costs such as socially inappropriate behavior (as in substance abuse or aggression), avoidance of problems (as in withdrawal), or self-deception (as in the use of some defense mechanisms). More effective ways of coping challenge the ways in which we think about stressors, view stressors as problems to be solved, and directly change our responses to stressors to cushion their impact.

Health Psychology in Action

Active Versus Passive Coping

What do you do when the pressures of work or school begin to get to you? What do you do when you feel that your instructor or your supervisor doesn't appreciate your performance? When your partner finds someone else? When you're uptight before a test or irritated because you're stuck in traffic? Is your manner of coping active or passive?

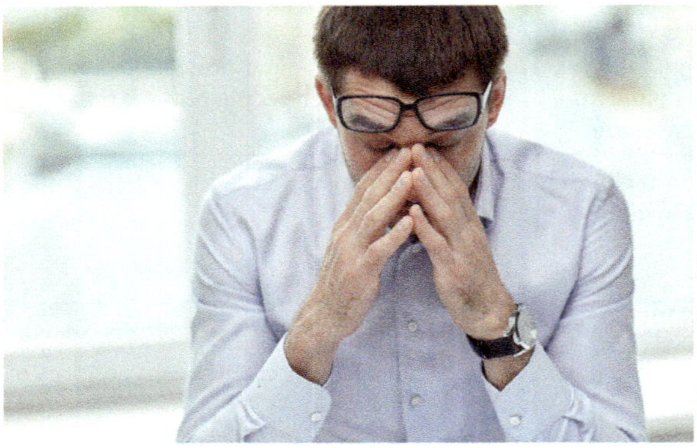

Syda Productions/Shutterstock.com

What's Your Coping Style? Do you embrace responsibility and confront stressors with appropriate targeted behavior, or do you avoid responsibility and allow external factors resolve—or fail to resolve—the situation?

In active coping, the person embraces responsibility for resolving a stressful situation, relies on internal resources, and attempts to confront a stressor through appropriate targeted behavior. In passive coping, people absolve themselves of responsibility for managing stressors, surrender control, and allow external forces to resolve—or fail to resolve—the problems. Passive coping may reduce the immediate impact of the stressor, but at a cost. Costs include socially inappropriate behavior (as in alcohol use disorder or regression), avoidance of problems (as in withdrawal), or self-deception (as in rationalization or denial).

Passive coping strategies have been shown to be unhealthy. For example, survivors of breast cancer with passive coping styles have been shown to have greater anxiety and depression, and also higher blood levels of cortisol, a biological marker for inflammation and psychological stress (Perez-Tejada et al., 2019).

Other researchers find that active and passive coping styles are associated with responses to organizational pressures and other stressors among police officers (Violanti et al., 2018). The study investigated active and passive coping strategies on the relationships among stressors impacting the officers (administrative and organizational pressures and physical and other psychological threats), presence of social support, and symptoms of posttraumatic stress disorder (PTSD). An active coping style mitigated the symptoms of PTSD. Moreover, social support mitigated the symptoms of PTSD among officers with either coping style.

Review 5.2

INTERACTIVE SELF-SCORING QUIZZES

Sentence Completion

1. __________ from a stressful situation can be emotional, as in loss of interest, or physical, as in moving or changing one's lifestyle.

2. The defense mechanism of __________ is defined as the use of self-deceiving justifications for unacceptable behavior.

3. The defense mechanism of __________ is defined as refusal to accept the real nature of a threat.

4. In __________ coping, people confront stressors using their internal resources.

Think About It

Do you know people who lie or deceived themselves about the reasons they engage in problematic behavior? Which defense mechanism are they employing? What other defense mechanisms are used by people you know? How do you think the mechanisms are helping these people cope with the stressors in their lives? Can you think of more productive ways for them to respond to stress?

Cognitive Appraisal and Coping

There is nothing either good or bad, but thinking makes it so.

—**Shakespeare, *Hamlet*, Act 2, Scene 2**

In order to understand variations among individuals under comparable conditions, we must take into account the cognitive processes that intervene between the encounter and the reaction, and the factors that affect the nature of this mediation. If we do not consider these processes, we will be unable to understand human variation under comparable external conditions.

—**Lazarus & Folkman, 1984, p. 23**

Philosophers and poets throughout history and health psychologists today recognize that the impact of a potentially stressful event reflects the meaning of the event to the individual (Carver, 2019; Folkman, 2011; Lazarus & Folkman, 1984; Meichenbaum, 2017). Pregnancy, for example, can be a positive or negative life change, depending on whether one wants and is prepared to have a child. We evaluate stressful events in terms of their perceived danger or risk, our values and goals, our beliefs in our coping ability, and the social support available to us. The same event is less taxing to someone who views it as an opportunity to master a challenge or develop new skills than to someone who lacks this perspective.

Self-Efficacy Expectations: "The Little Engine That Could"

According to social cognitive theory, our confidence in our abilities, our self-efficacy expectations, are linked to our ability to withstand stress (Meichenbaum, 2017; Schönfeld et al., 2016). People who believe in their abilities to meet the challenges they face are less likely to be disturbed by adverse events. People with higher self-efficacy are generally better able than their self-doubting counterparts to master life challenges, such as losing weight and not relapsing after quitting smoking, and they are also more likely to stick to a regimen of physical activity (Lim & Noh, 2017; Loprinzi et al., 2015). In the face of calamitous or traumatic events, people with higher levels of self-efficacy show better rates of recovery, perhaps because they take a more direct role in mending their lives (Benight & Bandura, 2004; Samuelson et al., 2017).

Optimism: Is the Glass Half Full or Half Empty?

Are you the type of person who sees the proverbial glass as half full or as half empty? People with more optimistic attitudes—who see the glass as half full—tend to be more resilient than others to the effects of stress, including stress associated with physical illness (Carver & Scheier, 2017; Hernandez et al., 2015). Investigators link optimism to lower levels of emotional distress among people with heart disease and cancer and to lower levels of reported pain, including pain among people with cancer (Basten-Gunther et al., 2019; Carver & Scheier, 2017). Optimism in pregnant women predicts better birth outcomes, as measured, for instance, by higher infant birth weights (Lobel & Ibrahim, 2018). Optimism in people undergoing coronary artery bypass surgery is also associated with fewer serious postoperative complications (Scheirer et al., 1999).

People with more pessimistic attitudes, in contrast, tend to have a greater risk of cardiovascular disease (Felt et al., 2020). Pessimistic people also report greater emotional distress in the form of depression and social anxiety (Carver & Scheier, 2017). More optimistic people tend to be healthier and to live longer, to sleep better, to be healthier as they age, and to have more satisfying and happier romantic relationships, and to be more successful in their careers (Koga et al., 2022; L. O. Lee et al., 2022; Weitzer et al., 2020; Carver & Scheier, 2017, and others).

Rozanski and his colleagues (2019) undertook an analysis of 15 studies on relationships among optimism and cardiovascular events and all-cause mortality. The combined studies had 229,391 participants who were followed over a period of 2–40 years (mean = 13.8 years). Overall, optimism was significantly associated with a lower risk of cardiovascular events and all-cause mortality. Other researchers concur, finding a lower incidence of cardiovascular events in people with more resilience resources they can draw upon to deal with life stress, such as ability to maintain an optimistic attitude (Park et al., 2022). The Rozanski group also reported studies showing that optimism moderates inflammation in the body (apparently buffering the effects of stress on the immune system to some degree) and high blood pressure—other signs that a positive mental attitude can benefit our physical health.

Optimism, Cardiovascular Disorders, and the Health Belief Model

Of course, the research on longevity, cardiovascular events, and other health issues is correlational, so it may also be the case that people who live longer generally feel healthier, contributing to their optimism. According to the HBM, being optimistic casts health challenges in a whole different light. Both people who are pessimistic and people who are optimistic may perceive themselves as being susceptible to potential cardiovascular disorders and other health challenges. They may both be aware of preventive measures they can take to try to ward off health problems. However, people who are optimistic may believe that engaging in healthful behaviors, including a healthy diet and exercise, will actually work, boosting their self-efficacy. As a result, they may be more likely to engage in these behaviors (Breland et al., 2020; Speck et al., 2020). Looking at it from the other side, a person who is pessimistic may not have faith that efforts to engage in healthful behaviors will pay off, so, why bother? Therefore, the health-related behaviors of people who are optimistic, and not simply their attitudes, may be the key predictors of healthy outcomes. That said, having more positive ideas may translate into making healthful behavior changes. Simply put, it's a win-win.

The nearby self-assessment will help you evaluate whether you are someone who sees the glass as half full or half empty.

Irrational Beliefs: Cognitive Doorways to Distress

Psychologist Albert Ellis (1913–2007), like Shakespeare centuries earlier, also believed that our beliefs about events we experience, as well as the events themselves, can be stressors that challenge our ability to adjust (Balkis & Duru, 2018; Ellis, 2008; Wirga et al., 2020). Consider a case in which a person is fired from a job and is anxious and depressed about it. It may seem logical that losing the job is responsible for the misery, but Ellis points out how the individual's beliefs about the loss are the determinants of personal misery.

Ellis looked upon the role of irrational beliefs with an A → B → C approach. Losing the job is an activating event (A). The eventual outcome, or consequence (C), is personal misery in the form of anxiety or depression, or both. Between the activating event (A) and the consequence (C), however, lie beliefs (B), such as these: "This job was the most important thing in my life," "What a no-good failure I am," "My family will starve," "I'll never find a job as good," "There's nothing I can do about it." Beliefs such as these foster and compound misery, as well as feelings of helplessness, and also divert us from planning and deciding what to do next. The belief that "There's nothing I can do about it" fosters helplessness. The belief that "I am a no-good failure" internalizes the blame and is exaggerated and distorted, the upshot of which is that the person may give up trying. The belief that "My family will starve" may also be an exaggeration. We can diagram the situation in this way

Activating events → Beliefs → Consequences
or
A → B → C

INTERACTIVE SELF-ASSESSMENTS

Self-Assessment

Are You an Optimist or a Pessimist?

Do you consider yourself to be an optimist or a pessimist? Do you expect good things to happen, or do you find the cloud around the silver lining? This questionnaire may provide you with insight into your general outlook on life.

Directions: Indicate whether each of the items represents your feelings by writing a number on the line according to the following code. Then check the scoring key at the end of the chapter.

1 = strongly disagree
2 = somewhat disagree
3 = neutral; neither agree nor disagree
4 = somewhat agree
5 = strongly agree

___ 1. I'm more of an optimist than a pessimist.
___ 2. You're born either lucky or, like me, unlucky.
___ 3. I generally expect things will turn out for the best.
___ 4. People who believe that "every cloud has a silver lining" are just fooling themselves.
___ 5. I believe I can succeed.
___ 6. I'm one of those realists who think the proverbial glass is half empty, not half filled.
___ 7. I generally believe that if things can go wrong, they will go wrong.
___ 8. I am very hopeful about my future.
___ 9. Life is just too uncertain to succeed even when you put in your best effort.
___ 10. The future looks good to me.

Anxieties about the future and feelings of sadness over a loss are normal and to be expected. However, the beliefs of the person who lost the job catastrophize or blow out of proportion the extent of the loss and contribute to anxiety and depression. By heightening the individual's emotional reaction to the loss and fostering feelings of helplessness, these beliefs transform sadness into despair and also impair coping ability. They also lower the person's self-efficacy expectations.

Ellis proposed that many of us adopt irrational beliefs that become our personal doorways to unhappiness. He argued that we make ourselves miserable by adopting the kinds of irrational beliefs shown in **Figure 5.2**. When we hold to these kinds of beliefs, we inevitably find that either we or the world at large comes up short, which can leave us feeling upset, angry, or depressed.

Ellis recognized that people want social approval, but he explained that the desire becomes irrational when we believe that we cannot possibly survive without it. It would be great to be competent in everything we do, but it's unreasonable to expect it. Sure, it would be nice to be able to serve and volley like a tennis pro, but most of us don't have the time or natural ability to perfect our game. Demanding perfection of ourselves prevents us from going out on the court on weekends and batting the ball back and forth just for fun.

1. The belief that it is necessary to have the love and approval almost all the time from people who are important to you
2. The belief that certain acts are awful or wicked and that people who perform such acts should be severely damned or punished
3. The belief that it is horrible when things do not go the way we want them to go. Life is awful when you don't get your first choice
4. The belief that human misery is externally caused and forced on us by outside people and events. Until these external pressures change, you must remain miserable
5. The belief that if something is or may be dangerous or fearsome, we should be terribly upset and endlessly obsess about it
6. The belief that it is easier to avoid than to face life's difficulties and assume responsibility for oneself
7. The belief that we need to rely on someone or something other, stronger, or greater than ourselves
8. The belief that we should be thoroughly competent, intelligent, and achieving in all possible respects
9. The belief that because something once strongly affected our life, it will indefinitely affect it
10. The belief that we must have perfect control over events
11. The belief that human happiness can be achieved by inertia and inaction
12. The belief that we have virtually no control over our emotions and that we cannot help feeling disturbed about things

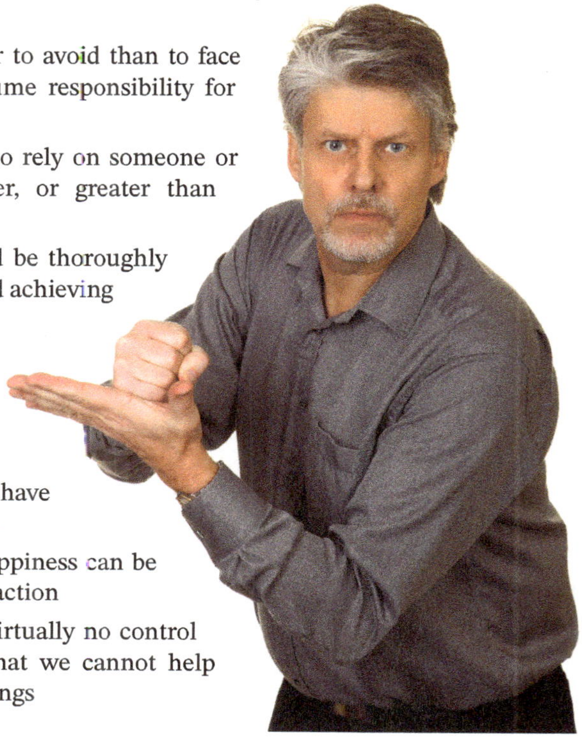

Mats Persz/Alamy Stock Photo

FIGURE 5.2 **Irrational Beliefs: Cognitive Doorways to Distress, as Identified by Albert Ellis**

Applying Health Psychology

Replacing Catastrophizing Thoughts with Rational Alternatives

How, then, do we change irrational thoughts? Cognitive behavioral psychologists present a challengingly simple answer: We change these thoughts by changing them. However, change can require some work. These irrational thoughts can become automatic, so before we can change them, we must first become aware of them (Buschmann et al., 2018). Cognitive behavioral psychologists suggest steps such as the following for controlling the irrational thoughts that often accompany feelings of anxiety, conflict, or tension.

1. Develop awareness of automatic self-defeating thoughts by careful self-examination. Check out the examples in Table 5.2 and ask yourself whether any of them ring true for you. And when you encounter anxiety or frustration, pay close attention to your thoughts. Negative thoughts are triggers for negative emotions.
2. Next, evaluate the accuracy of the thoughts. Are they guiding you toward a solution, or are they compounding your problems? Do they reflect reality, or do they blow things out of proportion? Do they misplace the blame for failure or shortcomings?
3. Then prepare thoughts that are incompatible with the irrational thoughts and practice saying them firmly to yourself. (If nobody is nearby, why not say them firmly aloud?)
4. Finally, reward yourself with a mental pat on the back for making adaptive changes in your thought patterns.

One category of stressful thoughts catastrophizes stressors; that is, it blows stressors out of proportion. Table 5.2 provides examples of catastrophizing thoughts and rational alternatives that help keep things in perspective.

TABLE 5.2 Catastrophizing Thoughts and Rational Alternatives

INTERACTIVE FIGURES, CHARTS, & TABLES

Catastrophizing Thoughts	Rational Alternatives
"Oh my God, it's going to be a mess! I'm losing all control!"	"This is annoying and upsetting, but I haven't lost all control and I don't have to."
"This is awful. It'll never end."	"It's bad, but it doesn't have to get the best of me. And upsetting things do come to an end, even if it's sort of hard to believe right now."
"I just can't stand it when Mom (Dad/my roommate/my partner) gives me that look."	"Life is more pleasant when everyone is happy with me, but I have to be myself, and that means that other people are going to disagree with me from time to time."
"There's no way I can get up there and perform/give that speech! I'll look like an idiot."	"So I'm not perfect; that doesn't mean I'm going to look like an idiot. And so what if someone thinks I look bad? It doesn't mean I am bad. And if I am bad, so what? I can live with that too. I don't have to be perfect every time. So stop being such a worrywart and get up and have some fun."
"My heart's beating a mile a minute! It's going to leap out of my chest! How much of this can I take?"	"Take it easy! Hearts don't jump out of chests. Slow down a minute—stop and think. I'll find a way out. And if I don't for the time being, I'll survive. Someday I'll look back on this and laugh at how upset I got myself."
"What can I do? I'm helpless! It's just going to get worse and worse."	"Take it easy. Just stop and think for a minute. Just because there's no obvious solution doesn't mean that I won't be able to do anything about it. There's no point to getting so upset. Why don't I just take it from minute to minute for the time being? If I can't think of anything to do, I can always talk to other people about it."

You have heard the expressions "blowing things out of proportion" and "making a mountain out of a molehill." As noted earlier, some cognitive psychologists refer to thoughts that blow things out of proportion as catastrophizing. Controlling catastrophizing thoughts reduces the impact of a stressor and gives you a chance to develop a plan for effective action. When effective action is not possible, controlling our thoughts increases our capacity to tolerate discomfort. So do meditation and relaxation, which we discuss later.

Benevolent Religious Reappraisal

A flight from Denver to Chicago encountered problems. An explosion in the plane's tail destroyed an engine and crippled the hydraulic systems. The crew fought to keep the plane in the air, but after an hour, it came in for a crash landing. As the airplane struggled in flight, passengers struggled with their thoughts, and many turned to religion. One woman reported:

After the flight attendant explained emergency landing procedures, we were left with our thoughts. That's when I began praying. I closed my eyes and thought, "Dear Lord, I pray that you'll guide the pilot's hands." I also thought that if God wanted to take my life, that it was O.K. with me. I was full of peace. Here I was sitting on the edge of eternity. I wasn't facing the end of my life.

Another person said:

I could see and smell death. It was like being at the doorstep of hell. I pulled my Bible out of my bag. That's all I wanted.

A man reported:

I wanted to be reborn into a family where I would be able to hear the teachings of Buddha.

But not all turned to religion. Another passenger said:

I don't believe there is a kindly Supreme Being who responds to people one to one. People ask me if I'm still a nonbeliever after my life was saved. If everybody had had his life saved except the bad people on the plane, maybe I'd believe a little more. But that's not what happened. Mothers of young children died.[1]

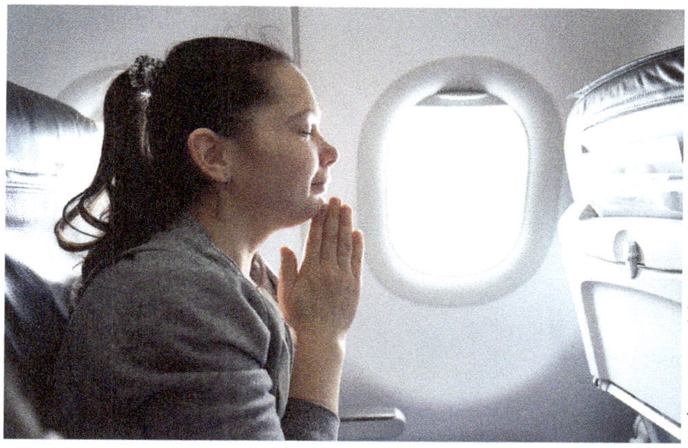

Andrey_Popov/Shutterstock.com

Praying for a Safe Landing The woman in the photo is frightened that the airplane may crash and is praying for it to land safely. Prayer helps her to regulate her emotions. She may also be praying to ask God to help her find meaning in her possible death. Prayer helps many people in times of need, but not everyone.

Tragedy and pain also make the threat of death very real, something that must be coped with in one way of another (Van Tongeren, 2020). Religious traditions use both problem-focused and emotion-focused methods to enable people to remain calm in the face of concern about their existence.

- One method is *problem-focused*: From this perspective, fear of death prompts greater belief in religious worldviews that see death as meaningful within a larger cosmic framework or as a leaping point into eternal life.
- The second method is *emotion-focused*: Religions endorse ways to manage human suffering, through prayer and through social gatherings, such as life events and funerals. The offering of specific thoughts and prayers, and ways in which to focus the body in prayer, help people regulate their emotions in the face of pain (Vishkin, 2020). Prayer itself is a way of coping with stressors and feeling relaxed (Ahmadi et al., 2019).

Religion also offers cognitive reappraisal of one's suffering—more specifically, **benevolent religious reappraisal** (Ahmadi et al., 2019). People under stress attempt to find meaning in their suffering (see nearby *Health Psychology in Action* feature).

benevolent religious reappraisal A method of reappraising one's travails such that one tries to find a lesson from God in them or to perceive that the trials are spiritually beneficial.

Health Psychology in Action

Benevolent Religious Appraisal as a Coping Skill

Health researchers find that benevolent religious reappraisal can help people cope with health problems. Investigators in Thailand observed the ways in which people with kidney disease coped with the discomforts of hemodialysis (Yodchai et al., 2017). People who used religious and spiritual explanations to make the onset of kidney disease meaningful and who used religious and spiritual practices to cope with hemodialysis found the procedure to be less stressful. In an American study of women with breast cancer and women with benign tumors, the women with cancer increased their use of benevolent religious reappraisal to deal with feelings of depression over the months following their diagnosis (Gall & Bilodeau, 2020). The women with benign tumors did not increase their use of benevolent religious reappraisal over the same period of time. Apparently, they did not need to do so.

An American study with 260 lesbian, gay, and bisexual adults found mixed usage of religious coping (Lauricella et al., 2017). Some found that a perceived connection with God through prayer and other religious activities helped them cope with the stigma they encountered in their larger communities. In contrast, some participants expressed anger and frustration toward their religious communities because they professed negative attitudes toward their same-sex sexual orientations. For the latter group, religion was not a path to adjustment.

[1]Excerpts are from K. I. Pargament (1997), *The psychology of religion and coping*. Guilford Press, pp. 1, 2.

What about the nonbelievers aboard the airplane? Nonbelievers vary in their response to stress. A review of the literature found that nonbelievers—atheists and agnostics—who firmly believe that their views are valid enjoy better psychological health than those whose views are uncertain (Weber et al., 2012). The reviewers of the literature did find one particular source of stress experienced by nonbelievers—the disapproval of acquaintances who do believe.

VIDEO CONTENT
Managing Stress

Cognitive Appraisal and Stress Management

Stimuli strike our sensory organs throughout the day and night. Many are familiar or below the threshold at which they would trigger conscious awareness. A car backfiring in the distance may catch our notice for an instant, but it probably won't distract us from what we're doing. However, a loud bang when we are driving or in an elevator will certainly capture our attention and demand rapid appraisal and perhaps a behavioral response.

According to Lazarus and Folkman (1984), there are several possible outcomes of the *primary appraisal* of a stimulus. In one case we appraise a stimulus, such as a distant backfiring, to be irrelevant to us and we get on with what we were doing. In a second case, we interpret the stimulus as being benign or positive, as we may do if we are on the beach and cloud cover gives way to sun or as we may do on a brutally hot day when we enter an air-conditioned building and feel welcome coolness on our skin. A third possible outcome is that primary appraisal identifies a stimulus or a situation as dangerous or seriously threatening. As we evaluate the threat, we undertake *secondary appraisal*, in which we assess our available and potential resources for coping with the stress. Then we generally choose either problem- or emotion-focused methods of coping (see **Figure 5.3**). When attempting to resolve complex stressors or a stressful situation that is in flux, we may combine both problem- and emotion-focused approaches.

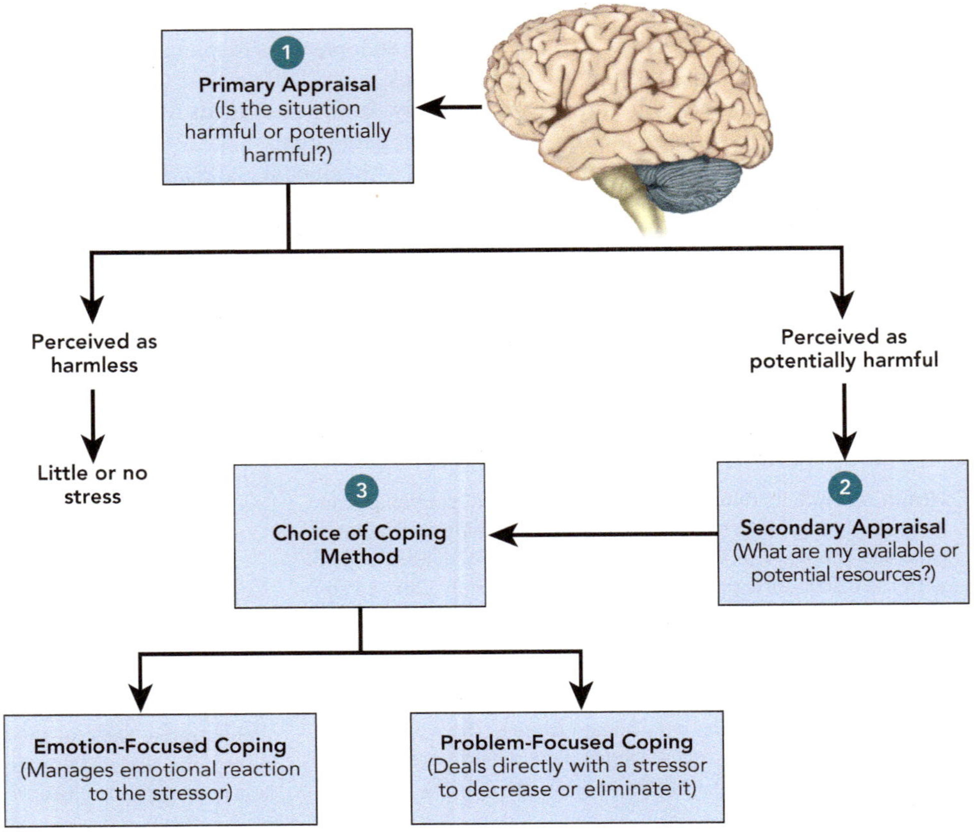

INTERACTIVE FIGURES, CHARTS, & TABLES

FIGURE 5.3 Cognitive Appraisal and Stress Management

Review 5.3

INTERACTIVE SELF-SCORING QUIZZES

Sentence Completion

1. Our confidence in our abilities is known as our __________-__________ expectations.
2. Researchers link (optimism or pessimism) to lower levels of distress among patients with cancer and heart disease.
3. Psychologist Albert Ellis noted a number of __________ beliefs that increase misery and compound the effects of stress.
4. Ellis's A → B → C scheme shows how __________ events can be exacerbated by our beliefs (B) to lead to negative consequences (C).
5. Viewing a catastrophe as a meaningful lesson from God is an example of __________ religious appraisal.

Think About It

Read through Ellis's list of irrational beliefs. Do you harbor any of these beliefs? How have these beliefs affected your life? If they have had a negative impact, what do you think you can do to change the beliefs?

Problem-Focused Coping

In order to get really creative in finding a solution, you have to be fearless in blowing up [the] current state [of things]. You can't be attached to, "This is how we've always done it." Then start asking anyone who will listen, even those not in the situation, how they would design the new process. I often will run ideas by my husband or other nonmedical people to get ideas that I may have never considered.

—Jennifer Johnson, D.O., Director of Medical Staff Quality, Mayo Clinic

What do the following have in common?

- You are repeatedly stuck in traffic on the way to school or work.
- You're not happy with what college life is doing to your waistline.
- You have frequent headaches.
- You're on a big campus, but you're lonely.
- Things aren't going the way you want them to go, and it's just plain awful.

These situations touch on different facets of your life, but what they have in common is that they are all problems to be solved. And it may well be that the best way to begin to cope with stress is to view stressors as problems to be solved rather than insurmountable obstacles. According to the American Psychological Association's *Stress in America* surveys, money and work are two of the major sources of stress we face (APA, 2017, 2018, 2019, 2020). If you don't have enough money to finish the school year, that's a problem to be solved. If you're having problems with your boss at work, that's a problem to be solved. If you're continually stuck in traffic getting back and forth to school or work, that's a problem to be solved. Then there are the problems concerning relationships. If you are in conflict with your family or your intimate partner, that's a problem to be solved. If you don't have friends or social support, that's another problem. Myriad other problems can assault us and stress us out. Some of them will be unique to individuals, as we sometimes create our own problems—as in the cases of irrational beliefs and the Type A behavior pattern (see Chapter 4).

Cognitive behavioral psychologists have developed methods for helping people become more effective problem solvers, such as **problem-solving therapy** (Bergström et al., 2017; Nezu et al., 2013). One approach to problem-solving adopts a seven-step procedure that is intended to help people create effective ways of coping with stressors (see **Figure 5.4**).

problem-solving therapy A cognitive behavioral method for solving problems that involves generating possible solutions, trying them out, and evaluating their effectiveness.

Step 1 is defining the problem, and psychologists encourage people to be as specific as possible so that concrete solutions can be developed. People often have a difficult time defining exactly what the sources of stress are. For example, someone might say, "Oh, it's school." But what does that mean? Is it grades? A specific course or two? Professors? Social situations? Someone else might say, "My family is driving me crazy." Again, what are the specifics? Who does or says what, and when? Thinking about the things that happen with one's family might yield answers, such as "My family doesn't approve of my major field. I love what I'm doing,

1. *Define the problem*. Be as clear and specific as possible. When and where does the problem occur?
2. *Set a realistic, achievable goal or Goals*. Seek measurable outcomes. Don't let the perfect be the enemy of the good—or the good enough.
3. *Generate or brainstorm multiple solutions*. The first idea may not be the best idea. List everything that comes to mind; be patient; seek help if you're coming up blank.
4. *Evaluate the pros and cons of each possible solution*. Be realistic. What can you actually do? (Are you underestimating your knowledge and skills? Are you expecting too much?)
5. *Select the preferred solution*. Use some cognitive filtering. Don't just select the easiest solution. Rank the possible solutions, with the most likely to work as number 1 (and keep some other plan at the ready).
6. *Implement a specific action plan*. What are the steps? What do you do first? (Twenty-five hundred years ago, the Chinese philosopher Laozi said that "a journey of a thousand miles begins with a single step.") Where will you try your solution? When?
7. *Evaluate the outcome*. Did you get there? If not, why not? What else can you try? View difficulties as opportunities, not insurmountable hurdles.

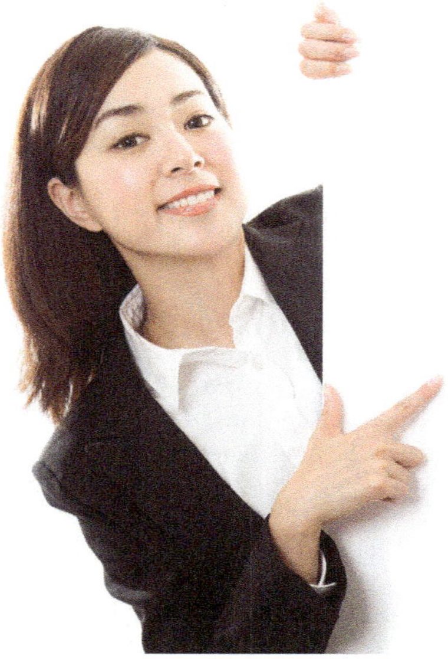

Yuichiro Chino/Alamy Stock Photo

FIGURE 5.4 Seven Steps toward More Effective Problem Solving

but they want me to do something that will make more money." Or "They disapprove of my boyfriend/girlfriend, who is from a different background." This is the point—what specifically are you, or people at school (or work), or your family doing and saying that defines the problem? Or you may think that the problem is anxiety when, in terms of what you actually do and say, it is a lack of assertiveness when people take advantage of you or try to make you conform to their expectations of what you should be.

Consider the problem of not having enough money (join the group). Are you aware of what you are bringing in and what you are spending? Do you understand what tuition and fees and books cost? Did you allow for snacks and entertainment and transportation, or for the supplies to wash your clothing? Do you understand what kinds of grants and loans are available? Is there a way to get by without mortgaging your future?

Do you have enough information to answer these questions? If not, where can you get the information?

Being specific also helps break a problem down into more manageable parts. A woman in middle adulthood in the authors' files—let's call her Maya—said that she had a problem with her "family relations." Breaking it down, she had a problem with role overload. She was working full time and also trying to cope with teenage children and keep the apartment clean. In addition, she was part of the "sandwich generation"—a group of people, generally of middle age, who are rearing their own children and at the same time trying to care for aging parents. Her brother lived in another city and was no help at all. Her sister, who lived nearby, claimed that she had her "own problems."

Step 2 is to set realistic, achievable goals. Goals are best described in observable and measurable behavioral terms. They should be achievable in a reasonable amount of time and with a reasonable amount of effort. If you want to lose 20 pounds, it probably isn't adequate to say that you will simply eat less and that you will exercise more. It is more useful to say that you will get a calorie counter and restrict your calorie intake to, say, 1,500 calories a day for one month and then see where you are. Or you could say you will join a specific aerobics class. Alternatively, you could explore why you want to lose the 20 pounds to help determine whether doing so is the wisest choice for you.

Maya was in the workforce, caring for the kids without much spousal help, and assuming the bulk of household chores while also assisting her aging parents. She needed to demand some assistance from her partner and her siblings. In order to avoid pointless resistance, Maya chose to channel her concerns using assertive communication rather than outward expressions of anger and frustration. One useful method she decided upon was not hosting the larger family on holidays until her siblings agreed to provide some assistance.

Step 3 is to generate multiple possible solutions—to brainstorm. When generating potential solutions, it is good to recognize that the first idea that pops into mind is not always the best idea. Also, the more potential solutions you are able to generate, the more likely it is that one of them will work. If you're repeatedly stuck in traffic, possible solutions might include using public transportation, leaving earlier (and returning later) to avoid rush hour, or taking the longer "scenic" route. If none of that is possible, listening to an audiobook while on the road may help.

If you're stumped, ask yourself how someone you know might respond to the problem. This is also where seeking professional help may be useful. Students concerned about money can stop by the college financial aid office for advice. Or if there is too much anxiety and confusion about the problem, maybe the first stop can be the college counseling center.

Step 4 is to compare the various possible solutions to consider the pros and cons of each. A student's family—let's call the student Tim—did not approve of his choosing to switch his major to the performing arts; they wanted him to remain a business major, which they believed would lead to greater financial security. Tim could have done as they wished, but he would have hated his coursework and felt that he was denying himself his true vocation in life. He considered not telling his family about the switch, but he felt that hiding the truth was not a good solution because he would feel bad about himself, and of course his lying would be discovered and lead to additional problems later on. He also thought he could avoid going home and avoid talking to his family. But he did not want to do that because he would miss his younger siblings. Maya also was in conflict as to how to confront her siblings and her partner because she did not want to risk tearing relationships apart.

Step 5 is to select the preferred solution or solutions, ones that will meet your goals. Tim decided that he would need to confront his family with his choice—find a way to discuss it with them directly. Maya decided she would need separate solutions for her partner and her siblings. With her therapist, she rehearsed making assertive but not aggressive requests. She avoided venting anger directly. For her siblings and her partner, the requests were variations on this theme: "I've been doing this all alone, and I need some help." She practiced the requests, actually looking at herself in the mirror to judge how well she was communicating.

Step 6 is to implement the selected solution or solutions. It is best for solutions to be specific action plans—precisely what one will do and say. Tim chose a weekend when he was largely free of academic demands to go home and talk with his family. He ran over what he would say repeatedly in his mind. He imagined what his parents would say and how he would respond. They would tell him that they wouldn't be around forever and that they only had his best interests at heart. He would acknowledge their concerns and try to provide a clear overview of what he was facing after graduation and how it could play out in the real world. (As he thought about that, he realized that it would be helpful if he had a backup plan—maybe some courses and internships in the businesses relating to the performing arts?) He also thought about his tone of voice.

Maya decided that she would have to have a discussion with her partner about dividing up the household chores and participating in child-rearing in additional ways. She chose the time and the day, where the kids would be, and what her and her partner's workdays would be like. She visualized the discussion and what she would say. And rather than deny the family a holiday get-together, she would use the meeting as a forum in which she could voice her concerns. She visualized sitting at the dining table, who would say what about this and that, and when and how she would make her requests. She visualized when she would take her sister aside for a one-on-one and when she would do so with her brother. And she followed the plan.

Step 7 is evaluating the outcome of the implemented plan. Tim found that his family was actually quite agreeable once he carefully outlined his goals to them and why striving to meet them would make him happy. Maya achieved mixed results. She got some cooperation from her partner in cleaning and shopping. She obtained some additional help from her sister in caring for their parents, but her brother kept his distance, further damaging his relationship with Maya.

The following are some questions to consider when evaluating the outcome of an attempted solution:

- What were the results? Was the implementation successful? If not, why not?
- If the solution concerned a social problem, who said what? Who did what?
- How do you feel about yourself as a result of having implemented the plan?
- What did you learn about yourself and the situation as a result of implementing the plan?
- If the solution was met with resistance or failed, were the goals defined clearly enough? Should the goals be modified?
- Did new obstacles arise? Does it seem that the problem is too difficult to tackle? If so, should a new solution be attempted?

There is much to be gained by seeing a difficult situation as a problem to be solved rather than an impossible roadblock. Working on a problem not only enhances coping skills; it also contributes to one's self-esteem.

Health psychologists find numerous advantages to problem-solving skills. A study of 500 Malaysian college undergraduates found that students who had little confidence in their abilities to solve their problems and control their emotions were more likely to report feeling stressed (Abdollahi et al., 2018). An African study found that depression suppresses adherence to obtaining antiretroviral therapy among people living with HIV. A problem-solving intervention lifted feelings of depression among a sample of people in Zimbabwe and also promoted their adherence to antiretroviral therapy (Nyamayaro et al., 2020). A Chinese study found that problem-solving skills in women helped them overcome feelings of loneliness and lift symptoms of depression (E. C. Chang et al., 2020). Returning to the United States, a problem-solving intervention among older adults with anxiety disorders reduced their risk of committing suicide (Lutz et al., 2020).

About Consulting That Helping Professional ... Here's a shocking bit of news: Your authors don't know everything. Fortunately, education teaches us to seek answers to problems by consulting others when we do not have the answers ourselves. When you do not know how to cope with the stressors in your life, it can be useful to consult a helping professional, such as a counselor in the college health center, a practitioner at a community mental health center, or someone in private practice. First you have to admit to yourself that you do not have the answers. Second, you need to tell yourself that there is nothing demeaning in seeking advice from other people. Many people think that there is stigma attached to seeking help from a psychologist, that it is an admission of weakness. Men in general are less willing than women to seek the help of a psychologist (Liddon et al., 2018; Wahto & Swift, 2016). The stereotype of the tough, independent male has a good deal to do with this attitude. Interestingly, when men do seek help, they have a slight preference for seeing a female psychologist (Liddon et al., 2018; Wahto & Swift, 2016). Asking for help apparently does not compromise a woman's sense of independence as much as it does a man's. When women seek help, they are much more likely to prefer a female psychologist because of concern that a male is less likely to be able to empathize with their situations (Liddon et al., 2018).

Review 5.4

INTERACTIVE SELF-SCORING QUIZZES

Sentence Completion

1. The first step in problem solving, according to the text, is to __________ the problem.
2. The final step is to __________ the outcome.

Think About It

Can you identify problems in your own life? (All right—try to limit it to just a couple.) How would the steps in problem solving outlined in the chapter help you cope with the problems? Are you willing to use the steps to get to work on them? Why or why not?

Emotion-Focused Coping

Sometimes people just need to turn down the alarm. If problem-focused coping seems to hit a wall, emotion-focused coping can bring down the level of alarm to the point at which people can return to problem-focused coping when some time has passed (Carver, 2019).

And sometimes emotion-focused coping offers pleasures and insights on its own. Think about your daily life. Do things run smoothly from day to day? Do you have enough time to "stop and smell the roses"? Or do you find yourself running frantically from place to place just to keep up with the many demands on your time? Does it seem that no matter how hard you try, there is still much more that needs to be done? If the demands on your time keep piling up, you may be facing more stress than you can handle.

In helping people manage stress more effectively, health psychologists and other helping professionals might begin with efforts to reduce the person's overall stress burden. They might draw upon the following suggestions, which you might find helpful in turning down the level of stress in your own life:

1. *Don't bite off more than you can chew.* Don't take on more tasks than you can reasonably accomplish, given the other demands on your time. Prioritize the tasks that remain, sorting them in priority order so that they become more manageable.
2. *Reduce daily hassles.* Might you be able to change your schedule to avoid the morning traffic jam? Can you carpool? Being stuck in traffic may be more tolerable if you are not the one behind the wheel and can use the time to catch up on your reading. What other daily hassles can you minimize or eliminate?
3. *Develop time-management skills.* Plan ahead and make a schedule that allows you to complete the tasks on a reasonable schedule before you reach the point of being overburdened at any particular moment.

Working It Out by Working Out

Exercise not only builds up physical resources but also helps us cope with stress by reducing the negative emotional effects of stress, such as anxiety and depression (Bernstein & McNally, 2018; Cooney et al., 2013; Schoenfeld et al., 2013).

Health Psychology in the Digital Age

"Calm"

Got Calm? More than 100 million people have already downloaded it, and more than 4 million are active users. More than just an app, there is a companion book called *Calm the Mind, Change the World* and even a "sleep mist" to spray on your pillow that is claimed to help you get to sleep. A Calm update addresses mindfulness for children. A competing meditation app, Headspace, has more than 2 million active users.

Psychologists working to tamp down the excess central nervous system activation have long employed methods such as meditation, distraction and fantasy, relaxation, and even—yes—problem solving. The Calm app provides the sounds and the visuals to assist in these methodologies—the crackling of wood in the fireplace (but watch that virtual carbon footprint!), flowing water, and crickets (assuming their rasping is a plus) to help you ease the muscles and the mind. There is a narrator who does voiceovers for calming images, and these mindful meditation programs: 7 Days of Calm, 7 Days of Sleep, and, simply, Breathe (which, considering the alternative, is not a bad idea).

The sleep tab offers the option of bedtime stories. There is a music tab, which enables you to access new-age electronics that are set to accompany images of waterfalls, seas, sunsets, and cityscapes—to each their own.

In short, Calm helps take you on that getaway you've been imagining. Now that you know how it works, can you fantasize your mental voyage on your own?

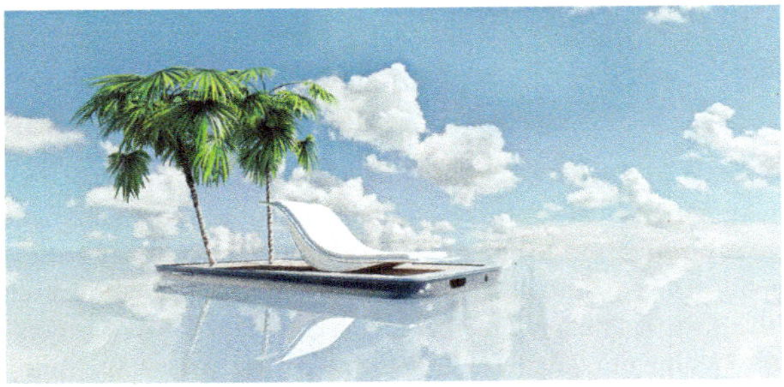

Donald Iain Smith/Photodisc/Getty Images

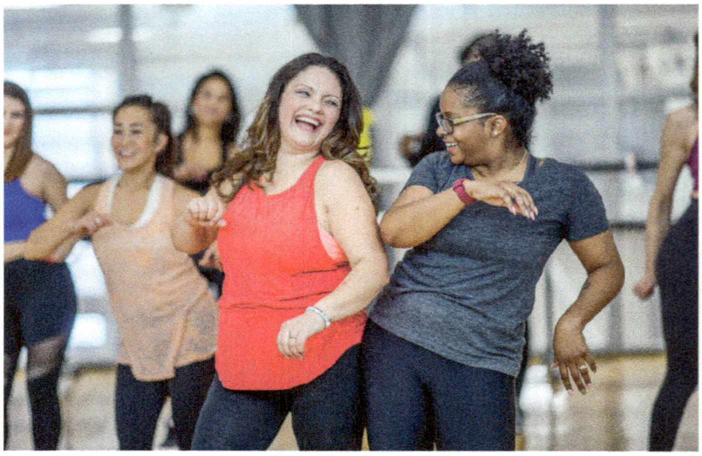
FatCamera/Getty Images

Working It Out by Working Out Exercise strengthens bodily systems, such as the cardiovascular system, that are affected by stress, and it may diminish negative thoughts, making us more resilient to stress.

Exercise is good for the brain as well as the body (Raichlen & Alexander, 2020). Health researchers find that when practiced regularly, aerobic or vigorous physical exercise (think of brisk-paced walking, biking, working out on treadmill or elliptical equipment) is associated with better mental health, clearer and sharper thinking, and better sleep (Ludyga et al., 2020; Park et al., 2021; Young et al., 2021).

Many people work off the tensions of the day with a vigorous game of racquetball, a run around the park, or a dozen laps in the pool. How does exercise help us cope with stress? One answer may lie in the fact that exercise promotes physical fitness. It strengthens bodily systems, such as the cardiovascular system, which are affected by stress. Vigorous exercise also raises the levels of pain-blocking endorphins in the bloodstream, helping us manage daily aches and pains. Exercise also reduces muscle tension and anxiety, at least for a few hours. As a result, it may help us achieve a more relaxed state of mind and body.

You need not push your body to extremes to benefit from the stress-reducing effects of exercise. Even mild levels of exercise—a gentle swim, a brisk walk in the park—can relieve stress. Regardless of the reasons that exercise relieves stress, exercise has a remarkable effect on our moods. It calms us down and improves our psychological outlook. Choose a physical activity that you enjoy. Pushing yourself to do something you detest will only increase the stress you experience.

Doing Something That You Enjoy Each Day

Stress is more manageable when you do something each day that brings you joy. Perhaps you would enjoy some leisure reading each day. Perhaps you would prefer to watch or participate in a sports event. Or maybe you would rather work on the car or surf the internet for a while.

As noted earlier, humor can help buffer the effects of stress. By making us laugh, humor can get our minds off our troubles, at least for a time. A regular dose of humor may make stress more bearable. Rewatch an old movie that makes you laugh, such as the classic movie, *Airplane*.

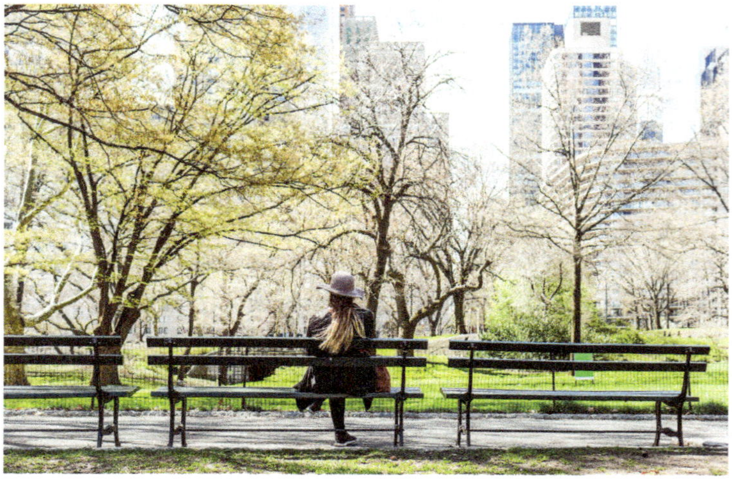
Astrakan Images/Getty Images

Finding Nature in the City Springtime! Does it just feel good or does it do something for you? Actually, sitting or walking in natural surroundings decreases the heart rate, normalizes the blood pressure, and lowers salivary cortisol. It restores feelings of vigor and decreases anxiety and depression. Frederick Law Olmsted, the principal designer of Central Park, wrote, "The enjoyment of scenery employs the mind without fatigue and yet exercises it; tranquilizes it and yet enlivens it; and thus, through the influence of the mind over the body gives the effect of refreshing rest and reinvigoration of the whole system."

City life is relatively new in human history, and in Chapter 4 we noted that it has its stresses. However, we can reverse some of that stress by returning to nature, even if for only a few minutes each day. Spending time outside can enhance a person's mood and also has positive effects on the brain (Kühn et al., 2021).

A research team at Cornell University (Meredith et al., 2020) reviewed more than 10,000 articles on the effects of spending time in nature on stress among college-age students. Only 14 met the criteria for well-designed studies. Some of the studies compared time sitting or walking outdoors in a natural setting rather than in an urban environment. Spending time in nature was associated with a number of markers indicative of more effective stress management, including decreased heart rate, lower levels of cortisol in the saliva, normalized blood pressure, decreased activity of the sympathetic nervous system, and increased activity of the parasympathetic nervous system. Ten to 50 minutes a day of spending time in nature was sufficient. Psychological health also improved. Participants who spent time in nature showed fewer feelings of anger and hostility and less anxiety and depression. They felt more vigor, calmer, more relaxed, and refreshed.

Many people take a back-to-nature approach to stress management, recognizing its restorative effects. They flock to green spaces on campus and sun themselves on warm days or walk or jog along rivers and in parks.

Meditation and Other Mind–Body Interventions

Meditation induces feelings of relaxation accompanied by lower levels of bodily arousal. There are many different forms of meditation, but all involve a narrowing of attention. Sometimes the practitioner narrows attention by repeating a word, thought, or phrase or by maintaining a steady focus on a particular object, such as a burning candle or the design on a vase.

One of the most widely practiced forms is Transcendental Meditation (TM), an Indian meditation practice distinguished by the repetition of mantras—relaxing, sonorous sounds such as *ieng* (pronounced EE-ENG) and *om* (pronounced OAM). TM was brought to the United States by Maharishi Mahesh Yogi in the 1960s and then popularized by the physician Herbert Benson in the 1970s, who saw it as a means to lower high blood pressure. The basic method of TM is to assume a relaxed position in a calm environment and engage in rhythmic thoughts, such as repeating a mantra, while passively ignoring distracting thoughts. The person does not fight the distracting thoughts but rather allows them to pass through. Research shows that the practice of TM decreases the consumption of oxygen, as well as the heart rate, the respiratory rate, and arterial blood pressure. It also increases the blood flow to the skeletal muscles, which is consistent with lessened sympathetic arousal (Benson, 1977; Dossett et al., 2020).

Another form of meditation long practiced by Buddhist monks is *mindfulness meditation*. Practitioners focus entirely on their thoughts and physical sensations on a moment-to-moment basis. In mindfulness meditation, you concentrate your attention completely on each moment in time, without analyzing, judging, or evaluating your unfolding mental experiences or analyzing how well you are doing it. The Dalai Lama, a Buddhist spiritual leader, described mindfulness as "a state of alertness in which the mind does not get caught up in thoughts or sensations, but lets them come and go, much like watching a river flow by" (quoted in Gyatso, 2003, p. A29).

Mindfulness mediation, like TM, produces a response that is characterized by a reduction in heart and respiration rates and in blood pressure. Research shows that the practice of meditation can help relieve chronic pain, lower high blood pressure, counter stress, lessen feelings of anxiety and depression, buttress the effectiveness of the immune system, and enhance emotional well-being (e.g., Burns et al., 2022; Galante et al, 2023; Goldberg et al., 2021; Lynch et al., 2018; Puhlmann et al., 2021; Strauss et al., 2023, among others). A study of Black people with heart disease found that daily practice of meditation reduced the risk of heart attacks as compared with a health education (control) condition (Schneider et al., 2018).

TM and mindfulness meditation also induce more frequent alpha waves—the brain waves associated with feelings of relaxation. Meditation also increases nighttime concentrations of the hormone melatonin, which induces sleepiness (George, 2015). Regular meditation is also linked to better memory functioning and coping with emotions, even at times the person is not meditating (Basso et al., 2019; Desbordes et al., 2015).

Health Benefits of Mind–Body Interventions Health professionals have increasingly enlisted mind–body therapies such as tai chi, qigong, yoga, and meditation in an effort to help people cope with stress and bolster the immune system (Bower & Irwin, 2016). By and large, the therapies have been shown to be effective improving people's quality of life, and continuing research is underway to determine their effects on biological markers of the alarm reaction, including the production of cortisol and cytokines. For example, a meta-analysis of 34 studies that assessed the effectiveness of tai chi, qigong, yoga, or mediation found that 7 to 16 weeks of these mind–body interventions reduced markers of inflammation in response to stress and also increased immune responses to vaccinations (Morgan et al., 2014). (See Chapter 3 for a further discussion of these kinds of complementary alternative medicine.)

Evidence also supports the value of techniques that integrate practices from Eastern and Western traditions. For example, use of an integrated treatment that combines mindfulness training with stress management techniques, called *mindfulness-based stress reduction* (MBSR), is associated with less arousal of the sympathetic division of the autonomic nervous system under stress, including stress relating to traumatic experiences (Chinh et al., 2020; Kearney & Simpson, 2020; McClintock et al., 2019).

Researchers continue to explore links between mindfulness and stress. One study assessed the relationship between mindfulness and stress in a sample of 59 undergraduate students. Stress levels were measured by the extent to which the participants sweated under stressful conditions (Hicks et al., 2019). Students who were more mindful about allowing stressful thoughts to pass through rather than ruminate on them were less likely to find stressful situations aversive and less likely to sweat under these conditions. Another study followed Cambridge University students in the United Kingdom as the exam period approached (Turner et al., 2020). The research group found that as stress increased, the proportion of B cells—a marker of immune system activity—increased. However, the group was *not* able to provide evidence that mindfulness training buffered the effects of stress on participants' immune systems, whether measured by levels of cytokines, serum cortisol, or B cells. Yet another study, which compared the effects of MBSR with a control intervention, did find that MBSR reduced the immune system's inflammatory response following exposure to a stressor (Rozenkranz et al., 2013). More research is needed to reconcile the effects of mindfulness on immune system functioning.

Studies of the effectiveness of mind–body interventions with specific health problems are also encouraging. Consider a study of patients with *fibromyalgia*, a syndrome characterized by musculoskeletal pain and associated cognitive and emotional symptoms (Andres-Rodriguez et al., 2019). The exact causes of fibromyalgia are unknown, although it is believed that it may, at least in part, reflect dysregulation of the immune system. Seventy women with fibromyalgia were randomly assigned to a treatment-as-usual group or a group that added MBSR to the treatment program. Blood levels of cytokines and other immune system markers were assessed at baseline and at a 12-month follow-up. The group receiving MBSR showed significantly greater reduction of the severity of their fibromyalgia symptoms; that is, they exhibited less pain and stiffness, and improved quality of sleep and level of energy. Women receiving MBSR also showed better immune system regulation. A limitation of the study was that MBSR was added to the treatment-as-usual regimen, so the MBSR group actually received more treatment than the control group did. Still, the results are encouraging and point to the need for further study.

Relax Yourself

There are many relaxation techniques, and some may work better for some people than others. Health professionals at your college or university counseling center can help you find a relaxation technique that works for you.

One method, called progressive muscle relaxation, was developed by the physiologist Edmund Jacobson in 1938. Jacobson noticed that people tend to tense their muscles when they are under stress, although they may not be aware of it. As muscle contractions are associated with emotional tension, Jacobson reasoned that relaxing muscles can reduce states of tension. Many of the people he worked with, however, didn't have a clue as to how to relax their muscles.

Jacobson taught people first to tense and then to relax specific muscle groups in the body. The method is "progressive" in that people progress from one group of muscles to another, literally from head to toe. You can get a feel for this technique by practicing on a particular muscle group, say the muscles in your right hand. First, make a tight fist in your right hand, but not so tight that you risk injuring your hand. Just tight enough to feel the tension. After tensing for a few seconds, let go of the tension completely. Study the difference between the states of tension and relaxation. Notice how the muscles in your hand seem to unwind and let go of the tension. As you gain experience with the technique, you may find that you can relax your muscles by "just letting them go" without first having to tense them.

Progressive muscle relaxation has been shown to decrease levels of stress hormones (Vander Wal et al., 2015) and, like meditation, to be helpful in the treatment of pain, high blood pressure, and anxiety (Chauhan & Sharma, 2017; Roozbahani et al., 2017; Wachholtz et al., 2017).

Applying Health Psychology

Practicing Meditation

The following suggestions will help you practice TM as a means of lowering the arousal connected with stress. TM employs a concentration aid, such as a mantra.

1. Begin by meditating once or twice a day for 10–20 minutes.
2. In meditation, what you don't do is more important than what you do do. Adopt a passive, "what happens, happens" attitude.
3. Create a quiet, nondisruptive environment. For example, don't face a light directly.
4. Do not eat for an hour beforehand; avoid caffeine for at least 2 hours.
5. Assume a comfortable position. Change it as needed. It's OK to scratch or yawn.
6. As a device to aid concentration, you could focus on your breathing or seat yourself before a calming object, such as a plant or burning incense. Try "perceiving" (rather than mentally saying) the word *out* on every outbreath. This means thinking the word but "less actively" than usual (good luck). Others suggest thinking or perceiving the word *in* as you are inhaling and *out*, or *ah-h-h*, as you are exhaling.
7. If you are using a mantra (such as the syllable *om*), you can prepare for meditation and say the mantra out loud several times. Enjoy it. Then say it more and more softly. Close your eyes and think only the mantra. Allow yourself to perceive, rather than actively think, the mantra. Again, adopt a passive attitude. Continue to perceive the mantra. It may grow louder or softer, disappear for a while, and then return.
8. If disruptive thoughts enter your mind as you are meditating, allow them to "pass through." Don't get wrapped up in trying to squelch them, or you may raise your level of arousal.
9. Allow yourself to drift. (You won't go far.) What happens, happens.
10. Take what you get. You cannot force the relaxing effects of meditation. You can only set the stage for them and allow them to happen.

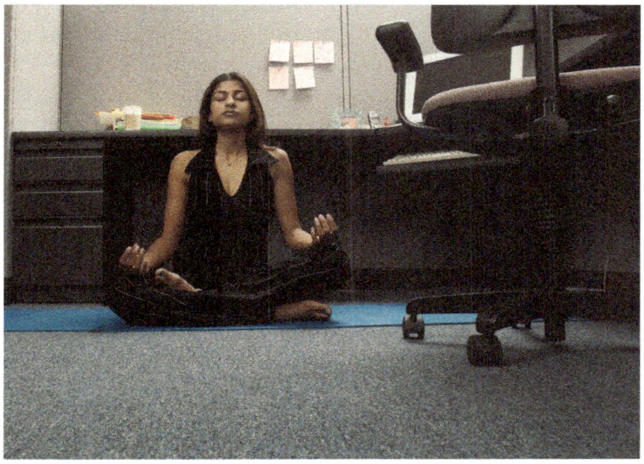

John M Lund Photography Inc/DigitalVision/Getty Images

Meditation Many people practice spiritual forms of meditation, but scientific researchers focus on the observable, measurable effects of meditation on variables such as muscle tension, blood pressure, and other measures of the physiological activity of the autonomic nervous system.

Breathing Calmly and Deeply

Has anyone ever told you to take a few deep breaths when you were feeling stressed or anxious? When we are tense, our breathing becomes shallow. We may hyperventilate or breathe more rapidly than usual. When we breathe, we exchange oxygen for carbon dioxide. But when we hyperventilate, we exhale too much carbon dioxide, which can cause feelings of dizziness or light-headedness. Breathing slowly and deeply from the diaphragm tones down the body's response to stress and restores a correct balance between oxygen and carbon dioxide in our bloodstream.

Deep breathing is a widely used relaxation technique. Breathing slowly and deeply counters arousal induced in times of stress by the sympathetic nervous system and helps restore balance by activating the parasympathetic nervous system (Chen et al., 2017; Hourani et al., 2020). One study enlisted a sample of people in the National Guard, Reserves, military veterans, firefighters, and police (Hourani et al., 2020). The research group used heart rate variability as the measure of monitoring stress and found that a breathing relaxation intervention lowered heart rate variability in the presence of stressors and curtailed dysregulation in breathing which, before treatment, was characterized by short periods of inhalation of air and prolonged exhalation. In practicing deep breathing relaxation,

- breathe through the nose only,
- take equal amounts of time to breathe in and out, and
- inhale and exhale continuously and leisurely.

Self-Assessment

INTERACTIVE SELF-ASSESSMENTS

The Brief COPE

Following is a shortened version of the COPE Scale, innovated by Charles Carver (1997), to provide people with insight into their coping styles. Now that you have completed the chapter and understand the various ways in which people cope with stress, why not complete the Brief COPE to see the approaches that best characterize the ways in which you handle stress?

Imagine that something unpleasant is happening. For example, you are doing poorly in your courses and there is no clear solution at the moment. Or you were in a relationship that came to an end, although you did not want it to do so, and you are feeling the pain. Or perhaps you are faced with financial difficulties. We apologize for placing you in this unpleasant situation, but use the code below to enter the number that you believe would best characterize your behavior to the left of the item. Then check the scoring key at the end of the chapter.

1 = I haven't been doing this at all
2 = I've been doing this a little bit
3 = I've been doing this a medium amount
4 = I've been doing this a lot

__ 1. I've been turning to work or other activities to take my mind off things.

__ 2. I've been concentrating my efforts on doing something about the situation I'm in.

__ 3. I've been saying to myself "this isn't real."

__ 4. I've been using alcohol or other drugs to make myself feel better.

__ 5. I've been getting emotional support from others.

__ 6. I've been giving up trying to deal with it.

__ 7. I've been taking action to try to make the situation better.

__ 8. I've been refusing to believe that it has happened.

__ 9. I've been saying things to let my unpleasant feelings escape.

__10. I've been getting help and advice from other people.

__11. I've been using alcohol or other drugs to help me get through it.

__12. I've been trying to see it in a different light, to make it seem more positive.

__13. I've been criticizing myself.

__14. I've been trying to come up with a strategy about what to do.

__15. I've been getting comfort and understanding from someone.

__16. I've been giving up the attempt to cope.

__17. I've been looking for something good in what is happening.

__18. I've been making jokes about it.

__19. I've been doing something to think about it less, such as going to movies, watching TV, reading, daydreaming, sleeping, or shopping.

__20. I've been accepting the reality of the fact that it has happened.

__21. I've been expressing my negative feelings.

__22. I've been trying to find comfort in my religion or spiritual beliefs.

__23. I've been trying to get advice or help from other people about what to do.

__24. I've been learning to live with it.

__25. I've been thinking hard about what steps to take.

__26. I've been blaming myself for things that happened.

__27. I've been praying or meditating.

__28. I've been making fun of the situation.

Source: Adapted from C. S. Carver (1997). You want to measure coping but your protocol's too long: Consider the Brief COPE. *International Journal of Behavioral Medicine*, *4*, 92–100.

In sum, stress is an inescapable part of life. We may not be able to eliminate all sources of stress, In fact, some stress is beneficial, helping to keep us alert and motivated (Oshri et al., 2022a, 2022b). Yet too much stress can overtax our ability to cope, causing personal or emotional distress and putting us at risk of stress-related health problems. Yes, stress may be a fact of life, but it is a fact we can learn to live with. We can view stress as an opportunity to take charge of our lives and solve problems—not as an unbearable burden to carry.

Review 5.5

INTERACTIVE SELF-SCORING QUIZZES

Sentence Completion

1. Exercise raises levels of pain-blocking __________ in the bloodstream.

2. A Cornell University research team found evidence that sitting or walking in a natural setting (decreases or increases) the level of cortisol in the saliva.

3. Sitting or walking in a natural setting also increases the activity of the __________ division of the autonomic nervous system.

4. Herbert Benson found that __________ meditation induced a relaxation response.

5. In __________ Meditation, you concentrate your attention completely on each moment in time, without analyzing, judging, or evaluating your unfolding mental experiences.

6. Tai chi, qigong, and meditation are examples of __________ body interventions to reduce stress.

7. A meta-analysis of 34 studies that assessed the effectiveness of tai chi, qigong, yoga, or mediation found that that these methods reduced markers of __________ in response to stress.

8. A Cambridge University group of researchers found that as student stress increased during an exam period, the proportion of __________ cells increased.

9. In the method of __________ relaxation, practitioners tighten muscles before relaxing them.

10. Researchers found that relaxation breathing lowered __________ rate variability.

Think About It

You have now read about several methods for coping with the emotional consequences of stress. Have you tried any of them? Do you think one of them might be of use to you? Explain why. Do you know people who meditate, practice yoga, or engage in other mind–body interventions? What do they have to say about the interventions?

Recite: An Active Summary

INTERACTIVE SELF-SCORING QUIZZES

Chapter 5 Practice Quiz

1. Identify factors that foster resilience to stress.

Factors that enhance our tolerance of stress include psychological hardiness (characterized by commitment, challenge, and control), positive self-efficacy expectations (thinking "I can" rather than "I can't"), a sense of humor and laughter, predictability and control, optimism, and social and emotional support. Loneliness is common, especially among older people, and is connected with higher morbidity (illness) and mortality rates. People placed in quarantine are prone to developing stress disorders. Timely information and perception of benefits of the quarantine help people cope.

2. Explain problematic ways of coping with stress.

Problematic ways of coping with stress include withdrawal from the stressful situation (behavioral disengagement), denial that stress exists (one of many defense mechanisms), substance abuse and aggression. These methods can lead to psychological problems, social problems, and health problems. In active coping, people confront stressors using their internal resources, as in changing maladaptive habits. In passive coping, people absolve themselves of responsibility for managing stressors, surrender control, and allow external forces to resolve—or fail to resolve—the problems.

3. Explain the role of cognitive appraisal in coping with stress.

Our confidence in our abilities, our self-efficacy expectations, are linked to our ability to cope with stress. People with more optimistic attitudes—who see the glass as half full—tend to be more resilient than others to the effects of stress, including stress associated with physical illness. Pessimistic people are more prone to health challenges, such as cardiovascular disorders. We sometimes create our own stressors with irrational beliefs, such as an excessive desire for social approval, perfectionism, or the idea that it is awful when things do not go as we want them to go. Psychologists help individuals replace irrational beliefs with rational alternatives. Many people turn to religion in trying times. Benevolent religious appraisal helps many individuals interpret their problems in ways that provide meaning, perhaps a lesson to be learned. Religion can also help stressed people regulate their emotions.

4. Describe problem-focused methods of coping with stress.

Problem-focused coping begins with viewing stress as a problem to be solved, not avoided or responded to in a maladaptive manner. Psychologists have identified a seven-step procedure for problem solving: (1) defining the problem, (2) setting realistic goals for solving it, (3) brainstorming multiple solutions, (4) evaluating the pros and cons of each possible solution, (5) selecting the preferred solution, (6) implementing a plan to apply the solution, and (7) evaluating the results.

5. Describe emotion-focused methods of coping with stress.

Emotion-focused coping involves ways of reducing the impact of stressors when they cannot be eliminated. Emotion-focused methods include engaging in regular exercise or physical activity to strengthen your body and help relieve feelings of anxiety and depression, pursuing activities that make you laugh, performing enjoyable activities each day, and turning down the volume in the sympathetic division of the autonomic nervous system through mind–body interventions, progressive relaxation, or relaxation breathing. Research shows that people who spend time sitting or walking in natural settings have fewer feelings of anxiety and depression.

Answers to Review Sections

5.1

1. commitment
2. are
3. decreases
4. instrumental
5. high
6. barrier
7. voluntary

5.2

1. Withdrawal
2. rationalization
3. denial
4. active

5.3

1. self-efficacy
2. optimism
3. irrational
4. activating
5. benevolent

5.4

1. define
2. evaluate

5.5

1. endorphins
2. decreases
3. parasympathetic
4. Transcendental
5. mindfulness
6. mind–
7. inflammation
8. B
9. progressive
10. heart

Scoring Key for "Are You an Optimist or a Pessimist?"

To arrive at your total score for the test, first reverse your score on items 2, 4, 6, 7, and 9. That is,

Change 1 to 5.
Change 2 to 4.
Leave 3 as it is.
Change 4 to 2.
Change 1 to 5.

Now sum the scores for all your responses. Your total score can vary from 10 to 50. The higher your score, the more optimistic you're likely to be. Scores of about 30 indicate more optimistic attitudes overall than pessimistic attitudes. Scores in the 30–40 range indicate a moderate level of optimism, whereas those in the 20–30 range indicate a moderate level of pessimism. Scores above 40 indicate a high level of optimism, whereas those below 20 indicate a high level of pessimism.

Scoring Key for "The Brief COPE"

Add the scores for the following items, as shown below.

Item 1 + Item 19 = ___ (Self-distraction)
Item 2 + Item 7 = ___ (Active coping)
Item 3 + Item 8 = ___ (Denial)
Item 4 + Item 11 = ___ (Substance abuse)
Item 5 + Item 15 = ___ (Use of emotional support)
Item 10 + Item 23 = ___ (Seeking support from others)
Item 6 + Item 16 = ___ (Behavioral disengagement)
Item 9 + Item 21 = ___ (Venting negative feelings)
Item 12 + Item 17 = ___ (Reframing or reevaluating the situation)
Item 14 + Item 25 = ___ (Planning)
Item 18 + Item 28 = ___ (Humor)
Item 20 + Item 24 = ___ (Acceptance)
Item 22 + Item 27 = ___ (Religious coping)
Item 13 + Item 26 = ___ (Self-blame)

Your score for each coping style can vary from 2 (if both were "I haven't been doing this at all") to 8 (if both were "I've been doing this a lot"). Simply eyeball the results. Where did you score relatively low, and where did you score relatively high? What do you believe that your scores tell you about the ways in which you usually handle stress? Are you satisfied with what you have learned? If not, what can you do to enhance your ability to tackle stressors as challenges and get to work on solving problems?

CHAPTER 6

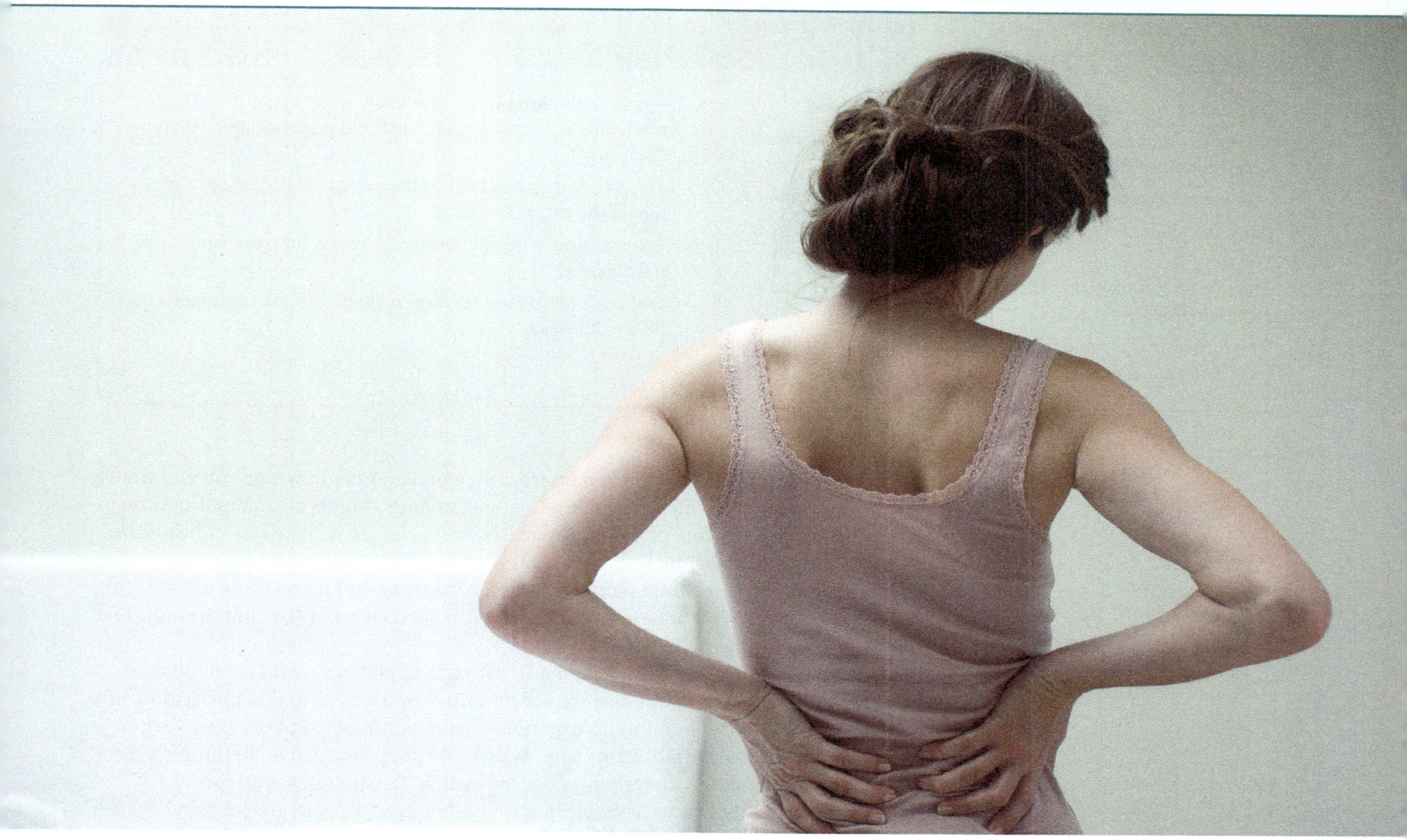

Tom Merton/Getty Images

Understanding and Managing Pain

LEARNING OBJECTIVES

After studying this chapter, you will be able to ...

1. **Describe** the ways in which the body processes pain.
2. **Describe** the biopsychosocial model of chronic pain.
3. **Describe** the role that health psychologists play in the management of chronic pain.
4. **Identify** and **describe** biomedical, psychological, and complementary health approaches for treating chronic pain.
5. **Describe** ways of coping with chronic pain.

Did You Know That ...

- Pain can be a good thing?
- The brain produces its own pain-killing chemicals that are similar in chemical structure to narcotics?
- Many people experience pain "in" limbs that have been amputated?
- More than half of adult Americans experience back pain each year?
- The risk of chronic pain differs across major racial and ethnic groups in the United States?
- People who catastrophize pain tend to report more intense pain than people who take it in stride?
- People with chronic pain are likely to do better by taking on more physical activity and household responsibilities than by doing less?
- The opioid crisis has become the worst epidemic of drug addiction in the nation's history?
- Transmitting a strong magnetic pulse into the brain may reduce pain?
- Cognitive behavioral therapy, a psychological treatment, can help reduce pain?

Imagine a life without pain. A life free of pain from paper cuts. A life in which you could stub your toe and not notice it. A life in which you could undergo surgery or dental treatment without anesthesia. Or a life free of pain from arthritis and cancer. A life without headaches, backaches, muscle pain, or toothaches.

It might seem that a life without pain would be a good thing, but if you think more deeply about it, a life without pain might be a short life indeed, a life colored by the continuous threat of wounds or injuries going unattended.

Pain means something is wrong in the body. Though unpleasant, pain is adaptive. Pain motivates us to do something about a source of an injury or a threat to our physical health (think chest pain). Without the ability to experience pain, you might not notice a burn or a splinter or bleeding from a wound. Pain is the body's warning sign that something requires attention—injuries, infections, underlying conditions that can threaten our survival if not addressed. There are isolated cases of children born without the capacity to feel pain because of defects in the body's processing of pain signals. Their parents watch them like hawks, lest they have a cut or accident that goes unnoticed.

If pain is adaptive, why should we be concerned about managing it? Unfortunately, millions of Americans live with chronic pain that continues after its function as a warning signal has passed. Health psychologists recognize that it takes a coordinated effort by different kinds of healthcare providers to help people manage pain more effectively. At the same time, healthcare providers face the challenge of seeking to relieve pain without addictive pain-killing medications. Behavioral interventions offer the promise of helping to relieve pain when used alongside nonaddictive medications or sometimes in place of them (National Institutes of Health, 2018).

In this chapter we consider the biological aspects of pain, the psychosocial factors involved, and the role of psychological interventions, especially cognitive behavioral therapy (CBT), in helping reduce discomfort and improve the quality of life of people living with chronic pain.

VIDEO CONTENT

The Psychology of Pain

Understanding Pain

Pain is part of a signaling system in the body that has clear survival benefits. Pain arises from tissue damage or bodily injury, as in the case of a burn or twisting your ankle or stubbing your toe. Pain also results from disease processes that damage internal organs, such as cancer, arthritis, or nerve damage. Pain receptors are located throughout the body, including in the skin and internal organs.

Health professionals distinguish between two types of pain, *acute pain* and *chronic pain.* Acute pain is triggered by the nervous system to alert you to a part of the body that may be injured or in need of medical attention. Acute pain tends to quickly diminish or disappear, but chronic pain continuously hurts as nerves carrying pain signals continue to fire. Although pain is a built-in biological response, pain is influenced by psychological as well as physiological factors.

Chronic pain can last months or years. It can drain the pleasure from life and sap vitality, even the will to live. For millions of Americans, persistent or chronic pain is an unwelcome daily presence. More Americans live with chronic pain than with diabetes, heart disease, and cancer combined (National Institutes of Health, 2018). Chronic pain is also the most common cause of long-term disability and elevates the risk of suicide (Kirtley et al., 2020).

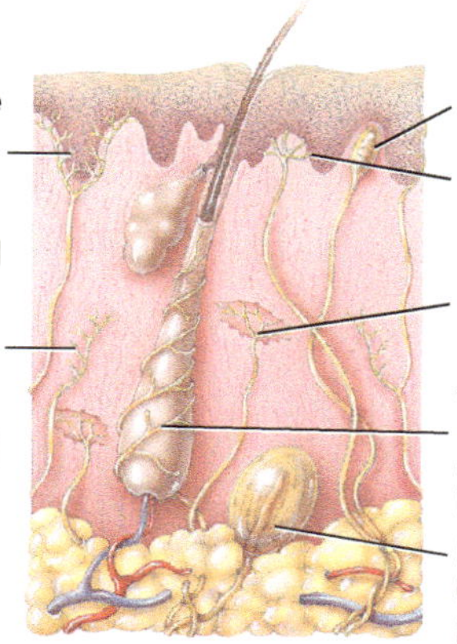

FIGURE 6.1 **Sensory Receptors in the Skin** Pain receptors lie close to the surface of the skin, making us sensitive to cuts, burns, and pinches.

Pain Signals: Knowing Where It Hurts

Pain usually originates at the point of contact, as with a stubbed toe. The pain message is relayed from the source of an injury to the spinal cord and from there to the brain, making us aware of the location and severity of tissue damage. In response to pain signals, the brain releases chemicals, including **prostaglandins**, which heighten circulation to the injured area, causing the redness and swelling that we call inflammation. Inflammation serves the biological function of attracting infection-fighting blood cells to the affected area to protect it against invading germs.

When you stub your toe, nerve signals from the injured area are transmitted from pain receptors in the skin to the spinal cord and from there to the brain for processing (see **Figures 6.1** and **6.2**). The technical term for a pain receptor is **nociceptor** (from the Latin *nocer*, meaning "to injure").

In the brain, pain signals pass through the **thalamus**, which functions as a kind of relay station for directing different types of sensory signals (sound, light, touch, etc.) to different parts of the brain's **cerebral cortex** for processing. The cerebral cortex is the brain's thinking, processing, and command center that is responsible for higher mental functions like thought, perception, language, and planning. The cortex is organized in four parts, called

prostaglandins Hormones that cause inflammation, pain, and fever, as part of the body's response to injury and illness.

nociceptor A sensory neuron that transmits pain signals.

thalamus A structure in the forebrain that serves as a relay station for directing sensory information to different parts of the cerebral cortex for processing.

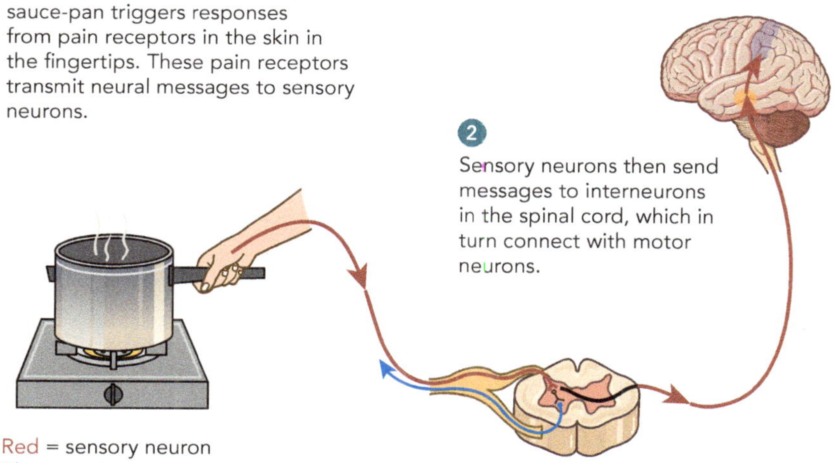

FIGURE 6.2 **Pain Pathways** Pain signals from the point of injury in the skin travel to the spinal cord and from there upward to the brain, where they are received by the thalamus, which functions as a relay station, and then to the cerebral cortex for processing, where the messages are interpreted as pain. In this case, however, even before the brain registers pain, a withdrawal reflex is triggered in the spinal cord, causing the individual to remove the hand from the pan, possibly dropping the pan in the process.

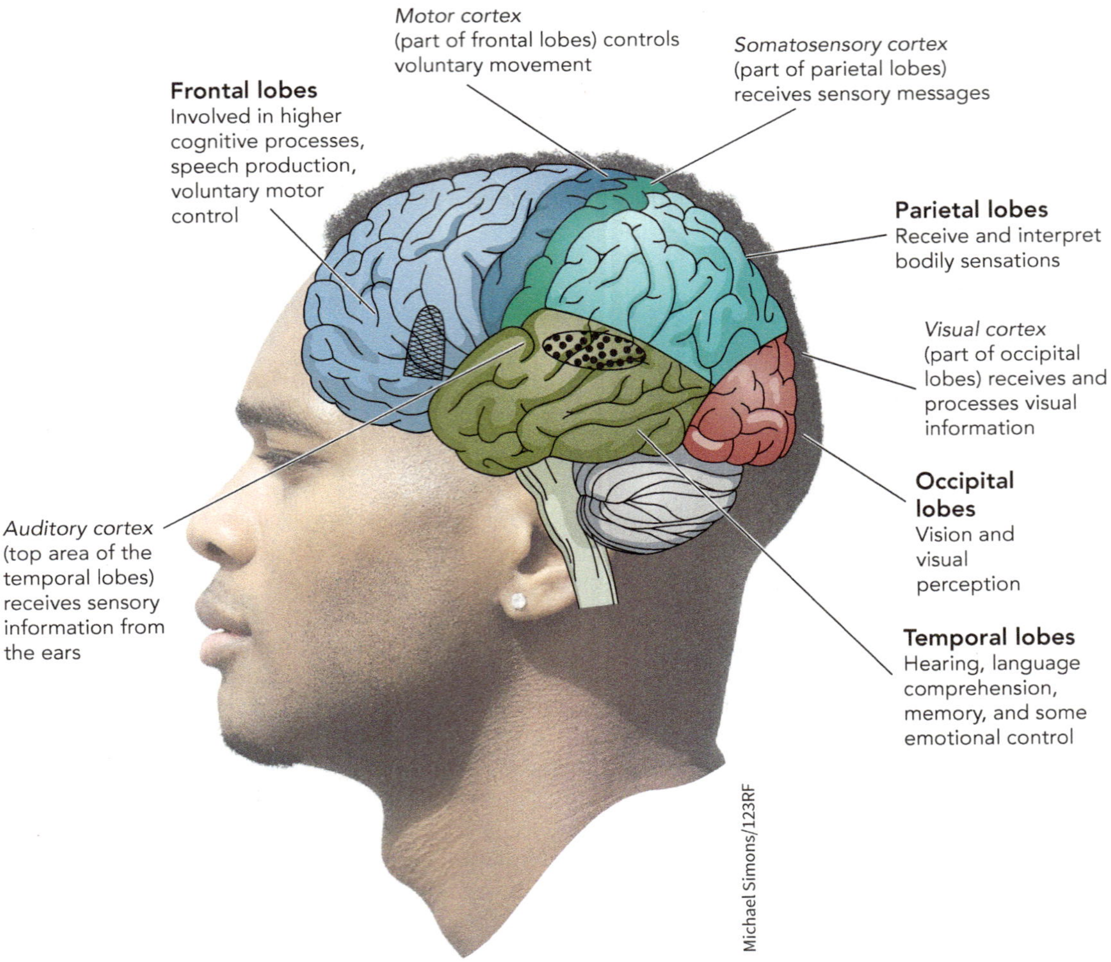

FIGURE 6.3 The Lobes of the Cerebral Cortex: Frontal, Parietal, Occipital, and Temporal Pain, along with touch and temperature are perceived in the somatosensory cortexes, which lie in the parietal lobes (see **Figure 6.4**).

cerebral cortex The thin, outer layer of the brain responsible for higher mental functions, such as thinking, perception, use of language, and problem solving.

frontal lobe The executive center of the brain, involved in thinking, planning, decision making, production of speech, and voluntary motor control.

occipital lobe The lobe at the back of the brain, involved in visual processing.

temporal lobe The lobe on the side of the brain, involved in hearing, language comprehension, and memory.

parietal lobe A part of the cerebral cortex that processes sensory information from various parts of the body.

lobes, each of which has distinctive functions: **frontal lobe** (thinking, calculating, planning, language functions, and body movement), **occipital lobe** (visual processing), **temporal lobe** (auditory processing), and **parietal lobe** (processing of sensory information from the skin senses and body awareness) (see **Figure 6.3**). The part of the cortex that processes pain signals and produces sensations of pain is the **somatosensory cortex**, an area in the parietal lobe that also processes signals for warmth, cold, touch, and pressure, as well as input from other parts of the body (see **Figure 6.4**).

Pain receptors are located not just in the skin but also throughout the body, in muscles, joints, ligaments, even the pulp of the teeth, which is the source of tooth pain. These sensors allow us to feel pain in most parts of the body. An exception is the brain, which contains no pain receptors, so it is possible to cut into brain tissue without anesthesia. Pain can be especially intense where nerve endings are closely bunched together, as in the fingers and the face, where any slight injury to the skin can be acutely felt.

Pain is a bodily signal that is hard to ignore, as it instantly draws your attention to the site of an injury that requires immediate attention. But pain normally shuts down once the message is received and the injury heals. For a minor injury like a stubbed toe, pain may cease within a matter of minutes, but for more serious injuries, it can continue for weeks or months as the healing process resolves.

Even before the affected area heals, the brain begins to turn off pain signals. It releases **endorphins**, the body's natural painkillers. Endorphins are **neurotransmitters** that block pain signals from getting through the spinal cord, blunting or deadening feelings of pain.

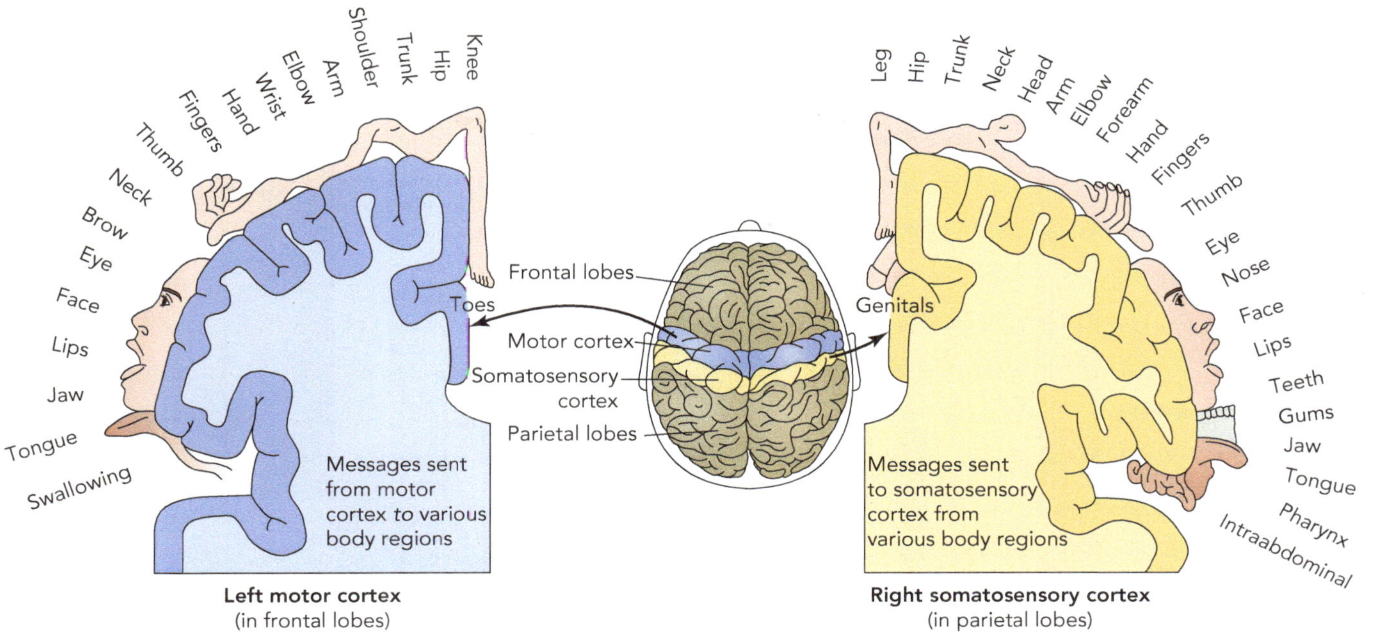

a. Note how larger areas of the *motor cortex* are devoted to body parts that need to be controlled with great precision, such as the hands, face, and tongue.

b. Similar areas of the *somatosensory cortex* are also disproportionately large because these body parts contain a high number of sensory receptors, which makes them particularly sensitive.

FIGURE 6.4 A Cross Section of the Somatosensory Cortex Pain signals, as well as other signals from sensory receptors in the skin, are processed in the somatosensory cortex, which is located in the parietal lobe of the cerebral cortex. The amount of "space" devoted to the face, hands and fingers, and genitals reflect the fact that these body areas contain many more receptors for pain (and other sensations) than do, for example, the legs. Therefore, these parts of the body are more sensitive to pain.

somatosensory cortex A part of the parietal lobe of the cerebral cortex that processes sensory information from the body.

endorphins Neurotransmitters produced in the brain that have pain-killing and pleasure-inducing effects.

Neurotransmitters are chemical messengers in the nervous system that ferry nerve impulses (messages or signals) from one nerve cell or neuron to another.

Before we consider the role of endorphins in pain relief, we review the functions of the **neuron**, or nerve cell, the basic unit in the nervous system. The nervous system is the body's communication network for transmitting sensory information from sensory receptors throughout the body to the brain for processing, which allows us to experience the world around us through the senses of vision, hearing, smell, taste, touch, and so on. The nervous system also carries commands from the brain to the muscles that control movement and to internal bodily organs, such as the pancreas, liver, and various glands. Some neurons control heart rate; others send commands to the liver to increase the secretion of glucose (blood sugar) in times of stress. Neurons in the brain allow us to think, solve problems, and use language.

The structure of the neuron is shown in **Figure 6.5**. The cell body, or **soma**, houses the genetic material of the cell and performs the cell's metabolic functions. Messages from other neurons and from external sources of stimulation (such as sound or light) are received by **dendrites** and then transmitted along a trunk-like structure called an **axon**, at the end of which are **terminal buttons** that hold neurotransmitters. Neurotransmitters are chemical messengers that carry the signal or message to the next neuron across a tiny gap, or **synapse**, that separates each neuron from another (see **Figure 6.6**).

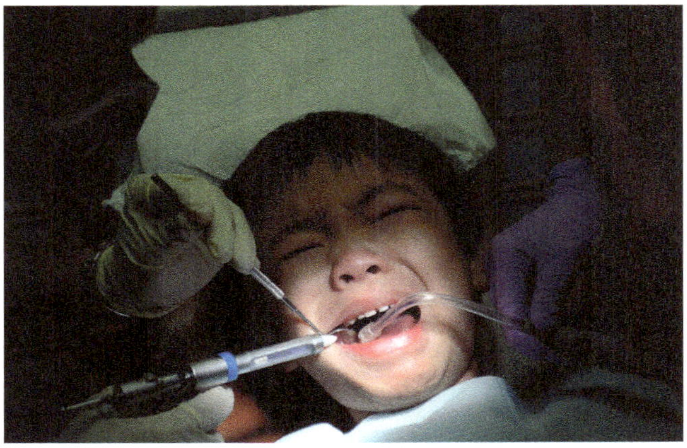

Kong Hon Loh/Alamy Stock Photo

Ouch! The injection provides some sharp pain, for a moment. However, is the boy making things worse for himself by telling himself that he is trapped in the seat and that the situation is awful? Is he remembering that the reason for the dental intervention is a cavity that has been plaguing him for weeks? Pain begins with biological stimulation, but our appraisal of the pain can amplify what we feel or tamp it down. Question: Why do many dentists offer earphones and ask you what type of music you would like to listen to?

neurotransmitters Chemical substances in the body that carry nerve signals from one neuron or nerve cell to another.

neuron Nerve cell, the basic unit of the nervous system.

soma The cell body that houses the nucleus containing the cell's genes and that performs the cell's metabolic functions.

dendrites Branch-like structures on the surface of the neuron that receive messages from transmitting neurons.

axon A tubelike structure along the cell membrane that transmits messages in electrochemical form down the length of the neuron.

terminal buttons The swellings at the ends of axons from which neurotransmitters are released into the synapse.

synapse A tiny, fluid-filled space between neurons. Also called the synaptic cleft.

receptor sites Structures on a receiving neuron where neurotransmitters dock (also called receptors).

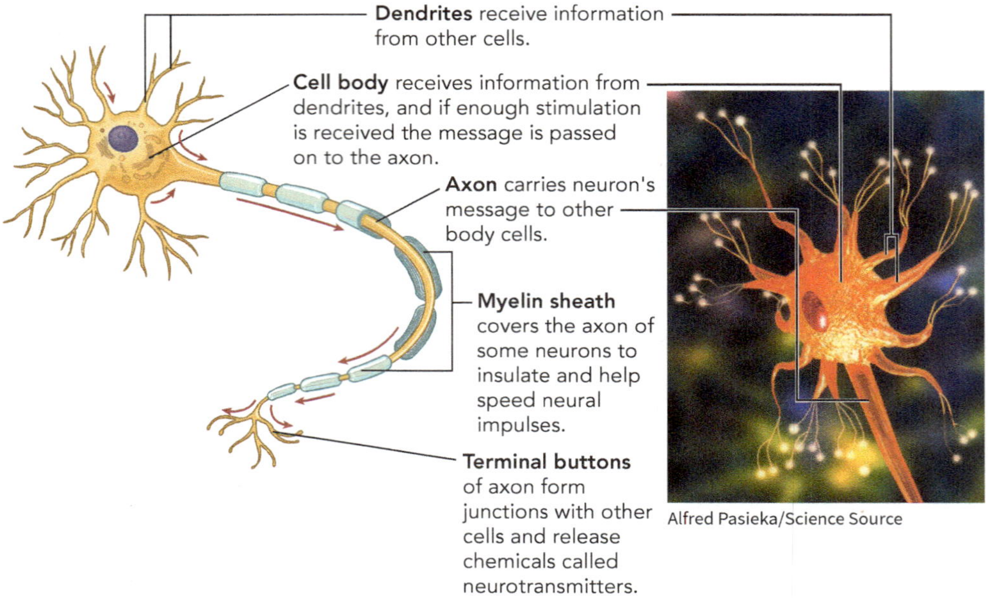

Alfred Pasieka/Science Source

FIGURE 6.5 Anatomy of a Neuron "Messages" enter neurons through dendrites, are transmitted along the trunk-like axon, and then are transmitted by axon terminal buttons to muscles, glands, and other neurons.

Neurotransmitter molecules dock at **receptor sites** (receptors) on receiving (post-synaptic) neurons, so that messages can be transmitted from one neuron to another neuron. Which brings us back to endorphins, which are types of neurotransmitters that play an important role in regulating sensations of pain and pleasure. (We'll encounter other neurotransmitters in later chapters.)

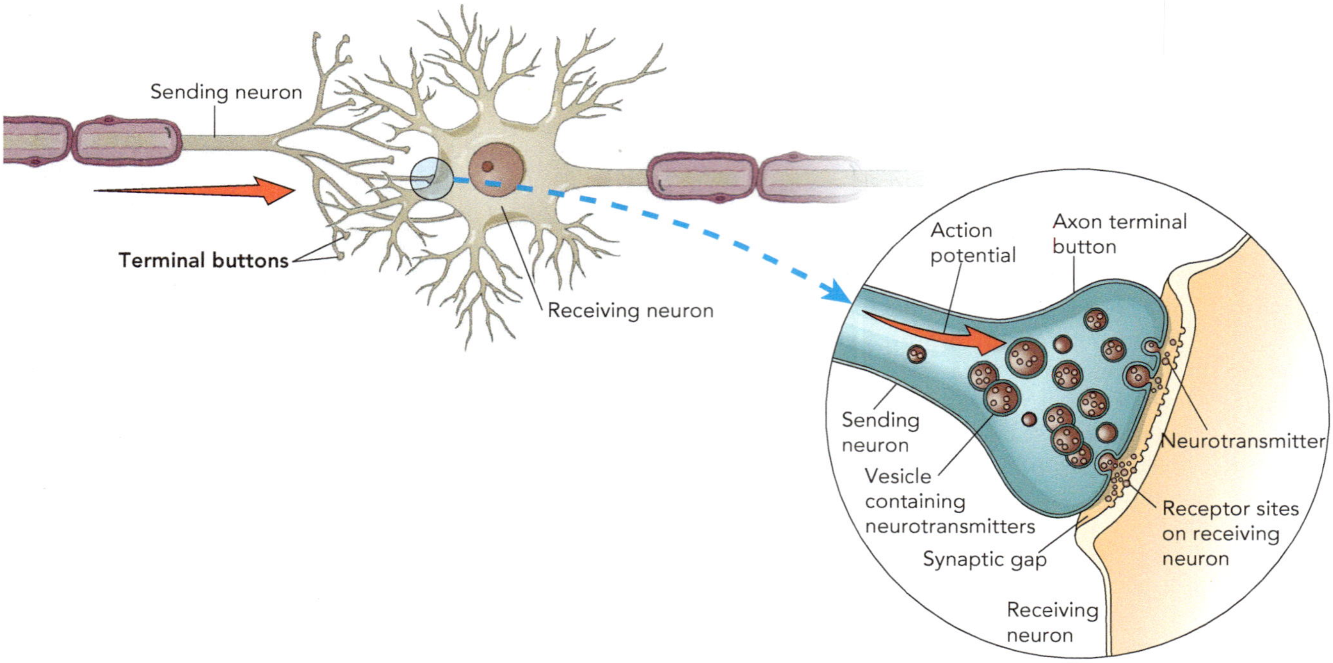

FIGURE 6.6 Closeup of an Axon Terminal Button, Synapse, and Receptor Sites on a Receiving Neuron Axon terminal buttons contain sacs of chemicals called neurotransmitters. Neurotransmitters are released into the synaptic cleft or gap, where many of them bind to receptor sites on the dendrites of the receiving neurons.

The word "endorphin" is a contraction of the words "endogenous" (meaning "coming from within") and "morphine" (a narcotic drug that deadens pain). Endorphins are similar in chemical structure to narcotic drugs like morphine and heroin that have pain-killing effects. Like these drugs, endorphins deaden pain by locking into receptor sites in the spinal cord that carry pain messages to the brain, thereby preventing pain messages from reaching the brain. Once the endorphin "key" is in the "lock," neurotransmitters that carry pain signals are prevented ("locked out") from transmitting pain messages. So if you stub your toe but the pain disappears after a few minutes, you can thank your brain for releasing endorphins.

Sources of Chronic Pain

Chronic pain is usually defined as pain lasting for more than 3 months (Murphy, Jackson, & Mishra, 2022). There are many sources of chronic pain, including the following: nagging back problems; migraines: pain in the joints connecting the jaw to the skull (temporomandibular pain); postsurgical pain; neurogenic or nerve pain; pain due to serious infection or illness, such as cancer, arthritis, and gastrointestinal disorders; injuries; and pain due to psychogenic (psychological) sources.

The most prevalent form of chronic pain is **musculoskeletal pain (MSP)**, which involves pain in the muscles, bones, ligaments, tendons, and nerves (Bonanni et al., 2022; van Dijk et al., 2023). MSP may be experienced in only one part of the body, such as the lower back, hips, or knees, or it may be widespread, as in fibromyalgia, a pain syndrome affecting muscles and soft tissues. People with fibromyalgia may look healthy, which may mislead others to question the severity and seriousness of their symptoms (Turk, 2018b).

musculoskeletal pain (MSP) Pain in the muscles, bones, ligaments, tendons, and nerves.

MSP typically lasts months or even years and is among the leading reasons for doctors' visits, days missed from work, and reduced quality of life. The most common type of MSP is back pain, especially lower back pain. Back pain affects more than 50% of adults in the United States each year and upward of 80% of adults during the course of their lifetime (Balderson et al., 2018).

Health Psychology in Action

Phantom Limb Pain—When What Hurts Isn't There

Some people detect sensations "from" missing limbs that have been amputated. Some of these sensations are of pain. As many as 80% of people with amputations report feeling tickling, itching, burning, or other symptoms of pain in the missing limb. There is clearly a mismatch between the physical reality of the body and what is experienced in the brain (Fan et al., 2016; Limakatso et al., 2019).

How can this happen? Normally, parts of the body that are in pain transmit sensory messages of pain to the somatosensory cortex, where it is perceived as pain. This messaging from the periphery of the body is no longer happening, but the part of the body that has been amputated is still represented in the brain. It appears that when the person with the missing limb sees what appears to be the amputated limb, that psychological event triggers neural activity in the part of the cortex that did experience sensations from the limb. It is then that the activity of these neurons results in the sensations of tickling and so on.

When people wear prosthetic limbs, phantom pain often subsides. Mirror visual therapy also affords relief from pain. Both methods appear to persuade the brain that there is no longer a missing limb (Thieme et al., 2016; Villa-Alcazar et al., 2019). The nervous system may in effect act as follows (Guo et al., 2016): The illusion of an intact limb is transmitted to the brain, in effect tricking the brain to function as though amputation has not happened. The person moves the remaining limb gently for several minutes a day. Sometimes the pain is not completely removed, but it is usually significantly reduced.

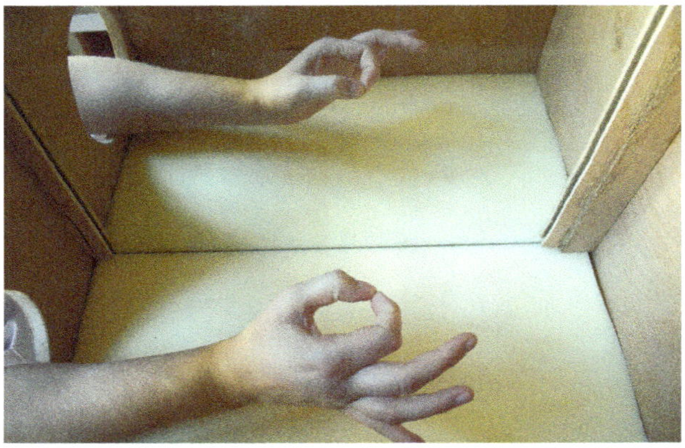

Media for Medical SARL/Alamy Stock Photo

Mirror Therapy for Phantom Limb Pain This method employs a mirror box or the positioning of a mirror across the midline of the body; in either case, the amputation site is hidden.

central pain syndrome (CPS) A neurological disorder involving damage or dysfunction of the central nervous system.

Central pain syndrome (CPS) involves a defect or dysfunction of the pain pathways in the central nervous system (brain and spinal cord) (Fink, 2019). CPS is often associated with stroke, multiple sclerosis, tumors, spinal cord injury, or Parkinson's disease. Typically, the pain in CPS is constant and falls within a moderate to severe range of intensity. Because the underlying cause of CPS differs among patients, the nature and severity of the pain also varies from person to person. Unfortunately, CPS is often difficult to treat, with the method of treatment depending on the specific cause of the condition.

rheumatoid arthritis (RA) A chronic inflammatory disease of the lining of the joints, causing pain, stiffness, and swelling and possible loss of function of the joints.

osteoarthritis (OA) A chronic degenerative disease of the joints, producing pain and restricting movement.

Arthritic diseases are also major causes of pain. There are two major forms of arthritic disease, **rheumatoid arthritis (RA)** and **osteoarthritis (OA)**. In RA, the disease predominantly involves inflammation of joints, leading to pain and destruction of cartilage and bone, which can result in disability if the deterioration is not controlled. OA, in contrast, is largely a degenerative process. For both types of arthritic disease, psychosocial approaches are important to help people function and manage their disease more effectively.

Who Hurts? Chronic Pain in America?

More than one in five American adults, more than 50 million people in total, suffer from chronic pain either most days or every day (Yong, Mullins, & Bhattacharyya, 2021). About 20 million U.S. adults experience pain severe enough to interfere with their daily functioning. Chronic pain also imposes significant economic costs to the nation, with estimates exceeding $600 billion annually with respect to costs for medical treatment and time lost from productive work (Castelnuovo & Schreurs, 2019; NCCIH, 2018).

Chronic pain is not limited to any particular group or age range, although it is more common among women and older adults (Bonanni et al., 2022). It is also more prevalent among people living in poverty, among adults with less than a high school education, and among adults who rely on public health insurance (Dahlhamer et al., 2018). Taking these factors into account can help health officials identify populations likely to be most in need of services providing pain management.

Racial and Ethnic Disparities in Chronic Pain

Who's in pain? Health researchers draw attention to disparities in the prevalence of pain among different racial and ethnic groups in our society. As shown in **Figure 6.7**, rates of chronic pain are highest among White (European) Americans. However, Black and Latino/Hispanic people over the age of 50 are more likely to have severe pain most of the time than are White Americans (Reyes-Gibby et al., 2007). These disparities may reflect the fact that White Americans tend to receive better-quality pain treatment than Black and Latino/Hispanic people (Wyatt, 2013).

biomedical model A traditional conception of disease as explained by disease processes.

Differences also exist in sensitivity to pain across groups, with lower thresholds for pain and pain tolerance reported among Black people than White people (Tait & Chibnall, 2014). Understanding racial and ethnic differences in the ways in which groups process pain may help treatment providers tailor treatment to members of particular groups. At the same time, we need to address disparities among racial or ethnic groups in their access to quality health care for pain management.

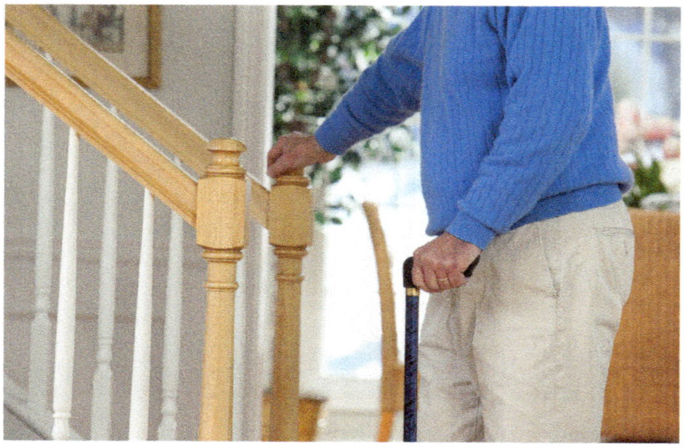

Huntstock/Getty Images

Chronic Pain It is estimated that more than 50 million U.S. adults live with chronic pain. What are the sex, age, racial/ethnic, and educational differences among people with pain?

The Biopsychosocial Model of Pain

Let's begin with a little historical context. The traditional model of pain, called the **biomedical model**, focused on the biological bases of pain (Salas et al., 2018; Turk & Murphy, 2019). In this view, pain is a symptom of an underlying disease, injury, or defect, and efforts to relieve pain take the form of medical interventions to treat or remediate the underlying medical condition and manage pain through medicine or other biomedical approaches.

This traditional model of pain adopted the mind–body dualism of Descartes (see Chapter 1), in which symptoms were considered either somatic (biological) or psychogenic

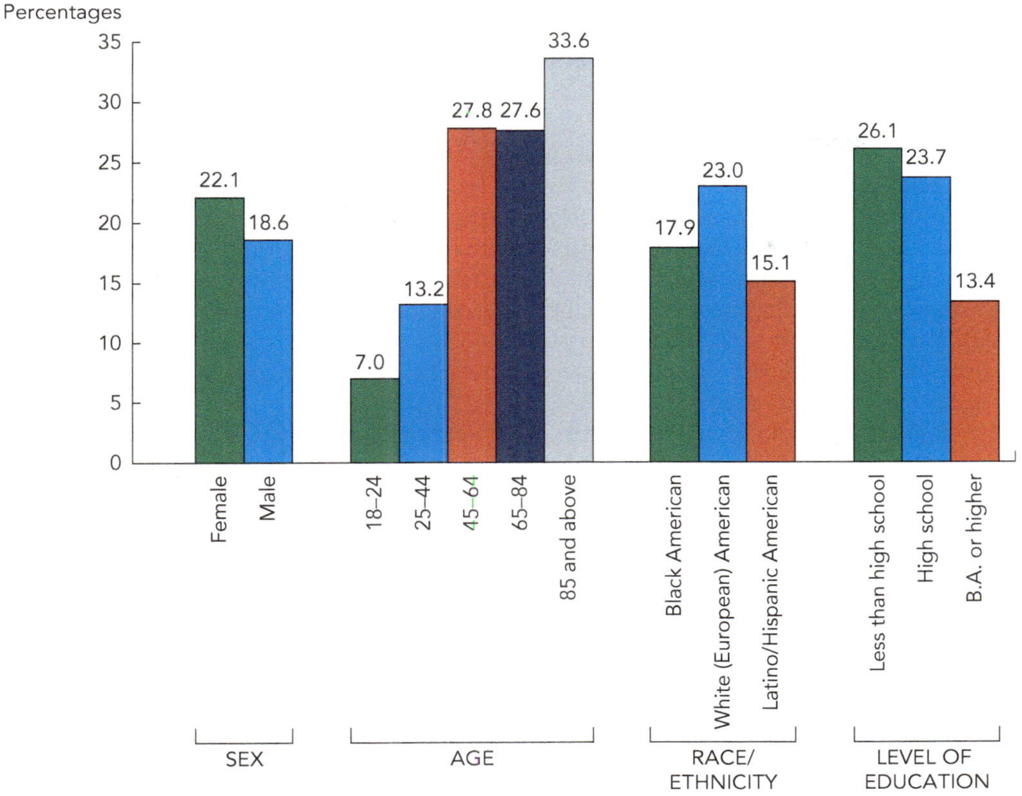

FIGURE 6.7 **Disparities Among People in Chronic Pain** Chronic pain is more common in women than men, among older people, among White (European) Americans, and among people with less education.

Source: J. Dahlhamer et al., 2016 J. Dahlhamer, J. Lucas, C. Zelaya, R. Nahin, S., Mackey, L. DeBar, L., ... C. Helmick. (2018). Prevalence of chronic pain and high-impact chronic pain among adults—United States, 2016. Morbidity and Mortality Weekly Report, 67(36), 1001–1006./U.S. Department of Health & Human Services / Public Domain.

(psychological) in origin (Turk & Gatchel, 2018). Physical pain was considered to be distinct from psychological or psychogenic pain, which was attributed to psychological factors, such as emotional trauma. Today, most clinicians recognize that pain cannot be easily broken down into psychological and physical components and that we need to take a more integrative view of pain that incorporates roles for biological, psychological, and social factors and their interactions (Lazaridou & Edwards, 2019; Salas et al., 2018). This conceptual framework, called the *biopsychosocial model* (see Chapter 1), is now the most widely accepted model for understanding and treating pain (Mescouto et al., 2022; Nicholas, 2022; Penlington, Urbanek, & Barker, 2022; Rosignoli et al., 2022).

Not only has our conceptual understanding of pain expanded to include a wider range of factors, but evidence shows that pain management is more effective when clinicians adopt a comprehensive, interdisciplinary approach based on the biopsychosocial model (Ray et al., 2018). This comprehensive treatment model includes both medical and behavioral interventions (Schütze et al., 2017). Psychological factors play a major role in how people cope with pain. For example, the availability of social support, of people showing concern and lending a helping hand, can help blunt the psychological effects of enduring pain. Treating chronic back pain often involves use of psychological techniques, such as relaxation training, mindfulness training, attentional distraction, and cognitive-behavioral therapy, along with physical therapy and other biomedical approaches (Burns et al., 2022; Ho et al., 2022).

Managing pain involves more than treating a physical symptom. Health professionals also need to focus on behavioral factors, such as the role of stress in the experience of pain and the role that pain-related behaviors play in a person's experience of pain, such as preoccupation with pain and avoidance of work and activities of daily living (Lumley & Schubiner, 2019; Turk & Gatchel, 2018). These approaches seek to improve the quality of life of people with pain, to reduce the fear of movement that can lead to withdrawal from life activities, and to help people learn coping skills to manage pain (Padovan et al., 2018).

gate control theory A conceptual model of pain that holds that a neural gate in the spinal cord opens to allow pain messages to reach the brain or closes to shut them out.

The Gate Control Theory of Pain

An example of a biopsychosocial approach to understanding pain is the **gate control theory** developed by psychologist Ronald Melzack and biologist Patrick Wall (1965, 1983). The theory holds that there is a gating mechanism in the spinal cord that opens to let pain signals pass through to the brain or closes to block them out. The "gate" is not a physical structure in the spinal cord but rather a neural mechanism for facilitating or blocking the flow of pain signals. People who have never heard of the gate control theory nonetheless apply it intuitively for temporary relief from pain. If you had a bruise or a strained ankle or knee, perhaps you found that gently rubbing or massaging the area, or applying an ice pack, provided some relief. Ice packs minimize swelling, reduce bleeding into the tissues surrounding the wound (i.e., bruising), and reduce muscle spasms. But these methods also provide competing sources of stimulation to the affected area, which sends nerve signals to the spinal cord that can create a "bottleneck" at the pain gate, blocking some pain signals from reaching the brain.

If you feel pain in a toe, for example, try squeezing all your toes. When you feel pain in your calf, rub your thighs. People around you may wonder what you're doing, but you're entitled to try to "flood the switchboard" so that some pain messages don't get through. But for sudden or persistent pain, see a healthcare professional. Again, pain is a sign that something is wrong, and it may require medical attention.

Neural impulses that code for throbbing or dull pain are carried by thinner and slower nerve fibers than those that carry sensory signals for warmth, cold, and touch. Therefore, gently rubbing the area, or applying ice to it, transmits signals to the spinal cord through thinner, faster nerve fibers, essentially competing for the same space as pain messages, temporarily blocking out signals that carry dull, throbbing pain messages (see **Figure 6.8**). Applying an ice pack to the injured areas transmits cold signals, helping create a bottleneck at the pain gate that may block some pain messages from reaching the brain. But sharp pain, the type of pain associated with cutting your finger or stubbing your toe, is carried along thicker, faster nerve pathways that take precedence in passing through the gate, which means you can't block the painful sensations they cause. Which, after all, is a good thing, as these signals quickly register in the brain, alerting you instantly to an injury that requires your immediate attention.

The nervous system is a marvel of engineering. We withdraw our hand from a hot object before we think about it. Then, when we experience the first pangs of pain, we are alerted to a source of danger to our health or survival. Then, by releasing endorphins, the brain tries to gradually shut the gate on pain. But in some injuries and chronic diseases, endorphins are not enough to shut the gate.

The gate control theory also recognizes the importance of psychosocial factors in modulating the experience of pain (Labott, 2018; Turk & Murphy, 2019). Anxiety or depression can exacerbate pain by, in effect, keeping the pain gate open long after the warning signal of pain has been processed by the brain. When we are depressed or anxious, we may believe we lack control over our life situations and avoid making active efforts to cope effectively with pain. We may withdraw from others

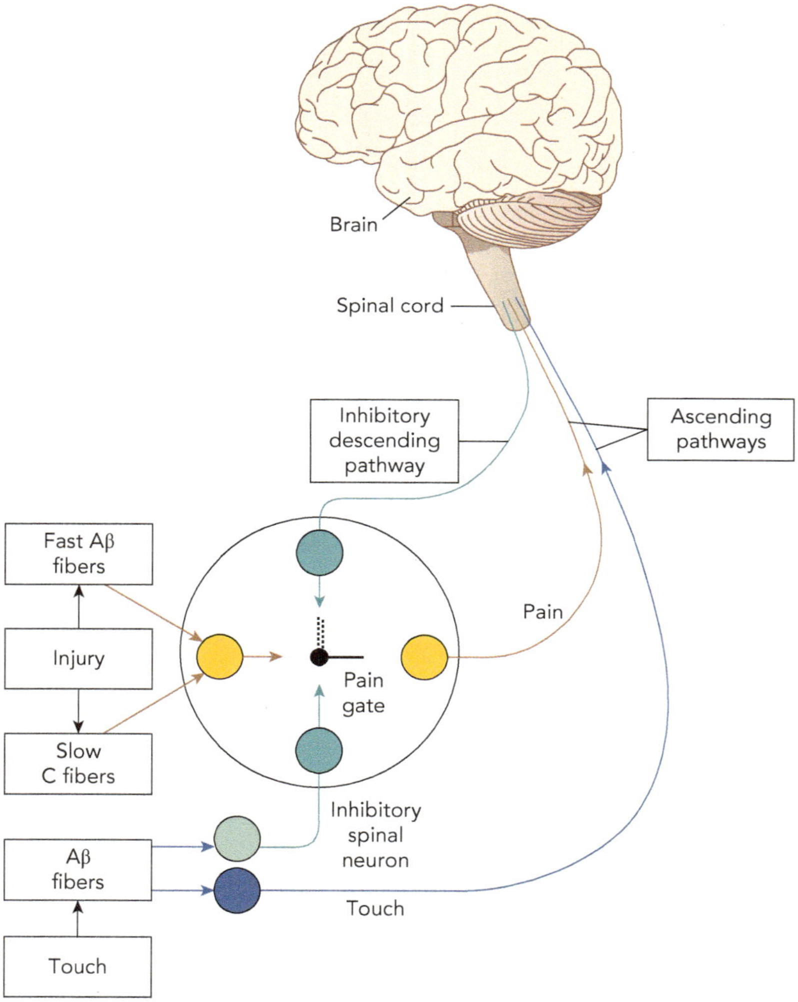

FIGURE 6.8 The Gate Control Theory of Pain Touching or gently rubbing an injured area sends relatively rapid signals up to the brain, whereas many sources of pain, especially dull or throbbing pain, use slower pathways. The brain may respond to the rapidly transmitted signals by sending inhibitory impulses down through the spinal cord to "shut the gate" on pain—or at least to "lean" against the gate.

and from daily activities, which may exacerbate pain by leading us to become preoccupied with it. Conversely, active coping responses can take our mind off the pain, as when we engage in distracting tasks, physical activities, or relaxation exercises. Practicing positive thoughts, such as reassuring ourselves that the pain will get better over time, can also help by creating more hopeful expectations.

Assessing Pain

Pain is a subjective experience, so we do not have precise objective standards of measurement. To know if you're in pain, you need to tell healthcare providers. The providers might ask you to rate your level of pain, such as by using a 10-point rating scale with (0) meaning "no pain at all" to (10) meaning "worst possible pain" (see **Figure 6.9**). Healthcare providers might also ask you to identify the location of the pain in your body or use a rating scale to distinguish between different types of pain, such as throbbing pain vs. shooting pain.

Of course, self-ratings of pain are limited by the fact that that one person's ratings may not reflect the same intensity of pain as those of another person who gives the same rating. In other words, Ayanna's rating of her pain as a "4" on a 10-point scale may not be equal in intensity to Mateo's "4" rating, as the felt experience of pain is ultimately subjective. Yet healthcare professionals and researchers need some way of measuring pain in order to track the intensity of people's symptoms over time and evaluate the efficacy of pain interventions. Comparing the same person's ratings of pain at different points in time provides a basis for knowing whether pain is changing over time for that individual.

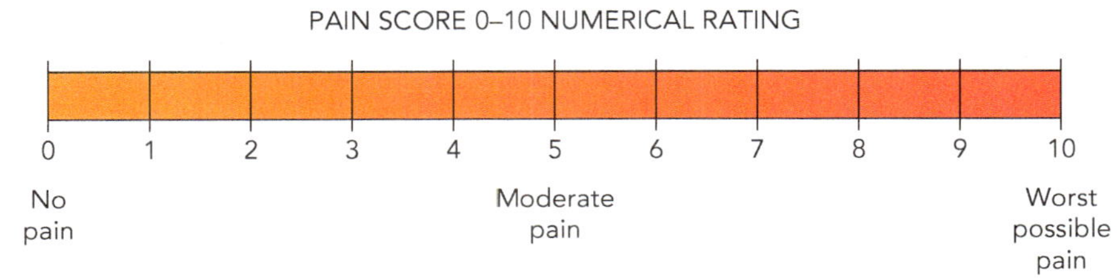

FIGURE 6.9 **Pain Intensity Ratings** Ten-point rating scales are often used to obtain subjective ratings from people in pain of the intensity of pain. Multiple ratings over time can give the healthcare provider—and the person—a sense of whether progress is being made.

Source: From Capitol Rehab of Arlington: https://capitolrehabofarlington.com/2015/12/why-doctors-ask-you-to-rank-how-you-feel-on-a-pain-scale/

Review 6.1

INTERACTIVE SELF-SCORING QUIZZES

Sentence Completion

1. Pain receptors are located throughout the body, including the __________ and internal organs.
2. More Americans live with __________ pain than with diabetes, heart disease, and cancer combined.
3. Pain receptors are called __________.
4. Pain signals are processed in the __________ cortex, an area in the parietal lobe of the cerebral cortex.
5. __________ are neurotransmitters that block pain signals.
6. The most prevalent form of chronic pain is __________ pain.
7. An estimated one in (two or five) adult Americans lives with chronic pain.
8. Chronic pain is (more or less) prevalent among people living in poverty.
9. The __________ model is now the most widely accepted conceptual model for understanding and treating chronic pain.
10. Neural impulses that code for throbbing or dull pain are carried by (thinner and slower, or thicker and faster) nerve fibers than those carrying sensory signals for warmth, cold, and touch.

Think About It

Why is it a misconception to think of pain as necessarily a bad thing?

Self-Assessment

INTERACTIVE SELF-ASSESSMENTS

The Short-Form McGill Pain Questionnaire

One commonly used standardized measure of pain is the McGill Pain Questionnaire, a short version of which is shown here. Using this scale, clinicians can evaluate the type of reported pain (e.g., throbbing, sharp, hot-burning, etc.) and the level of intensity of each type. The scale is widely used in evaluating patients' reports of pain following surgery or physical injury.

This questionnaire provides a list of words that describe some of the different qualities of pain and related symptoms. To complete the questionnaire, put an X through the numbers that best describe the intensity of each of the pain and related symptoms you felt during the last week. Use the 0 if the word does not describe your pain or related symptoms.

1. Throbbing pain	*none*	0	1	2	3	4	5	6	7	8	9	10	*worst possible*
2. Shooting pain	*none*	0	1	2	3	4	5	6	7	8	9	10	*worst possible*
3. Stabbing pain	*none*	0	1	2	3	4	5	6	7	8	9	10	*worst possible*
4. Sharp pain	*none*	0	1	2	3	4	5	6	7	8	9	10	*worst possible*
5. Cramping pain	*none*	0	1	2	3	4	5	6	7	8	9	10	*worst possible*
6. Gnawing pain	*none*	0	1	2	3	4	5	6	7	8	9	10	*worst possible*
7. Hot-burning pain	*none*	0	1	2	3	4	5	6	7	8	9	10	*worst possible*
8. Aching pain	*none*	0	1	2	3	4	5	6	7	8	9	10	*worst possible*
9. Heavy pain	*none*	0	1	2	3	4	5	6	7	8	9	10	*worst possible*
10. Tender	*none*	0	1	2	3	4	5	6	7	8	9	10	*worst possible*
11. Splitting pain	*none*	0	1	2	3	4	5	6	7	8	9	10	*worst possible*
12. Tiring-exhausting	*none*	0	1	2	3	4	5	6	7	8	9	10	*worst possible*
13. Sickening	*none*	0	1	2	3	4	5	6	7	8	9	10	*worst possible*
14. Fearful	*none*	0	1	2	3	4	5	6	7	8	9	10	*worst possible*
15. Punishing-cruel	*none*	0	1	2	3	4	5	6	7	8	9	10	*worst possible*
16. Electric-shock pain	*none*	0	1	2	3	4	5	6	7	8	9	10	*worst possible*
17. Cold-freezing pain	*none*	0	1	2	3	4	5	6	7	8	9	10	*worst possible*
18. Piercing	*none*	0	1	2	3	4	5	6	7	8	9	10	*worst possible*
19. Pain caused by light touch	*none*	0	1	2	3	4	5	6	7	8	9	10	*worst possible*
20. Itching	*none*	0	1	2	3	4	5	6	7	8	9	10	*worst possible*
21. Tingling or 'pins and needles'	*none*	0	1	2	3	4	5	6	7	8	9	10	*worst possible*
22. Numbness	*none*	0	1	2	3	4	5	6	7	8	9	10	*worst possible*

Source: R. H. Dworkin, D. C. Turk, D. A. Revicki, G. Harding, K. S. Coyne, S. PeirceSandner, S., ... R. Melzack (2009). Pain, 144, 35–42. http://www.westicu.cn:8880/ UpFile/201406/2014062643591953.pdf./with permission of International Association for the Study of Pain (IASP).

Psychosocial Factors in Chronic Pain

The biopsychosocial model recognizes that chronic pain impacts many aspects of daily life, affecting psychological, physical, social, and occupational functioning (Portenoy & Dhingra, 2017). Pain can interfere with sleep, make it difficult to function at school or on the job, reduce the quality of life, even sap the will to live. About 9% of recorded suicides occur among people in chronic pain (Petrosky et al., 2018; Roy-Byrne, 2018). People with chronic pain also show high rates of psychological disorders, principally major depression, panic disorder, and generalized anxiety disorder (Bamonti et al., 2018; Salas et al., 2018).

Psychological factors play a significant role in how a person copes with chronic pain and determining whether pain turns into a disabling condition (Hruschaka & Cochran, 2018; Labott, 2018; Linton, 2018; Turk & Gatchel, 2018). Ronald Melzack (1999a) notes that believing there is nothing we can do to handle pain can increase our perception of its intensity. But if we are confident in our ability to manage stress, including the stress of chronic pain, perceptions of pain may diminish.

People living with chronic pain may become fearful of what the pain means and what it portends for the future. Fear and anxiety about the meaning of the pain and its future course can increase sensitivity to pain signals, which may in turn exacerbate the felt experience of pain. People in pain may also become demoralized or depressed as pain drags on, especially if they feel they lack control over the pain or believe it will never end, which can dampen their motivation to take a more active role in managing their pain. Depression and feelings of helplessness may further weaken their motivation. The double burden of pain and depression may lead people with pain to withdraw from their usual life activities, even if they are encouraged by their healthcare providers to remain as active as possible. They can wind up spending much of their time preoccupied with their pain, which sets the stage for pain to become a disabling condition.

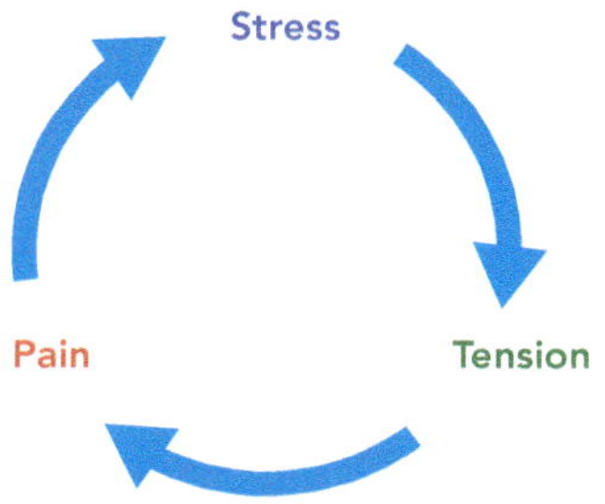

FIGURE 6.10 The Stress–Pain Cycle In a vicious cycle, pain causes stress and tension, which, in turn, can exacerbate the experience of pain.

Source: Adapted from Mayer and Gatchel (1988).

Stress and Pain

Stress can be both a trigger of pain and a consequence of pain. Pain may intensify when stress increases, as during times of financial hardship or when coping with the loss of a family member (Rios & Zautra, 2011). Pain itself is a source of stress that exacts a significant toll on our ability to meet our daily responsibilities. Pain can become a constant source of worry, concern, and preoccupation, overtaxing one's ability to cope and just get through the day.

When we are under significant stress, we may contract the muscles in our shoulders, neck, forehead, and scalp, creating musculoskeletal tension that can result in headache pain or worsen an existing headache (see **Figure 6.10**). One common type of pain aggravated by stress is the *muscle-tension headache*, the most frequent kind of headache. Tension headaches usually develop gradually, as the muscles in the head and neck tighten or contract. These headaches are associated with a dull, steady pain on both sides of the head with feelings of tightness or viselike pressure throughout the head.

Cognitive Appraisal of Pain

As noted in Chapter 5, the Lazarus and Folkman (1984) model of coping with stress holds that in response to stress, people form an appraisal (an evaluation or judgment) of the source of the stress, such as persistent pain. Their appraisal of the stressor then determines which, if any, coping responses they employ. For example, if a person appraises pain as a looming catastrophe over which they have no control, they will likely experience significant emotional distress, which may intensify their feelings of pain and reduce their ability to cope with it (Burston et al., 2019; Slawek et al., 2022). Pain catastrophizing is found in upwards of 30% of patients with chronic pain (Slawek et al., 2022).

Maladaptive coping approaches can lead to demoralization, passivity, inactivity, and preoccupation with painful sensations (Turk & Gatchel, 2018). People who catastrophize pain tend to report more intense pain, have more pain-related disability and higher rates of anxiety and depression, are at increased risk of suicide, and show a poorer response to medical treatment (e.g., Schütze et al., 2017; Slawek et al., 2022). By appraising the pain as a manageable problem, however, the person is more likely to seek ways of coping with it, such as finding ways to remove the pain or, if the pain cannot be completely eliminated, practicing emotion-focused coping methods, such as meditation, or engaging in distracting activities.

Believing that nagging pain is a sign of a deteriorating physical problem rather than a stable problem that might improve in the future can (Turk & Gatchel, 2018):

- Increase the intensity of pain,
- Increase preoccupation with the source of pain and what it means,

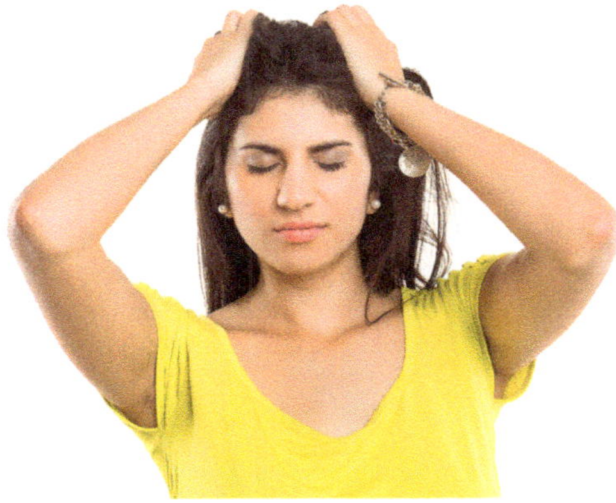

Hugo Felix/Alamy Stock Photo

Muscle-Tension Headache When we are under stress, we tend to contract the muscles in our shoulders, neck, forehead, and scalp—responses that can lead to the development of a muscle-tension headache. Therapies that help us relax are muscles, such as biofeedback, relaxation training, and visualization of calming scenes, may help relieve the pain associated with this type of headache.

- Restrict daily activities, and
- Reduce efforts to use active coping strategies for managing pain.

Social cognitive theory posits that a cognitive factor closely related to one's level of pain is self-efficacy. People who believe that they are powerless to make positive changes in their lives may become resigned to severe pain and fearful of what is to come. But people who believe in their ability to manage pain tend to report less pain intensity (Turk & Gatchel, 2018). Evidence also shows that boosting people's self-efficacy can reduce their feelings of pain (Gandy et al., 2018).

Another cognitive factor relating to the degree of pain is catastrophizing, which is a pattern of exaggerated, distorted thinking as represented in thoughts such as these:

"I can't stand this. I won't be able to live with this much longer."

"I can't stop thinking about the pain. I know it's only going to get worse."

"There's nothing I can do about this pain. It's just hopeless."

Fortunately, catastrophizing pain can often be treated successfully with cognitive-behavioral therapy (CBT), a form of therapy that helps people—including people suffering pain—to identify and correct distorted ways of thinking, as in the following case:

Carlos complained of excruciating facial pain that left him feeling terrified and helpless. He cared for a sick wife with multiple sclerosis and feared that the pain would prevent him from providing her with the care she needed. He also worried about whether anyone would care for him. When his pain became unbearable, he would go to the emergency room, where he would be prescribed opioid drugs. The opioids temporarily reduced the pain, but it would always return. Carlo began working with a health psychologist, who taught him about the negative effects of pain catastrophizing. He learned to identify his catastrophizing thoughts and used several cognitive behavioral techniques for managing pain, including distraction and correcting maladaptive beliefs. He learned to calm down his bodily arousal rather than ramping it up by focusing on worst-case scenarios. Instead, he focused on what could do to help himself and his wife.[1]

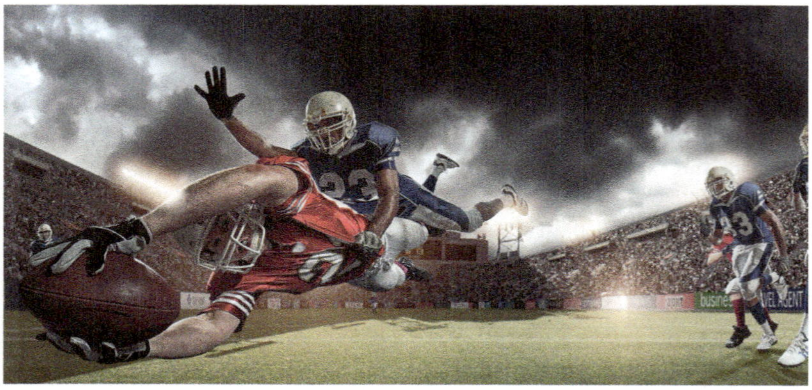
peepo/Getty Images

Crunch Professional athletes, especially those in hard contact sports, need to learn to cope with injuries suffered on the playing field. How does pain catastrophizing play a role in their ability to cope with nagging pain?

Professional athletes need to learn to cope with injuries sustained on the playing field and the resulting pain. Athletes who compete in hard contact sports like football are most at risk. A recent study focused a lens on pain catastrophizing in a group of 90 retired NFL players, who averaged 58 years of age at the time of the study (Mannes et al., 2020). Many of these ex-players continued to suffer from chronic pain for many years and even decades after their playing days were over. The health psychology researchers found that greater pain catastrophizing was linked to more severe pain intensity, more depression, greater interference of pain in daily life, and higher levels of opioid use, among other findings. These results suggest that healthcare professionals should pay close attention to pain catastrophizing in athletes, even well after their playing days are over, in order to help them cope with the long-term physical and emotional effects of chronic pain.

Sports Injuries

Professional athletes, especially those in hard contact sports, need to learn to cope with injuries suffered on the playing field. How does pain catastrophizing play a role in their ability to cope with nagging injuries?

[1] Adapted from Darnell (2019).

Self-Assessment

INTERACTIVE SELF-ASSESSMENTS

Pain Catastrophizing Scale

Do you catastrophize pain? The Pain Catastrophizing Scale assesses the types of thoughts and feelings that you have when you are in pain. Listed below are 13 statements describing different thoughts and feelings that may be associated with pain. Using the scale, please indicate the degree to which you have these thoughts and feelings when you are experiencing pain. Then consult the scoring key at the end of the chapter.

		Not at all	To a slight degree	To a moderate degree	To a great degree	All the time
1.	I worry all the time about whether the pain will end.	0	1	2	3	4
2.	I feel I can't go on.	0	1	2	3	4
3.	The pain is terrible and I think it's never going to get any better.	0	1	2	3	4
4.	The pain is awful and I feel that it overwhelms me.	0	1	2	3	4
5.	I feel I can't stand the pain anymore.	0	1	2	3	4
6.	I become afraid that the pain will get worse.	0	1	2	3	4
7.	I keep thinking of other painful events.	0	1	2	3	4
8.	I anxiously want the pain to go away.	0	1	2	3	4
9.	I can't see to keep thoughts of pain out of my mind.	0	1	2	3	4
10.	I keep thinking about how much I hurt.	0	1	2	3	4
11.	I keep thinking about how badly I want the pain to stop.	0	1	2	3	4
12.	There's nothing I can do to reduce the intensity of the pain	0	1	2	3	4
13.	I wonder whether something serious may happen.	0	1	2	3	4

Source: Adapted from M. J. L. Sullivan, S. R. Bishop, & J. Pivik (1995). The Pain Catastrophizing Scale: Development and validation. *Psychological Assessment*, *7*(4), 524–532. https://doi.org/10.1037/1040-3590.7.4.524

The Fear-Avoidance Model of Pain The **fear-avoidance model** of pain further explains how catastrophizing leads people with pain to engage in self-defeating behavior that decreases their ability to cope productively with pain (see **Figure 6.11**). For example, they may avoid physical activity from fear of reinjury or exacerbating the pain (Scott & McCracken, 2019). Avoidance, however, leads to inactivity, disability, and depression, which can intensify pain and create a vicious cycle in which fear of pain drives avoidance and avoidance leads to more pain (Markfelder & Paul, 2020).

fear-avoidance model A conceptual model of chronic pain that posits that fear of movement leads to avoidance of physical activity, which in turn leads to disability, depression, and more pain.

Anticipation of negative consequences about working while in pain is a major factor accounting for pain-related disability and loss of work (Gatchel et al., 2016). Over time, lack of physical activity may lead to loss of strength and flexibility, which can exacerbate the underlying condition causing the pain (Turk & Gatchel, 2018). Exaggerated misconceptions about the nature of chronic pain may lead a person with pain to think "I must avoid any activity to let my body heal and not aggravate the pain." Pain-related avoidance may generalize to other activities (Glogan, Liu, & Meulders, 2023). For example, someone suffering from pain resulting from an injury sustained on a treadmill may fear using a vacuum cleaner or walking in the neighborhood. You can appreciate how fear can spread to affect many aspects of our daily lives.

These beliefs run counter to the advice that people with pain are likely to receive from healthcare providers, who may advocate following a structured exercise program to strengthen muscles, improve flexibility, and promote cardiovascular fitness (Meade et al., 2019). To break the cycle, cognitive behavioral therapists help people cognitively restructure pain as a

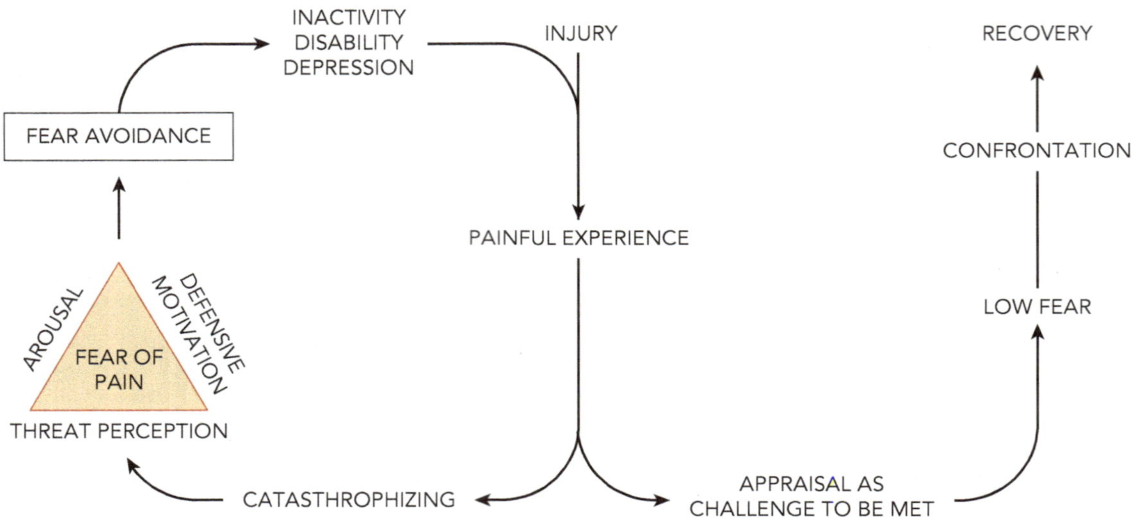

FIGURE 6.11 **The Fear-Avoidance Model** According to this model, a person's appraisal of a painful experience can lead to inactivity, disability, and depression or to recovery.

challenge that can be met rather than an impossible hurdle. They aim to help people reduce their fear and avoidance, enabling them to confront their pain and get on with their lives (Igwesi-Chidobe et al., 2020; Salas et al., 2018).

Family Factors

Family interactions also affect pain-related behavior. Family members may unintentionally reinforce pain-related behaviors of people living with chronic pain by releasing them from their usual household or childcare responsibilities (Tonkha et al., 2018; Turk & Gatchel, 2018). When people are reinforced for complaining about symptoms, they are encouraged to adopt a sick role, fostering inactivity and withdrawal from usual daily activities. A person may become preoccupied with the pain and what it means, increasing the likelihood of overemphasizing or misinterpreting pain symptoms and perceiving oneself as disabled (Turk, 2018).

When other family members chip in by assuming a greater share of household chores, the sick role of the person living with pain is reinforced. Health psychologists seek to change these reinforcement patterns. They assist family members to reinforce people for engaging in productive activities and adhering to medical advice (Balderson et al., 2018). Family members are usually well advised to use praise as a positive reinforcer when the person performs adaptive behaviors, such as smiling, exercising, and assuming family responsibilities (Sanders, 2018).

Successful rehabilitation is more likely to occur when people in pain believe in their ability to function despite their discomfort (Turk, 2018). Health psychologists play an important role in helping these people challenge self-defeating beliefs and replace them with more adaptive ways of thinking. Through these efforts, people living with pain come to recognize that even if they cannot be as helpful as they were before, there are still things they can do to assist others. Psychologists may work with the person and family members to identify small chores the person in pain can do to help around the house the best they can.

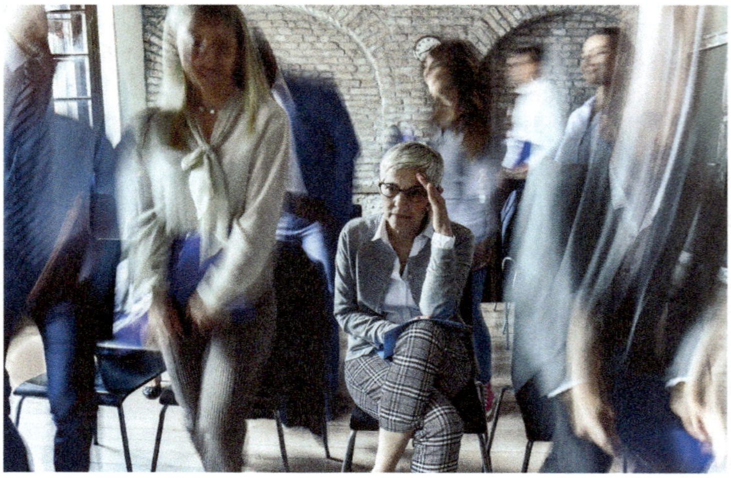

skyneshers/Getty Images

Will She or Won't She Join the Group? She's afraid that by pushing herself into physical and social activity, she may experience intense pain or reinjure herself. Her healthcare provider tells her that she needs to get out and do as much as she can rather than focus on her discomfort.

Review 6.2

INTERACTIVE SELF-SCORING QUIZZES

Sentence Completion

1. Psychologists help people living with chronic pain change ________-related beliefs and behaviors about daily activities.

2. Stress can be both a trigger for pain and a ________ of pain.

3. Tension headaches usually develop (quickly or gradually), as the muscles in the head and neck tighten or contract.

4. Boosting ________ often results in reduction of reported pain.

5. Family members in pain may be ________ for complaining about symptoms by garnering attention and support.

6. People living with pain are (more likely or less likely) to show improvement in managing pain if they remain actively engaged in their daily lives as much as possible.

Think About It

How does stress relate to pain? Do you experience pain more intensely when you are under a lot of stress? What role does controlling stress play in managing chronic pain?

Treating Chronic Pain

Treatment of chronic pain remains a major challenge to healthcare providers, especially in the aftermath of the nation's opioid epidemic (see the Closer Look feature). A range of biomedical, rehabilitation, and psychological service providers may be needed to help reduce pain and improve the ability to function of people with chronic pain.

Biomedical Treatments

Biomedical therapies are first-line treatments for pain. These treatments focus on providing relief from the physical symptoms of pain and on medical interventions, such as surgery, to treat the underlying cause.

Medicine Medical care specialists, such as doctors and nurses, use various types of pain medication to help relieve pain. The most commonly used medications are analgesic drugs, such as aspirin, acetaminophen, ibuprofen, and naproxen. These pain-relieving medications reduce inflammation and fever as well as pain. Several belong to a family of drugs called **nonsteroidal anti-inflammatory drugs (NSAIDs)** that vary in strength and are used to treat inflammatory conditions, such as arthritis. These medications also inhibit production of hormones called prostaglandins, which are involved in transmission of pain messages to the brain. Although they often help reduce or relieve pain, they are not always effective, and they also carry a risk of side effects, such as gastrointestinal problems. Stronger painkillers, including **opioids**, may be prescribed when nonaddictive analgesics such as ibuprofen and related drugs are unable to control pain effectively. The problem is that opioids are highly addictive and carry a high-risk potential for overdoses, which often have fatal consequences.

nonsteroidal anti-inflammatory drugs (NSAIDs) A class of pain-relieving and fever-reducing anti-inflammatory medications, including aspirin, acetaminophen, ibuprofen, and naproxen.

opioids A class of highly addictive narcotic drugs having pain-killing and pleasure-inducing effects.

When opioids are prescribed, they should be used for the shortest possible period of time and only if nonaddictive alternatives are not feasible. The CDC advises prescribing therapies other than opioids for the treatment of chronic pain (Dowell et al., 2016). Despite the guideline, statistics show that people who complain of musculoskeletal pain are often prescribed opioids, and more so than alternative treatment approaches, such as physical therapy and nonpharmacological approaches (NIH News Release, 2020). When opioids are used in treatment, the need for continuing opioid treatment should be evaluated periodically in light of the associated risks. The broadened conceptualization of pain represented in the biopsychosocial model highlights the value of psychological interventions as a treatment alternative.

Deep Brain Stimulation Among the newer advances in medical treatment of pain is **deep brain stimulation (DBS)**. DBS involves the transmission of an electrical current to parts of the brain involved in processing pain signals. Electrodes are implanted in these parts of the brain, delivering electrical impulses controlled by a pacemaker-like generator surgically inserted under the skin in the upper chest (see Figure 6.12). While many people have reported

A Closer Look

The Opioid Epidemic

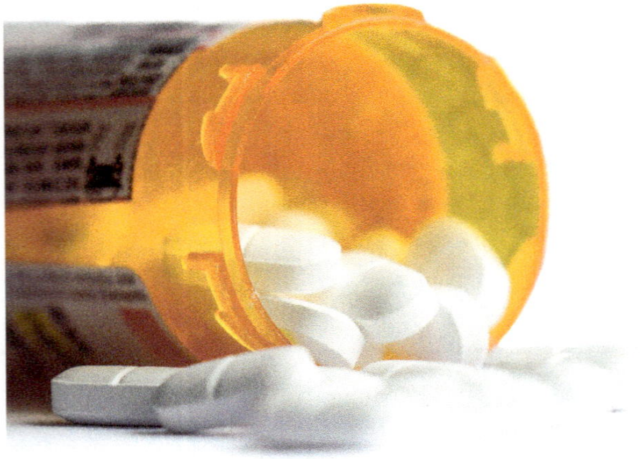

Charles Wollertz/Alamy Stock Photo

The opioid crisis is the worst epidemic of drug addiction in the nation's history. Record numbers of opioid overdose deaths have been reported in recent years (Bechara et al., 2019). Opioids are highly addictive drugs, whether they are derived naturally from the poppy plant in the form of morphine, heroin, codeine, or opium, or synthesized in the laboratory to have opioid-like effects, such as the synthetic opioids OxyContin and Vicodin. Consider some facts about the opioid epidemic:

- Overdose rates are highest among people aged 25–54, non-Hispanic White people, and men in general (Hedegaard et al., 2017).
- More than 80,000 Americans died from opioid overdoses in 2021 (NIDA, 2023). That is a about a tenfold increase in deaths from overdose since 2000. The number is higher than that for deaths from car accidents, firearms, or HIV/AIDS.
- Among the major contributors to the opioid epidemic is the incredible rise in use of prescription opioids for pain relief (Peltz & Südhof, 2018). Millions of people are routinely prescribed opioids for pain; one in four of them struggles with addiction (Powell et al., 2020; Strickler et al., 2020). Opioid prescriptions jumped by a third in the first 15 years of the new millennium (Strickler et al., 2020).
- A particularly powerful synthetic opioid is fentanyl, which poses an even greater risk of death from overdose than heroin (Goodnough, 2019). Synthetic opioids have become the leading cause of drug overdose deaths in the United States (NIDA, 2019).

The risk of death from opioid overdoses occurs because stimulation of opioid receptors in deeper parts of the brain causes drowsiness and depresses respiration. Remember, too, that the body normally produces its own opioid-like substances (endorphins), which are largely responsible for the so-called runner's high and also help us cope naturally with discomfort. However, repeated use of narcotics decreases production of endorphins, explaining in part why people experience discomfort when they discontinue using narcotics.

Physicians may cut off people for whom they have prescribed narcotics once they believe that it is time for their dependence on the drug to come to an end. If people who have become dependent of opioids can no longer obtain them legally, they may turn to the black market. Unfortunately, they cannot know the doses of the street versions or whether they are laced with even more harmful substances, such as fentanyl.

Greater efforts are needed to develop and disseminate non-pharmacological treatment alternatives, such as transcranial magnetic stimulation (TMS) and other forms of brain stimulation (Bechara et al., 2019; Iglesias, 2020). The biopsychosocial model offers an alternative framework to the traditional biomedical approach to pain management by broadening the availability of treatment alternatives to include psychosocial techniques, such as cognitive behavioral therapy (CBT), relaxation training, distraction techniques, physical therapy, and exercise programs (Gandy et al., 2022; Ho et al., 2022; Martin et al., 2021; McCracken, Yu, & Vowles, 2022).

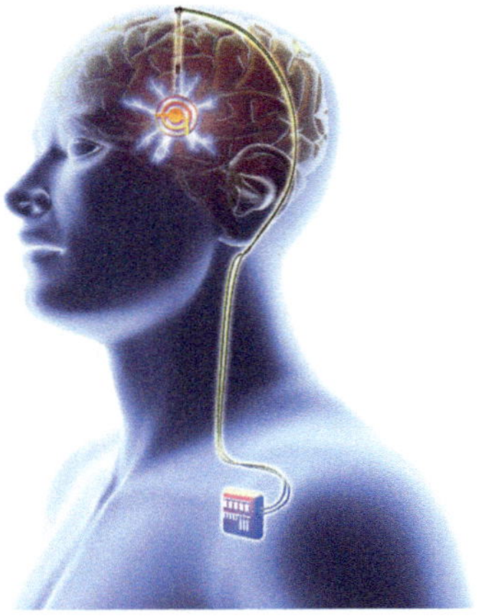

ALFRED PASIEKA/Science Source

FIGURE 6.12 Deep Brain Stimulation In DBS, an electrode is implanted in the brain and delivers electrical impulses that are controlled by a pulse generator that has been surgically inserted in the chest.

that DBS offers significant benefits in reducing chronic pain, research evidence of the effectiveness of the procedure is mixed (Frizon et al., 2020; Leplus et al., 2022; Wang et al., 2023).

The word transcranial means "across the cranium," or skull. *Transcranial magnetic stimulation* (TMS) is a noninvasive form of brain stimulation in which a magnetic field is used to stimulate nerve cells in the brain (see **Figure 6.13**). The magnetic stimulation generates a strong magnetic field that passes through the skull and affects electrical activity in underlying brain structures, such as the parts of the cerebral cortex involved in processing pain signals. TMS shows some promising results, such as in the treatment of some forms of nerve pain and migraines (Iglesias, 2020). It also shows benefits in cases of severe depression and obsessive-compulsive disorder that have failed to respond to more conventional treatments (Denys et al., 2020; Kaster et al., 2019).

Transcutaneous Electrical Nerve Stimulation Other types of electrical stimulation, such as spinal cord stimulation, may also provide relief from pain. "Transcutaneous" means "across the skin." In transcutaneous electrical nerve stimulation (TENS), low-voltage electrical stimulation is applied directly to nerves (see **Figure 6.14**). Electrodes are placed in various sites on the body to conduct electric currents to nerve fibers that carry pain messages. A battery-operated TENS unit modulates the current. However, research evidence supporting the effectiveness of TENS in relieving chronic pain, such as lower back pain and knee pain, remains inconclusive (Aiyer, Johnson, & Poli, 2022; Binny et al., 2019).

Complementary Approaches

Many people seek help outside the mainstream of medical practice for relieving chronic pain. They may turn to other treatment providers because traditional medical approaches have proved ineffective or because they do not want to rely on drugs. These alternative techniques are generally classified as complementary health approaches because they are intended to complement, not replace, traditional medicine.

Evidence supporting the effectiveness of alternative health approaches is mixed. The government agency overseeing research on alternative treatments, the National Center for Complementary and Integrative Health (NCCIH), a division of the National Institutes of Health, points to a growing body of evidence supporting some of these approaches. The alternative approaches to pain relief receiving some support in the research literature include acupuncture, yoga, relaxation, tai chi, hypnosis, massage, mindfulness meditation, spinal manipulation, and music (yes, listening to music may help relieve pain) (NCCIH, 2018).

Although these techniques may be helpful to some people with chronic pain, they typically provide a small to moderate benefit in relieving pain, and their effects may be short-lived (Chou et al., 2017). Although alternative therapies are generally safe, we shouldn't assume they are risk free for everyone. Even "natural" methods aren't always free of side effects or interactions with medications. It's best to consult with a qualified healthcare professional before trying them.

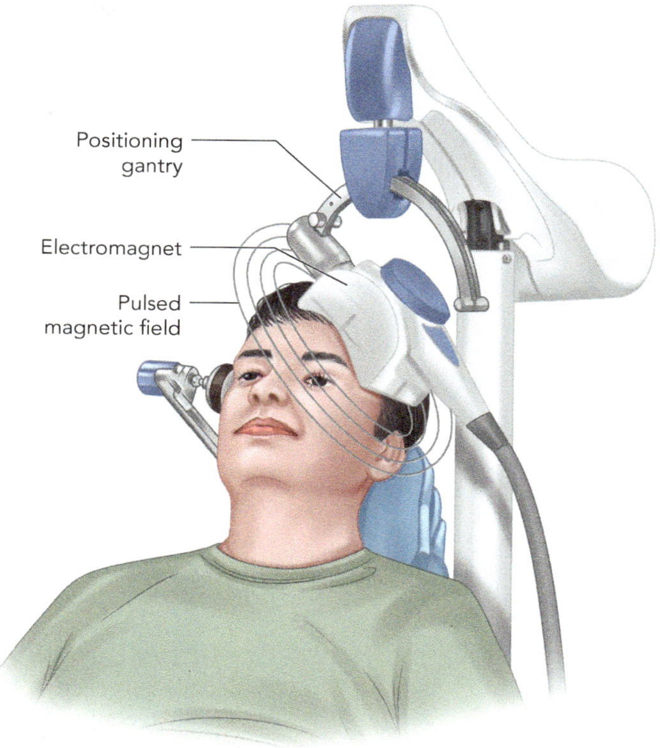

FIGURE 6.13 Transcranial Magnetic Stimulation TMS transmits a magnetic pulse to the head through the use of a powerful electromagnet. TMS is used to treat pain and, sometimes, depression, typically when other treatments have not been effective.

There is some evidence that acupuncture can reduce a person's need for opioids (NCCIH, 2018). Acupuncture is a traditional Chinese medical practice in which thin needles are placed at selected points in the body, called acupuncture points, and then rotated by the acupuncturist. In traditional Chinese folklore, rotation of the needles is believed to release the body's own healing energy, leading to relief from pain. People undergoing acupuncture may report a lessening of pain, but questions remain about the nature of "natural healing energy" and whether the benefits of acupuncture are due to the technique or to a placebo effect.

There is also evidence of the effectiveness of acupuncture in treating headaches and other types of pain, as well as nausea (Cummings, Hróbjartsson, & Ernst, 2018). However, the evidence also shows that some benefits of acupuncture may be explained by a placebo effect (Colloca, 2019). Supporting the placebo effect explanation, researchers fail to find that acupuncture provided benefits beyond those of fake (sham) procedures in which needles were inserted in areas that are *not* designated as acupuncture points (Hinman et al., 2014; Young, 2014).

Although we generally don't think of exercise as an alternative treatment technique, a compelling body of evidence shows that physical exercise may provide relief from pain, such as lower back pain (Chou et al., 2017). In the treatment of MSP, the leading cause of chronic pain, exercise programs with structured, repetitive movement have been shown to help relieve pain and improve musculoskeletal functioning (Meade et al., 2019). Physicians treating lower back pain and other forms of MSP often recommend exercise programs for their patients, or have them work with physical or occupational therapists who oversee structured physical exercise programs for back, hip, or knee pain as well as problems with balance and muscular coordination (see the Health Psychology In Action feature below).

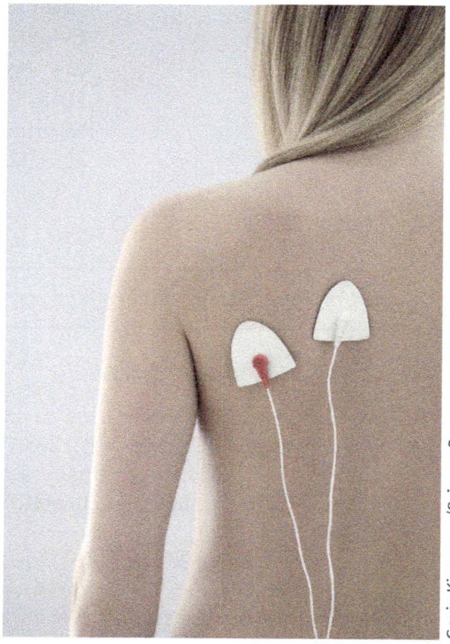

Gavin Kingcome/Science Source

FIGURE 6.14 Transcutaneous Electrical Nerve Stimulation The woman is using TENS to relieve pain in her upper back. The main TENS unit produces minute electrical impulses that are passed into the skin by the two electrode pads. The pulses are intended to block the nerve signaling pathway, thus preventing pain signals reaching the brain and being felt.

Psychological Techniques in Treating Chronic Pain

The shift from a biomedical model to a biopsychosocial model has led to the adoption of integrative models of care that incorporate psychological interventions, such as CBT (Arnold et al., 2016; Hruschaka & Cochran, 2018). Taking an integrative approach recognizes that chronic pain conditions may not be adequately managed by medications alone (Gauntlett-Gilbert & Brook, 2018). Treatment providers use psychological methods that focus on behaviors and coping styles to help improve clients' ability to function, to relieve pain symptoms, and to enhance clients' overall quality of life (Kent et al., 2023). A general consensus has emerged that the most effective treatment approach for chronic pain typically involves a multidisciplinary team approach with psychologists and other behavior health specialists taking roles in treatment (Balderson et al., 2018; Sharpe et al., 2020).

Adopting a comprehensive treatment model, a multidisciplinary treatment team that includes a physician, a nurse, a psychologist, and perhaps a physical therapist or occupational therapist may work with people who suffer from chronic pain. Each team member is tasked with different roles, but they work best when they are under the same roof so that they can consult frequently with each other to meet the multifaceted needs of people who have chronic pain (Ray et al., 2018).

Psychological interventions have been shown to be helpful in reducing the intensity of pain and the interference of pain in people's lives (Castelnuovo & Schreur, 2019).

Cognitive Behavioral Therapy for Pain CBT has emerged as the leading psychological approach in treating chronic pain. CBT involves a combination of cognitive and behavioral techniques to help people change maladaptive beliefs and attitudes about pain and adopt healthier behaviors. The therapist focuses on a person's experience of pain and what they tell themselves about the pain, not on just the physical symptoms (Turk & Murphy, 2019). Cognitive distortions can set the stage for feelings of helplessness and hopelessness, including catastrophizing pain. Psychologist Dennis Turk identified several types of cognitive distortions often seen in people with chronic pain, including those shown in **Table 6.1**.

A large and growing body of research evidence supports the efficacy of CBT in treating chronic pain (e.g., Darnall, 2019; Niknejad et al., 2018; Turk, 2018; Turk & Murphy, 2019). Evidence shows that CBT helps reduce the intensity of pain, the catastrophizing of pain, and depression while also increasing self-efficacy for managing pain (Darnall, 2019; Lami et al., 2018; Lumley & Schubiner, 2019). Researchers also find that CBT reduces the risks of long-term disability associated with chronic pain and the need for opioid medication (Garland et al., 2019; Linton, 2018; Schwenk, 2019; Turk, 2018a).

Health Psychology in Action

Exercise for Relief of Pain

Exercise programs are widely used to help relieve pain and improve functioning. People with chronic pain should begin exercise routines slowly and gradually increase their intensity, consistent with constraints recommended by their healthcare providers.

How does exercise relieve pain? One leading theory is that vigorous exercise leads to the release of endorphins, the brain's own pain-killing chemicals (Bechara et al., 2019; Turk, 2018a).

Regardless of whether exercise programs help, most people do not adhere to them consistently. Many either drop out or exercise infrequently. But health psychologists have made inroads in adapting behavior change techniques to increase regular participation in exercise by people with MSP. Social support (encouragement from others), the setting of realistic goals, and the development of self-efficacy (people's belief that they can perform the behaviors they see others practicing) all help to promote adherence (Meade et al., 2019).

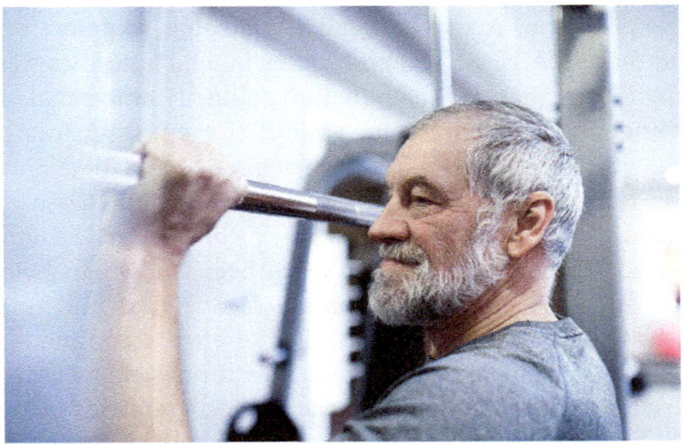

Jozef Polc/Alamy Stock Photo

INTERACTIVE FIGURES, CHARTS, & TABLES

TABLE 6.1 Common Types of Cognitive Distortions in People with Chronic Pain

Type of Cognitive Distortion	Description	Examples
Black-or-white (dichotomous) thinking	Thinking in all-or-nothing terms	• "After one session, there was no reduction in my pain. This treatment isn't any good."
Catastrophizing	Exaggerating negative outcomes or consequences	• "This pain is never going to get better." • "I'm going to be an invalid for the rest of my life." • "I'm never going to be able to work and then what? I'll be desperate."
"Should" statements	Imposing unreasonable expectations on self or others	• "I should be able to do everything I was able to do before the injury, pain or no pain." • "I shouldn't allow my pain to affect me the way it does."
Emotional reasoning	Believing that because it feels a certain way, it must be that way	• "I'm so afraid this pain is never going away."
Negative focusing	Focusing only on the negatives	• "When I'm in pain, nothing else matters. I can only think about the pain."
Entitlement fallacy	Believing one is entitled to a pain-free life	• "It's so unfair I have to live with this pain." • "I feel I've been cheated in life and life shouldn't be this way."

Source: Adapted from Turk (2018a, 2018b).

Cognitive behavioral therapists challenge these maladaptive ways of thinking. They encourage people with chronic pain to evaluate their thoughts in light of evidence. They might ask whether a thought is grounded in reality or is distorted or exaggerated. They identify thinking patterns that focus only on the negative and dismiss any positives. People with chronic pain may be asked to shift their perspective by considering how others might view what they are going through differently or what they might say to help someone in a similar situation. Therapists gently guide clients to consider whether there might be alternative ways of thinking and acting. They propose mini-experiments as homework assignments, such as encouraging people to increase their level of physical activity and evaluate the results to see if their preconceived negative beliefs were borne out.

People also learn to adjust their expectations of themselves, understanding that they need to distinguish what they would like to do ideally from what they can do realistically without incurring a flare-up (Darnall, 2019). The saying "Do not let the perfect be the enemy of the good" applies. People with chronic pain also learn to pace themselves in their physical activities, adopting a gentle, steady pace rather than pushing themselves too aggressively.

Evidence suggests that CBT also alters brain functioning of people with pain. Researchers took brain scans of people with chronic pain before and after 11 weekly CBT group therapy sessions (Seminowicz et al., 2013). After treatment, the brain scans showed significant increases in activity levels of brain regions associated with pain control, and these changes correlated with people's reports of pain relief. Other research showed that a course of CBT helped normalize connectivity among neurons in resting-state brain networks, and these changes were linked to reduced pain intensity (Yoshino et al., 2017).

Helping people with chronic pain make positive behavioral changes often requires building motivation to change as well as self-efficacy (Jensen, 2018). People with high levels of self-efficacy tend to have a lower risk of disability due to pain. Therapists also help people identify the types of changes in their daily activities they can make that allow them to do more and hurt less. But therapists must be alert to each person's level of motivation to change and use methods of gentle persuasion, such as those shown in Table 6.2, to help them build their motivation to put behavioral changes into effect.

Mindfulness/Acceptance Approaches **Mindfulness meditation** is a widely used form of meditation in which people learn to be fully aware of their present-focused experiences without judging or evaluating them. We can liken it to watching the continuous flow

mindfulness meditation A form of meditation in which one focuses on the moment-tomoment unfolding of experience without imposing judgment or evaluation on the experience.

TABLE 6.2 Building Motivation in Working with People in Chronic Pain

Treatment Aims	Examples of Clinician Responses
Encourage adaptive thinking	Reflect back the client's adaptive thoughts or change talk (e.g., "You're saying you want to start exercising in order to feel better and that you think it may be possible to tolerate a higher level of activity. Is that about right?").
Point out discrepancies	Gently point out discrepancies between the goals the client sets (e.g., relief from pain, getting back to usual activities) and the client's current behavior (e.g., cutting back on activity, relying only on pain medications that don't seem to provide long-term relief).
Avoid arguing with clients	If the client begins arguing, change the focus to return to listening and reflecting what the client is saying rather than lecturing or debating.
Boost self-efficacy	Focus on how the client has met challenges before by saying something like "Tell me about how you were able to function before when you were hurting. What can you learn from that experience you can put into effect today?"
Validate the client	Use praise and compliments tied to specific health behaviors, as, for example, "I see you're really trying to spend more quality time with your son. Tell me how that's going."
Build an action plan for change	Develop a realistic action plan that fits the client's goals and lifestyle. Be flexible in providing different options to achieve these goals. Be specific in the steps the client can take to achieve these change goals and review progress periodically, offering suggestions and alternatives when obstacles arise.

Source: Adapted from Jensen (2018).

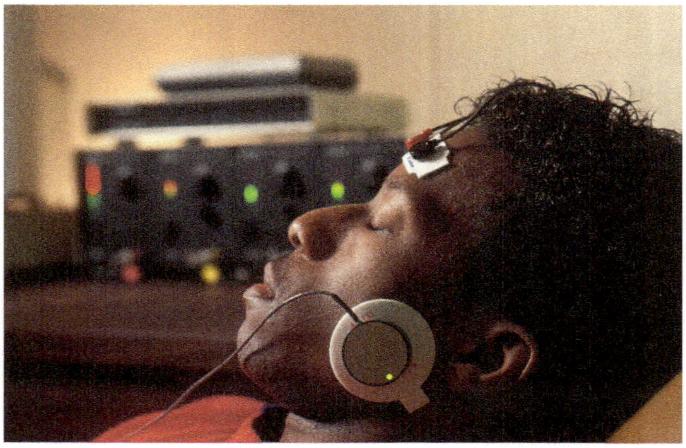

Will & Deni McIntyre/Science Source

Biofeedback Training to Relieve Tension in the Forehead and Jaw He sought treatment for muscle-tension headaches and painful clenching of his jaw. BFT is helping him learn to monitor and relax the muscles involved in the headaches and jaw pain.

of a river in which the person is trained to become keenly aware of the ever-flowing "river" of bodily sensations, emotions, and mental experiences. Unlike cognitive behavioral techniques that encourage people to identify and correct distorted thoughts, mindfulness approaches encourage people to become aware of bodily sensations, including painful ones, but to regard them with a sense of detachment—without catastrophizing them. Mindfulness is often blended with an acceptance approach to therapy in which people are instructed to accept the pain rather than try to make it go away, while not letting the pain prevent them from getting on with their lives. This approach involves a shift in mental attitude from "I can't stand this pain and I can't do anything until it goes away" to "I may be in pain, but I can tolerate it and do what I need to do in my life."

Mindfulness techniques yield significant benefits in treating chronic pain (Nigol & Di Benedetto, 2020; Sturgeon & Darnell, 2018; Zorn et al., 2020). In one research example, investigators found that a meditation/acceptance approach produced even greater reduction in reports of daily pain than a CBT approach in treating people with rheumatoid arthritis (Davis et al., 2015).

biofeedback training (BFT) A psychological treatment in which physiological monitoring equipment is used to provide feedback about bodily functions so that individuals can gain some degree of control over them.

Biofeedback Training

Biofeedback training (BFT) is a treatment technique in which information (feedback) about internal bodily responses helps people gain some degree of control over those responses. It is a psychological intervention because participants use the feedback as a cue in learning to alter physiological responses. BFT helps people gain some degree of control over bodily functions, such as heart rate, blood pressure, muscle tension, body temperature, and brain wave patterns (Weir, 2016). BFT is useful in relieving pain, especially headache pain, lower back pain, and jaw pain (Ezenwa et al., 2018; Gatchel & Noe, 2019; Kondo et al., 2019; Stubberud et al., 2018). In BFT, people are connected to physiological monitoring equipment that provides them with a continuous stream of information about their internal bodily states, such as muscular tension and heart rate. Changes in the pitch of an auditory tone or beep indicates (and thereby reinforces) changes in the desired direction—for example, a slower heart rate. (Knowledge of results is a powerful reinforcer.) A rising tone may indicate increasing heart rate or muscle tension, while a lower tone indicates changes in the opposite direction. People use these biofeedback signals as cues to help them learn to modify bodily responses. How do they do it? The answer may vary from person to person, but most people apply some form of self-relaxation or pleasant mental imagery to reduce muscle tension and states of bodily arousal, using the feedback to gauge their progress.

One form of BFT, called **electromyographic (EMG) feedback**, monitors states of muscle tension, especially in the forehead. It is used to treat muscle-tension headache, which in many cases is associated with tensing or tightening of muscles in the head and neck.

electromyographic (EMG) feedback A form of biofeedback training that provides information about muscle tension in selected parts of the body, typically the forehead; used in treatment of muscle tension headaches.

In using EMG feedback for muscle-tension headaches, electrodes are placed on the forehead to monitor muscle tension in the head. Changes in the pitch of an auditory tone indicate increases or decreases in muscle tension. People use the feedback to learn to relax their forehead muscles, helping reduce pain associated with tension headaches. About 50% of people with tension headaches experience significant improvement using BFT (Arena & Tankersley, 2018). EMG biofeedback also shows benefits in treating other forms of pain, including lower back pain and temporomandibular joint or jaw pain (Labott, 2018; Sadora et al., 2023).

BFT can also be helpful in treating **migraine headache**, a type of severe headache affecting about 37 million Americans (Voelker, 2020). Migraines are intense, throbbing headaches that often affect one side of the head and can last for hours or days. Sensory and motor disturbances often precede the pain; a warning aura may include vision problems and the perception of unusual odors. Migraines are often accompanied by sensitivity to light, loss of appetite, nausea, vomiting, sensory and motor disturbances such as loss of balance, and changes in mood.

migraine headache A severe, throbbing or piercing headache that may be accompanied by nausea and visual disturbances.

Migraines are a complex condition in which a genetic tendency or predisposition interacts with other factors, including triggers that make attacks more likely to occur (Klenofsky et al., 2019; Rosignoli et al., 2022). These triggers include emotional stress, bright lights and fluorescent lights, menstruation, stressful work environments, sleep deprivation, altitude, pollen, certain drugs, the chemical monosodium glutamate (MSG, sometimes used to enhance the flavor of food), alcohol, hunger, and weather and seasonal changes. Women are as much as three times more likely to be affected by migraines. Hormonal changes before and during menstruation may be involved in migraines in women. Pain catastrophizing is often a feature of frequent migraines and may become a target for treatment using cognitive-behavioral therapy (CBT) (Rosignoli et al., 2022).

A form of BFT called **thermal feedback** is widely used to relieve pain associated with migraine headaches that are associated with irregularities in the blood flow to the brain. A temperature-sensing device is attached to a finger. It beeps more slowly (or more rapidly, depending on how it is set) as the temperature in the finger rises. Raising the temperature in a finger, as by imagining the finger getting warmer, is accompanied by increased blood flow (vasodilation) to the limbs and away from the head. The standard psychological treatment of migraine headache involves a combination of relaxation training and thermal biofeedback (Arena & Tankersley, 2018). Prescription medications may also be helpful in treating migraines, including ones that help regulate brain levels of the neurotransmitter serotonin, a neurotransmitter implicated in migraines.

thermal feedback A form of biofeedback training that provides information about changes in body temperature in specific parts of the body; used in the treatment of migraine headaches.

Let us note that the benefits of BFT may be achieved in some cases through simpler forms of relaxation training that do not require electronic equipment, such as relaxation training and relaxation breathing, both discussed in Chapter 5.

Hypnosis

Many people think of **hypnosis** in terms of shows in which hypnotists induce people to do funny things on stage. As it turns out, hypnosis can also be good medicine. We have abundant evidence that hypnosis has positive effects in treating both chronic and acute pain (Adachi et al., 2014; Heap, 2019; Schwenk, 2019).

hypnosis A method of inducing a state of focused attention, deep relaxation, and heightened susceptibility to suggestion.

The use of hypnosis in health care has a long history. In 1842, London physician W. S. Ward amputated a man's leg after using hypnosis as the anesthetic. According to reports, the man experienced no discomfort. Several years later, operations were being performed routinely under hypnosis at Ward's infirmary. Today, hypnosis is used to help people stop smoking or lose excess weight or reduce chronic pain; it also is used as an anesthetic in dentistry, childbirth, and some forms of surgery (Jensen, 2008; Manworren et al., 2018; Wang et al., 2020). People being prepped for surgery may undergo hypnosis and given the suggestion that when they notice certain cues, such as a particular doorway leading to the surgical suite, they will allow themselves to feel deeply relaxed, and their relaxed feelings will further deepen as they start changing into their hospital gown and when they feel a line being inserted in their arm (Heap, 2019). Keeping these mental expectations in mind can help replace anxiety and tension with feelings of calmness.

Scholars debate what hypnosis is and why it works. Hypnosis was once seen as an altered state of consciousness called a trance—a state in which the person is highly responsive to suggestions. Psychologists generally reject the view that hypnosis involves a special state of consciousness or a trance. But they do use it to help people cope with pain.

When hypnosis is used for pain relief, a person is first deeply relaxed and is then given suggestions by the hypnotist with the aim of changing their experience of painful sensations. For example, people with chronic pain may be given a suggestion that the sensation of pain in an affected area will lessen or be replaced by feelings of warmth, coolness, or relaxation (McKernan, et al., 2018). Or they might be given a suggestion that although the pain remains, it is not very bothersome. The hypnotist might also employ distraction and fantasy by, for example, directing the person to visualize relaxing on a warm, exotic shore.

Health Psychology in Action

Preventing the Development of Chronic Pain in Children

Health psychologists who specialize in pain management typically work within multidisciplinary teams of physicians, physical therapists, nurses, and other healthcare professionals. One example of a multidisciplinary approach is at Dupont Hospital for Children in Wilmington, Delaware, where pediatric health psychologists work closely with primary healthcare providers, including pediatricians and family physicians, in multidisciplinary teams (Salamon & Cullinan, 2019). Team members oversee an integrated pain management program for children with pain-related disorders. Dealing with chronic pain is demanding in itself and can significantly impair a child's functioning, leading to poor school attendance, social withdrawal, and reduced participation in extracurricular activities.

The integrated pain management program focuses on preventing the development of chronic pain in children, such as those with pediatric cancer, or limiting its impact. Early intervention is the key. The model embodies three levels of prevention focusing on universal, targeted, and clinical treatment interventions (see **Figure 6.15**). The treatment model combines medical and psychological interventions designed to help children and their families manage pain more effectively. Here we outline the three levels of care in this comprehensive prevention model:

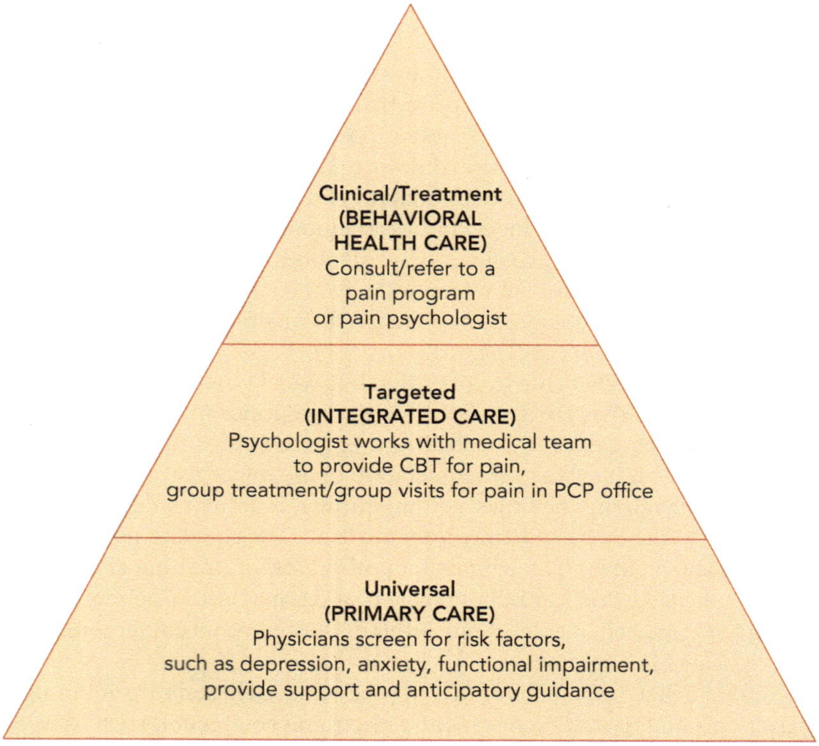

FIGURE 6.15 The Integrated Model for Pain Clinical health psychologists developed this treatment model to tailor treatment interventions to the level of care of children living with pain.

Source: Salamon & Cullinan (2019). Reproduced with permission of American Psychological Association.

1. *Universal level:* The universal level focuses on *primary prevention*, which involves the prevention of pain-related problems through early screening and intervention. Pediatricians and other treatment team members identify risk factors that might set the stage for development of chronic pain and target resources to help prevent the pain or minimize its impact. Screening includes questions about the frequency of various types of pain, such as headaches or stomachaches, and whether they interfere with the child's daily functioning (e.g., "Do you get pain frequently? Does pain get in the way of doing the things you enjoy?").
2. *Targeted level:* The aim of the targeted level is *secondary prevention*, which involves identifying problems at an early enough stage that intervention might forestall the development of more serious pain-related conditions. An integrative

approach to treatment services includes medical and psychosocial interventions. For example, children at this level might participate in brief CBT interventions to help them develop skills for handling pain and its emotional impacts, such as anxiety and depression. Or the family might be provided with referrals to community mental health providers who can provide more extensive treatment. The goals of treatment at this level include educating the child about the nature of pain, helping the child develop self-relaxation skills, encouraging the child to participate in pleasurable or pleasant activities, and identifying and countering negative ways of thinking.

3. *Clinical/Treatment level:* At this level, the full impact of a pain-related disorder is felt, and the treatment team seeks referral to specialized pediatric pain management programs. The American Pain Society (2018) lists outpatient, day treatment, and inpatient pediatric chronic pain programs in the United States and Canada. Liaisons or nurse advocates may reach out to these programs to gather additional information on services and the referral process and to inquire about educational seminars for primary care providers in the office.

This integrated pain management program is a model for tailoring treatment services to the child's level of care. Health psychologists play important roles in developing and implementing these types of integrated healthcare programs.

Applying Health Psychology

Coping with Pain

Coping with that age-old enemy—pain—has traditionally been a medical issue. The primary treatment has involved use of pain-killing medications, but psychological factors also play a major role in how people cope with pain. For example, the availability of social support, of people showing concern and lending a helping hand, can help blunt the psychological effects of enduring pain.

Treatment of chronic pain has become a team effort that involves medical care providers, health psychologists, and other behavioral health professionals, such as physical and occupational therapists. But the person in pain should also be a team member. Here are some ways in which people can help themselves to manage pain more effectively.

Obtain Accurate Information

Many people in pain try to avoid thinking about it and its implications. But remaining in the dark about the source of their pain may prevent them from obtaining the medical treatment needed to properly diagnose and treat the underlying problem. One of the most effective psychological methods for managing pain is obtaining factual, thorough information. Obtaining accurate medical information can reduce stress by helping people maintain a sense of control over their situation. They feel they are doing something about their medical condition rather than simply trying to ignore it.

Use Distraction and Fantasy

Experimenters find that people tend to report lower levels of pain if they focus their attention away from their pain (Ho et al., 2022). Dascal et al., 2017). If one is faced with a painful medical or dental procedure, one might keep one's mind off their pain by focusing on a pleasing picture on the wall or letting one's mind become absorbed in a pleasant fantasy. The simple technique of counting your breaths can also distract your attention from pain and help block disturbing thoughts.

People with chronic pain may find they are better able to cope with their pain if they distract themselves by engaging in activities that take their mind off the pain, such as exercising, becoming immersed in a good book or video, engaging in hobbies or other enjoyable tasks, having a conversation, or playing games (Labott, 2018). Laboratory research shows that people tend to report lower levels of pain when they focus attention away from their pain (Coderre et al., 2003). Distraction doesn't simply redirect attention away from pain; it actually reduces the frequency of pain signals transmitted through the spinal cord to the brain (Coderre et al., 2003; Sprenger et al., 2012).

Practice Relaxation Training and Biofeedback Training

When we are in pain, we often tense up. Tensing muscles is uncomfortable in itself and focuses attention on the pain. Relaxation training is an important component of a multifaceted treatment for pain. Deep breathing exercises or use of relaxing imagery can distract the person from the pain and deepen feelings of relaxation. Some people prefer practicing meditation to enter a deeply relaxed state. Alternatively, relaxation breathing may help distract people from pain and discomfort.

When people practice relaxation or meditation, their muscles unwind, which can help stem pain stemming from muscle tension. Even when pain arises from other sources, relaxation can help people get their minds off their pain and avoid aggravating the pain by tensing up.

Take Control of Your Thoughts

Taking control of your thoughts is an important coping skill for dealing with persistent pain. What you think has a bearing on how much pain you feel and how well you cope with it. Thinking pessimistic or hopeless thoughts ("This will never get better") and catastrophic thoughts ("I can't take this anymore. I'm going to fall apart!") can heighten pain (Pinto et al., 2011). More generally, maintaining a sense of control—seeing ourselves as taking an active role in managing pain rather than becoming helpless victims—can enhance our ability to cope with pain.

Health psychologists find that helping people with chronic pain counter catastrophic thinking with rational alternative thoughts helps reduce the intensity of the pain and improves daily functioning (Turner et al., 2006). Here are some suggested alternatives to negative thoughts about pain:

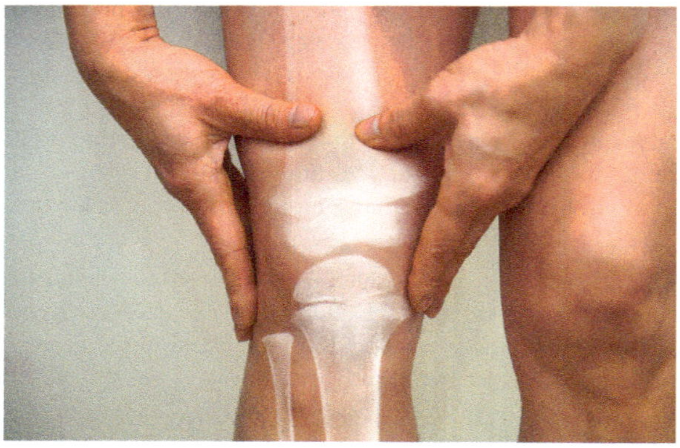

Peter Dazeley/Getty Images

Hold That Thought! Pain is a sign that something is wrong, but now that you've gotten the message, why catastrophize the pain by assuming the worst will happen?

Change	to
"This is the worst thing in the world"	"Yes, this is bad, but other things would be so much worse."
"I can't cope with this anymore"	"It's a struggle, but I can deal with this. I've managed to deal with pain like this before, and I can do so again."
"What's the use of trying? This pain will never end"	"Don't give in to hopelessness. Think in the present. Focus on what you need to do today to cope with the pain."

Findings from brain-scanning studies show higher levels of catastrophizing or thinking the worst are associated with greater levels of pain-related brain activity (Edwards et al., 2009). Even if changing thoughts and attitudes does not eliminate pain, it can help people manage their pain more effectively. Adopting more hopeful, optimistic attitudes and maintaining a sense of control—seeing ourselves as taking an active role in managing pain rather than becoming helpless victims—can increase our ability to cope with pain.

Close the Gate on Pain

Simple remedies like applying an ice pack or rubbing the injured area frequently help relieve pain. The gate control theory of pain holds that a gating mechanism in the spinal cord opens and closes, letting pain messages get through to the brain or shutting them out. One may be able to create a traffic jam at the gate by lightly rubbing an irritated area or applying an ice pack to the injured area, transmitting stimulation to the spinal cord that can compete with pain signals. (Icing the area may also reduce inflammation.)

"Flood the gate" so that some pain messages don't get through. But for sudden or persistent pain, don't simply treat the symptoms—see a physician. Pain is a sign that something is wrong in the body that requires medical attention.

Reach Out and Touch Someone (or Be Touched by Someone)

It turns out your mother was right (*Isn't she always?*). Researchers find that a loved one's touch can ease pain. Touch may be the most basic form of human connection, from the tender stroking of an infant's skin to lovers holding hands while out for a stroll.

In the lab, health researchers tested the power of touch. They randomly assigned romantic partners to a pain condition in which mild heat was applied to the arm of one of the partners or a control condition in which no painful stimulus was administered (Goldstein et al., 2018). Both groups were instructed to either touch their partner by holding hands or not touch each other during the experiment. The experimenters measured reports of pain and brain wave patterns of both partners during the experiment. The results showed that holding hands during the administration of a painful stimulus increased synchronization of brain wave patterns between the partners and, further, that brain syncing was associated with lower levels of reported pain by the pain recipient. The investigators speculate that a supportive touch may make the person being touched feel understood and connected, which might trigger pain-dampening processes in the brain

The simple act of touching may play a role in helping people cope with pain, as when a parent holds a child's hand when the child is receiving a painful injection. Touch is indeed more than skin deep; it creates a personal connection that brings into sync brain wave activity of two individuals, which in turn may relieve pain. The lesson here is that to help reduce the pain of another person, share a touching moment.

Take a Problem-Solving Approach

Effective problem solvers generate alternative solutions to problems, evaluate the pros and cons of each solution, and then try out the most feasible solution to see how it works. Even if the solution fails, the experience is an opportunity to learn what they might do differently going forward. They recognize that failure is not fatal; it is feedback.

Keep Abreast of New Developments

Pain management is a rapidly growing science. New technologies and approaches to pain management are being introduced to clinical practice each year. If you have chronic pain, keep abreast of new developments by regularly consulting your healthcare provider or pain management specialist.

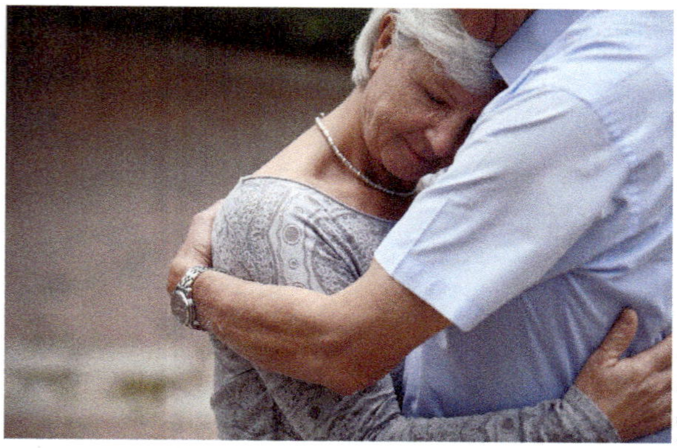

laflor/Getty Images

A Touching Experience Researchers find that holding someone in pain, even holding hands, dampens the experience of pain.

Review 6.3

INTERACTIVE SELF-SCORING QUIZZES

Sentence Completion

1. The most commonly used medications for pain are __________ drugs, such as aspirin and ibuprofen.
2. If __________ are used in treating pain, they should be used for the shortest possible period of time.
3. The CDC recommends that therapies other than __________ are preferred for treatment of chronic pain.
4. More Americans die from opioid overdoses than from either firearms or __________ accidents.
5. In __________ stimulation, electrodes are implanted in certain parts of the brain to deliver electrical impulses.
6. A noninvasive form of brain stimulation in which electric current is passed through a coil to produce a magnetic pulse is called __________ magnetic stimulation.
7. In __________ electrical nerve stimulation, low-voltage electrical stimulation is applied directly to nerves through an electrical stimulator.
8. __________ techniques may be helpful to some patients but typically provide a small to moderate benefit in relieving pain, and their effects may be short-lived.
9. The most effective treatment approach for chronic pain typically involves a __________ team approach.
10. __________ interventions have been shown to be helpful in reducing both pain intensity and interference of pain in people's lives.
11. One form of the BFT, called __________ feedback, monitors states of muscle tension, especially in the forehead.
12. A form of the BFT called __________ feedback is widely used to relieve pain associated with migraine headaches.
13. Three levels of preventive efforts targeting chronic pain in children are __________, targeted, and clinical/treatment levels.

Think About It

Do you or someone close to you live with chronic pain? What steps can you take to help yourself or another person with chronic pain? What techniques discussed in the text might you find helpful?

Recite: An Active Summary

INTERACTIVE SELF-SCORING QUIZZES

Chapter 6 Practice Quiz

1. Describe the ways in which the body processes pain.

Pain is detected by pain receptors in the skin and other parts of the body, which transmit pain signals to the spinal cord and from there to the somatosensory cortex in the brain for processing. Scientists believe that a gating mechanism in the spinal cord allows pain signals to reach the brain or blocks them out.

2. Describe the biopsychosocial model of chronic pain.

The biopsychosocial model of chronic pain takes a broader perspective than the traditional biomedical model by accounting for the effects of pain on psychological, emotional, physical, social, and occupational functioning. Psychological factors play important roles in how people cope with chronic pain, including avoidance-related beliefs and behaviors that are often associated with living with chronic pain.

3. Describe the role that health psychologists play in the management of chronic pain.

Health psychologists work as team members on interdisciplinary teams in helping people with chronic pain develop more adaptive behaviors in dealing with pain, change maladaptive patterns of thinking, such as catastrophizing, and cope with stress, as well as helping family members provide constructive support.

4. Identify biomedical, psychological, and complementary health approaches in treating chronic pain.

Biomedical approaches involve the use of pain medications and, in some cases, deep brain stimulation. Psychological approaches typically involve the use of cognitive behavioral therapy to assist people with chronic pain in developing more adaptive behaviors and thinking patterns. Complementary treatments include such techniques as mindfulness and acceptance approaches, biofeedback training, relaxation training, exercise, hypnosis, and acupuncture.

5. List ways of coping with chronic pain in daily life.

Ways of coping with chronic pain include obtaining accurate information, using distraction and fantasy, practicing relaxation training and biofeedback training, taking control of your thoughts, creating a bottleneck at the pain gate, taking a problem-solving approach, and keeping abreast of new developments.

Answers to Review Sections

6.1

1. skin
2. chronic
3. nociceptors
4. somatosensory
5. Endorphins
6. musculoskeletal
7. 5
8. more
9. biopsychosocial
10. thinner and slower

6.2

1. avoidance
2. consequence
3. gradually
4. self-efficacy
5. reinforced
6. more likely

6.3

1. analgesic
2. opioids
3. opioids
4. car
5. deep brain
6. transcranial
7. transcutaneous
8. CAM
9. multidisciplinary
10. Psychological
11. electromyographic
12. thermal
13. universal

Scoring Key for Short-Form McGill Pain Questionnaire

Simply add your scores across the 22 items and then divide the sum by 22. That will give you a mean (average) score for each item. By comparison, a sample of 882 people with chronic pain obtained a mean score of 6.93. These participants had experienced chronic pain for an average of more than 8 years.

Scoring Key for the Pain Catastrophizing Scale

The Pain Catastrophizing Scale helps people with chronic pain evaluate their tendencies to exaggerate or catastrophize their pain, which can make it more difficult to cope with pain or even intensify the pain they experience. To score the scale, add up your responses on the 13 items. Scores can range between 0 and 52. A total score of 30 or higher is indicative of a level of catastrophizing that corresponds to the 75th percentile of scores of people with chronic pain. That is, a score of 30 equals or exceeds that of three out of four test-takers. Health psychologists help people with chronic pain replace catastrophizing thinking with more adaptive ways of thinking that can help them manage pain more effectively.

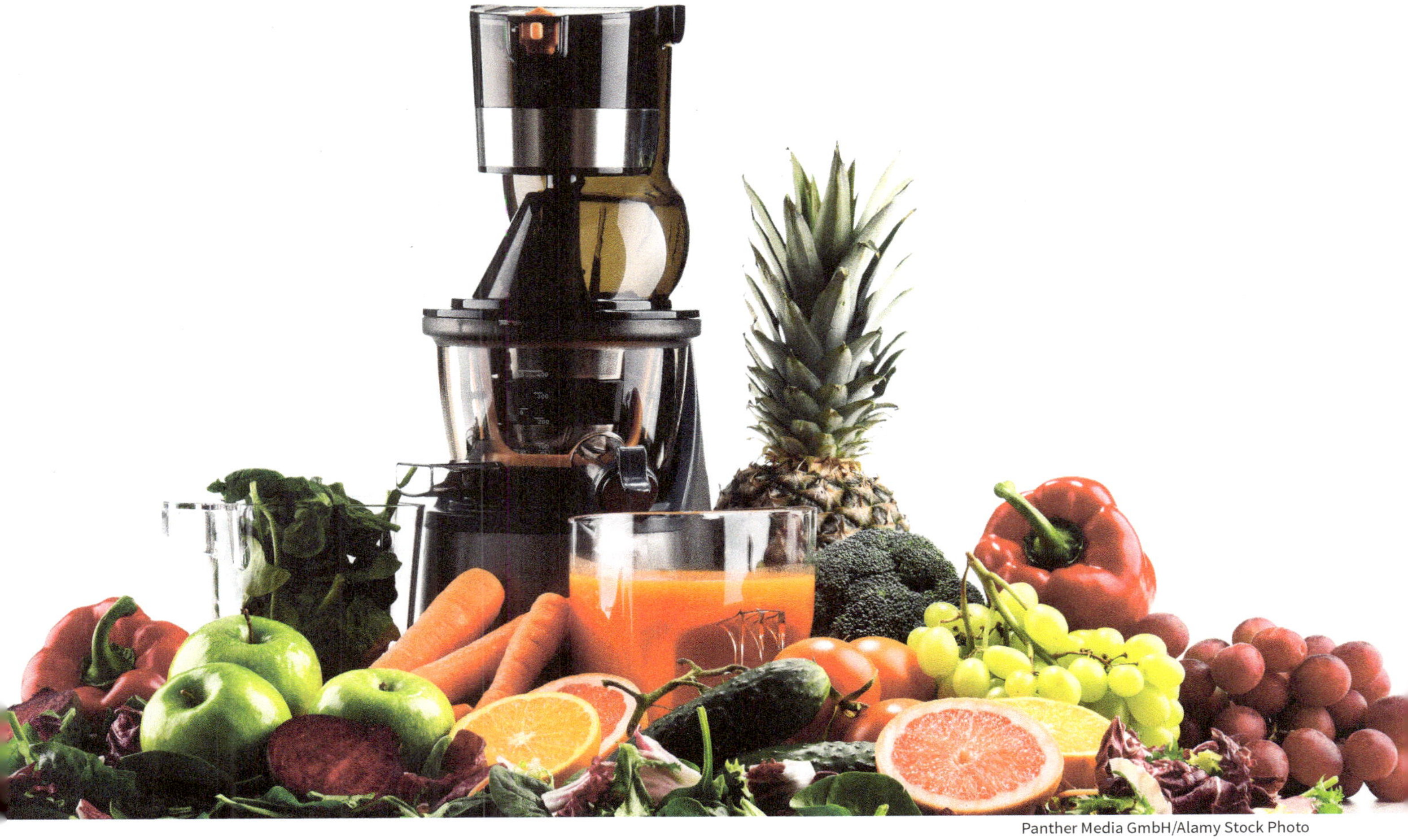

Panther Media GmbH/Alamy Stock Photo

Healthy Living: Nutrition, Weight Management, and Physical Activity

LEARNING OBJECTIVES

After studying this chapter, you will be able to ...

1. **Describe** the parts of the digestive system and explain how the hunger drive works to maintain a steady state.
2. **Define** the essential nutrients and explain their roles in health.
3. **Define** overweight and obesity, and discuss their origins.
4. **Discuss** the role of health psychology theories in weight control.
5. **Define** anorexia nervosa and bulimia nervosa, and discuss their origins.
6. **Describe** USDHHS guidelines for physical activity.
7. **Describe** the physical and psychological health benefits of exercise.
8. **Explain** how to get a move on—how to safely develop a personal fitness program.

Did You Know That ...

- As many as one cancer death in three is linked to poor nutrition?
- The majority of American adults are overweight?
- Many overweight people are victims of severe fat shaming?
- When people are obese, some physicians attribute almost any health complaint to their weight?
- Suburbanites are more likely than city-dwellers to be overweight?
- Health psychologists find that people tend to eat more when food is served on larger plates?
- Dieting has become the normal way of eating for women in the United States?
- Prolonged sitting is a recognized health risk?
- You don't have to exercise 30 minutes a day, 5 days a week in order to reap the benefits of exercise?
- Exercise may boost your brain power?
- Exercise helps combat feelings of anxiety and depression?

Let food be thy medicine and medicine by thy food.

—Hippocrates

Hippocrates (460 B.C.E.–370 B.C.E.) was the ancient Greek physician in whose honor newly graduated physicians to this very day swear an oath to uphold a set of ethical professional standards. Hippocrates recognized that what we eat has an important bearing on our health and well-being. Food can be good medicine, as the body depends on food for the nutrients it needs to function at its best and sustain good health.

Hippocrates would not have been surprised to learn about recent evidence pointing to healthful benefits of a food product you probably have sitting in your kitchen cabinet or pantry—olive oil. As reported in 2020 in the *Journal of the American College of Cardiology*, researchers examined links between olive oil intake and heart disease (Guasch-Ferré et al., 2020). The investigators surveyed more than 61,000 women who participated in the Nurses' Health Study and more than 31,000 men drawn from another large survey of health professionals, the Health Professionals Follow-up Study.

Based on an average follow-up period of 24 years, the investigators found that people who reported higher levels of consumption of olive oil had significantly fewer cardiovascular events, such as heart attacks and strokes, than those reporting lower levels of consumption. In fact, participants who consumed, on average, more than half a tablespoon of olive oil daily had a 14% lower risk of cardiovascular incidents than those who consumed olive oil less than once a month. The investigators also estimated that people who had switched from margarine to olive oil showed a lower risk of cardiovascular disease.

Survey research does not have the experimental controls needed to demonstrate cause-and-effect relationships, so we cannot say for certain that consuming olive oil, or substituting olive oil for other types of fats, such as butter or margarine, will reduce our risk of developing cardiovascular problems. But this type of correlational evidence can point us in the direction of possible causal factors deserving of further experimental study. Meanwhile, we may want to consider the dietary choices we make in our daily lives, including the kinds of fats we typically use.

Olive oil is a staple of the Mediterranean diet, which you'll learn about in this chapter. Health professionals are exploring whether the foods we consume and the diets we adopt might benefit or harm our health. This is a developing area of research, so we don't have all the answers. In this chapter we take a closer look at the health effects of diet on health outcomes and the role of health psychology in furthering our understanding of the psychosocial factors that contribute to healthier nutrition.

This chapter is about life choices, and how health psychologists help people make healthier choices—the key choices involved in nutrition. The chapter also applies theories of health psychology to how we can adopt a healthier diet and manage our weight more effectively. Healthy nutrition is one component of the bodily energy equation, the component involved in consuming food that supplies the body with the energy and nutrients it needs. The other part of the bodily energy equation is the expenditure of energy through physical activity and body metabolism. We will see how regular physical activity is a key part of a healthy lifestyle and the role that health psychologists play in getting us moving in our daily lives.

The Digestive System and the Hunger Drive

Think about the last thing you ate. What happened to it after it slid down your throat? This chapter is about the bodily system that takes the food you consume and converts it into sources of energy the body needs to perform all of its various functions. This system is called the **digestive system**. Let's have a look at the inner workings of your digestive system to find out.

digestive system The system by which food eaten is broken down mechanically and chemically to provide the body with absorbable nutrients and to eliminate waste products. The system contains the GI tract, the liver, the pancreas, and the gallbladder.

The digestive system consists of the gastrointestinal (GI) tract (the pathway by which food enters the body and solid wastes are eliminated from the body: the mouth, pharynx, esophagus, stomach, small intestine, large intestine, and anus), the liver, the pancreas, and the gallbladder (**Figure 7.1**). Your GI tract is curled up and would stretch out to about 20 feet if it were straightened.

The digestive system is a laboratory, and you are both a food processor and a chemist. As a food processor, you break up much of the food you eat mechanically by chewing, but you use chemistry to further break it down and convert it to heat, energy, and chemicals you need to grow and repair your body. This conversion process is what we mean by **digestion**. The system breaks food down mechanically (by chewing) and chemically by means such as salivation, gastric juices, and enzymes. Your body expels what is left over through the rectum, which is the final section of the large intestine and terminates at the anus.

digestion The mechanical and chemical processes involved in breaking food down into absorbable nutrients.

You salivate when food enters your mouth. You may also salivate when you smell food, see other people eating, or even think about food. The Russian scientist Ivan Pavlov trained dogs to salivate when they heard a bell by pairing food with the sounding of the bell. What learned stimuli cause you to salivate? (Perhaps "The pizza's here!"?)

Salivation lubricates food, making it easier to swallow, protects your teeth from bacteria, and contains chemicals that help break food down. The salivary glands may become swollen

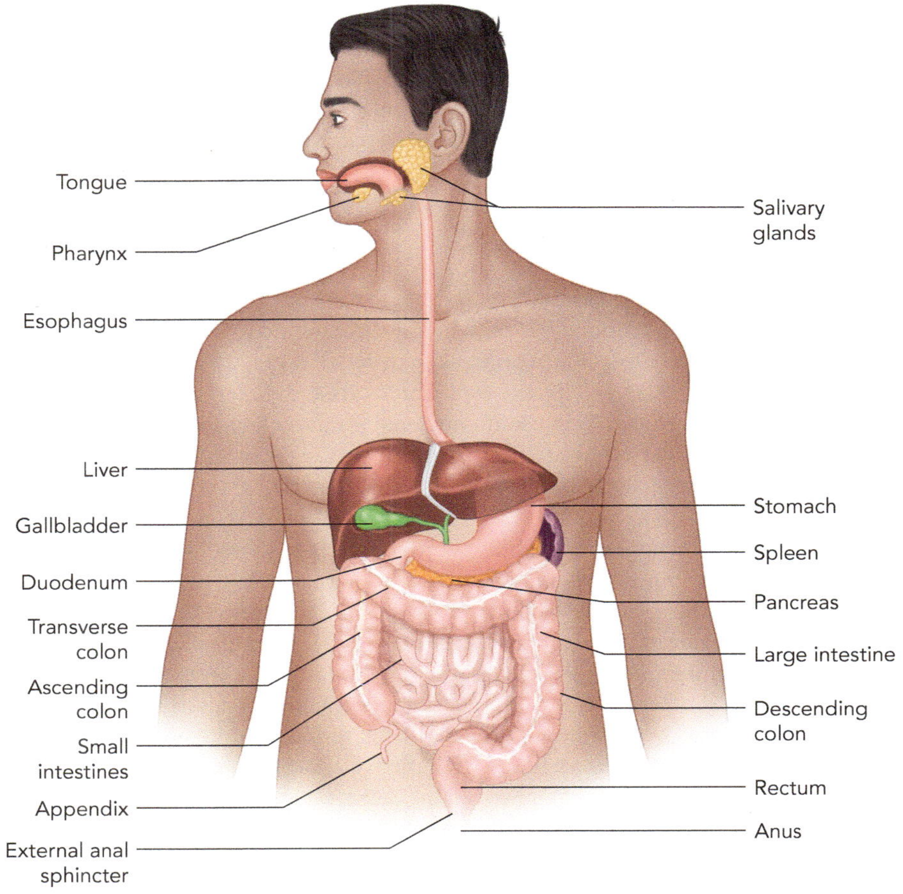

FIGURE 7.1 The Parts of the Digestive System

because of buildups of crystallized saliva or by bacterial infections, both of which can be painful and cause a fever. A dry mouth may affect us as we age. Consult a physician or dentist if you suspect you have these conditions.

Food passes through the esophagus to the stomach and then the intestines. The esophagus and stomach push food along by wavelike muscular contractions called **peristalsis**. In the stomach, gastric juices mix with the food to break it down. It isn't just gravity that pushes food down, although you will digest your food better if you are sitting or standing rather than lying down. Gastric juices may start flowing when you think about food, and they may cause nausea if you don't put some food into your stomach. But it may surprise you to know that because of the work done in the small intestine, you can survive without a stomach.

peristalsis The wavelike involuntary contraction and relaxation of muscles in a hollow organ, such as the intestine, to propel food onward.

Food passes from the stomach to the first part of the small intestine, the duodenum. The pancreas secretes **enzymes** that further break down protein, carbohydrates, and fats. Proteins are broken down into amino acids, carbohydrates into sugars, and fats into glycerol and fatty acids. The pancreas also secretes **insulin**, a hormone that aids in the absorption of sugar. You will learn more about insulin in the discussion of diabetes in Chapter 14. The liver produces bile, which helps break down fats in the duodenum. The gallbladder stores bile between meals, and as you eat, your gallbladder squeezes bile through bile ducts into your small intestine. Most of this mixture is absorbed into the bloodstream through the lining of the small intestine.

enzymes Substances produced by an organism that facilitate specific biochemical reactions.

insulin A pancreatic hormone that regulates the amount of sugar in the blood. Lack of insulin causes a type of diabetes (see Chapter 14).

What is left of what you ate then continues its journey into the large intestine. Water may be absorbed by the first half of the part of the intestine, which is called the colon, but bacteria convert the remaining food material into feces, giving them their signature odor. Feces collect in the rectum and are expelled when you defecate (have a bowel movement or, as a child might say about the pet dog, "poop"). Defecation for infants is automatic or involuntary. For older children and adults, defecation is usually voluntary unless the person cannot "hold it." Toilet training involves helping children to gain control over defecation and urination.

In Chapter 4 we noted that the autonomic nervous system (ANS) plays a role in digestion. The parasympathetic division of the ANS promotes digestion. The sympathetic division of the ANS prepares you to fight or flee a predator, but it might also prompt you to throw up your food in the process. Moreover, when the sympathetic division dominates, your mouth will be dry because of lack of salivation.

Physicians recommend colonoscopies to check for colon cancer in people who are middle aged or older. During a colonoscopy, a doctor inserts a flexible instrument through the anus to inspect the colon for cancer or precancerous **polyps**, which can be removed during the procedure.

polyps Small growths protruding from mucous membranes. They are normally benign but can develop into cancerous growths.

The Hunger Drive

For food to enter the digestive system, you have to eat it first. You and 7 billion other people and countless animals are prompted to eat when the hunger drive is stoked.

Psychologists refer to hunger and thirst as **primary drives**, which are based on our biological makeup. We also acquire drives—called **acquired drives**—through experience. We may acquire a drive for money because money enables us to buy food and various kinds of drinks, as well as nights out on the town. Drives such as hunger and thirst trigger arousal (tension) and activate behavior. We learn to engage in behaviors that reduce the tension associated with the drives.

primary drives Motives to behave in a certain way because of the biological makeup of the organism.

acquired drives Learned drives.

Primary drives such as hunger and thirst are normally triggered when we are in states of deprivation—that is, when we haven't eaten or taken in fluids for some time. Sensations of hunger motivate us to behave in ways that restore the bodily balance. There is thus a tendency to maintain a steady state, which is called **homeostasis**. Homeostasis is like a biological thermostat. When the temperature in a room falls below the **set point** on the thermostat, the heat turns on to raise the temperature until the set point is reached. Similarly, animals tend to eat until the tension created by the hunger drive has been reduced to the point when they are no longer hungry. This doesn't always work for humans, unfortunately. Many of us eat recreationally, as when we see or sniff out an appealing dessert. We may also keep on raising the set point for the hunger drive by overeating, especially by overeating sugars and fats.

homeostasis The tendency of a living organism to maintain a relatively stable balance or equilibrium among the conditions inside it.

set point The target value for a variable, such as weight.

We might think that hunger is controlled by the stomach if we experience hunger pangs on an empty stomach. But medical research shows the brain is in control of regulating hunger and appetite. A key part of the brain involved in regulating the hunger drive is the **hypothalamus**,

hypothalamus A gland in the brain that is involved in many bodily processes, including hunger, sleep, emotions, aggression, and body temperature.

comfort food Food that provides emotional comfort and feelings of satiety during the processes of eating and digestion, including foods with high sugar content and psychologically associated with one's childhood and home cooking.

a pea-sized gland involved in many aspects of motivation, including the sex drive, aggression, and hunger. When we haven't eaten for a while, the blood sugar (glucose) level drops. The hypothalamus detects the falloff in blood sugar and then triggers a cascading series of bodily processes that results in hunger and appetite. When we eat, the body uses the food we digest to restore our blood glucose levels. (The role of the hypothalamus in responding to stress is discussed in Chapter 4.)

Psychologists have shown that psychological as well as biological factors play important roles in determining hunger and eating behavior. How many times have you become hungry by the sight or aroma of food? How many times have you eaten not because you were hungry but because you were at a relative's home or hanging around a cafeteria or coffee shop? Or because you were anxious or depressed and you were looking for **comfort food**? Or just because you were bored?

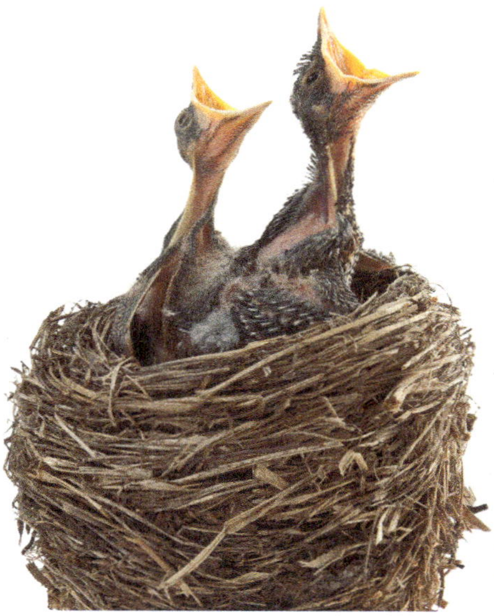

stanley45/Getty Images

Disorders of the Digestive System

Problems of the digestive system are generally treated medically by specialists such as *gastroenterologists* (GIs). However, these problems are also of interest to health psychologists because behavioral factors play an important role in their development, such as dietary habits and exposure to harmful substances, such as tobacco. Here we focus on several of the major types of digestive problems.

GERD and Constipation

The most common digestive disorders are acid reflux disease (known more technically as **gastroesophageal reflux disease [GERD]**), constipation, and diarrhea. GERD is characterized by burning in the chest (heartburn) after eating, nausea, and a feeling of a lump in the throat. GERD can be triggered by smoking, eating meals late at night, fatty or fried foods, alcohol or coffee, or pain medicines such as aspirin, ibuprofen, and naproxen. Antacids and prescription medications can help, but also consider your diet. Constipation can be caused by a diet low in fruits, vegetables, and whole grains and by taking certain medications, especially opioids. Over-the-counter medicines can help with constipation.

gastroesophageal reflux disease (GERD) A condition in which acidic gastric juices flow upward into the esophagus, causing nausea and heartburn.

electrolytes Substances that can dissolve into ions (atoms that have lost electrons) in solutions and can conduct electricity, such as sodium, potassium, chloride, calcium, and phosphate.

dysentery A dehydrating intestinal inflammation, mostly of the colon, which leads to cramping and severe diarrhea with blood or mucus in the feces.

peptic ulcers Sores on the lining of the stomach (gastric ulcers) or small intestine (duodenal ulcers).

Diarrhea and Dysentery

Diarrhea can be caused by bacteria, viruses, and parasites, and is a major killer of children in developing nations. Most of the time, in developed countries, diarrhea is a transient disease. However, if diarrhea is caused by pathogens (bacteria, viruses, or parasites), the infection should be eradicated. Treatments for diarrhea can include antibiotics in case of bacteria. Because chronic diarrhea dehydrates the body, it is important to take in liquids, especially liquids containing **electrolytes**. An over-the-counter medicine, loperamide, helps with diarrhea by calming the digestive system, allowing it to absorb the fluids and salt it needs.

Dysentery has been called bloody diarrhea. Visible red blood and mucus are found in the feces. It is also characterized by abdominal cramps and fever. Dysentery is usually spread by contaminated food or water and most often is caused by a bacterial or parasitic infection of the intestines, but it may also result from a viral infection. Treatment usually involves eradication of the infectious organism. Like diarrhea, dysentery is a common cause of death in developing countries and efforts to control these diseases focus on developing sanitation systems and providing people with healthy food choices and clean water.

Peptic Ulcers

Peptic ulcers are sores on the lining of the stomach (gastric ulcers) or the small intestine (duodenal ulcers). Symptoms include burning stomach pain, heartburn, nausea, belching, and intolerance of fatty foods. Peptic ulcers may be caused by *Helicobacter pylori* bacterium or an excess of gastric juices that eat away at the lining of the stomach or duodenum in the absence of food.

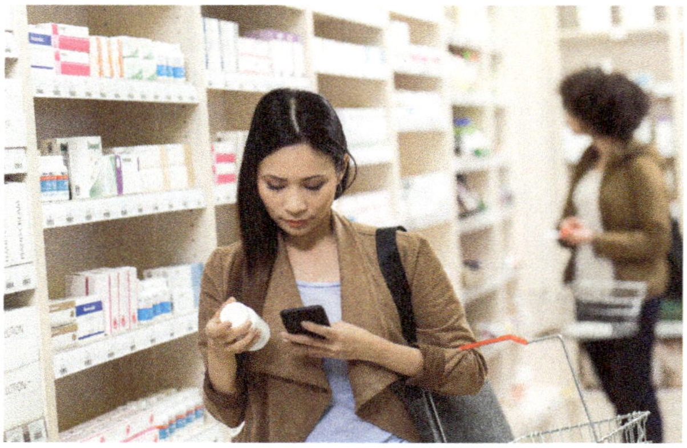

Tashi-Delek/Getty Images

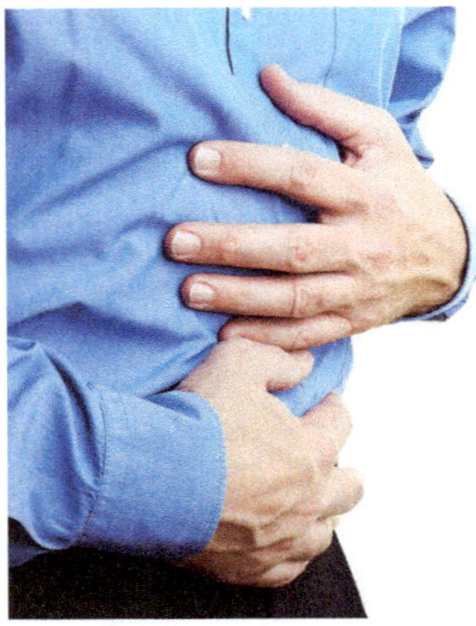

Robert Kneschke/Alamy Stock Photo

Persistent abdominal pain and cramping are symptoms of a number of digestive disorders. If they become a regular feature of life, a person needs to consult a healthcare professional.

Behavioral factors also play a role. High levels of stress, consuming spicy foods, smoking, and drinking alcohol may contribute to peptic ulcers. Over-the-counter preparations can help soothe the stomach, but if a bacterial infection is present, it needs to be treated with an aggressive course of antibiotics.

Inflammatory Bowel Disease There are two types of inflammatory bowel disease (IBD)—ulcerative colitis and Crohn's disease. Ulcerative colitis, as the name implies, causes inflammation and sores on the lining of the innermost part of the large intestine, the colon, and the rectum. **Crohn's disease** most often affects the lower part of the small intestine and the colon. Symptoms of both disorders include diarrhea, abdominal pain and cramping, bloody stools, fever, fatigue, reduced appetite, unintended weight loss, and abnormal changes in the menstrual cycle. It was once thought that IBD was caused by stress and diet, but these hypotheses have not been borne out by research. But there are known risk factors. One is age; unlike all those health problems that appear among older people, IBD is likely to develop before the age of 30 years. Non-Hispanic White Americans are most likely to develop IBD. Family history, smoking, and use of nonsteroidal anti-inflammatory medicines (NSAIDs) such as ibuprofen (e.g., Advil) and naproxen (Aleve), all elevate the risk. People with IBD are more likely to develop colon cancer later in life.

Crohn's disease Chronic inflammation of the lower part of the small intestine and the colon.

Despite the fact that over-the-counter NSAIDs heighten the risk of IBD, IBD is usually treated with other anti-inflammatory medications that are available only by prescription. Health professionals may also prescribe antibiotics, when infection is of concern, and drugs that suppress an overactive immune system. Other treatments include anti-diarrheal medicines, acetaminophen (e.g., Tylenol) for pain, iron supplements, and calcium and vitamin D supplements. Surgeons sometimes remove damaged portions of the digestive tract.

Health psychologists have a role to play in IBD because lifestyle changes involving adoption of healthier behaviors are also recommended, such as limiting use of dairy products and consuming low-fat foods. Researchers also find that psychological factors, such as anxiety and depression, can affect the course of the disease and frequency of relapse (Eugenicos & Ferreira, 2021). Psychological treatments, such as cognitive-behavioral therapy (CBT), may also help curb gastrointestinal symptoms and reduce associated emotional distress (Eugenicos & Ferreira, 2021).

Health psychologists also focus on the emotional effects of living with digestive disorders. A survey of 903 people with IBD and 170 physicians found that most people with IBD experience profound anxiety and depression, yet three in ten say that their health professionals are not interested in treating their emotional responses (Marín-Jiménez et al., 2017). Half the doctors said they asked people with IBD about their emotional responses, but the patients themselves said that inquiries about their feelings occurred only one-quarter of the time. The research group recommends that psychologists be included on the treatment teams of IBD patients (Barreiro-de Acosta et al., 2018; Marín-Jiménez et al., 2017).

Disorders of the Liver Disorders of the liver include hepatitis and cirrhosis. Unhealthy behavior patterns often play a role in contracting these diseases, such as unsafe sexual and injection practices in the case of hepatitis, and alcohol abuse in the case of cirrhosis.

hepatitis An inflammation of the liver that can impair the function of the organ and is usually caused by a virus.

Hepatitis refers to inflammation of the liver. There are three primary forms of hepatitis caused by different strains of the hepatitis hepatitis A, B, and C. Hepatitis A is highly contagious and usually transmitted by means of contaminated food or water or close contact with an infected person or object. Symptoms of hepatitis A can include fatigue, nausea, abdominal discomfort, joint pain, clay-colored bowel movements, dark urine, itching, low-grade fever, loss of appetite, and yellowing of the skin and the whites of the eyes (jaundice). The symptoms are usually mild and end in a few weeks, but some cases are more severe and endure for months. You can protect yourself from hepatitis A by washing your hands regularly. There is a vaccine for the disease.

Hepatitis B is a more serious infection of the liver, caused by the hepatitis B virus. Symptoms are like those for hepatitis A. Hepatitis B is more likely than hepatitis A to become a chronic condition, and it can lead to liver failure. There is a vaccine for the disorder.

Hepatitis C is also a viral infection. It is transmitted by means of contaminated blood and inflames the liver and can cause serious liver damage. The symptoms include bleeding and bruising easily, fatigue, poor appetite, jaundice, spider-like blood vessels in the skin, muscle aches, confusion and fatigue, and fluid buildup in the abdomen. About half of people who are infected are symptom-free, sometimes for decades. The disease responds well to antiviral medication.

In **cirrhosis** of the liver, healthy liver tissue is replaced by fibrous tissue, or scarring. Cirrhosis is most often a result of chronic drinking of alcohol. Excessive drinking damages the liver, and as the liver tries to heal itself, scar tissue forms. Symptoms include fatigue; easy bruising; nausea and loss of appetite; swelling in the legs, feet, or ankles; itchy skin; and jaundice. There is really no alternative—people with cirrhosis of the liver should make every effort to stop drinking.

cirrhosis Scarring of the liver.

Cancer

Cancer may develop in any part of the digestive system. Dentists screen you, or should screen you, for cancers of the mouth and oral cavity at every visit. Human papillomavirus (HPV) can lead to cancer in the throat of people who engage in oral–genital sex with women whose reproductive systems have HPV. The HPV vaccine may guard against throat cancer due to HPV and cervical cancer. Cancers of the esophagus are uncommon, afflicting about 1 man in 130 and 1 woman in 450. Pancreatic cancer affects about 1 person in 70, but it is particularly deadly to some degree because people are not regularly screened for the disease. That means it is rarely caught early. Cirrhosis is a risk factor for cancer of the liver. Colon and rectal cancers afflict about 1 person in 20–25, and about half that number die from it. Again, regular screening is imperative. As we'll see in the text, health psychologists play important roles in promoting cancer screening efforts.

Review 7.1

INTERACTIVE SELF-SCORING QUIZZES

Sentence Completion

1. The esophagus propels food along with wavelike contractions called __________.

2. __________ juices may start to flow when you fantasize about food and may cause nausea if you don't eat.

3. The pancreas secretes the hormone __________, which aids in the absorption of sugar.

4. The __________ division of the ANS facilitates the processes of digestion in the small intestine.

5. The body's tendency to maintain a steady state is called __________.

6. The __________ is a gland in the brain that stokes the hunger drive and is also involved in regulation of sleep cycles, the sex drive, and aggression.

7. A colonoscopy can remove precancerous growths called __________.

8. Because chronic diarrhea dehydrates the body, it is important to take in liquids, especially with __________.

Think About It

Have you experienced any of the digestive disorders discussed in the section? If so, what did you do about them? Did your choices help? If not, what else can you do?

Nutrients: The Stuff of Life

Food is an important part of a balanced diet.

—Fran Lebowitz

We are what we eat—literally. Our bodies convert what we consume into bones, muscles, nerves, and other bodily tissues. What we consume also affects our health. Researchers have established strong links between proper nutrition and avoidance of serious chronic diseases, such as cardiovascular disease and some forms of cancer. As many as one in three deaths due to cancer, and many other deaths due to heart disease, diabetes, or stroke, are linked to poor nutrition, especially consumption of a high-fat, high-calorie diet (Schwingshakl et al., 2019). But many of us don't watch what we eat. For some busy college students, out of sight is out of mind. They skip meals, especially breakfast. Many students eat on the run—catch as catch can. Others are attracted to the colorful trays of food that line the glass cases at the cafeteria. Still others chomp through bags of potato chips and jars of peanuts while they are studying. Others heed the call when someone suggests going out for pizza—even if they are not hungry.

nutrition The process by which plants and animals consume and utilize foods (from the Latin root *nutria*, meaning "to feed").

nutrients Essential food elements that provide energy and the building blocks of muscle, bone, and other tissues: protein, carbohydrates, fats, vitamins, and minerals.

proteins Organic molecules that comprise the basic building blocks of body tissues.

amino acids Organic compounds from which the body manufactures proteins.

carbohydrates Organic compounds that form the structural parts of plants and that are important sources of nutrition for animals and humans.

fiber Complex carbohydrates that form the structural parts of plants, such as cellulose and pectin, that cannot be broken down by human digestive enzymes.

fats Organic compounds that form the basis of fatty tissue of animals, including humans (body fat) and are also found in some plant materials.

Nutritional matters are on the back burner for many college students. But adopting healthy nutritional habits is not just a problem for college students. Americans eat far too much junk food that is laden with sugar and fat—foods such as high-fat meats, French fries, potato chips, and cheese. We may also fool ourselves into thinking we are eating well when we order fish or chicken—but then eat these foods deep fried or baked in butter.

The word **nutrition** refers to the process by which organisms consume and utilize foods. Foods provide **nutrients** that furnish energy and the building blocks of muscle, bone, and other tissues. Essential nutrients include protein, carbohydrates, fats, vitamins, and minerals.

Proteins **Proteins** are **amino acids** that build muscles, blood, bones, fingernails, and hair. Proteins also serve as enzymes, hormones, and antibodies. We obtain several proteins from food; others we manufacture for ourselves. The most popular sources of protein are meat, poultry, eggs, fish, and dairy products such as milk and cheese. Legumes (beans, lentils, and peas) and grains are also fine sources of protein. Americans tend to eat more protein than they need. Protein deficiencies are rare in well-fed societies, such as the United States and Canada. But any excess protein we consume is converted into fat.

Carbohydrates **Carbohydrates** ("carbs") are the major sources of energy in our diet. There are two major types of carbs—simple and complex. Complex carbohydrates include starches and dietary fiber. They provide a steady source of energy as well as vitamins and minerals. By contrast, simple carbohydrates, which comprise various types of sugars, offer little more than a spurt of energy and many incur health risks when used in excess (see nearby Health Psychology in Action feature).

Many nutritionists recommend that starches account for 50–60% of our daily calorie intake. Foods rich in complex carbohydrates include whole grains and cereals; citrus fruits; crucifers such as broccoli, cabbage, and cauliflower; leafy green vegetables; legumes; pasta (also high in protein, low in fats); root vegetables such as potatoes and yams; and yellow fruits and vegetables, including carrots and squash. Many starches are also rich in dietary **fiber**, which aids digestion and may have other health benefits, such as helping to protect us from heart disease (Harvard Health Letter, 2014). Many health experts recommend that we consume 20–35 grams of dietary fiber a day (some recommend 25 grams minimum). Yet only half of Americans consume more than 10 grams of fiber a day.

In recent years, many people have adopted "high-protein, low-carb" diets to control body weight. Leading health organizations, including the American Heart Association, take issue with these diets, including the once-popular Atkins diet (American Heart Association, 2018). They point to the lack of nutritional balance and emphasis on high-fat sources of protein (meat, eggs, and cheese) that can contribute to coronary heart disease (CHD), the major form of cardiovascular disease and the leading cause of death of Americans, mostly as the result of heart attacks (see Chapter 13). Although these diets may promote quick weight loss, much of the loss may be in the form of water weight (bodily fluids) as the result of cutting carbohydrates. We lack conclusive evidence that these diets are safe and effective in the long term.

Fats **Fats** provide stamina, insulate us from extremes of temperature, nourish the skin, and store vitamins A, D, E, and K. Most Americans, however, especially those who are addicted to fast food, consume far more fat in their diets than they need. Saturated fat, which comes from animal sources such as meat and dairy products, greatly increases levels of unhealthy blood cholesterol, setting the stage for heart disease. Monounsaturated and polyunsaturated fats (check the food labels), such as those found in vegetable oils such as olive oil and canola oil, are healthier forms of fat (e.g., Fernandes et al., 2020; Massaro et al., 2020).

Health professionals recommend that adults limit their total fat intake to 20–35% of their daily calorie consumption. Many people are paying heed; evidence shows that Americans, on the average, are cutting back on saturated fat and cholesterol and reducing their calorie consumption (Beck & Schatz, 2014). **Table 7.1** shows the recommended limits for total daily fat intake; **Table 7.2** decodes some high-fat food choices that are definitely not heart-healthy. Eating well on campus can be quite a challenge. In some places overeating seems to be a competitive sport; the aptly named "Octuple Bypass Burger" at the Las Vegas Heart Attack Grill boasts 19,900 calories (Wei, 2017). (We don't recommend a visit.)

Health Psychology in Action

Knowing the Facts About Sugar and Health

If you follow discussions in the media about nutrition, you probably know that sugar consumption is often identified as Public Enemy #1 when it comes to unhealthy eating. There's good science to back up the claim that excess sugar intake contributes to serious health concerns, such as diabetes and cardiovascular disorders, as well as tooth decay and obesity. But just how much sugar is too much?

Health scientists applied the scientific method of *meta-analysis* to find out. Meta-analysis is a statistical technique which averages the findings of large numbers of studies. So instead of basing scientific claims on the results of any one study, no matter how well designed it may be, meta-analysis groups the findings of large numbers of studies judged to meet scientific standards. Recently, a group of Chinese and U.S. investigators conducted an umbrella meta-analysis, which as the term implies, combines the results of many meta-analyses, in this case 73 meta-analyses comprising 8,601 studies (Huang, Fan, & Hu, 2023).

Most of these studies were observational. This means the investigators measured statistical relationships between sugar intake and health outcomes but did not conduct controlled trials in which some people were randomly assigned to consume either high or low quantities of the independent variable (sugar). In a controlled trial, we can infer whether there is a causal link, or cause-and-effect relationship between the independent variable and the dependent variable (the measure or measures of interest).

Observational studies allow us to identify factors linked to health risks, but they don't determine that these factors are causally responsible for the observed effects. In other words, we can observe whether people who report high sugar intake stand an increased risk of disease, but we can't say whether sugar plays a causal role in disease. It is possible, likely even, that people who consume high levels of sugar also have other health habits that lead to chronic diseases like diabetes or heart disease, such as inactivity or unhealthy diets, but that sugar itself is not a causative factor (we might say that sugar "goes along for the ride" but does not drive the bus, if you follow this metaphor).

The Chinese and U.S. researchers compiled results based on 8,601 studies, finding evidence of at least a moderate level of quality linking higher sugar intake to a greater risk of cardiovascular disease, childhood obesity, and interestingly, depression. Might sugar make you depressed? We can't claim a causal link between sugar and depression, as we lack evidence from controlled trials. But we can speculate that people who struggle with depression may look to soothe their feelings with sweets; in other words, perhaps depression leads to increased sugar consumption rather than the reverse. Or perhaps people who are depressed just tend to be less concerned about following a healthy diet.

The investigators drilled down in their data set, finding that for every additional sugar-sweetened beverage people consumed, the risk of coronary heart disease increased 17% and the risk of death from all causes combined increased 4%. The general finding is that consuming high amounts of dietary sugar from foods and beverages is associated with increased risk of serious chronic diseases, such as diabetes and heart disease (Harris, 2023a). Evidence linking dietary sugar intake to cancer remains inconclusive, so more research is needed, as are controlled trials in which sugar consumption is directly manipulated so that we can observe its possible effects on health outcomes (Huang et al., 2023). In the meantime, it is prudent to be aware of links between what we eat and drink with our health and well-being.

What, then, is the recommended daily limit on added sugar in our diet? The answer, according to government health officials, is that added sugars should comprise no more than 10% of daily calorie consumption, which amounts to about 12 teaspoons (or some 48 grams) per day for an average person on a 2,000 calorie per day diet plan (CDC, 2021). We can make it a healthy habit to check food labels of foods and beverages for amounts of added sugars to help us keep below the recommended limit. Let's also be aware that added sugars are found in many foods and beverages, such as snacks, desserts, and sweetened beverages.

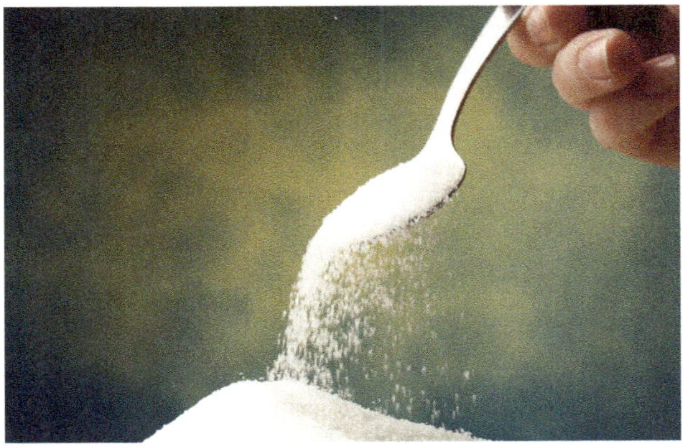
stocksnapper/Getty Images

Added Sweetness Comes with a Cost High sugar intake is linked to many significant health problems. Do you know the sugar content of the foods you consume? Should you become a label reader?

TABLE 7.1 Recommended Daily Totals of Dietary Fat at Specified Calorie Levels

Calories per Day in the Diet	Amount of Fat (in Grams) That Provides 30% of Calories
1,500	33–58
2,000	44–78
2,500	56–97
3,000	67–117

Note: A gram of fat provides nine calories.

TABLE 7.2 Find That Fat!

If you are selecting a meal from a restaurant menu, beware of dishes described with the following terms. They are super high in fat—sort of a heart attack on a plate.

• Alfredo—a basic cream sauce	• Hollandaise—a cream sauce
• Au gratin—a dish with a crusted top, usually composed of cheese and bread crumbs	• Creamed—notes use of a fat (usually butter) whisked with sugar rapidly to incorporate air
• Au fromage—with cheese	• Buttered—with extra fat
• Au lait—with milk	• Crispy—fried
• A la mode—with ice cream	• Basted—with extra fat
• Bisque—cream soup	

When you find these terms on the menu, you can ask for the dish to be prepared in a healthier way. Instead of cooking in butter, you can ask that a dish be prepared with the least amount of olive oil possible. You can also request that fried dishes be grilled, poached, or baked.

Source: Adapted from U.S. Department of Agriculture, Dietary Guidelines for Americans 2005.

vitamins Organic substances needed by the body in small amounts to maintain essential bodily processes.

free radicals Metabolic waste that may damage cell membranes and genetic material.

osteoporosis A bone disorder primarily affecting older people in which the bones become porous, brittle, and more prone to fracture.

Vitamins and Minerals **Vitamins** are essential organic compounds that need to be eaten regularly. Vitamin A is found in orange produce, such as carrots and sweet potatoes, and in deep green vegetables. It is also abundant in liver, but organ meats like liver are extremely high in cholesterol. (Find healthier sources.) Vitamins A and D are found in fortified dairy products. B vitamins are abundant in legumes, vegetables, nuts, and whole-grain products. Fruits and vegetables are rich in vitamin C. Vitamins A, C, and E are antioxidants; that is, they deactivate substances in some foods, called **free radicals**, that might otherwise contribute to the development of cancer. (Don't let those radicals go free.) Health psychologists recognize the need to separate fact from fiction and to ground nutritional advice in scientific evidence. Take a look at **Table 7.3**, which debunks some common myths about vitamins and health.

We also need minerals such as calcium (for conducting nerve impulses and making bones and teeth), iron, potassium, and sodium. Calcium and vitamin D help maintain good bone health and reduce the risk of **osteoporosis** later in life.

Applying Health Psychology

Eating Right on Campus

Here are some suggestions for making healthier food choices on campus. Plan to refuel every few hours to help you keep up your concentration and avoid a headache or nagging hunger pangs.

- For breakfast, choose whole-grain breads, high-fiber cereal, granola bars, fresh fruit, whole-grain crackers, and low-fat milk or milk alternatives (soy milk) rather than muffins, doughnuts, and refined grains (white bread or rolls).
- For lunch or dinner, choose grilled fish or chicken breast or lean beef, veggie burgers, vegetable wraps, the salad bar, sushi, turkey breast on whole-wheat bread, fish, beans (but not refried beans), brown rice, baked potato without the toppings, hummus, low-fat yogurt, low-fat milk or milk alternatives (soy milk), whole-wheat pita sandwiches with veggies or lean meat and salsa topping (not mayo or sour cream) rather than fried entrees, high-fat foods such as burgers and fries, rich pasta sauces, white rice, French fries, whipped cream, syrups, added sugar and salt, cheesy foods, high-fat dressings, or giant-sized portions.
- For between-meal snacks, choose healthful snack bars, low-calorie snacks, granola bars, peanut butter crackers, trail mix, fruits, veggies, nuts, or whole-wheat crackers rather than candy bars, potato chips, cookies, or salted pretzels.

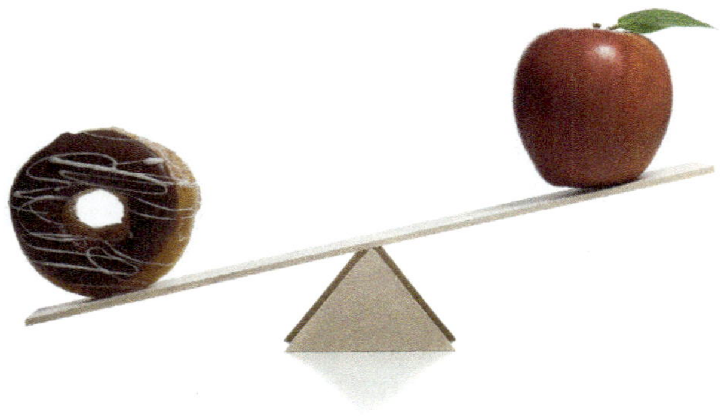

Rubberball/Mike Kemp/Rubberball Productions/Getty Images

INTERACTIVE FIGURES, CHARTS, & TABLES

TABLE 7.3 Vitamin Myths Versus Facts

Myth	Fact
Popping a vitamin pill can correct a poor diet.	Vitamin pills do not compensate for a poor diet. A multivitamin pill can ensure that you receive essential vitamins, but it does not provide the other nutrients you need.
The more vitamins you take, the better.	Excess doses of some vitamins can be harmful. Overdoses of vitamin D and niacin (vitamin B3) can lead to liver damage, for example. Check with your healthcare provider before taking vitamin supplements.
Vitamin supplements help boost athletic performance.	Vitamins do not improve your game or increase your performance in sports.
Taking "stress vitamins" will help me to cope better with my emotional problems.	So-called stress vitamins help the body counter the effects of physical stress, such as changes in temperature. There is no evidence that vitamins help people cope with emotional stress.
Natural vitamins are better than synthetic vitamins.	There is no evidence that the body responds differently to natural and synthetic vitamins.

Taking care of our health involves an active effort to educate ourselves about good nutrition. To that end, we can consult with physicians, pharmacists, and dieticians about daily requirements for vitamins and minerals and other nutrients. It also involves debunking personal beliefs that can be outright dangerous. For example, we need to recognize that overdoses of vitamins and minerals can be harmful. Don't assume that more is better and mindlessly pop megavitamin pills.

Applying the critical thinking skills discussed in Chapter 1 can help us make healthier food choices. We are bombarded daily with health-related claims in television commercials, product advertisements, or product packaging. Take a casual walk through any supermarket or health-food store and begin counting the many health claims on product boxes.

Critical thinkers maintain a healthy skepticism toward advertising and product information. They carefully consider the source of any claim and demand evidence that supports its validity. For example, they recognize that saying a product "may boost the immune system" is not the same thing as saying "does boost the immune system." (You *may* win the lottery, but don't count on it.) Claims that a food or supplement "boosts the immune system" or "protects against heart attacks" may stem from a copywriter's imagination, not hard scientific evidence, or may ignore the qualifiers that researchers address in scientific publications that temper the conclusions drawn from their findings.

Relationships between nutritional patterns and health have grown clearer in recent years. For example, many cases of heart disease and cancer are linked to poor diet (see Chapters 12 and 13). Adopting a healthier diet helps reduce the risk of some forms of cancer. Following a diet low in saturated and trans fats and rich in fruit, vegetables, fish, and whole grains also reduces the risk of CHD (American Heart Association, 2018a).

Stress is also linked to dietary quality. In a recent study, adolescents who reported higher levels of life stress and more daily negative life events reported stronger cravings for tastier foods and greater difficulty resisting these foods (Hsu & Raposa, 2021). The researchers commented that eating is often used by adolescents (and let us add, older people as well) as a means of coping with the stress of difficult emotions.

Although the United States is generally an affluent country, about 1% of children in the country are chronically malnourished (Johns Hopkins Medicine, 2018). They tend to be short for their ages, bloated or thin, physically weak, and have poor immune systems. They bruise easily, develop rashes, and have soft bones. Their condition is a national—and inexcusable—tragedy. Even though the majority of Americans obtain enough food, their food choices are often unhealthy. Moreover, about two in three U.S. adults are overweight, and more than 40% are obese.

Food companies typically use labels on their products to spur sales. By contrast, public health campaigns use food warning labels (FWLs) to nudge people to avoid unhealthy food choices. But do warning labels actually work or do they just add to the background noise of modern life, like those annoying links on websites that people tend to just ignore? Examples of

Health Psychology in Action

Which Cue to Action Would You Choose: "Healthy Choice Turnips" or "Herb n' Honey Balsamic Glazed Turnips"?

There is a song titled "Accentuate the Positive." Unfortunately, when it comes to promoting healthful foods, the tendency is to accentuate the negative (Talati et al., 2019). Thus we may see unhealthful foods referred to as high in "food energy" rather than sugars. Vegetables are healthful, but there is a tendency for people to avoid vegetables or to fry them in butter or oil to make them more palatable.

Health psychologists recognize that personal food choices may be influenced more by product labels and advertising that emphasize taste than nutritional value. Consider a recent experiment that found that taste-focused labels (e.g., "Ambrosial Zucchini a l'Italienne") increased vegetable intake more than health-focused labels that simply listed the ingredients of vegetable dishes (e.g., "zucchini, bread crumbs, Parmesan"). The research was conducted at private and public university dining halls across the United States—in the West, the Northeast, and the South (Turnwald et al., 2019). There were some 135,000 students in total, half of whom were female, and various racial and ethnic groups were represented in the study sample (Turnwald et al., 2019).

In the experimental manipulation, health-focused labels that touted the nutritional values of the vegetables competed with taste-focused labels, many of which were products of vivid and even poetic imaginations.

- "Herb n' Honey Balsamic Glazed Turnips" vs. "Healthy Choice Turnips"
- "Sizzlin' Szechuan Green Beans with Toasted Garlic" vs. "Nutritious Green Beans"

The psychologists used exciting words ("twisted," "splashed") as additional cues to action, indulgent words ("glazed," "mouthwatering"), traditional words ("old-fashioned," "Mama's"), and location-based words ("New Orleans," "Thai"). All of these themes boosted expectations of an enjoyable taste experience.

Figure 7.2 shows that students at School A (a private Western suburban university) selected and ate significantly more of the taste-focused vegetables. Students at all schools were also asked to indicate their taste expectations of vegetable dishes based on the label, using a scale that ranged from 1 ("not at all delicious") to 5 ("very delicious"). Again, the foods with the taste-focused labels were associated with greater expectations of positive taste experiences. The message is that food choices and expectations about the tastiness of foods may be influenced more strongly by referencing taste than health.

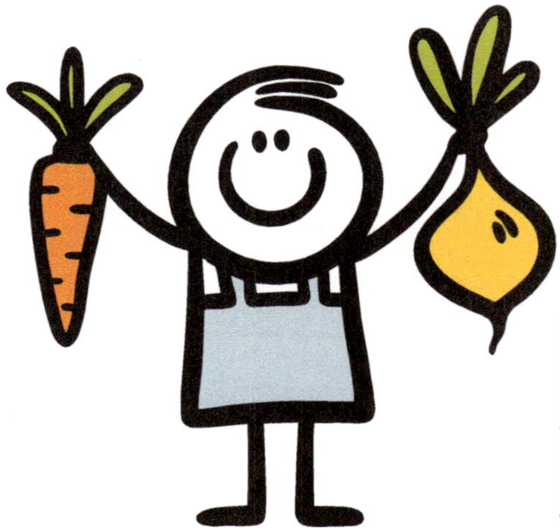

ekapanova/ Getty Images

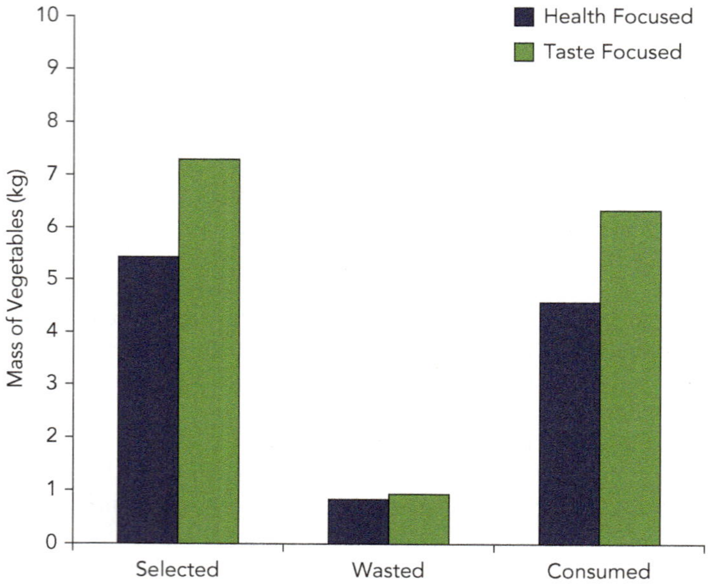

FIGURE 7.2 Mean vegetable mass (in kilograms, kg) selected, wasted, and consumed per day at School A in the Turnwald multisite study for each labeling condition. Error bars represent 95% confidence intervals of the estimate for each condition.

Source: Adapted from Turnwald et al. (2019, p. 1608).

food warning labels include those that point to health risks posed by sugar-sweetened beverages, caffeinated energy drinks, and energy-dense (read high calorie) snacks. A recent review article of scientific evidence showed that in laboratory settings, warning labels decreased choices of unhealthy foods and alcohol products by about 25% (Clarke et al., 2020). The problem is we don't yet know whether such effects apply to the real-world, that is, to the supermarkets where people make their food and beverage choices. But this is a reminder to us all to pay attention to food warning labels, as they are meant to help guide us to make more nutritious and healthier choices.

Review 7.2

INTERACTIVE SELF-SCORING QUIZZES

Sentence Completion

1. _____ are amino acids that build muscle, blood bones, fingernails, and hair.

2. The nutrient _____ provides the body with energy.

3. _____ provide stamina, insulate us from extremes of temperature, nourish the skin, and store vitamins.

4. Vitamin _____ is found in orange produce, such as carrots and sweet potatoes, and in deep green vegetables.

5. Many starches are rich in dietary _____, which aids digestion and may protect us from heart disease.

Think About It

Do you pay attention to the nutrients in your diet? Which nutrients do you eat in excess, if any, and might you profit from increasing your intake of one or more other nutrients?

Health Challenges of Excess Weight

More Americans are overweight or obese than ever before. Nearly 70% of adult Americans are overweight, and about 42% of adults are obese (Elmaleh-Sachs et al., 2023; Hales et al., 2020; Ogden et al., 2020). If current trends continue, it is estimated that half the U.S. population will be obese by 2030 (Ward et al., 2019). **Figure 7.3** shows the trends in obesity and severe obesity over the past two decades for adults aged 20 and above. **Figure 7.4** shows the prevalence of obesity in the United States by sex and by race/ethnicity. Asian Americans are least likely to be obese. Non-Hispanic Black Americans are most likely to be obese.

The prevalence of obesity *decreases* with level of education (Adult Obesity Prevalence Maps, 2019; see **Table 7.4**). Age is also a factor. Young adults aged 18–24 years have the lowest prevalence of obesity (18.1%), and adults aged 45–54 have the highest prevalence (36.9%) (Adult Obesity Prevalence Maps, 2019).

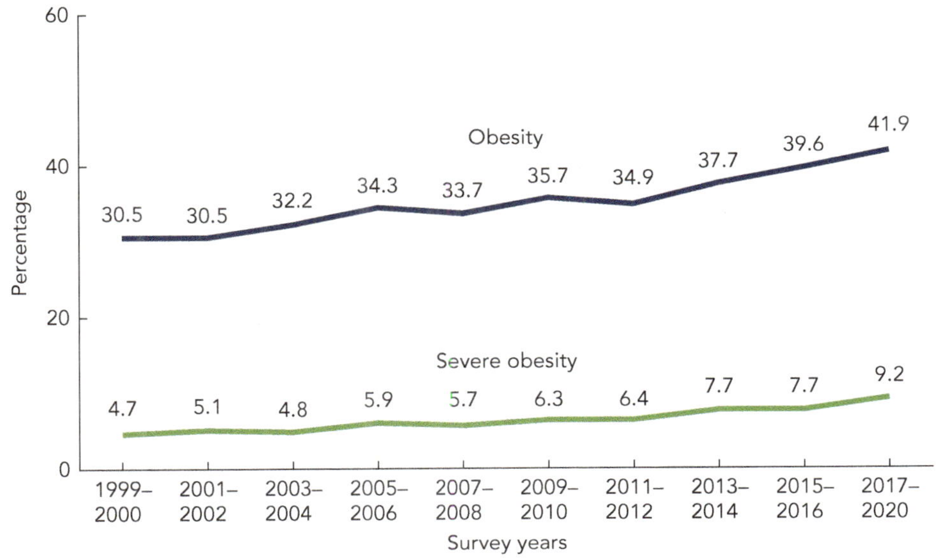

FIGURE 7.3 Trends in Obesity and Severe Obesity Among Adults Aged 20 and Over Obesity is defined as a body mass index (BMI) of 30 or above. Severe obesity is defined as a BMI of 40 or above.[1]

Sources: https://www.cdc.gov/nchs/data/databriefs/db360-h.pdf; CDC, Overweight and Obesity, 2022. https://www.cdc.gov/obesity/data/adult.html / Centers for Disease Control and Prevention / Public Domain.

LDL (bad) cholesterol Acronym for low-density lipoprotein, a combination of lipids (fat) and protein, which collects on the walls of blood vessels, potentially causing blockages and coronary heart disease.

HDL (good) cholesterol Acronym for high-density lipoprotein, a combination of lipids and protein with a high proportion of protein, which cruises in the bloodstream and removes LDL, thereby reducing the risk of CHD.

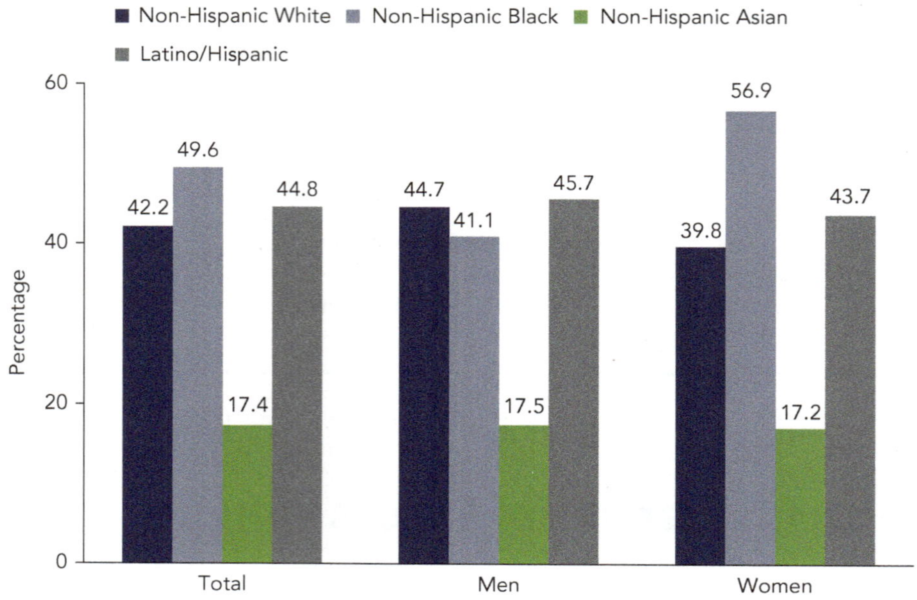

FIGURE 7.4 Obesity Among Adults by Sex and Race/Ethnicity, in Percentages

Source: https://www.cdc.gov/nchs/data/databriefs/db360-h.pdf / Centers for Disease Control and Prevention / Public Domain.

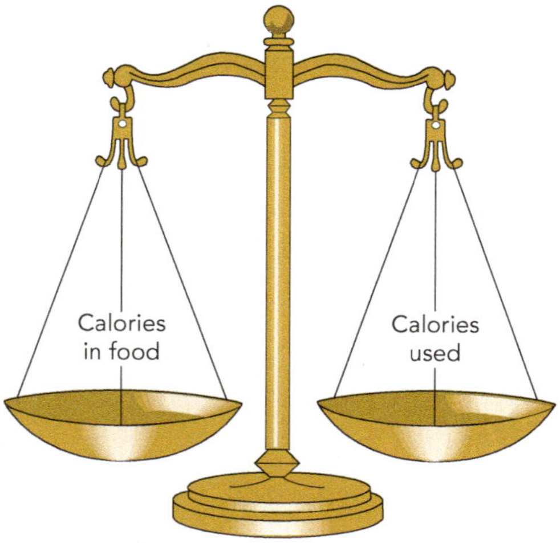

FIGURE 7.5 Weight: A Balancing Act Our body weight is determined by the balance between calories (food energy) consumed and calories used in the course of the day.

Source: Modified from National Institutes of Diabetes and Digestive and Kidney Diseases (NIDDK). (n.d.). Physical activity and weight control. http://win.niddk.nih.gov/publications/physical.htm.

Why is obesity such a concern? From a health standpoint, it is not a matter of physical appearance. Obesity is a major health risk that reduces life expectancy by an average of 6–7 years (Sarwer & Grilo, 2020; Taksler et al., 2018). Obesity is linked with a wide range of serious, even life-threatening medical conditions as well as psychological disorders, including the following (Elmaleh-Sachs et al., 2023; Hadi et al., 2020; Jian, Cifu, & Sam, 2022; Lindberg et al., 2020; Sarwer & Grilo, 2020; Sharafi et al., 2020, and others):

- High blood pressure (hypertension)
- High **LDL (bad) cholesterol** and low **HDL (good) cholesterol**
- Type 2 diabetes
- Coronary heart disease (CHD)
- Stroke
- Gallbladder disease
- Osteoarthritis (a breakdown of cartilage and bone within a joint)
- Sleep apnea and breathing problems
- Some kinds of cancer, including cancers of the endometrium, breast, colon, kidney, gallbladder, and liver
- Lower quality of life
- Psychological disorders, such as depression and anxiety in both children and adults
- Chronic pain and difficulty with physical functioning

ANIMATION CONTENT

Environmental Factors in Eating and Obesity

Determinants of Obesity

Why are so many Americans overweight and obese? The answer is simple enough—we take in too many calories and engage in too little vigorous activity. And did you know that living in the suburbs increases the risk of obesity? The reason, health researchers believe, is an over reliance on the automobile and the corresponding reduction in walking and physical activity as compared with city-dwellers (Gordon et al., 2018).

TABLE 7.4 Prevalence of Obesity Among Adults by Level of Education

Percentage Who Are Obese	Level of Education
35.0	No high school diploma
33.1	High school graduate
33.0	Some college
24.7	College graduate

Source: C. M. Hales, M. D. Carroll, C. D. Fryar, & C. L. Ogden (2020). Prevalence of obesity and severe obesity among adults: United States, 2017–2018, *NCHS Data Brief No. 360,* February 2020 / U.S. Department of Health & Human Services / Public Domain.

Health Psychology in Action

Fat Shaming

In her book *Fat-Talk Nation*, Susan Greenhalgh (2015) reminds us that in the wake of the 9/11 attack, which brought the World Trade Center down, the Surgeon General of the United States said that the rise in the prevalence of childhood obesity was "every bit as threatening to us as is the terrorist threat we face today." If the attack on the World Trade Center represented the threat from without, childhood obesity was "the threat from within" (p. 8).

Childhood obesity poses a significant health threat to children and sets the stage for obesity later in life. Moreover, children and adolescents who are overweight or obese are often taunted by peers in the form of fat shaming. Greenhalgh (2015) refers to fat shaming as a form of "biobullying" and states that biobullying is found not only among peers in school and on the playground. It is also perpetrated by teachers and parents. Nor is fat shaming limited to children. It is also practiced by adults and even healthcare professionals who express concern about the physical well-being of their patients but sometimes voice or imply disgust toward those who are obese (Kasardo & McHugh, 2015; Kinzel, 2018). Further reinforcing the need for the slender body are all the forms of media—television, films, print ads, brochures—showing "perfect" bodies (Lupton, 2017; Stanford et al., 2018). The TV reality show *The Biggest Loser* rewards people for shedding pounds, not for their self-worth as individuals.

Fat shaming is everywhere in our society and—in fact—in many parts of the world (Brewis et al., 2018; Shehu et al., 2016). Individuals who intend to be helpful often feel that they are faced with a dilemma—how do they balance the psychological well-being of people who are overweight or obese with their desire to help them avoid the physical dangers of excess body weight (Cain et al., 2017)?

People who are obese may be at greater risk for some health problems than other people, but fat shaming is a health hazard in itself. Overweight and obese people commonly face discrimination and fat shaming (Dakkak, 2023; Gerend et al., 2022). Heavier people face a near constant barrage of offensive comments, social rejection, unwanted attention, and bullying. Like other forms of discrimination, weight-based discrimination is linked to a range of adverse health consequences, with evidence suggesting that it can increase both psychological problems (depression, substance abuse) and physical health problems, increasing the risk of diabetes and even heart attacks (Gerend et al., 2022). Discrimination in whatever form is stressful and carries the risk of negative health effects.

Fat shaming also discourages heavier people from visiting physicians; when they do muster up the courage for a visit, they are frequently subject to misdiagnoses because many symptoms are attributed to excess weight rather than to other potential causes that go overlooked (Chrisler & Barney, 2017).

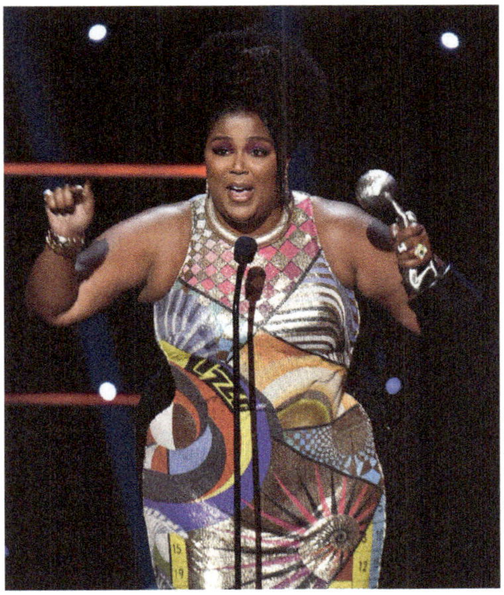

Aaron J. Thornton/Getty Images

Lizzo Accepts Entertainer of the Year Award During the 51st NAACP Image Awards. Many activists point out that real women (and real men) have curves and that it is basic to a person's self-esteem to be able to embrace their body.

In an effort to fight fat shaming, many contemporary authors and television talk-show hosts speak about the need for people of different shapes and sizes to adopt positive attitudes toward their bodies. According to a *Psychology Today* article (Schreiber, 2016), nearly half of the users of the Whisper app suggest that heavy people supporting each other is one of the best ways to cope with fat shaming. About 3 in 10 users of the app say that more attention needs to be paid to oversized models, and about 1 in 4 says the media should hire people of all sizes. Four in 10 users of the app say that heavy people should wear "great clothes" and tell themselves that they are "awesome" (25.3%). Even the swimsuit issue of *Sports Illustrated* has begun to use some plus-sized models.

Body weight is basically a balancing act between calories consumed and calories expended through physical activity and maintenance of bodily processes (see **Figure 7.5**). When calorie intake exceeds calorie expenditure, we gain weight. To lose weight, we need to reduce the number of calories consumed or increase the calories expended. Maintaining a stable weight involves balancing calories consumed with calories used.

body mass index (BMI) A widely used measure of weight that takes into account a person's height.

How would you characterize your own height and body shape? Health authorities gauge overweight and obesity by a measure called the **body mass index (BMI)**, which considers a person's weight as it relates to their height (see **Figure 7.6**). The same chart applies to women and men. The National Institutes of Health classifies people with a BMI of 25–29 as overweight. Those with a BMI of 30 or higher are classified as obese (see Figure 7.6). The causes of obesity are complex and involve many factors, including biological and psychosocial factors (Golding et al., 2022). Let's take a closer look.

Biological Factors Excess body weight is a complex issue with multiple causes. Evidence from kinship studies, including twin studies and adoption studies, shows that heredity plays a major role in determining body weight (Qasim et al., 2018; Roy et al., 2018). Some people may inherit a tendency to burn up extra calories, whereas others may inherit a tendency to turn extra calories into fat.

fat cells Cells that contain fat; known more technically as adipose tissue.

Genetics is an important major factor in overweight and obesity (Karlsson Linnér et al., 2021). However, genes do not tell the whole story. Environmental factors (diet and exercise patterns) are also major contributors. Another factor undermining efforts of overweight people to manage their weight is a form of internal sabotage by microscopic units of life called **fat cells**. No, fat cells are not cells that are overweight. They are *adipose tissue*, or cells that store fat. As time passes after a meal, blood glucose concentrations drop. Fat is then drawn from fat cells to provide further nourishment. The hypothalamus detects the depletion of fat from fat cells, as well as the falling of blood sugar levels, and triggers the hunger drive. Overweight people have more fat cells—many billions more—than people of normal weight (Barquissau et al., 2018; Serbulea et al., 2018). People with more adipose tissue (fat cells) than others feel food-deprived earlier, even though they may be equal in weight. This might occur because more fat-depletion signals are sent to the brain from the body's fat cells. Unfortunately, when we lose weight, we do not lose fat cells; they just sort of shrivel up. Thus, many people who have lost weight complain that they are always hungry when they try to maintain normal weight levels (MacLean et al., 2015).

calories Food energy; scientifically, units expressing the ability to raise temperature or give off body heat.

adaptive thermogenesis A cluster of metabolic, endocrine, and autonomic nervous system responses that attempt to maintain stores of body energy at a consistent "ideal" level despite changes in calorie consumption.

Fatty tissue also metabolizes ("burns") food more slowly than muscle does. People vary in the rate at which their bodies convert **calories** to energy, largely as a result of genetic differences. In addition, people who carry excess body weight—who have a high fat-to-muscle ratio—metabolize food more slowly than people of the same weight with a lower fat-to-muscle ratio. That is, two people who are identical in weight may metabolize food at different rates, depending on the distribution of muscle and fat in their bodies. People who are obese therefore are doubly handicapped in their efforts to lose weight—not only by their extra weight but also by the fact that much of their body is composed of adipose tissue.

The efforts of overweight people to maintain a slender profile may be further hindered by an adaptive mechanism that would help preserve life in times of famine—**adaptive thermogenesis**. This mechanism involves survival mechanisms in the autonomic nervous system and the endocrine system that cause the body to expend less energy (burn fewer calories) when calorie intake from food consumption is reduced (as when people diet) (Bray & Bouchard, 2014; de Oliveira et al., 2017). This does not mean that people who restrict their calorie intake will not lose weight; it *does* mean that losing weight might take longer than expected and be quite frustrating at times. Adaptive thermogenesis might have aided the survival of ancestral humans who had to endure times of famine, but it has become a liability to people who attempt to lose weight and

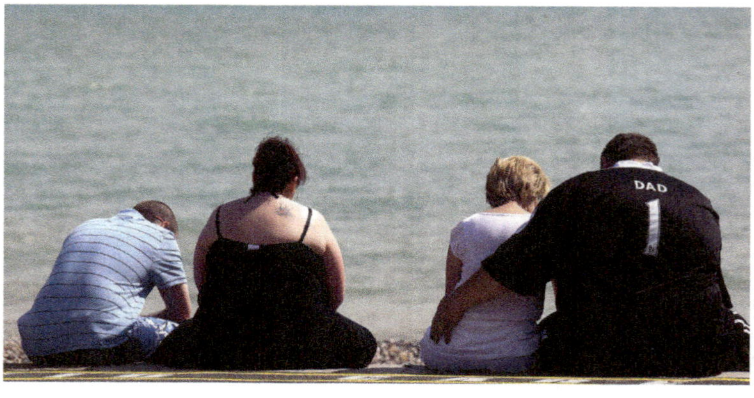

Neil Setchfield/Alamy Stock Photo

All in the Family? Genetic factors play an important role in overweight and obesity, but so do a sedentary lifestyle and a diet high in calories and saturated fats.

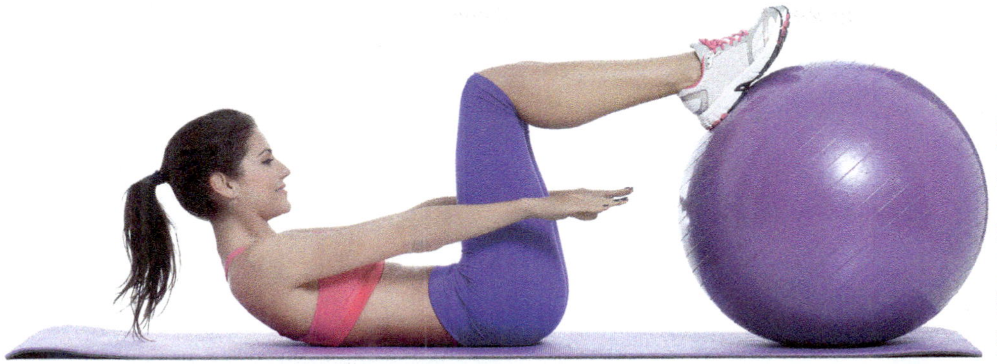

Mihai Blanaru/Alamy Stock Photo

Height (inches)	BMI 19	20	21	22	23	24	25	26	27	28	29	30	31	32	33	34
58	91	96	100	105	110	115	119	124	129	134	138	143	148	153	158	162
59	94	99	104	109	114	119	124	128	133	138	143	148	153	158	163	168
60	97	102	107	112	118	123	128	133	138	143	148	153	158	163	168	174
61	100	106	111	116	122	127	132	137	143	148	153	158	164	169	174	180
62	104	109	115	120	126	131	136	142	147	153	158	164	169	175	180	186
63	107	113	118	124	130	135	141	146	152	158	163	169	175	180	186	191
64	110	116	122	128	134	140	145	151	157	163	169	174	180	186	192	197
65	114	120	126	132	138	144	150	156	162	168	174	180	186	192	198	204
66	118	124	130	136	142	148	155	161	167	173	179	186	192	198	204	210
67	121	127	134	140	146	153	159	166	172	178	185	191	198	204	211	217
68	125	131	138	144	151	158	164	171	177	184	190	197	203	210	216	223
69	128	135	142	149	155	162	169	176	182	189	196	203	209	216	223	230
70	132	139	146	153	160	167	174	181	188	195	202	209	216	222	229	236
71	136	143	150	157	165	172	179	186	193	200	208	215	222	229	236	243
72	140	147	154	162	169	177	184	191	199	206	213	221	228	235	242	250
73	144	151	159	166	174	182	189	197	204	212	219	227	235	242	250	257
74	148	155	163	171	179	186	194	202	210	218	225	233	241	249	256	264
75	152	160	168	176	184	192	200	208	216	224	232	240	248	256	264	272
76	156	164	172	180	189	197	205	213	221	230	238	246	254	263	271	279

Body weight (pounds)

FIGURE 7.6 Body Mass Index The BMI is a measure of weight that takes height into account. To calculate your own BMI, first find your height and then move your finger across the table to find your weight. The number in the top row shows your BMI. Health authorities classify people with BMIs of 25–29 as overweight and those with BMIs of 30 or higher as obese.

avoid regaining it today. As the body inches downward toward the individual's desired range, the pounds may come off more and more slowly. Of course we can continue to shed pounds by continued exercise and calorie reduction, but it helps to understand what we are up against and why "the battle of the bulge" is so difficult for so many people.

Adopting the biopsychosocial model, health psychologists and other health professionals recognize the importance of environmental and psychosocial factors roles in determining excess body weight. Adults and children in the United States are exposed to thousands of food-related environmental cues, such as commercials for fast-food restaurants that emphasize high-fat menu selections. Environmental cues can trigger hunger even when our bodies are satiated. Maintaining a healthy weight may also be impeded by stress and negative emotions such as depression and anxiety, which can serve as cues leading to excess eating or bingeing (Tomiyama, 2019).

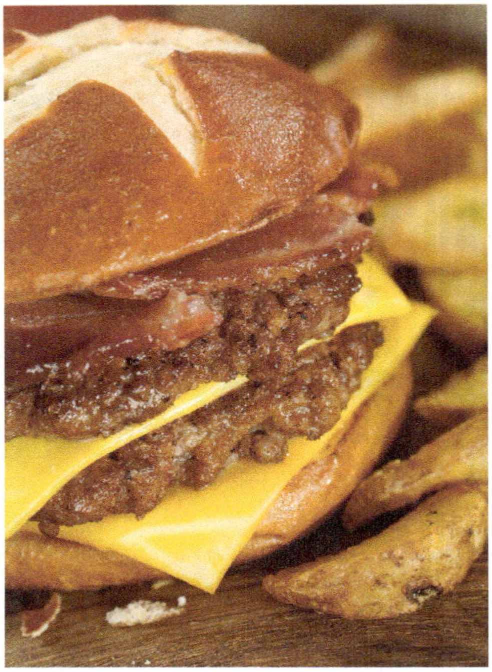

LauriPatterson/E+/Getty Images

Restaurants today are using larger dinner plates and piling on the food, pizzerias are using larger pans, and fast-food restaurants are offering huge soft drinks that pack 800 calories into a 64-ounce cup! (New York City recently passed a law restricting "supersizing" of sugary drinks.)

Unfortunately, people generally eat larger amounts of food when it is served in larger portion sizes (Keenan et al., 2018; Keller et al., 2018). Even the size of the plate can affect food intake. A study showed that people dining at a Chinese buffet who were given large plates ate—now get this—45% more food than those who were given smaller plates (Wansink & van Ittersum, 2013).

Ever notice how well lit supermarkets are? Or that you need to walk to the back of the store even if the only thing you need is a container of milk? Or that high-calorie snacks are usually positioned at a child's eye level at the checkout counter?

None of these environmental factors are random. Health psychologists recognize that supermarkets are carefully designed shopping environments intended to get you to buy in abundance, especially tempting but unhealthy snacks and other high margin products. Well, health psychologists are seeking to turn the tide in favor of healthier nutrition. For example, in one study, researchers were able to increase purchases of healthy snack foods in a café by posting signs highlighting healthier snack options at point of purchase locations (Allan, Johnston, & Campbell, 2015). Other health psychologists reviewed evidence on whether healthier purchases can be influenced by various in-store interventions (Golding et al., 2022). They found that what didn't work was simply providing nutritional information about products. What seemed to work better are price promotions and discounts for healthier food choices as well as prompts or cues, such as shelf tags that highlight healthier food choices.

Media exposure to tasty foods also influences food choices. Recently, health psychologists analyzed 244 top-grossing Hollywood movies released from 1994–2018 (Turnwald et al., 2022). They found the foods that characters consumed and seemed to like typically were unhealthier food choices (greasy fries, anybody?).

Might obesity be catching? Might it be a kind of social disease? Well, not quite. But evidence shows that obesity tends to be shared among people in social networks involving friends, neighbors, spouses, and family members (Datar et al., 2020; Smith et al., 2020). The people with whom we interact in our social networks may influence how much we eat, and what we eat, and affect our judgments about the acceptability of obesity. Investigators suspect that social networks may be an even stronger determinant of obesity than genes (Barabási, 2007).

What's the bottom line on maintaining a healthy weight? Health experts suggest that quickie fad diets and weight-loss pills are not the answer to long-term weight management (Hensley, 2018). They recommend, instead, making healthy eating and exercise habits a part of one's lifestyle so that calories consumed are balanced by calories expended through exercise and daily activities (Butryn et al., 2021; Hill et al., 2023; Wadden, Tronieri, & Butryn, 2020; Yanovski & Yanovski, 2021).

Health Psychology in the Digital Age

Texting Your Way to a Slimmer Figure

A health psychology study at Duke University used texting to help people keep tabs of their weight-loss efforts (Steinberg et al., 2013). Each morning, participants in a weight-loss program received a text that prompted them to enter the number of steps they had taken the previous day (the target was 10,000 steps as measured by a pedometer), along with the number of sugary drinks they consumed and whether they ate at a fast-food restaurant. Based on this input, participants received a personalized reply with a weight control tip for the day. The researchers found that texting was a convenient way of helping participants stay on track. More than 85% of participants texted every day, and most said that texting was easy and helped them meet their program goals. If you are committed to a weight-loss goal, you might look for a program that provides this type of personalized feedback, or you can check out apps to download to help you keep track of your daily food intake and physical activity.

Review 7.3

INTERACTIVE SELF-SCORING QUIZZES

Sentence Completion

1. About _____ adults in three in the United States are overweight or obese.

2. The body _____ index is a measure of whether one's body weight is too low, in the normal range, or overweight or obese.

3. A BMI of above _____ is considered obese.

4. Obese people are subjected to _____ shaming by society and, often, by their own physicians.

5. People gain weight when they take in more __________ than they "burn."

6. A small structure in the brain, the __________, detects fat depletion and triggers the hunger drive.

7. The mechanism of adaptive __________ causes the body to produce less energy (burn fewer calories) when someone restricts food intake.

Think About It

Where do you fit in on the BMI chart? How do you feel about it? What about your family and friends? What factors appear to have contributed to your body shape and your weight?

Health Psychology Theories Applied to Weight Control

Health psychologists suggest that weight management does not require drastic and dangerous fad diets, such as fasting, eliminating all carbohydrates, or emphasizing specific foods, such as grapefruit or rice. Successful weight management can be achieved based on applying principles embedded in theoretical frameworks in health psychology, especially the Theory of Planned Behavior, social cognitive theory, and the operant conditioning model (Macready et al., 2018; Wadden et al., 2020):

- The *Theory of Planned Behavior* (TPB) focuses on understanding intentions to act in changing one's dietary and exercise habits. Intentions can be influenced by providing information about the connections between diet and health and about the consequences of unhealthy diets. Evidence shows that providing nutritional knowledge can have beneficial effects on efforts to control weight (Pillai et al., 2019). The TPB also recognizes that our expectations of whether other people, such as friends and family members, will approve of our weight control efforts have an important bearing on our intention to carry through on a weight-loss plan.
- *Social cognitive theory* focuses on the social context of behavior, including the need for social support for behavioral change, and encouragement to change. Both the TPB and social cognitive theory stress the importance of positive beliefs that one can change one's behavior for the better (i.e., self-efficacy). Behavior can be changed by setting weight-loss goals, self-monitoring (keeping track) of one's efforts toward achieving those goals, and making smarter food choices to meet these goals (Garcia-Silva et al., 2018). Evidence supports the value of self-monitoring for improving dietary quality and weight management (Spring et al., 2021).
- The *operant conditioning model* focuses attention on identifying cues that trigger unhealthy eating (or healthy eating), the behaviors involved in eating (e.g., eating rapidly or pausing between bites), and the consequences or reinforcements that maintain patterns of eating (Garcia-Silva et al., 2018; Wadden et al., 2020).

Let us see how health psychologists apply these theories and principles to help individuals manage their own weight.

Putting Theory into Practice to Achieve Weight Control

These three theoretical models focus on setting reasonable goals, improving nutritional knowledge, decreasing calorie intake, exercising, modifying eating behavior, and tracking progress (Wadden et al., 2020). It has been shown that the methods help individuals adhere to their diets (Garcia-Silva et al., 2018; Wadden et al., 2020). Putting theory into practice involves examining eating habits and making changes in behavior. Here our focus is on setting reasonable goals and then changing the ABCs of eating behaviors to accomplish these goals.

Setting Reasonable Weight-Loss Goals Select a reasonable weight-loss goal. You can use the BMI chart (**Figure 7.6**) if you like, but your ideal weight also depends on your body composition—your muscle-to-fat ratio—because muscle weighs more than fat and burns more calories. That is why a running back in professional football can be 5'8" tall but weigh 190 lbs and look thin. Your physician may be able to help you assess your fat-to-muscle ratio by using (painless!) skinfold calipers as a measuring tool.

Psychologists recognize that gradual weight loss is generally more effective than crash dieting. Set a reasonable goal of losing about a pound or two a week and focus on the long-term outlook. Eating fewer calories is the key factor to weight loss, so we first need to do some simple math. One pound of body weight roughly equals 3,500 calories. As a rule of thumb, if you eat 3,500 more calories than your body requires to maintain its current weight, you will gain a pound or so. If you consume 3,500 fewer calories than you burn, you will lose a pound or so. That breaks down to about 500 calories daily you will need to shave off your baseline level to lose about a pound a week. How many calories do you burn in a day? Your calorie expenditure is a function of your activity level and, yes, of your weight. Gender and age figure in somewhat, but not as much.

The general guidelines in **Table 7.5** will help you arrive at an estimate of daily calories expended. Let's follow a hypothetical example of Alejandro, a rather sedentary office worker, through his day. He weighs 150 pounds. First, he records 8 hours of sleep a night. As we see in **Table 7.6**, that's 8 × 60, or 480 calories. He spends about 6 hours a day at the desk, for another 900 calories. He eats for about an hour (120 calories) and drives for an hour (143 calories). He admits to himself that he spends about 5 hours a day in quiet sitting, watching television or reading (525 calories). He has begun an exercise program of walking rapidly for an hour a day—that's 300 calories. Another couple of hours of desk work at home—working on his stamp collection and other hobbies (300 calories)—accounts for the remainder of the day. In this typical weekday, Alejandro burns up about 2,768 calories. If you weigh less than Alejandro, your calorie expenditure will probably be less than his, unless you are more active.

To lose weight, you need to take in fewer calories, burn more calories through vigorous physical activity, or do both. The information in **Table 7.5** can help you estimate the number of calories you burn each day.

To lower calorie intake, consult a calorie counter and a healthcare provider. The counter will provide calorie information to help you track your calorie intake. The healthcare provider can tell you how much you can safely reduce your calorie intake in light of your general health

TABLE 7.5 Calories Expended in 1 Hour According to Activity and Body Weight

	Calories Expended, by Body Weight (in Pounds)				
Activity	100	125	150	175	200
Sleeping	40	50	60	70	80
Sitting quietly	60	75	90	105	120
Standing quietly	70	88	105	123	140
Eating	80	100	120	140	160
Driving, housework	95	119	143	166	190
Walking slowly	133	167	200	233	267
Walking rapidly	200	250	300	350	400
Swimming	320	400	480	560	640
Running	400	500	600	700	800

TABLE 7.6 Approximate Number of Calories Burned by Alejandro* on a Typical Weekday

Activity	Hours/Day		Calories/ Hour		Subtotal
Sleeping	8	×	60	=	480
Desk work	6	×	150	=	900
Driving	1	×	143	=	143
Eating	1	×	120	=	120
Sitting quietly	5	×	105	=	525
Hobbies	2	×	150	=	300
Walking rapidly	1	×	300	=	300
Totals	24				2,768

*Based on a body weight of 150 pounds.

condition. Establish specific weight-loss plans, including daily calorie intake goals. If the daily goal sounds forbidding—such as consuming 500 calories a day fewer than you do now—you can approach it gradually. For example, reduce daily intake by, say, 100 calories for a few days or a week, then 200 calories, and so on.

Before cutting down on your calorie intake, you may wish to determine your calorie-intake baseline. Track the calories you consume throughout the day by jotting down the following:

- What you have eaten or drunk (everything that passes your lips)
- Estimated number of calories (use the calorie counter)
- Time of day, location, and activity

Your record may suggest foods that you need to cut down on or eliminate; places you should avoid; activities associated with unwanted snacking (such as talking on the telephone or watching TV); and times of day, such as midafternoon or late evening, when you are particularly vulnerable to snacking. You can plan small, low-calorie snacks (or distracting activities) for these times so that you won't feel deprived and then go on a binge.

Once you have established your baseline, maintain a daily record of calories consumed throughout your weight-loss program. You may weigh yourself regularly (we suggest once a week), but use calories, not weight, as your guiding principle. By meeting your calorie reduction goals, your weight will eventually follow suit.

Health Psychology in the Digital Age

Calorie Counters

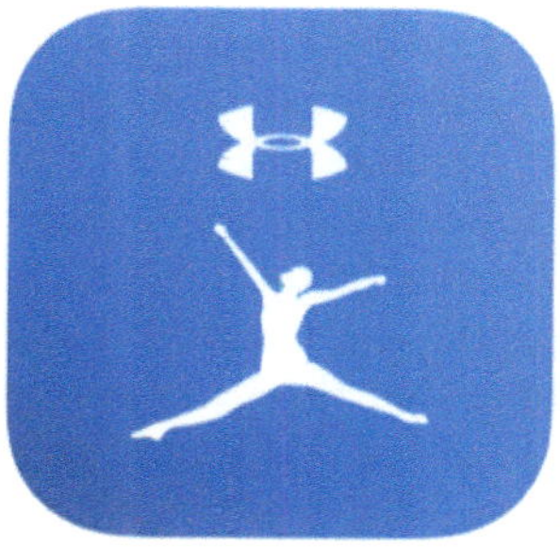

PREMIO STOCK/Shutterstock.com

There are many calorie-counting apps, and some also track your activity levels and link you to (endless) advice. MyFitnessPal has been rated positively by *Consumer Reports* (which makes no money from advertising) and *PC Magazine*. Like other apps of the type, it helps you track what you're eating, adds up the calories, and scans barcodes on food packages to access nutritional information. The database contains more than 6 million foods—a bit more than you're likely to need. Other calorie counters include

- Fitbit Built-In Calorie Counter
- Fooducate
- Lose it! (also an exercise log)
- Lifesum
- My Diet Coach
- MyPlate
- Calorie Count
- Jawbone UP
- Cron-o-meter
- SparkPeople

Modifying the ABCs of Eating

> **The odds of going to the store for a loaf of bread and coming back with only a loaf of bread are three billion to one.**
>
> **—Erma Bombeck**

The ABCs of weight control, as outlined in **Table 7.7**, put principles of operant conditioning into practice. They are designed to help people seeking to lose excess weight gain better control over the A's (the antecedent cues or stimuli that trigger problematic eating behaviors), the B's (problematic eating behaviors themselves), and the C's (the consequences of desirable and undesirable eating behaviors). Use these suggestions or rely on your ingenuity to develop your own strategies to modify your eating behaviors to achieve your weight-loss goals.

Diets

When people consider starting a diet, their knowledge of the connections between diet and health are of paramount importance. For most people, dieting simply means eating less so that they burn up more calories than they take in. Doing so will work, at least up to a point. Low-calorie diets tend to be effective at first, but long-term adherence and long-term effectiveness are more challenging (Koliaki et al., 2020). Remember that as you restrict your food intake, your body tends to go into adaptive thermogenesis; that is, you need fewer calories to retain your weight, so weight loss slows down or plateaus for a while.

The Weight Watchers Diet adopts a calorie-reduction approach but encourages users to consume a balanced diet along with foods that they actually want to eat, so that dietary changes become part of the person's lifestyle. Participants also attend Weight Watchers meetings in which people encourage each other and offer advice to help others surmount hurdles. The meetings alter the social context of eating for many dieters. The meetings provide information on how individuals can resist tempting treats and provide sources of social approval for weight control. Does the diet work? Evidence shows that people who adhere to the diet tend to lose weight (Koliaki et al., 2020).

Part of the rationale for following a low-fat diet is that a gram of fat has more than twice the calories of a similar weight of carbohydrates or protein. Fat, especially the kinds of saturated fats that are found in red meat, is also not heart-healthy (Zheng et al., 2019). Unfortunately, however, foods that are low in fat may not be as satisfying as those that are higher in fact—thus the cravings for meat, ice cream, and cookies experienced by many low-fat dieters. Cravings are also linked to cognitive dysfunction, as they can impair a person's ability to carefully assess longer-term consequences of overeating versus the immediate pleasures of consuming desirable foods (Gunstad et al., 2020). As with other diets, the ability to lose weight on a low-fat diet depends on the person's ability to stick with it. But therein lies the problem, as many people find it difficult to make these diets a regular part of their lifestyle.

ketogenic Giving rise to ketosis, a metabolic process that breaks down stores of fat in the body to obtain energy.

Then there are **ketogenic** diets, which are based on severely restricting the intake of carbohydrates, especially at first. The metabolic process, *ketosis,* breaks down stores of fat in the body when there is insufficient blood glucose circulating in the body. People on a ketogenic diet can eat the hot dog or the hamburger, but not the bun. They also must go easy on the ketchup. Ketogenic diets have been popular for half a century, but do they work? Yes. They actually seem to be more effective than low-fat diets in head-to-head comparisons (Li & Heber, 2020; Tobias et al., 2015). However, consuming foods high in cholesterol, especially red meats, raises blood levels of low-density lipoproteins (LDL), the "bad cholesterol" that increases the risk of cardiovascular disease (Zheng et al., 2019). People who advocate the diet argue that the increased LDL is more than offset by the reduction in weight. Researchers find that this is not necessarily the case (Mansoor et al., 2016; Tobias et al., 2015). It's important to first consult with a healthcare provider when considering ketogenic diets or other diets that alter the nutritional balance of the foods you consume.

TABLE 7.7 Strategies for Modifying the ABCs of Eating

Method	Strategy	Examples of Use of the Strategy
Changing the A's of Overeating—The *Antecedents* or Stimuli That Trigger Problematic Eating Behaviors		
Limit your exposure to cues that trigger overeating.	Controlling external stimuli associated with eating	• Avoid settings that trigger overeating. (Eat at The Celery Stalk, not The Burger Palace.) • Don't leave tempting treats around the house. • Serve food on smaller plates. Use a lunch plate rather than a dinner plate. • Don't leave seconds on the table. • Serve preplanned portions. Do not leave open casseroles on the table. • Immediately freeze leftovers. Don't keep them warm on the stove. • Avoid the kitchen as much as possible. • Disconnect eating from other stimuli, such as watching television, talking on the telephone, or reading. • Establish food-free zones in your home. Imagine there is a barrier at the entrance to your bedroom that prevents the passage of food.
Learn to cope with upsetting feelings in more constructive ways than overeating.	Controlling internal stimuli associated with eating	• Don't bury disturbing feelings in a box of cookies or a carton of ice cream. • Relabel feelings of hunger as signals that you're burning calories. Practice saying to yourself "It's OK to feel hungry. It doesn't mean I'm going to die or pass out. Each minute I delay eating, more calories are burned." • Practice relaxation or meditation when feeling tense rather than turning to food.
Changing the B's of Overeating—Changing Problematic *Behaviors* Related to Consumption of Food		
Put your fork down after every bite to allow your brain to catch up to your stomach.	Slow down the pace of eating	• Put down utensils between bites. • Take smaller bites. • Chew thoroughly. • Savor each bite. Don't wolf each bite down to make room for the next. • Take a break during the meal. Put down your utensils and converse with your family or guests for a few minutes. (Give your rising blood sugar level a chance to signal your brain.) • When you resume eating, ask yourself whether you need to finish every bite. If the answer is no, stop eating.
Prepare a shopping list before grocery shopping.	Modify shopping behavior	• Shop from a list. Don't browse through the supermarket. • Shop quickly. Don't make shopping the high point of your day. • Treat the supermarket like enemy territory. Avoid the aisles containing junk food and snacks. If you must walk down these aisles, put on mental blinders and look straight ahead. • Never shop when hungry. Shop after meals, not before.
Substitute a nonfood activity for a food activity.	Competing responses	• Substitute non-food-related activities for food-related activities. When tempted to overeat, leave the house, take a bath, walk the dog, call a friend, or walk around the block. • Substitute low-calorie foods for high-calorie foods. Keep lettuce, celery, or carrots in the middle of the refrigerator so they are available when you want a snack. • Fill spare time with non-food-related activities: volunteer at the local hospital, play golf or tennis, join exercise groups, read in the library (rather than the kitchen), take long walks.
Set a kitchen timer to delay snacking.	Chain breaking	• Stretch the overeating chain. Before allowing yourself to snack, wait 10 minutes. Next time wait 15 minutes, and so on. • Break the eating chain at its weakest link. It's easier to interrupt the eating chain by taking a route home that bypasses the bakery than to exercise self-control when you're standing in line waiting to place your order.
Changing the C's—or *Consequences*—of Overeating		
Reward yourself for meeting your calorie-reduction goals.	Self-reward	• Reward yourself for meeting weekly calorie goals by buying yourself small treats (not food!). • Reward yourself with gifts you would not otherwise purchase for yourself, such as a new sweater or tickets to a show. • Repeat the reward program from week to week. If you deviate from your dietary program, don't lose heart. Get back on track next week.
Punish yourself (mildly) for failing to meet calorie-reduction goals	Self-punishment	• Delay getting the new smartphone for a week or downloading a desired app for a week or a month. • Don't allow yourself to Facebook, Instagram, or Snapchat if you have not met your daily calorie goal. • Review the reasons you're controlling calorie intake for 5 minutes.

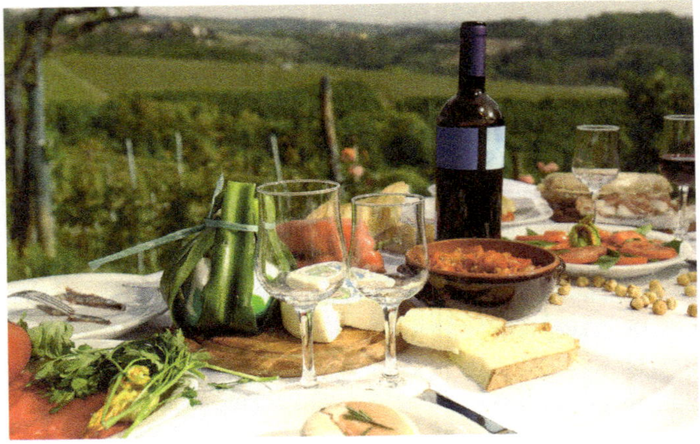

Image Source/Getty Images

Some Elements of the Mediterranean Diet. *Alla vostra salute!*

The Mediterranean diet derives its name from the food styles in Italy and Greece. It emphasizes plant-based foods, including whole grains, fruits and vegetables, nuts, and legumes. As noted at the beginning of the chapter, the diet replaces butter with olive oil or canola oil; it relies on herbs for flavor rather than salt; it focuses on fish and poultry—and on a glass of red wine. The weight-loss results are as impressive as those obtained following low-fat and low-carbohydrate diets, and the diet enhances heart health (Koliaki et al., 2020; Mayo Clinic, 2019b). Yes, you may crave some gelato, a cannoli, sfogliatelle (I'm taking a break and running to the kitchen!), or baklava, of course, but as the Greek philosopher Aristotle said, "Moderation in all things." The Mediterranean diet also lowers blood levels of LDL—that is, bad cholesterol (Michielsen et al., 2019; Sialvera et al., 2018).

Medical Approaches to Weight Control

metabolic rate The rate of metabolism, that is, the amount of energy used by an organism over a unit of time.

morbid obesity Obesity characterized by a BMI of 40 or above or at least 100 pounds of weight above that which is considered normal.

bariatric surgery Surgical techniques performed on the stomach or intestines, or both, to induce weight loss.

One of the great advantages to psychological methods is that they contribute to the development of self-efficacy. People who effectively modify their eating behaviors see themselves as being in charge of their behavior and capable of achieving their weight-loss goals. Some people may also benefit from using biomedical approaches to help them lose excess weight.

Weight-Loss Drugs and Medications There has been progress of late in the development of anti-obesity drugs, with five drugs now approved for use, including *semaglutide* (brand name Ozempic) (see Ge et al., 2020; Yanovski & Yanovski, 2021). Some people may find one or more weight-loss drugs to be helpful in weight management, at least in the short-term. People committed to healthy weight loss should discuss various choices with a healthcare professional. It also remains to be seen whether any of the newly approved drugs stand-up over time in helping people lose weight and keep it off.

Despite the continuing efforts to combat overweight and obesity through medication, many health experts recognize that the key to long-term success in losing excess weight and keeping it off requires lifestyle adjustments, including adopting a sensible, low-calorie but nutritionally sound diet and exercising regularly (e.g., Baer et al., 2020; Hill et al., 2023; Wadden et al., 2020, and many others). Health psychologists work with overweight and obese people to change their exercise and eating habits to foster long-term weight reduction.

Might coffee be of help in fighting the "battle of the bulge"? Caffeine is a stimulant drug found in coffee, tea, chocolate, and some other foods. As a stimulant, it may work as a mild appetite suppressant. It also boosts the **metabolic rate**, meaning that people burn calories more rapidly when they consume caffeine (Tabrizi et al., 2018). As with other stimulants, caffeine can also boost the heart rate and cause jitteriness and insomnia.

Green tea fans may be pleased to know that green tea, especially in the form of green tea extract, may boost the body's ability to metabolize fat, particularly in the abdomen (Alonso-Castro et al., 2019; Figueira, 2019). But green tea extract may cause constipation and also stomach pain and nausea.

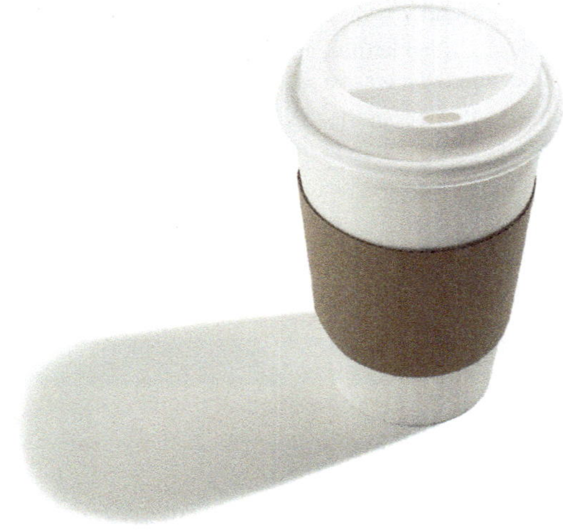

Big Pants productions/Alamy Stock Photo

Coffee for Weight Reduction? Why not? Coffee contains the stimulant caffeine, and stimulants not only boost the metabolic rate, they also suppress the appetite (unless you're used to having a doughnut with your morning brew).

Surgery Some people have **morbid obesity**, meaning that they weigh at least 100 pounds more than they should weigh or have a BMI of 40 or higher. The BMI standard may drop to 35 or above for people who have serious weight-related conditions such as (very) high blood pressure, type 2 diabetes (see Chapter 14), heart disease or stroke (see Chapter 12), or unrelenting GERD.

When weight-loss programs based on diet and exercise fail, **bariatric surgery** may be recommended. Bariatric surgery involves the use of various surgical procedures that either restrict the amount of food that a person's stomach can hold or that a person can absorb into the body. The procedures may reduce the size of the stomach by using a gastric band or removing part of the stomach. Gastric bypass surgery creates a small pouch from the stomach and connects the "new" pouch to the small intestine, which reduces the amount of food that is absorbed into the body (Figure 7.7).

Evidence shows that bariatric surgery not only leads to dramatic reductions in weight but also increases people's quality of life, both in adolescents and adults (Hachem & Brennan, 2016; Paulus et al., 2015). Other research shows that women who underwent bariatric surgery had lower rates of pregnancy-induced diabetes and high blood pressure during pregnancy (Kwong et al., 2018).

There are risks and drawbacks to bariatric surgery. There are risks of leakage where the cuts are made and the stomach pouch is joined to the intestine (Chang et al., 2018). There are other potential serious complications, even the risk (however rare) of subsequent heart attacks. Moreover, people who have had gastric bypass surgery show lower absorption of vitamins and need to take vitamin supplements for the rest of their lives (Chaktoura et al., 2016). It is important for a person considering bariatric surgery to carefully weigh the potential risks and benefits in consultation with a surgeon. It may also be advisable to seek a second opinion before undertaking a surgical procedure.

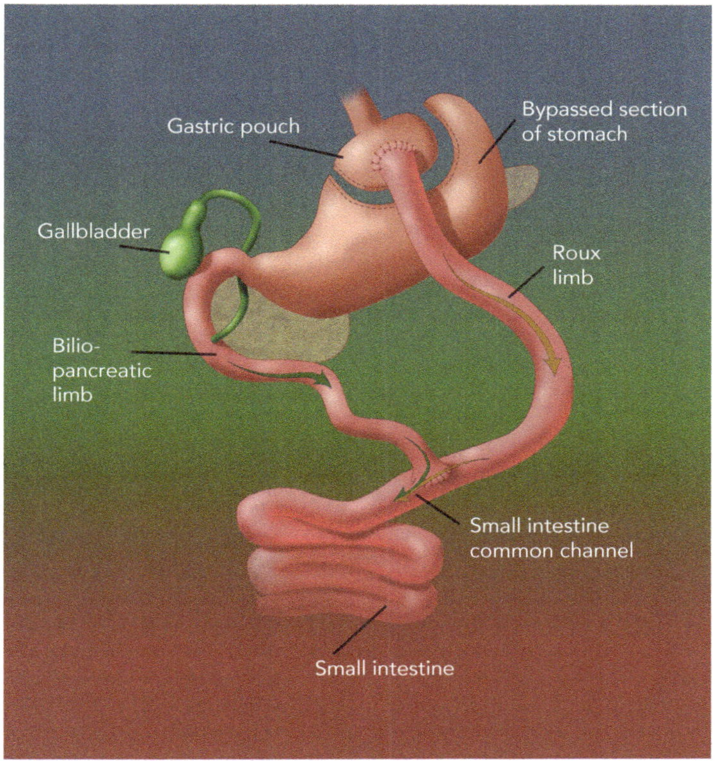

FIGURE 7.7 **Gastric Bypass Surgery** In this weight control method, a small pouch is created from the stomach, and food is directed from that pouch to the lower part of the small intestine, preventing absorption of the food by the larger part of the stomach and the upper part of the small intestine.

Review 7.4

INTERACTIVE SELF-SCORING QUIZZES

Sentence Completion

1. Healthy methods for weight control include setting reasonable __________, improving nutritional knowledge, decreasing calorie intake, exercising, modifying eating behavior, and tracking your progress.
2. One cognitive behavioral technique for eating less is to __________ external stimuli that are associated with eating.
3. The Atkins diet is an example of a low-__________ diet.
4. The __________ diet emphasizes, fruits and vegetables, nuts, whole grains, fish, and olive oil.
5. It is useful to pause when eating or to eat slowly to allow your rising blood __________ level to signal your brain.
6. Stimulants help people reduce or maintain their desired body weight by boosting the __________ rate.
7. Orlistat may help some people lose weight by impairing the absorption of dietary __________.
8. __________ tea extract may help people lose weight by boosting the body's ability to metabolize fat.
9. Bariatric surgery is sometimes recommended for people who are __________ obese and for whom diet and exercise have failed to produce positive results.
10. Gastric bypass surgery creates a small pouch from the __________ and connects the "new" pouch to the small intestine

Think About It

Have you tried to lose weight? If so, what have you tried? What has been effective? What has been ineffective? What suggestions in this section sound as if they might be helpful to you?

Eating Disorders

VIDEO CONTENT
Hunger and Eating

Did you know that dieting is now the normative pattern for young women in the United States? Young women today have come of age in an American culture obsessed with thinness, especially thinness in women. However, eating disorders are not normal; in many cases they arise from distorted eating behaviors that are grounded in excessive dieting or the pursuit of unrealistic standards of thinness. Two major types of eating disorders are *anorexia nervosa* and *bulimia nervosa*. According to recent estimates, eating disorders affect about 5% of women and about 2% of men in the United States (Attia & Guarda, 2022).

Anorexia and bulimia typically affect young women during adolescence and young adulthood, when social pressures to conform to an unrealistically thin ideal are at their peak. Estimates of the prevalence of these eating disorders vary widely across cultures and disproportionally occur in Western countries, including the United States and Canada. We should also recognize that a great many more people, men as well as women, develop problematic eating behaviors that are not severe enough to merit a diagnosis of an eating disorder. Eating disorders are disturbing in themselves, but they often co-occur with anxiety and depressive disorders (Brownell & Walsh, 2017; Levinson et al., 2017).

Anorexia Nervosa

There is a saying that you can never be too rich or too thin. We can't say whether you could ever be too rich (though we'd like to try it for a while), but, as in the case of Karen, we can certainly say that you can be too thin.

Karen was the 22-year-old daughter of a renowned English professor. She had begun her college career full of promise at the age of 17. But 2 years ago, after "social problems" occurred, she had returned to live at home and taken progressively lighter course loads at a local college. Karen had never been overweight, but about a year ago her mother noticed that she seemed to be gradually "turning into a skeleton."

Karen spent hours every day shopping at the supermarket, butcher, and bakeries as well as in the kitchen conjuring up gourmet treats for her parents and younger siblings. Arguments over her lifestyle and eating habits had divided the family into two camps. The camp led by her father called for patience. The camp headed by her mother demanded confrontation. Her mother feared that Karen's father would "protect her right into her grave" and wanted Karen placed in residential treatment "for her own good." The parents finally compromised on an outpatient evaluation.

At an even 5 feet, Karen looked like a prepubescent 11-year-old. Her nose and cheekbones protruded crisply. Her lips were full, but the redness of the lipstick was unnatural, as if too much paint had been dabbed on a corpse for the funeral. Karen weighed only 78 pounds, but she had dressed in a stylish silk blouse, scarf, and baggy pants so that not one inch of her body was revealed. More striking than her mouth was the redness of her rouged cheeks. It was unclear whether she had used too much makeup or whether minimal makeup had caused the stark contrast between the parts of her face that were covered with makeup and those that were not. Karen vehemently denied that she had a problem. Her figure was "just about where I want it to be," and she engaged in aerobic exercise daily. A deal was struck in which outpatient treatment would be tried as long as Karen lost no more weight and showed steady gains back to at least 90 pounds. Treatment included a day hospital with group therapy and two meals a day. But word came back that Karen was artfully toying with her food—cutting it up, sort of licking it, and moving it about her plate—rather than eating it. After 3 weeks, Karen had lost another pound. At that point her parents were able to persuade her to enter a residential treatment program where her eating could be carefully monitored.

—Authors' files

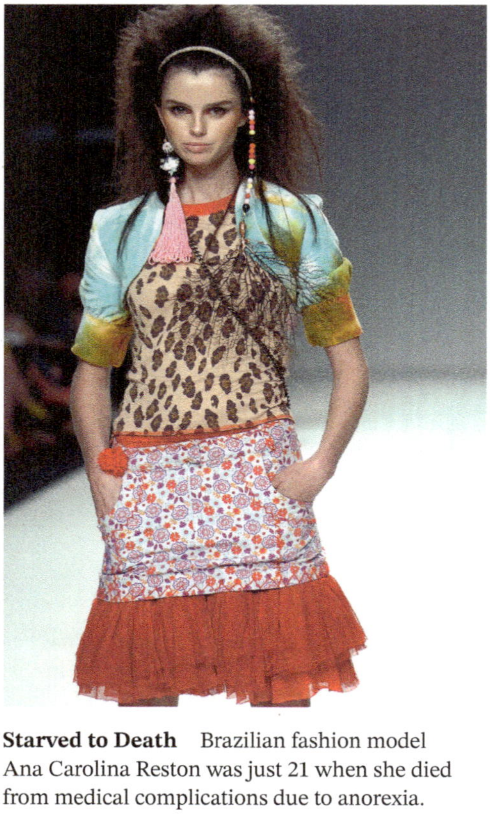

Fernanda Calfat/Getty Images Entertainment/Getty Images

Starved to Death Brazilian fashion model Ana Carolina Reston was just 21 when she died from medical complications due to anorexia. Unfortunately, the problem of anorexia and other eating disorders among fashion models is widespread, as it is in other situations in which pressure is imposed to attain unrealistic standards of thinness.

Karen was diagnosed with anorexia nervosa, a potentially life-threatening psychological disorder characterized by a pattern of self-starvation leading to a severely unhealthy body weight, and associated with an intense fear of being overweight and a distorted body image. The great majority of cases of anorexia, about three in four, occur among females, predominantly young women (Foreman, 2022).

Women with anorexia nervosa may lose 25% or more of her body weight in a year. They may become so emaciated that they succumb to medical complications (Mitchell & Peterson, 2020), as in the case of the Brazilian supermodel Ana Carolina Reston who died at the age of 21 (see nearby photo).) At the time of her death, the 5'7" woman weighed only 88 pounds. Unfortunately, this is not an isolated case. Anorexia nervosa is associated with higher death rates than any other psychological disorder (Foreman, 2022).

Sadly, between 5% and 20% of cases of anorexia nervosa result in death, either from suicide or malnutrition due to starvation (Bodell, Cheng, & Wildes, 2019; Franko et al., 2013). In the typical anorexic pattern, a young woman notices some weight gain after menarche (first period) and decides that it must come off. However, dieting—and often exercise—continues at a fever pitch, even after the girl reaches an average weight and even after family members and others tell her that she is losing too much weight. Girls with anorexia almost always adamantly deny that they are wasting away. They may point to their extreme exercise program as proof of their fitness. But their body images are distorted (Mitchell & Peterson, 2020). Others may perceive them as "skin and bones," but the women themselves frequently sit before the mirror and see themselves as still having unsightly pockets of fat.

Many people with anorexia become obsessed with food. They study cookbooks, take on the family shopping chores, and prepare elaborate dinners—for others.

Bulimia Nervosa

The case of Nicole is a vivid account of a young woman who was diagnosed with bulimia nervosa:

> *Nicole awakens in her cold dark room and already wishes it was time to go back to bed. She dreads the thought of going through this day, which will be like so many others in her recent past. She asks herself the same question every morning: "Will I be able to make it through the day without being totally obsessed by thoughts of food, or will I blow it again and spend the day [binge eating]"? She tells herself that today she will begin a new life, today she will start to live like a normal human being. However, she is not at all convinced that the choice is hers. It turns out that this day Nicole begins by eating eggs and toast. Then she binges on cookies; doughnuts; bagels smothered with butter, cream cheese, and jelly; granola; candy bars; and bowls of cereal and milk—all within 45 minutes. When she cannot take in any more food, she turns her attention to purging. She goes to the bathroom, ties back her hair, turns on the shower to mask any noise she will make, drinks a glass of water, and makes herself vomit. Afterward she vows, "Starting tomorrow, I'm going to change." But she knows that tomorrow she will probably do the same thing. (Adapted from Boskind-White & White, 1983, p. 29)*

Nicole's problem, bulimia nervosa, is characterized by recurrent cycles of binge eating followed by dramatic measures to purge the food. Binge eating frequently follows food deprivation—for example, severe dieting. Purging includes self-induced vomiting, fasting or strict dieting, use of laxatives, and/or vigorous exercise (Jin, 2022). Some people with bulimia purge only after a binge, but others purge regularly after meals.

Like those with anorexia, people with bulimia have an underlying fear of gaining weight and are typically unhappy with their bodies. But unlike anorexia, people with bulimia tend to be of average weight or overweight (Jin, 2022). The disorder typically begins in late adolescence as a young woman (the great majority of cases are found in young women) begins to practice compensatory behaviors to control her body weight, such as self-induced vomiting (Stice et al., 2021). A repetitive pattern becomes established in which binge eating alternates with periods of strict dieting. About 1.5% of adult women, and about 0.5% of adult men, are affected by bulimia nervosa (Jain & Yilani, 2023).

Like young women with anorexia, those with bulimia tend to hold perfectionistic views about body shape and weight and express unhappiness with their own body shape. But unlike women with anorexia, those with bulimia generally maintain a relatively normal weight level.

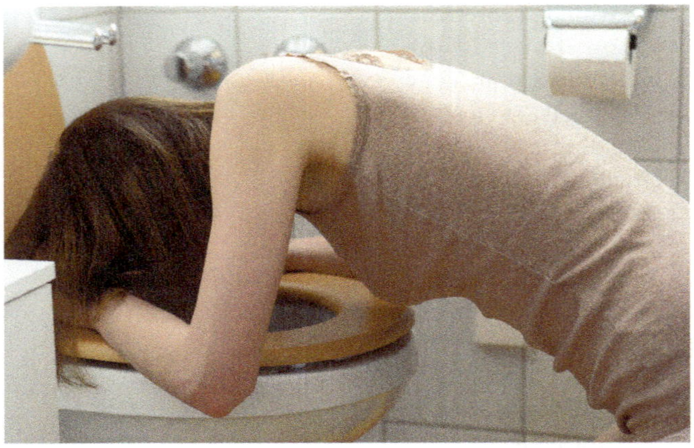
Michael Heim/Alamy Stock Photo

After the Binge The psychological disorder bulimia nervosa is characterized by recurrent cycles of binge eating and dramatic measures to purge the food, such as self-induced vomiting. Binge eating often follows strict dieting, and people with the problem—nearly all young women—tend to be perfectionistic about their body shape and weight.

Why Do People Develop Eating Disorders?

Understanding the roots of eating disorders is best approached from the biopsychosocial model, as the underlying causes are complex and involve biological and psychosocial factors, including body dissatisfaction (not liking your body), which is closely linked to social pressure to adhere to an unrealistically thin body ideal (Ordaz et al., 2018; Tatangelo & Ricciardelli, 2017). Some psychodynamic theorists suggest that anorexia represents a female's effort to revert to **prepubescence**. In this view, anorexia allows her to avoid growing up, separate from her family, and assume adult responsibilities. Because of the loss of fat tissue, her breasts and hips flatten. In her fantasies, perhaps, a woman with anorexia remains a child, sexually undifferentiated.

Adolescent girls may use refusal to eat as a weapon against their parents. Evidence points to disturbed relationships within the family in many cases. For example, parents of adolescents with eating disorders were relatively more likely to be unhappy with their family's functioning, to have problems with eating and dieting themselves, to think that their daughters should lose weight, and to consider their daughters to be unattractive (Brownell & Walsh, 2017). Adolescents may develop eating disorders as a way of coping with feelings of loneliness and alienation they experience in the home. Could binge eating symbolize the effort to gain parental nurturance? Does purging symbolically rid one of negative feelings toward the family?

prepubescence The years just prior to puberty.

Social cognitive theorists suggest that young women with anorexia set unreasonable demands on themselves in the pursuit of perfection, including what in their minds is the "perfect body" (Deas et al., 2011; J. Johnston et al., 2018). Yet "perfection" is an impossible goal, even for fashion models, who are themselves prone to develop eating disorders because of pressures to match an idealized image.

Many young women with eating disorders have issues of control as well as perfectionism (Egan et al., 2013; Menatti et al., 2013). These women may feel that eating is the only part of their lives over which they can exercise control.

Let's also take into account the larger sociocultural context. A revealing study showed that the quintessential U.S. role model, Miss America, has been slimming down over the years. Since the beginning of the pageant in 1922, the winner of the contest has gained 2% in height but lost 12 pounds in weight. In the 1920s her weight as compared to her height was in what is today considered the "normal" range, according to the World Health Organization (WHO)—that is, a BMI of 20 to 25. The WHO considers people with a BMI lower than 18.5 to

Health Psychology in the Digital Age

How Do I Shape Up ... on Facebook?

Facebook may be a great way to connect to others, but there is a psychological risk when you use it to compare yourself to others. A study of 232 college women tracked their Facebook use for about 4 weeks (Smith et al., 2013). Those who used Facebook to compare themselves with others showed higher levels of body dissatisfaction, which was linked to a greater frequency of bulimic symptoms and overeating. Another recent study of 960 college women found those who spent more time on Facebook showed higher levels of disordered eating (Mabe et al., 2014). The take-away message is that limiting use of Facebook may help reduce the risk of problems with body image and disturbed eating behaviors.

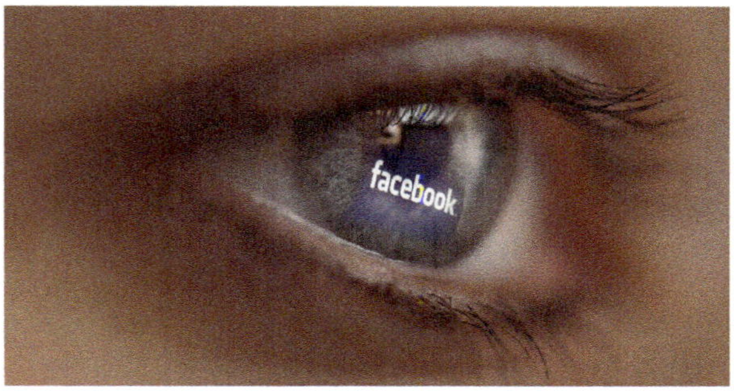

Bernhard Classen/Alamy Stock Photo

be undernourished, and many recent Miss Americas have had a BMI of about 17 (Rubinstein & Caballero, 2000). Miss America has become another undernourished role model. In 2018 the Miss America contest dropped its swimsuit competition, in part to help prevent young women from "joining the competition" by means of excessive dieting (Yahr, 2018).

As the cultural ideal slims down, women with average or heavier-than-average figures feel more pressure to shed pounds. Investigators found that 5- to 8-year-old girls exposed to images of Barbie dolls felt worse about their bodies and had a greater desire for a thinner body shape than did girls who were exposed to more realistically proportioned dolls (Dittmar et al., 2006). Another study compared body dissatisfaction among a sample 1,515 preadolescent children (Dion et al., 2016). They found that 50.5% of the girls wanted to be thinner as compared with 35.9% of the boys. More of the boys (21.1%) than the girls (7.2%) wanted a larger body shape. Of children who were weighed and measured as being underweight, 58% of girls (!) and 41.6% of boys were content with their bodies.

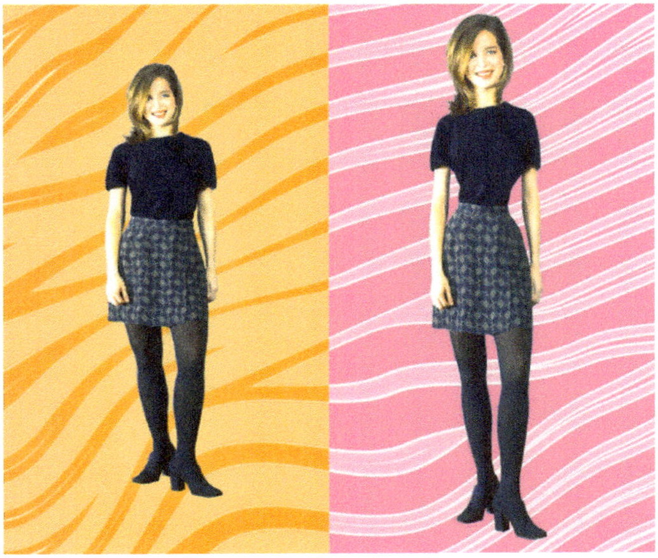

Oh, to Be Barbie? People recognize that the Barbie doll is an absurd representation of the female figure, yet it does suggest that women want or need to be tall, buxom, and slender. Were women's bodies to be proportioned like those of the Barbie doll, they would look like the figure on the right. To achieve those proportions, however, the slender woman on the left would have to gain a foot in height, slim her waistline by 5 inches, and add 4 inches to her bustline. Is this one of the reasons that women with normal bodies often think of themselves as being heavy?

Gender differences in weight perceptions also occur among college students. In a survey that reported data from 26,139 college students drawn from 52 schools, a greater percentage of college females believed they are either slightly or very overweight (39%) as compared with college males (31%) (American College Health Association, 2018) (see Table 7.8). Fifty-eight percent of the women respondents said they were trying to lose weight, as compared with only 34% of the men. For women in college, dieting is clearly the norm, despite the fact that at least in this sample, the majority of women (54%) said they were at about the right weight! That is, for some, the right weight is not good enough.

Eating disorders predominantly affect young women from Western cultures who are repeatedly exposed to images promoting an ultrathin feminine ideal, especially in the United States (Bell & Dittmar, 2011). Women ballet dancers are also at special risk of developing eating disorders. Eating disorders seem to be much less common among Black women and other minority women, for whom body image and body satisfaction are not tied as closely to body weight as they are among White women (Overstreet et al., 2010; Rodgers et al., 2018). For ethnic minority women, a strong positive ethnic identity is apparently protective against the "thinspiration" of the dominant culture (Rodgers et al., 2018).

Let's not lose sight of the fact that some men develop eating disorders. Many of these men compete in sports, such as wrestling and ice skating, or pursue dance or modeling, all of which place pressures on them to keep their weight within a limited range. Other factors linked to

TABLE 7.8 How College Students Describe Their Body Weight, in Percentages

	Male	Female
Very underweight	2	1
Slightly underweight	14	7
About the right weight	54	54
Slightly overweight	27	33
Very overweight	4	6

Source: Adapted American College Health Association. (2018). *American College Health Association—National College Health Assessment II—Reference Group Data Report*, Fall 2017. American College Health Association, 2018. Reprinted by permission of The American College Health Association. https://www.acha.org/documents/ncha/NCHA-II_FALL_2017_REFERENCE_GROUP_EXECUTIVE_SUMMARY.pdf.

eating disorders in men are excessive concerns about leanness and muscularity (Murray et al., 2020). Images in the media and on social media sites of overly masculinized men may lead to obsessive concerns about muscularity, which in some men may lead to disordered eating behaviors that set the stage for development of eating disorders (Murray et al., 2017; Seekis, Bradley, & Duffy, 2021).

Biological factors, such as genetic influences and brain mechanisms that control feelings of hunger and satiety, play roles in eating disorders. For example, irregularities in how the brain utilizes the neurotransmitter serotonin are implicated in bulimia, based in part on evidence that antidepressant drugs that increase the availability of the chemical often help curb bingeing episodes (Hildebrandt et al., 2010). The connection with serotonin is not surprising because the neurotransmitter functions like a behavioral seat belt in constraining impulsive behaviors—and bingeing certainly qualifies as an impulsive act.

Although eating disorders are difficult to treat and relapses are common, promising results have been reported in using psychological treatments and psychoactive medications. Cognitive behavioral therapy (CBT) has shown promise in helping patients challenge and change distorted beliefs about weight and body image and learn to tolerate dietary lapses without catastrophizing or bingeing (Agras & Bohon, 2021). One study, for example, found that cognitive behavioral therapy helped 42% of people with bulimia nervosa stop binge eating (Poulsen et al., 2014). Gains remained at a 2-year follow-up. However, treatment gains have proved more difficult with anorectic patients and evidence supporting the effectiveness of CBT in treating anorexia nervosa remains lacking (Agras & Bohon, 2021).

Medical treatments are also available, either with or without psychotherapy. Antidepressants are the most widely used. They increase the activity of the neurotransmitter serotonin in the brain, which tends to improve appetite in people with anorexia and may help people with bulimia control their urges to binge (e.g., Galsworthy-Francis, 2014; Mitchell et al., 2013; Thompson-Brenner, 2013). The mood stabilizer lamotrigine also holds some promise (Trunko et al., 2017).

Review 7.5

INTERACTIVE SELF-SCORING QUIZZES

Sentence Completion

1. Eating disorders are usually characterized by a _____ body image.

2. _____ nervosa is symptomized by cycles of binge eating and purging.

3. Irregularities in how the brain utilizes the neurotransmitter _____ are implicated in bulimia nervosa.

4. A study found that women who spent more time on Facebook were (more or less) likely to develop symptoms of eating disorders.

Think About It

Do you have any thoughts on why women are more likely than men to develop eating disorders? Do you know anyone with an eating disorder? What do they say about it?

Physical Activity

physical activity Any bodily movement produced by the contraction of skeletal muscles that increases the expenditure of energy.

exercise Planned, structured, and repetitive physical activity that is intended to produce fitness.

fitness A state of health, well-being, and ability to perform in sports and daily activities.

Physical activity refers to any bodily movement produced by the contraction of skeletal muscles that increases energy expenditure above a base level. **Exercise** is a type of physical activity that is planned, structured, repetitive, and performed in order to promote fitness, such as jogging, biking, or fast walking. All exercise fits within the definition of physical activity, but not all physical activity is exercise. Then, too, there is the concept of **fitness**. Fitness broadly refers to health, well-being, and the ability to perform in sports and daily activities. Fitness is gradually achieved by means of adequate nutrition, moderate to vigorous exercise, and sufficient rest.

Fitness is an essential component of a healthy lifestyle. We will see that becoming physically fit through regular exercise tones and builds muscles, increases stamina and flexibility, strengthens the heart, improves lung capacity, combats stress, helps relieve depression and anxiety, sheds excess pounds, and reduces the risk of serious health problems, such as coronary heart disease (CHD), diabetes, and even some forms of cancer. Regular exercise may even lengthen life. Exercise also gives you the energy and sense of well-being that you need to "keep on pushing" and meet the challenges of life.

Cardiovascular fitness means that the heart, lungs, and blood vessels are able to efficiently supply enough oxygen to the muscles to enable sustained exercise or physical activity. Fitness is not directly a matter of how strong you are or whether you can run an 8-minute mile. Rather, it is your body's ability to withstand stress and pressure. People who are physically fit are able to perform moderate to vigorous levels of physical activity without undue fatigue. If you can't climb the stairs to your office or walk uphill without losing your breath or exhausting yourself, consider yourself unfit.

USDHHS Guidelines for Physical Activity

The United States Department of Health and Human Services issued the following guidelines to Americans to help them reap the health benefits of regular physical activity (USDHHS, 2018):

Guidelines for Children and Adolescents Children and adolescents should be encouraged to participate in physical activities that are appropriate for their age, are enjoyable, and offer variety. One hour or more of daily moderate to vigorous physical activity is recommended for children and adolescents aged 6–17 years. The activity should be aerobic (using large muscle groups in sustained rhythmic activity) for at least 3 days a week and muscle-strengthening for at least 3 days a week. Some of the time should be spent in activity that also strengthens bones, such as running, lifting weights, jumping rope, gymnastics, tennis, and basketball.

Guidelines for Adults To obtain substantial health benefits, adults should engage in 150 minutes (2 hours 30 minutes) to 300 minutes (5 hours) a week of moderate-intensity, or 75 minutes (1 hour and 15 minutes) to 150 minutes (2 hours 30 minutes) a week of vigorous-intensity aerobic physical activity, or an equivalent combination of moderate- and vigorous-intensity aerobic activity. Aerobic activity is best spread throughout the week. Adults should also engage in muscle-strengthening activities that involve all major muscle groups on 2 or more days a week. For adults who cannot engage in recommended levels of activity, note that some physical activity is better than none. Table 7.9 shows the percentages of adults who meet the USDHHS guidelines.

Guidelines for Older Adults The guidelines for adults also apply to older adults. Older adults are also advised to engage in activity that includes balance training to help prevent falls as well as aerobic and muscle-strengthening activities. Examples of balance

TABLE 7.9 Percentages of U.S. Adults Aged 18 and Above Who ...

Activity	Percent*
Engage in no leisure physical activity	25.4
Meet minimum aerobic physical activity guideline—moderate intensity for ≥150 minutes/week or more, or vigorous intensity for ≥75 minutes/week	54.2
Meet high aerobic physical activity guideline—moderate intensity for >300 minutes/week or vigorous intensity for >150 minutes/week	37.4
Meet muscle-strengthening guideline—muscle-strengthening activities ≥2 days/week	27.6
Meet guidelines for aerobic physical activity and muscle-strengthening activity	24

Source: Adapted from Centers for Disease Control and Prevention (2020). Trends in meeting the 2008 Physical Activity Guidelines, 2008–2018. https://www.cdc.gov/physicalactivity/downloads/trends-in-the-prevalence-of-physical-activity-508.pdf / U.S. Department of Health & Human Services / Public Domain.
*For year 2018.

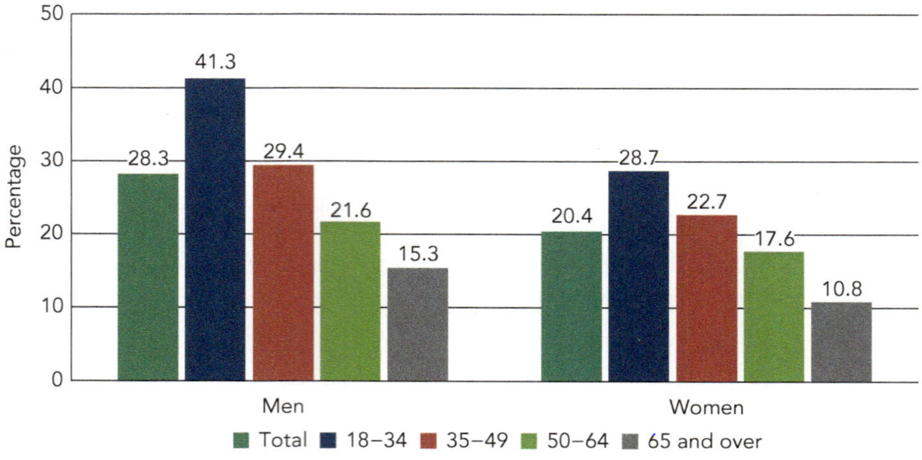

FIGURE 7.8 **Percentages of Adults Aged 18 and Above Who Meet Federal Guidelines for Both Aerobic and Muscle-Strengthening Leisure-Time Activity**

Source: National Center for Health Statistics, National Health Interview Survey, 2020 / U.S. Department of Health & Human Services / Public Domain.

training include yoga, tai chi, and balance classes. When older adults cannot do 150 minutes of moderate-intensity aerobic activity a week because of chronic conditions, they should be as physically active as their abilities and conditions safely allow.

Slightly more than half (54.2%) of American adults meet minimum guidelines for aerobic physical activity (see Table 7.9). **Figure 7.8** shows that men are more likely than women to meet minimum guidelines for both aerobic and muscle-strengthening activities and that male and female emerging adults (people aged 18–24 years) are most likely to do so. Then, not surprisingly, engaging in sustained physical activity drops off with age. Of the three largest racial and ethnic groups in the United States, non-Hispanic White people are most likely to meet the guidelines for both aerobic and muscle-strengthening activities, (see **Figure 7.9**).

The American College Health Association (2022) has also surveyed the extent of physical activity among its sample of college undergraduates, who mostly fall in the 18 to 22 age range. They found that 75.4% of the men and 67.9% of the women met the guidelines for aerobic activity (150 minutes of moderate physical activity or 75 minutes of intense physical activity per week). They also found that 54% of the men and 41.3% of the women engaged in both aerobic activity and strength training (two or more days per week of moderate or intense muscle strengthening).

Types of Physical Activity

The types of physical activity that contribute to our health include various kinds of exercise: aerobic exercise, muscle-strengthening exercise, exercise that enhances flexibility, and exercise that improves one's balance. Exercise may be used to build and maintain fitness and improve health. It is also used in physical rehabilitation, to help people manage and, when possible, overcome disabilities.

aerobic exercise Brisk, sustained exercise that makes demands on the heart and lungs to circulate more oxygen through the body, thereby strengthening the heart and lungs. (The roots of *aerobic* mean "with oxygen.")

Aerobic Exercise

Aerobic exercise refers to brisk, sustained exercises, such as jogging, rowing, swimming, or cycling, that promote the circulation of oxygen through the body and stimulate and strengthen the heart and lungs. When we are physically active, our heart and lungs need to work harder to supply oxygen-rich blood to our muscles. In people with good cardiorespiratory (aerobic) fitness, the heart and lungs are able to sustain vigorous activity for extended periods of time. If you can engage in vigorous whole-body activities, such as swimming, jogging, or walking briskly, for a period of at least 20 minutes without feeling overcome by breathlessness, consider yourself to have at least a moderate level of aerobic fitness.

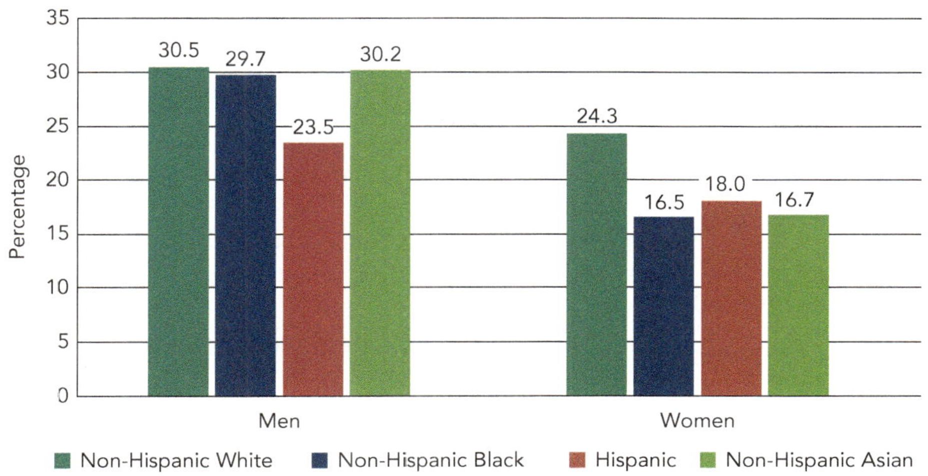

FIGURE 7.9 Percentages of Adults Aged 18 and Above Who Meet Federal Guidelines for Both Leisure-Time Aerobic and Muscle-Strengthening Leisure-Time Activity—by Race and Ethnicity

Source: National Center for Health Statistics, National Health Interview Survey, 2020 / U.S. Department of Health & Human Services / Public Domain.

According the USDHHS (2018), aerobic activity has three components: intensity, frequency, and duration. If your chosen exercise is jogging, that means that you should jog faster as time goes on, do it more frequently (as in four times a week rather than two), and for a longer amount of time (as in 40 minutes rather than 20). Aerobic exercises use large muscle groups in repetitive, rhythmic body movements. The heart pumps more rapidly to meet the needs of working muscles for increased supplies of oxygen. Muscles engaged in aerobic exercise may require as much as 10 times the amount of oxygen they need at rest. For example, if you are sitting quietly while reading this book, your heart is pumping about 5 quarts of blood through your body each minute, but if you were running around a track, your heart would need to pump at least 4 times as much blood, or 20 quarts or more, per minute. People in excellent aerobic condition, such as conditioned athletes, have a cardiac output as high as 30 quarts or more per minute. People who are aerobically fit have a resting heart rate below that of their less fit peers. The trained heart works more efficiently, even at rest. It can pump the same amount of blood with fewer beats.

Aerobic exercise also increases the rate at which the body metabolizes fat. This means that people who exercise aerobically burn more calories than those who don't, even when they're watching television. Beginners are advised to *start easy.* Whether you opt for jogging, cycling, or an aerobic dance class, don't overdo by making yourself breathless. Progress gradually. At first, perhaps, jog a quarter mile (a lap on a track) and then walk a quarter mile. After a few days or a couple of weeks, jog half a mile, and so on. Give your body time to adjust. No pain—yes, gain.

Table 7.10 provides examples of moderate and vigorous aerobic activities.

Muscle-Strengthening Activity

Muscle-strengthening activity includes resistance training and weight lifting. Like aerobic activity, it has three components (USDHHS, 2018): intensity, frequency, and—in this case—sets and repetitions. If you are lifting weights, intensity refers to the amount of resistance or weight (as in doing chest presses with 20 pounds or 40 pounds), frequency refers to the number of times you train, and repetitions and sets might mean two sets with 15 repetitions each, with a couple of minutes to rest between sets. As you progress, you will

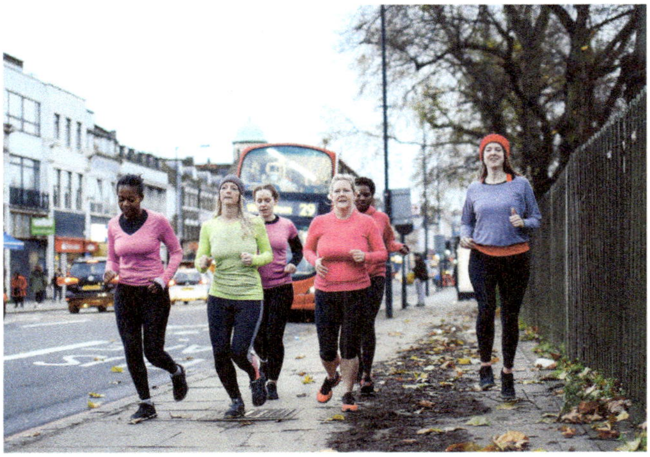

Cultura Creative (RF)/Alamy Stock Photo

Do I Jog Better "With a Little Help from My Friends?" Exercising with friends provides social and emotional support, which increase the probability of adherence.

TABLE 7.10 Examples of Moderate and Vigorous Aerobic Exercise

Moderate Aerobic Exercise	Vigorous Aerobic Exercise
1. Walking at a moderate or brisk pace (4–4.5 mph on a level surface)	1. Race-walking and aerobic walking (5 mph or faster)
2. Bicycling 5–9 mph on level terrain or with a few hills	2. Jogging/running
3. Light calisthenics	3. Swimming laps
4. Gymnastics	4. Bicycling (more than 10 mph or on a steep uphill climb)
5. Dancing (ballroom, line, square, folk, modern, disco, or ballet)	5. High-impact aerobic dancing or step aerobics
6. Tennis (doubles)	6. Tennis (singles)
7. Shooting baskets	7. Playing active sports (basketball, football, soccer, lacrosse, racquetball, ice hockey)
8. Using a stair-climber at a light-to-moderate pace	8. Cross-country skiing or downhill skiing (with vigorous effort)
9. Downhill skiing with light effort	9. Ice skating (fast pace or speed-skating)
10. Ice skating at a leisurely pace	10. Gardening (heavy or rapid shoveling, digging ditches, carrying heavy loads, or felling trees)
11. Gardening and yard work (raking, digging, hoeing, light shoveling, weeding while standing or bending)	

Exercise Benefits in CVD: Key Points - American College of Cardiology. (2023, April 10). American College of Cardiology. https://www.acc.org/Latest-in-Cardiology/ten-points-to-remember/2023/04/10/15/09/exercise-benefits-in-cvds

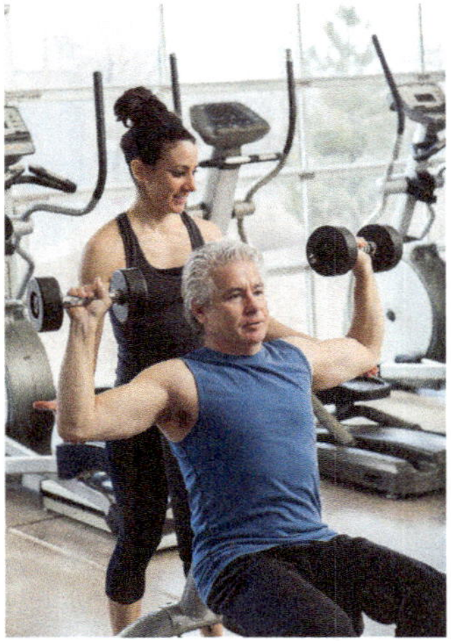
Marc Romanelli/Getty Images

usually increase the number of pounds or kilograms in a given exercise, and you might increase the number of repetitions. Again, start easy, with low weights. Build your strength gradually. Pain is a signal that you are pushing too hard and may injure yourself. There is no reason that muscle-strengthening exercise should be painful.

There is some aerobic gain with prolonged muscle-strengthening activity, but muscle strengthening is not a substitute for aerobic activity. We need to engage in aerobic exercise to build aerobic or cardiorespiratory fitness, but muscle strengthening builds muscle tone and strength. The USDHHS (2018) recommends a combination of aerobic exercise and muscle strengthening.

Guidelines for Exercising Safely[1] Note the following guidelines for exercising safely and reducing the risk of injuries and other adverse events:

1. Understand the risks, yet be confident that physical activity can be safe for almost everyone.
2. Choose types of physical activity that are appropriate for your current fitness level and health goals, because some activities are safer than others.
3. Increase physical activity gradually over time to meet key guidelines or health goals.
4. Inactive people should "start low and go slow" by starting with lower intensity activities and gradually increasing the frequency and duration of their activities.
5. Protect yourself by using appropriate gear and sports equipment, choosing safe environments, following rules and policies, and making sensible choices about when, where, and how to be active.
6. Consult a healthcare provider if you have chronic conditions or symptoms. People with chronic conditions and symptoms can consult a healthcare professional or physical activity specialist about the types and amounts of physical activity that are appropriate for them.

The Physical Benefits of Physical Activity

Inactivity is a key risk factor in many chronic diseases that cut lives short, including CHD, adult-onset diabetes, and some cancers. Regular exercise, especially vigorous exercise, can

[1]U.S. Department of Health and Human Services (USDHHS) (2018). *Physical activity guidelines for Americans*, 2nd ed. Author. https://health.gov/sites/default/files/2019-09/Physical_Activity_Guidelines_2nd_edition.pdf

increase lung capacity (the amount of air the lungs can hold). Increased lung capacity is associated with greater longevity, and that is only the beginning.

Reduced Risk of Cardiovascular Disease Inactive people have nearly twice the risk of developing CHD as their more active peers. By becoming more active, even seasoned couch potatoes can reduce their risk of diseases of the cardiovascular system, the system that circulates blood throughout the body. Regular vigorous exercise has many healthy effects on the heart and circulatory system, including reducing hypertension, lowering risks of heart attacks and strokes, and boosting levels of good cholesterol (HDL), which sweeps away fatty deposits from artery walls (Bach, 2023; Franczyk et al., 2023). Even moderately intense activity, such as gardening or brisk housework, can reduce the risk of cardiovascular disease when performed for at least 30 minutes a day. But to better condition your heart and lungs, it is advisable to engage in 20 minutes or more of vigorous (aerobic) activity at least three times a week. Aerobic dancing, bicycling, cross-country skiing, hiking uphill, running, rowing, stair climbing, and fast walking all fit the bill. Aerobic exercise, which requires a sustained increase in the use of oxygen, widens blood vessels, allowing blood to circulate more freely. Better circulation reduces high blood pressure (hypertension), a risk factor for CHD. Exercise, along with stress management training, even improves the cardiovascular risk profile of people with established heart disease.

Regular exercise boosts the level of the good form of cholesterol, high-density lipoproteins (HDL). High blood levels of HDL are associated with lower risk of heart disease. A landmark study of 7,000 male runners showed that the more miles the men ran, the higher their HDL levels were (Kokkinos et al., 1995). Even men who logged only 7 miles per week showed significantly higher HDL levels than people who did not exercise. Regular exercise also helps lower the blood levels of triglycerides, a type of fat associated with increased risk of heart disease, especially in people with low levels of HDL.

Exercise helps maintain an adequate supply of oxygen to the heart, which is vital to health. Regular vigorous (aerobic) exercise also lowers the resting heart rate, enabling the heart to pump with less wear and tear.

Weight Management and Improved Body Composition Regular exercise helps people maintain a healthy body weight and avoid obesity, yet another risk factor for cardiovascular disease, as well as for diabetes and other health problems. Exercise takes weight off directly by burning *calories* (units of food energy released during metabolism). It also improves body composition by increasing the muscle-to-fat ratio. At rest—for example, when we're relaxing and watching TV—muscle tissue burns about 75 calories per hour, compared to a mere two calories burned by a pound of fat. Finally, regular exercise increases the metabolism, the rate at which the body burns calories.

Improved Immune System Functioning Regular exercise helps boost the functioning of the immune system, the body's line of defense against disease-causing pathogens such as bacteria and viruses (Fernandez-Ruiz, 2020). People who exercise regularly show higher levels of natural killer (NK) cells, a type of white blood cell that destroys invading pathogens (Wennerberg et al., 2020).

Reduced Risk of Cancer A physically active lifestyle reduces the risks of certain types of cancer, especially colorectal cancer and breast cancer (Papadimitriou et al., 2020; Vulczak et al., 2020). A European study found that women who exercised regularly had a 40% lower risk of breast cancer than sedentary women (Bellocco et al., 2016). The sharpest reductions are found in women who run, swim, or play tennis about 4 hours a week. Even women who exercised 2 or 3 hours a week showed a reduced risk.

What accounts for the cancer-preventive role of exercise? For colorectal cancer, one possibility deserving further study is that exercise helps propel waste material through the colon, allowing less time for cancer-causing substances to affect the colon lining. We know that breast cancer is linked to length of exposure to the sex hormone estrogen, and exercise lowers the level of estrogen. In addition, one of the functions of the immune system is to help rid the body of cancerous cells before they turn into malignant growths, and, as noted, exercise strengthens the immune system.

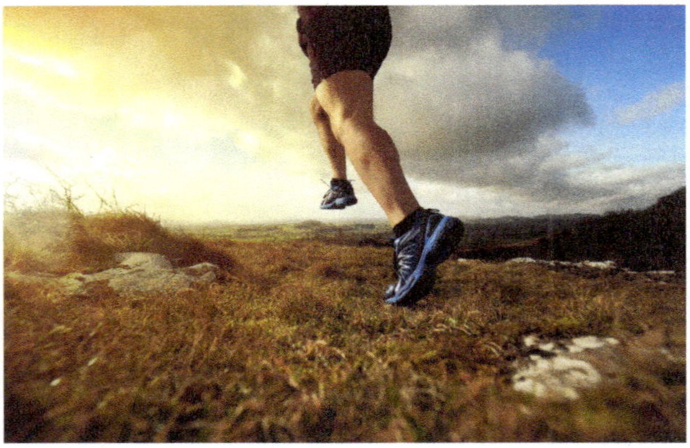

Regular Exercise Builds Endurance Aerobic exercise increases the body's utilization of oxygen, which improves stamina and circulation.

osteoarthritis Degeneration of joint cartilage and the underlying bone.

osteoporosis A condition in which the bones become brittle and fragile from loss of tissue, typically as a result of hormonal changes, or deficiency of calcium or vitamin D.

resistance training A form of exercise in which people move muscles against weights or other forms of resistance to build strength.

Increased Endurance

Regular exercise helps boost endurance and combats fatigue (Hjalmarsson et al., 2020; Miya et al., 2020). People often report feeling energized and more alert after a brisk walk, swim, or workout. Exercise may boost energy by inducing changes in brain chemicals or in the brain's electrical output. Exercise also increases the body's utilization of oxygen, which improves stamina and circulation.

However, moderate exercise seems to work best as an energy booster; too much exercise can be exhausting, both physically and mentally (Meeusen et al., 2020). As we build our fitness, what was originally too much exercise can become "moderate exercise," but it is best to build fitness gradually and to monitor our feelings as we improve.

Prevention of Osteoarthritis and Osteoporosis

Muscles are bundles of fibers that contract to move the body. Maintaining strong muscles improves mobility, reduces the likelihood of injury, and helps prevent lower back problems. Muscle strengthening is also important to healthy bones. Bone is living tissue composed of a lacelike matrix of the protein collagen and the mineral calcium. Bones grow in length until about age 21 years but continue to change in density or thickness throughout life. Density gives bones their strength; stronger bones are less vulnerable to fractures or breaks. Unless bones are worked, especially through weight-bearing activity, they become thinner and more brittle.

Important physical benefits of muscle strengthening exercise include reduced risks of both osteoarthritis and osteoporosis. **Osteoarthritis** is a chronic, degenerative disease of the joints. It is linked to wear and tear on the joints and can result in painful and restricted movement. Muscle strengthening and stretching helps keep joints and tendons flexible (Ellegaard et al., 2020).

When bones are not stressed through repeated use, they begin to lose density (i.e., they become demineralized) due to loss of calcium. Loss of bone density is a sign of **osteoporosis**, a bone disease that makes bones more vulnerable to fractures. Weight-bearing exercise—also called **resistance training**—helps maintain bone density and improves resistance to fractures (Aquino et al., 2020; Stanghelle et al., 2020). Bone mass (a measure of the density or strength of bones) is typically greater among regular exercisers than inactive people, but some types of exercise appear to be better than others for building bone mass and reducing the risk of fractures.

Increased Sensitivity to Insulin

Regular exercise can also increase insulin sensitivity—the body's ability to utilize insulin. Insulin is a hormone produced by the pancreas that stimulates cells to absorb blood sugar (glucose) and other nutrients from the bloodstream. Insulin is essential to maintaining blood sugar at a proper level. By increasing insulin sensitivity, regular exercise helps the body regulate blood sugar levels. In *diabetes mellitus,* the pancreas either produces too little insulin or insulin is not used efficiently. Even people who show early warning signs of diabetes can significantly cut their risk of developing the disease by engaging in 30 minutes of moderate physical activity per day (Bergman & Goodpaster, 2020; Sjøberg et al., 2017).

Table 7.11 summarizes health benefits for people with chronic disease or disabilities, according to the USDHHS (2018).

The Psychological Benefits of Physical Activity

Physical activity is not only good for physical functioning. It also enhances psychological functioning, with respect to ability to process information, learning, memory, executive functions (e.g., planning and self-regulation), and managing anxiety and depression.

Cognition—The Braininess of "Gym Rats"?

People who engage in greater amounts of moderate to vigorous physical activity may experience improvements in cognition,

TABLE 7.11 Health Benefits Associated with Regular Physical Activity for People with Chronic Health Conditions and Disabilities

Condition or Disability	Benefits
Survival of cancer	• Improved health-related quality of life • Improved fitness
Survival of breast cancer	• Lower risk of dying from breast cancer • Lower risk of all-cause mortality
Survival of colorectal cancer	• Lower risk of dying from colorectal cancer • Lower risk of all-cause mortality
Survival of prostate cancer	• Lower risk of dying from prostate cancer
Osteoarthritis (knee and hip)	• Decreased pain • Improved physical function • Improved health-related quality of life • No effect on disease progression at recommended physical activity levels
Hypertension	• Lower risk of cardiovascular disease mortality • Reduced cardiovascular disease progression • Lower risk of increased blood pressure over time
Type 2 diabetes	• Lower risk of cardiovascular disease mortality • Reduced progression of disease indicators—hemoglobin A1c, blood pressure, body mass index, and lipids
Dementia	• Improved cognition
Multiple sclerosis	• Improved physical function, including walking speed and endurance • Improved cognition
Spinal cord injury	• Improved walking function, muscular strength, and upper extremity function
Disease or disorders that impair cognitive function (including ADHD, schizophrenia, Parkinson's disease, and stroke)	• Improved cognition

Source: USDHHS (2018). *Physical activity guidelines for Americans*, 2nd ed. Author, Table 2.4. https://health.gov/sites/default/files/2019-09/Physical_Activity_Guidelines_2nd_edition.pdf#page=43 / U.S. Department of Health & Human Services / Public domain.

Notes: Some physical activity is better than none. For most health outcomes, additional benefits occur as the amount of physical activity increases through higher intensity, greater frequency, and/or longer duration.

including performance on academic achievement tests and on tests involving speed of mental processing, memory, and executive functioning. Physical activity may be especially helpful in improving cognitive functioning among older adults (Ludyga et al., 2020; USDHHS, 2018).

Consider a couple of studies with "gym rats." The first involves aerobic training (Nokia et al., 2016). One group of rats was simply supplied with running wheels in their cages, whereas a control group was not. Most of the rats given the opportunity—that is, the wheels—jogged at moderate paces for several miles a day. It was found that the joggers showed greater creation of new cells in a brain region called the hippocampus. The hippocampus is involved in the regulation of emotions, the formation of long-term memories, and spatial navigation. The fact that exercise promotes the development of new brain cells in the organ is intriguing, to say the least.

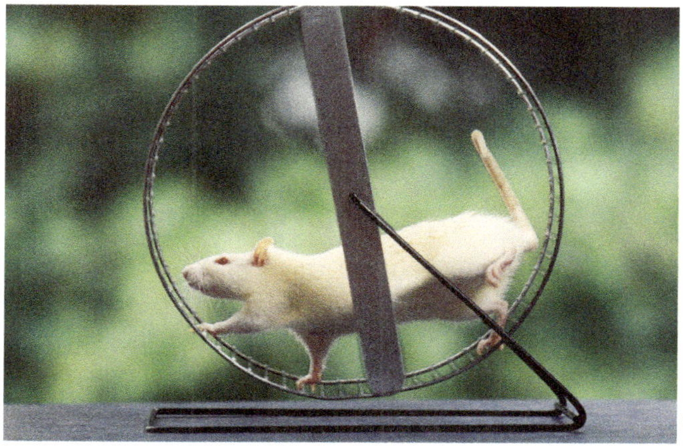

Will & Deni McIntyre/Science Source

A "Gym Rat" Researchers found that aerobic training in rats led to the creation of new cells in parts of the brain associated with the regulation of emotions, formation of memories, and spatial navigation.

Health Psychology in Action

Prolonged Sitting Is a Recognized Health Risk

Did you know that you may be putting your health at risk by doing something that virtually every college student does much of the time—sitting? That's right, the simple act of sitting is a known health risk when it occupies a large part of your day, especially long bouts of uninterrupted sitting (think bingeing on Netflix). Frequent sedentary behavior (SB), which includes sitting, increases the risk of serious health consequences such as diabetes and heart disease (Katzmarzyk et al., 2019). But health psychologists find that taking even brief breaks from sitting, such as walking, standing, and stretching for at least a minute at a time can have beneficial effects on several health indicators, including blood pressure, insulin levels, and HDL cholesterol levels (Dillon et al., 2022).

These researchers used texting to help university students break the pattern of uninterrupted sitting. First they held behavioral counseling sessions online with students to help them develop an action plan, essentially how they planned to break up their sitting time. For example, a student might set a timer or alarm on their phone to buzz them every 45 minutes to take a 2-minute walk while studying. The participants also received daily text messages to reinforce their action plans. Compared to students who received no intervention, those in the (planning and texting) intervention group showed significantly less sitting time and more time walking and stretching. So the message here can be boiled down to two things: have a plan to get yourself up from sitting too long and send a daily reminder to yourself.

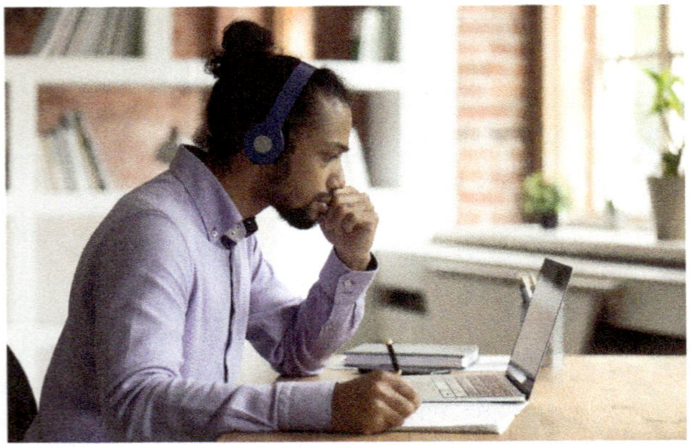

fizkes/Adobe Stock

The second experiment with rats involves resistance training. The researchers assigned a group of rats to weight training as defined by taping bags of weighted pellets to their backs and having them climb 3-foot ladders. The ladder-climbing was not forced; rather, the rats were reinforced with Froot Loops when they reached the top, and they were soon buzzing up and down the ladder with (apparent) glee. Other rats were injected with a substance that causes slight inflammation of the brain and some cognitive deficits akin to the early stages of dementia in humans. But then half of the injected rats began the resistance-training routine. All rats were then compared in maze learning with a control group that was neither injected nor weight-trained. The injected but trained rats soon equaled the performance of the control animals, whereas the injected but untrained group never caught up. Microscopic examination of the brain tissue of the trained animals found that their brains teemed with genetic markers and chemicals that prompt the creation and maintenance of new neurons. The study was run with rats and not with people, so we cannot be certain that we can generalize the results to humans. Nevertheless, the findings do suggest that resistance training in humans might also boost learning and memory, perhaps even delaying the progress of dementias.

In another study, 55- to 85-year-old (human) participants either rested for 30 minutes prior to a memory discrimination task or rode a stationary bicycle for 30 minutes (Won et al., 2019). Those who rode the bicycles showed greater activation in parts of the brain associated with memory functioning, and they were significantly better at discriminating between the names of "famous" and nonfamous people. Other researchers reported that for older adults age 60 or older, engaging in more than 10 hours a day of sedentary behaviors like sitting or driving significantly increased the risk of dementia (Raichlen et al., 2023).

Gray matter in the brain consists of cell bodies of brain cells, and its volume is associated with cognitive abilities and skills. A Mayo Clinic research study of more than 2,000 adults found that those with greater cardiovascular fitness, as defined in part by higher levels of uptake of oxygen during periods of exertion, had a larger volume of gray matter in their brains (Petersen et al., 2020; Wittfeld et al., 2020). Other investigators find that physical activity and fitness appear to protect cognitive functioning in late adulthood as well as build physical endurance (Mendez Colmenares et al., 2021; Opel et al., 2019).

Anxiety and Depression Regular physical activity can elevate the mood and help people feel less tense, anxious, and depressed, not only during workouts but also throughout the day (Henriksson et al., 2022; Pearce et al., 2022). The connection between improved mood and exercise is so strong that mental health professionals often encourage their patients who are struggling with anxiety or depression to exercise regularly.

One study examined the effects of physical activity on anxiety and depression in people with multiple sclerosis, muscular dystrophy, spinal cord injury, and postpoliomyelitis syndrome (Battalio et al., 2020). The study assessed relationships between physical activity and scales that measured self-reported feelings of anxiety and depression over a period of four years. People who engaged in vigorous physical activity showed decreases in anxiety and depression, but changes in mood were not associated with mild physical activity.

Another study drew data from the U.S. Behavioral Risk Factor Surveillance System to assess the relationships between moderate to vigorous physical activity among 17,839 adults aged 18–85 years (Bennie et al., 2019). About 18% of the participants met government guidelines for both aerobic exercise and strength training. Aerobic fitness and strength training were each associated with a lower prevalence of depression than that found among people who met neither guideline, but the lowest prevalence of depression was found among people who met both guidelines.

Aerobic exercise helps normalize the levels of the neurotransmitters that play key roles in regulating our moods, which is apparently one path to combating depression (Kandola et al., 2019). Exercise can also be enjoyable, providing a break from the strains of everyday life, another reason that it may help combat depression. Furthermore, exercise can give us a sense of mastery and accomplishment, boosting our self-image and self-confidence and helping to combat the sense of helplessness that is often associated with depression (Kandola et al., 2019).

Physical Activity Interventions and Adherence

Adherence to an exercise program can be as important as adherence to taking prescribed medicines. Motivation is the key factor in determining whether you will begin an exercise program and stick with it long enough to reap the benefits. Nearly half of people who start an exercise program drop out within a few months. Why? Among the more common reasons are scheduling difficulties, competing demands on time, lack of affordable or accessible programs, lack of confidence in one's ability to keep pace, and lack of visible progress. Health psychologists have learned that factors such as the following promote adherence:

1. Set realistic goals and realistic expectations for progress (Lock et al., 2020). Don't fall into the trap of losing motivation by expecting too much too soon.
2. Avoid comparing yourself to others on social media, especially elite athletes. Psychologists find that viewing idealized images of toned athletes and fitness stars can dampen a person's mood and increase their dissatisfaction with their own body (see A Closer Look below; Prichard et al., 2020).
3. Bring a friend or join a group of people like yourself. If you're a beginner, don't attend a group for elite athletes. Appropriate groups and friends provide all-important social and emotional support.
4. Select enjoyable exercise activities, preferably activities you can continue for a lifetime.
5. Use music to accompany the exercise routine. You'll pick your own playlist, but consider fast music with a beat that propels you forward. Psychologists conducted a meta-analysis of 139 studies that examined the effects of music on exercise and found that music elevates the mood, enhances physical performance, reduces the sense of exertion, and actually improves physiological efficiency, as measured by the consumption of oxygen (Terry et al., 2020).
6. Choose exercise that fits the individual. Older women are particularly subject to problems associated with high-impact exercises, such as fast walking or jogging. A Mexican study used low-impact exercising in a pool for a sample of older women over a 17-week period. As compared with a matched control group who did not exercise, the "aquafit" women lost more excess weight and body fat, decreased their body mass index, and became more optimistic (Perkins et al., 2020).

7. Make exercise so regular that it becomes a habit (Phillips & Gardner, 2016). Habits can work for people as well as against them.
8. Make a commitment to exercise (Pears & Sutton, 2020). Tell people about it and live up to it.
9. Develop intrinsic motivation by focusing on the continued benefits of exercising and the health risks of being sedentary. Intrinsic motivation (motivation that comes from within) is a better predictor of adherence to exercise than extrinsic motivation (as in being told to exercise by a healthcare provider) (Thøgersen-Ntoumani et al., 2016).

Physical Activity and Theories of Health Behavior Change

The Theory of Planned Behavior (TPB) predicts health behaviors on the basis of attitudes, subjective norms, intentions, planning, and perceived behavioral control. A review of the research focused on the relationships among these factors in the prediction of healthful physical activity (Rhodes et al., 2018). The probability of engaging in physical activity was increased when:

1. The participants believed that physical activity would improve their health and well-being (attitudes);
2. Others known to the participants were engaging in physical activity and would approve of their doing so (subjective norms);
3. Participants expressed the intention to be physically active (as in "I will go to the gym");
4. Participants had concrete plans for engaging in the physical activity (as in "on Monday, Wednesday, and Friday of this week"); and
5. Participants perceived that they had behavioral control over the physical activity; that is, the activity was controllable and they had the self-efficacy to carry it out.

A Closer Look

Is Strong the New Skinny? On #Fitspiration Images

Fitspiration images showing lean and muscular bodies have been used to promote exercise and healthful foods (Tiggemann & Zaccardo, 2018). However, the use of idealized images creates negative social comparisons concerning body image with virtually all viewers (Seekis et al., 2020; Tiggemann & Zaccardo, 2018).

For example, a study with 106 female college undergraduates randomly assigned participants to view one of three sets of images of women (Robinson et al., 2017)—the thin ideal, the athletic ideal, and the muscular ideal. Exposure to the thin ideal and the athletic ideal (the fitspiration images) increased the students' dissatisfaction with their own bodies. The purely muscular images did not discourage them, apparently because they were not considered to be attractive. After viewing the fitspiration images and the thin ideals, the women engaged in a bout of exercise. Although the thin ideal and fitspiration images increased the women's body dissatisfaction, they did not motivate the women to engage in higher levels of exercise. Conclusion? The fitspiration images made the women feel worse about themselves and did not encourage them to change their behavior. A similar experiment confirmed that women exposed to fitspiration imagery had more negative moods and dissatisfaction with their bodies (Prichard et al., 2020). But it also found that a brief bout of exercise following exposure to the fitspiration imagery made their moods yet more negative. The message seems clear—idealized fitspiration images may only make matters worse for people (men and women) who are already anxious about their body images (Seekis et al., 2020).

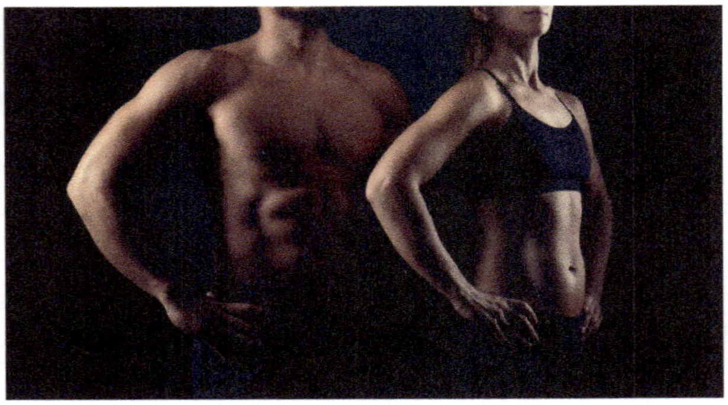

TeamDAF/Getty Images

"Fitspiration" Images Who has a body like this? Very few of us do. Comparing oneself to elite athletes or models is a sure way to dampen the mood and increase dissatisfaction with one's own body. And no, there is no evidence that the social comparison inspires us mere mortals to exercise more.

A study of the TPB in Hong Kong found that perceived behavioral control was the main factor in university students' intentions to walk for purposes of exercise (Sun et al., 2015). Belief that walking would be beneficial for their health (attitudes) and subjective norms (believing that other students walked for exercise and would approve of their joining in) also enhanced the predictive power of the model.

According to the Health Belief Model (HBM), people are motivated to undertake a course of action if they perceive benefits in doing so and if they are not discouraged by perceived barriers. They are further motivated by perceived vulnerability to a health problem—in this case, the health problems associated with a sedentary lifestyle. People also respond to cues to action, such as a troubling news from a healthcare provider or seeing themselves adding on the pounds.

The following benefits and barriers concerning exercise are informed by the Exercise Benefits/Barriers Scale developed at the University of Michigan by Karen R. Sechrist, Susan N. Walker, and Nola J. Pendler.[2] They also reflect research into benefits and barriers concerning exercise with people with heart failure (Adsett et al., 2019), HIV/AIDS (Neff et al., 2019), chronic obstructive pulmonary disease (Meshe et al., 2020), major depressive disorder (Monteiro et al., 2020), and other health problems.

Benefits of Exercise

Exercising feels good.

Exercise is good for my blood pressure.

Exercise helps me keep my body trim and fit.

I sleep better at night when I exercise.

Getting out and exercising helps me meet new people.

Exercising increases my endurance.

Barriers to Exercise

Exercising takes too much time out of my day.

Exercising is difficult for me.

Exercising is too costly.

I am embarrassed when other people watch me exercising.

Exercising is too tiring.

There are no nearby facilities for exercising.

Lower Extremity Injuries and Theories of Health Behavior Change

Leg injuries are common among physically active people, especially joggers, runners, and players in sports such as tennis, skiing, and basketball. They account for more than half of the injuries experienced by college students and the general adult population. As a result, exercise-related injury prevention programs (ERIPPs) have been developed as an aid to participants. Because of low enrollment in these programs, health psychologists have studied the enrollment issue from the perspectives of various theories of health behavior change. One of the few studies on the matter found that the following TPB factors were significantly correlated with the intention to enroll in an ERIPP (Gabriel et al., 2019):

1. Attitudes (concerning the value of avoiding injury),
2. Subjective norms (e.g., believing others will enroll and would approve of one's choices), and
3. Perceived behavioral control (the perceived ability to carry out the intended behaviors).

[2]Retrieved from https://deepblue.lib.umich.edu/bitstream/handle/2027.42/85354/EBBS-English_Version.pdf?sequence=2

The following HBM factors also correlated significantly with the intention to enroll:

1. Perceived benefits (avoiding pain and forced time off from exercising),
2. Self-efficacy (similar to perceived behavioral control), and
3. Cues to action (e.g., learning of another person's injury).

Perceived susceptibility to injury was less crucial a determinant of intention to enroll. Nor were perceived barriers, such as taking the time to participate in ERIPPs and engaging in the injury-prevention exercises.

Before moving on, consider the following questions: Do you engage in regular physical activity? How does your exercise program relate to the federal guidelines? Thinking of starting to exercise? Which of our suggestions for getting a move on might be of use to you? Is it time to get moving? If not, why not? If you are ready, why not get started today?

Review 7.6

INTERACTIVE SELF-SCORING QUIZZES

Sentence Completion

1. __________ exercise requires a sustained increase in the consumption of oxygen.
2. __________-__________ activity involves short bursts of muscle activity, as in resistance or weight training.
3. Regular exercise raises the level of (LDL or HDL) cholesterol.
4. Of the racial/ethnic groups discussed in this section, __________ Americans are most likely to meet federal guidelines for engaging in physical activity.
5. Adults in the __________ age group are most likely to meet federal guidelines for physical activity.

Think About It

Do you engage in regular physical activity? How does your exercise program adhere to the USDHHS guidelines? Are you thinking of starting to exercise? How do your beliefs about the costs and benefits of exercise affect your intention to exercise regularly? Which of the suggestions for getting a move on might be of use to you?

Recite: An Active Summary

INTERACTIVE SELF-SCORING QUIZZES

Chapter 7 Practice Quiz

1. Describe the parts of the digestive system, and explain how the hunger drive works to maintain a steady state.

The digestive system consists of the mouth, pharynx, esophagus, stomach, small and large intestines, and anus. Food deprivation causes the hypothalamus to trigger the hunger drive, which motivates eating behavior to restore a steady blood sugar level. Feedback mechanisms from the mouth through the intestines provide sensations of satiety. Common disorders of the digestive system include acid reflux, constipation, irritable bowel disease, and diarrhea. Diarrhea and dysentery are major causes of death in developing nations. Various forms of hepatitis are caused by different strains of the hepatitis virus. There are vaccines for hepatitis A and B. Cancers may develop in any part of the digestive system.

2. Define the essential nutrients, and explain their roles in health.

People need to consume a balanced diet that provides sufficient quantities of proteins, carbohydrates, fats, vitamins, and minerals. But Americans tend to eat too much protein and fats. Complex carbohydrates (starches) are better sources of nutrients than simple carbohydrates (sugars). Consumption of large amounts of dietary cholesterol and saturated fat, along with obesity, heightens the risk of cardiovascular disorders.

Define overweight and obesity, and discuss their origins. Overweight is defined as a body mass index (BMI) of 25–29.9, and obesity is defined as a BMI of 30 or higher. Obesity is a complex health problem involving an interplay of biological factors, such as heredity, amount of adipose tissue (body fat), and metabolic rate (the rate at which the individual converts calories to energy), as well as psychological factors, such as stress and the use of food to alleviate negative emotions.

3. Discuss the role of health psychology theories in weight control.

Effective weight control involves acquiring knowledge of the relationships between calories, food intake, and physical activity, along with making behavioral changes in eating behavior, such as reducing one's exposure to stimuli that trigger eating, changing the pace of eating behavior itself, and altering the consequences of eating so that overeating becomes punitive rather than rewarding. Anti-obesity medications may be of help to some people, but long-term weight management involves making healthy lifestyle changes. In cases of morbid obesity, bariatric surgery may be recommended.

4. Define anorexia nervosa and bulimia nervosa, and discuss their origins.

Anorexia nervosa is characterized by refusal to eat and maintenance of an unhealthy low body weight. Bulimia nervosa is characterized by cycles of binge eating and purging. Women are more likely than men to develop these disorders. Most researchers point to the cultural ideal of the slender woman as a key cause of eating disorders. A distorted body image and the need for perfectionism play roles.

5. Describe USDHHS guidelines for physical activity.

The guidelines recommend 150–300 minutes/week of moderate intensity physical activity or 75–150 minutes/week of vigorous activity for adults. It is recommended that children engage in an hour or more of daily physical activity. Older adults should be as active as their health conditions permit. Physical activity should include aerobic exercise and muscle-strengthening activity.

6. Describe the physical and psychological health benefits of exercise.

Physically speaking, exercise reduces the risks of cardiovascular disease, cancer, osteoarthritis and osteoporosis, and diabetes. Exercise helps manage weight, improves the functioning of the immune system, and increases stamina. Psychologically, exercise appears to boost mental processing speed, memory, and executive functioning. Exercise may also decrease feelings of anxiety and depression.

7. Explain how to get a move on—how to safely develop a personal fitness program.

Start gradually. Set realistic goals. Select enjoyable activities, preferably activities you can continue for a lifetime. Make exercise a regular routine. Focus on the benefits of exercise to help foster adherence.

Answers to Review Sections

7.1

1. peristalsis
2. Gastric
3. insulin
4. parasympathetic
5. homeostasis
6. hypothalamus
7. polyps
8. electrolytes

7.2

1. Proteins
2. carbohydrates
3. Fats
4. A
5. fiber

7.3

1. two
2. mass
3. 30
4. fat
5. calories
6. hypothalamus
7. thermogenesis

7.4

1. goals
2. avoid, limit, remove, etc.
3. carbohydrate
4. Mediterranean
5. sugar
6. metabolic, heart
7. fats
8. Green
9. morbidly
10. stomach

7.5

1. distorted
2. Bulimia
3. serotonin
4. more

7.6

1. Aerobic
2. Muscle-strengthening
3. HDL
4. White
5. 18–24 year age range

CHAPTER 8

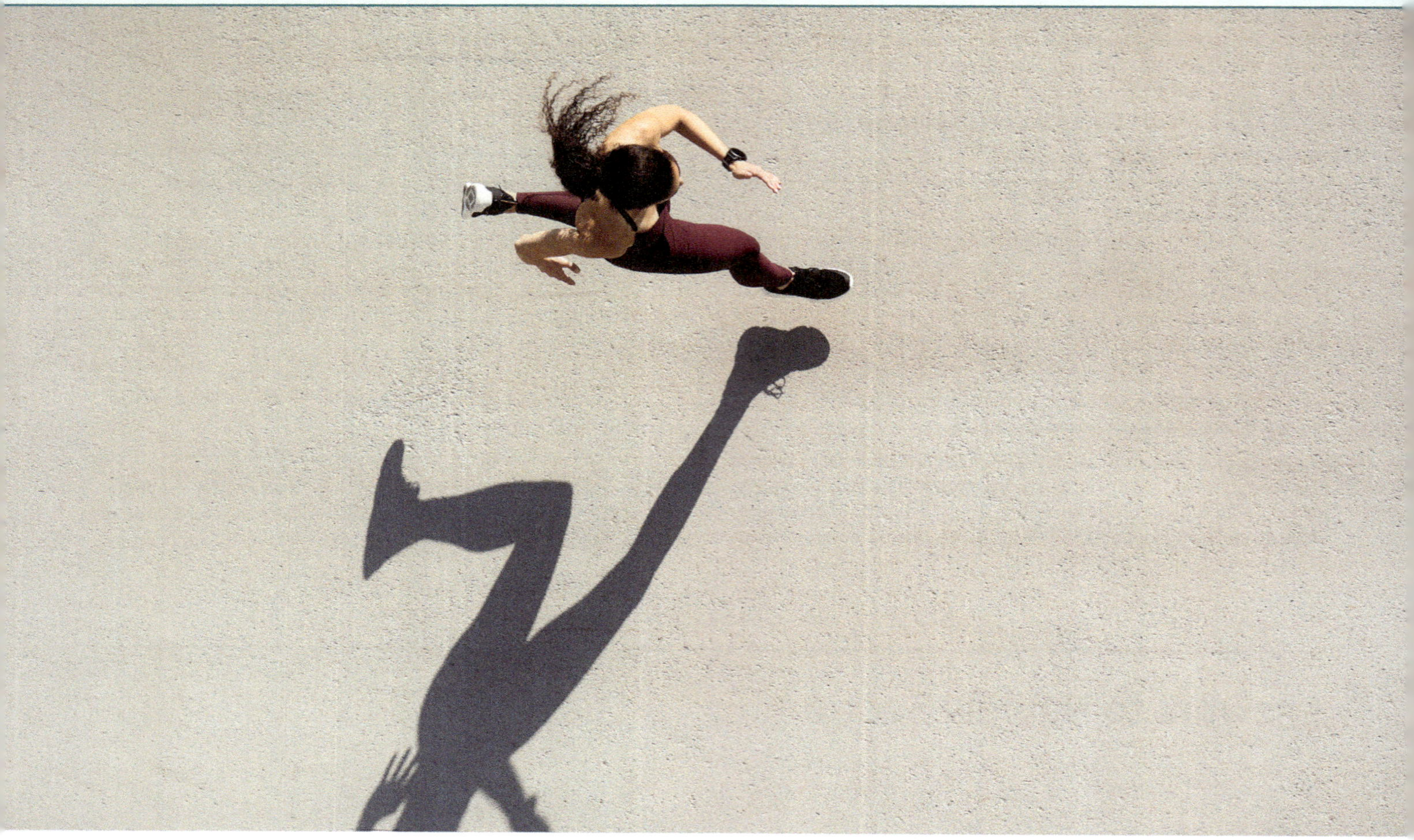

Tempura/Getty Images

Playing It Safe: Reducing Health Risks by Practicing Safety Behaviors

LEARNING OBJECTIVES

After studying this chapter, you will be able to …

1. **Discuss** crimes of violence in the United States.
2. **Discuss** factors involved in rape and rape prevention.
3. **Discuss** myths that support rape, and why rape often goes unreported.
4. **Discuss** underlying factors involved in violent behavior.
5. **Discuss** various kinds of unintentional injuries, factors that contribute to them, and ways of preventing them.

Did You Know That ...

- Nearly 50,000 Americans die each year from firearm-related causes?
- Fewer than 4% of violent crimes are committed by mentally ill people?
- One in six victims of homicide in the United States is killed by an intimate partner, including nearly half of all female homicide victims?
- The great majority of rapes are not reported to authorities?
- Women are much more likely to be raped by someone they know than by a stranger?
- There's no place like home—for accidents, that is?
- Wearing seat belts saves about 15,000 lives a year?
- More than 3,500 lives are lost annually in the United States due to distracted driving?
- For the average person, the chances of dying from a fall are about 1,000 times greater than dying in a flood or earthquake?

People often say the only certainties in life are death and taxes. Life is filled with uncertainty. We might even say that uncertainty is a fact of life. Just about everything in life entails some degree of risk, whether it is traveling by car or airplane, crossing a street, walking up or down the stairs, or even taking a bath (you could trip or fall). You could even fall even getting out of bed. The world is filled with yet more uncertainties that pose varying degrees of risk, from political turmoil to threats of terrorism to international conflicts and to crime in the streets, to name but a few. We cast a wary eye toward fellow travelers at airports and when boarding trains and many of us live behind triple-locked doors or equip our residences with state-of-the-art electronic security systems.

People vary in how they deal with risks. Some have a nonchalant, "whatever happens, happens" attitude. Others sequester themselves at home, ever fearful of venturing outside, especially at night. Between these extremes lies the alternative of living a full but careful life. Putting safety first is more than a catchphrase; it is a prescription for living that acknowledges the need to take reasonable steps to protect ourselves from the many risks we may face in daily life.

Adopting safer behaviors involves making reasonable accommodations to living with uncertainty. We can't guarantee you will ever be perfectly safe, no one can. But with a little planning and organized effort we can greatly reduce the risks we may face. This chapter is about the efforts of health psychologists, safety experts, and government officials to keep us informed about risks we face on the roads, in the streets, and even in our own homes and the ways in which each of us can play it safe to reduce the risks to our personal safety we might face.

Violence

Columbine . . . Aurora . . . Sandy Hook . . . Charleston . . . El Paso . . . Tree of Life Synagogue. . .

These names may forever be linked with mass shootings. But these are only a few of the many locales in which innocent people, many of whom were children, lost their lives to gun violence.

America the beautiful? Yes, but also America the violent. Concerns about crime and violence, including mass shootings, have become a staple of American life, and for good reason. A very concerning, indeed shocking, statistic is that more than half of U.S. adults or their family members have experienced gun violence in one form or another. They either have personally been threatened by someone with a gun, witnessed a shooting, or had a relative killed by firearms, such as by homicide or suicide (Harris, 2023b). Gun violence is not an equal opportunity destroyer, as about twice as many Black Americans as White Americans have had a relative killed by a gun or witnessed a shooting.

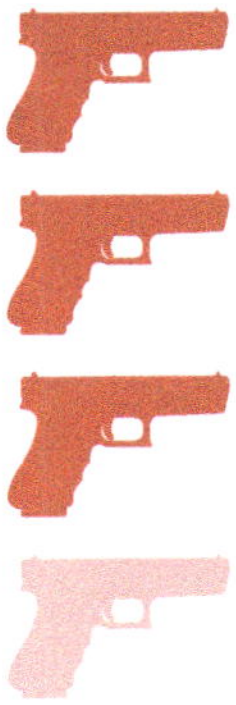

Three in four of Gen Zs report mass shootings as a significant source of stress.

Many people today live behind triple-bolted doors, invest thousands in home security systems, and avoid parks at night. The daily wail of car alarms and the sirens of ambulances and police cars remind city dwellers how crime affects their lives. Reports of crime dominate the headlines. The more sensational the crime, the greater the media feeding frenzy. Violent police dramas dot the prime-time landscape of commercial television, and reality police

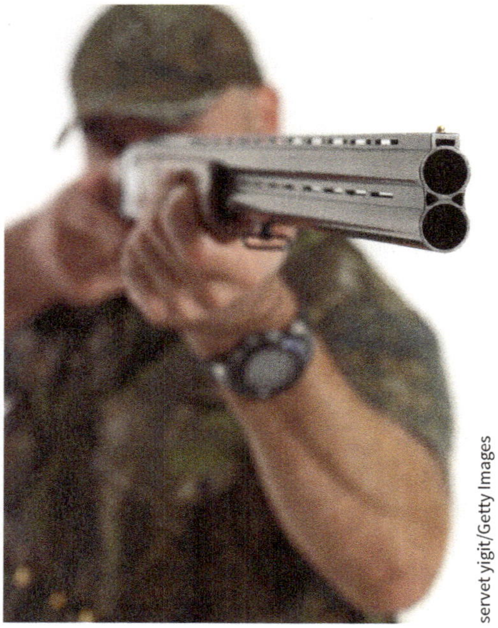

Violent Gun Death Nearly 50,000 people are killed by guns in the United States each year as the result of homicide or suicide. Violent gun deaths are all but absent in other developed nations such as Japan, South Korea, and the United Kingdom.

shows pull in huge revenues. Movies feature a never-ending diet of stabbings, slashings, shootings, and ever more inventive methods of mayhem.

First some good news. According to the U.S. Bureau of Justice Statistics (2022), the rate of violent crimes in the United States fell during the 10-year period of 2012 to 2021 (Thompson & Tapp, 2022). Tempering this downward trend, however, the rate of crime in urban areas increased from 2020 to 2021. Overall, some 4.6 million Americans over the age 12 or older were victims of violent crime in 2021. Men and women were about equally likely to be victims of violent crime, but men committed more violent crimes, proportionally speaking, than women. Most violent incidents involving White victims were committed by White people, and likewise, most violent incidents involving Black victims were committed by Black people. Young adults in the 18- to 29-year age range were more likely to be victimized than older adults.

Violent Gun Death: As American as Apple Pie?

Although no one factor accounts for the high rate of homicide in the United States, the availability of firearms is a major contributing factor. Consider these grim statistics:

- According to recent statistics, more than 26,000 Americans lose their lives to homicide annually, with about 21,000 of these deaths linked to the use of firearms (CDC, 2023d).
- Teenage boys are more likely to die from the use of firearms than from all natural causes combined.
- Firearm-related deaths among children and adolescents in the United States has been rising and now accounts for a record number of deaths in this age group, more than 4,700 in total annually (Lovelace, 2023).
- Firearms are used in about four of five homicides in the United States, as compared to fewer than one in four in other industrialized countries.

Gun violence in the United States reached a record level in 2021 (McPhillips, 2023). All told, there are more violent gun deaths in the United States, proportionally speaking, than in any other affluent, developed nation (Aizenman, 2018) (see **Figure 8.1**). Violent gun deaths are all but absent in Japan, Indonesia, China, South Korea, the United Kingdom, and Iceland.

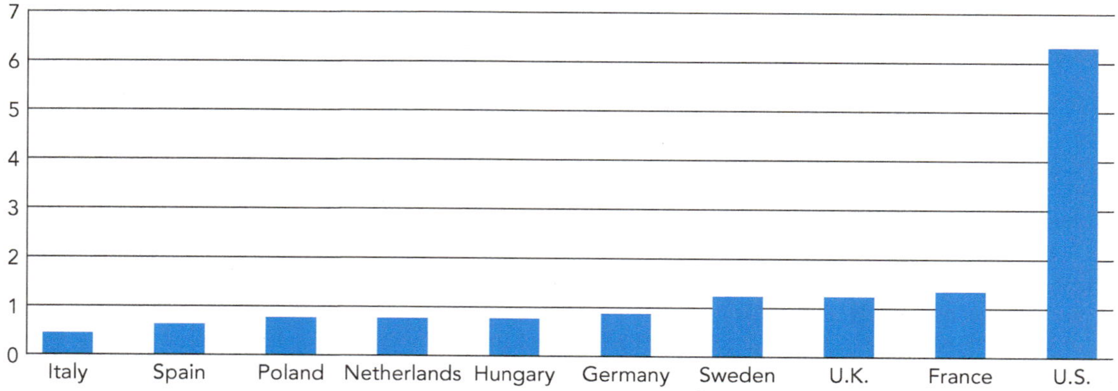

FIGURE 8.1 Homicide Rates in the United States in Comparison to European Countries (per 100,000 people) Homicide rates in other developed countries in Europe pale in comparison to the rate in the United States.

Source: Adapted from Buchholz, 2023 Based on data from Eurostat and U.S. Centers for Disease Control and Prevention; Adapted from https://www.worldatlas.com/articles/murder-rates-by-country.html.

A recent and highly influential Johns Hopkins University report cited additional statistics to underscore the risks of gun-related deaths (Davis, Kim, & Crifasi, 2023):

- Nearly 50,000 Americans died in 2021 from firearms-arms related causes of deaths, resulting from homicides and suicides.
- The increase in firearms-related deaths in 2021 was the largest increase in a single year in four decades.
- An average of 134 people die from gun violence (homicides and suicides) every 11 minutes in the United States, which amounts to one life lost in the nation every five minutes.
- More people in America die from firearms than from motor vehicle crashes.

To put the health-related concerns about gun violence in the sharpest but also bleakest terms, the Johns Hopkins report found that the leading cause of death in children and teens in 2021 was not cancer, not COVID, not motor vehicle crashes, but guns. With concern, we note that the homicide rate among young Americans aged 10 to 24 years, which had declined from 2006 to 2014, has since increased by 60% (Curtin & Garnett, 2023). Moreover, young people in this age group are nearly as likely to die from homicide as suicide. Homicide now stands as the third leading cause of death in this age group, after accidents and suicide.

Generation Z—people born in the 1990s or early 2000s—report gun violence to be a significant source of stress (American Psychological Association, 2018). Three out of four Gen Zs referred to mass shootings as a major source of stress; 72% mentioned school shootings; and 21% said that they were constantly or often concerned about a shooting at their own school. Three out of four (74%) of their parents agreed that school shootings were a significant source of stress.

Handguns are the most commonly used weapon in murders in the United States, followed by other kinds of firearms (Statista, 2019). Then, in descending order, come knives and other cutting instruments; personal weapons such as hands, fists, and feet; blunt objects such as clubs and hammers; and asphyxiation. Use of narcotics as a murder weapon, fire, strangulation, drowning, and poisonings are relatively rare. Although we may see people and buildings regularly blown up in films and TV shows, only a handful of murders in the United States can be attributed to the use of explosives.

Most murders occur among people who know each other and are often members of the same family or household. The great majority of perpetrators are males and most homicides occur among people of the same race or ethnic group (FBI, 2019). However, the homicide rate for Black victims is the highest among all the major ethnic/racial groups in the United States (Chamie, 2023) (see **Figure 8.2**). Mindful of all these grim statistics, we can see how violence, especially gun violence, is a major health threat to us all.

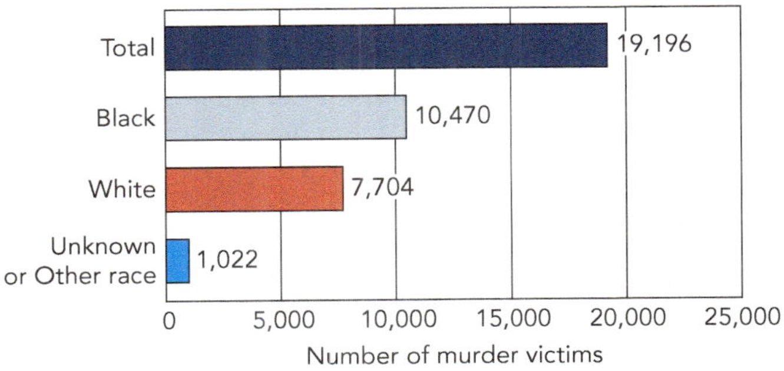

FIGURE 8.2 **Number of Homicide Victims in U.S. in 2022 by Race**

Source: https://www.statista.com/statistics/251877/murder-victims-in-the-us-by-race-ethnicity-and-gender/.

Violent Behavior and Mental Illness

Researchers find that the great majority of mental patients, even those with severe disorders like schizophrenia do not commit any violent acts at all, even among those who remain untreated (DeAngelis, 2021; Whiting et al., 2022). While there certainly are cases in which mental illness plays a part in violent behavior, these actually represent but a small percentage of violent crimes. According to the U.S. Department of Health and Human Services (USDHHS), only about 4% of violent crimes are committed by emotionally disturbed people and in fewer than 10% of cases of violent behavior can we trace the violence to psychological or mental disorders of assailants (Kolker, 2022; Peterson et al., 2014). Moreover, people with severe psychological or mental disorders stand a higher risk of becoming a victim of violent crime themselves than do people in the general population (Teplin et al., 2005).

Drilling deeper into the data, researchers identify several factors tied to an increased risk of violent behavior among people with emotional disorders. For example, patients with more severe disorders, such as schizophrenia and bipolar disorder, have higher risk profiles for committing acts of violence in comparison to the general population (Friedman, 2014; Whiting et al., 2021). The risk for violent behavior is even greater for patients during acute psychotic episodes (breaks with reality) who remain untreated and suffer from delusions of persecution and have a past history of violent behavior (Buchanan et al., 2019; Keer et al., 2013).

We shouldn't overlook the relatively few cases of violent behavior committed by emotionally disturbed people. We need to ensure that emotionally disturbed people get the help they need, especially those in acute psychotic states who may be left to essentially fend for themselves. But we should not confuse perception with reality by subscribing to the false belief that mental disorders are a major cause of violent behavior. Health psychologists play important roles in exploring links between mental illness and violent behavior and developing interventions targeting violent behavior in people with mental or psychological disorders. Media reports are replete with examples of violent crimes committed by people with diagnosable mental disorders, many of whom have fallen between the cracks of the mental health system and may not be receiving active treatment or taking prescribed medication. We hear about the person standing on the subway platform who is pushed on the tracks by someone with schizophrenia or of people with psychiatric histories attacking or aggressively accosting people on city streets. These are very concerning incidents, but they need to be put in context.

Health psychologists recognize the importance of perceptions as drivers of health-related behaviors, such as the perceived risk of contracting a disease and the perceived benefits of practicing disease-preventive behaviors. What about public perceptions of the risks of violent behavior posed by people with mental disorders? Public perception does not square with the facts but is exaggerated by media reports that place disproportionate attention on a few highly publicized cases. Media reports of sensationalistic crimes committed by mental patients only reinforce stereotypes of dangerousness of mental patients, leading to fear and stigmatization of people in need of compassionate care. Factors driving violent behavior are more strongly linked to alcohol and substance abuse and a history of child maltreatment than to mental illness (DeAngelis, 2021). Violence takes many forms, and certainly one of its most pernicious manifestations are crimes motivated by hate.

Hate Crimes in the United States

In 2015, a White supremacist shot and killed nine Black Americans who were engaged in Bible study at the Emanuel African Methodist Episcopal Church in Charleston, South Carolina. A year later, a gunman opened fire in a crowded gay nightclub in Orlando, killing 49 people and wounding 29. In 2018, a gunman killed 11 people and wounded six at the Jewish L'Simcha Congregation in Pittsburgh. In 2019, a gunman entered an El Paso Walmart with an AK-47 rifle and multiple magazines and killed 22 people. He said that he was targeting Mexicans.

These are not only mass murders. They are also hate crimes. The term "hate crime" can be misleading. It does not mean anger, rage, or general dislike. It refers specifically to bias against people or groups having certain characteristics, as defined by law. At the federal level, hate crimes are those committed on the basis of a person's race, color, religion, national origin, sexual orientation, gender, gender identity, or disability. The Federal Bureau of Investigation (FBI) reported more than 9,000 hate crimes nationwide in a recent year (FBI, 2023). The actual numbers are surely much higher, as many violent acts don't go down on the books as hate crimes but may be classified as simple assaults, rapes, or murders.

Any group can be the target of hate crimes. But statistics shows that seven in 10 victims of race-related hate crimes are Black Americans. Seven in 10 victims of crimes based on religious bias are Jews. Nearly one in five crimes is motivated by anti-LGBTQ bias, and the number of hate crimes against LGBTQ individuals is on the rise (U.S. Department of Justice, 2019). **Figure 8.3** shows the categories of bias motivation for victims of hate crimes, according to government statistics.

More than half (53.6%) of perpetrators of hate crimes are White people, and 24% are Black people (Department of Justice, 2019). The largest number of hate crimes (25.7%) occurs in or near the homes of the victims. Nearly one in 10 (8.9%) occurs at schools or colleges. Despite the fact that hate crimes at churches, synagogues, and mosques make the headlines, only 3.7% of hate crimes occur at those sites.

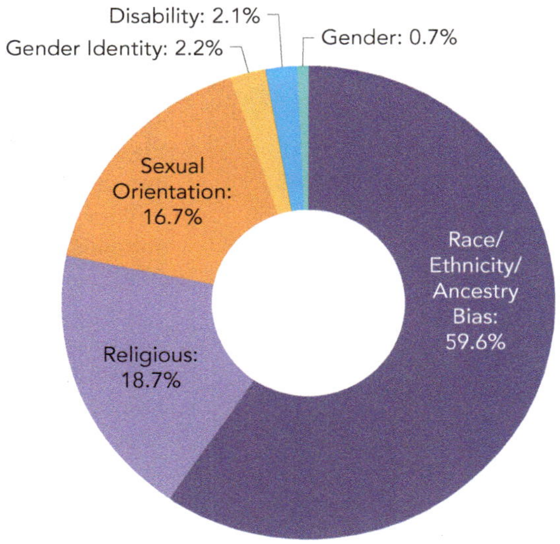

FIGURE 8.3 Bias Motivation Categories for Victims of Hate Crimes

Source: U.S. Department of Justice (2023, March 13). FBI Releases Supplemental 2021 Hate Crime Statistics. https://www.fbi.gov/news/press-releases/fbi-releases-supplemental-2021-hate-crime-statisticsn/Public Domain.

Crimes on Campus The idyllic view of a college campus as a safe refuge from the social ills of society unfortunately doesn't measure up to the facts. Crime statistics tell a different story. As we can see in **Table 8.1**, reported crimes on the nation's campuses add up in the thousands. Many other crimes, especially sexual assaults, go unreported. By far the greatest number of crimes on campus are burglaries, typically involving property stolen from door rooms or college offices. If someone breaks into your dorm room, or enters without your permission or knowledge, and takes your laptop or cell phone, it is considered a burglary. Although campus crime is an all too familiar experience on the nation's campuses, college students in the 18- to 24-year age range are less likely to be victims of crime than their noncollege counterparts in the community (NCES, 2023).

People often say that safety begins at home. For college students, putting safety first begins in the dorm or off-campus apartment, such as ensuring that rooms (and windows) are properly locked or secured, entry is restricted to people you know and trust, and an inventory is kept of all valuables in case a theft should occur. But safety on campus also involves becoming familiar with the campus, noting the locations of college buildings and campus security and taking note of lighting conditions, and along campus walkways and in parking lights. It also involves charting a secure path between campus buildings and residential halls.

TABLE 8.1 Most Widely Reported Crimes on Campus

Type of Crime	Number	Percentage of Total
Forcible sexual offenses	11,800	43%
Robbery	8,000	3%
Aggravated assault	2,200	8%
Burglary	9,000	33%
Motor vehicle theft	3,100	11%

Source: Criminal Offenses. U.S. Department of National Center for Education Statistics, 2022/Public Domain.

Intimate Partner Violence

intimate partner violence Acts of physical or psychological aggression, stalking, or physical or sexual violence perpetuated by someone with whom one has an intimate relationship (also called domestic violence).

Nearly one woman in five and about one man in seven have experienced **intimate partner violence** (IPV; also called *domestic violence*) in the form of severe physical violence (see **Figure 8.4**). Women in the United States experience at least 5 million acts of domestic violence annually, with more than 3 million suffering domestic violence involving men. About 1.5 million women intimate partner rapes and physical assaults against women are committed annually, and men experience about 800,000 sexual assaults from their intimate partners (Huecker et al., 2023). Various forms of IPV are listed in **Table 8.2**.

More than 43 million women and 38 million men in the United States have encountered psychological aggression by an intimate partner during their lifetime. Psychological aggression is defined as the use of verbal and nonverbal forms of communication with the intention of harming the other person mentally or emotionally or to exert control over the other person. As many as 11 million women and 5 million men who report being victimized by intimate partner sexual violence, physical violence, or stalking said they initially experienced these behaviors before they turned 18. Stalking is defined as a pattern of repeated, unwanted attention and contact by a partner, or former partner, that causes concern about one's safety or the safety of someone close to the victim, such as a child.

While most acts of IPV are relatively minor, as for example grabbing, shoving, pushing, and slapping, many involve serious and even fatal injuries (Huecker et al., 2023). Overall, 1 in 6 victims of homicide in the United States is killed by an intimate partner, but nearly half of all female homicide victims die at the hands of an intimate partner (CDC, 2019e). Tragically,

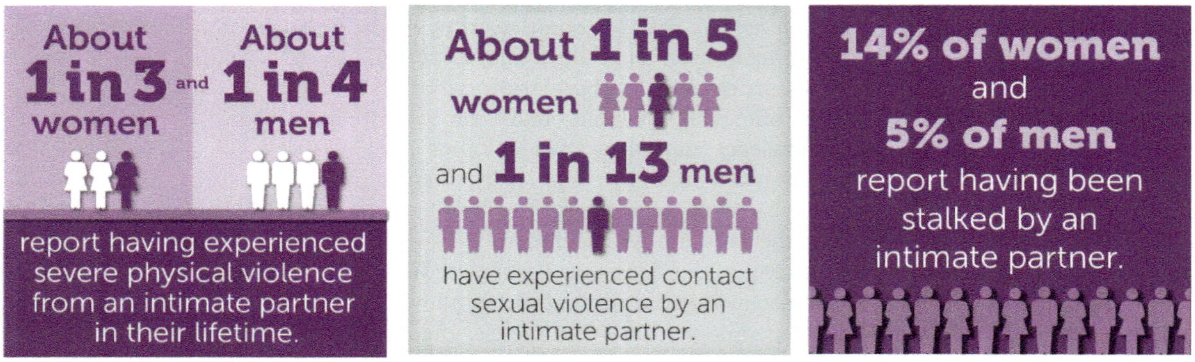

FIGURE 8.4 **Intimate Partner Violence in America** Violence at the hands of an intimate partner is unfortunately far too common in our society. What can society do to reduce the occurrence of IPV?

Source: Centers for Disease Control and Prevention (CDC) (2019). https://www.cdc.gov/violenceprevention/intimatepartnerviolence/fastfact.html/Public Domain.

TABLE 8.2 **Types of Intimate Partner Violence**

Types	What It Is
Physical violence	A person hurting or trying to hurt a partner by hitting, kicking, or using another type of physical force
Sexual violence	Forcing or attempting to force a partner to take part in a sex act, sexual touching, or a nonphysical sexual event (e.g., sexting) when the partner does not or cannot consent
Stalking	Repeated, unwanted attention and contact by a partner that causes fear or concern for one's own safety or the safety of someone close to the victim
Psychological aggression	Verbal and nonverbal communication with the intent to harm another person mentally or emotionally and/or to exert control over another person

Source: Centers for Disease Control and Prevention (CDC) (2019e, February 26). Preventing intimate partner violence: What is intimate partner violence? https://www.cdc.gov/violenceprevention/intimatepartnerviolence/fastfact.html/Public Domain.

more than 1,000 women die each year at the hands of their partners and husbands. To put these statistics in perspective, women are more likely to be beaten, raped, and killed by men they live with than by any other type of assailant.

Domestic violence is not limited to male partners. Many women in intimate relationships also attack their male partners, but it is important to note that women are much more likely to sustain serious bodily harm at the hands of their male partners, including broken bones and damage to internal organs. Bruises and broken bones are the visible signs of abuse, but the psychological effects can linger and include post-traumatic stress disorder (PTSD), depression, low self-esteem, alcohol and substance abuse, risky sexual behavior, even suicide.

Many batterers have problems with anger control and are impulsive, antisocial, and hostile (Bouchard & Wong, 2020). Many have drug abuse problems and low self-esteem as well. They may feel personally inadequate, which leads them to feel threatened when they perceive their partners as growing distant, more independent, or developing interests of their own (such as school or work). Violence may then be triggered by criticism or rejection by their partner. As in so many other instances of violence, the use of alcohol or other substances heightens the risk.

There is also an unequal power distribution between men and women in our society. Young men are socialized to play dominant roles and may expect women to bend to their wishes (Hamel, 2020). Men may enter relationships believing that force is appropriate when their needs are not met or their power is challenged.

More than 3 million children in the United States witness partner abuse each year, and they too experience psychological effects, such as depression and anxiety. Children with aggressive parents may learn that violence is an acceptable means of solving conflicts. The lesson may "transmit" domestic violence from generation to generation.

How Does Society Respond to Violence by Intimate Partners? How do police react when they are called to stop domestic violence? Too often they take a male perpetrator aside and "have a talk" with him rather than arrest him. Even if the man is arrested, he may only receive a slap on the wrist—a lesser sentence than he would have received if he had attacked a stranger. This leniency is based on old-fashioned idea that men somehow "own" their wives. After all, in traditional weddings, women are "given" away by their fathers to their husbands-to-be. The implications of this symbolic act may be that the bride becomes the groom's property. From a safety standpoint, we need to ensure that the justice system protects the rights of all victims of violent behavior, ensuring that one partner in a domestic relationship does not have the right to exert control over the other or resort to violence when their needs are not met.

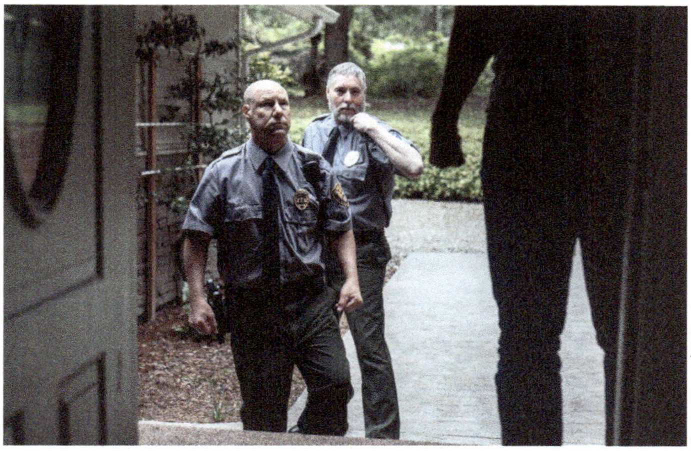

RyanJLane/Getty Images

Will He Be Arrested? How might incidents of domestic violence be treated differently by law enforcement than other types of violent crime?

Preventing domestic violence requires that parents demonstrate zero tolerance of domestic violence. Young men can be encouraged to respond to conflict with their heads, not their fists. The criminal justice system should deal with domestic violence as it deals with other acts of violence, and not make exceptions because the victim lives under the same roof as the assailant.

Roots of Violent Behavior

There are many forms of violence, from violent street crimes to actions of a mob enforcer to political violence in the form of upheavals, revolts, and acts of terror, as well as interpersonal violence such as intimate partner violence and rape. The problem of violence in all its many forms has no single cause. Understanding the roots of violence is best approached by the biopsychosocial model, which takes into account biological, psychological, and sociocultural factors. Let's take a closer look.

Biological Influences

The biological roots of aggression remain under study. One line of approach focuses on gaining a better understanding of the brain circuitry involved in regulating anger, as anger is often a catalyst for impulsive aggressive or violent behavior. As we will explore in Chapter 12, health psychologists play important roles in developing anger management programs, in part to reduce the risks that persistent anger poses with respect to cardiovascular health, but also to help people with anger problems learn to curb tendencies to lash out in anger. Relatedly, another line of research focuses on the possible roles of neurotransmitters involved in regulating anger. Toward this end, researchers have focused largely on the neurotransmitter serotonin, which works to "put the brakes" on impulsive behaviors, including impulsive anger. Serotonin has been described as a "behavioral seat belt" or an "emergency brake" that helps us restrain our impulsive behaviors (Raine, 2008). These are promising leads, but we lack solid evidence tying either abnormal brain circuitry or irregularities in neurotransmitters directly to violent behavior.

Then there is the possible role of the male sex hormone testosterone. We might hear someone say that overly aggressive men are pumped up with testosterone. However, the scientific evidence to date is not as clear-cut. A recent scientific review concluded that there is no strong evidence supporting a causal role of testosterone in fostering aggressive behavior in humans (Geniole et al., 2020). We should also note that not all, nor even most, men with high testosterone levels are aggressive, nor do all aggressive or violent men have high testosterone levels. What is clear is that human aggression in all its many forms is too complex a problem to be explained simply by the levels of circulating hormones in the bloodstream.

Alcohol is a psychoactive drug that affects the body's physiological functioning and mental processes and is associated with many acts of violence, including domestic violence, homicide, and rape (Kuypers et al., 2020; Robertson et al., 2020; Sontate et al., 2021). Alcohol does not directly cause violence, but it can set the stage for it. Alcohol impairs judgment and decision-making, reducing the ability to weigh the consequences of behavior. Alcohol may also affect brain processes controlling impulsive behavior, including impulsive acts of aggression or violence. From the social-cognitive perspective, we recognize that alcohol affects how people interpret social situations, for example, leading people to misperceive the motives of others as malevolent, which in turn might prompt aggressive responses on their part. However, it is important to consider that not everyone who consumes alcohol, even those who consume high levels of the drug, become aggressive.

Sociocultural Influences

The sociocultural perspective places aggressive and violent behavior in a broader social and cultural context. From this vantage point, we recognize the violent behavior often takes place against a backdrop of social stressors such as poverty, prolonged unemployment, lack of opportunity, child abuse and neglect, family breakdown, and exposure to violence in the family and community.

Exposure to violence in the home during childhood can have lasting impact. Growing up in a family wracked by violence exposes one to parenting figures as role models who may scream or punch first and discuss differences later—if at all (Hou et al., 2016; Valgardson & Schwartz, 2019). Becoming a target of violent rage at the hands of family members may build reservoirs of hostility that later become tapped at unpredictable times. The abused child may well become child abuser in adulthood in what we might describe as the intergenerational transmission of violence.

In many distressed neighborhoods, we find gangs that garner prestige for their members and offer young people a twisted sense of belonging. They provide a source of social approval that can rival the approval of parents and schools, as gang members offer rewards and privileges that young people cannot find in other aspects of their lives (Gravel et al., 2018). Gang violence is a way of protecting turf, of establishing power structures, and exerting control. Effective social interventions that provide alternatives to gang culture often involve efforts focused on networking with community organizations and stakeholders, building relationships with gang members and helping them resolve their problems, and providing them with resources and advocacy to cope with the underlying social problems that lead to gang membership (Free, 2020).

Violent behavior may also be a social influence tactic in which coercion, or threat of violence, is used to get people to comply with one's wishes. Examples of this form of violence are seen in the strong-arm tactics of a "mob enforcer" and also in cases of domestic abuse in which a husband uses violent behavior against his wife to compel her to accede to his demands.

Religious and sectarian violence between warring factions or between warring countries is a scourge that has caused the death of untold hundreds of millions of people throughout the millennia. Terrorism is a sociopolitical form of violence that unfortunately has touched our shores and remains a continuing threat here as well as across the world.

Anger and Frustration

Strong negative emotions, like anger and frustration, can provoke aggressive responses, especially when alcohol is part of the picture. But in humans, an aggressive response to a provocation is not automatic. Provocative behavior invokes a process of cognitive appraisal that can either prolong or defuse feelings of anger and the likelihood of aggression (Novaco, 2017). That is, the way in which a person appraises a provocation, such as treating it as an affront that must be met in kind, or merely an unwelcome act, has a determining effect on their response. The values the individual brings to bear in confrontative situations and the freedom to make choices interact to influence the likelihood of aggressive behavior. A history of reinforcement for acting violently, however, can increase the likelihood of aggression.

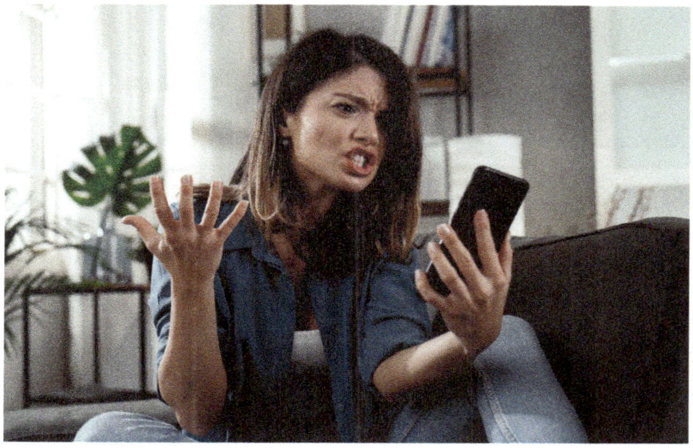

JustLife/Adobe Stock

Anger and Aggression What role does cognitive appraisal play in determining whether we act out in anger?

Anger is another negative emotion that can incite violence. The husband who is angered by something his wife says or does may act out violently in anger, or the child abuser may turn to physical violence when a child is slow to comply with parental demands. Psychologists recognize that angering thoughts trigger expressions of anger (e.g., "I can't let him/her get away with this . . .") as do tendencies to exaggerate the meaning of minor provocations out of all proportion to reality. Cognitive behavior therapists utilize techniques, such as those outlined in the discussion of anger management (see Chapter 12), to help people with anger management issues practice calming, alternative thoughts in conflict situations.

Frustration is an emotional reaction to situations in which your needs or goals are thwarted. While frustration often leads to aggression, other outcomes are possible. For example, picture yourself sitting behind someone in a movie theater who is talking throughout the show. You might feel frustrated because the person's behavior interferes with your ability to enjoy the movie, which in turn might prompt a state of readiness to respond aggressively either verbally or physically if the person doesn't heed requests to be silent. However, whether you act aggressively may depend on factors grounded in social-cognitive theory, especially your expectation about whether aggressive responses are likely to yield positive outcomes and whether you have been reinforced ("getting your way") in the past for aggressive behavior, among other factors.

All in all, violent behavior is best understood in terms of a complex matrix of factors.

Rape and Rape Prevention

The number of rapes is shockingly high. According to recent statistics, there are about 325,000 reported forcible rapes annually in the United States (Thompson & Tapp, 2022). But the number of reported rapes is but the tip of the iceberg, as only about one out of four or five rapes is reported to authorities.

To further explore how many women are sexually assaulted in the United States, we need to turn to surveys conducted by respected polling organizations. The National Intimate Partner and Sexual Violence Survey reported that one in five women experience **rape** or

rape Illegal sexual intercourse or any other sexual penetration of the vagina, anus, or mouth of another person, by force or threats, using a sex organ, another body part, or a foreign object without the consent of the victim.

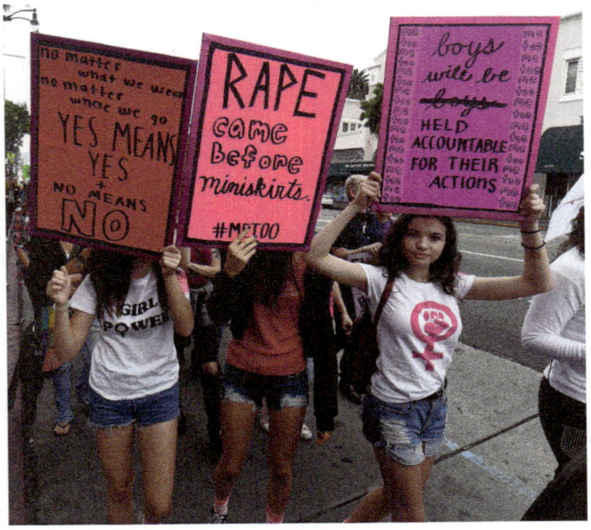

MARK RALSTON/Getty Images

attempted rape at some point in their lifetime (Smith et al., 2018). About 1% or 2% of men experience rape or attempted rape (Huecker et al., 2023).

In about 8 of 10 cases of rape, the victim knew the perpetrator. Of course, one rape by anyone, including a stranger, is one rape too many. One girl in 4 and 1 boy in 6 is sexually abused before their 18th birthday. Three in 10 females who are raped are between the ages of 11 and 17 years. It should go without saying, but let's say it anyway: It is illegal for men to force sex on their wives. However, many married women, as many as 1 in 7, have been raped by their husbands (National Sexual Violence Resource Center, 2018).

Twenty percent of women respondents to a *Washington Post*–Kaiser Family Foundation (2015) poll, aged 17–26, reported they had been sexually assaulted in college. So did 5% of the men. The women told pollsters things such as "We were kind of wrestling around. Things turned more sexual. I told him to stop. He thought I was joking. I froze. There was no question about consent. I said 'no' and he didn't care."

The effects of rape can be devastating, including depression, anxiety, and fear of social situations. Often women who have been raped develop sexual problems and sexual dysfunctions that are difficult to communicate to partners or spouses. Rape survivors may also find less pleasure in their daily lives.

Rape on Campus The *Washington Post*–Kaiser Family Foundation telephone survey provides a snapshot of rape on campus. To make sure participants represented the target population, interviewees were contacted by both land lines and mobile phones. A random nationally representative sample of adults aged 17–26 years who were in college or had recently been in college was recruited.

Overall, 20% of the women and 5% of the men reported that they had been sexually assaulted. Nine percent of the women reported they were overcome by physical force, and 14% said they were assaulted while incapacitated, most often by alcohol, although some women thought they had been slipped a drug. The sample all but universally (96%) agreed that having sex with a person who was incapacitated by alcohol or passed out was sexual assault. Only about 20% of women and 30% of men thought that students would claim that they had been sexually assaulted when it was not true.

Many states have enacted laws stating that college students must provide affirmative consent for sexual activity to be legitimate. We have all heard the expression that "No means no," but this standard means that only "Yes means yes." Couples are encouraged to pause while making love to ascertain that they are in agreement that they can go farther.

By and large, sexual assailants on campus are not strangers. One in 4 or 5 (22%) female victims of rape or other unwanted sexual contact said they knew the attacker very well, and 25% said they knew him fairly well. Only 28% said they didn't know the attacker at all.

Nearly 3 in 4 (71%) of women who survive a rape on campus told someone about the assault, but only 12% of these reported the incident to the police or college authorities. Why do they avoid telling the authorities? Reporting a sexual assault is embarrassing for many or most victims, and the process of following up with testimony or physical evidence can also be embarrassing, even humiliating. There is also the question as to whether the complaint will go anywhere; only 1 attacker in 10 was ever held responsible or punished for the assault.

A majority of students felt that the following measures might prevent sexual assault at their school: harsher punishments for perpetrators, training students how to defend themselves and to intervene to defend others, and requiring all students, male and female, to attend prevention programs. To be fair, colleges are paying more attention to the problem of sexual assault; 71% of respondents felt that their schools were doing enough to try to prevent sexual assault.

Most students also felt it would help if men paid women more respect, if there were less drinking, and if students avoided casual hookups.

Self-Assessment

INTERACTIVE SELF-ASSESSMENTS

Cultural Myths That Create a Climate That Supports Rape

Here are some examples of myths about rape that help create a cultural climate that increases the likelihood of rape in the United States. Place a checkmark in front of those myths you believe—or did believe—before reading this section of the text. Then check the retorts at the end of the chapter that help to debunk these beliefs.

___ Myth 1: A woman who would go to a man's home or apartment on a first date is implying that she is willing to have sex.

___ Myth 2: Many women claim that they have been raped only to call attention to themselves.

___ Myth 3: A healthy woman can resist a rapist if she sincerely wants to do so.

___ Myth 4: Women who don't wear bras or who wear short skirts and other sexually appealing clothing are asking for trouble.

___ Myth 5: Most women who have been raped are promiscuous or have a bad reputation.

___ Myth 6: A girl who engages in necking or petting is letting things get out of hand, so you can't blame her partner if he forces sex on her.

___ Myth 7: Women who are hitchhiking get what they deserve.

___ Myth 8: Women who think they're too good to talk to men they pass on the street need to be taught a lesson.

___ Myth 9: Many women have an unconscious desire to be raped.

___ Myth 10: Many women who report a rape are angry with the men they accuse and want to punish them, or they find themselves pregnant and don't want to be blamed.

Why Do Men Sexually Assault Women? According to Emily Rothman (2017), codirector of the Violence Prevention Research Unit at the Boston University School of Public Health, there are at least four reasons that men sexually assault women. Some people have trouble controlling impulses—in this case, sexual impulses. However, let us note that some professionals argue that sexual harassment and assault are more often about power and aggression than sex (Quick, 2018). Other attackers have deviant ideas about what intimate relationships ought to be. A third reason is a sense of entitlement—the feeling that people can do as they wish because, as suggested by James Campbell Quick (2018) of the University of Texas, they are in positions of power. And, fourth, some perpetrators are sexually excited by deviant sexual stimuli, including aggressive sex and other acts perpetrated without the consent of the victim.

Evolutionary psychologists suggest that among ancestral humans, males who were more sexually aggressive were more likely to transmit their genes to future generations (Gladden & Cleator, 2018; Huppin & Malamuth, 2017). Thus, men may have a genetic tendency to be more sexually aggressive than women. However, evolutionary psychologists do not condone rape or sexual aggression. Human beings have also evolved complex brains that give us the ability to regulate our emotions and behavior; we can choose whether or not to behave aggressively (Davis, 2020).

Many social critics, however, contend that American culture socializes young men— including perhaps that "nice" young man next door—into sexually aggressive roles by reinforcing them for aggressive and competitive behavior (Krivoshchekov et al., 2022; O'Dea et al., 2022). Boys are often exposed to coaches who emphasize winning at all costs. They are taught to be dominant and to vanquish their opponents, even if winning means injuring or taking out the opposition. Might this philosophy carry over from the playing field into relationships with women?

The lessons learned in competitive sports may predispose young men to dominate and overpower their opponents, even to the point of viewing the women they date as opponents in a game in which "winning" is everything and "scoring" sexually is the goal. Sexual behavior and sports in our culture are also linked through common idioms. A young man may be taunted by his friends after a date with a woman with such questions as "Did you score?" or more bluntly, "Did you get it in?" Unfortunately, these lessons may carry over when women resist their sexual overtures. Many young men view their dating partners as opponents whose resistance must be overcome by whatever means is necessary, even if it requires force. The addition of alcohol to the mix impairs judgment and ability to weigh the consequences of behavior, further increasing the risk of sexual aggression (Bonomi et al., 2018). Then too, gender stereotyping may socialize young men to reject traditionally feminine traits such as tenderness and empathy which might otherwise curb aggressive behavior (Tian, 2023).

We also need to consider the cognitive underpinnings of rape. Men may misread a woman's resistance as a coy form of game-playing on her part, thinking that "no" means "maybe" and "maybe" means "yes." When it comes to reading signals, men generally have blurrier social perceptions than do women. Men tend to overestimate the sexual interest of women they have just met, especially when the men think of themselves as "hot" even if they're not, and also when men find women more sexually attractive (Treat et al., 2017). Women, in contrast, tend to underestimate men's sexual interest.

The Role of Beliefs About Rape

The aptly named Health Belief Model (HBM) focuses on the role of beliefs in determining health-related behaviors—beliefs regarding health threats and the benefits of making healthy changes in behavior, such as getting screened for cancer or obtaining vaccinations. Personal beliefs are also important in determining the likelihood of engaging in sexually coercive behaviors or legitimizing these behaviors.

Rape myths are a set of erroneous beliefs that create a social climate that serves to legitimize rape and sexual assaults (Milesi et al., 2020). Although both men and women are susceptible to believing myths about rape, researchers find that men are more accepting of rape myths than women (Barnett et al., 2017; Ryan, 2019; Stoll et al., 2017). College men also cling more stubbornly to myths about date rape than women do, even following date rape education classes designed to challenge these views.

Rape myths tend to blame the victim rather than the rapist. An example is the belief that women who don't fight back or appear to "freeze in place" actually want to be raped. Yet scientists argue that a freezing response to trauma (and a sexual attack certainly qualifies as a trauma) represents an involuntary defensive response in humans and other animals (Percy, 2023).

Adopting a set of false beliefs about rape might lead to making excuses for acts of sexual violence and even creating a mindset that increases the likelihood of committing these acts. Rape myths do not occur in a social vacuum. They are related to other social attitudes, including gender-role stereotyping, perception of sex as adversarial, and acceptance of violence in relationships. Widely held social attitudes serve to sanction sexual aggression, such as beliefs that women who say "no" really mean "yes" and that women prefer men who are pushy and forceful (Lilley at al., 2023; Wilson & Newins, 2023). In the nearby Self-Assessment, we take a closer look at examples of commonly held rape myths.

Rape Prevention The responsibility and fault for a sexual crime lies entirely with the perpetrator—the rapist. But we also understand that there are steps each of us can take to reduce our personal vulnerability to sexual assault and address the larger social context that creates an environment that supports sexual violence. It is encouraging that many colleges and universities now require students to attend rape awareness lectures and seminars. Many of these programs are also directed at men from traditionally "masculinized" college groups: members of fraternities and athletes (Ruvalcaba et al., 2022). More generally, rape prevent programs address both men and women and seek to promote more respectful sexual attitudes, dispel myths about rape, and teach men that "no" means "no" (Koss, 2018; Winerman, 2018).

On a societal level, we need to encourage the enacting of laws and policies that will make it easier for rape survivors to come forward and participate in the prosecution of sex criminals. The criminal justice system can be a nightmare for people who survive rape. Many women fear coming forward because of the widespread acceptance of rape myths, all of which have the effect of blaming the victim. Moreover, in court, defense attorneys may trot out a woman's entire sexual history to show that she can hardly be considered a victim of a man's sexual advances. It is not surprising that the majority of women who survive rape tell friends about the assault but do not bring it to the attention of authorities.

Stopping sexual violence before it starts is an important national health goal (CDC, 2023e). Accomplishing this goal requires coordinated efforts between government health officials, healthcare providers, the criminal justice system, and educational and cultural institutions.

Applying Health Psychology

Now What? Will She Report It to the Authorities?—Benefits and Barriers of Reporting

Consider the following hypothetical scenario:

She was sexually assaulted by someone she knows. She had been drinking but was far from drunk. They had been "clowning around," but things took a serious turn. She said no but he didn't listen. She is overwhelmed and she is angry. She believes that her assailant committed a crime, but will she report it to authorities?

The Health Belief Model (HBM) can help us better understand the underlying factors involved in reporting a sexual assault. According to the model, people are more likely to engage in a course of action when they determine that the perceived benefits of taking action outweigh the costs that they may face. In the aftermath of a rape, women often struggle with weighing the perceived costs and benefits, as well as the barriers, of reporting the rape to authorities.

Another HBM factor that can tip the scale toward reporting the rape is self-efficacy, which is one's belief in their ability to successfully carry out a course of action, such as knowing whom to contact and how to follow through with filing a report. And then there are cues to action, another HBM factor. A person who survives rape might be more likely to act if she had been visibly injured as the result of the assault. She might also be more likely to act if she told a friend about it and the friend urged her to report the act. On the other hand, what if a friend told her she would only be wasting her time and embarrassing herself by reporting the incident? All of these factors may be weighed in consideration of whether to file a report of a sexual assault.

Women who are raped may perceive a benefit of reporting it to be the need for justice to be served. They may believe that the perpetrator should be punished, that he should not be allowed to get away with his crime of violence and continue his life as if nothing had happened. Yet only about 1 rape in 5 or 6 is reported to authorities (O'Donohue, 2019), and many women who report rape wait a month or more after the incident to do so. For many that month is filled with reflection on the barriers to reporting the assault (Abavi et al., 2020; O'Donohue, 2019):

1. Many women who survive rape feel overwhelmed and tend toward avoidance-based coping, such as trying to put it out of mind and avoiding the stimuli—such as the locale—where the rape took place.
2. Women who survive rape may be uncertain as to where to draw the line between sexual advances and crimes of violence (Schwarz et al., 2017).
3. Fear and embarrassment. Many women who survive rape report fear of backlash from others, of being in the spotlight, of not being believed or supported (Schwarz et al., 2017). They may also fear backlash from friends and family, or social and legal consequences. Some may report, "The risks seem greater than any reward."
4. Personal relationship with the perpetrator. They may say, "He was my friend (or boyfriend)," or, simply, "I knew him."
5. Alcohol. Drinking alcohol often leads women who survive rape to think that they and their assailants are both to blame or that she should have known better or been better able to stop the assault (Hahn et al., 2020; Mouilso & Wilson, 2019).
6. The ideas of "victim blaming" and "slut shaming" are built into U.S. culture, and women who survive rape may not be willing to expose themselves to these pernicious slurs (Bhuptani & Messman-Moore, 2019; Grandgenett et al., 2020).
7. Some women report being unsure about the details of the incident and that they might not be able to effectively report them.

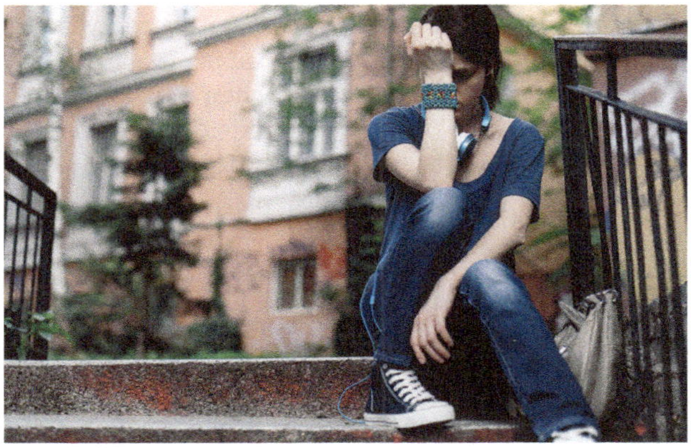

martin-dm/E+/Getty Images

She Has Been Sexually Assaulted. Now What? We hope that she had a medical checkup and took precautions about the possibilities of becoming pregnant or infected with sexually transmitted diseases. Unfortunately, she is likely to be overwhelmed with anxiety, fear, and feelings of depression, and may have difficulty coping with the assault. Will she report the rape? She may tell friends but be more hesitant about bringing in the authorities. The criminal justice system and society at large have a way of blaming and humiliating survivors of rape.

Informed by the best available evidence, the CDC promotes a multipronged strategy to prevent sexual violence, which includes the following preventive measures:

- Promoting social norms that protect against violence
- Teaching skills to prevent sexual violence
- Supporting victims/survivors to lessen harms
- Providing opportunities to empower and support girls and women
- Creating protective environments

In addition to such efforts at the societal level, there is much we can do as individuals to protect ourselves from sexual violence perpetrated by strangers and acquaintances.

First let us consider sexual violence by strangers. Some measures are common sense. Put only your first initials on the apartment mailbox and in phone or email listings. Use deadbolt locks on doors and keep windows locked. Have your keys ready for the car and the door. Check the car's rear seat before getting in; drive with windows up and doors locked. Don't pick up hitchhikers, including women. Shout "Fire!," not "Rape!" Most people will be inclined to help victims of fire but shy away from violent situations. Take self-defense training. Research evidence suggests that there are some situations in which it is helpful to physically resist a would-be assailant (Dardis et al., 2018).

There are also reasonable ways to lessen the likelihood of date rape:

1. *Be clear about your sexual limits.* If your date touches you in ways that make you uncomfortable, you might say something like "Please stop doing that. I hardly know you." Look your date in the eye. The more definite you are, the less likely it is that the man will misinterpret your wishes.
2. *Meet new people in public places, and don't get in a car with a stranger or a group of people you've just met.* It's safest to take your own car or take public transportation and meet your date in a public place.
3. *Respond to your fears.* Is your assertiveness stifled by concern about displeasing your date? If your partner is respectful of you, you need not fear an angry or demeaning response. But if your partner is not respectful, get out of the situation as soon as you can. (Hit the panic button on your app?)
4. *Trust your "vibes"—your gut-level feelings.* Many women who survive rape by acquaintances had strange feelings about the man but ignored them.
5. *Be cautious if you are in a new environment, such as starting college or visiting a foreign country.* Rapists may target newcomers. You may be especially vulnerable to exploitation when you are becoming acquainted with a new environment, different people, and different customs.
6. *If you have broken off a relationship with someone you don't trust, don't let him into your place.* Change locks if necessary. Many acquaintance rapes are committed by angry or frustrated ex-boyfriends.
7. *Stay sober and see that your date does too.* Alcohol loosens inhibitions, clouds the judgment, and makes one more vulnerable.

Health Psychology in the Digital Age

Rape Prevention? There's an App for That (Actually, There Are Several)

After a colleague raped her, Nancy Schwartzman rode home with him (Lapowsky, 2014). She was 24 years old, living alone in a foreign city, and she didn't know exactly where she was. Living so far from friends and family at home, she didn't have anyone to call to pick her up. So, after enduring the most frightening and violating experience of her life, she wound up with her assailant driving her back to her apartment.

Now Schwartzman works on technology to ensure that no woman ever feels stranded before or after an assault. Schwartzman is the CEO of a company that makes Circle of 6, a free app that recruits six trusted friends whom users can easily alert in case of emergency. Users enter their circle into the app, and with a simple press of a button the contacts will be texted. Users can send texts that ask members of the circle to come for them or call them. The app can also connect national rape support lines. For college students, Circle of 6 can come programmed with the phone numbers of the college's support resources.

Several other apps also help a woman prevent a sexual assault—On Watch, Safety Siren, Panic Guard, and My Force. Most of them are free.

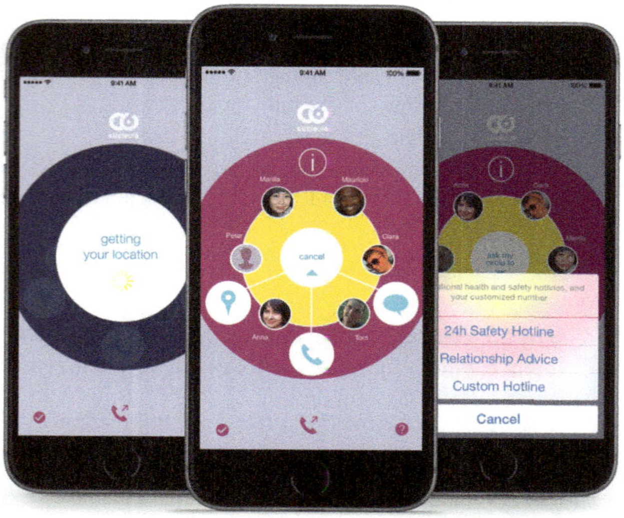

Source: Circleof6.com

Circle of 6 The free rape-prevention app is an excellent method for preventing sexual assault. It can have your friends use GPS to pick you up or to call you *right now*.

Review 8.1

INTERACTIVE SELF-SCORING QUIZZES

Sentence Completion

1. Victims of violence are usually of the (same or different) race of the assailant.

2. __________ are the most commonly used weapons in murder in the United States.

3. Nearly __________ people in the United States are killed by firearms each year.

4. Black adults are (more or less) likely to be victims of homicide than other major ethnic/racial groups in the United States.

5. More than half of perpetrators of hate crimes are __________ Americans.

6. Nearly 1 woman in __________ has experienced severe physical violence at the hands of an intimate partner.

7. __________ percent of women respondents to the *Washington Post* poll reported that they had been sexually assaulted in college.

8. Cultural myths create a social climate that (supports or inhibits) rape.

9. Blaming the __________ is a barrier experienced by women who are considering reporting a rape to authorities.

Think About It

As you considered the cultural myths that support a climate that encourages rape, did you find any that rang true to you? Now that you think about it, can you see how these items blame the victim? Why do you think that women are reluctant to go to the authorities when they have been sexually assaulted? Can you think of any case in which a woman has been publicly humiliated when she has claimed that a man sexually assaulted her?

Accident Prevention

Accidents or unintentional injuries account for nearly 225,000 deaths in the United States, representing the fourth leading cause of deaths in the nation (CDC, 2023c). There are notable sex differences. Unintentional injuries were the third leading cause of death for males, accounting for 7.6% of deaths but the sixth leading cause of death for females, accounting for 4.4% of deaths. Age differences are even more notable. Unintentional injuries are the number one leading cause of death for Americans between the ages of 1 through 44, accounting for 40.6% of deaths for 10- to 24-year-olds. Accidents then become less likely causes of death for older age groups, accounting for 8.8% of deaths for 45- to 64-year-olds and 2.7% for people aged 65 years and above.

What do you suppose is the most frequent type of fatal accident? If you guessed motor vehicle accidents, take this opportunity to guess again. Number one on the list of fatal accidents is poisoning, with more than 64,000 deaths per year (CDC, 2017c). Next come motor vehicle accidents with about 40,000 deaths per year. Third are falls, claiming the lives of more than 36,000 people per year, often older people.

Nonfatal accidents affect millions of people in the United States each year, with many of these often avoidable accidents causing serious injuries and leading to chronic pain. Nearly 4 of 10 emergency department visits result from accidents. About one person in nine seeks medical attention for an accidental injury each year. Accidentally being struck by people or objects accounts for another 1 in 10 accident-related visits, as do cuts or puncture wounds.

It may come as a surprise to learn that you stand a much greater chance of drowning in your bathtub than dying in a lightning strike. Yet under the threat of lightning, people will scurry for cover, as they well should, but very few people express fear of taking a bath.

We're not suggesting living in fear of daily life experiences, but it would be prudent to ensure that our homes and cars are safe and that we exercise appropriate care when driving, biking, swimming, and boating. Practicing safety behaviors is an important topic of interest to health psychologists and to us all.

Let us start our search for safety where most of us get up in the morning—at home.

Playing It Safe at Home

"There's no place like home"—for accidents, that is. Home is where we face the greatest risk of serious or disabling injuries. In fact, accidents in the home account for more than twice

Applying Health Psychology

Preventing Repetitive Stress Injuries

Many college students complain of pain from using a keyboard. Continual keyboard use can lead to carpal tunnel syndrome, an inflammation of the tissue that covers nerves in the wrist. As the tissue becomes inflamed, it presses on nerves, causing pain and impairing functioning. Use of ergonomically designed keyboards can help relieve stress on the wrist and hand, reducing the pain.

Other suggestions:

1. Adjust the height of the keyboard so that your forearms remain parallel to the floor.
2. Adjust the height of your chair so that your thighs are also parallel to the floor.
3. Keep your wrists parallel to the floor—don't rest them on the desk.
4. Use your arms to move your fingers around the keyboard. Don't let your fingers do all the stretching.
5. Sit straight up in your chair and avoid leaning toward the keyboard.
6. Take frequent breaks to stretch and move about the room or office.

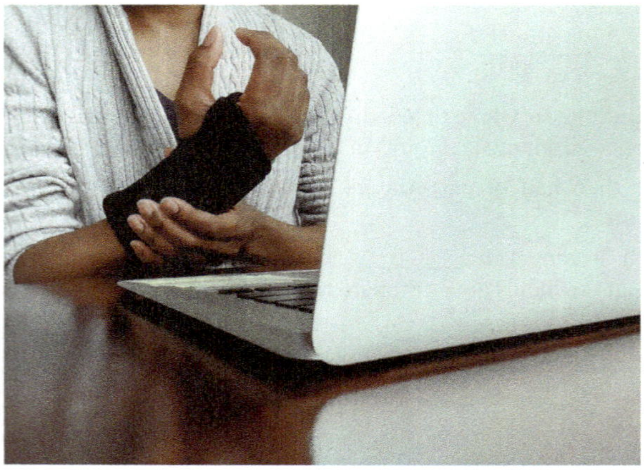

Grace Cary/Getty Images

the number of disabling injuries as motor vehicle crashes. Accidents in the home account for some 13 million disabling injuries and about 54,000 deaths each year in the United States (National Vital Statistics Reports, 2019). By contrast, accidents in the workplace account for some 4,300 deaths and 3.2 million disabling injuries annually.

More than 200 children die annually in the United States as the result of accidents involving firearms. In total, more than 500 Americans lose their lives each year from the accidental discharge of firearms, and many thousands more are severely injured (National Safety Council, 2023b).

Most household accidents are preventable. How do we make our homes safer? Here are some ideas:

1. **Store household chemicals and cleansers in their proper containers.** Follow the product instructions for use and storage.
2. **Avoid falls.** Accidental falls are the leading cause of preventable deaths in the home. Use slip-resistant strips in bathtubs and under area rugs. Provide adequate lighting on stairs. Avoid leaving small objects on the floor or stairs where people may trip over them and keep steps and handrails in good condition.
3. **Child-proof the home.** Secure windows with window guards. If there are small children, install gates at the tops and bottoms of stairways to prevent accidental falls. Use outlet covers for exposed electrical outlets. Keep matches, lighters, household chemicals, over-the-counter or prescription medications or drugs, or any objects with sharp edges, such as knives or scissors out of the reach of children.
4. **Prevent fires.** Keep candles away from furniture or flammable materials. Have a fire extinguisher handy. Install smoke detectors and check the batteries regularly. Never smoke in bed (better yet, never smoke). Do not leave cooking food unattended; most household fires start in the kitchen. Develop a fire-escape plan.
5. **Protect your family from firearms:**
   a. Take a gun safety course.
   b. Store firearms in such a way that children cannot access them. Lock them in a safe or gun storage cabinet.
   c. Store ammunition and guns in separate, locked locations.
   d. Use trigger locks.

Preventing Injuries on the Road

What do you suppose is the leading cause of death of young Americans in the 16- to 20-year-old age range? Infectious diseases like COVID-19 or HIV/AIDS? Cancer? Or is it homicide or suicide? The answer is motor vehicle accidents. The greatest numbers of incidents on the road involving serious injuries or fatalities are found among young, inexperienced or newly licensed drivers.

The good news is that improvements in car safety and efforts of government at the local, state, and federal levels to curb risky driving have saved thousands of lives.

One of the key safety measures resulting in fewer deaths and serious injuries on the nation's roads is the use of seat belts. Seat belts save about 15,000 lives and prevent about 300,000 serious injuries each year. Nearly half of all front row passengers killed in motor vehicle crashes were not wearing seat belts at the time of accident (Kidd & Singer, 2019).

Owing in large part to public health campaigns promoting the use of seat belts and legal requirements imposed on drivers and front-seat passengers, seat-belt use has been consistently rising, and is now up to more than 90% of all car occupants (National Safety Council, 2023a). However, seat-belt use is lower among young people in the 16- to 24-year-old age range than among older groups (NHTSA, 2020). Young men are at greatest risk. Among 18- to 34-year-old men involved in fatal crashes, 60% were not wearing seat belts.

Although we have made much progress in promoting safety on the nation's roads, more than 42,000 Americans still die each year in motor vehicle accidents (NHTSA, 2023a). Many of these deaths could have been prevented. Another 3 million people annually sustain serious injuries from motor vehicle accidents (NHTSA, 2020).

According to the National Highway Traffic Safety Administration (NHTSA), buckling up is the single most effective way to protect oneself in a crash (NHTSA, 2020). Air bags are designed to work with seat belts, not to replace them. Don't assume that you needn't wear seat belts if you're only going a few miles; the majority of fatal crashes occur within 25 miles from home and at speeds under 40 miles an hour.

What can *you* do to avoid becoming another statistic? A number of things:

1. **Buckle up:** Use your seat belt and make sure children are securely buckled or, if young enough, placed in a car safety seat.
2. **Obey the speed limit:** Each month more than 1,000 Americans are killed in crashes involving speeding.
3. **Stay sober:** Impairment of driving skills begins with the first drink and increases with each drink.
4. **Do not engage in distracted driving:** Don't text, eat, or drink while driving. Just drive.

Health Psychologists Take to the Road Think for a moment about the role of health psychology in promoting seat-belt use. This is a major health preventive behavior that for most people has become as routine a habit as turning on the car radio, maybe more so. But a generation or two ago, many drivers simply ignored safety instructions to buckle up. Consistent with the Health Behavior Model (HBM; see Chapter 2), the perceived risk (threat) of accidents is among the major psychological factors predicting self-reported use of seat belts (Sheveland et al., 2020). But we can also take a lesson from automobile manufacturers about putting principles of behavior change discussed in Chapter 2 into practice.

You'll recall that reinforcers are stimuli or events that increase the likelihood of the behaviors they follow. So when we praise children for brushing their teeth and they begin brushing more regularly, we would consider praise to be an effective reinforcer. In particular, it is a positive reinforcer because it is introduced after a desired behavior (tooth brushing) occurs. By contrast, a negative reinforcer involves the removal of an unpleasant or aversive stimulus after a desired response occurs. Like positive reinforcement, negative reinforcement strengthens behavior. For example, when faced with the unpleasant stimulus of raindrops falling on our head, we learn to raise an umbrella, which removes the unpleasant stimulus—an example of negative reinforcement in daily life (assuming we remember to bring an umbrella with us). Raising an umbrella when pelted with rain quickly becomes a learned habit.

Let's apply the concept of negative reinforcement to seat-belt use. A successful public health campaign in the 1960s, "Buckle Up for Safety," raised awareness about the safety benefits of using seat belts. Many people buckled up, but some held fast to unrestrained driving. To encourage greater use of seat belts, automobile manufacturers began installing auditory chimes and annoying alarms that were automatically activated whenever a car was started while seat belts remained unfastened. These auditory signals served as reminders to buckle up but also as negative reinforcers. That is, people who didn't first fasten their seat belts before starting the car soon learned to do so to avoid the annoying warning sound or they quickly buckled themselves up to turn off the unpleasant stimulus if they had neglected to do so. From the standpoint of learning theory, stopping an annoying sound after performing the desirable act of fastening the seat belts makes the practice of using seat belts more likely to occur, to a point now that people buckle up without giving it a second thought. This simple behavioral nudge in the form of a seat-belt warning sound has likely saved many lives.

Behavioral researchers have also turned their attention to identifying factors linked to the risk of accidents. For example, British researchers studied the perceptions of risk factors for traffic accidents among a sample of 210 drivers (Smith & Smith, 2017). Two of 3 participants (66.2%) identified driving after having four drinks as the single greatest risk. Half (50.5%) identified having lapses of concentration. Nearly half (48.5%) identified driving when tired, and 4 in 10 (41.9%) identified speeding. More than 1 in 4 (27.2%) identified "indicating hostility" to other drivers. The group did not find driving with the radio on, driving with a passenger, or driving with the window open to be notable risks.

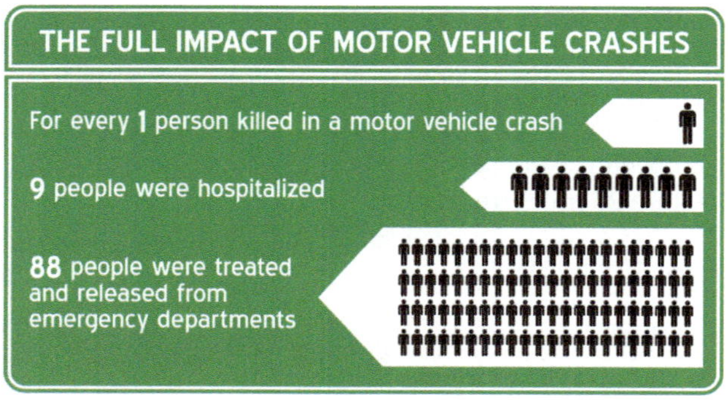

Source: https://www.cdc.gov/motorvehiclesafety/index.html / Public Domain.

(Avoid) Driving While Distracted

Nineteen-year-old Aaron was driving home from a weekend with his girlfriend at 75 miles an hour when he felt he had to express his love by sending her a text message. He wound up pinned beneath a truck with two broken legs and an injured kidney, liver, and spleen.

Twenty percent of motor vehicle accidents resulting in injuries are due to distracted driving (Distracted Driving, 2019). The main risk faced by driving and phoning is loss of concentration, not fumbling with the phone. According to Dr. Amy Ship of Harvard Medical School, "Driving while distracted is roughly equivalent to driving drunk."

The U.S. Government Website for Distracted Driving lists the following distractions:

1. Texting
2. Talking on a cellphone
3. Eating and drinking
4. Talking to passengers
5. Grooming
6. Reading
7. Setting a navigation unit
8. Watching a video
9. Adjusting the radio station, DVD, or MP3 player

Drivers under the age of 20 years are most likely to have distraction-related fatal crashes (Distracted Driving, 2019). The Youth Risk Behavior Surveillance System of the Centers for Disease Control and Prevention found that 42% of high school drivers sent a text or email while driving within the past month. Students who texted while driving were also less likely to wear seat belts, more likely to ride with drivers who have been drinking alcohol, and more likely to drink and drive themselves.

Eating or drinking while driving distracts your attention from the road, but foods that drip, spill, and ooze are most likely to divert our attention (see **Table 8.3**). Coffee may be the most dangerous, in part because of fiddling with the cup. Even cups with coffee lids tend to spill. Hot coffee can cause painful burns, but coffee is not the only serious offender.

TABLE 8.3 Top 10 Food Offenders While Driving

Offender	Comment
1. Coffee	Always finds a way to spill from the cup
2. Hot soup	High spill potential, which burns
3. Tacos	Messy, messy, diverting attention to keep contents from falling out
4. Chili	Ditto—potentially dangerous drips
5. Hamburgers	Drips, especially grease, mustard, ketchup
6. Barbecue	Ditto—only more so, and grease on steering wheel may cause hands to slip
7. Fried chicken	Grease again, on fingers, steering wheel, etc.
8. Jelly or cream-filled doughnuts	Ooze, causing a distracting mess
9. Soft drinks	Spill from containers, especially over bumps in the road
10. Chocolate	Gets on fingers and steering wheels, tempting drivers to clean it off, creating a dangerous risk of swerving or losing control

Source: Strillacci, L (2005). 10 Most Dangerous Foods to Eat on the Road. *Insure.com.* http://moneycentral.msn.com/content/Insurance/P51290.asp

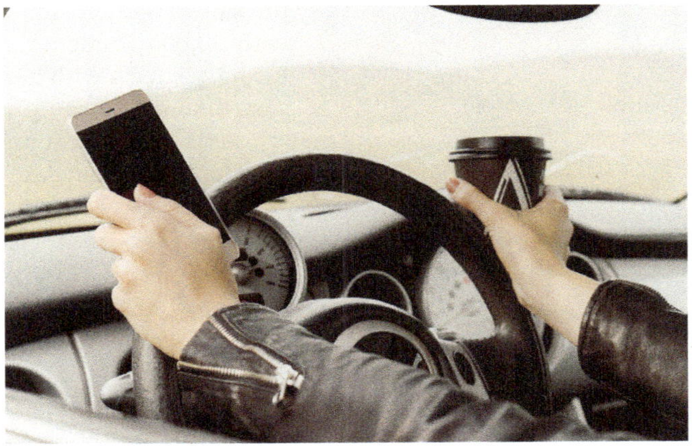

yanik88/Shutterstock.com

Keeping Your Eyes on the Road, Not on Your Shirt Here is a math problem for you that can have real world consequences, sadly tragic consequences. Don't worry, we'll do the computations. Assume that a car traveling 60 miles an hour covers the length of a football field in less than 4 seconds. If you are distracted from your driving by eating, the car may be traveling blindly for 5, 10, or more seconds. Now assume that your car is 17 feet long and your car is five car lengths behind the car in front of you. Imagine that the car ahead of you suddenly slows down while you are trying to clean the ooze from a taco that has stained your shirt. If you're traveling 60 miles an hour, you will cover the distance between your car and a rapidly slowing car ahead in about a second. A mere one second can make the difference between a preventable disaster and a tragic accident.

Would you agree that you and other drivers and passengers would be better off if you left the taco ooze on your shirt or, better yet, not ever facing such a situation by eating a taco or anything else while your car is parked? The HBM posits that perceptions of a health threat or risk, combined with beliefs about the benefits of practicing safer behaviors, influence the types of behaviors people are likely to practice on the road. For your safety and those of other drivers on the road, consider the risks of distracted driving against the benefits of driving safely.

Driving While Drowsy The government estimates that nearly 800 people die on the nation's roads, and more than 50,000 are injured, as the result of drivers who are drowsy or asleep at the wheel (NHTSA, 2023b). Accidents are most likely to occur in the early morning hours when drivers are most fatigued. You can protect yourself and others from distracted driving by modifying your behavior—yet another example of how changing behavior can save lives and lead to healthier outcomes.

Drowsy driving is a common problem in many parts of the world. An Indonesian health psychology study found that factors that influenced drowsy driving were consistent with the Theory of Planned Behavior (TPB; see Chapter 2) and included perceived behavioral control and perceived barriers to performing safer behaviors (Rahmadiyani & Widyanti, 2023). Think about putting the TPB model into practice. Consider what behaviors you can directly control to avoid drowsy driving and the barriers that might interfere with performing these safety behaviors, such as the suggestions described in the nearby Applying Health Psychology feature.

Applying Health Psychology

How to Stay Alert (and Alive) on the Road

To prevent distracted driving, keep in mind when driving that you are operating a potentially deadly weapon. Here are some safety behaviors you can practice to reduce the risk of becoming yet another statistic in the tally of motor vehicle fatalities and injuries (NHTSA, 2023b):

1. Getting adequate sleep on a daily basis is the only true way to protect yourself against the risks of driving when you're drowsy.
2. Before starting a long family car trip, get a good night's sleep, or you could put your entire family and others at risk.
3. Avoid drinking any alcohol before driving. Consumption of alcohol interacts with sleepiness to increase drowsiness and impairment.
4. Always check your prescription and over-the-counter medication labels to see if drowsiness could result from their use.
5. If you take medications that could cause drowsiness as a side effect, use public transportation when possible.
6. If you drive, avoid driving during the peak sleepiness periods (midnight–6 a.m. and late afternoon). If you must drive during the peak sleepiness periods, stay vigilant for signs of drowsiness, such as crossing over roadway lines or hitting a rumble strip, especially if you're driving alone.
7. Bear in mind that drinking coffee or energy drinks may not be sufficient to keep you alert and their effects may only last a short time. But if you are feeling sleepy while driving, drinking one to two cups of coffee and pulling for a short 20-minute nap in a safe place may increase alertness, but only for a short time.

Crossing the Street While Distracted—Are We Experiencing a Smartphone Zombie Apocalypse? If ever there was a reason to stop (on the sidewalk!) and think, the smartphone apocalypse is it. Rexburg, Idaho, is a small city with 30,000 residents that has an unsought distinction: Five pedestrians died crossing Rexburg streets with a lethal lesson in distracted behavior; their noses were buried in their smartphones.

As a result, Rexburg banned crossing streets with pedestrians' attention glued to their smartphones. Montclair, California, officials have also had their fill of what the city manager dubbed "cellphone zombies," and the city has made it illegal to cross streets while texting, wearing music buds, or talking on a smartphone. Repeat offenders can be served with $500 fines. Honolulu also has the ban. New York and other cities are contemplating it.

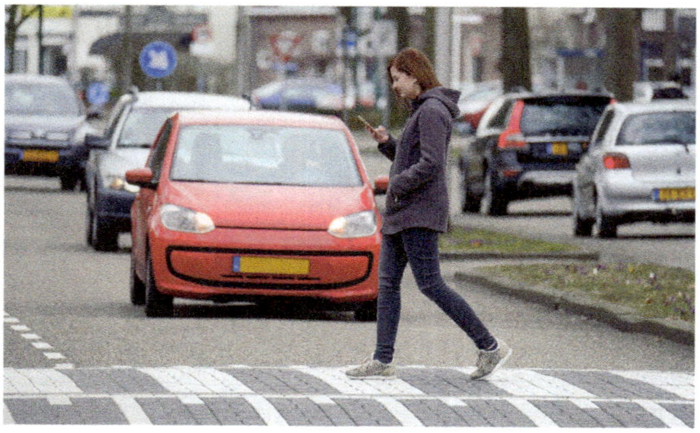
itsajoop/Shutterstock.com

We generally recognize the dangers of distracted driving, but distracted walking is also a threat, especially when pedestrians with plugged ears assume they own the street once the light turns green—if they notice the light at all. Nearly 6,000 U.S. pedestrians die each year, and another 68,000 are injured, apparently because they assumed that all potentially deadly moving objects will find their ways around them (Barton et al., 2016). Or perhaps they don't think about that at all—their attention was elsewhere.

Health Psychology in Action

The TPB and Distracted Walking

A study by Benjamin Barton and his colleagues (2016) at the University of Idaho tested the applicability of the TPB to pedestrians who cross streets while distracted. The participants in this study considered various scenarios in which, for example, they would cross a street while answering a phone call from a friend, while texting or reading a text or email, or while listening to music that blotted out the sounds of traffic. Participants who said they would cross the street under these types of conditions explained their behavior by indicating that walking would go by faster and be more pleasant if they crossed the street under one or more of these scenarios. Moreover, they perceived themselves to have control over the situation (they believed they could cross without getting hit by a car or another vehicle).

The researchers speculated that the short-term payoff (greater enjoyment of the walk) outweighed the relatively remote possibility of being stuck down in the street. Social norms were not an issue, apparently because the participants were not aware of others who would frown intensely on their behavior. Two things are particularly worth noting. First, participants who knew people who had been injured when crossing traffic because they were distracted, or who had been injured themselves, were more likely to avoid being distracted. The risk was more real for them. Second, males were more likely than females to perceive that they had control over the situation.

Motorcycling, Bicycling, Rollerblading, and Skateboarding

More than 5,000 people are killed in motorcycle accidents each year, and some 96,000 are injured (NHTSA, 2020). Motorcycles lack many of the safety features of cars and trucks. Unlike occupants of four-wheeled vehicles, the motorcyclist has no protective barrier of steel and padding.

Motorcyclists can take steps to minimize their chances of being included in these statistics. According to the NHTSA, the helmet is the motorcyclist's most important piece of safety equipment. Helmets do not prevent crashes, but they reduce the risk of death by more than a third (37%). Health behavior research shows that public health campaigns on motorcycle safety, such as promoting use of helmets, can increase use of helmets by both motorcycle riders and passengers (Akbari et al., 2021).

The health advantages of wearing a helmet also apply to bicycling, rollerblading, and skateboarding. Wearing a bicycle helmet reduces the risk of serious injuries to the head and brain injury by 85%. However, a national study in the United States found that only 42% of children 5 through 17 years of age always wore a helmet while biking and 31% never wore a helmet (Jewett et al., 2016).

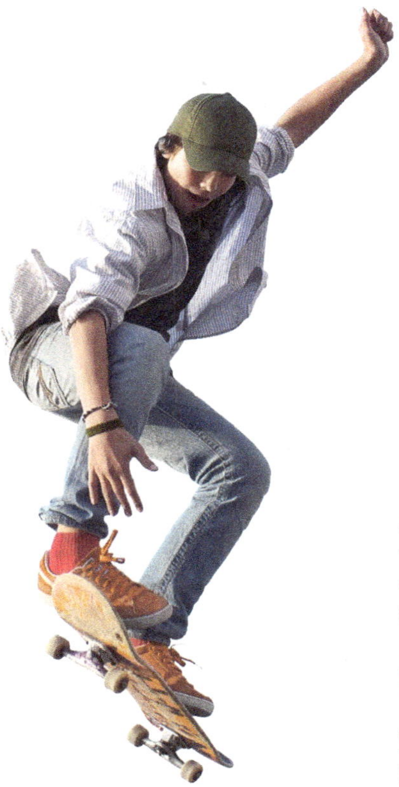

biletskiyevgeniy.com/Shutterstock.com

Health psychologists are interested in factors that either increase or decrease these types of health preventive behaviors. Researchers find some consistent patterns (Jewett et al., 2012). Children are more likely to wear a bicycle helmet when they are accompanied by an adult who wears a helmet. Helmet use is also lower among lower-income households. Among the more common reasons people give for not wearing a helmet are cost, discomfort, and the belief that it is not necessary to prevent an injury (Lee et al., 2022). Viewed through the lens of the HBM, we can see how degree of perceived risk of injury and perceived benefits of wearing a helmet converge in helping determine helmet use among bicyclists. Legislation can also be a powerful tool to increase safety behaviors, such as requiring use of a bicycle helmet. Evidence shows that helmet legislation decreased both head injuries and fatalities associated with bicycling (Lee et al., 2022). Bicycle safety also includes obeying traffic signals, signaling before turning, using reflectors, and wearing brightly colored reflective clothing at night.

The NHTSA also recommends that motorcyclists participate in motorcycle safety programs, which include rider training and motorist awareness. Aggressive driving and use of alcohol figure prominently in many motorcycle crashes, as they do in automobile and boating accidents.

Health Psychology in Action

The Theory of Planned Behavior and Risky Subway Riding—Chinese Style

The Chinese subways, called metros, are efficient and environmentally friendly. They are not so friendly to the passengers, as interruptions of service and even rider casualties are all too common and are mainly attributable to the behavior of passengers—particularly male passengers. Pressing into people attempting to board cars at the last second, elbowing others in cars to make space, and pushing into people attempting to leave cars when the doors open are all too frequent in China's metros and are seen less often in the United States, even during rush hour. One problem is the extreme crowding. Sardines are not packed in as tightly as many Chinese metro passengers.

The passengers themselves are responsible for many of the injuries that befall them. A study applied the TPB to try to arrive at explanations as to why passengers crammed into cars at the last moment, shoved each other repeatedly in the effort to get in or out or just make a little breathing space, and tried to force doors open to get in or out at the last moment (Wan et al., 2016). To do so researchers surveyed a total of more than 1,500 regular passengers. The most significant factor was perceived behavioral control—the finding that pushy passengers generally believed that they could be in control of the situation. Subjective norms and perceived risk were also predictive factors. Concerning subjective norms, it certainly appears as if (almost) everyone is doing it. And men, as health researchers often find, frequently underestimate the risks of their behavior.

And so, as the metros push through their tunnels, their passengers will likely continue to push and shove within, sometimes with tragic (and preventable) results.

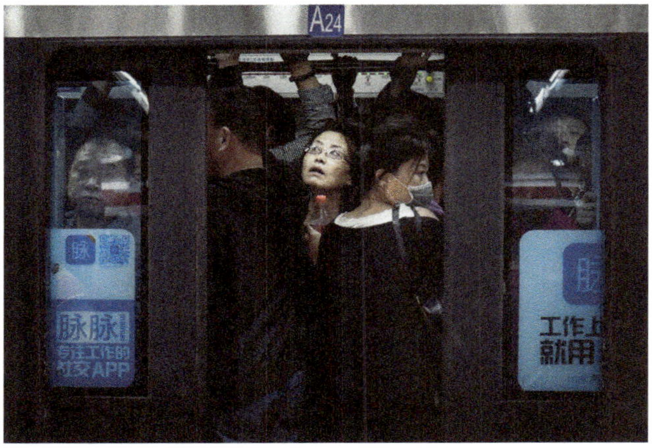

Kevin Frayer/Getty Images

"Am I really here?" Yes, it's a Chinese Metro.

Review 8.2

INTERACTIVE SELF-SCORING QUIZZES

Sentence Completion

1. Unintentional injuries are the __________ leading cause of death in the United States.
2. Continual keyboard use can lead to __________ tunnel syndrome—inflammation of the tissue that surrounds nerves in the wrist.
3. Accidents in the home account for some __________ million disabling injuries each year.
4. The leading cause of death for 16- to 20-year-olds is __________.
5. Twenty percent of motor vehicle crashes are associated with __________ driving.
6. Participants in a University of Idaho study said they would cross the street while listening to music because it would make walking more enjoyable and they believed they had __________ __________ over the situation.

Think About It

Do you ever cross the street while you are distracted by texting someone, answering a phone call, or listening to music that is loud enough to blot out the sounds of traffic? Do you think about why you do it? Do you believe that taking the chance of crossing while distracted is worth possible injury or death? Do you believe that you have control over the situation? Explain.

Recite: An Active Summary

INTERACTIVE SELF-SCORING QUIZZES

Chapter 8 Practice Quiz

1. Discuss crimes of violence in the United States.

Nearly 50,000 people are killed by firearms each year. Black Americans are the most likely victims of hate crimes, and Jews are most likely to be victimized by hate crimes based on religion. Nearly one woman in 5 and about one man in 7 experienced severe physical violence from a partner in an intimate relationship.

2. Discuss factors involved in rape and rape prevention.

Many factors are implicated in rape, including problems with impulse control, possible biological influences, socialization of men into sexually aggressive roles, desire to exert power over victims, adoption of rape myths and beliefs that create a mindset that sanctions sexually coercive behavior. Rape prevention involves efforts to change societal attitudes toward sexual aggression, enactment of laws and policies that more fully support rape victims in coming forward to report and prosecute offenders, and debunking widely held rape myths. Individuals can also reduce their personal risk of sexual assault by practicing safety behaviors.

3. Discuss myths that support rape, and why rape often goes unreported.

Cultural myths blame the victim and create a social climate that supports rape. Barriers that center around blaming the victim prevent many women from reporting rape to authorities.

4. Discuss underlying factors involved in violent behavior.

Violent behavior is not explained by any one factor but by a matrix of factors that vary from case to case. Exploration of the root causes of violent behavior focuses on biological influences, possibly involving brain processes involved in regulating impulsive anger and hormonal influences, as well as use of psychoactive drugs, such as alcohol, that affect brain function. We also need to consider sociocultural factors, such as the family environment in the home of origin, neighborhood characteristics, gang culture, use of violence as a social influence tactic, religious and sectarian violence, and terrorism. Strong negative emotions such as anger and frustration also play an important role in this matrix of factors.

5. Identify various kinds of unintentional injuries and factors that contribute to them.

Unintentional injuries from accidents are the fourth leading cause of death in the United States. Many accidental deaths result from household chemicals, falls, fires, and use of firearms. Yet motor vehicle accidents account for more than 42,000 deaths per year. Seat belts save some 15,000 lives per year. Many motor vehicle accidents are caused by distracted driving. Thousands of Americans each year are struck by motor vehicles as they cross the street—many of these pedestrians are texting, talking on the phone, or listening to music at the time of the accident. A common theme is that many people feel they have behavioral control of their situations when they actually do not.

Answers to Review Sections

8.1

1. same
2. Handguns
3. 50,000
4. more
5. White
6. 5
7. Twenty
8. supports
9. victim

8.2

1. fourth
2. carpal
3. 13
4. motor vehicle accidents/crashes
5. distracted
6. behavioral control

Debunking Rape Myths (as numbered in Self-Assessment)

1. A woman has a right to feel comfortable in a man's residence without fearing she will be sexually assaulted.
2. Nonsense! One could be just as suspicious anytime anybody complained about anything, such as complaining about a painful toe.
3. Men are often physically stronger and can physically overpower the woman.
4. Don't confuse a current style or choice with a sexual invitation.
5. It's not true, and even if it were, it wouldn't give men a license to commit rape.
6. Yes, you can. Any person has the right to say "no" at any time.
7. It may be a sign of poor judgment to hitchhike, but rape is never justified. Period.
8. This myth is a perfect example of hatred of women. Women walking on the street should not be victimized by catcalls, leering, and sexual invitations.
9. Some people, men as well as women, may have occasional rape fantasies; it does not mean they actually want to be raped and certainly doesn't give anyone an excuse to violently assault them.
10. Again, this is just blaming the victim.

CHAPTER 9

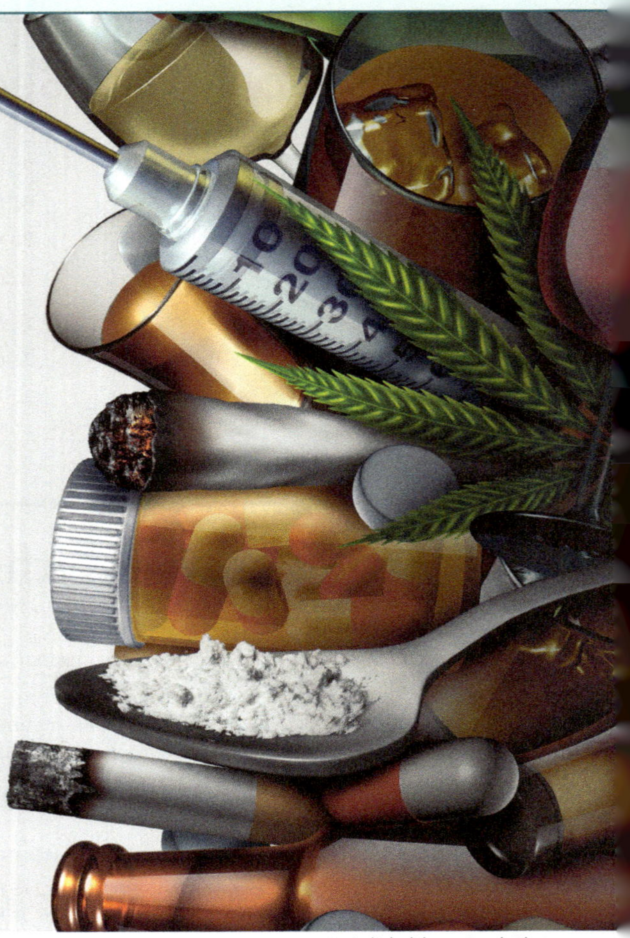

Brain light/Alamy Stock Photo

Substance Use and Abuse

LEARNING OBJECTIVES

After studying this chapter, you will be able to ...

1. **Define** substance abuse and substance dependence, and explain how you can know whether you are dependent on a substance.
2. **Discuss** psychological and biological factors in substance use and dependence.
3. **Discuss** depressants, focusing on alcohol and opioids.
4. **Discuss** stimulants, focusing on nicotine, amphetamines, cocaine, and caffeine.
5. **Discuss** hallucinogens, focusing on marijuana and LSD.
6. **Discuss** self-guided strategies for cutting down and quitting substance abuse.
7. **Discuss** the role of medication in the treatment of substance abuse.
8. **Discuss** ways in which psychologists help people with substance abuse problems.
9. **Discuss** strategies for relapse prevention.

Did You Know That …

- Alcohol is the BDOC (Big Drug on Campus)?
- People who black out from drinking may never wake up if they fail to receive prompt medical attention?
- More people in the United States die each year from smoking-related illnesses than from motor vehicle accidents, alcohol and drug abuse, suicide, homicide, and HIV/AIDS combined?
- Coca-Cola® once "added life" by using the stimulant cocaine as an ingredient?
- Preterm infants are typically treated with the stimulant caffeine?
- A stimulant is frequently prescribed to treat children who are already hyperactive?
- Most people who are dependent on substances manage to cut down or quit on their own?
- A highly addictive opioid is frequently prescribed to help people quit using two other highly addictive drugs, morphine and heroin?
- People may relapse when quitting a substance because they believe that one slip means they have lost the battle?

One friend had been struck by Leslie's piercing green eyes. Another recounted how Leslie had loved to dance barefoot at parties. A roommate remembered how Leslie ate handfuls of chocolate chips straight from the bag and picked the marshmallows out of Lucky Charms cereal. She even remembered the time that Leslie baked a tuna casserole without removing the Saran Wrap. Leslie had been an art major, and her professors described her work as promising (Winerip, 1998). Her overall GPA at the University of Virginia had been 3.67, and she had been preparing her senior essay on a Polish-born sculptor. But she did not finish the essay or graduate. Instead, Leslie died from falling down a flight of stairs after binge drinking alcohol. Some said Leslie had been doing her "fourth-year fifth," consuming a fifth of liquor for the final home football game. While deaths from opioid and cocaine overdoses get more publicity, more than a thousand college students die from alcohol-related causes (overdoses, accidents, and the like) each year.

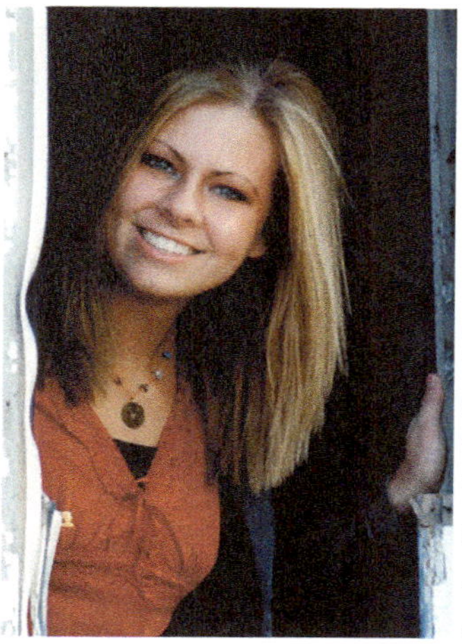

Courtesy Sam Spady Foundation

Death by Alcohol Alcohol overdoses claim the lives of many U.S. college students each year. Nineteen-year-old Samantha Spady of Colorado State University, shown here, died after a night of heavy drinking with her friends.

Why do people choose to drink alcohol? Perhaps no drug has meant so much to so many. Alcohol is our dinnertime relaxant, our bedtime sedative, our cocktail party social facilitator. We use alcohol to celebrate holy days, applaud our accomplishments, and express joyous wishes.

Alcohol is just one of many substances that many people use and sometimes abuse. This chapter is about the use and misuse of these substances and the factors involved in the development of problematic use of **psychoactive substances**. Some of these factors involve biochemical effects that drugs have on the body. But adopting a biopsychosocial model brings us to recognize the role of social factors, such as ethnicity and gender, and psychological factors, including positive and negative reinforcement and attitudes toward and expectancies about drugs. Health psychologists are concerned about the problem of substance abuse because it is linked to negative health and life outcomes.

psychoactive substances A drug or other substance that affects the functioning of the brain to cause changes in awareness, thoughts, feelings, mood, or behavior.

Use and Misuse of Psychoactive Substances

VIDEO CONTENT

Consciousness Altered: Drugs

The world is a supermarket of psychoactive drugs. The United States is flooded with drugs that distort perceptions and change mood—drugs that let you down, scoop you up, and scoot you across town. Some people get started using drugs because their friends do or their parents tell them not to. Make Ł Some are seeking pleasure; others, relief from pain; still others, inner truth. For better or for worse, drugs are part of life in the United States.

Other than alcohol, marijuana is the most widely used drug—whether by young people or adults. More than 48 million Americans, some 18% of the population, report using marijuana at least once in the past year (CDC, 2022). Nearly 70% of 12th graders report using alcohol, despite the fact that all states prohibit drinking by people under the age of 21 (L. D. Johnston et al., 2018). A majority of high school students report getting drunk at least once in their lives.

Then there is the increasing prevalence of illicit use of prescription medications, such as tranquilizers and sleeping pills, on many high school and college campuses. The nonmedical use of prescription drugs, such as the painkillers Vicodin and OxyContin, is limited to about 4.2% of teenagers (L. D. Johnston et al., 2018). In case you think of substance abuse as mainly a trap for the young, the opioid epidemic—which has also been called the opioid crisis—involves people of all age groups.

attention-deficit/hyperactivity disorder A disorder characterized by problems focusing on tasks, excessive activity or restlessness, and impulsivity.

Stimulants used in the treatment of **attention-deficit/hyperactivity disorder** (ADHD), such as Adderall and Concerta, have become drugs of abuse on college campuses. Adderall is used by as many as 1 in 10 college students who are seeking to boost their attention and alertness for studying and test taking. Usage is highest (about 12%) among 21- to 24-year-olds (Schulenberg et al., 2019). These young adults may not realize the drug can have adverse side effects, such as loss of appetite, headaches, increased blood pressure, and difficulty falling asleep. Yet the most popular drugs on campus remain the perennial favorites: alcohol and tobacco. Tobacco contains the highly addictive stimulant nicotine.

Alcohol remains the big drug on campus (BDOC) by a wide margin, with 58% of students reporting alcohol consumption in a 30-day period (National Institute on Alcohol Abuse and Alcoholism, 2018). A growing problem on college (and high school) campuses is use of prescription drugs that are not prescribed by a doctor—drugs such as prescription painkillers, antidepressants, and stimulants. More than 1 in 10 college students (11.8%) report using prescription drugs without a prescription in the past 30 days.

substance use disorders A diagnostic category comprising patterns of problematic use of psychoactive substances. For example, *alcohol use disorder* is a substance use disorder involving problematic use of alcohol.

substance abuse Continued use of a substance despite knowledge that it is dangerous or that it is linked to social, occupational, psychological, or physical problems.

substance dependence Dependence is shown by signs such as persistent use despite efforts to cut down, marked tolerance, and withdrawal symptoms.

tolerance The body's habituation to a drug, so that with regular use, increasingly higher doses of the drug are needed to achieve similar effects.

withdrawal syndrome A typical pattern of unpleasant symptoms accompanying the elimination of, or a sharp decrease in the usage of, a substance (also called an abstinence syndrome).

alcohol use disorder (AUD) A diagnostic category that applies to problematic use of alcohol.

delirium tremens A condition characterized by sweating, restlessness, disorientation, and hallucinations (also known as the DTs).

disorientation Gross confusion; loss of sense of time, place, and the identity of people.

Crossing the Line Between Use and Abuse

The American Psychiatric Association (2022) uses a diagnostic category of **substance use disorders** to classify patterns of problematic use of psychoactive substances. These disorders encompass problems of substance abuse and substance dependence. Unfortunately, substance use disorders are all too common in the United States, affecting some 46 million people according to recent estimates (Larkin, 2023).

The term **substance abuse** refers to repeated use of a substance despite the fact that it causes or compounds social, occupational, psychological, or physical problems. People who miss school or work because they are drunk or sleeping it off are abusing alcohol. The amount they drink is not the critical feature; rather, it is a pattern of use that disrupts their lives in significant ways.

Substance dependence is a more severe form of problematic substance use that has both psychological and biological aspects. Psychologically, dependence is often characterized by cravings and impaired control over the use of the substance. People with problems of substance dependence may organize their lives around obtaining and using the substance. Signs of biological or physiological dependence may be characterized by the development of tolerance, withdrawal symptoms, or both.

Tolerance is the body's habituation to a substance, so that with regular usage, higher doses are required to achieve similar effects. Addictive drugs have characteristic withdrawal symptoms when the level of usage suddenly drops off. A typical **withdrawal syndrome** (also called an abstinence syndrome) is encountered by people who suffer from **alcohol use disorder (AUD)**. The term "alcoholism" is not an official diagnosis but corresponds to severe forms of alcohol use disorder. The abstinence syndrome from alcohol may involve **delirium tremens** ("the DTs"). The DTs is characterized by heavy sweating, restlessness, **disorientation,** and terrifying hallucinations—often of creepy, crawling animals.

Factors in Substance Abuse and Dependence

Substance abuse and dependence frequently begin with experimental use in adolescence. Why do people experiment with drugs? The reasons are many—curiosity, conformity to peer pressure, parental modeling of drug use, rebelliousness, temporary escape from boredom, pressing personal problems or negative emotions, and the seeking of states of pleasure or personal enlightenment. Drug use patterns established during adolescence foreshadow future problems. For example, drinking in early adolescence is a risk factor for alcohol abuse in adulthood. Let us take a closer look at factors involved in substance abuse and dependence.

Psychosocial Factors Social cognitive theorists posit that positive and negative reinforcement play important roles in drug use and misuse (Bechara et al., 2019). Positive reinforcement—the principle that positive consequences or rewards strengthen the behaviors they follow—plays a primary role with respect to initiating drug use, as people learn that taking certain drugs produces desirable effects, such as feelings of euphoria, commonly described as a "high." Use of a substance may also be positively reinforced by drug-using peers.

Negative reinforcers strengthen behaviors that lead to the removal of an unpleasant or aversive stimulus. In terms of negative reinforcement, once a person becomes dependent on a drug, further use of the drug is negatively reinforced by the removal (cessation) of unpleasant cravings or withdrawal symptoms. Moreover, continued use of the drug may also become a form of self-medication when it is negatively reinforced by reduction of unpleasant feelings or sensations, such as pain, anxiety, fear, tension, and even depression.

We shouldn't be surprised that a pattern of solitary drinking is linked to the development of alcohol use disorders, as people who drink alone may be using alcohol to numb negative emotions or cope with stress or chronic pain (Skrzynski & Creswell, 2020). Both negative and positive reinforcers increase the probability that the behaviors that lead to reinforcement will be more likely to recur in the future, so a combination of positive and negative reinforcement can quickly lead to development of drug habits.

Cognitive factors such as positive expectations about the effects of a substance are powerful predictors of its use. In one study researchers studied a diary of stress, expectations about alcohol, and drinking (Armeli et al., 2000). They found that men who expected that alcohol would lessen feelings of stress were more likely to drink on stressful days. In contrast, men who expected that alcohol would impair their coping ability drank less on stressful days.

Gender is a psychosocial construct that plays an important role in problems of substance use and abuse. Men are about twice as likely as women to develop severe problems with alcohol, which is not surprising as men are also twice as likely to become heavy users of alcohol (NCHS, 2023). One reason for this gender differences is that heavy drinking may be more readily tolerated in men than women, as tighter cultural constraints tend to be placed on alcohol use by women. Another factor is biological, that alcohol tends to affect ("hit") women harder, and not simply because they typically weigh less than men. Alcohol may "go to a woman's head" faster than is the case with men, in part because women don't have as much of an enzyme that metabolizes alcohol in the stomach than men do. As a result, women tend to absorb more alcohol directly into their bloodstreams and so may become more intoxicated on less alcohol than men.

Our psychological expectancies about the effects of drugs, which psychologists call *outcome expectancies*, has a major bearing on our use of drugs. These expectancies are strongly influenced by other people's beliefs, such as attitudes of friends and family members toward drugs, as well as by first experiences with drugs such as alcohol (e.g., Padovano et al., 2022). For example, positive expectancies about alcohol use, such as believing that drinking will boost one's popularity or control states of tension or anxiety, can lead to frequent and perhaps problematic use of the drug. Negative outcome expectancies, such as the belief that psychedelics lead to terrifying hallucinations, are likely to curb their use. Health psychologists investigate the roles that these types of expectancies have on drug use, especially among teens who may be strongly influenced by their peers and media exposure to drug use.

Another psychosocial factor, observational learning, also comes into play. Parents who use drugs may model drug-using behavior for their children (McCutcheon et al., 2018; Wilsnack et al., 2018). In effect, they may be showing their children when and how to use drugs—for example, to drink alcohol to reduce tension or to "lubricate" social interactions.

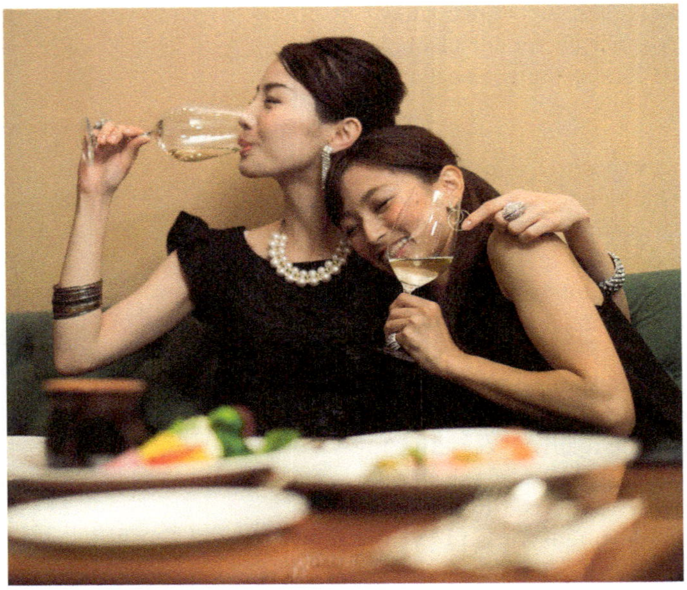

Michael H/DigitalVision/Getty Images

How Well Will They Hold Their Liquor? Our biological makeup is connected with our responses to various substances. For example, women and Asians have less of the enzyme aldehyde hydrogenase, which metabolizes alcohol in the stomach. As a result, they may not "hold their liquor," which may place a biological constraint on excess drinking.

Biological Views The **cognitive-dysfunction view of drug abuse** and dependence posits a dysfunction in the control of drug cravings or urges by the *prefrontal cortex*, the executive or decision-making center of the brain (Bechara et al., 2019). People with impaired executive control are more likely to give in to drug cravings than to carefully weigh the consequences of using drugs. Drug use behavior may be based on the short-term pleasures of using drugs, or on relief from negative feelings that drugs may provide, rather than on the long-term health and social benefits of exercising self-control.

Evidence also points to genetic factors that contribute to problematic use of drugs such as alcohol, cocaine, opioids, amphetamines, and nicotine in the form of tobacco products (Deak & Johnson, 2021; Karlsson Linnér et al., 2021; Saunders et al., 2022). But what is the inherited component? There may be several factors to consider.

Consider an Iranian study of people with opioid dependence (Tolami et al., 2019). Cells in the nervous system have opioid receptors where opioids dock. The genomes of 404 individuals undergoing methadone treatment to end their dependence on more harmful opioids were typed. The researchers isolated four genes linked to opioid dependence that are involved in strengthening the docking of opioids to receptors on neurons in the nervous system.

cognitive-dysfunction view of drug use The view that executive functioning becomes impaired with drug use such that short-term pleasure and relief from negative feelings outweighs longer-term considerations.

Clues have also emerged in the case of alcohol dependence (Cope et al., 2017; Wang et al., 2018). Researchers using evidence from the Minnesota Twin Study have found that monozygotic (MZ) twins, who share 100% of their heredity, are more likely than dizygotic (DZ) twins, who share 50% of their heredity, to be concordant (in agreement) for alcohol dependence (Legrand et al., 2005). Lisa Legrand and her colleagues (2005) estimated that about half of the difference between the two groups (MZ and DZ twins) was due to heredity, but environmental factors also played a role in alcohol dependence.

Other investigators have pointed out that people may inherit a tendency to reap greater pleasure from alcohol and have a reduced sensitivity to the negative effects of excessive alcohol use, such as upset stomach, dizziness, and headaches (Heath et al., 1999). That is, people may inherit a tendency to be able to better hold their liquor, which may place them at greater risk of developing drinking problems. Think of it this way: People whose bodies more readily put the brakes on excess drinking because they experience more negative effects of alcohol may be less likely to develop problems with excess drinking.

There are also ethnic and gender differences in susceptibility to problems with alcohol. For example, due to genetic factors, Asians and women have lower levels of the enzyme aldehyde dehydrogenase, which metabolizes alcohol in the stomach; thus they are likely to experience unpleasant effects from excessive drinking (Matsushita & Higuchi, 2017; McHugh et al., 2017; Petrosino et al., 2014). Asians and Asian Americans are also more likely than Europeans and non-Hispanic White Americans to show a *flushing*—face reddening—response to alcohol (Matsushita & Higuchi, 2017). A flushing response may help inhibit excess drinking.

dopamine-sensitization hypothesis The view that use of a substance, particularly a stimulant, triggers spikes in dopamine activity, causing users to want or crave the substance.

dopamine A chemical that functions as a hormone and a neurotransmitter; it is involved in various bodily functions, including reward-motivated behavior and producing pleasurable sensations.

According to the **dopamine-sensitization hypothesis** of substance dependence, usage of a psychoactive substance, especially strong stimulants and opioids, triggers increased release of the neurotransmitter **dopamine** in the brain, resulting in pleasurable sensations (Bechara et al., 2019). The influx of dopamine from regular use of these drugs, such as cocaine and heroin, sensitizes nerve pathways in the brain to the chemical, resulting in a steady flow of pleasurable sensations that makes it difficult for users to focus on anything other than obtaining and using these drugs (Wise & Robble, 2020).

The major classes of psychoactive drugs are depressants, stimulants, and hallucinogens.

Review 9.1

INTERACTIVE SELF-SCORING QUIZZES

Sentence Completion

1. __________ is the most widely used psychoactive substance.

2. Substance __________ is repeated use of a substance despite the fact that it is causing or compounding social, occupational, psychological, or physical problems.

3. Psychologically, substance __________ is often characterized by craving and loss of control over use of the substance.

4. __________ dependence on a substance is typified by tolerance, withdrawal symptoms, or both.

5. Addictive drugs have characteristic __________ syndromes when the level of usage suddenly drops off.

6. Once a person has become dependent on a drug, use of the drug is __________ reinforcing in that it is followed by the individual's avoidance of cravings for the drug and withdrawal symptoms.

7. According to the __________-__________ view of drug dependence, the prefrontal region of the cerebral cortex declines in its capacity to govern behavior.

8. According to the dopamine-sensitization hypothesis, regular use of certain drugs increases the amount of __________ available in the brain, increasing the sensitivity of reward pathways to the chemical and producing intense feelings of pleasure.

Think About It

As you read through the chapter, consider whether you or people you know have abused substances or become dependent on them. Which one or ones? What factors led to the dependency? Has dependency impaired your—or their—physical, academic, or interpersonal functioning? How so?

Depressants

Depressants are not called by that name because they cause depression. Rather, they are drugs that depress or slow down the activity of the **central nervous system (CNS)**. In high doses, these drugs can slow down the CNS to such an extent that death may result from respiratory (breathing) arrest or cardiovascular collapse. Psychologically, these drugs have relaxing or sedating effects and may induce feelings of euphoria. Here we focus on the major types of depressants: alcohol, barbiturates, and opioids.

depressants Drugs that decrease the rate of activity of the central nervous system.

central nervous system (CNS) The part of the body's nervous system that consists of the brain and spinal cord.

Alcohol: The "Swiss Army Knife" of Psychoactive Substances

People use alcohol like a Swiss Army knife—It does it all. Alcohol is the all-purpose medication you can buy without prescription. Some people use it as a form of self-medication to curb negative feelings, such as social anxiety, depression, or loneliness (Cludius et al., 2013; Hogarth et al., 2018; McCaul et al., 2017; Patrick et al., 2017). Most people use alcohol because of its positively reinforcing effects, such as pleasure or relaxation, or because it is linked to enjoyable social occasions.

But the army knife has a blade. It is also the case that no drug has been as abused as alcohol. According to the National Institute on Alcohol Abuse and Alcoholism, nearly 29 million adults age 18 and over in the U.S. currently suffer from a diagnosable substance use disorder called *alcohol use disorder* (AUD) (NIAAA, 2023). Excessive drinking is linked to many negative social, economic, and health outcomes, including lower productivity, loss of employment, and downward movement in social status. The commonly used term *alcoholism* (or *alcohol dependence*) is not a diagnostic term but is generally applied to people with more severe forms of AUD.

Overall, about 11% of the population is currently affected by AUD, making it one of the most common psychological disorders (Kranzler, 2023). But problems with alcohol are age-related. As you can see in **Figure 9.1**, the likelihood of alcohol dependence

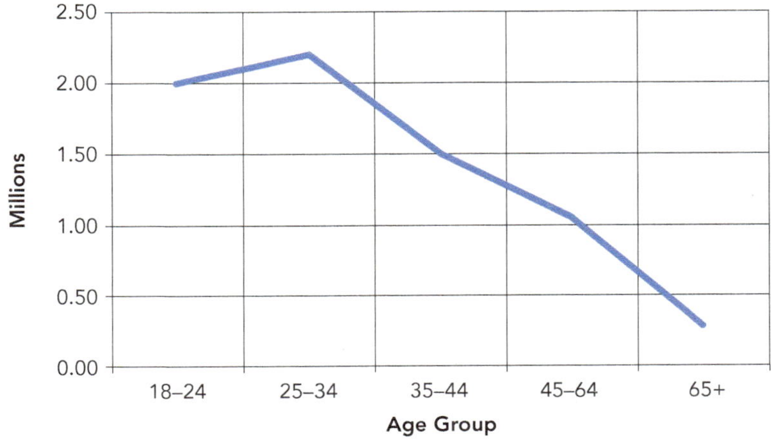

FIGURE 9.1 **Approximate Number of People Dependent by Age Group**
Source: Bishop (2018), p. 3 / with permission of Sage Publications.

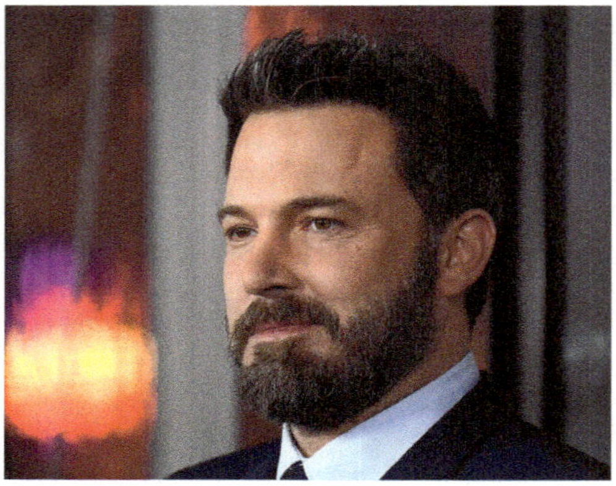

Frazer Harrison/Getty Images

Actor Ben Affleck, Speaking About Addiction "People with compulsive behavior, and I am one, have this kind of basic discomfort all the time that they're trying to make go away. You're trying to make yourself feel better with eating or drinking or sex or gambling or shopping or whatever. But that ends up making your life worse. Then you do more of it to make *that* discomfort go away. Then the real pain starts. It becomes a vicious cycle you can't break. That's at least what happened to me" (in Barnes, 2020).

increases from about 2 million Americans aged 18–24 years to about 2.3 million Americans aged 25–34 years. The incidence of alcohol dependence then decreases with age, falling to about 280,000 people aged 65 years and above (Bishop, 2018). Some of the decrease among older people is likely due to mortality, but many dependent people gain control over their drinking; most formerly dependent drinkers becoming abstinent, and a smaller number—perhaps 10%—becoming drinkers who can control or limit their alcohol intake (Bishop, 2018).

Positive expectancies about the effects of alcohol are a major determinant of alcohol use, especially among young people (Doran et al., 2011; Smit et al., 2018). People may use alcohol because they expect it will make them more popular or fun to be around. Alcohol may induce feelings of elation and euphoria that may wash away self-doubts. Alcohol is also associated with a liberated social role in our culture. Drinkers may place the blame for misbehavior on alcohol ("It's the alcohol, not me"), even though they choose to drink.

Regardless of how or why one starts drinking, regular drinking can lead to physiological dependence. Once dependence develops, people maintain their alcohol intake to avoid withdrawal symptoms. Still, even when people with AUD have dried out—withdrawn from alcohol—many return to drinking. Perhaps they still seek to use alcohol as a way of coping with stress or escaping from it.

Alcohol has effects on the mind and body, varying with dose and duration of use. Although alcohol is a depressant, low doses can be stimulating. However, higher doses have a relaxing or sedating effect. Alcohol relaxes people and deadens minor aches and pains. It impairs cognitive functioning, slurs speech, and reduces motor coordination. Overall, alcohol is involved in about half of all fatal automobile accidents in the United States. Alcohol lowers inhibitions and impairs our ability to weigh the consequences of our behavior. Consequently, when we drink, we may say or do things we later regret, take excessive risks, or act impulsively without thinking (Baumeister & Alghamdi, 2015; Maisto & Simons, 2016).

Effects of Chronic, Heavy Drinking

Chronic, heavy drinking is also linked to coronary heart disease, ulcers, hypertension, osteoarthritis, kidney disease, and pancreatitis—painful inflammation of the pancreas. Alcohol affects brain cells, can trigger bleeding, and can lead to hormonal changes that dampen the sex drive and disrupt the menstrual cycles of women. Heavy consumption of alcohol increases the risk of neurological disease and dementia. Heavy drinking may have its most damaging effects on the liver, the main organ that metabolizes alcohol. Chronic heavy drinking is the single most important cause of illness and death from liver disease (alcoholic hepatitis and cirrhosis) in the United States. Alcohol-related liver diseases include fatty liver disease, hepatitis, and cirrhosis (Y. Chang et al., 2020).

fatty liver A condition characterized by accumulation of fat in the liver, causing enlargement of the organ.

alcoholic hepatitis Inflammation of the liver.

cirrhosis of the liver A disease in which healthy cells of the liver are replaced by scar tissue.

Fatty liver disease refers to a buildup of fat that enlarges to liver. **Fatty liver** is relatively benign and can often be reversed by abstinence from alcohol (Lamuela-Raventos et al., 2020). **Alcoholic hepatitis** is inflammation of the liver. It can be life threatening, but like fatty liver, is often reversed by abstinence; however, there may be permanent scarring of the liver. **Cirrhosis of the liver** is the most harmful liver disease, claiming more than 22,000 lives in the United States each year. Alcohol-related deaths are highest among people aged 45–74 years, males, and Native Americans (White et al., 2020). In cirrhosis of the liver, scar tissue replaces healthy liver cells. The more chronic and heavier the drinking, the greater the risk of cirrhosis. Unlike fatty liver and alcoholic hepatitis, cirrhosis of the liver is not reversible, but abstinence may prevent further damage. Some 10–25% of heavy, chronic drinkers develop cirrhosis of the liver.

A Closer Look

A Snapshot of College Drinking

The consequences of excessive and underage drinking affect virtually all college campuses, college communities, and college students, whether they are younger or older than the minimum legal drinking age and whether or not they choose to drink.

- Alcohol consumption: About 58% of full-time college students report drinking in the past month.
- Binge drinking: Approximately 38% of college students report binge drinking at least once during the past month.
- Deaths and injuries: About 2,000 college students between ages 18 and 24 years die each year from alcohol-related unintentional injuries, including motor vehicle crashes (about half among students under 21).
- Assaults: It is estimated that nearly 700,000 students each year between the ages of 18 and 24 years are assaulted by another student who has been drinking.
- Sexual abuse: More than 97,000 students between the ages of 18 and 24 years are victims of alcohol-related sexual assault or date rape each year.
- Risky sex: More than 400,000 students between the ages of 18 and 24 years had unprotected sex as a result of their drinking, and 97,000 students between the ages of 18 and 24 years report having been too intoxicated to know whether they consented to having sex each year.
- Academic problems: About 25% of college students report academic consequences of their drinking, including missing class, falling behind, doing poorly on exams or papers, and receiving lower grades overall.

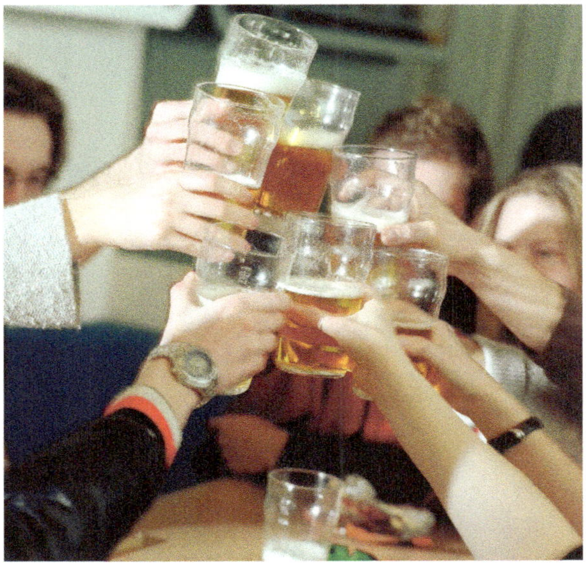

Image Source/Getty Images

- Vandalism: About 11% of college student drinkers report that they have damaged property while under the influence of alcohol.

Source: Adapted from National Institute on Alcohol Abuse and Alcoholism (NIAAA) (2018). Alcohol facts and statistics. https://www.niaaa.nih.gov/alcohol-health/overview-alcohol-consumption/alcohol-facts-and-statistics.

Alcohol is high in calories and carbohydrates but lacking in other nutrients. Alcohol also makes it more difficult for the body to absorb certain vitamins, such as vitamin B1 (thiamine). As a result, people with AUD are prone to health problems associated with vitamin and protein deficiencies, such as cirrhosis of the liver and a psychological disorder called **Wernicke-Korsakoff's syndrome** (due to a deficiency in thiamine). People with Wernicke-Korsakoff's syndrome experience confusion, disorientation, and memory loss for recent events.

Wernicke-Korsakoff's syndrome A form of cognitive impairment related to AUD and deficiency of vitamin B1 (thiamine).

The physical and cognitive effects of heavy drinking are indicated in **Figure 9.2**.

Binge Drinking Binge drinking is an epidemic in the United States. Binge drinking is defined among men as having five or more drinks on a single occasion and among women as having four or more drinks. Twice as many men as women binge drink (Kanny et al., 2018). Binge drinkers show increased rates of aggressive behavior, poor grades, missed classes, absences from work, unprotected promiscuous sex (and sexually transmitted infections), and motor vehicle accidents (NIAAA, 2018). Enrolling in college is a trigger for binge drinking among many adolescents (Leech et al., 2020). About one college student in four report engaging in binge drinking episodes during the past month (NIAAA, 2023). Overall, some 38% of

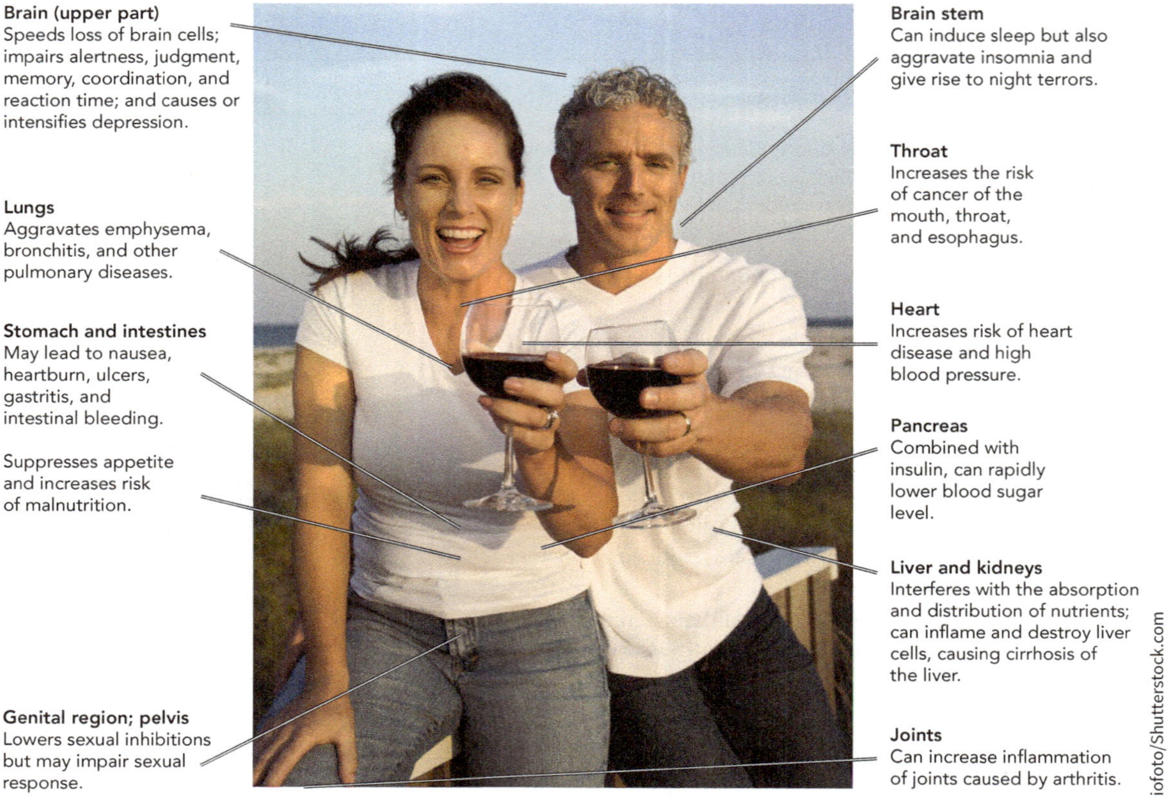

FIGURE 9.2 **Effects of Heavy Drinking**

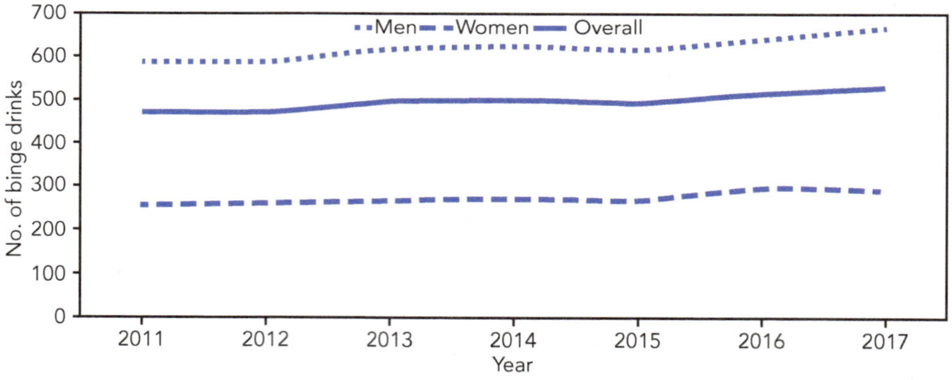

FIGURE 9.3 **Number of Binge Drinks Reported Annually, by Sex, United States**

Source: D. Kanny, T. S. Naimi, Y. Liu, H. Lu, & R. B. Brewer (2020). Trends in total binge drinks per adult who reported binge drinking—United States, 2011–2117. *Morbidity and Mortality Weekly Report, 69*(2), p. 32 / US Department of Health and Human Services / Licensed under CC BY 3.0.

American college students report engaging in binge drinking in the past month. Turning 21 has become an occasion for binge drinking on many campuses (Garcia et al., 2022). Yet this is only the tip of the iceberg. Approximately 1 American in 5 (60–70 million people) reports at least one episode of binge drinking per month. Although binge drinking can lead to dependence on alcohol, most people who binge drink or drink heavily are not dependent on alcohol (Bishop, 2018). Therefore, most of them see no need for treatment. What they may not realize is that binge drinking often leads to chronic problems with alcohol.

Figure 9.3 shows the number of binge drinks, by sex, that they reported annually (Kanny et al., 2020). Men who binge drink reported more than twice the number of drinks reported by women who binge drink. Moreover, the number of binge drinks appears to be rising among men, whereas it appears to have leveled off among women. **Figure 9.4** breaks down binge drinking by age (Bohm et al., 2021). Binge drinking is most common among young adults in the 18–34 years age group. The incidence then drops off as people progress through middle and late adulthood.

Binge drinking and other forms of excessive drinking, such as drinking games (e.g., beer chugging or downing a series of shots), can put drinkers at immediate risk of coma or death from overdose (Roberts, 2017). In fact, binge drinking is responsible for half of alcohol-related deaths (Kanny et al., 2018). Some of these deaths are caused by people choking on their own vomit. Although drinking heavily can induce vomiting, the drug's depressant effects may suppress the normal vomiting response. Consequently, vomit may accumulate in the air passages, possibly leading to asphyxiation and death. Unfortunately, people who play drinking games may not stop until they're too drunk or sick to continue. Alcohol overdosing is a serious medical condition that requires immediate medical attention. Don't assume a friend who falls asleep in a stupor will sleep it off. Some friends never wake up.

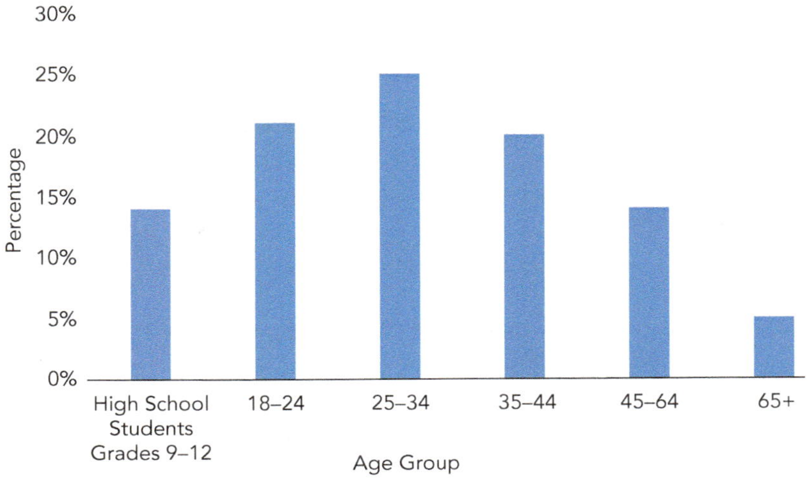

Source: Adapted from Youth Risk Behavior Surveillance System, 2019 and Behavioral Risk Factor Surveillance System, 2021.

FIGURE 9.4 **Who Binge Drinks?**

What should you do if a friend blacks out from drinking? Are they just sleeping it off? Should you let them do so? Do you have the expertise to determine the extent of the danger? Should you dial 911?

Here are some general guidelines. First, look for signs of overdose, which include:

- Failure to respond when talked to or shouted at
- Failure to respond to being pinched, shaken, or poked
- Inability to stand up on their own
- Failure to wake up
- Purplish color or clammy skin
- Rapid pulse rate or irregular heart rhythms, low blood pressure, or difficulty breathing

Do not leave an unresponsive or unconscious person alone. Treat the situation as a medical emergency. Stay with the person until you or someone else can obtain medical attention. (Dial 911 on your smartphone.) Place the person on their side or, if possible, have the person sit up with head bowed. Do not give the person food or drink. Do not induce vomiting. If the person vomits, you may want to reach (carefully) into their mouth and clear the airway; provide artificial respiration or CPR if necessary—if you know how. (Not a bad skill to learn!) Most important, call a medical care provider or 911 and ask for advice.

Is a Drink a Day Good for You? Given the health risks of heavy consumption of alcohol, it seems ironic that light to moderate drinking might have positive effects. There is some evidence suggesting that up to two drinks a day for men and a drink a day for women may reduce the risk of heart attacks and lower the death rate (Nova et al., 2019). However, other research casts serious doubt on the health benefits of modest alcohol use, so we need to await the results of yet further studies to clarify these mixed findings (Biddinger et al., 2022; Schutte, Smith, & Wannamethee, 2022).

How might modest drinking bestow a health benefit? One explanation is its effects on raising levels of high-density lipoproteins (HDL, or good cholesterol). HDL reduces the risk of blockage of blood vessels by low-density lipoproteins (LDL, or bad cholesterol) and decreases the tendency of platelets in the blood to clump together (Nova et al., 2019; Vogel, 2019).

Self-Assessment

INTERACTIVE SELF-ASSESSMENTS

Is Drinking Becoming a Problem for You?

Do you have a problem with alcohol? Are you concerned that you might have one? Here are some questions to ask yourself. In the past year, have you:

- Had times when you ended up drinking more or longer than you intended?
- More than once wanted to cut down or stop drinking, or tried to, but couldn't?
- Spent a lot of time drinking? Or being sick or getting over the aftereffects?
- Experienced craving—a strong need, or urge—to drink?
- Found that drinking—or being sick from drinking—often interfered with taking care of your home or family? Or caused job troubles? Or school problems?
- Continued to drink even though it was causing trouble with your family or friends?
- Given up or cut back on activities that were important or interesting to you, or gave you pleasure, in order to drink?
- More than once gotten into situations while or after drinking that increased your chances of getting hurt (such as driving, swimming, using machinery, walking in a dangerous area, or having unsafe sex)?
- Continued to drink even though it was making you feel depressed or anxious or adding to another health problem? Or after having had a memory blackout?
- Had to drink much more than you once did to get the effect you want? Or found that your usual number of drinks had much less effect than before?
- Found that when the effects of alcohol were wearing off, you had withdrawal symptoms, such as trouble sleeping, shakiness, irritability, anxiety, depression, restlessness, nausea, or sweating? Or sensed things that were not there?

If you have engaged in any of these behaviors, your drinking may already be a cause for concern. The more items you endorsed, the more urgent the need for change. A health professional can conduct a formal assessment of your drinking behavior to evaluate the nature of the problem and ways of addressing it.

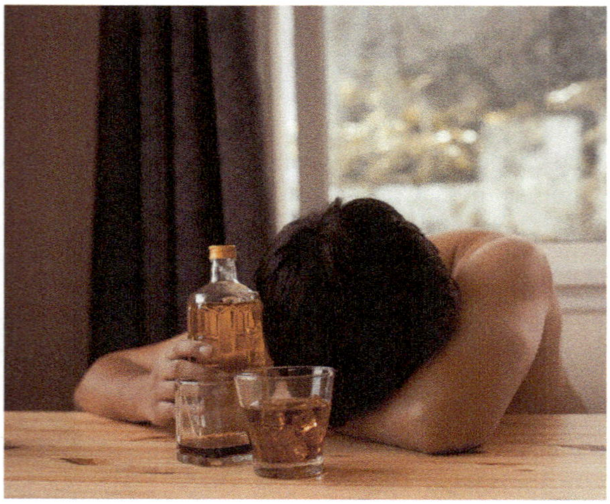

skaman306/Moment/Getty Images

Source: Adapted from National Institute on Alcohol Abuse and Alcoholism (2023). Alcohol use disorder. https://www.niaaa.nih.gov/alcohol-health/overview-alcohol-consumption/alcohol-use-disorders.

However, responsible health practitioners do not suggest that people who do not currently drink take up light or moderate drinking as a way of promoting cardiovascular health. For one thing, research does not support such an approach. This research involves people who already consume alcohol, not abstainers who are encouraged to drink. Second, the research is observational, not experimental. It would not be feasible or ethically responsible to randomly assign nondrinkers to continue to abstain, or drink moderately, or drink heavily to determine the possible outcomes of alcohol use on cardiovascular health and mortality. Moreover, encouraging nondrinkers to start consuming alcohol would likely lead to increased rates of AUD.

Opioids

No tongue or pen will ever describe ... the depths of horror in which my life was plunged at this time; the days of humiliation and anguish, nights of terror and agony, through which I dragged my wretched being.

—A former Union soldier (cited in Carroll, 2016, pp. 68–69)

opioids Drugs derived from the opium plant or synthesized in the laboratory to have opiate-like effects, they are classified as depressants because they slow the activity of the central nervous system.

The Union soldier just quoted was a veteran of the U.S. Civil War, who was despairing at his difficulty in attempting to overcome addiction to an opioid. **Opioids** include opiate drugs derived from the opium plant, which include morphine, heroin, opium, and codeine, and drugs synthesized in the laboratory that produce opiate-like effects, such as Vicodin and

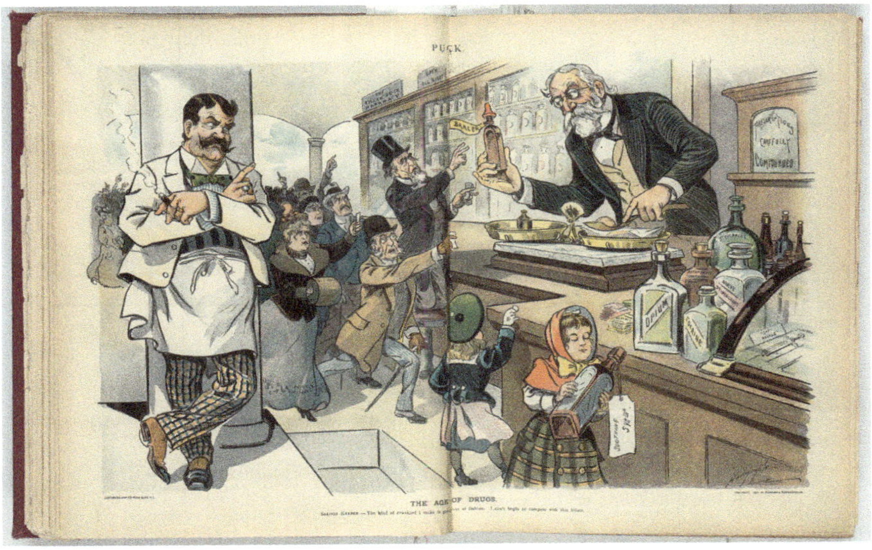

The Library of Congress/Public domain

"The Age of Drugs," by Louis Dalrymple, 1900.

OxyContin. Some opioids are widely prescribed for pain, but all are highly addictive **narcotics.** About 2 million adults in the United States suffer from opioid use disorder (Kalin, 2020).

narcotics Addictive drugs such as opioids that have pain relieving and sleep inducing properties, along with producing feelings of euphoria.

Heroin is a generally illegal drug known for its euphoric "rush." The pleasure it provides is reported to surpass the pleasures of sex, food, and other life experiences. Although morphine and synthetic opioids—Vicodin, OxyContin, Percodan, fentanyl—are prescribed to relieve pain, they can also induce feelings of euphoria. As with other depressants, opioids slow the activity of the CNS. Opioids are also widely abused as street drugs. Illicit use of prescription opioids as painkillers has become a significant drug abuse problem in the United States, as discussed in Chapter 6.

Morphine was introduced in the United States in the 1860s, at about the time of the Civil War, and in Europe during the Franco-Prussian War (1870–1871). It was used to deaden pain from wounds. Physiological dependence on morphine therefore became known as the soldier's disease. Hundreds of thousands of Americans were addicted to opium and its derivatives in the 1860s—an era that can be said to have been defined at least in part by the nation's first opium crisis. Heroin, which is derived from opium, was so named because it made people feel "heroic." It was also hailed as the "hero" that would cure physiological dependence on morphine. Yet heroin proved to be just as addictive as morphine. Regular users of opioids develop tolerance, leading them to take higher doses and potentially life-threatening overdoses.

The use of opioids knows no geographical boundaries. Opioids are used and abused in cities, in suburbs, and in small towns and villages. Non-Hispanic Black Americans and Latino/Hispanic people show a higher prevalence of heroin use, whereas most users entering substance abuse treatment programs are non-Hispanic White Americans who were introduced to opioids by prescription (Pouget et al., 2018).

As this book is being written, heroin remains illegal in 49 states. Because the penalties for possession or sale are high, it is also expensive. Many people who become dependent on heroin support their habit through dealing (selling drugs), prostitution, or selling stolen goods. Heroin addiction is associated with extreme withdrawal syndromes, which may begin with flu-like symptoms and progress through tremors, cramps, chills alternating with sweating, rapid pulse, high blood pressure, insomnia, vomiting, and diarrhea. However, these syndromes are variable from one person to another and can be managed medically.

Opioids act on opioid receptors in the brain (Bechara et al., 2019). These receptors usually target **endogenous** opioids, such as endorphins, which are released by the brain during exercise (giving rise to the "runners' high"), orgasm, excitement, and pain. Opioids such as heroin, morphine, oxycodone, and fentanyl can produce intense feelings of pleasure when they bind to opioid receptors. While the painkilling properties of opioids are associated with pain

endogenous Originating from or grown within the person.

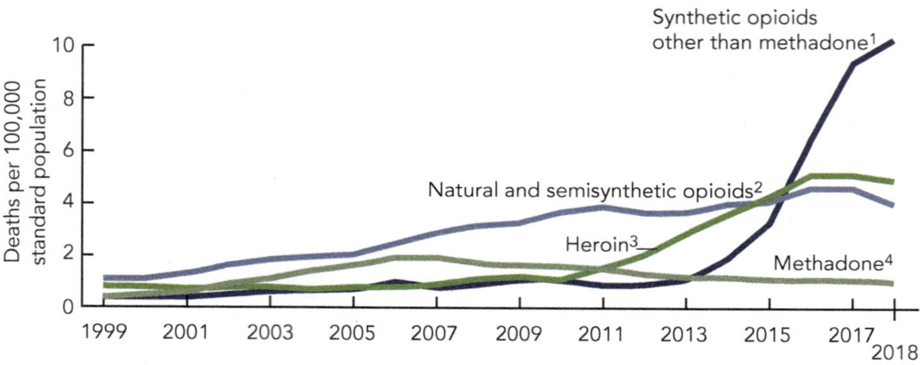

1. Fentanyl is the strongest and most deadly synthetic opioid.
2. Natural opioid painkillers include morphine and codeine. Semisynthetic opioid painkillers include oxycodone (OxyContin), hydrocodone, and some others.
3. Heroin is also a semisynthetic opioid that is made from morphine.
4. Methadone is used to treat addiction to heroin.

FIGURE 9.5 **Drug Overdose Death Rates Involving Opioids, United States, 1999–2018**

Source: H. Hedegaard, A. M. Minino, & M. Warner (2020). Drug overdose deaths in the United States, 1999–2018. *NCHS Data Brief, 356*, p. 3. https://www.cdc.gov/nchs/data/databriefs/db356-h.pdf / US Department of Health and Human Services / Public Domain.

pathways in the brain, the addictive properties of opioids can be attributed to increased release of dopamine in the brain (Wise & Robble, 2020).

The repeated use of opioids results in changes in brain reward circuitry, involving dopamine, that cause physiologically dependent individuals to crave the use of the drug (Bechara et al., 2019; Wise & Robble, 2020). Because of the physiological changes, people may find themselves craving an opioid even after they have been "successfully" withdrawn from the drugs—especially when they find themselves in situations in which they have used the drugs or in emotional states in which the drugs have (temporarily) led them to feel better. Even reflecting on the euphoria of the drug-induced high can lead to craving.

The death toll from opioid overdoes has been increasing (Hedegaard et al., 2020; see Figures 9.5 and 9.6), with the synthetic opioid fentanyl responsible for much of the surge. The drug overdose death rate is about twice as high for men as for women.

Barbiturates

barbiturates Addictive depressants used to relieve anxiety or induce sleep.

Barbiturates are a class of sedating medications that have calming and relaxing properties. Some common examples of barbiturates include amobarbital, pentobarbital, phenobarbital, and secobarbital. These drugs have some legitimate medical uses, including relief from pain and treatment of epilepsy. However, barbiturate use can quickly lead to physiological and psychological dependence. Barbiturates are popular as street drugs not only because of their relaxing effects but also because they produce a state of mild euphoria. High doses of barbiturates result in drowsiness, motor impairment, slurred speech, irritability, and poor judgment. A physiologically dependent person who is withdrawn abruptly from barbiturates may experience severe convulsions that can lead to death. Thus it is important that withdrawal be carefully monitored. Barbiturates have additive effects with other drugs, which makes them especially dangerous when mixed with alcohol and other depressants.

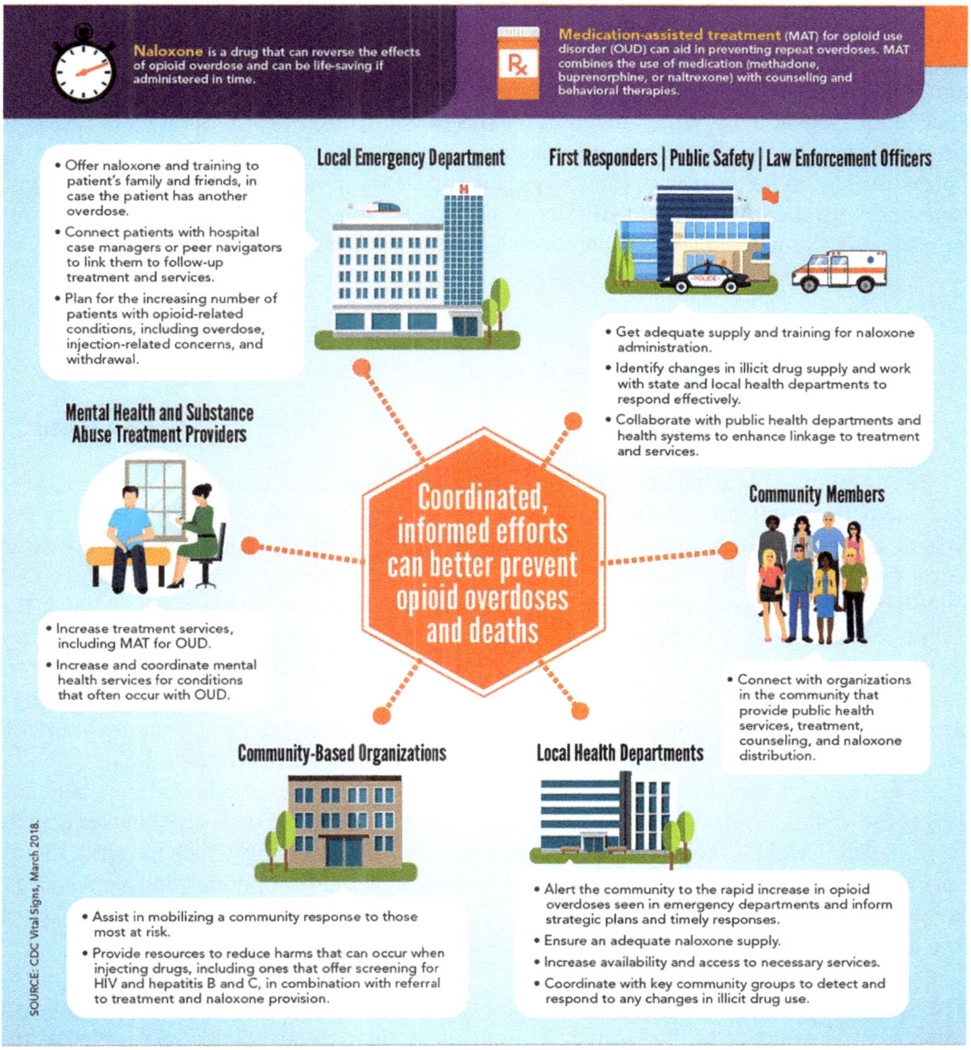

FIGURE 9.6 **A Rise in Opioid Overdoses. What Now?**

Source: Centers for Disease Control and Prevention (2018). Opioid overdoses treated in emergency departments. https://www.cdc.gov/vitalsigns/opioid-overdoses/infographic.html / US Department of Health and Human Services / Public Domain.

Review 9.2

INTERACTIVE SELF-SCORING QUIZZES

Sentence Completion

1. According to the text, depressants slow the activity of the __________ nervous system.

2. Alcohol is also associated with a __________ social role in our culture.

3. Alcohol is involved in about __________ of all fatal automobile accidents in the United States.

4. Nearly __________ college students between the ages of 18 and 24 are victims of alcohol-related sexual assault or date rape each year.

5. __________ of the liver, the most harmful liver disease related to excessive drinking, claims more than 20,000 lives in the United States each year.

6. (Women or men) are more likely to engage in binge drinking.

7. Light drinking appears to raise the level of __________-density lipoproteins in the bloodstream.

8. During the 1860s, physiological dependence on __________ became known as the soldier's disease.

9. Opioids act on receptors in the brain that usually target __________.

10. People who have been withdrawn from opioids may still crave the drugs due to changes in brain __________ circuitry.

11. Phenobarbital belongs to a class of sedating drugs known as __________.

Think About It

How would you describe your own experiences with alcohol? How does drinkers' behavior on social occasions differ from their usual behavior as a result of drinking? Have you or they said, "Don't blame me, it was the alcohol"? Should people be blamed for behaving badly when drinking? Why or why not?

Stimulants

Stimulants have effects on the CNS opposite to those of depressants. Stimulants accelerate, or speed up, CNS activity, which heightens states of bodily arousal and mental alertness. But stimulants such as amphetamines and cocaine can also lead to a powerful "rush," or feelings of pleasure, which helps explain their powerful appeal and potential for abuse. We begin our discussion with nicotine—a mild stimulant that poses a grave threat to our health and well-being because of the means by which it is usually administered: smoking.

Nicotine

Giving up smoking is the easiest thing in the world. I know because I've done it thousands of times.

—**Mark Twain**

nicotine The highly addictive stimulant found in tobacco.

Giving up smoking is *not* easy because tobacco smoke and e-cigarettes contain **nicotine**—a highly addictive stimulant. People who smoke regulate their smoking to maintain fairly even levels of nicotine in their bloodstream. Addiction develops quickly, often within the first few weeks of smoking.

When dependence develops, people who smoke experience withdrawal symptoms if they abruptly stop smoking. These symptoms include nervousness, drowsiness, loss of energy, headaches, irregular bowel movements, lightheadedness, insomnia, dizziness, cramps, palpitations, tremors, and sweating. People who smoke and are nicotine-dependent often resume smoking to control these withdrawal symptoms. They may quit, then suffer withdrawal symptoms, and then resume smoking—a pattern that may occur repeatedly in the form of a vicious cycle.

As a stimulant, nicotine speeds up bodily processes, such as heart rate and metabolic rate; curbs appetite; and increases concentration, alertness, and arousal. Some people smoke cigarettes to control their weight. Others tend to eat more when they stop smoking, which may lead them to return to smoking. Nicotine also produces mild feelings of pleasure (euphoria), and, paradoxically, it may induce feelings of mental calmness or relaxation. Consequently, people who smoke may come to depend on nicotine to lift them up and settle them down.

The Leading Preventable Cause of Death ...

Smoking is the leading preventable cause of death in the United States, causing nearly 480,000 deaths each year from smoking-related illnesses (CDC, 2023g). This is the equivalent of three jumbo jets colliding in midair each day, with all passengers lost. Each year more Americans die from smoking-related diseases than from motor vehicle accidents, alcohol and drug abuse, suicide, homicide, and HIV/AIDS combined.

All in all, cigarette smoking accounts for about 1 in 7 deaths worldwide, cutting life expectancy by about 10 years for the average person who smokes (Hodson, 2023a; Jha et al., 2013; Renteria et al., 2016). Smoking *triples* the likelihood of dying between the ages of 25 and 79 (Jha et al., 2013).

Although nicotine is the addictive substance in tobacco, it is not the most dangerous constituent of cigarette smoking; that dishonor falls on such other ingredients as carbon monoxide and "tars." The carbon monoxide in cigarette smoke impairs the blood's ability to carry oxygen, causing shortness of breath and compromising the cardiovascular system. The tars (actually chemical compounds called hydrocarbons) in cigarette and cigar smoke are largely responsible for causing lung cancer. Smoking is a factor in 80% of the deaths from lung cancer in women and in 90% of men (American Lung Association, 2020). Women who smoke are 13 times as likely to develop lung cancer as women who do not smoke. The figure rises to 23 times for men.

Black people are more likely to develop and die from lung cancer than any other racial group in the United States

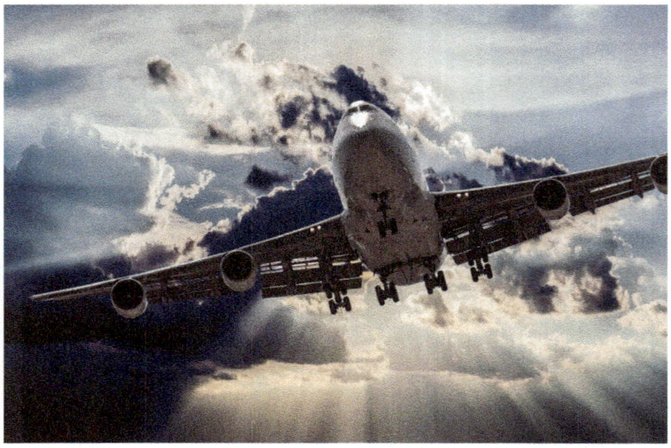

guvendemir/E+/Getty Images

Jumbo Jets Would jumbo jets be allowed to continue to fly if three of them crashed every day, with all passengers lost? Would you continue to fly? Yet just as many people in the United States die each day from smoking-related causes.

(American Lung Association, 2020). Although Blacks smoke fewer cigarettes than other groups, Black men are 30% more likely to develop lung cancer. Black American women who smoke are as likely to develop lung cancer as other groups of women who smoke, even though they also tend to smoke less.

You may be aware that smoking causes lung cancer. But it turns out that smoking damages nearly every organ and system in the body. It is a major contributor to cardiovascular disease (heart and artery disease); emphysema and other chronic lung disorders; and many cancers other than lung cancer, including cancer of the cervix, kidney, pancreas, and stomach (U.S. Surgeon General, 2010). Moreover, women who smoke have reduced bone density, increasing the risk of fractures of the hip and other bones. Pregnant women who smoke have a higher risk of miscarriage, preterm births, low-birth-weight babies, and stillborn babies.

People who smoke cigars are less likely to inhale than are those who smoke cigarettes, so some cigar smokers have assumed (wrongly) that cigar smoking was relatively safe. However, regular cigar smoking is linked to an increased risk for cancers of the lip, tongue, mouth, and throat as well as lung cancer (Centers for Disease Control and Prevention, 2020), even when the people do not inhale. If they do inhale, they are just as prone to the diseases incurred by people who smoke cigarettes.

Passive smoking is also linked to respiratory illnesses, asthma, and other health problems. Prolonged exposure to household tobacco smoke during childhood is a risk factor for lung cancer. Because of the effects of secondhand smoke, smoking has been banned in many public places, including as airplanes, restaurants, elevators, and even parks and apartment complexes.

passive smoking Inhaling smoke from other people's tobacco products (also known as secondhand smoking).

Why, then, do people smoke? For many reasons—such as the desire to look sophisticated (although these days people who smoke are more likely to be judged foolish than sophisticated), to quell nervousness, to have something to do with their hands, and—of course—to regulate their intake of nicotine.

But there is some positive news on the nonsmoking front. The percentage of American adults who smoke cigarettes has been declining steadily for the past 50 years, from more than 40% in 1966 to about 11.4% today (NCHS, 2023). Moreover, 3 out of 4 (74%) 12th graders believe that smoking a pack or more of cigarettes a day is harmful (Miech et al., 2019). By contrast, fewer than 1 in 5 (18%) 12th graders believes that regular vaping is harmful. Though substantial progress has been made in getting Americans to quit smoking, some 39 million adults in the United States continue to smoke cigarettes (VanFrank & Presley-Cantrell, 2021).

A Closer Look

Stopping Smoking? Good Idea! After You Quit Smoking ...

20 minutes: Heart rate drops

12 hours: Carbon monoxide level in blood returns to normal

2 days: Ability to smell and taste improves

2–3 weeks: Heart attack risk begins to drop; lung function improves; walking becomes easier

1 month: Coughing and shortness of breath decrease

1 year: Risk of heart disease is cut in half

5 years: Risk of stroke is reduced to that of a person who doesn't smoke

10 years: Risk of dying from lung cancer is about half that of a person who continues to smoke

25 years: Risk of coronary heart disease approximates that of people who have never smoked

Source: NYC Health Department (2018) and Duncan et al., 2019.

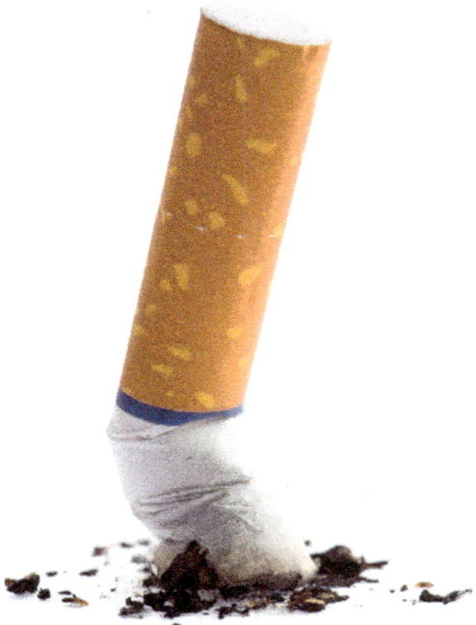

pkline/E+/Getty Images

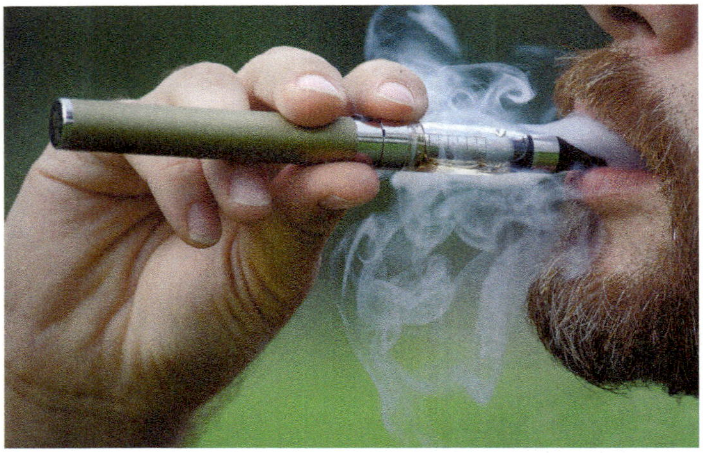

Marc Bruxelle RF/Alamy Stock Photo

Vaping

And Then Came ... Vaping

What do Walgreens, 7-Eleven stores, and Shell gas stations have in common? They and 1,100 other retailers received severe warning letters from the federal Food and Drug Administration in 2018, demanding that they stop selling e-cigarettes (e-cigs) to minors (Kaplan & Hoffman, 2018). Companies which make e-cigarettes that look like sleek flash drives, were also warned.

Nicotine-laced e-cigarettes were introduced to help cigarette smokers curb withdrawal symptoms when they quit smoking (Hajek et al., 2019; Rigotti, 2020). E-cigs provide a dose of nicotine, which helps quell withdrawal symptoms when nicotine-dependent smokers stop using tobacco products. E-cigs do not contain any tobacco; nor do they have the hydrocarbons or tars, the substances that are most harmful to bodily organs, However, they are powered by batteries and heating elements that produce a nicotine-containing vapor the user inhales that has been shown to be harmful to the lungs and the cardiovascular system (Abbasi, 2020; Diaz et al., 2020; Marsden et al., 2020). The nicotine in the vapor is as addictive as the nicotine in cigarettes. Minors are not permitted to purchase or use e-cigs, but they are readily available to most adolescents. Unfortunately, e-cigs are creating a new generation of adolescents who are addicted to nicotine.

Many students vape in bathrooms. Some sneak vaping in class. A school official said that students can pin Juuls "on to their shirt collar or bra strap and lean over and take a hit every now and then" (Zernike, 2018 p. A1). Because Juuls and similar devices leave little in the way of telltale plumes, the official added, "Who's to know?"

Surveys of high school students show that use of vaping exceeds that of cigarette smoking (Wang et al., 2020). Nearly 20% of high school students, more than 3 million in total, report using e-cigs or vaping (Wang et al., 2020). With millions of young people vaping, concerns are raised that we may see a generation of young people addicted to nicotine (Drazen, Morrissey, & Campion, 2019).

According to the National Health Interview Survey (Vahratian et al., 2018), vaping has not caught on all that much among adults—yet (see **Figure 9.7**). And the prevalence of vaping declines sharply with age. Older people are presumably less interested in finding something new to draw into their lungs.

When we compare the vaping and smoking of 8th, 10th, and 12th graders, we see that vaping nicotine is more popular among 10th and 12th graders (see **Table 9.1**). High school students are apparently becoming increasingly involved with vaping nicotine.

It would thus appear that the practice of vaping nicotine is undergoing a spurt in popularity. Although, as mentioned, nicotine-containing vapors do not have hydrocarbons, the great majority of them are flavored with the chemical *diacetyl*, which is associated with several respiratory diseases, including bronchiolitis (Allen et al., 2016), a viral infection characterized by a runny and stuffy nose, a cough, difficulty breathing, and, sometimes, a fever.

Another issue is illustrated by a study in which adolescent users of e-cigs who did not smoke tobacco cigarettes and adolescents who used neither e-cigs or tobacco cigarettes provided samples of saliva and urine (Rubinstein et al., 2018). Participants were on average 16.4 years old. The teens who vaped were found to have significantly higher levels of a number of cancer-causing chemicals in their saliva and their urine than the teens

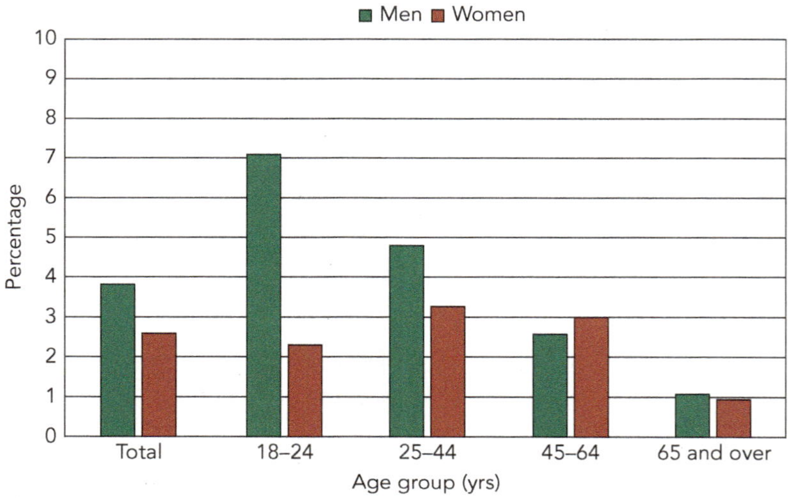

FIGURE 9.7 Percentage of Adults Aged 18 and Above Who Use E-Cigarettes

Source: Adapted from M. A. Villarroel, A. E. Cha, & A. Vahratian (2020). Electronic cigarette use among U.S. adults, 2018. *NCHS Data Brief, 365*. https://www.cdc.gov/nchs/data/databriefs/db365-h.pdf.

TABLE 9.1 Lifetime Prevalence of Vaping Nicotine and Smoking Tobacco Cigarettes in Grades 8, 10, and 12, in Percentages

	8th Graders	10th Graders	12th Graders
Vaping nicotine	21	36	41
Tobacco cigarettes	9	21	25

Sources: Adapted from R. Miech, L. Johnston, P. M. O'Malley, J. G. Bachman, & M. E. Patrick (2019). Trends in adolescent vaping, 2017–2019. *New England Journal of Medicine, 381*, 1490–1491; R. A. Miech, L. D. Johnston, P. M. O'Malley, J. G. Bachman, J. E. Schulenberg, & M. E. Patrick (2019). Monitoring the future: National survey results on drug use 1975–2018: Volume I, *Secondary school students*. Institute for Social Research, The University of Michigan. Figures 6-20 and 6-22.

who used neither e-cigs nor tobacco cigarettes. Therefore, although some people who smoke tobacco cigarettes switch to vaping, we should not assume that vaping is safe. Remember that vaping has only recently arisen; we do not have longitudinal evidence of the long-term effects of vaping.

contingency management A therapeutic approach in which meeting certain desirable behavioral goals are reinforced or rewarded, such as remaining abstinent from drugs.

Amphetamines

Amphetamines were first used by soldiers during World War II to help them remain alert through the night. Truck drivers have used them to stay awake all night, students have used them to stay up for all-night cram sessions, and dieters have used them to quell feelings of hunger. These drugs can be taken orally, smoked, snorted, or injected.

amphetamines A class of stimulants, including methamphetamine, that can increase states of alertness and induce pleasurable feelings.

Called speed, uppers, bennies (for Benzedrine), and dexies (for Dexedrine), these drugs are often used for the euphoric rush they can produce in high doses. Regular users may stay

Health Psychology in Action

Vape No More: The Use of Contingency Management in Quitting Vaping

As the health risks of vaping have become clearer, health researchers have begun to focus on intervention programs to help young people break their dependence on vaping products. Though use of tobacco products has declined among teens and young adults, vaping has become a disturbing trend. Along with health information disseminated in schools and by healthcare providers raising awareness about the risks of addiction and physical health damage caused by vaping, greater efforts are needed to prevent young people from getting hooked on vaping products and assisting those who are vaping to quit.

One promising approach involves **contingency management**, a technique that applies the principle of positive reinforcement to reward efforts to reduce or eliminate unhealthy habits, such as vaping. In contingency management programs, monetary incentives are often used as rewards for healthy behaviors. Stop for a moment to consider how rewards in the form of money, praise, good grades, and social approval influence virtually everything you do, from studying for exams to working for a paycheck, to helping out around the house.

Recently a group of health researchers at the Medical College of South Carolina evaluated a pilot program that used contingency management to target vaping among young adults (Palmer et al., 2022). The program, which was run through a smartphone app, involved 25 young adults age 17 to 21 who vaped regularly but expressed an interest in quitting. The key component of the program was the use of incentives (small monetary rewards) for producing negative (drug-free) saliva test samples after a scheduled quit day. Participants in the CM group received cash payments of $20 for each clean saliva sample, up to a maximum of $200 for 10 clean samples over a 4-week period. Participants mailed in their saliva samples which were tested for the presence of a metabolite of nicotine. Clean samples showed no detectable levels of the metabolite, indicating abstinence from nicotine from vaping or tobacco products. Control participants in a monitoring condition also received $20 cash payments for each saliva sample, irrespective of whether it showed abstinence or not. The key difference between the conditions was the contingency in the CM program in which payments were made contingent on submitting clean samples, indicating abstinence from vaping.

The researchers found that 55% of the saliva samples from CM participants showed abstinence, as compared to only 8% from the monitoring-only control group. The results of this small, pilot program are encouraging, as they show that incentives can increase healthy behavior.

CM is not limited to vaping or tobacco interventions. For example, other health researchers find contingency management programs boost the frequency of other positive health outcomes, such as achieving abstinence in substance abuse treatment programs (Bolívar et al., 2021; Ginley et al., 2021). But such programs do raise important ethical and practice questions that need to be addressed, such as whether we should pay people to change their unhealthy behaviors and about where the money to fund such programs would be drawn. But the evidence is clear: Rewarding desirable behavior works.

awake and "high" for days on end. Such highs must come to an end. People who have been on prolonged highs sometimes crash, or fall into a deep sleep or depression. Because of tolerance, many of them take very high doses.

People can become psychologically dependent on amphetamines, especially when they are routinely used to cope with stress or depression. Tolerance develops rapidly. Regular use of methamphetamine, a particularly powerful amphetamine, can also lead to physiological dependence or addiction (Takashima & Mandyam, 2018). High doses of amphetamines may cause restlessness, insomnia, loss of appetite, and irritability. Amphetamine use can also induce a form of psychosis ("break with reality") characterized by hallucinations and delusions that mimic the symptoms of paranoid schizophrenia.

Fewer than 1% of people in the United States have used methamphetamine in the past month; 6–7% have used it during their lifetimes (Johnston et al., 2018; National Institute on Drug Abuse, 2020). Use of "meth" as well as meth overdoses are on the rise in the United States (Han et al., 2021). Heavy use of methamphetamine—also known as meth, chalk, ice, crystal, and glass—is also linked to cognitive and emotional problems as well as to possible neurological damage. Brain imaging studies show that methamphetamine use can damage the brain, causing problems with learning, memory, and other cognitive functions (Dean et al., 2018; Li et al., 2018).

Many psychoactive drugs, such as amphetamines, alcohol, opioids, and cocaine, increase levels of the neurotransmitter dopamine in brain pathways that produce feelings of pleasure (Flagel et al., 2011). Over time, heavy use of methamphetamine reduces the brain's production of dopamine. As a result, habitual users of speed (or cocaine) come to rely on having the drug in their bodies in order to experience any pleasure in life.

Another stimulant, methylphenidate (Ritalin), has a legitimate clinical use in the treatment of ADHD in children. It works by stimulating the executive center of the brain to exercise control over hyperactivity. However, Ritalin may also become a drug of abuse when used by adolescents or adults for its stimulating effects.

Ecstasy

Ecstasy An amphetamine-like drug that has mild euphoric and hallucinogenic effects.

Ecstasy is synthetized in the laboratory. It produces mild euphoric and hallucinogenic effects. The formal name for the drug is MDMA (3,4-methylenedioxymethamphetamine). It is a chemical cousin of amphetamine and established a foothold in late-night dance clubs, or raves, in American cities in the 1990s and early 2000s.

Many users, especially teens, believe it to be relatively safe, but health officials warn that the drug poses both serious physical and psychological risks. It raises blood pressure and heart rate—physiological reactions that can be dangerous to people with cardiovascular conditions. It can also lead to a tense or chattering jaw and in high doses can be deadly. Psychologically, it can produce unpleasant symptoms such as depression, anxiety, insomnia, and even paranoia. Heavy use of the drug can lead to problems with learning, memory, and attention and may cause brain damage (Di Iorio et al., 2011). If you think this cleverly named drug will leave you ecstatic, think again.

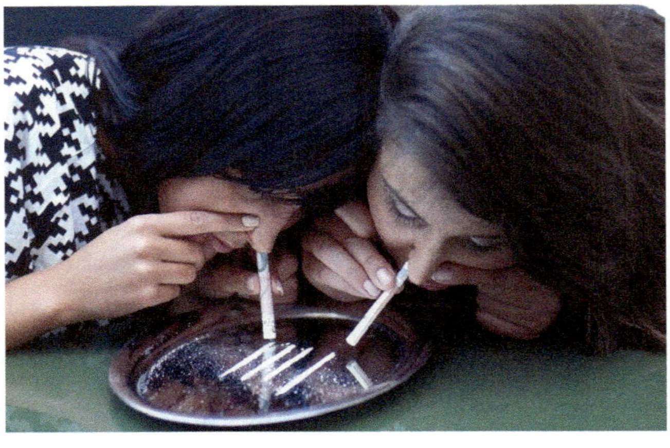
hiphunter/E+/Getty Images

Snorting Cocaine

Cocaine

One of cocaine's early enthusiasts was a Viennese physician by the name of Sigmund Freud (Markel, 2020). Freud heard of cocaine hydrochloride, a supposed medical cure-all. He used it in the form of a white powder so frequently that he became dependent on the drug. His drug-induced elation prompted him to talk endlessly about what he thought were repressed memories, and he prescribed the drug for some clients in the development of his "talking cure" for psychological problems. However, after a decade or so of use, he experienced bouts of depression and difficulty concentrating, and his nose became so congested from snorting the drug that he required an operation to cut a hole between his nostrils. Eventually, he cut back on his use of cocaine.

The beverage Coca-Cola® (Coke) was originally brewed with an extract of cocaine and was marketed at the time as a "brain tonic." But Coca-Cola® hasn't been "the real thing" since 1906, when the company discontinued the use of the stimulant.

Cocaine is a powerful stimulant derived from coca leaves. It can produce feelings of euphoria, curb hunger, deaden pain, and bolster self-confidence. Cocaine apparently works by binding to sites on transmitting neurons that would normally reuptake molecules of the neurotransmitters norepinephrine, dopamine, and serotonin. With cocaine "locking the doors" of the receiving neurons, molecules of these transmitters remain longer in the synaptic cleft, enhancing the molecules' mood-altering effects and producing their euphoric "rush." But when cocaine levels drop, lower absorption of neurotransmitters by receiving neurons causes the user's mood to crash. According to the *dopamine-sensitization hypothesis*, repeated use of cocaine may sensitize the nervous system to dopamine by disrupting reuptake of dopamine on a long-term, possibly irreversible basis.

Cocaine may be brewed from coca leaves as a "tea," snorted in powder form (as taken by Freud), or injected in liquid form. Repeated snorting constricts blood vessels in the nose, drying the skin and sometimes exposing cartilage and perforating the nasal septum. These problems require cosmetic surgery. A hardened form of cocaine, called crack, is sold in small, ready-to-use smokable doses that are affordable to many adolescents, leading many of them to quickly become regular users.

About 5% of young adults, in the United States uses cocaine each year (Mustaquim, Jones, & Compton, 2021). Cocaine is a highly addictive drug that gives rise to a withdrawal syndrome characterized by intense cravings, depressed mood, fatigue, insomnia, increases in appetite, and loss of ability to obtain pleasure from the ordinary enjoyable experiences of daily life. Users may also become psychologically dependent on the drug, using it compulsively to deal with life stress.

Cocaine is also a highly dangerous drug. As shown in **Figure 9.8**, the rate of death from cocaine overdoses more than tripled between the years of 2012 and 2018 (Hedegaard et al., 2020). Cocaine stimulates spikes in blood pressure, constricts the coronary arteries and thickens the blood (both of which decrease the oxygen supply to the heart), and quickens the heart rate. Overdoses may result in respiratory and cardiovascular collapse, leading in some cases to sudden death. Overdoses can also cause restlessness and insomnia, tremors, headaches, nausea, convulsions, and psychological symptoms, such as hallucinations and delusions. Over time, use of cocaine damages brain circuits that regulate feelings of pleasure. This may account for the fact that cocaine abusers often become depressed and unable to reap pleasure from ordinary life experiences when they stop using the drug.

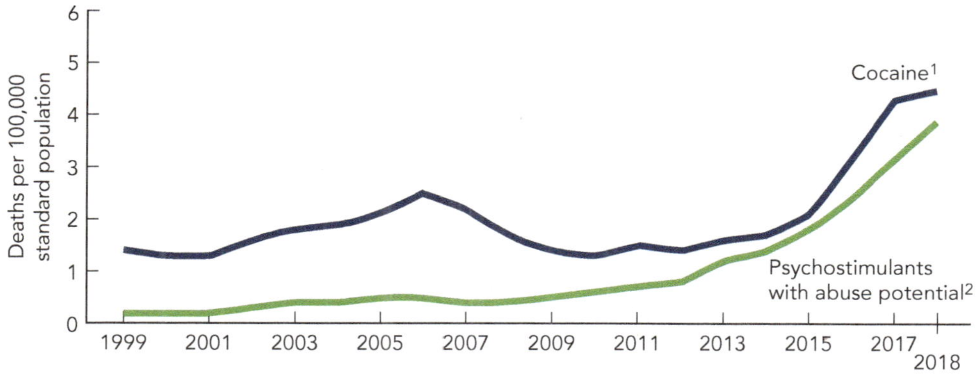

[1]Significant increasing trend from 1999 through 2006, decreasing trend from 2006 through 2012, and increasing trend from 2012 through 2018 with different rates of change over time, $p < 0.05$.
[2]Significant increasing trend from 1999 through 2005, 2008 through 2012, and 2012 through 2018 with different rates of change over time, $p < 0.05$.

FIGURE 9.8 **Drug Overdose Death Rates Involving Stimulants, United States, 1999–2018**

Source: H. Hedegaard, A. M. Minino, & M. Warner (2020). Drug overdose deaths in the United States, 1999–2018. *NCHS Data Brief, 356*, p. 4. https://www.cdc.gov/nchs/data/databriefs/db356-h.pdf / US Department of Health and Human Services / Public Domain.

TYPE OF COFFEE	CAFFEINE (MILLIGRAMS)
Dunkin' brewed, 16 oz (480 mL)	143–206
Generic brewed, 8 oz (240 mL)	95–200
Generic brewed, decaffeinated, 8 oz (240 mL)	2–12
Generic instant, 8 oz (240 mL)	27–173
Generic instant, decaffeinated, 8 oz (240 mL)	2–12
Starbucks Vanilla Latte, 16 oz (480 mL)	150
TYPE OF TEA	**CAFFEINE (MILLIGRAMS)**
Black tea, brewed, 8 oz (240 mL)	40–120
Black tea, decaffeinated, brewed, 8 oz (240 mL)	2–10
Starbucks Tazo Chai Tea Latte, 16 oz (480 mL)	100
Stash Premium Green, brewed, 6 oz (180 mL)	26

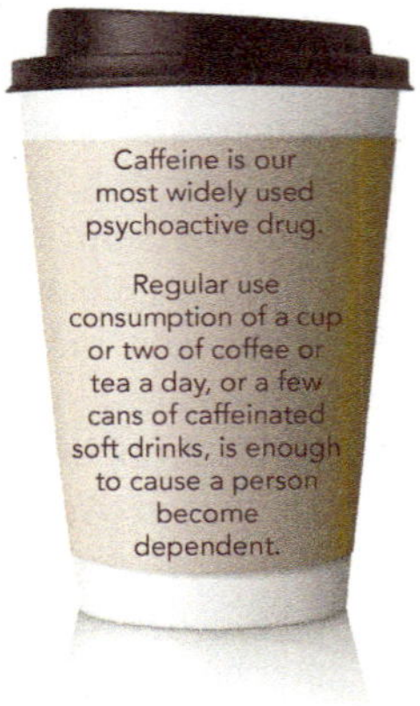

artcyclone/DigitalVision Vectors/Getty Images

FIGURE 9.9 **Amount of Caffeine in Coffee and Tea Products**

Caffeine

Would it surprise you to learn that many, perhaps most, people who lead perfectly normal lives never realize that they may by chemically dependent on a mind-altering drug? That drug is available in any supermarket, is likely sitting in a kitchen cabinet near you or on your desk, and is the reason that Starbucks and Dunkin' stores have inundated the world. It is caffeine, the mild stimulant found in coffee, tea, cola beverages, and chocolate (**Figure 9.9**). As a mild stimulant, caffeine does not produce the intense effects or euphoric highs of stronger stimulants such as cocaine and methamphetamine. Yet it is our most widely used psychoactive drug. More than half of American adults drink coffee, averaging more than three cups a day. And given the cups we see people carrying on city streets, many people would not leave home (or the coffee bar) without it.

If you regularly drink caffeinated beverages, you are probably dependent on caffeine. One sign of dependence is waking up with a headache (sometimes a severe headache) that is relieved by drinking coffee. Caffeine may be among the least harmful of psychoactive substances, but it still carries risks. Some studies have connected caffeine intake by pregnant women with giving birth to babies who are preterm (Okubo et al., 2015) or small for gestational age, but a Norwegian study of more than 67,000 mother–infant pairs suggests that moderate caffeine intake (< 200 mg/day) apparently does not lead to neonates who are small for gestational age or otherwise impair neonatal health (Modzelewska et al., 2019).

For most healthy (nonpregnant) adults, moderate caffeine intake (200–300 mg per day, or about two to three cups of coffee daily) does not appear to pose significant health problems. However, caffeine, like other stimulants, can increase blood pressure by activating arousal of the sympathetic division of the autonomic nervous system (Yu et al., 2016).

Like other stimulants, caffeine increases alertness and learning (Tully et al., 2020). It also enhances athletic performance as measured by cycling power and other endeavors (Lara et al., 2019). A study found that laboratory rats receiving moderate doses of caffeine performed significantly better than controls and than those receiving extremely high doses of caffeine on measures of learning and memory, and of motor coordination (Almosawi et al., 2018). As the ancient Greek poet Hesiod wrote: "Observe due measure, moderation is best in all things."

Review 9.3

INTERACTIVE SELF-SCORING QUIZZES

Sentence Completion

1. The most widely used stimulant is __________.

2. Stimulants are used in the treatment of __________ because they stimulate the executive center of the brain to exercise control.

3. e-cigarettes are least likely to be used by people aged __________.

4. The __________ in cigarette smoke are most likely to be responsible for causing lung cancer.

5. Overdoses of the stimulant __________ have caused respiratory and cardiovascular collapse, leading to sudden death in some cases.

6. Women who smoke have reduced __________ __________, making them more vulnerable to fractures of the hip and other bones.

7. The stimulant __________ is a treatment of choice for preterm infants, in whom it is intended to prevent temporary cessation of breathing.

8. The soft drink Coca-Cola® once contained the stimulant __________.

9. The stimulant __________ is used by as many as 1 in 10 college students to boost their attention and alertness for studying and test taking.

Think About It

Which stimulants have you used or have been used by people you know? If you are dependent on caffeine to get going in the morning, do you consider that dependence an example of substance abuse? Why or why not? Do you know people who have successfully quit smoking? What strategies did they use to do so?

Hallucinogens

Hallucinogens (also called hallucinogenic drugs or **psychedelics**) induce sensory distortions and **hallucinations**. The most widely used hallucinogen is marijuana.

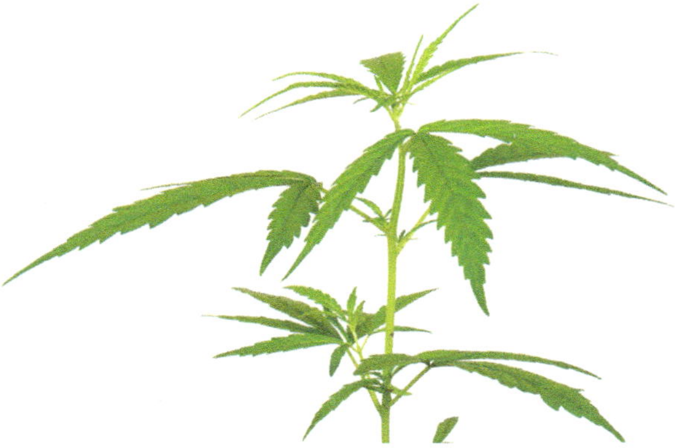

Panther Media GmbH/Alamy Stock Photo

Cannabis sativa **Plant**

Marijuana

We find ourselves in a new environment concerning **marijuana**. The substance, which was illegal and whose use was widely seen as immoral, is now legalized in many states for recreational purposes. Moreover, medical marijuana has been prescribed by physicians to help patients control chronic pain. Psychiatrist Richard Friedman (2018) argues that marijuana is not only an effective pain reliever but may help many who might otherwise turn to opioids to reduce pain. Yet we will see that there are concerns about the use of marijuana.

Marijuana is derived from the *Cannabis sativa* plant, which grows wild in many parts of the world. Today, with marijuana legal in a growing number of states and countries, it is also cultivated in hothouses. Marijuana has complex psychological effects. It can induce feelings of relaxation, elevate the mood, and produce mild hallucinations, such as distortion of the passage of time. The active psychoactive substance in marijuana is delta-9-tetrahydrocannabinol (THC). THC is found in the branches and leaves of the plant, but it is highly concentrated in the sticky resin. **Hashish** is derived from the resin and is more potent than marijuana.

In the 19th century, marijuana was used as much as aspirin is used today for headaches and minor aches and pains. It could be bought without a prescription in any drugstore. But the drug became illegal in every state by the 1930s, and it was outlawed for any use, including medical uses, in 1970.

Until it became legal in many states, marijuana was the most widely used illicit drug in the United States. About 1 young adult in 4 currently uses marijuana, as do nearly as many 12th graders (NCHS, 2023). Nearly half of all adult Americans have tried marijuana at some point in their lives. With the legalization of marijuana in many states, young people have come to perceive the drug as less risky (Johnston et al., 2018). Parental disapproval has also

psychedelics Drugs that cause hallucinations and delusions or heighten perceptions.

hallucinations Perceptions in the absence of sensation that are confused with reality.

marijuana The dried vegetable matter of the *Cannabis sativa* plant.

hashish A more potent form of marijuana, a drug derived from the resin of the *Cannabis sativa* plant (also called hash).

declined. Some 80–90% of high school seniors say that marijuana would be easy to get if they wanted to use it. Approximately 40% of 12th graders report having done so in the past year (Johnston et al., 2018).

Like alcohol, marijuana affects motor coordination and thus impairs driving ability (Moreno-Rius, 2019). Short-term use can sap focus and motivation, making it more difficult for college students to complete that term paper after using marijuana the night before. Although many users report positive mood changes, others experience disturbing feelings of anxiety and confusion and, occasionally, even psychotic reactions, such as a heightened state of anxiety, confusion, and paranoia. Heightened awareness of bodily sensations may lead some people who use marijuana users to fear that their heart will "run away" with them. Some people who smoke marijuana find the disorientation that often occurs to be frightening or threatening. Smoking marijuana also introduces cancer-causing substances into the body. Marijuana also has negative effects on both physical and mental functioning. It elevates the heart rate and, in some people, the blood pressure. This higher demand on the heart and circulation poses a threat to people with hypertension and cardiovascular disorders. Evidence also shows that regular use of marijuana can lead to problems with learning and memory (Ellingson et al., 2020; Niloy et al, 2023).

People can become psychologically dependent on marijuana, and about 4 million people in the United States have been diagnosed with marijuana use disorder (National Institute on Drug Abuse, 2020). However, marijuana has not been classified as an addictive drug because the presence of an identifiable withdrawal syndrome continues to be debated. Yet recent evidence points to the presence of a withdrawal syndrome in long-term regular users who abruptly quit using the drug (Connor et al., 2022; Zehra et al., 2019). The characteristic signs of this withdrawal syndrome include nausea, cramps, headaches, insomnia, anxiety, and sweating and chills.

LSD and Other Hallucinogens

LSD The acronym for lysergic acid diethylamide, a hallucinogenic drug.

flashbacks Distorted perceptions or hallucinations that mimic the LSD "trip" but occur days, weeks, or longer after usage.

LSD, or "acid," is the acronym for lysergic acid diethylamide, a synthetic hallucinogenic drug. LSD is not nearly as popular with young people as marijuana, as only about 4% of 12th graders have tried it (Miech et al., 2023). Some users claim that it expands consciousness and opens up new worlds to them. Sometimes people believe they have achieved great insights while using LSD, but when it wears off, they don't seem able to apply or exactly recall these discoveries. As a powerful hallucinogen, LSD produces vivid and colorful hallucinations. Some LSD users experience **flashbacks**.

Other hallucinogens include mescaline (derived from the peyote cactus) and phencyclidine. Regular use of hallucinogens may lead to tolerance and psychological dependence. But hallucinogens are not known to lead to physiological dependence. High doses may induce frightening hallucinations, impaired coordination, poor judgment, mood changes, and paranoid delusions.

A survey of 3,525 university students found that about 11% had used hallucinogens and nearly 5% had done so during the past year (Grant et al., 2019). Use of hallucinogens was associated with use of many other substances, including alcohol and opioids; mental health issues; risky sexual behavior; low self-esteem; and impulsivity but not with compulsive behavior. In that study, it did not appear that use of hallucinogens led to use of other substances or behavioral problems but rather that personality issues were connected with the substance use and behavioral problems.

Health Psychology in the Digital Age

Internet Addiction

How much time do you spend on the internet each day? Excessive use of the internet can become a compulsive form of behavior called internet addiction (IA). IA is found more commonly among adolescents and young adults and is believed to affect as many as 10% of college students (Lozano-Blasco et al., 2022; Starcevic & Aboujaoude, 2017).

Are you at risk of becoming addicted to the internet? Here are some common signs:

- Do you feel compelled to check the internet every chance you get?
- Do you check your e-mail or your Facebook page every few minutes?
- Are you spending 3, 4, or more hours a day in chat rooms or participating in virtual communities?
- Is this behavior creating distance between yourself and the real world? Is it interfering with your functioning at school, at home, on the job, or in relationships?
- Can you imagine being without access to the internet for a week? A day? If that's too painful to contemplate, how about only 3 or 4 hours?

People who become addicted to the internet may neglect their studies or work and their real (unlike virtual) social lives. Estimates of the prevalence of internet addiction on college campuses range between 1% and 10% (Starcevic & Aboujaoude, 2017). Internet addiction may take different forms. Some heavy users become involved in excessive gaming and competition, whereas others become preoccupied with internet porn. Still others compulsively participate in virtual communities, to a point that their self-esteem hinges on creating fictional assets in the form of avatars as alter-egos they can use to compensate for their perceived deficits—to become taller or more attractive than they really are. And yet others compulsively use social networking and chat rooms to satisfy emotional needs or combat loneliness or boredom in the real world. Health psychologists are concerned about internet addiction because, like other compulsive behavior problems such as pathological gambling and compulsive shopping, it is connected to emotional problems of anxiety and depression, impulsivity, and substance abuse. Below are some suggestions for combating internet addiction. But as with other forms of addiction, should the problem persist, it would be worthwhile to consult a helping professional:

- Strictly limit the amount of time you allow yourself to spend online for recreational use. Reward yourself for sticking to the limit by putting away money toward something you really want.
- Shut your computer off (don't just let it go to sleep) after you have spent your allotted amount of time online or finished with your legitimate purposes.
- Engage in a competing activity. Read a book, go for a walk, check your assignments, or chat (offline!) with a friend.
- Limit internet use to public places. For example, use the library or the student center or the cafeteria.
- Develop relationships in the real world. Join clubs and campus organizations, and expand your friendships rather than substitute virtual relationships.

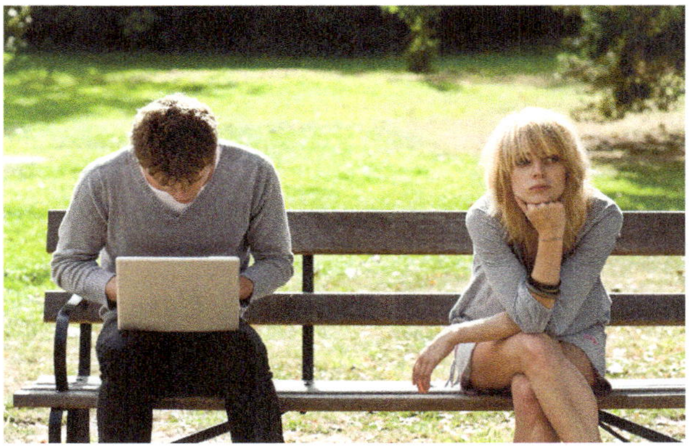

Tino Tedaldi/Cultura/Getty Images

Review 9.4

INTERACTIVE SELF-SCORING QUIZZES

Sentence Completion

1. The psychoactive substance in marijuana is __________.

2. Some users of __________ experience flashbacks to the drug experience.

3. Marijuana is classified as a hallucinogenic drug because it can produce __________.

4. Heavy, regular use of marijuana can damage __________ tissue.

5. It is clear that people can become __________ dependent on marijuana.

6. Marijuana impairs __________ coordination, thus impairing driving ability.

Think About It

Marijuana is the most widely used "recently illegal" drug in the United States. Do you believe that regular use of marijuana is harmful? Why or why not? Has the fact that recreational use of marijuana is now legal in many states affected people's perceptions of its possible harmfulness? What do you think?

Health Psychology and Behavioral Change

Psychologists have shown that certain substances require specific strategies for curtailing abuse, whereas there are some general principles that apply to a number of substances. Treatments and strategies run the gamut from medical supervision for withdrawal or replacement of a substance to self-guided change, therapeutic groups, apps and online methods. We will also see that B. F. Skinner's theory of operant conditioning offers useful advice for using the ABCs of behavior to cut down or discontinue substance abuse.

Detoxification

For those who are physiologically dependent on drugs, the first step in treatment may be detoxification, or the ridding of the body of the substance. "Detox" may occur in a hospital setting so that people can be medically supervised as they withdraw. Depending on the substance, a detox program may last as long as 28 days, during which time people who are recovering receive counseling to prepare them for remaining substance-free upon discharge. Counselors attempt to break through the layers of denial that often cloud abusers' recognition of the need to come to grips with the consequences of their usage. Counselors also advise avoiding people and situations associated with abuse of the substance.

Strategies for Change

Psychologists have developed many strategies to promote long-term changes in health-related behavior, but so have laypeople (Bishop, 2018). In fact, the majority of people who have quit or cut down on substance abuse have looked to their own resources to gain control.

Alcohol People with alcohol use problems are often motivated to change their level of alcohol consumption for a number of reasons, including health problems, social costs such as the loss of a marriage or a relationship, and financial loss due to loss of employment (Bishop, 2018).

The strategies they use for changing are similar to those developed by cognitive behavioral therapists. For example, they learn to say "no" when they are offered a drink. They alternate drinking alcoholic with nonalcoholic beverages. (This is a method of cutting down gradually.) They reduce the number of drinks they have during the day and the number of days they drink per week. (Another approach to cutting down gradually.) They maintain their self-control by thinking about the negative consequences of their drinking and by thinking about the positive consequences of not drinking.

Health Psychology in the Digital Age

Apps That Help People Change Their Drinking Habits

People who are attempting to control their alcohol intake can turn to a number of mobile apps for motivation and reminders to think about their alcohol intake. Examples of mobile apps include:

- Happify, which focuses on the feelings of depression and anxiety that are often associated with AUD
- SoberTool, which provides daily motivational messages and a tool that helps users prevent relapse when they have cravings
- Twenty-Four Hours a Day, which provides inspirational messages and meditations to help users cope with cravings
- Leaf, an alcohol tracker application that not only tracks alcohol intake but also provides alerts when the individual is going over planned consumption
- Daybreak, which provides an emotionally supportive network with set notifications concerning check-ins
- 12 Steps Companion, an app tailored to the 12-step program of Alcoholics Anonymous (AA), which tracks the extent of the individual's sobriety
- Drunkalyzer, an app that not only helps track alcohol intake, but also calculates blood alcohol level according to the number of drinks registered by the user
- Drink Tracker, which tracks not only the number of drinks consumed by the user but also estimates the number of calories from alcohol that the user is ingesting

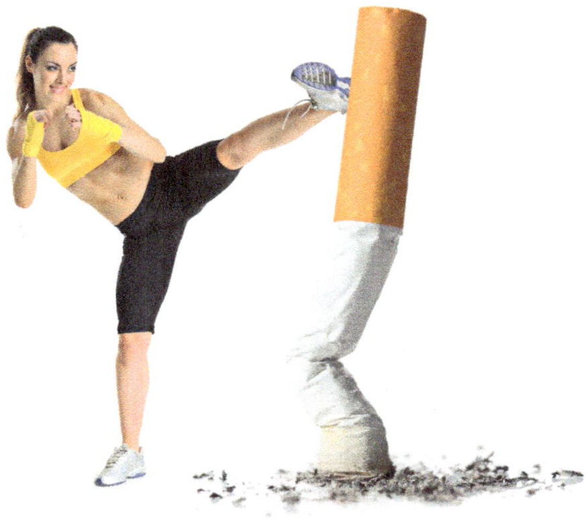

Kicking the Habit The majority of people who quit smoking do so on their own, focusing on the harmful effects of smoking.

Opioids It is a myth that people who are dependent on opioids such as heroin cannot quit. It is true that many thousands die each year from overdoses of opioids, but it is also true that most people who are dependent on them eventually quit. Many of these people do it without professional intervention, but many others rely on professorial help. One study found that half of users quit within 4 to 5 years of becoming dependent (Blanco et al., 2013). About 3 in 4 people addicted to heroin who become dependent in their teens or 20s quit by the time they reach their 30s. This phenomenon has been referred to as "maturing out."

Sometimes a change of environment is involved in breaking drug use patterns. Interviews were with conducted 898 servicemen returning from the war in Vietnam (Robins et al., 1975). Heroin was readily available to troops in Vietnam, and 20% of the troops tested positive for opioids. We don't know what percentage of those who tested positive were dependent on heroin, but we do know that only 1 year later, after returning home, only 1% still tested positive. In Vietnam, there was "R & R" (rest and relaxation), which, for many men, meant alcohol and drugs. With the change in environment when the men returned home, there was finding work, seeking advancement, building families and a home life.

Studies find that the primary strategies people use to moderate their usage or to abstain from heroin and opioids include changing the amount of the drug used (cutting back) and the frequency of usage (Bishop, 2018). Of course, many people who use these drugs do not know whether they can get by on a smaller dose. Or they may be given to all-or-nothing thinking, which cognitive behavioral therapists see as a cognitive error, and believe that they must simply quit cold turkey rather than cut down gradually (Beck et al., 1993; Lee & O'Malley, 2018). They can try taking half a dose or half a pill and wait to see whether it is effective. After a few days they can then go to one-quarter of a dose. Cutting down may cause some discomfort, but cognitive behavioral therapists point out that it is irrational to believe that one cannot abide some discomfort, and the individual can be prompted to focus on the pros of cutting down and the cons of not doing so (Beck et al., 1993).

Nicotine Quitting smoking is fiercely difficult for many. Most people who smoke try to quit repeatedly, and the number of attempted quits reported in a Canadian study of 1,277 people who smoked ranged from 6 to 142 (Chaiton et al., 2016). A majority of relapses occur within a year of quitting (Peterson & Marek, 2017).

Yet most people who quit—or attempt to quit—do not seek professional assistance or believe that it would be helpful. Nearly 4 in 5 people who smoke believe that they can quit on their own and do so by themselves (Bishop, 2018). Motives for quitting include the cost of tobacco (governments have been increasing the taxes on cigarettes) and concerns about health in the present and in the future. One of your authors had attempted to quit six or seven times and finally did so after awaking one morning with a hacking cough and difficulty catching his breath. He went cold turkey at that point, and a powerful craving lasted for a week. During that time he was irritable and anxious (more so than usual), had headaches, found it difficult to concentrate on his work, and substituted sweets for cigarettes. All of the withdrawal symptoms and the craving subsided in less than 2 weeks. However, over the years he would have nightmares in which he was smoking, realized what he was doing, and despaired that all was lost.

Going cold turkey is a common approach. Some smokers set a quit date and adhere to it, or attempt to do so. Some use nicotine replacement therapies (NRTs), which help reduce withdrawal symptoms. NRTs are available in the form of gum, inhalers, lozenges, nasal sprays, and skin patches. Cigarette users seeking to quit may use e-cigs as an NRT to help quell withdrawal symptoms when they quit smoking (Barbeau et al., 2013). However, in adolescents e-cigs (vaping) often function as a gateway to smoking tobacco cigarettes (Berry et al., 2019). E-cigs also provide the biobehavioral feedback that people who smoke seem to enjoy when they are attempting to quit, such as putting something in the mouth, holding something in the hands, the experience of inhaling, and experiencing the vapor hit the back of the throat (the "throat hit") (Barbeau et al., 2013).

Cocaine Some people who use cocaine, including fit athletes, die from constriction of blood vessels and heart damage. Some people's noses and faces become disfigured. The drug provides a sense of overconfidence that can be associated with risky behavior. However, the good news is that nearly half of people who have become dependent on cocaine quit the drug within 5 years. Eventually, well over 90% of users stop using the drug (Lopez-Quintero et al., 2011). Research suggests that only about 1 in 10 people who need treatment to quit cocaine receive it, but more than 90% of these individuals do not think they need help (Lipari et al., 2016).

From a health psychology standpoint, the decision to choose to stop using cocaine is based on factors such as the cognitive process of weighing the pluses and minuses of continuing to use cocaine as well as pressure from family and friends and financial difficulties associated with use of the drug (Bishop, 2018). Those who change or end their cocaine usage report using strategies such as the following to maintain abstinence:

- Finding ways of boosting self-esteem and self-confidence in living without drugs
- Focusing on all the negative consequences of using cocaine
- Obtaining professional assistance
- Avoiding social contact with drug-using companions and friends, thereby avoiding social pressures and situations in which others are using cocaine
- Focusing on building mature behaviors, such as a career and family life
- Learning to tolerate cravings for the drug without resuming use, letting them pass through or toughing them out
- Seeking social and emotional support from family and friends
- Changing one's environment to avoid stimuli associated with drug use
- Turning to religion or spirituality as sources of support

Self-Help Groups

The most widely used program for AUD is AA, a self-help program in which individuals provide mutual support in a context in which people progress through 12 designated steps toward sobriety. Members meet regularly and call other members between meetings when they are tempted to drink. The 12 steps require admitting to the group that one's drinking is out of control, calling upon a higher power for strength, examining the injurious behavior (physical, psychological, or financial) that one has inflicted on others, and attempting to make amends. A buddy system encourages members to seek the support of other members when they feel tempted to drink. AA appears to be most effective when members struggling with alcoholism remain in treatment for many years, when they make a commitment to remain abstinent, when it helps them alleviate feelings of depression, and when it increases their confidence that they can navigate life's challenges and high-risk situations (like parties) without drinking (Breuniger et al., 2020; MacKillop et al., 2018). However, the strong spiritual focus of AA may not be suited to every individual. Evidence shows that a variety of other group approaches may be as effective as AA (Breuniger et al., 2020; Zemore, 2017).

The National Institute on Alcohol Abuse and Alcoholism funded a large-scale study in which more than 1,700 problem drinkers were randomly assigned to the 12-step program, cognitive behavioral therapy, or "motivational-enhancement therapy" (Ouimette et al., 1997). The cognitive behavioral treatment taught problem drinkers how to cope with temptations and how to refuse offers of drinks. Motivational enhancement was designed to enhance the desire of people who drink to help themselves. The treatments worked equally well for most people, with some exceptions. For example, people with psychological problems fared somewhat better with cognitive behavioral therapy. People who participate in AA typically do better when they make a commitment to abstinence, have a strong intention to avoid high-risk situations associated with alcohol use, and stick with the program longer (Moos & Moos, 2004; Zemore, 2017).

Narcotics Anonymous is another 12-step program that encourages members to share their drug-related experiences and problems, including the challenges they face and the successes they find. Cocaine Anonymous is a self-help group for people seeking to recover from dependence on cocaine. Group members help each other handle their cravings for cocaine and avoid the situations that can lead to relapse. Cocaine Anonymous, unlike AA, does not call upon a higher power to give members insight and strength.

Therapeutic Medications

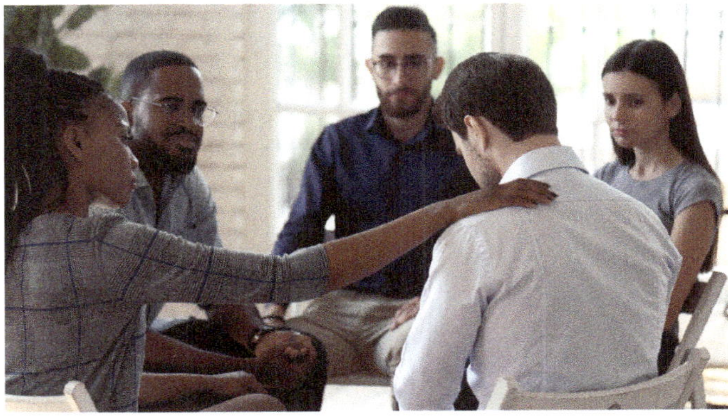

fizkes/Shutterstock.com

Group support often helps individuals cope with substance abuse. At the very least, they learn that they are not alone in their quest to gain control of their lives.

Ironically, therapeutic medications may be used to treat people with problems of substance abuse or dependence. In effect, one drug may be used to break a destructive pattern of use of another drug.

The medication *disulfiram* (trade name Antabuse), which is used to curb dependence on alcohol, was discovered when workers at a rubber manufacturing plant inadvertently inhaled it and discovered that they couldn't drink alcohol without feeling sick (De Sousa, 2019a). It turns out that disulfiram impairs the functioning of acetaldehyde by locking into its receptors, thus causing the flushing response, abdominal discomfort, nausea, and headaches experienced by many Asians and women who drink alcohol. For Antabuse to be effective, people must take it daily and be aware of the negative consequences that will ensue when consuming alcohol. In this way Antabuse reaffirms people's decisions to stop drinking. Some problem drinkers who take Antabuse drink anyway, and when they become ill from consuming alcohol, they decide to stop taking the medication rather than abstain from alcohol. Therefore, people for whom Antabuse is prescribed profit from treatment or self-guided strategies that encourage them to make a public commitment to quit drinking and provide emotional and social support for doing so (De Sousa, 2019b).

Another medication, *naltrexone* (trade name ReVia), blocks the high people normally get from alcohol, which may help break the vicious cycle in which one drink creates a strong desire for another, leading to binge drinking in people who are alcohol dependent (Avery, 2022; Kranzler, 2023; Santos et al., 2022). But, again, investigators recognize that medications are usually more effective when they are combined with psychological approaches to help people with alcohol and other drug problems learn to cope more effectively without relapsing (Runarsdottir et al., 2017).

Methadone, a synthetic opioid, is used widely in treating heroin addiction because it prevents the highly unpleasant withdrawal symptoms that follow withdrawal from the drug. When used as prescribed, it does not produce the rush associated with heroin, so people maintained on methadone often hold jobs and get their lives back on track. But methadone, like other opioids, is highly addictive, so it is only distributed at clinics. Methadone too leads to withdrawal symptoms upon going cold turkey. However, people can be weaned gradually from methadone by cutting the dose down gradually with proper supervision. *Levomethadyl acetate* is similar to methadone but is longer acting. Users may thus visit a clinic three times a week rather than the daily visits recommended for methadone users.

It is also to be noted that a key issue in the substitution of methadone for heroin is compliance with treatment. People who miss appointments to receive methadone start to experience withdrawal symptoms and cravings that may lead them back to heroin or other opioids. One study found that telephone delivery of incentives for clinic visits, including use of praise and modest financial rewards, helps bring users back (Metrebian et al., 2020). Some might question the moral basis of paying people who use drugs to attend their methadone treatment sessions; however, one might also ask whether the costs of missing appointments and returning to the use of illicit drugs are higher for the individual and for society at large.

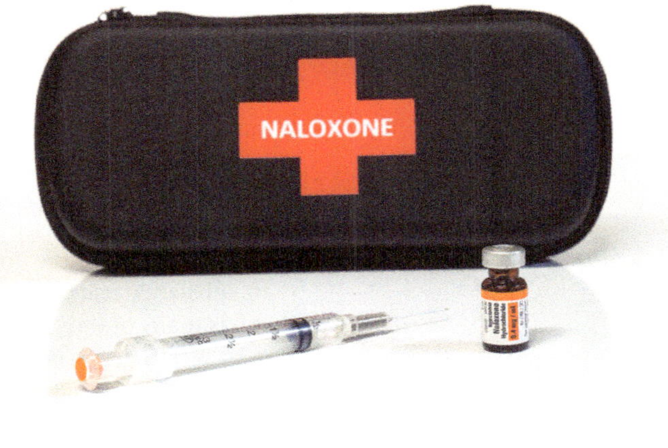

Tomas Nevesely/Shutterstock.com

An Overdose Rescue Kit The kit includes naloxone and a syringe for nasal atomization of the drug. Naloxone can block the effects of opioids. It is also available as a nasal spray and a tablet that is placed under the tongue.

The medication *naloxone* (trade name Narcan) blocks the effects of opioids as well as those of alcohol (Carpenter et al., 2019). It is used in emergency situations to rapidly reverse the effects of an opioid overdose, including overdoses of the powerful synthetic (Carpenter et al., 2019).

Having noted the difficulty of discontinuing use of opioids, it must also be noted that withdrawal symptoms are harsher for some people than for others. For example, a 14-day double-blind study of the effectiveness of various medications for addiction found that women tend to undergo more severe symptoms than men (Dunn et al., 2020). Additional research is recommended to further explore individual and group differences in experiences during withdrawal (Dunn et al., 2020).

NRTs such as the nicotine patch can provide a steady supply of nicotine to the body, which can help wean nicotine-dependent smokers from dependence. However, fewer than one in five smokers who use NRT become abstinent by a 6-month follow-up (USPSTF, 2021). Antidepressant medications that increase the availability of serotonin in the brain (e.g., sertraline, fluvoxamine, and paroxetine) help normalize serotonin activity, which may help bring cravings for cocaine, nicotine, or other drugs under control (Coleman & Gouaux, 2018; Rigotti et al., 2022). Deficiencies of the neurotransmitter serotonin are not only connected with psychological problems such as depression; they also may contribute to cravings for drugs. However, use of therapeutic drugs should be combined with behavioral counseling to help people developing coping skills and change problem behaviors that lead to drug use and abuse.

Relapse Prevention

In medicine, the term "relapse" means deterioration in one's health after a period of improvement. More broadly, relapse means falling back into a previous state, as in returning to harmful behavior, such as smoking, drinking, or using another substance, after a period of abstinence.

According to G. Alan Marlatt's cognitive behavioral model of relapse prevention, one of the keys to relapse prevention is learning how to avoid and manage the various triggers of relapse (Hendershot et al., 2011; Larimer & Marlatt, 2004). The ability to regulate one's emotions is connected with the ability to prevent relapse (Clarke et al., 2020). As we saw in **Table 9.2**, the triggers of relapse include socializing with people who engage in substance abuse and managing internal triggers to relapse, such as cravings, by using self-relaxation or mediation. Responses to being offered a drink, or a cigarette, or a hit of marijuana require some social skills training, as in assertiveness training, which can be used in a group setting, and rehearsing polite ways of saying "Thanks, but I'd rather not." According to the cognitive behavioral model, **self-efficacy**, or the belief that one is in charge of one's behavior and can achieve one's goals, is also connected with the ability to prevent relapses (Bandura, 2010; Larimer & Marlatt, 2004).

self-efficacy According to Albert Bandura, one's belief in one's ability to achieve success in specific situations or to accomplish a task.

A goal of relapse prevention training is to prevent a lapse from becoming a full-blown relapse. One of the problems with preventing relapse in the case of AUD is the widespread belief that just one drink is destined to trigger a full-blown relapse. However, cognitive behavioral therapists such as Marlatt argue that one drink does not necessarily mean that one has "fallen off the wagon" and cannot just climb back on. A momentary lapse need not spell complete failure or disaster.

The belief that a single slipup is a catastrophe is an example of a cognitive distortion that cognitive therapist Aaron Beck referred to as "all-or-nothing thinking" (Beck et al., 1993; Dobson et al., 2018). The question is what people attempting to abstain from alcohol or nicotine or another substance tell themselves when they have a drink or take a puff. Do they tell themselves that they are "doomed" or "fated" to experience a total relapse, or do they say to themselves, "OK, I messed up this time, but it doesn't mean that all my efforts are down the drain. I go on from here"? Therapists are also well advised to inform people with substance use disorders that slipping up and not experiencing cravings does not necessarily mean that one can safely have another drink or another cigarette.

Although peer-based programs like AA may not be well suited for everyone or succeed in every case, there is little doubt they can have positive effects for many people attempting to cope with substance use disorders (Ashford et al., 2020). Sober Grid, a recovery social network site that has many of the features of Facebook, is an example of a smartphone app that has replaced face-to-face therapy and live social groups with digitized supporters. A study of the utility of Sober Grid found that 3 of 5 users were male, with a mean age of 39 (Ashford et al., 2020). The men using the app had a mean sobriety length of 196 days and experienced 4.5 relapses since signing on, but they continued to use the app. Statistical analysis showed that the numbers of connections and numbers of check-ins were positively related to the length of sobriety.

It is perhaps easy to recognize that strategies for relapse prevention also apply to weight management. In Chapter 7 we noted that dieters fare better when they avoid the triggers of

Applying Health Psychology

Applications of Operant Conditioning to Substance Abuse

Most people use psychoactive drugs in one way or another. They may start their day with a cup of coffee or tea (which contains the mild stimulant caffeine) and end it with a nightcap (which contains alcohol). Or they may use cigarettes or vaping products, or illicit drugs. Helping professionals, including health psychologists, develop behavior change strategies to help people to control (or to avoid) the use of harmful substances, including tobacco, illicit drugs, and excessive or inappropriate use of alcohol.

Cognitive behavioral psychologists note that an important step in changing patterns of substance abuse lies in raising our awareness of what we tell ourselves and other people about our behavior. For example, if you're going to quit smoking, why not tell your family and friends that you're quitting? Making a public commitment shores up your resolve. Also plan a target date for quitting, perhaps a date when you will be on vacation or away from the usual settings in which you smoke. You can use a nicotine substitute like a skin patch to help cut down before the target date and to prove to yourself that you can survive on fewer (and, ultimately, on no) cigarettes. You can plan specific things to tell yourself when you feel the urge to smoke: how you'll be stronger, free of fear of cancer, ready for the marathon, and so on. Once you have stopped, you can remind yourself repeatedly that the first few days are the hardest. After that, withdrawal symptoms weaken dramatically. And don't be afraid to pat yourself on the back by reminding yourself that you are accomplishing something that may literally be a lifesaver.

Principles of operant conditioning are applied in the development of behavioral techniques outlined in **Table 9.2**, which modify the ABCs of substance abuse—the A's, or antecedent cues, that trigger drug use behavior; the B's, or drug use behaviors themselves; and the C's, or reinforcers or consequences of drug use behavior.

TABLE 9.2 Strategies for Modifying the ABCs of Substance Abuse

Control the A's (Antecedent Cues) That Trigger Cravings by

- Removing drinking and smoking paraphernalia from the home, including alcoholic beverages, beer mugs, ashtrays, lighters, and so on.
- Dealing with triggers for using the substance: for example, if you smoke with your morning coffee or tea, have your first coffee at work where smoking is probably not permitted. If you smoke after meals, plan to get up and out after meals, perhaps for a brisk walk.
- Restricting the environment in which drinking or smoking is permitted. Limit use of the substance to a stimulus-deprived area of the home, such as the garage, bathroom, or basement.
- Avoiding socializing with people who have substance abuse problems and avoiding situations linked to use of the substance, such as bars or certain kinds of parties.
- Socializing more with people who abstain from the substances. (One man who had had AUD switched jobs because his co-workers at the first job had drinks at lunch and after work.)
- Frequenting substance-free environments, such as lectures or concerts, a gym, or museums.
- Managing internal triggers for abuse, as by practicing self-relaxation or meditation to ease stress or states of tension.

Prevent or Interrupt the B's (Behaviors) of Substance Abuse by

- Physically preventing the undesired behavior from occurring or making them more difficult, such as by not having the harmful substances in your home or at work.
- Using competing responses when tempted, such as chewing mints or sugar-free gum. Putting other (healthful) things in your mouth when oral cravings strike, such as raw vegetables (e.g., carrot sticks). Other competing responses include brushing your teeth, taking a bath or shower, walking the dog, walking around the block, taking a drive, practicing meditation, or exercising.
- Making abuse labor-intensive, such as buying one can of beer at a time; storing matches, ashtrays, and cigarettes far apart. Keep only the smallest amounts of marijuana at home.
- Pausing for 10 minutes when struck by the urge to drink, smoke, or use another substance and asking oneself, "Do I really need this one?"

Control the C's (Consequences) of Substance Abuse by

- Switching to brands of beer or cigarettes you don't like.
- Setting gradual substance-reduction schedules and rewarding yourself for sticking to them.
- Punishing yourself for failing to meet substance-reduction goals, as in assessing yourself a monetary penalty for each slip and donating the cash to an unpalatable cause, such as an in-law's birthday present—assuming that you're not crazy about your in-law.
- Rehearsing motivating thoughts or statements you can write down or key in and have available when temptations arise. For example: "Each day I don't smoke adds another day to my life." People who smoke can carry 20–25 such statements and read several at various times throughout the day. They can become parts of one's daily routine, a constant reminder of one's goals.

overeating or of eating unwanted foods and when they regulate their emotions so that they can cope with their cravings. And with weight management, too, a single slip-up, such as eating a piece of cake at a family gathering or celebration, need not mean that one is forever doomed to fail. The next day is, well, the next day.

Review 9.5

INTERACTIVE SELF-SCORING QUIZZES

Sentence Completion

1. The most widely used group for treating alcohol dependence is Alcoholics __________.

2. For those who are physiologically dependent on a drug, a method of withdrawing them in a hospital setting is called __________.

3. About __________ in 4 heroin addicts who became dependent in their teens or 20s quit by the time they reach their 30s.

4. In a study of Vietnam veterans returning home, it was found that about 20% tested positive for opioids. A year later the figure was ______%.

5. Nearly __________ in 5 people who smoke believe that they can quit on their own and do not seek professional assistance.

6. __________ provides a sense of overconfidence that can lead to risky behavior.

7. People with alcohol use disorder who use the drug __________ cannot drink without feeling ill.

8. The drug __________ is used in overdose rescue kits to block the effects of opioids.

9. __________ is used widely in treating heroin addiction because it prevents the withdrawal symptoms and does not produce the euphoric rush associated with heroin.

10. According to __________'s cognitive behavioral model of relapse prevention, one of the keys is learning how to avoid and manage the various triggers of relapse.

11. The belief that a single slipup in the effort to avoid use of a drug is a catastrophe is an example of a cognitive distortion that cognitive therapist __________ refers to as "all-or-nothing thinking."

Think About It

Mark Twain said it was easy to quit smoking; he'd done it thousands of times. Why is relapse so common when it comes to quitting substance abuse? Why is viewing a single slipup as a catastrophe make relapse more likely? What strategies are available to help prevent relapse? Why do you think that the great majority of Vietnam veterans who tested positive for opioids on return from the war showed abstinence a year later?

Recite: An Active Summary

INTERACTIVE SELF-SCORING QUIZZES

Chapter 9 Practice Quiz

1. Define "substance abuse" and "substance dependence," and explain how you can know whether you are dependent on a substance.

Substance abuse is the continued use of a substance despite the fact that usage is causing personal, social, and financial problems. Substance dependence is recognized by tolerance and the presence of a withdrawal syndrome.

2. Discuss psychological and biological factors in substance use and dependence. Both positive and negative reinforcement are involved in drug use and abuse.

Cognitive factors such as positive expectances about drug use, also figure prominently. Observational learning plays a role in that people learn about the effects of substances from other people. The cognitive-dysfunction view of dependence is that with repeated usage of a substance, the executive center of the brain declines in its ability to govern behavior. People differ in their genetic vulnerabilities to various substances, as in one's level of the enzyme aldehyde dehydrogenase, which metabolizes alcohol. Substances may also lead to spikes in dopamine, which in turn can lead to long-term cravings.

3. Discuss depressants, focusing on alcohol and opioids.

Depressants slow the activity of the CNS although alcohol initially provides stimulating effects by dilating blood vessels. Alcohol is the most widely used depressant and is associated with a liberated social role and risky behavior. Millions of people have alcohol use disorder, and millions—men more so than women—engage in binge drinking, which can be lethal. Alcohol is associated with many thousands of automobile accidents. Opioids are highly addictive and are often prescribed for pain, although high doses can create euphoria. Repeated use of opioids can change brain circuitry so the people experience powerful cravings.

4. Discuss stimulants, focusing on nicotine, amphetamines, cocaine, and caffeine.

Nicotine is the highly addictive stimulant in cigarettes and other tobacco products. It is also available through electronic cigarettes and nicotine replacement therapies, such as skin patches. Nicotine itself is dangerous to the cardiovascular system, but the hydrocarbons (tars) in tobacco smoke cause cancer of the lungs and elsewhere. Many students use amphetamines to help with studying and test taking, but amphetamines may also cause insomnia, agitation, and irritability. Methamphetamine is associated with brain damage. Other stimulants, such as Ritalin, are often prescribed for children with ADHD to enable the executive centers of their brains to gain control over more primitive centers of the brain. Cocaine is highly addictive; it can produce feelings of euphoria and self-confidence, but it can also cause spikes in blood pressure and constriction of coronary arteries, sometimes leading to cardiovascular collapse and death. Many people become physiologically dependent on the mild stimulant caffeine, found, for example, in coffee, tea, and chocolate.

5. Discuss hallucinogens, focusing on marijuana and LSD.

Marijuana can produce feelings of pleasure and mild hallucinations, as of time passing more slowly than it is. Medical marijuana is an effective pain reliever that also helps people with cancer who are undergoing chemotherapy. Marijuana, like alcohol, impairs driving ability and other tasks that require motor coordination. Users can become psychologically dependent on marijuana, but it is unclear whether they become physiologically dependent. LSD produces more intense hallucinations and is not known to be addictive.

6. Discuss self-guided strategies for cutting down and quitting substance abuse.

Most people cut down on and quit harmful substances on their own. They report thinking about health, social, and financial problems connected with substance abuse. Some switch to vaping or nicotine replacement therapies. Some people use self-help groups, such as Alcoholics Anonymous.

7. Discuss the role of medication in the treatment of substance abuse.

Detoxification from opioids and alcohol is often conducted under medical supervision. People with alcohol use disorder may use disulfiram, which prevents them from drinking without becoming ill. Users of heroin may be switched to methadone, an addictive opioid that does not provide the rush of heroin but quells withdrawal symptoms, enabling people to function in the workplace and in society. Overdose rescue kits for opioid overdose use the drug naloxone, which blocks the effects of the other drugs.

8. Discuss ways in which psychologists help people with substance abuse problems.

Psychologists are involved in helping people with substance abuse problems adhere to disulfiram or methadone treatment and conduct research on the use of telephone reminders, texts, and apps. Psychologists also apply behavioral principles to help people who abuse substances modify the ABCs of their problematic behavior—the antecedents (stimuli that trigger problem behavior), the behavior itself, and the consequences (reinforcers) for wanted and unwanted behavior. Psychotherapy also helps people who abuse substances understand their behavior, regulate their emotions, and interact more productively with other people.

9. Discuss strategies for relapse prevention.

According to Marlatt, a key to relapse prevention is learning to avoid situations in which one has used the substance. Another is regulating one's emotions to deal with cravings. According to Beck, people are advised to avoid all-or-nothing thinking, which may catastrophize a lapse as a relapse.

Answers to Review Sections

9.1

1. Alcohol

2. abuse

3. dependence

4. Biological, or physiological

5. withdrawal

6. negatively

7. cognitive-dysfunction

8. dopamine

9.2

1. central

2. liberated

3. half

4. 100,000

5. Cirrhosis

6. Men

7. high

8. morphine

9. endorphins

10. reward

11. barbiturates

9.3

1. Caffeine

2. attention-deficit/hyperactivity disorder, ADHD, hyperactivity

3. 65 and above

4. hydrocarbons, "tars"

5. cocaine

6. bone density

7. caffeine

8. cocaine

9. Adderall (or caffeine)

9.4

1. delta-9-tetrahydrocannabinol, THC

2. lysergic acid, LSD

3. hallucinations

4. brain

5. psychologically

6. motor, or visual-motor

9.5

1. Anonymous

2. detoxification (or detox)

3. 3

4. 1

5. 4

6. Cocaine

7. disulfiram (Antabuse)

8. naloxone

9. Methadone

10. G. Alan Marlatt

11. Aaron Beck

CHAPTER 10

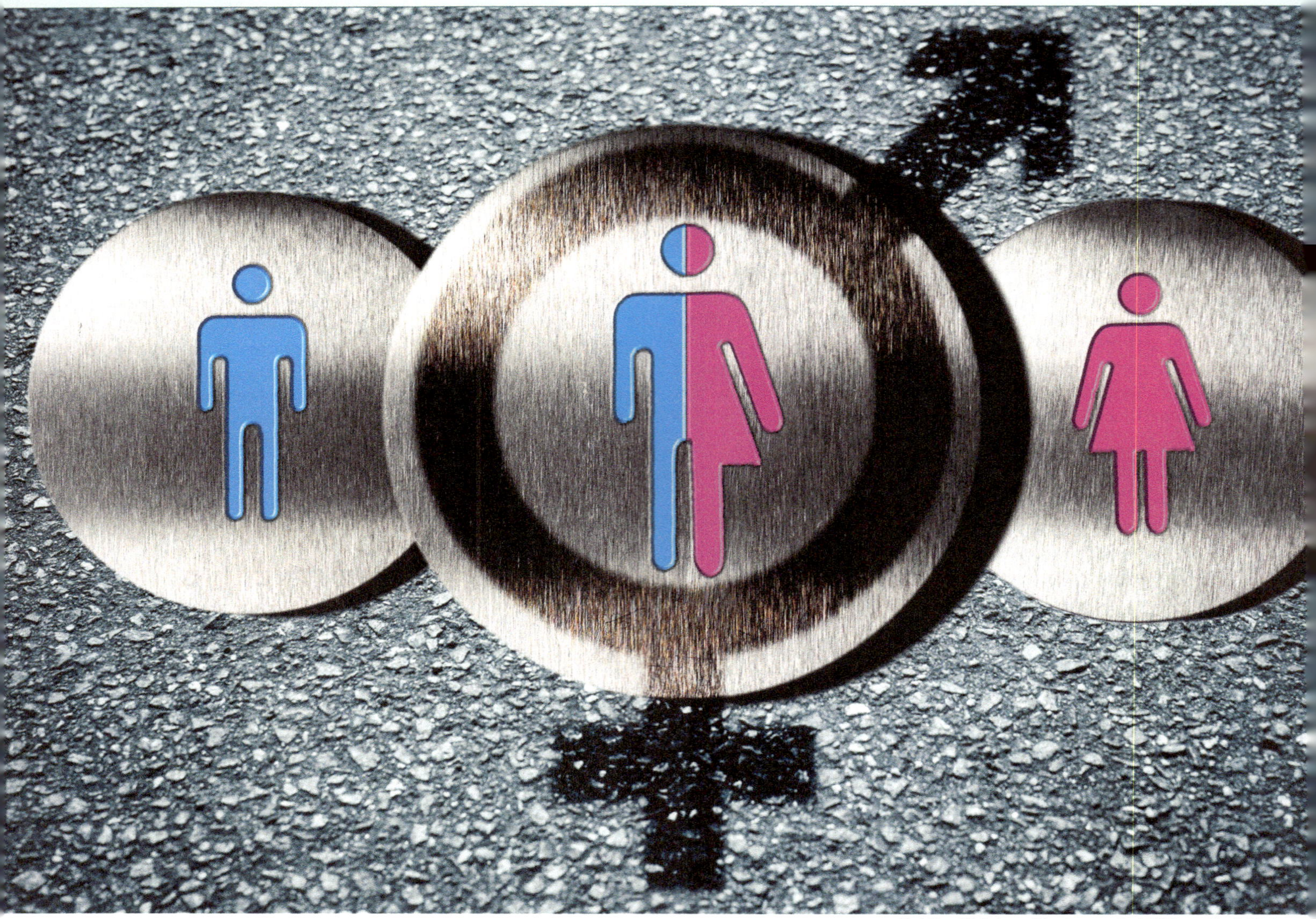

Christian Ohde/mauritius images GmbH/Alamy Stock Photo

Reproductive and Sexual Health

LEARNING OBJECTIVES

After studying this chapter, you will be able to ...

1. **Identify** and **describe** the parts of the female and male reproductive systems.
2. **Discuss** ways in which health psychologists help women with menstrual problems, postpartum depression, and menopause.
3. **Explain** how theories of health behavior can help people make reproductive choices.
4. **Identify** and **discuss** sexually transmitted infections, focusing on HIV/AIDS, and how the Health Belief Model applies to people's decisions as to whether or not to use PrEP.
5. **Identify** and **discuss** the origins of sexual dysfunctions and **explain** how psychologists help people overcome sexual dysfunctions.
6. **Define** sexual orientation and gender identity and **discuss** the health challenges of LGBTQ individuals.

Did You Know That ...

- The majority of women experience premenstrual discomfort?
- It is normal for women feel let down and irritable following childbirth?
- People can have gratifying sex lives after menopause?
- You can carry the genes for an illness yet not become ill yourself?
- Most people who are infected with HIV remain symptom-free and seem to be healthy for years?
- Although PrEP can prevent users from being infected with HIV, many people at risk for being infected do not use it because they do not perceive themselves to be at risk?
- The same medicines that help older people control high blood pressure and high levels of cholesterol can make it extremely difficult to become sexually aroused?
- Around 8% of Millennials identify as being lesbian, gay, bisexual, or transgender?

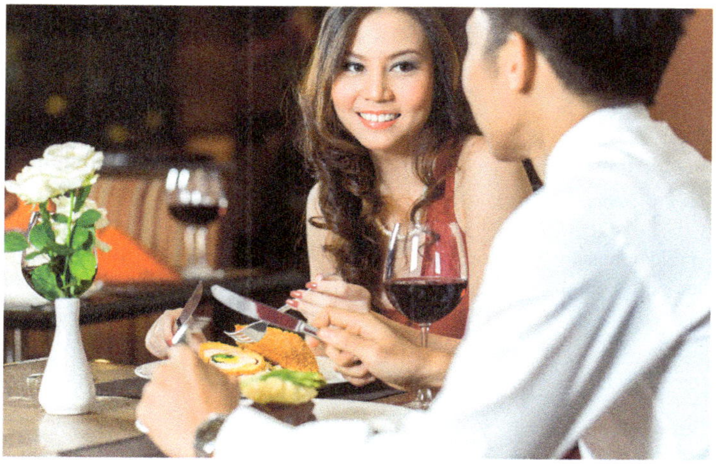

Kzenon/Shutterstock.com

They are enjoying a romantic dinner, having dated for a few weeks. Although nothing explicit is said at the dining table, they are both thinking about taking the relationship "to the next level." What considerations are they taking into account?

Consider the question from the point of view of the Health Belief Model (HBM). How are they weighing the potential benefits and barriers to having sexual relations? For her, the potential benefits include sexual pleasure and the possible deepening of the relationship. Barriers might include concerns about whether she and her partner will enjoy sexual relations and whether she can trust that he is free of sexually transmittable infections. He, like his date, is also looking forward to pleasure, but a barrier looms—Will he be able to perform, or will he feel humiliated as he did some months ago with another woman he was dating? As another barrier, he is also afraid that she might be more experienced than he is.

Health psychologists recognize that decisions we make about our sexual behavior, including whether to engage in sexual activity or to use condoms if we do, involves a cognitive process of weighing perceived health threats and perceived benefits and costs of practicing protective behaviors. Health psychologists find that people who perceive greater health threats from unprotected sex are more likely to form intentions to use condoms (Rodrigues et al., 2018). But whether they carry through with these intentions may depend on factors that affect their judgment, such as their use of alcohol and their level of emotional or sexual arousal.

VIDEO CONTENT

Sexuality and Sexual Motivation

How does our sexual behavior impact our health? Why do people engage in some sexual behaviors, such as **unprotected sex**, even though they know it is risky? The Theory of Reasoned Action (TRA, discussed in Chapter 2) suggests that the best predictor of sexual behavior is our intentions, which are determined by factors such as our own attitudes toward the behavior and social norms (Montano & Kasprzyk, 2015). The Theory of Planned Behavior (TPB) (also discussed in Chapter 2) adds the factor of whether we perceive ourselves to have control over the behavior. Despite the "best of intentions," the sex drive is so powerful in adolescence and early adulthood that our intentions might, as the saying goes, fly out the window. Other factors affect the likelihood of engaging in risky sexual behaviors, such as having unprotected sex. Health psychologists find that lack of sleep may increase sexual risk-taking in adolescents, perhaps because it impairs judgment and the ability to weigh the consequences of behavior (Troxel et al., 2019).

unprotected sex Sexual activity that poses increased risks of sexually transmitted infections or unwanted pregnancies, such as not using a condom.

In this chapter we discuss theories of behavior change to help us better predict and explain health behaviors involved in our sexual experiences. We touch upon the contraceptive choices we make, whether to use a condom during sexual relations, and the steps we are taking or should be taking to protect ourselves from HIV/AIDS and other sexually transmitted infections. We will also consider a range of sexual problems many people experience involving difficulties with sexual arousal and response—patterns of behavior classified within a category of psychological disorders called *sexual dysfunctions*. We will see that these problems, like some many other health issues we find in the pages of this text, are best understood from the broad conceptual framework we have discussed earlier, the biopsychosocial model.

Before we begin our exploration of reproductive and sexual health, let us first review our reproductive anatomy, the bodily structures that make it possible for humans to reproduce. As we do so, consider the question of how well you know your own body.

The Reproductive System

Although we may consider ourselves knowledgeable about sex, based on what we may have learned in sex education classes, from the internet, from friends and family members, or from personal experience, how much do we really know about the internal workings of our bodies and, in particular, our reproductive systems?

vulva The female external reproductive organs.

pudendum Another term for the vulva.

urethral opening The tube that conducts urine from the body and, in males, the ejaculate.

mons veneris The mound of fatty tissue that covers the joint of the pubic bones and cushions the female while having sex.

The Female Reproductive System

The external female reproductive organs are called the **vulva** (Latin for "covering"). The vulva is also known as the **pudendum**, derived from roots "something to be ashamed of"—a clear reflection of sexism in ancient Western culture. The vulva has several parts (see Part A of **Figure 10.1**)—the *mons veneris*, the *clitoris*, and the *major and minor lips*, and the vaginal opening. Females urinate through the **urethral opening**. The **mons veneris** (Latin for "hill of love") is a fatty cushion that lies above the pubic bone and is covered with short pubic hair. The mons and pubic hair cushion the woman's pelvis during sexual intercourse.

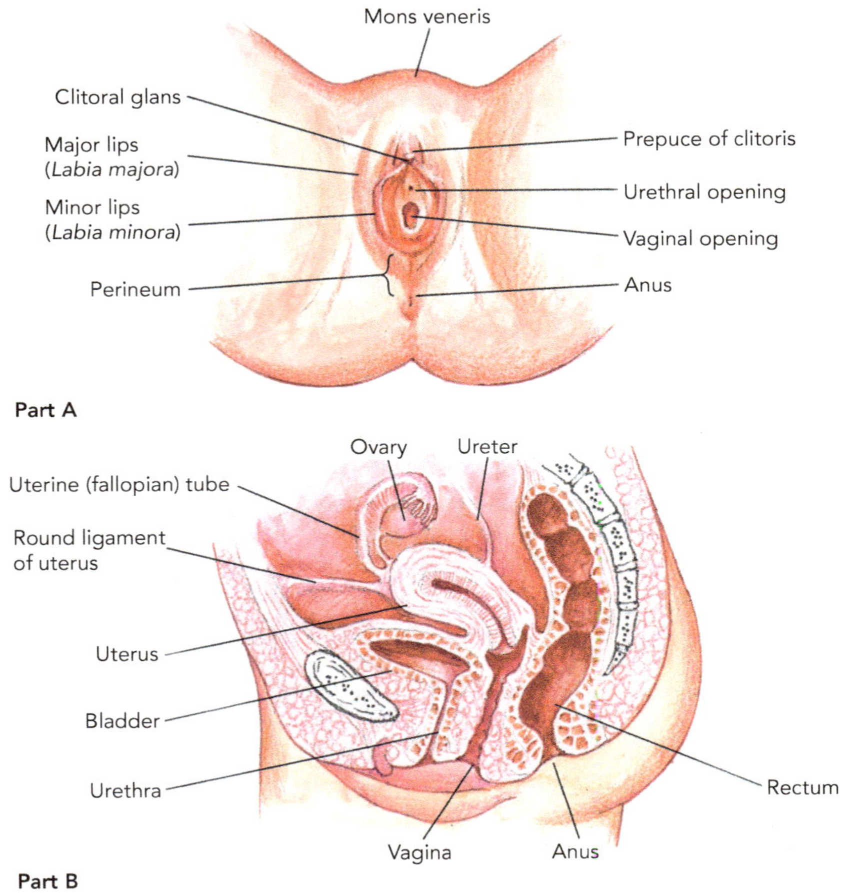

FIGURE 10.1 **Female Sexual Anatomy** Part A is an external view of the vulva. Part B is a cross section of the female internal reproductive organs.

The woman's sexual organ, the **clitoris**, lies below the mons and above the urethral opening. The clitoris is not a reproductive organ per se, but it plays an important motivational role in reproduction in that it is primarily responsible for the pleasurable sensory input that triggers orgasm in women (Herbenick et al., 2018). The clitoris consists of a shaft and a tip, or **glans**. The glans is the more sensitive of the two and may become irritated by too much direct sexual stimulation. Two layers of fatty tissue, the outer or **major lips** and the inner or **minor lips**, line the entrance to the vagina. The outer lips are covered with hair and are less sensitive to touch than the inner lips.

The woman's internal reproductive organs include the vagina, cervix, fallopian tubes, and ovaries (see Part B of **Figure 10.1**). The **vagina** houses the penis during intercourse. When a woman becomes sexually aroused, her vaginal walls produce moisture that serves as lubrication during sexual activity.

High in the vagina is a small opening called the **cervix** that connects the vagina to the **uterus**. Slender **fallopian tubes** lead from the uterus to the abdominal cavity. **Ovaries**, which produce ova and the sex hormones estrogen and progesterone, lie near the uterus and the fallopian tubes. When an egg cell, or **ovum**, is released from an ovary, it normally finds its way into the nearby fallopian tube and makes its way to the uterus. Conception usually takes place in the tube, but the embryo becomes implanted and develops in the uterus. During labor the cervix dilates, and the baby passes through the distended cervix and the vagina.

The ovaries produce the sex hormone **estrogen**, a term that actually refers to a number of sex hormones that foster the development of the female reproductive organs and female sex characteristics, such as accumulation of fatty tissue in the breasts and hips. The ovaries also produce the sex hormone **progesterone**, which fosters the development of the reproductive organs and helps maintain pregnancy. Levels of estrogen and progesterone vary throughout the menstrual cycle and regulate the cycle. Following menstruation—the monthly sloughing off of the inner lining of the uterus—estrogen levels increase, leading to the ripening of an ovum and the growth of the **endometrium**. Sharp abdominal pain during this time of the month may be a symptom of *endometriosis*—inflammation of the endometrium. Endometriosis has become a more common cause of infertility as women are delaying childbearing to further their educations and to establish careers. What happens is this—each month, tissue develops to line the uterus in case the woman conceives. This tissue, called the endometrium, is normally sloughed off during **menstruation**. However, some of it may back up into the abdomen through the same fallopian tubes that provide a duct for an ovum. Endometrial tissue then collects in the abdomen, where it can cause pain and reduce the chances of conception. Physicians may treat endometriosis with hormones that temporarily prevent menstruation or through surgery.

Ovulation—the release of an ovum by an ovary—occurs halfway through the menstrual cycle, when estrogen blood levels reach their peak. Then, in response to secretion of progesterone, the inner lining of the uterus thickens so that it can support an embryo if fertilization occurs. If the ovum is not fertilized, estrogen and progesterone levels drop suddenly, triggering menstruation once again.

Menstruation

Menstruation is the cyclical bleeding that stems from the shedding of the uterine lining (endometrium). Menstruation takes place when a reproductive cycle has not led to the fertilization of an ovum. The word "menstruation" derives from the Latin *mensis,* meaning "month." The menstrual cycle averages 28 days, but variations among women, and in the same woman from month to month, are common.

Ovulation may not occur in every menstrual cycle. *Anovulatory* (without ovulation) cycles are most common in the years just after **menarche** (the first menstrual period). They may become frequent again in the years prior to menopause, but they may also occur irregularly at any age.

Although menarche is a biological event, in many cultures it is also a rite of passage imbued with cultural traditions passed from mothers to daughters across the generations. Therefore, menarche is also suffused with psychological meanings. One study interviewed three generations of women about their experience with menarche—grandmothers, mothers, and daughters (Field-Springer et al., 2018). Virtually all of the grandmothers reported that there had been a lack of communication between themselves and their mothers about

clitoris The female erogenous organ whose only known function is the reception and transmission of sensations of sexual pleasure.

glans Tip or head.

major lips The large folds of skin that run along the sides of the vulva (in Latin, *labia majora*).

minor lips The folds of skin that lie within the major lips and enclose the urethral and vaginal openings (in Latin, *labia minora*).

vagina The tubular female sexual organ that receives the penis during sexual intercourse and through which the baby passes during childbirth.

cervix The lower part of the uterus that opens into the vagina.

uterus The pear-shaped female reproductive organ in which the fertilized ovum implants and develops until childbirth.

fallopian tubes The straw-like tubes through which the ovum passes between the ovaries and the uterus.

ovaries Female reproductive organs that produce ova and the female sex hormones—estrogen and progesterone.

ovum An egg cell (plural: ova).

estrogen A generic term for several female sex hormones that foster growth of female sex characteristics and regulate the menstrual cycle.

progesterone A female sex hormone that promotes growth of the reproductive organs, helps maintain pregnancy, and is also involved in regulation of the menstrual cycle.

endometrium The tissue forming the inner lining of the uterus.

menstruation The monthly shedding of the inner lining of the uterus by women who are not pregnant.

ovulation The release of an ovum from an ovary.

menarche The first occurrence of menstruation.

menarche. The grandmothers also mentioned that there were many myths about menstruation in their day, as expressed here by one of the participants: "Like when you started your period, you couldn't get in water, you weren't supposed to take a bath in the bathtub, you couldn't go swimming and all this stuff that you find out later that, yes, you can do that" (Field-Springer et al., 2018). The grandmothers as well as the mothers shared that being reared in a culture of silence influenced them to be more open in discussing menarche with their own daughters.

Menstrual Problems Although menstruation is a natural biological process, the majority of women experience some discomfort prior to or during menstruation. Pain or discomfort during menstruation—called **dysmenorrhea**—is the most common menstrual problem. Most women have at least mild menstrual pain or discomfort, so it is perfectly normal, even if annoying. Pelvic cramps are the most common manifestation of dysmenorrhea. They may be accompanied by headache, backache, nausea, or bloating. Women who develop severe cases of dysmenorrhea usually do so within a few years of menarche. Endometriosis, pelvic inflammatory disease, and ovarian cysts are some of the organic disorders that can give rise to dysmenorrhea.

dysmenorrhea Painful menstruation, usually involving abdominal cramps.

Dysmenorrhea appears to be related to hormonal changes that regulate the menstrual cycle. For example, menstrual cramps sometimes decrease dramatically after childbirth, as a result of the massive hormonal changes that occur with pregnancy. Women who have been pregnant report a lower incidence of menstrual pain but a higher incidence of premenstrual symptoms and menstrual discomfort.

Headaches frequently accompany menstrual discomfort. Most headaches (in both females and males) stem from simple muscle tension, notably in the shoulders, the back of the neck, and the scalp. Pelvic discomfort may cause muscle contractions, contributing to the tension that produces headaches. Women who are tense about their menstrual flow are candidates for muscle tension headaches. Migraine headaches may also arise from changes in the blood flow in the brain, however. Migraines are typically limited to one side of the head and are often accompanied by visual difficulties.

Amenorrhea is the absence of menstruation and is a primary sign of infertility. Amenorrhea has various causes, including abnormalities in the structures of the reproductive system, hormonal abnormalities, growths such as cysts and tumors, and psychological issues, such as stress. Amenorrhea is normal during pregnancy and following menopause. Hormonal changes that accompany emaciation, which may occur in women with anorexia nervosa, are believed to be responsible for the cessation of menstruation.

amenorrhea The absence of menstruation.

Behavioral Factors in Menstrual Problems Menstrual discomfort is of interest to health psychologists for several reasons. One is that behavioral factors may contribute to menstrual problems. For example, amenorrhea may be a symptom of anorexia nervosa, the eating disorder discussed in Chapter 7. Amenorrhea may also occur in women who exercise strenuously, such as competitive long-distance runners (Kerns et al., 2022; Maya & Misra, 2022). It is unclear whether the cessation of menstruation in female athletes is due to the effects of strenuous exercise itself, to related physical factors such as low body fat, to the stress of intensive training, or to a combination of factors

Although hormones regulate the menstrual cycle, psychological factors can affect the secretion of hormones, as in amenorrhea, and lead to menstrual irregularities. Stress can also delay or halt menstruation. The term **premenstrual syndrome (PMS)** describes the combination of biological and psychological symptoms that may affect women during the 4–6-day interval that precedes their periods each month. It is characterized by physical symptoms, such as cramps and bloating, but also by psychological symptoms, such as depressed mood and irritability. For many women, premenstrual symptoms persist during menstruation.

premenstrual syndrome (PMS) A cluster of mood-related and physical symptoms, such as cramps, bloating, depression, and irritability, that may affect women for the 4–6-day interval that precedes menstruation.

Premenstrual dysphoric disorder (PMDD) is a more severe disorder which is characterized by the following (American Psychiatric Association, 2022):

premenstrual dysphoric disorder (PMDD) A more severe form of PMS, characterized by a range of symptoms such as mood swings or depressed mood, irritability, anxiety, and anger.

- Depressed mood, as evidenced by crying and feelings of sadness, hopelessness, or worthlessness
- Withdrawal from activities that are usually sought out and enjoyed
- Difficulty concentrating and paying sustained attention to tasks
- Fatigue, lack of energy

- Feelings of tension and anxiety, being on edge
- Feelings of irritability or anger, possibly causing conflict with family members and others
- Feeling overwhelmed, that life is out of control
- Significant changes in appetite that can lead to binge eating or the craving of particular foods and often result in weight gain
- Problems in sleeping—sleeping too much (hypersomnia) or too little (insomnia)
- A variety of other physical problems, such as swelling or tenderness of the breasts, pain in muscles, pain in joints, migraine headaches, and feeling bloated

Unlike PMS, PMDD is a persistent problem. The diagnosis does not apply unless the woman has experienced the problem during most menstrual cycles over a period of a year. The diagnosis also requires that the symptoms impair the woman's life experiences, perhaps her functioning at work or in academic pursuits, perhaps in her social or family relationships.

The causes of PMS and PMDD are unclear, but researchers are looking to possible relationships between menstrual problems, including PMS and PMDD, and chemical imbalances in the body. PMS and PMDD appear to be linked with imbalances in neurotransmitters such as serotonin (Studd & Nappi, 2012). Serotonin imbalances are also linked to fluctuations in appetite, usually increases in appetite. Another neurotransmitter, gamma-aminobutyric acid (GABA), also appears to be involved in premenstrual problems; medicines that affect the levels of GABA help many women with these problems (Bäckström et al., 2003). PMS and PMDD may well be caused by a complex interaction between ovarian hormones and neurotransmitters (Itriyeva, 2022; Nappi et al., 2022).

A couple of generations ago, premenstrual disorders were seen as "a woman's lot"—something women must put up with. No longer. Today there are many treatment options, as we see in the next Applying Health Psychology feature. Though there is much we can do on our own to safeguard our health, informed health consumers recognize the need to bring troubling, persistent, or severe symptoms to the attention of their healthcare provider.

Postpartum Psychological Adjustment

The term "postpartum" derives from Latin roots meaning "after" and "birth." The postpartum period consists of the weeks following delivery, but there is no specific time limit. The immediate postpartum period can be a joyous time for the new mother. The long wait is over, concerns about pregnancy and labor are history, and, despite some local discomfort, the mother's "load" has been lightened—literally.

Yet many mothers are beset by postpartum depression (PPD). Although PPD is used as a catch-all phrase, it is recognized as a subtype of clinical depression by the American Psychiatric Association (2022). It is one of several significant psychological health problems that new mothers may experience.

About half of new mothers have periods of tearfulness, sadness, and irritability that are often referred to as the "baby blues" (Rezaie-Keikhaie et al., 2020). The baby blues are characterized by feelings of sadness, crying for no apparent reason, irritability, restlessness, anxiety, and impatience. They are common in the first weeks after delivery but tend to disappear on their own. The baby blues are reported around the world, in places as far flung as China, Turkey, Guyana, Australia, and South Africa, and in similar frequencies as in the United States (American Psychiatric Association, 2022).

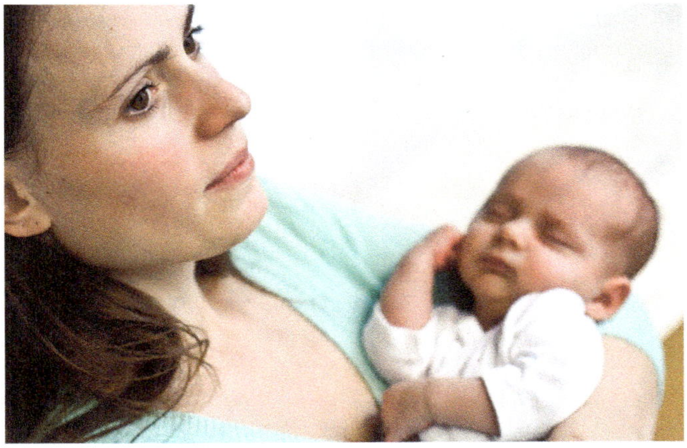

Phanie/Alamy Stock Photo

Baby Blues About half of new mothers experience the baby blues—feelings of being let down, irritability, anxiety, and restlessness, apparently due to the plummeting of steroids and sex hormones following delivery. The baby blues tend to pass for most new mothers in a few days or weeks, but some women develop a postpartum mood disorder, such as postpartum depression (PPD), which is a subtype of major depression.

Researchers believe that the baby blues are so common because of hormonal changes that follow delivery. Levels of steroids peak during labor and then drop off within a few hours, creating a period of emotional vulnerability (Rasmussen et al., 2023). Moreover, estrogen and progesterone levels plummet, further contributing to emotional disturbances.

Applying Health Psychology

Managing Menstrual Discomfort

Nearly 3 women in 4 experience some premenstrual symptoms (Studd & Nappi, 2012). Women with persistent menstrual distress may profit from the suggestions listed here. Researchers are exploring the effectiveness of these techniques in controlled studies. You might consider trying the suggestions that sound right for you. Try them for a few months to see if you reap any benefits, but as always, persistent or troubling health concerns should be brought to the attention of a healthcare provider.

- Don't blame yourself! Menstrual problems were once erroneously attributed to women's "hysterical" nature. This is nonsense. Menstrual problems appear to mainly reflect hormonal variations or chemical fluctuations in the brain during the menstrual cycle.
- Keep a menstrual calendar so that you can track your symptoms systematically and identify patterns.
- Develop strategies for dealing with the days on which you experience the greatest distress—strategies that will help enhance your pleasure and minimize stress. Go to a movie or get into that novel you've been meaning to read.
- Consider whether you harbor self-defeating attitudes toward menstruation that might compound distress. Do close relatives or friends see menstruation as an illness, a time of "pollution," a "dirty thing"? Have you adopted any of these attitudes—if not fully consciously, then in behavior, as in restricting your social activities during your period?
- See a gynecologist about your concerns, especially if you have severe symptoms. Severe menstrual symptoms can be secondary to medical disorders such as endometriosis and pelvic inflammatory disease.
- Ask your gynecologist about oral contraceptives that reduce the number of menstrual periods per year. Still others shorten periods.
- Develop nutritious eating habits—and continue them throughout the entire cycle (that means always). Consider limiting intake of alcohol, caffeine, fats, salt, and sweets, especially during the days preceding menstruation. A low-fat, vegetarian diet may reduce the duration and intensity of premenstrual symptoms.
- Eat several smaller meals (or nutritious snacks) throughout the day rather than a few big meals.
- Some women find that vigorous exercise—jogging, swimming, bicycling, fast walking, dancing, skating, even jumping rope—helps relieve premenstrual and menstrual discomfort. Research evidence supports the benefits of exercise in reducing premenstrual symptoms in women with PMS (Saglam & Örsal, 2020).
- Check with your healthcare provider about vitamin and mineral supplements, such as calcium and magnesium.
- *Ibuprofen* (brand names Advil, Motrin, etc.) and other medicines available over the counter may help with cramping. Prescription drugs such as anti-anxiety medications (e.g., alprazolam) and antidepressant medications (selective serotonin reuptake inhibitors) may also be of help. Antidepressants affect levels of neurotransmitters in a way that can be helpful for women with PMS or PMDD. Ask your doctor for a recommendation.
- Remember that menstrual discomfort is time limited. Don't worry about getting through life or a career. Just get through the next couple of days.

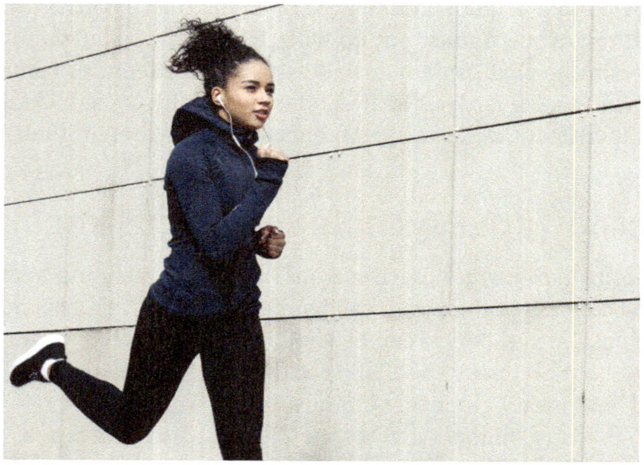

Artem Varnitsin/Shutterstock.com

Some women find that vigorous physical activity helps them on discomforting days of the menstrual cycle—and throughout the month as well!

The baby blues are not a psychiatric disorder and no treatment is usually necessary. New mothers may be reassured knowing that their feelings fall within the normal spectrum of responses following childbirth. As with other stressful situations, emotional and social support are of help in those first few weeks.

The baby blues typically last about 10 days and generally are not severe enough to impair the mother's functioning. That said, the emotions the new mother experiences should not be trivialized or brushed off or dismissed, as by saying "Oh, you're just experiencing what most women experience. It'll pass." Providing support and understanding can help her cope more effectively.

Some women develop a more severe and persistent form of depression following childbirth, which is classified as a form of major depression. According to the American Psychiatric Association (2022), this form of PPD is labeled *major depression with perinatal onset*. It affects

1 new mother in 9 or 10. The phrase "perinatal onset" refers to the period just before or after birth. The disorder most often begins about a month after delivery and may linger for weeks or months. PPD, like other forms of major depression (see Chapter 11), is characterized by sadness, crying, feelings of helplessness and inadequacy, irritability, frightening thoughts and panic, difficulty concentrating, and possible thoughts of suicide. Symptoms may also include fatigue, insomnia (or too much sleep), and lack of feeling for the baby or excessive concern about the baby. Concern or lack of concern about the baby may occasion feelings of guilt and shame.

Which new mothers are most likely to be affected by PPD? Several biomedical factors are associated with increased risk, such as gestational diabetes, a form of diabetes that can develop during pregnancy, and having a low birthweight baby. Here we see the interface between physical health and psychosocial factors, as the demands of coping with these types of stressors—diabetes and meeting the special needs of low birthweight babies—can add to the stress burden that new mothers carry. Behavioral researchers also identify various psychosocial factors associated with increased risk of PPD, including the following (Huang, Fan, & Hu, 2023; Payne, 2021; Zacher Kjeldsen et al., 2022):

- Financial problems or marital conflict
- Exposure to domestic violence
- First time motherhood and single motherhood
- Stressful life experiences
- Lack of social support from the partner or family members
- Coping with a sick or temperamental child or having an unwanted child
- Past history of an anxiety or mood disorder or family history of a psychiatric disorder

Major depression with perinatal onset is generally treatable by psychological interventions, especially cognitive behavioral therapy (CBT), or biomedical treatment, such as antidepressant drugs or the drug *brexanolone*, which is a steroid that mimics the effects of progesterone and seems to have a stabilizing effect on mood states after childbirth (Jarman et al., 2020; Reddy, 2021). In 2023, the drug, *zuranolone*, a steroidal drug that works on a different neurotransmitter than conventional antidepressants, became the first pill specifically approved for treating PPD (Marcus, 2023).

Why CBT? Because our thinking patterns underlying beliefs and thoughts affect our feeling states and can either help us cope with the stressful challenges we face or make matters worse for ourselves. Psychotherapy also has the advantage of not having physical side effects (Choudhary et al., 2020).

Much rarer still, affecting perhaps 1 woman in 1,000, is *postpartum psychosis*, which involves a psychotic episode or "break with reality" (American Psychiatric Association, 2022). Postpartum psychosis is considered an emergency because of high suicide and infanticide rates (about 4% each) (McEvoy, 2020). Women with postpartum psychosis may have delusional thoughts about their infant that may place the infant at risk with their infants that may place them at risk. Some women with postpartum psychosis experience delusions that the infant is possessed by the devil, and some experience "command hallucinations" in which a voice or voices inside their heads command them to kill their infants. Women with postpartum psychosis frequently have a history of serious psychological disorders or substance abuse and clearly are in need of immediate treatment (McEvoy, 2020).

Menopause

Menopause, or the "change of life," is the cessation of menstruation. The ovaries no longer ripen egg cells or produce the sex hormones estrogen and progesterone. Menopause most commonly occurs between the ages of 46 and 50 years and lasts for about 2 years. However, it may begin any time between the ages of 35 and 60 years.

Perimenopause refers to the beginning of menopause and is usually characterized by 3–11 months of amenorrhea (lack of menstruation) or irregular periods. Perimenopause ends with menopause. Menopause, in other words, is a specific event in a longer-term process

menopause The point in time when menstrual cycles come permanently to an end.

perimenopause The term means "around menopause" and refers to the time during which a woman's body makes the natural transition to menopause, marking the end of the reproductive years.

climacteric A period of decreased reproductive capacity culminating in menopause.

known as the **climacteric** (critical period). The term "climacteric" specifically refers to the gradual decline in the reproductive capacity of the ovaries. The climacteric generally lasts about 15 years, from about ages 45 to 60 years. After age 35 years or so, the menstrual cycles of many women shorten, from an average of 28 days to 25 days at age 40 years and to 23 days by the mid-40s. By the end of her 40s, a woman's cycle may become erratic, with some periods close together and others missed.

Estrogen deficiency may lead to a number of unpleasant symptoms, such as night sweats and hot flashes (suddenly feeling hot) and hot flushes (suddenly looking reddened). Hot flashes and flushes may alternate with cold sweats, in which a woman feels suddenly cold and clammy. Anyone who has experienced cold feet or hands from anxiety or fear will understand how dramatic the shifting patterns of blood flow can be. Hot flashes and flushes stem largely from waves of dilation of blood vessels across the face and upper body. All of these sensations reflect *vasomotor instability*. That is, there are disruptions in the body mechanisms that dilate or constrict the blood vessels to maintain an even body temperature. Additional signs of estrogen deficiency include dizziness, headaches, pains in the joints, sensations of tingling in the hands or feet, burning or itchy skin, and heart palpitations. The skin usually becomes drier. Women may also encounter sleep problems, such as awakening more frequently at night and having difficulty falling back to sleep. Many perimenopausal women also experience migraine headaches.

There is some loss of breast tissue, vulvovaginal atrophy (loss of tissue in the genital region), and decreased vaginal lubrication during sexual arousal (see **Figure 10.2**). In a survey conducted by the North American Menopause Society (2013), women reported that vaginal discomfort affected them as follows:

- 80% reported that it negatively affected them
- 25% said it reduced their quality of life
- 36% reported that it made them feel old
- 26% said it lowered their self-esteem
- 75% said that vaginal discomfort impaired their sex life
- 33% reported that it impacted their marriage or primary relationship
- 29% said that it disrupted their sleep patterns

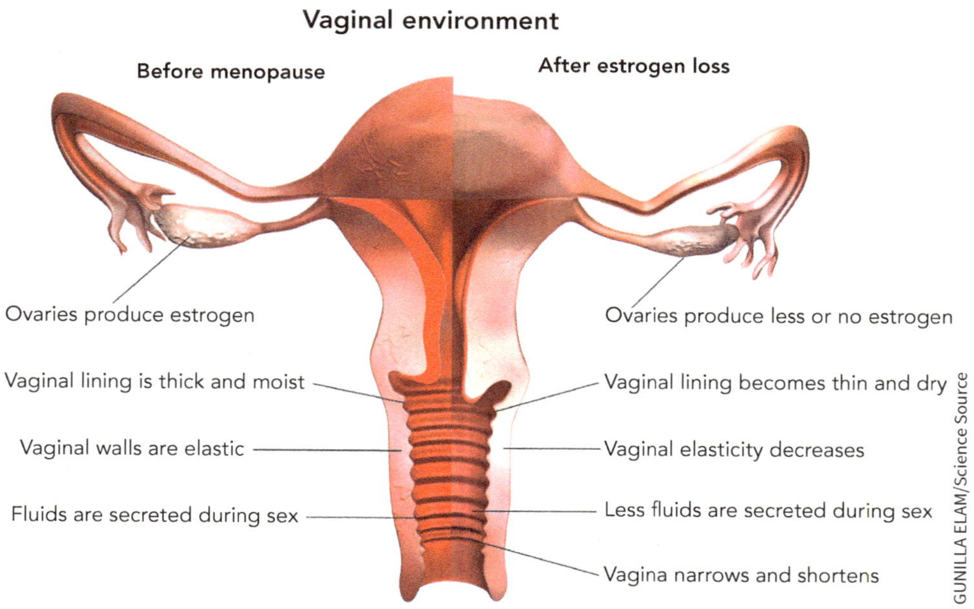

FIGURE 10.2 **Effects of Menopause on the Internal Female Reproductive System** The illustration shows the effects of a decrease in the production of the hormone estrogen by the ovaries, leading to cessation of menstrual periods. The lining of the vagina changes from thick and moist to thin and dry; the vaginal wall becomes less elastic; less lubrication is secreted during sexual activity; and the vagina narrows and shortens.

A more recent study found that many women experience such vaginal discomfort that they develop fear of visiting the gynecologist (Naumova & Castelo-Branco, 2018).

Behavioral Aspects of Menopause Menopause is a perfectly natural occurrence, not an illness or physical disorder. But as health psychologists recognize, the meaning the woman ascribes to the changes brought about by menopause contributes to or exacerbates the physical symptoms she is likely to encounter (Süss & Ehlert, 2020). The change of life can be especially troublesome for women whose identities were closely connected to childbearing. Some women may no longer see themselves as feminine or attractive. Moreover, menopause is an obvious marker of aging. The physical changes of menopause can also have psychological effects. For example, estrogen deficiency can impair cognitive functioning and feelings of psychological well-being. Psychological problems associated with menopause are quite common; evidence shows that about 20% of menopausal women experience symptoms of anxiety and depression (Süss & Ehlert, 2020).

For all these reasons, cognitive behavioral therapy can be used to help menopausal women adjust to the many changes they may face during menopause, such as vasomotor symptoms (hot flashes and flushes), depression, anxiety, sleep disturbances, and sexual concerns (Cho et al., 2023; Crandall et al., 2023). Cognitive behavioral therapy helps women evaluate their beliefs and attitudes about the change of life and encourages them to engage in activities they enjoy, including social activities.

Cognitive behavioral therapy also tackles myths about menopause, such as the idea that it means the end of a woman's sex life. For the few women who believe that sexual activity is acceptable only in the context of procreation, menopause may indeed be the end of their sex lives. However, women with such strong beliefs probably avoided sexual activity for many years before menopause as well. Sexual activity can be pleasurable at any age as long as individuals and their partners shape their expectations to fit the realities of their changing bodies.

The Male Reproductive System

The major male reproductive organs consist of the **penis**, the **testes** (or testicles), the **scrotum**, and the series of ducts, canals, and glands that store and transport **sperm** and produce **semen**.

penis The male organ that serves as a conduit for sperm during ejaculation and for urine during urination.

testes Male reproductive organs that produce sperm cells and male sex hormones. Also called *testicles*.

scrotum A pouch of loose skin that houses the testes.

sperm Male germ cell (from a Greek root meaning "seed").

semen The whitish fluid that carries sperm. Also called the *ejaculate*.

Health Psychology in the Digital Age

Symptoms of Menopause? There's an App for That—Actually, There Are Several

As the American population has been aging, the numbers of women encountering menopause is also on the rise, increasing by about 2 million per year. Yet there are few centralized sources of information about menopausal symptoms and what to do about them. Treatment possibilities are also controversial as they may carry health risks, as in the case of hormone replacement therapy, which is linked to increased risks of cardiovascular problems and some forms of cancer.

In an effort to provide support to menopausal women, the North American Menopause Society created a free app called MenoPro that works with smartphones and computers. A sister app is available to aid physicians in diagnostic work and in sifting through treatment options. In using the app, women answer a number of questions to determine, first of all, whether their symptoms are connected with menopause, and to help assess symptom severity. Based on the responses, women may receive information about behavioral approaches, such as changes in lifestyle, or about prescription medications, including hormone replacement therapies. By the way, women considering hormone replacement therapy may be encouraged to make lifestyle changes for a few months before seeking medical treatment. These behavior changes may help them make the adjustment to menopause more successfully.

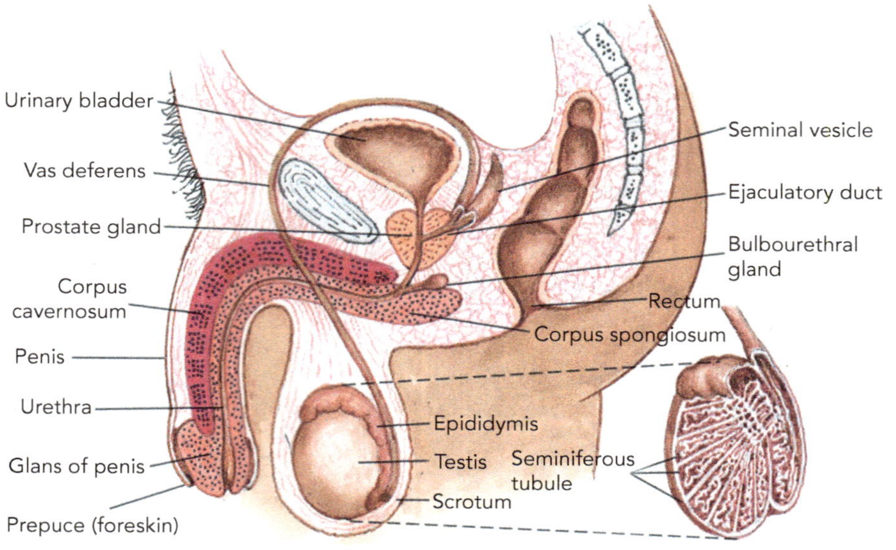

FIGURE 10.3 **Male Sexual Anatomy** A cross section of the internal and external reproductive organs of the male.

testosterone A generic term for a number of male sex hormones that promote the development of male sexual characteristics and have activating effects on sexual arousal.

prostate gland A male reproductive organ that produces semen.

The testes produce sperm and the male sex hormone **testosterone**. The scrotum allows the testes to hang away from the body (sperm require a lower-than-body temperature). Sperm travel through ducts up over the bladder and back down to the ejaculatory duct (see **Figure 10.3**), which empties into the urethra. In females, the urethral opening and the orifice for transporting the ejaculate are different; in males, they are one and the same. Although the male urethra transports urine as well as sperm, a valve shuts off the bladder during ejaculation. Thus, sperm and urine do not mix.

Several glands, including the **prostate gland**, produce semen. The prostate is responsible for producing most of the seminal fluid in the ejaculate that carries sperm cells. It is normal for the prostate gland to enlarge as men reach middle and late adulthood, which may cause problems, such as slowed urination, most of which can be treated with medication. Semen transports, activates, and nourishes sperm, enhancing their ability to swim and fertilize the ovum. Like the clitoris, the penis has a shaft and tip, or glans, which is highly sensitive to sexual stimulation, especially on the underside. The testes are also highly sensitive to sexual stimulation, but rough stimulation can be painful. Following sexual stimulation—within just a few seconds in adolescent and young adult males—blood rushes reflexively into caverns within the penis, just as blood engorges the clitoris. Despite the slang term "boner," it is engorgement with blood—and not bone—that produces erection. Men cannot will an erection. It is an involuntary reflex. They or their partners can only set the stage for erection by applying sexual stimulation. As adolescents and young men know very well, just a little bit of psychological stimulation—seeing or thinking about an attractive person—often is more than enough.

Testosterone plays an important role in human sexuality by energizing or activating sexual desire in both men and women. Testosterone is produced in women's bodies by the ovaries and the adrenal glands, but in smaller amounts than the amounts produced by the testes. (Men, like women, also produce small amounts of testosterone in their adrenal glands.) Women normally produce testosterone in the adrenal glands and ovaries, so women whose adrenal glands and ovaries have been removed may gradually lose sexual interest and the capacity for sexual response. Medical treatment with testosterone can increase sexual interest and desire in both men and women whose bodies produce too little of the hormone (Aydogan et al., 2023; Loeb et al., 2023).

Health Psychology and Prostate Cancer

Prostate cancer (cancer of the prostate) is the second most common form of cancer in men, after skin cancer, and the second leading cancer killer, after lung cancer. In the United States, nearly 35,000 men die annually from prostate cancer and nearly 300,000 receive a prostate cancer diagnosis (NCI, 2023). About one man in eight will eventually develop prostate cancer.

Prostate cancer typically produces few noticeable symptoms in its early stages, which helps explain why many men are unaware that they have the disease. Because prostate cancer tends to affect older men and often grows slowly in the body, many men die with prostate cancer rather than from prostate cancer. Nonetheless there is an aggressive form of prostate cancer that grows rapidly and can cause death in men of any age, unless it is detected early and treated effectively. However, due in large part to increased screening rates and improvements in cancer treatment, nearly all men in the United States who have prostate cancer can expect to survive for at least 5 years, in contrast to about a 30% survival rates some 30 years ago.

Recommended Screenings The American Cancer Society recommends that men consult with their primary healthcare provider to make an informed decision about whether to be screened for prostate cancer. The decision should be based on the man's age and risk level. Men at average risk should be screened at age 50, but those that higher risk because of a family history of prostate cancer in a first-degree relatively (father or brother) should be screened at younger ages based on consultation with their healthcare provider. Prostate cancer screening typically consists of a blood test called the *prostate-specific antigen* (PSA) *test* and possibly a *digital rectal exam* (DRE) in which the medical care provider manually uses a finger inserted in the rectum to feel for bulges or hardness in the prostate. The PSA tests for the level of a substance naturally produced in the prostate that may indicate the presence of a developing cancer that can't be felt manually.

Treatment for prostate cancer depends on the stage of development of the cancer, the man's age, and his general health condition. Surgery may be used to remove the cancerous growth, and while it reduces the risk of the cancer spreading in the body, it can carry a risk of significant side effects, such as urinary incontinence and problems with erection. Radiation

Health Psychology in Action

Role of Health Psychology in Prostate Cancer Screening

Health psychologists play several important roles in prostate cancer prevention and treatment. Coping with a diagnosis of prostate cancer can take an emotional toll, leading to emotional problems like anxiety and depression (Fervaha et al., 2020). A recent scientific review showed that psychological interventions, such as cognitive behavior therapy (CBT), can improve psychological functioning in men with prostate cancer (Mundle et al., 2021). Health psychologists also recognize that stigma associated with cancer screening is often a barrier to obtaining recommended screenings (Foster et al., 2021).

Black men have a higher risk of developing prostate cancer during the lifetime than other men, so efforts directed to increasing screening among Black men becomes an urgent priority. Recently, health psychologists investigated the role of self-efficacy in determining the likelihood of seeking prostate cancer screening. As you may recall from our discussion of social-cognitive theory in Chapter 2, self-efficacy refers to our belief in our ability to successfully carry-out behaviors we attempt to perform. Health psychologists recently measured intentions to seek prostate cancer screening in a sample of Black men in Northeast Ohio and the Southeastern United States (Qin et al., 2022). The researchers found that men with high levels of self-efficacy, or a strong belief their ability to go ahead and obtain recommended screenings, were more than two times as likely to form an intention of getting screened as were men who doubted whether they could follow through with screening.

Other researchers applied the Health Belief Model (HBM) in predicting prostate cancer screening behaviors. Among a sample of Black men in Florida, researchers found that those of lower socioeconomic level and younger men (under 50 years of age) perceived low levels of behavioral control (not believing they could do anything to lower their personal risk of prostate cancer) (Odedina et al., 2011). This brings to mind that healthcare providers can be especially helpful in raising awareness in Black men about racial disparities in cancer detection and treatment and addressing questions about the benefits and risks of prostate cancer screening (Shungu & Sterba, 2021).

What we take away from these studies is the importance of focusing on beliefs men hold about the need to be screened for prostate cancer. Whether a man obtains prostate cancer screening may depend on addressing such questions as, "Do I need to be screened? . . . Am I at significant risk? . . . . How do I obtain screening? . . . Can I afford it? . . . What do I need to do? . . Will I be able to do it? . . . (and) Will it make a difference?"

There remains a need to raise awareness about the risks and benefits of prostate cancer screening and the need to adopt a "can do" attitude toward obtaining cancer screening and following other health recommendations. One promising lead in health psychology that requires some further investigation involves the use of social media as a means of promoting cancer screening and early diagnosis in men at risk of the disease (Benedict et al., 2023; Plackett et al., 2020).

may be used as an alternative treatment to kill or shrink cancerous tissues. In some cases, men with early prostate cancer, especially if they are older, may be advised to follow a "watchful waiting" approach to monitor the growth of the cancer in lieu of surgery or radiation. In some cases, hormone therapy may also be used.

Review 10.1

INTERACTIVE SELF-SCORING QUIZZES

Sentence Completion

1. The ovaries produce ova and the sex hormones estrogen and __________.
2. Conception normally takes place in a __________ tube.
3. Levels of estrogen and progesterone regulate the __________ cycle.
4. Tissue called the __________ is normally sloughed off during menstruation.
5. __________ is the release of an ovum by an ovary.
6. Pain during menstruation is called __________.
7. The term __________ syndrome describes a cluster of biological symptoms that occur during the 4–6-day interval that precedes menstruation.
8. About __________ of new mothers have periods of tearfulness, sadness, and irritability that are referred to as the baby blues.
9. Researchers believe that the baby blues are common because of the __________ changes that follow delivery.
10. __________ refers to the beginning of menopause and is usually characterized by 3–11 months of amenorrhea (lack of menstruation) or irregular periods.
11. The __________ refers to the gradual decline in the reproductive capacity of the ovaries, which may last about 15 years.
12. Hot flashes and flushes stem largely from dilation of __________ vessels across the face and upper body.
13. The testes produce sperm and the male sex hormone __________.
14. It is normal for the __________ gland to enlarge as men age.
15. Erection is caused by engorgement of the penis with __________.
16. Testosterone is produced in women's bodies by the ovaries and the __________ glands.

Think About It

What is the role for health psychology in helping women manage menstrual discomfort? The discomfort is real, but how might health psychologists use cognitive behavioral therapy to help women manage the discomfort? What types of self-defeating things do people tend to say to themselves when they are experiencing discomfort?

Decision-Making About Reproductive Options

Familiarity breeds contempt—and children.

—Mark Twain

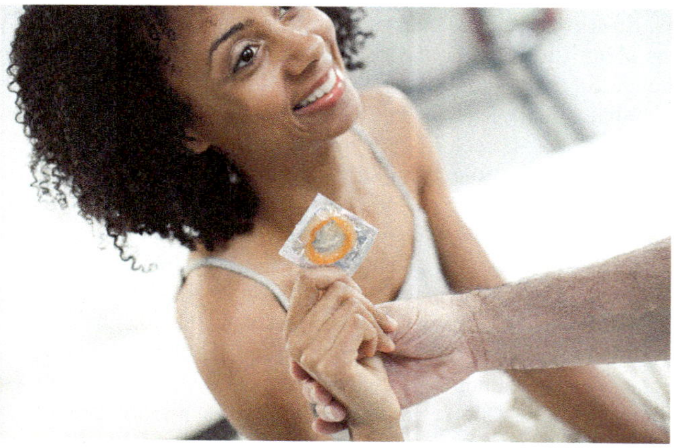

Image Source/Getty Images

Taking a Break? She is interested in having sex, but not without protection. The condom, used properly, protects against unwanted pregnancies and sexually transmitted infections.

Health psychologists study decision-making about various types of health behaviors, including decisions about contraceptive choices. One couple in 6 faces the frustration of attempting to conceive children and failing. Other couples run the risk of unwanted pregnancy. Perhaps they become involved in impassioned lovemaking and engage in condomless sex. Perhaps they had a bit too much to drink. And a woman may have been sexually assaulted.

Contraception (the prevention of pregnancy) has a fascinating history. For example, ancient Egyptians douched with wine and garlic after sex; they also soaked crocodile dung in sour milk and stuffed the mixture into the vagina. The dung blocked the passage of many—if not all—sperm and also soaked up sperm. A social mechanism may also have been at work. Perhaps the crocodile dung discouraged all but the most ardent suitors.

TABLE 10.1 Effectiveness and Reversibility of Methods of Contraception

	Percentage (%) of Women Who Have Unplanned Pregnancy Within First Year of Use			
Method	**Typical Use[1]**	**Consistent, Correct Use**	**Reversible?**	**Protects Against Sexually Transmitted Infections (STIs)?**
None	85	85	Yes	No
Spermicides	29	18	Yes	No
Rhythm methods	20		Yes	No
Calendar		9		
Ovulation method		3		
Basal body temperature		3		
Post-ovulation		3		
Withdrawal	27	4	Yes	No
Cervical cap[2]	20–40	10–30	Yes	Some
Diaphragm[2]	16	6	Yes	Some
Female condom	21	5	Yes	(Scarce information)
Male condom	15	2	Yes	Yes
Contraceptive pills	8	0.3	Yes	No
Progestin only		0.5		
Combined		0.1		
Intrauterine device	0.2–0.8	0.2–0.6	Yes, except if fertility is impaired	No
Depo-provera	3	0.3	Yes	No
Injectable contraceptives	0.5	0.5	Yes	No
Female sterillization	0.5	0.5	Questionable	No
Male sterilization	0.15	0.10	Questionable	No

[1] Accidental pregnancies among typical couples.
[2] With spermicide.
Sources: American Family Physician (2022); Hatcher et al. (2018); Zieman (2021–2022).

In any event, sexually active individuals need to face the question of contraception, and today's methods are more reliable—if not more interesting—than those of the ancient Egyptians. Here we consider a number of methods of contraception. **Table 10.1** summarizes the reliability, reversibility, and degree of protection against sexually transmitted infections (STIs) provided by various methods. Reliability is generally higher among people who use the methods carefully. For example, some women forget to take the pill regularly, and condoms can tear or slip. The nearby Applying Health Psychology feature invites you to evaluate your own decision-making process in the context of the HBM.

About 3 of 5 college women were on the birth control pill during their most recent sexual encounter (American College Health Association, 2023). Two of 3 males and 3 of 5 females report using condoms the last time they had sex. About 1 college man in 4 and 3 college women in 10 report using the withdrawal method. As you can see in Table 10.1, the withdrawal method is far from reliable. And as you can see in **Figure 10.4**, once women and men

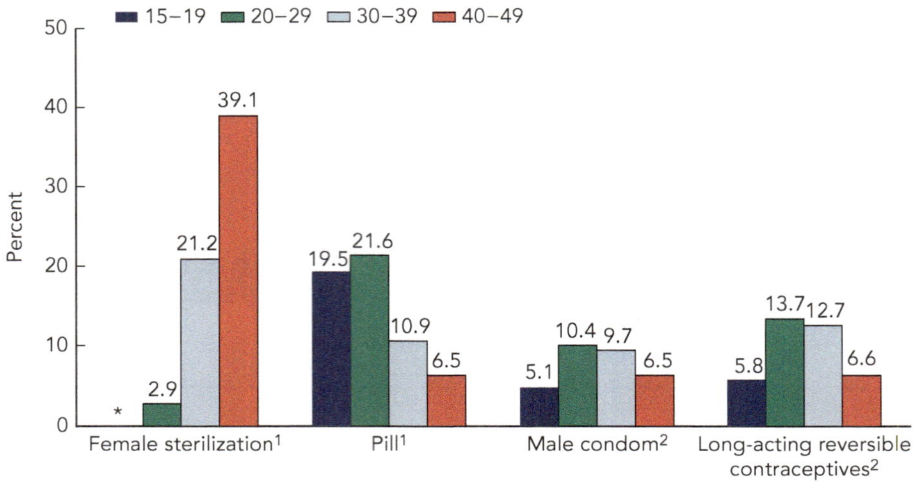

FIGURE 10.4 Percentage of All Women Aged 15–49 years Who Are Currently Using Female Sterilization, the Pill, Male Condoms, or Long-Acting Reversible Contraception, by Age Group, United States

Source: Daniels & Abma (2018). https://www.cdc.gov/nchs/data/databriefs/db327-h.pdf./US Department of Health and Human Services / Public Domain.

have had their children, or decided that they will not be having children, female and male sterilization is more likely to enter the picture. Sterilization does not affect the sex drive or sexual response. Nor does it affect the production of sex hormones or, in women, the menstrual cycle. Sperm cells and egg cells (ova) are simply reabsorbed by the body. It is prudent for people considering sterilization to assume that it is not reversible, although there are occasional successes in reversing the procedures.

Health Psychology in the Digital Age

Apps That Predict Safe Periods for Sex

Women can become pregnant only when they are ovulating. There are many ways to predict ovulation. Women who wish to become pregnant will aim to have sex for a couple of days before ovulation and during ovulation. Women who wish to avoid pregnancy will limit sex to days more distant from ovulation. A number of apps can help women identify "safe" periods by counting days, tracking body temperature, and the like. The apps are friendlier and probably more accurate than jotting things down on a paper calendar or in a notebook. They include:

- Clue (relies on the calendar method)
- Kindara (comprehensive charting app that tracks cervical mucus and basal temperature, and provides a social platform for charting questions)
- Ovia (tracks cervical mucus)
- Glow (combines the calendar method, the temperature method, and the cervical mucus method)

The illustration is from the Kindara.com website. It's what you'll be looking at on your mobile phone if you use the app. Go to https://www.kindara.com/avoid-pregnancy.

Source: Kindara.com. Reproduced with permission of Kindara.

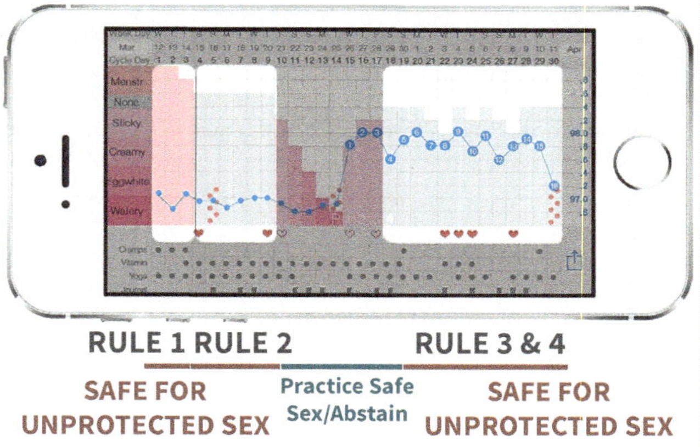

It is also prudent to use a backup birth control method, such as condoms, when you're testing out a birth control app. You can also check out how well you are using your app by buying an ovulation test kit or a fertility monitor and using it for a while along with the app.

Applying Health Psychology

The Health Belief Model and Benefits and Barriers in Selecting a Method of Contraception

You and your partner will likely apply the HBM to decide whether you need contraception and, if so, which methods to choose. To begin with, you would not be considering contraception unless you saw yourself as being susceptible to unwanted pregnancy. A cue to action may be hearing that someone you know became pregnant due to carelessness. Here are other matters to consider:

- *Convenience.* Convenience can be a benefit in the case of long-acting, affordable methods, but inconvenience can be a barrier to use. Is the method you are considering convenient? Does it require a device that must be purchased in advance? If so, is a prescription required? Will the method work at a moment's notice, or, as with the birth control pill, will it require time to reach effectiveness?
- *Self-efficacy.* Do you and your partner have confidence that you can use the method properly?
- *Moral acceptability.* According to the HBM, religion can be a modifying variable. A method that is morally acceptable to one person may be objectionable to another. For example, those who strictly follow the teachings of the Roman Catholic Church may object to artificial means of contraception.
- *Cost.* Within the HBM, cost can be a barrier to action. Methods of contraception vary in cost. Some more costly methods involve devices (such as the diaphragm, the cervical cap, and the intrauterine device [IUD]) or hormones that require medical visits in addition to the cost of the devices themselves.
- *Sharing responsibility.* Most forms of birth control place the burden of responsibility largely, if not entirely, on the woman. The woman must consult with her doctor to obtain birth control pills or other prescription devices, such as diaphragms, cervical caps, and IUDs. The woman must take birth control pills reliably or check to see that her IUD remains in place. Some couples prefer methods that allow for greater sharing of responsibility, such as alternating use of the condom and the diaphragm. A man can also share the responsibility for the birth control pill by accompanying his partner on her medical visits and sharing the expense.
- *Safety.* How safe is the method? What are the side effects?
- *Reversibility.* Lack of reversibility would be a barrier to those who may want children in the future. Sterility, of course, is usually irreversible.
- *Protection against STIs.* Hormonal methods such as the pill protect against pregnancy, but not against STIs.
- *Effectiveness.* Techniques and devices vary widely in their effectiveness in actual use. The failure rate for a particular method refers to the percentage of women who become pregnant when using the method for a given period of time, such as during the first year of use. Failure rates among typical (rather than highly conscientious) users may be considerably higher because of incorrect, unreliable, or inconsistent use. See Table 10.1 for the failure rates, reversibility, and degree of protection against STIs afforded by various contraceptive methods.

Review 10.2

INTERACTIVE SELF-SCORING QUIZZES

Sentence Completion

1. In typical use, the withdrawal method of contraception fails in about 1 out of __________ cases in a year of use.

2. The best method to protect against both conception and sexually transmitted infections is the __________.

3. In the great majority of cases, the burden of contraception is placed on the (woman or man).

4. The __________ is the most widely used method of female contraception.

5. __________ becomes a widely used method of contraception once people have had the children they want to have or decided that they do not want children.

6. Use of __________ as a means of contraception should not be considered to be reversible.

Think About It

Why do women most often shoulder the responsibility for contraception? What methods of contraception also place responsibility on the man?

Sexually Transmitted Infections

There has been a recent surge of **sexually transmitted infections (STIs)** in the United States, especially among adolescents and young adults, and nearly two-thirds of cases are among youth of color (Feldstein et al., 2020). Overall, the Centers for Disease Control and Prevention (CDC) estimates that nearly 68 million Americans had an STI on any given day; 26 million Americans contracted an STI each year; and about half of these new cases were contracted by people aged 15–24 (CDC, 2021b).

sexually transmitted infections (STIs) Infectious diseases that are transmitted by means of sexual contact.

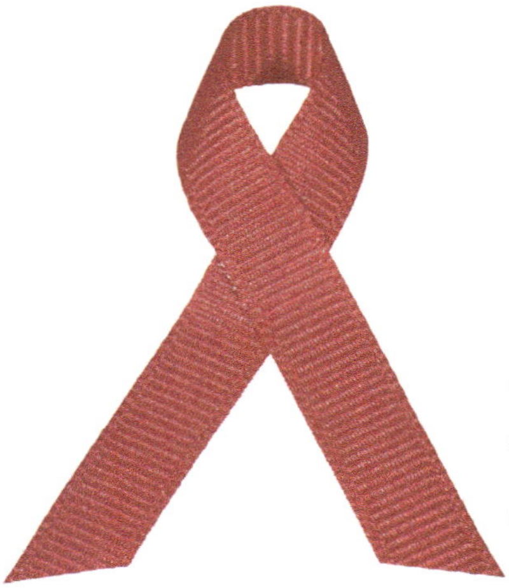

Amos Morgan/Getty Images

Although media attention has focused largely on HIV/AIDS, other STIs are far more widespread. Whereas about 1.2 million Americans are living with HIV/AIDS, some 50 to 60 million are infected with other STI-causing viruses, such as those causing herpes, hepatitis, and cervical cancer. More than 42 million Americans have human papillomavirus (HPV), the organism that causes genital warts and cervical cancer, and the virus infects some 13 million Americans each year (CDC, 2022c). HPV can also lead to throat cancer in men or women who engage in cunnilingus with an infected woman. To put this in context, there are more new cases of HPV infection each year, some 13 million cases, than there are of syphilis, genital herpes, and HIV/AIDS combined (HPV Infection, 2023). Most sexually active people can expect to contract HPV at some point in their lives (HPV Infection, 2023). Although most people infected with HPV clear the disease on their own, in some cases the infection remains dormant for many years and may eventually lead to cancer. Many young people, especially young men, have little awareness of the health risks posed by HPV (Jenkins et al., 2023).

Consider too that while more than 1 million Americans are infected with HIV, 1 in 6 Americans aged 14–49 years are believed to be infected with genital herpes (herpes simplex virus). Most people with genital herpes don't know they have it because they are free of symptoms. But even without symptoms, they can still transmit the virus to their sexual partners. Nearly 1.6 million cases of chlamydia, a sexually transmitted bacterial infection, are reported annually (CDC, 2022b). Most people infected with chlamydia also don't know it because of the absence of telltale symptoms.

Knowledge, so they say, is power, but lack of knowledge can be lethal. Remaining unaware of the risks posed by unsafe sexual practices can lead to potentially lethal infections, such as HIV/AIDS. Moreover, between 15% and 30% of cases of infertility in women are the result of damage to reproductive organs caused by chlamydia and gonorrhea. In addition to the physical health issues caused by STIs, there are untold numbers of people suffering the emotional anguish associated with STIs, not to mention relationships strained to the breaking point. Anyone can contract STIs. In fact, the majority of people will contract an STI at some time in their lives. What will you do to learn about them and protect yourself?

Most college students seem to be reasonably well informed about HIV/AIDS, but many remain unaware that chlamydia can go undetected for years. If chlamydia is not treated, in women it can produce a serious infection of the internal reproductive system and can lead to pelvic inflammatory disease and infertility. In men it can lead to reduced fertility. Yet most people with chlamydia have no symptoms, which underscores the need for regular medical screening (Chlamydia, 2017). The bacterial STI gonorrhea also heightens the risk of developing pelvic inflammatory disease and infertility (Reekie et al., 2018).

Women bear a heavier burden than men when it comes to STIs. They are more likely to be affected by chlamydia and gonorrhea and to develop infertility if an STI spreads through their reproductive system. In addition to their biological effects, STIs take an emotional toll and strain relationships.

Throughout the remainder of this section we focus on HIV/AIDS, but readers seeking more information about other STIs are advised to talk to their healthcare provider or visit their college health centers.

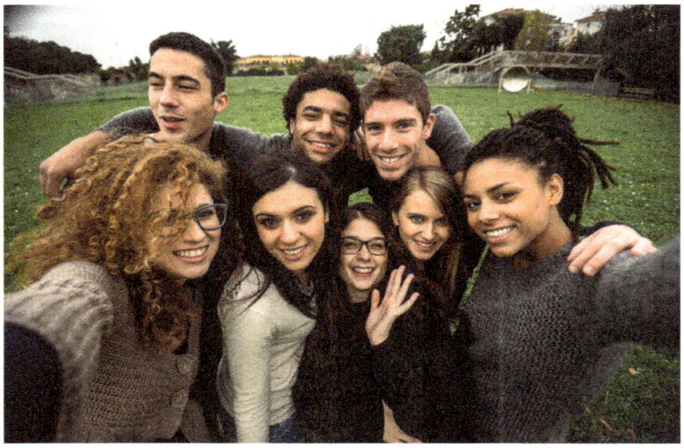

franckreporter/Getty Images

Who Is at Risk? Anyone can contract STIs. In fact, the majority of people will contract an STI at some time in their lives. What will you do to learn about them and protect yourself?

HIV/AIDS

HIV/AIDS is a life-threatening viral disease in which a virus, the *human immunodeficiency virus* (HIV), invades the immune system, the very system that defends against disease-causing agents such as bacteria and viruses. More than 38 million people worldwide and more than 1.2 million in the United States are believed to be living with HIV/AIDS (World Health Organization, 2020a). A majority of cases of HIV/AIDS worldwide, and about 1 in 4 in the United States, occur through heterosexual (male–female)

Health Psychology in Action

The Health Belief Model and the Decision to Get the HPV Vaccine

Health behavior change models help inform our understanding of factors determining disease-preventive behaviors, such as getting vaccinations. On the one hand, a highly effective vaccine is available that protects women from the strains of HPV that cause most forms of cervical cancer (Brotons & Bruni, 2020; Drolet et al., 2019; Palmer et al., 2019). On the other hand, many young people remain unvaccinated.

The Advisory Committee on Immunization Practices (ACIP) recommends that multiple doses be given routinely to 11- or 12-year-olds (Petrosky et al., 2015). The ACIP also recommends that the vaccine be given to females aged 13–26 if it has not been given previously. The vaccine should also be given to boys routinely at ages 11 or 12 to prevent health problems, such as cancer of the anus (contracted via anal sex with an infected partner) and cancer of the throat (contracted by oral sex with an infected partner) later in life. Since the ACIP recommends that people can be given the vaccine through the ages of 26 for women and 21 through men, people who have not received it previously can choose to obtain it as adults. The Food & Drug Administration has actually approved use of the vaccine through the age of 45 (ACIP, 2019). (Does one of these age categories include you?)

Women are more likely than men to have received the HPV vaccine, and among women, non-Hispanic White women are more likely to have been vaccinated than Latino/Hispanic or Black women (Boersma & Black, 2020; see **Figure 10.5**). Among men, Black people are most likely to have been vaccinated against HPV. Despite public health efforts to vaccinate adolescents against HPV, many remain unvaccinated. Because the HPV vaccine is typically given to minors, parents can determine whether or not their preteens and younger teenagers will receive it.

The Health Belief Model (HBM) can help identify the points of resistance to getting the vaccine. The model teaches that a combination of factors converge on whether people participate in vaccination programs or other health-preventive measures. *First* is perceived threat or susceptibility. A parent may not believe their child is at risk because are sexually inactive or believed to be too young to be sexually intimate. *Second* is the perceived seriousness of the threat. Many people are unaware that HPV is the major cause of cervical cancer, a potentially deadly disease. *Third* is the belief that the benefits of the vaccine may be outweighed by the risks. Some parents voice are concerns that making a "sexual" vaccine to their children could expose them to greater risks by encouraging them to engage in sexual activity more freely (Kim et al., 2018; Reno et al., 2018). This same concern has led many parents to object to sex education in the schools, despite evidence that sex education does not encourage sexual activity and does help prevent teenage pregnancy (Breuner et al., 2016; Hell et al., 2016; Secor-Turner et al., 2017). Nor is there any evidence that HPV vaccination increases sexual activity in adolescents or young adults.

Evidence from a recent scientific review on parental factors associated with HPV vaccination rates pinpointed several important factors that dovetail with the HBM (Rodriguez et al., 2020). Parental factors associated with a greater likelihood of initiation or completion of HPV vaccination of both female and male adolescent children included the following:

- Knowledge about HPV vaccination
- Perceived effectiveness of the vaccine
- Interaction with the healthcare system
- Health provider recommendation (a cue to action)
- Reminders (another cue to action)

Parental factors associated with reduced likelihood of HPV vaccination were something of a mirror image, including the following:

- Lack of knowledge about the HPV vaccine
- Low perceived susceptibility of child to HPV or related diseases
- Concerns about vaccine safety and side effects
- Concerns about costs (a perceived barrier)
- Lack of healthcare provider recommendations (absence of a cue to action)

Pediatricians and other healthcare professionals need to better educate parents that the vaccine is safe and effective (Wong, 2016). Healthcare providers also need to dispel myths about the vaccine so that parents can make decisions based on the evidence, not on misinformation. The concern about the vaccine especially impacts parents of boys, for whom the vaccine may prevent throat cancer 30 or 50 years in the future. Some young people whose parents are resistant to providing vaccines seek them on their own, and there is public debate about whether minors should be able to obtain vaccinations without parental consent (Haddad et al., 2018).

sex (**Figure 10.6**). However, 2 of 3 diagnoses (66%) in the United States are found in men who have sex with men (MSM). Although the annual number of new HIV diagnoses in the country States has been decreasing, more than 38,000 people in the United States are diagnosed with HIV each year (World Health Organization, 2020b).

As you see in **Figure 10.7**, the burden of HIV/AIDS is not borne equally by various racial and ethnic groups in the United States. Although (non-Hispanic) White Americans comprise the majority of the population, they account for only 1 in 4 new HIV diagnoses (25.6%). Latino/Hispanic Americans account for slightly more (29%), and non-Hispanic Black/African American Americans account for 41%. Non-Hispanic Asian Americans and those of other racial and ethnic groups are least likely to be afflicted.

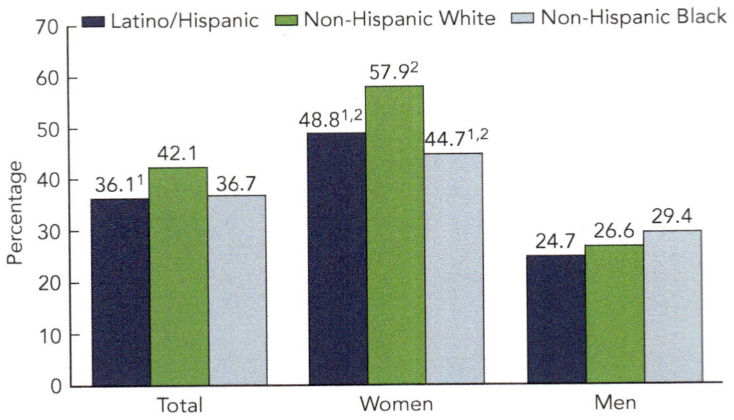

FIGURE 10.5 **Percentage of Adults Aged 18–26 Who Received One or More Doses of HPV Vaccine, by Sex, Race, and Ethnicity: United States**

Source: P. Boersma, & L. I. Black (2020). Human papillomavirus vaccination among adults aged 18–26, 2013–2018. *NCHS Data Brief, 354.* https://www.cdc.gov/nchs/data/databriefs/db354-h.pdf./US Department of Health and Human Services / Public Domain.

HIV and the Immune System

Spikes on the surface of HIV allow it to bind to sites on cells in the immune system. Like other viruses, HIV uses the cells it invades to spin off copies of itself. HIV uses the enzyme *reverse transcriptase* to cause the genes in the cells it attacks to make proteins that the virus needs to reproduce.

HIV attacks the immune system by destroying a type of lymphocyte called the CD4 cell. These CD4 cells, also known as T-cells or helper T-cells, "recognize" invading pathogens and signal B-lymphocytes (B-cells) to produce antibodies that inactivate pathogens and mark them for annihilation. CD4 cells also signal another class of T-cells, called killer T-cells, to destroy infected cells. By attacking and destroying helper T-cells, HIV disables the cells on which the body relies to fend off diseases. As HIV cripples the body's defenses, the individual develops *opportunistic infections*, infections that would not otherwise take hold or be so severe. Cancer cells might also proliferate.

Human blood normally contains about 1,000 CD4 cells per cubic millimeter. The numbers of CD4 cells may remain at about this level for years following HIV infection. Many people show no symptoms and appear healthy while CD4 cells remain at this level. Then, for reasons that are not clearly understood, the levels of CD4 cells begin to drop off, although symptoms may not appear for a decade or more. People become most vulnerable to opportunistic infections when the level of CD4 cells falls below 200 per cubic millimeter.

internalized homophobia Negative stereotypes, beliefs, stigma, and prejudice about LGBT people that a person with same-sex attraction turns inward on themselves, whether or not they identify themselves as being LGBT.

Progression of HIV/AIDS

HIV follows a complex course once it enters the body. A recently infected individual may experience mild flu-like symptoms—fatigue, fever, headaches, muscle pain, lack of appetite, nausea, swollen glands, and possibly a rash. Such symptoms usually disappear within a few weeks, and people may dismiss them as a case of the flu. People who enter this symptom-free or carrier state generally look and act well and do not realize that they are infectious. Thus, they can unwittingly pass the virus to others.

Even during the years when HIV appears to be dormant, billions of viral particles are being spun off. In a seesaw battle, most of them are wiped out by the immune system, but eventually, in almost all cases, the balance tips in favor of HIV. Then the numbers of the virus swell. Perhaps a decade or more after the person is infected with HIV, the virus begins to overtake the immune system. It obliterates the cells that house it and spreads to other immune system cells. About half of the people with HIV develop AIDS within 10 years of initial infection. For this reason, people who know that they are infected with HIV may feel that they are carrying time bombs within them.

AIDS is called a syndrome because it is characterized by a variety of different symptoms. The beginnings of full-blown cases of AIDS are often marked by swollen lymph nodes, fatigue, fever, night sweats, diarrhea, and weight loss (a "wasting syndrome") that cannot be attributed to dieting or exercise. AIDS is connected with the appearance of diseases such as tuberculosis, Pneumocystis carinii pneumonia (PCP); Kaposi's sarcoma (a form of cancer), toxoplasmosis of the brain (a parasitic infection); or herpes simplex with chronic ulcers. These are termed opportunistic

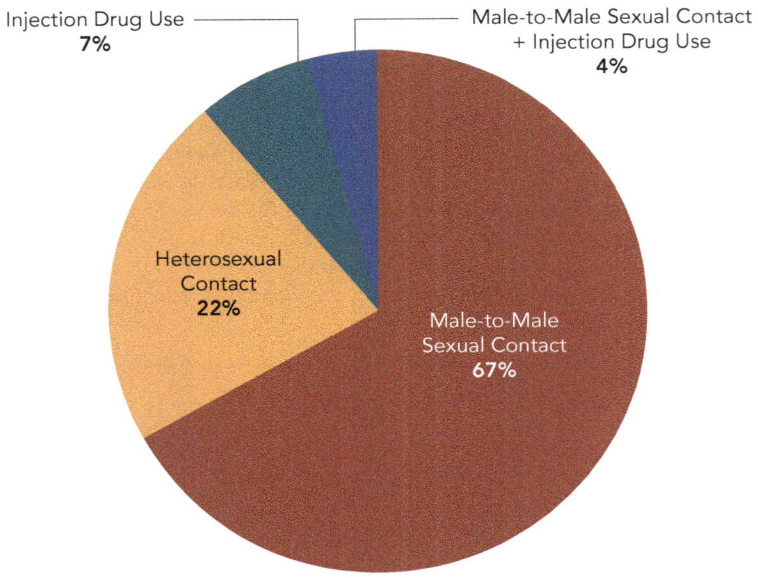

FIGURE 10.6 **New HIV Diagnoses in the United States, by Transmission Category**

Source: Centers for Disease Control and Prevention (CDC). Diagnoses of HIV infection in the United States and dependent areas, 2021. HIV Surveillance Report, 34/US Department of Health and Human Services / Public Domain.

diseases because they are not likely to emerge unless a weakened immune system grants the opportunity.

About 10% of people with AIDS have the wasting syndrome—the unintentional loss of more than 10% of a person's body weight that is connected with HIV/AIDS, some other infections, and cancer. As HIV/AIDS progresses, people become thinner and more fatigued. They become unable to perform ordinary life functions. If left untreated, AIDS almost always results in death within a few years.

Transmission HIV is transmitted by infected blood, semen, vaginal and cervical secretions, and breast milk. The virus can be contracted through vaginal, anal, or oral sex with an infected partner. It may also be transmitted from an infected mother to fetus during pregnancy or from mother to child during childbirth or breastfeeding. Other means of infection include sharing a hypodermic needle with an infected person and transfusion with contaminated blood. There is no evidence that public toilets, insect bites, holding or hugging an infected person, or living or attending school with an infected person transmits HIV.

Theories of Health Behavior and the Low Level of Perceived Risk Among the Heterosexual Population The HBM predicts that people are more likely to engage in healthy sexual behavior when they perceive a risk in failing to do so. The Theory of Reasoned Action posits that fear of consequences, such as contracting a sexually transmitted infection, may prompt healthful behavior, although people may throw caution to the winds if those they socialize with do not practice safer sex.

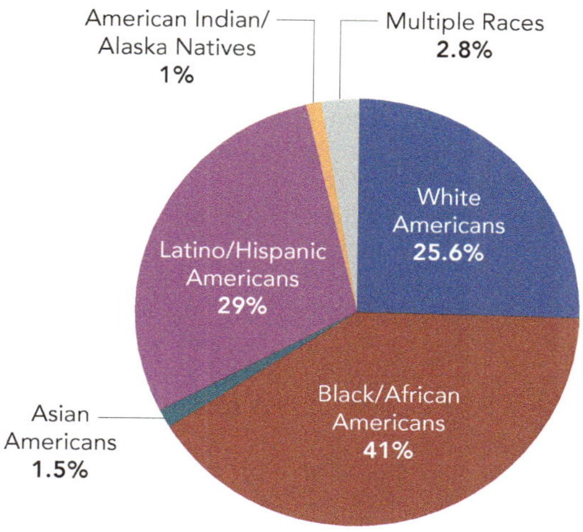

FIGURE 10.7 **New HIV Diagnoses in the United States by Race/Ethnicity**

Source: Centers for Disease Control and Prevention (CDC) (2023). HIV in the United States by Race/Ethnicity: HIV Incidence. Centers for Disease Control and Prevention. https://www.cdc.gov/hiv/group/racialethnic/other-races/incidence.html/US Department of Health and Human Services/Public Domain.

Health Psychology in Action

PrEP—Perceived Benefits and Barriers of Using the HBM as a Plan for Action

Researchers have investigated the use of antiretroviral drugs to lower the risk of being infected with HIV. The method is called pre-exposure prophylaxis, or PrEP, and it employs a combination of antiretroviral drugs. Jonathan Volk and his colleagues (2015) at Kaiser Permanente's San Francisco Medical Center followed 657 men who had sex with men (MSM) for more than 2 years. The men took PrEP as prescribed but made no effort to limit their number of sexual contacts. Not one contracted HIV during the trial.

However, the use of PrEP apparently encouraged many MSM in the study to think that they no longer needed to be cautious in their sexual encounters. The researchers found that MSM taking PrEP were less likely to use condoms, even with strangers. Their lower use of condoms was associated with a higher incidence of contracting other STIs. Other researchers bear out the finding that use of PrEP is connected with less use of condoms and a higher incidence of STIs other than HIV/AIDS (Barreiro, 2018; Burrell et al., 2019).

All the men in the Volk study received PrEP; none received a placebo. Therefore, the study does not qualify as a random controlled trial. However, a British study of the benefits of PrEP did randomly assign some participants to a placebo, and some of those who took the placebo became infected with HIV (McCormack et al., 2016). The English study was stopped early, because it became clear that PrEP was effective and that there was no scientific reason to expose the men taking the placebo to further risk. Evidence favoring the use of PrEP is now clear and leading medical experts recommend the use of PrEP for MSM who are at increased risk of HIV infection (Barry et al., 2023). The problem is getting people at high risk of acquiring HIV to take advantage of PrEP. PrEP offers the following benefits: lowered risk of being infected with HIV, protection in case of inconsistent use of condoms, protection even if their sex partners misrepresent their HIV status (i.e., say they are seronegative but actually be seropositive for HIV), low cost, insurance coverage, and ease of adding PrEP to their daily health and medication regimes. One study observed the relationships among use of PrEP, casual sex without condoms, and the psychological factors of depression, anxiety, and **internalized homophobia** (Moeller et al., 2020). Use of PrEP lowered the discomforts of all three psychological factors. Moreover, rates of anxiety were higher among those non-PrEP users who reported unprotected sex with greater numbers of sex partners.

We can use the HBM model as a lens through which to look at factors that increase the likelihood of using the PrEP preventive model to reduce the spread of HIV. The HBM consists of various elements that predict and help explain health-preventive behaviors, such as getting recommended vaccines and practicing safer sex techniques. Several of these elements come into play with PrEP, including perceived risk, barriers to use, and cues to actions. Let's apply the model to the likelihood of using PrEP.

Perceptions of low risk work against using PrEP. So too do a lack of cues to action, such as not being offered PrEP by a healthcare provider, barriers to use, such as potential side effects, taking too many other medicines, the cost, and simply the additional burden of taking PrEP daily (Hughto et al., 2019). Lack of education is another barrier (Pette, 2019; Raifman et al., 2019). Moreover, many men who have anal sex with men have internalized the widespread cultural stigma directed against anal sex. Because of the stigma, they are often unwilling to disclose their sexual practices to others. As a result, some are unwilling to seek health care (Kutner et al., 2020).

We see that it is one thing to have PrEP available; it is another thing to make use of it. Julia Raifman and her colleagues (2019) identified women who visited an STI clinic in Rhode Island who were at risk of contracting HIV from a sexual relationship with men who might be infected with HIV. Only one-third of women were aware of the availability of PrEP. White American women were more likely to be aware of PrEP than Black women or Latino/Hispanic women. Three in 5 men who attended the same clinic and who had sex with men were aware of PrEP. In a related study with MSM who attended the same clinic, Raifman and her colleagues (2018) found that an education program increased awareness of PrEP by 63% and use of PrEP by 159%.

There's much that the health community can do to increase use of this potentially life-saving program, such as by raising awareness of the risks of HIV infection, reducing barriers to use, reducing cost and increasing accessibility, and perhaps most importantly, providing cues for action by using educational campaigns to call attention to the need

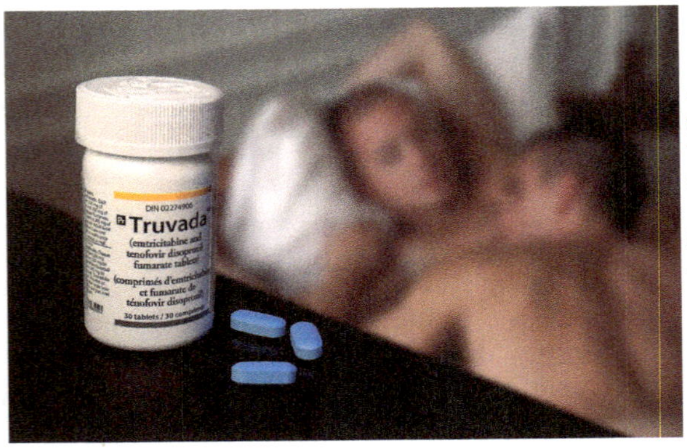

Marc Antoine Saucier/Alamy Stock Photo

PrEP Viagra isn't the only blue sex-related pill on the block. Truvada is one of the antiretroviral medication cocktails that help prevent users from becoming infected with HIV. But men who use PrEP are less likely to use condoms, thereby exposing themselves to the risk of contracting other STIs.

Because HIV/AIDS has been characterized as mainly transmitted by anal intercourse (a practice that is fairly common among gay men) and the sharing of contaminated needles, many heterosexual Americans who do not use drugs may not perceive themselves at being of risk of infection with HIV and may dismiss the threat. Yet male–female sexual intercourse can transmit the disease and accounts for the majority of cases around the world. Although gay men and people who abuse drugs and their partners have been hit hardest by the epidemic in the United States, HIV cuts across all boundaries of gender, sexual orientation, ethnicity, and socioeconomic status.

There is no safe, effective vaccine against HIV/AIDS. However, a combination of antiretroviral drugs (ART or antiretroviral therapy) has transformed HIV/AIDS into a manageable chronic disease for most people, not a terminal one. The combination may be taken as a daily pill or a bimonthly injection, and patients generally report preferring the injection (Currier, 2020; Swindells et al., 2020). However, having patients come in to a clinic on a bimonthly basis can be burdensome, and some people probably will miss injections. Health psychologists can be of help in establishing methods to bolster adherence, such as phone calls, texting, and so forth. Because we still do not know what happens with people who use antiretroviral drugs for many decades, the most effective way of dealing with HIV/AIDS is prevention. For people who are seropositive for HIV, prevention currently entails careful choice of partners, using condoms, using medications that keep the virus at low nontransmissible blood levels, and avoiding sharing needles when using illicit drugs.

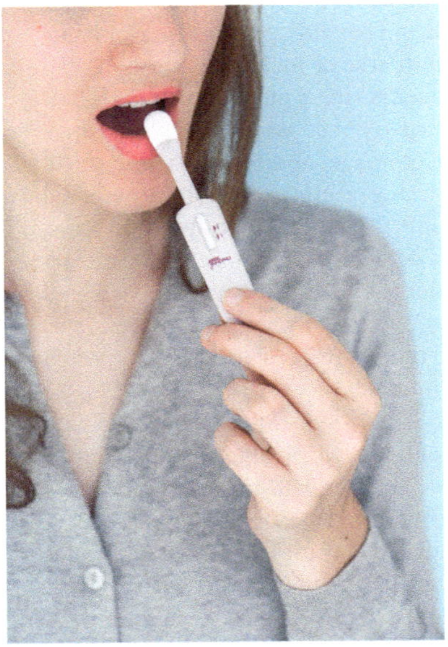

Phanie/Alamy Stock Photo

OraQuick The over-the-counter OraQuick test informs people within a few minutes as to whether they have HIV antibodies in their saliva. Can you apply the HBM to discuss the psychological barriers to testing oneself?

Health Belief Model or Theory of Planned Behavior? Adolescents and Sexual Risk-Taking

The Health Belief Model (HBM) seems to have met its match in trying to account for high-risk sexual behavior among adolescents (O'Dwyer et al., 2019). The HBM predicts health behavior change based on a person's assessment of perceived health threats, their perceived vulnerability to the threat, and the benefits and costs of making behavioral changes to address those threats. But in the case of adolescents and sex, the HBM may

Applying Health Psychology

Prevention of STIs in the Age of HIV/AIDS

It can be clumsy to try to protect yourself from STIs such as HIV/AIDS. How do you request a conversation about STIs in the heat of the moment? How do you recommend that you both be tested for ... everything?

Because of the difficulties in discussing STIs with sex partners, some people admit that they "wing it." That is, they assume that a partner does not have an STI, or they hope for the best. Don't wing it. The risks are too high. The only sure way to prevent sexual transmission of HIV and other STIs is either abstinence from sexual activity or maintaining a monogamous relationship with an uninfected partner. However, partners of HIV-positive people who are HIV-negative can take oral *PrEP (pre-exposure prophylaxis)* to prevent becoming infected themselves (World Health Organization, 2018a).

What can you do to prevent the transmission of HIV and other STIs? A number of things:

- *Don't ignore the threat.* Many people try to put HIV/AIDS and other STIs out of their minds. Do not ignore STIs or assume that they will not affect you.
- *Consider abstinence or "outercourse."* One way to curb the sexual transmission of HIV and other organisms that cause STIs is sexual abstinence. Kissing, hugging, and petting to orgasm (without coming into contact with semen or vaginal secretions) are generally considered safe in terms of HIV transmission. Petting to orgasm is often referred to as outercourse, in contrast to intercourse. However, kissing can transmit oral herpes (as shown by the development of cold sores) and some bacterial STIs.
- *Limit sex to a monogamous relationship with someone who is not infected.* Sexual activity within a monogamous relationship with an uninfected person is safe.
- *Be selective.* If you're going to have more than one partner, have sex only with people you know well.
- *Wash your own genitals before and after contact.* Washing beforehand helps protect your partner. Washing promptly afterward with soap and water helps remove germs. But consider douching to be ineffective.
- *Don't rely on spermicides for additional protection.* They won't prevent transmission of STIs.
- *Use condoms.* Latex condoms (but not condoms made from animal membrane) protect women from having HIV-infected semen enter the vagina and men from contact with HIV-infected vaginal (or other) body fluids. Condoms also prevent transmission of bacterial STIs. Despite concerns among some that condoms will negatively affect sexual pleasure, participants in a nationally representative probability sample did not report that condoms diminished sexual arousal or pleasure (Baldwin et al., 2019).
- *Don't assume that oral sex is a safe alternative.* Although it is unlikely that HIV can be spread by oral sex, other STIs, such as syphilis and HPV, can.
- *If you fear that you have been exposed to HIV or another infectious organism, talk to your doctor about it.* Early treatment is most effective. It is also possible to be exposed to HIV but not yet be infected. Ask your doctor about *post-exposure prophylaxis (PEP)*, which should begin within 72 hours after exposure to HIV.
- *When in doubt, stop.* If you are not sure that sex is safe, stop and think things over or seek expert advice.

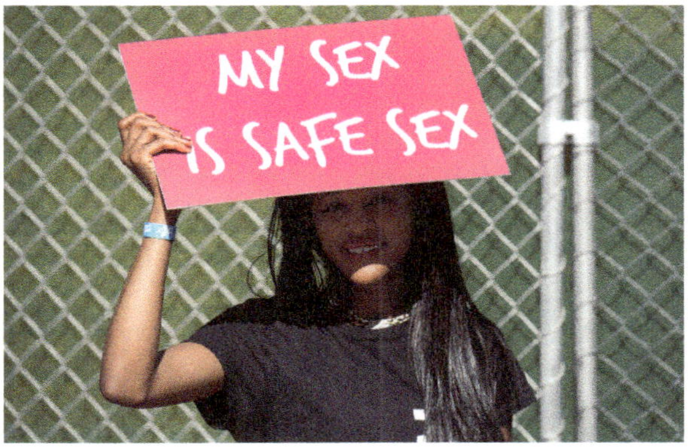

Ronen Tivony/NurPhoto/Getty Images

miss the mark. In adolescents, willingness to abstain from sex or to use condoms when they have sexual intercourse may not directly reflect their cognitive appraisal of perceived threats and benefits. In the heat of the moment, deliberate cognitive appraisal may fly out the window. Adolescents may engage in risky sexual behaviors even if they are aware of the risks, such as unwanted pregnancy, HIV/AIDS, and other STIs.

What factors, then, account for adolescent sexual risk-taking? The Theory of Planned Behavior (TPB; see Chapter 2) points to a key role for subjective norms. Health psychologists find that subjective norms in the form of peer values influence the use of condoms; that is, adolescents are more likely to use condoms and initiate sex at younger ages when they believe that their peers are doing so (O'Dwyer et al., 2019).

Other factors in the TPB also play a role. In a study with college students, researchers found several components of the TPB—positive attitudes (about

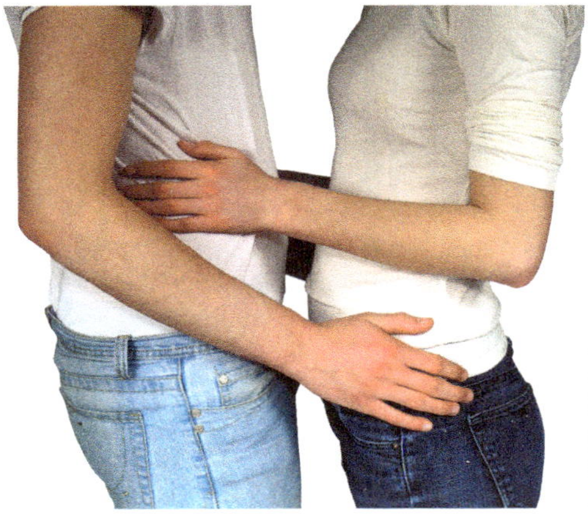
LisaValder/Getty Images

using condoms), perceived behavioral control (belief that one is capable of using condoms and able to obtain them), and subjective norms (beliefs that peers are using them)—predicted intentions to use a condom, which in turn predicted actual condom use (Asare, 2015). In deciding whether to use a condom, sexually active couples weigh the perceived benefits (preventing pregnancy and transmission of sexually transmitted infections) against the perceived barriers (cost of condoms, lessened sexual sensations, or fears of being rejected by asking a partner to use them) (Gehlert & Ward, 2019).

Emotional factors also come into play in sexual risk-taking, such as love (perhaps a crush) and fear of disappointing a partner. Then, too, lack of parental involvement or oversight may be a factor. Researchers believe that the components of the TPB (attitudes toward the behavior, subjective norms, and perceived behavior control) act synergistically, in effect rubbing off on each other to produce behavior change, such as use of condoms (Montanaro, Kershaw, & Bryan, 2018).

Applying Health Psychology

Using the Health Belief Model in Weighing Decisions About Condom Use

The Heath Belief Model (HBM) was originally developed to help explain and predict health-related prevention behaviors such as vaccination against tuberculosis (see Chapter 2). But the model can extend to other health-related behavior, including sexual risk-taking. We can consider how the components of the HBM relate to condom use, which is an important component of safer sexual practices to guard against sexually transmitted infections as well as unwanted pregnancies.

You can apply the model to your decision-making process. We're not telling you what you should do, whether you or your partner should use condoms or not, but we are suggesting it may be helpful to weigh the following factors in making a personal decision.

1. *Perceived susceptibility*. This factor focuses on the person's appraisal of their personal vulnerability to a health risk, such as contracting a sexually transmitted infection. A male partner who is more concerned about his own or his partner's infection status would be more likely to use a condom than one who is confident that he and his partner are free of infection. Also, the person's belief about the likelihood of contracting an infection from an infected partner, or passing one to a partner, would be more likely to use a condom.
2. *Perceived severity*. Here the focus is on the person's perceptions of the severity or seriousness of the consequences of not using a condom. The HBM would predict that a couple would be more likely to use a condom if they believed the risks posed by not using one would involve a potentially dangerous or life-threatening STI, like AIDS, or a lifelong infection, like genital herpes, than a more manageable infection that could be easily cured by a round of antibiotics or if they believed the consequences would be relatively mild or temporary. Similarly, condom use would be more likely if the couple perceived an unwanted pregnancy to be a serious concern.
3. *Perceived benefits*. The HBM considers how people perceive the advantages or benefits of practicing preventive behaviors, such as use of condoms. If people believe that using condoms would benefit the relationship and lead to healthier outcomes, they would be more likely to use them. How, if they doubted whether condom use would produce any positive outcomes, perhaps because they believe that not very effective in preventing disease, they would be unlikely to use them.
4. *Perceived barriers*. The HBM predicts that people are less likely to engage in a health-preventive behavior if they perceive significant barriers or obstacles to their use. In predicting condom use, we might consider factors such as cost (are they affordable?), availability (are they handy when the couple engages in sexual relations?), and degree of effort involved and intrusivenessness (are they difficult to use correctly, how much do they interrupt the sexual act?)
5. *Self-efficacy*. Self-efficacy refers to the confidence we have in our own ability to carry out intended actions, which in this case would involve the couple's belief that they can successfully engage in the preventive behavior (condom use). Self-efficacy estimations are based on skills, experience, and knowledge. A couple who doubt their ability to fit the condom or use it properly, to know which type of condom to purchase, or where to purchase it, would be less likely to use one.
6. *Cues for action*. This component of the HBM refers to triggers that prompt health preventive behaviors. In the case of condom use, a cue for action might be having the condom readily available at the appropriate moment, or a nudge from a partner, or it may involve exposure to a health recommendation from a medical care provider, a friend, or a public health campaign.

Now that we've considered the elements that comprise the HBM and considered how they might relate to the decision to use a condom, take a moment to examine your own attitudes and beliefs in the light of the HBM. Which of these factors, or which combination of these factors, is likely to determine your decision whether or not to use a condom?

Review 10.3

INTERACTIVE SELF-SCORING QUIZZES

Sentence Completion

1. The Centers for Disease Control and Prevention estimates that nearly __________ million Americans contract a sexually transmitted infection each year.

2. Most people with genital __________ don't know they have the disease because they are free of symptoms.

3. Human __________ is the organism that cause genital warts and cervical cancer.

4. HIV/AIDS is caused by the human __________ virus.

5. __________ is the most common bacterial infection.

6. HIV is transmitted by infected blood, __________, vaginal and cervical secretions, and breast milk.

7. Partners of HIV-positive people who are HIV-negative can take oral PrEP (pre-exposure __________) to prevent becoming infected themselves.

Think About It

Consider the methods presented for preventing STIs. Now imagine yourself in a new relationship that could become sexual. Which method or methods of prevention make sense for you? Do they involve communication with your partner? How would you handle that?

Sexual Dysfunctions

VIDEO CONTENT

Sexual Dysfunction and Paraphilias

One important aspect of our sexual health is our ability to perform sexually in the context of mutually satisfying intimate relationships. The belief that sexual fulfillment just comes naturally flies in the face of problems encountered by untold millions, probably hundreds of millions, or people across the world who encounter persistent problems with sexual interest, arousal, or response. When these problems prevent desired sexual activity and are persistent or recurrent, they are classified within a category of mental or psychological disorders called **sexual dysfunctions**. A glance at Table 10.2, which pulls in data from epidemiological studies around the world, will give you an idea of how many people have sexual problems or dysfunctions. The table suggests that nearly half of women and 1 man in 3 or 4 can be diagnosed with a sexual dysfunction today. With the exception of premature ejaculation—that is, ejaculating too soon—these problems tend to arise or increase as we grow older.

sexual dysfunctions Persistent, recurring problems with sexual desire, arousal, or orgasm.

Diagnosis of sexual dysfunctions is organized in terms of types of disorders that correspond to problems of sexual interest, arousal, and responses. Table 10.3 shows the four major categories and also the technical names for the problems, as defined by the American Psychiatric Association (2022).

TABLE 10.2 Prevalence of Sexual Problems Based on Epidemiological Studies from Around the World (Percentages)

	Women	Men
At least one current sexual problem	40–45	20–30
Low sexual interest or desire	20–30	8–25
Arousal and lubrication problems in woman; erectile disorder (ED) in males	25	15–80*
Difficulty reaching orgasm†	16–37‡	12–19
Premature (early) ejaculation		8–30
Sexual pain	1–27	1–6

* The potential high prevalence of erectile disorder reflects the fact that many studies find that the majority of older men may develop erectile problems.
† Difficulty reaching orgasm in women; delayed ejaculation in men.
‡ Some estimates put the percentage as high as 80% for older women.
Sources: Adapted from American Psychiatric Association (2022); McCabe et al. (2016).

INTERACTIVE FIGURES, CHARTS, & TABLES

TABLE 10.3 Sexual Problems and Their Corresponding Diagnostic Terms

Sexual Problem	Diagnostic Term*
Low sexual interest or desire	Male hypoactive sexual desire; female sexual interest/arousal disorder
Difficulty becoming sexually aroused	Male erectile disorder; female sexual interest/arousal disorder†
Difficulties in reaching orgasm	Female orgasmic disorder; in the male: premature ejaculation or delayed ejaculation
Painful sex	Genito-pelvic pain/penetration disorder

* According to the American Psychiatric Association (2022).
† The American Psychiatric Association combines problems in sexual interest and sexual arousal in the case of women. (This labeling has met with criticism within the professional and lay communities.)

In women, problems with sexual arousal are characterized by too little vaginal lubrication to prepare the vagina for penile penetration. Too little lubrication is also the major reason for painful sex in women. Sexual arousal in the male is characterized by erection. Almost all women have difficulty now and then becoming or remaining lubricated. Almost all men have occasional difficulty attaining an erection or maintaining an erection throughout intercourse. These occasional problems are normal and are considered sexual dysfunctions only when they become persistent or recurrent.

Biopsychosocial Factors in Sexual Dysfunctions

Like many of the health issues we encounter in this text, sexual dysfunctions are complex problems that reflect multifaceted causes. The biopsychosocial model of disease is especially helpful in understanding these problems, as they often involve an interaction of biological, psychological, and sociocultural factors.

Women who have difficulty becoming aroused or reaching orgasm most often do not receive adequate sexual stimulation, although it is also possible that they do not find their partners appealing, are tired, or have been drinking heavily. If women have not lubricated adequately, pain may prevent them from reaching orgasm or wanting to continue with sexual stimulation. Men with difficulty reaching orgasm may similarly not find their partners appealing, be tired, be drinking too much, or just aging (not an issue for most college students!). In some cases, people can reach orgasm readily by masturbating or by having sex with one partner but not another. These types of problems, as well as problems of low sexual interest, are more common among women than men. Men in adolescence and early adulthood are more commonly troubled by premature ejaculation. They ejaculate with minimal sexual stimulation, often frustrating their partners.

Many sexual problems have biological causes, reflecting chronic health conditions, which tend to accumulate as we age. Lack of sexual desire in either men or women may result from low levels of testosterone. (Yes, women do secrete testosterone in the ovaries, adrenal glands, and elsewhere, and it is connected with their sex drive.) Low levels of estrogen, as following menopause, seriously hamper female lubrication. Diabetes can damage blood vessels and nerves, including those that provide blood to the penis, leading to erectile disorder. Erectile dysfunction may also involve other medical problems affecting the flow of blood to and through the penis or damage to nerves involved in erection.

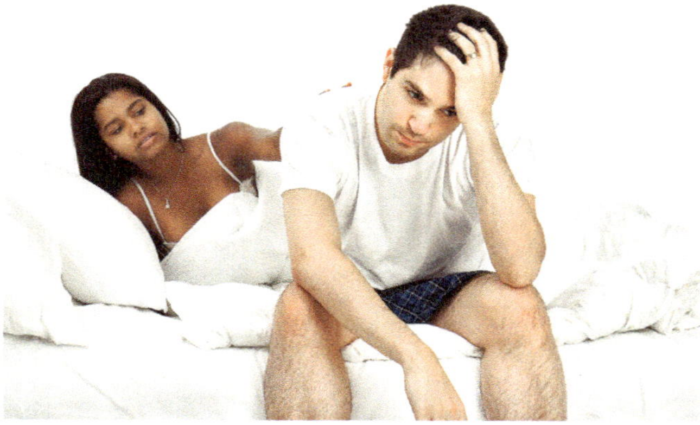

jhorrocks/Getty Images

A Problem It didn't go according to script tonight—or last night. A sexual problem can become exacerbated when couples become anxious about it, because anxiety interferes with sexual response. A person can fall into a vicious cycle in which sexual failure on one occasion leads to anxiety on the next occasion, which further dampens sexual response, and so on. A sex therapist can help couples break the cycle.

Obesity increases the risks not only of heart disease and diabetes but also of erectile disorder (Liu et al., 2023). The underlying process may involve high blood cholesterol levels. Cholesterol leads to formation of fatty deposits (plaque) in blood vessels that can impede the flow of blood to the penis just as it impedes the flow of blood to the heart. Health psychology interventions that help obese men lose weight and increase their activity levels can lead to better erectile functioning (Mulhall et al., 2018).

Fatigue can reduce sexual desire and inhibit sexual response. Depressants such as alcohol, narcotics, and tranquilizers can also impair sexual response. Lack of sexual drive or interest may be connected with mental health problems, such as depression. Health problems, including coronary heart disease, multiple sclerosis, spinal cord injuries, and complications from certain surgical procedures, such as prostate surgery, can cause sexual problems in both men and women. The use of medications to treat high blood pressure and high levels of cholesterol can severely dampen sexual response.

In other cases, sexual trauma is implicated. Physically or psychologically painful sexual experiences, such as child sexual abuse or sexual assault, can block future sexual response (Meston & Stanton, 2017). Survivors of child sexual abuse or sexual assault often find it difficult to respond sexually to their partners or may respond to sexual stimulation with deep feelings of revulsion or disgust; feelings of helplessness, anger, or guilt; or even flashbacks to the abuse or assault rather than pleasure.

Cultural beliefs can also affect sexual response and sexual behavior. For example, one traditional stereotype suggests that men find sex pleasurable but that sex is a duty for women. In this "liberated" day and age, it may seem hard to imagine that some Americans are unaware of women's potential for experiencing sexual pleasure. But remember that this is a nation with literally hundreds of subcultures. People reared in some traditions may acquire attitudes toward sexuality that differ from those we regularly see in the popular media. Even if they have cognitive awareness of their sexual potential from the media, sex education programs, or peers, conflicting attitudes and anxiety may make it difficult for them to act on their knowledge.

Sex Therapy

If people bring sexual problems to the attention of a helping professional, sex therapy may be recommended, especially when the problems do not have obvious biological causes. Sex therapy is a form of psychological treatment that generally incorporates educational, cognitive, and behavioral components. Sex therapy is largely indebted to the pioneering work of Masters and Johnson (1970), but other therapists have developed techniques to help couples improve their sexual functioning. Sex therapists typically use the following techniques:

- *Reducing performance anxiety.* Anxiety is associated with sympathetic nervous system activity, which inhibits sexual arousal (see Chapter 4). Unfortunately, people with sexual problems often develop **performance anxiety** when they contemplate their next sexual opportunities (see **Figure 10.8**). One man with erectile dysfunction said that on a date he kept thinking about how disappointed his partner would be if he failed to perform sexually. He went on to say "By the time we did go to bed, I was paralyzed with anxiety." Therapists therefore often begin sex therapy by asking couples to touch, massage, or stroke each other in nongenital areas of the body in order to diminish performance anxiety. Lessened performance anxiety allows natural reflexes, such as erection, lubrication, and eventually orgasm, to occur.
- *Changing irrational beliefs and expectations.* If we believe that we need a lover's approval at all times, we may view a disappointing sexual episode as a catastrophe. If we demand that every sexual encounter be perfect, we set ourselves up for failure. Clients are shown how expectations of failure can increase anxiety and become self-fulfilling prophecies. The irrational belief that a man somehow knows what he is doing sexually—or ought to know—places great demands on couples. For one thing, it discourages many men from seeking (scientific) knowledge about sex or even asking their partners what they like. The belief also leads many women to be reluctant to guide their partners in sexually arousing them. They may think that if they are "forward," or express their sexual likes and dislikes, they will be viewed as "sluttish." But it is irrational for people to expect that their lovers can read their minds.

performance anxiety Fear as to whether or not one will be able to carry out a task or behavior adequately.

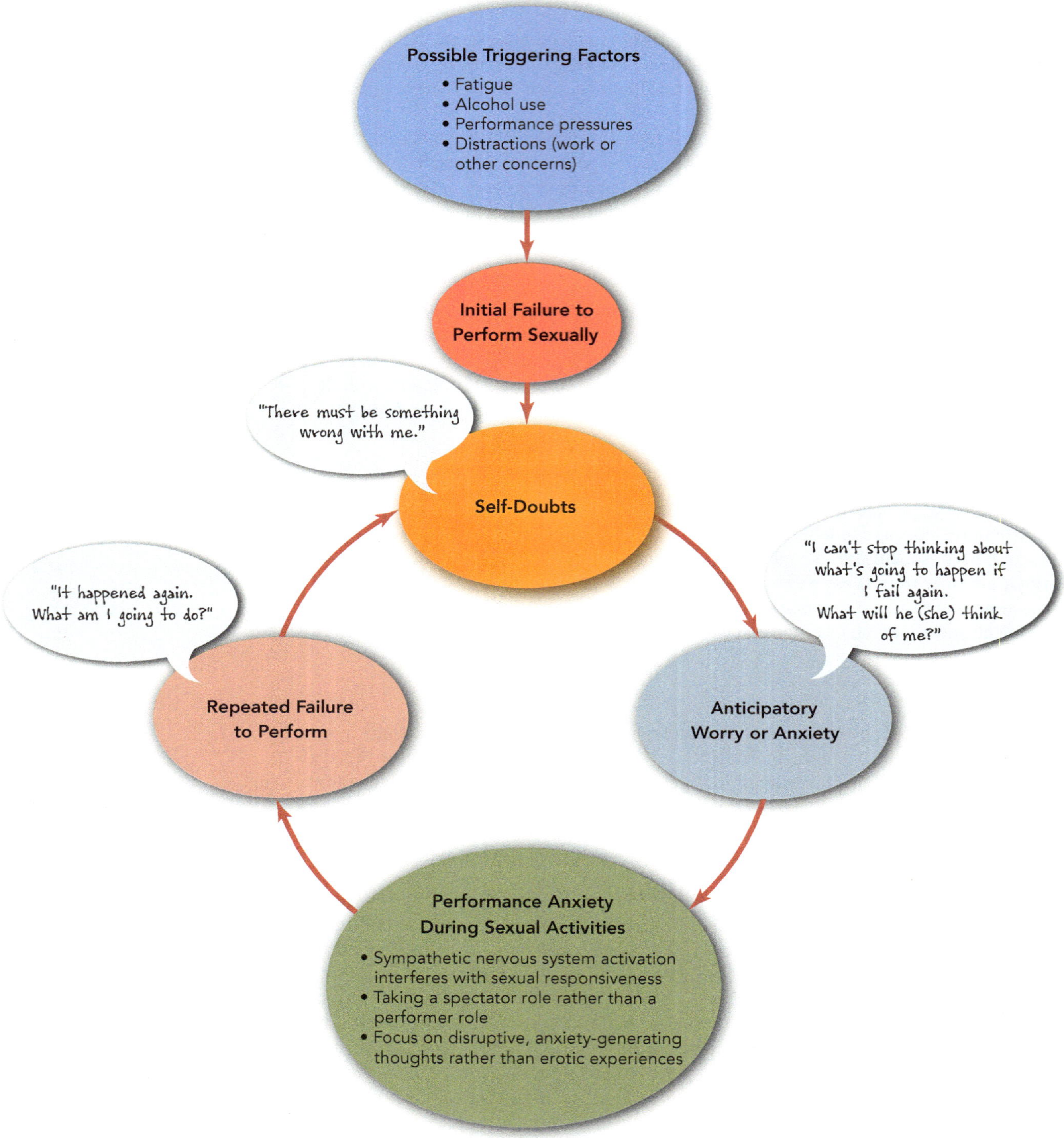

FIGURE 10.8 **The Vicious Cycle of Performance Anxiety and Failure**

- *Teaching sexual skills.* Sexual competencies, like other competencies, are based on knowledge and skill and derive largely from learning experiences. Although sex is a natural function, we learn what makes us and others feel good through trial and error, by talking and reading about sex, and perhaps by watching erotic films. In therapy, clients lacking sexual skills may be taught how to provide each other with adequate sexual stimulation.

In the case of premature ejaculation, they may also be shown how to delay ejaculation by means such as the *stop-and-go* method (repeatedly pausing as the man becomes highly aroused and then restarting, so that the man becomes better able to gauge the level of stimulation, or point of no return, that triggers ejaculation).

- *Enhancing sexual knowledge.* Some problems are connected to ignorance or misinformation about biological and sexual functioning.
- *Focusing on the relationship.* A sexual relationship is usually no better than other aspects of a relationship (Maxwell & McNulty, 2019). Problems in the relationship may not be left at the bedroom door. Deep-seated feelings of anger and resentment may be difficult to turn off in bed. In therapy, partners are taught ways of coping with problems in the relationship and of enhancing sexual communication by showing each other what they like and do not like.

The Good-Enough Sex Model

> *With the Good-Enough Sex model, intimacy is the ultimate focus, with pleasure as important as function, and mutual emotional acceptance as the environment. Sex is integrated into the couple's daily life and daily life is integrated into their sex life to create the couple's unique sexual style.*
>
> **—Metz & McCarthy (2007, p. 351)**

As women and men age, it is normal for their sexual performance to decline in various ways. It may take longer for men to obtain an erection and for women to lubricate. Erections may not be as firm as they used to be, and women may encounter vaginal discomfort. Men, especially aging men, may turn to the use of erectile drugs such as Viagra or Cialis to restore their performance. Efforts to find a "female Viagra" that might compensate for age-related changes have not been as successful. A different approach, sometimes called the good-enough sex model, brings reality into the picture. The focus is on intimacy, not performance. Good-enough sex need not always involve penile penetration. Good-enough sex need not always culminate in orgasm for either or both partners. The pursuit of perfectionism is an obstacle to true intimacy, as is nostalgia for the years gone by. Reasonable expectations buffer feelings of disappointment and overreactions to sexual problems. Sexuality is viewed as a means to relieve stress, to reap pleasure from physical contact, and, perhaps most important, to strengthen and reaffirm the importance of the relationship.

Review 10.4

INTERACTIVE SELF-SCORING QUIZZES

Sentence Completion

1. (Women or men) are more likely to experience painful sex.
2. Women with female sexual interest/_____ disorder have difficulty lubricating.
3. A sexual __________ is a persistent or recurrent sexual problem that is of concern to the individual or the couple.
4. __________ anxiety is fear as to whether or not one will be able to carry out a task or behavior adequately.
5. Men with persistent difficulty attaining or maintaining an erection are said to have __________ __________.
6. Males who ejaculate too quickly may be diagnosed with __________ __________.
7. __________ __________ generally focuses on reducing performance anxiety, changing irrational beliefs, teaching sexual skills, enhancing sexual knowledge, and improving relationships.

Think About It

Think of family, friends, teachers, and religious leaders who have been a part of your life. Also think about your favorite movies, TV shows, and books. What messages about sex have you received from these sources? Do they mesh together, or do they contradict? How do you think they have contributed to your own attitudes toward sex and whether you are likely to develop sexual problems?

The Health of LGBTQ+ Individuals

LGBTQ An acronym for lesbian, gay, bisexual, transgender, queer or questioning.

The health of **LGBTQ+** individuals has emerged as a key area of research and practice for health psychologists, other health professionals, and researchers. Health psychologists are intimately involved in studying and attempting to lower the barriers to the diagnosis, treatment, and prevention of health problems among LGBTQ+ individuals. Healthcare providers need to be sensitive to the historical stigmatization experienced by LGBTQ+ individuals, their experiences (frequently negative) with healthcare providers, and the prevalence of certain risk factors and health problems in these individuals (Baldwin et al., 2018).

sexual orientation The directionality of one's erotic and romantic interests—toward members of the same sex, the other sex, both, or neither.

gay Men who are sexually attracted to and desire to form romantic relationships with other men.

lesbian Females who are sexually attracted to and interested in forming relationships with other females.

heterosexual The sexual orientation in which a person experiences erotic attraction to and preference for developing romantic relationships with members of the other sex.

bisexual The sexual orientation in which a person experiences erotic attraction to and preference for developing romantic relationships with members of either the same or the other sex.

Sexual Orientation

Miley Cyrus became well known to the public through her role in *Hannah Montana*, a Disney Channel series. She played Miley Stewart, who was your average American schoolgirl during the day but led a double life as teen idol recording artist Hannah Montana at night. When the series ended, Miley could be said to have embarked upon another double life—she shot dramatically from wholesome teenager to a flesh-baring pop star under her own name.

Is Miley Cyrus leading a third double life in terms of her sexual orientation? She is an LGBTQ+ activist who reports having romantic and sexual relationships with people of any gender. She reports romantic relationships with women that were as serious as the relationships with men such as actor Liam Hemsworth. "I'm very open about it," she told a British magazine. "I'm pansexual." She elaborated on her sexual orientation and gender identity in an interview with *Paper* magazine:

> *I am literally open to every single thing that is consenting and doesn't involve an animal and everyone is of age. Everything that's legal, I'm down with ... I'm down with any adult—anyone over the age of 18 who is down to love me. I don't relate to being boy or girl, and I don't have to have my partner relate to boy or girl. I've had [relationships with women] but people never really looked at it, and I never brought it into the spotlight.*
>
> **—Miley Cyrus, cited in Petrusich (2015)**

The term **sexual orientation** refers to an enduring emotional, romantic, or sexual attraction toward members of one's own sex, the other sex, both, or neither. The American Psychological Association (2015) defines sexual orientation as

> *A component of identity that includes a person's sexual and emotional attraction to another person and the behavior and/or social affiliation that may result from this attraction. A person may be attracted to men, women, both, neither, or to people who are genderqueer, androgynous, or have other gender identities. Individuals may identify as lesbian, gay, heterosexual, bisexual, queer, pansexual, or asexual, among others.*

People who are generally attracted to people of their own sex identify as **gay** or **lesbian**. People who are **heterosexual**, or "straight," are generally attracted to people of the other sex. It's not just about sexual behavior, however. Lesbians, gay men, and heterosexuals also prefer to develop romantic relationships with, respectively, people of their own sex or people of the other sex. People who are **bisexual** are generally attracted to both women and men.

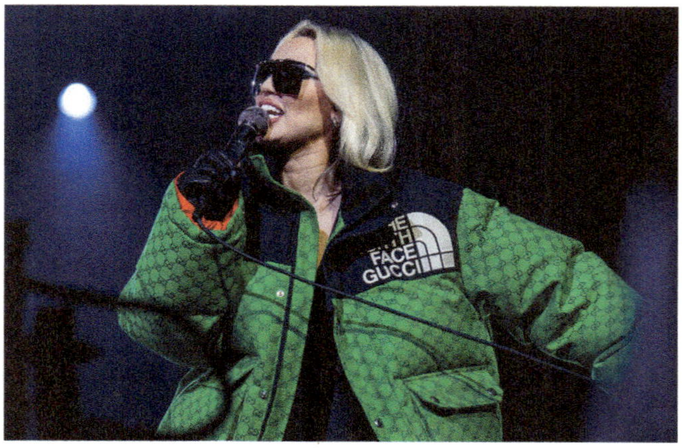

Mauricio Santana/Getty Images

Miley Cyrus

We commonly hear the term "gay marriage" used as being synonymous with "same-sex marriage," and in this case "gay" refers to lesbians as well as to gay men.

In Western culture, few sexual practices have been met with such widespread censure as sexual activities with members of one's own sex. In the Bible, the Book of Leviticus (20:13) is also clear in its condemnation:

> ***If a man lies with a man as with a woman, both of them have committed an abomination; they shall be put to death, their blood is upon them.***

Same-sex sexual behavior has been outlawed or frowned upon in nearly every society for thousands of years. Some nations, including Saudi Arabia, Afghanistan, and Iran, consider male–to-male sexual behavior to be a crime punishable by death. Yet after decades of debate, public opinion in the United States has shifted. About 70% of people in the United States now support same-sex marriage (McCarthy, 2023). The shift preceded the Supreme Court ruling of 2015 that people of the same sex have a constitutional right to get married. Why the change? Many reasons. LGBTQ+ characters were populating TV shows and movies. Greater acceptance has also come from more people knowing or working with LGBTQ+ individuals. As more LGBTQ+ people disclose their sexual orientations and gender identities, those around them realize that they are friends, family, coworkers, and public role models. It is inconsistent to enjoy the work of public personalities such as Kate McKinnon, Ellen DeGeneres, Anderson Cooper, Elton John, and Neil Patrick Harris and to condemn their sexual orientations. We also have many openly gay politicians, including Secretary of transportation Pete Buttigieg and Colorado governor Jared Polis.

Gender and Gender Identity

Yes, my teenage son is transgender. No, you may not ask about his genitals.

I am the mother of a 16-year-old transgender boy. For years, our child, whom we had thought was our daughter, suffered from depression, anxiety, an eating disorder, self-cutting and suicidal thoughts before he came to us with his big secret. He was, in fact, male and he had hidden this through episodes of bullying and transfers to five different schools in three years. His life had been painful and he had wanted to end it at times. Finally, with the help of a kind and understanding therapist, he'd decided at the age of 15 to share with us who he truly was inside. We immediately showered him with love and support and watched with amazement as his anxiety and depression all but disappeared. Living as his true self was the blessing he'd been looking for, and our family was so much better off with a happy and more adjusted son.

—**Sharon Dunski (2015)**

Why would Sharon Dunski be referring to her son's genitalia? The answer is that many **transgender** (or "trans") individuals undergo gender affirmation surgery to provide the appearance of the genitals of people of the anatomic sex with which they identify. But many others do not. While some transgender individuals wish to possess the anatomic features of people of the other sex, others do not. Further, some transgender individuals identify as transgender whereas others identify as men or women or another identity, such as genderqueer, nonbinary, or somewhere else along (or outside of) the gender spectrum.

According to the American Psychological Association's *Dictionary of Psychology*, **gender** is defined as "the condition of being male, female, or neuter. In a human context, the distinction between gender and SEX reflects the usage of these terms—Sex usually refers to the biological aspects of maleness or femaleness, whereas gender implies the psychological, behavioral, social, and cultural aspects of being male or female (i.e., masculinity or femininity)."

The American Psychological Association (2015) then goes on to define gender identity as "A person's deeply-felt, inherent sense of being a boy, a man, or male; a girl, a woman, or female; or an alternative gender (e.g., gender queer, gender nonconforming, gender neutral) that may or may not correspond to a person's sex assigned at birth or to a person's primary or secondary sex characteristics. Since gender identity is internal, a person's **gender identity** is not necessarily visible to others."

Gender identity is one of the most obvious and important aspects of our self-concept. **Sex assignment** reflects the child's anatomy, and it refers to a process that typically occurs at birth, although with the use of blood tests and imaging techniques in developed nations, it frequently occurs during prenatal development.

When a person's gender identity is consistent with their sexual anatomy, they are said to be **cisgender**. When a person's gender identity is at odds with their sexual anatomy, as is the case with Sharon Dunski's son, they are said to be transgender. Significant distress that may occur when one's gender identity is not consistent with their sexual anatomy is termed **gender dysphoria** by the American Psychiatric Association (2022).

transgender An umbrella term for people whose gender identity is different from their sex assigned at birth.

gender The psychological state of being female or male (or somewhere else along the gender spectrum), as influenced by cultural concepts of stereotypical gender-appropriate traits and behavior. Contrast the concept of gender with that of *anatomic sex*, which is based on the physical differences between females and males.

gender identity One's sense of being male or female (or somewhere else along or outside of the gender spectrum).

sex assignment The labeling of a newborn (or fetus) as a male or female.

cisgender Relating to or denoting a person whose gender identity is consistent with his or her assigned sex at birth.

gender dysphoria According to the American Psychiatric Association, gender dysphoria is conflict between people's assigned sex and the gender with which they identify, which may lead to discomfort with their bodies and the social roles commonly associated with their assigned sex.

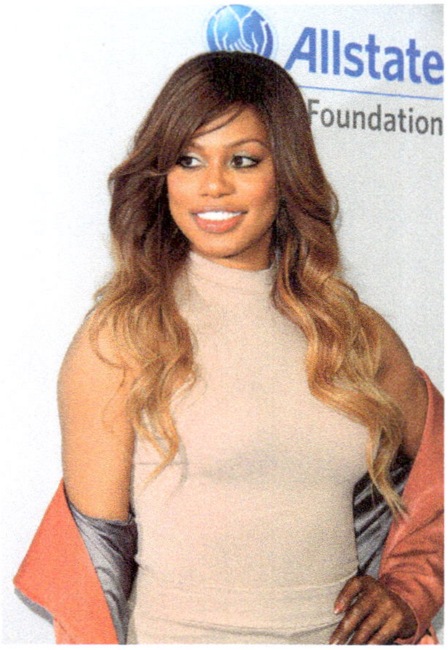

Everett Collection Inc/Alamy Stock Photo

Orange Is the New Black Actress Laverne Cox The appearance of transgender celebrities, such as Caitlyn Jenner, Chas Bono, and Laverne Cox, has familiarized many Americans with matters of gender identity. In an interview, Cox told Katie Couric, "The preoccupation with transition and surgery objectifies trans people. And then we don't get to really deal with the real lived experiences. The reality of trans people's lives is that so often we are targets of violence. We experience discrimination disproportionately to the rest of the community."

Many transgender individuals undergo hormone treatments and surgery to create a facsimilie of the external genitals typical of the other sex. This can be done more readily with male-to-female than female-to-male individuals. After the decision to have surgery is reached, hormone treatments, which must be taken for a lifetime, are begun. Male-to-female transgender women receive estrogen, which fosters the development of fatty deposits in the breasts and hips, softens the skin, and inhibits growth of facial hair. Female-to-male transgender men receive male sex hormones, which deepen the voice, distribute hair according to the male pattern, enlarge muscles, and lessen fatty deposits in the breasts and hips.

As noted, many transgender individuals retain their reproductive organs, but others undergo gender-affirming surgery. In female-to-male transitions, the internal sex organs (ovaries, fallopian tubes, uterus) are removed, along with the fatty tissue in the breasts. Some transgender men engage in a series of operations to construct an artificial penis, called metoidioplasty. After surgery some transgender women can participate in sexual intercourse and even attain orgasm, assuming that the muscles that originally surrounded the base of the penis—and which now surround the constructed vaginal barrel—remain undamaged (Barcelos et al., 2022). Metoidioplasty does not often create a penis that is large enough for sexual intercourse; nor can transgender men ejaculate.

Reviews of the literature confirm that gender-affirmation surgeries are generally safe and that complication rates are low. An analysis of date from 27,715 individuals throughout the United States who had obtained gender affirmation surgery found that they were less likely than transgender people who had not had surgery to experience distress in the past month (Almazan & Keuroghlian, 2021). Those who obtained gender-affirmation surgery were also less likely to have binged on alcohol, smoked cigarettes, or considered suicide within the past year.

Having noted these generally positive results for gender reassignment, we should add that practitioners in the field urge caution when it comes to treating children and adolescents. Not all children and adolescents with gender dysphoria develop into adults who desire gender reassignment. Therefore, a common medical practice among adolescents who identify as transgender is to start a regimen of puberty blockers—hormones that suppress secondary sex characteristics—in order to delay the gender-affirmation surgery decision-making process. Secondary sex characteristics include growing facial hair and enhance distress among transgender adolescents who identify as female, for instance. However, some individuals may eventually choose to retain the gender identity consistent with their assigned sex at birth and identify as gay men or lesbians. Once puberty blocking has taken place, it cannot be reversed; therefore, many parents of transgender children who desire gender affirmation hormone treatments and eventual surgery are in deep conflict because they wonder whether their children's wishes and decisions will remain constant for their lifetimes.

How Many People Are "LGBTQ+"?

Numerous surveys and polls have attempted to define the numbers of LGBTQ individuals in the general population. One of the most reliable of these is the Gallup Organization Daily Tracking Survey of sexual orientation and gender in the United States (Jones, 2022). The results are based on some 340,000 interviews, and the results show that since 2012, when the tracking poll began, the overall percentage of adults identifying as LGBT (lesbian, gay, bisexual, or transgender) has risen steadily from 3.5% to 7.1%.[1]

It is particularly fascinating to break down the results by age group. **Figure 10.9** shows that about 20% of members of Generation Z, born between 1997 and 2003, the youngest group in the survey, are likely to identify as LGBT. About 10% of Millennials, born between 1981 and 1996, self-report as LGBT, as compared with 4.2% of people born between 1965 and 1983, 2.6% of "Baby Boomers," who were born between 1946 and 1964, and 0.8% of people who were

[1] The Gallup survey used LGBT, not LGBTQ; therefore, we can only report results for people who identified as lesbian, gay, bisexual, or transgender (LGBT).

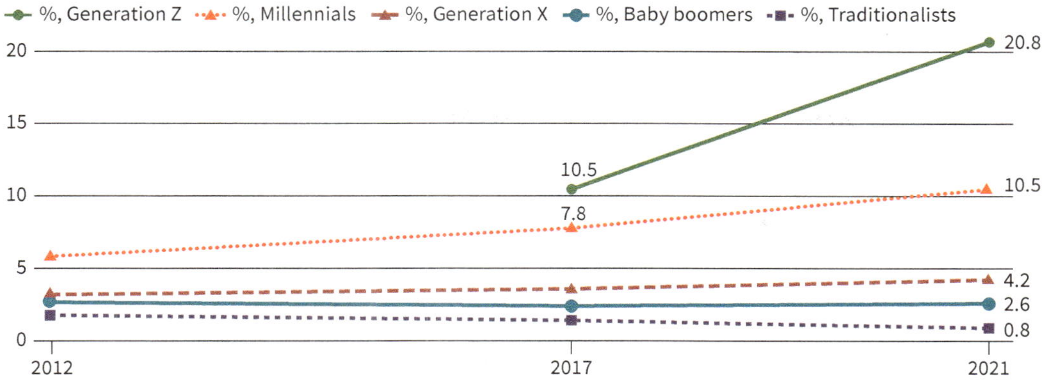

FIGURE 10.9 **Percentage of Americans Identifying as LGBT, by Birth Cohort**

Source: F. Newport (2018). In U.S., estimate of LGBT population rises to 4.5%. https://news.gallup.com/poll/234863/estimate-lgbt-population-rises.aspx © 2018. Gallup, Inc.

born before 1946. The older the group, the less likely they are to report identifying as LGBT. There are at least two possibilities for the age differences, and both may be at work. First, people belonging to older age groups, who grew up in an atmosphere in which there was more prejudice against LGBTQ individuals, may be less willing to report their LGBT status. Second, younger people—perhaps due to a more accepting social atmosphere and to the visibility of LGBTQ people in the media—are more likely to discover their sexual orientation and gender identities at an early age. It is unlikely that the actual incidence of an LGBTQ identity has changed significantly over the past decades.

The majority of LGBT individuals surveyed by the Gallup poll are lesbian, gay, or bisexual. About 1.8% of a population-based survey from 10 state and 9 urban school districts identified as transgender (Johns et al., 2019). If that percentage is accurate, millions of Americans are transgender.

Biological Perspectives on LGBTQ+ Individuals

Here is a question for heterosexual and cisgender readers of this book—Did you *choose* to be heterosexual? Did you choose whether you saw yourself as being a female or being a male? Can you remember a time in childhood or adolescence when you surveyed the people around you and decided that you would be attracted to members of the other sex? Can you remember a time when you decided you were really a member of the other sex?

The answer will most likely be "no." The answer is the same for LGBTQ+ individuals. They do not *choose* to whom they will be attracted. Why, then, in a society that has not yet fully accepted LGBTQ+ people, do people become lesbian, gay, bisexual, transgender, queer, or questioning? The answer may have something to do with sex hormones.

Sex hormones govern the mating behavior of other species (Hines et al., 2015; Pradhan et al., 2015). Researchers have looked into possible hormonal factors in determining sexual orientation in humans. The male sex hormone testosterone is essential to the prenatal development of male reproductive organs. Thus, levels of testosterone and its by-products in the blood and urine have been studied as possible influences on sexual orientation, but research has failed to connect sexual orientation in people of either sex with hormone levels *in adulthood* (Hines et al., 2015).

What of prenatal development, however (Baum & Bakker, 2017; Reinisch et al., 2017)? Swedish neuroscientists Ivanka Savic and her colleagues (2010) report evidence that one's gender identity as being male or being female and one's sexual orientation (heterosexual, lesbian, gay, or bisexual) can develop during pregnancy. They note that sexual differentiation of the sex organs occurs during the first 2 months of pregnancy, whereas sexual differentiation of the brain begins later, during the second half of pregnancy. Sexual differentiation of the genitals and the brain both depend on surges of testosterone, but because they happen at different times, they can occur independently. Therefore, it is possible that an individual's sex organs can develop in one direction while the biological factors that may underlie an individual's sexual orientation develop in another direction.

Some transgender women (i.e., male-to-female women) recall that, as children, they preferred playing with dolls, enjoyed wearing dresses, and disliked rough-and-tumble play (Zucker, 2005a, 2005b). They were often perceived by their peers as "sissy boys." Some transgender men (female-to-male men) report that, as children, they disliked dresses and acted like "tomboys." They preferred playing "boys' games" and playing those games with boys. These behavior patterns may well be rooted in prenatal development of the brain.

The Health and Healthcare of LGBTQ+ Individuals

Even though the social climate has been improving for LGBTQ+ individuals, they are much more likely than the general population to develop psychological disorders. Most often, negative psychological and health outcomes among LGBTQ+ individuals can be attributed to discrimination, harassment, and stigma (Lee et al., 2016). Michael King and his colleagues (2008) analyzed 476 articles on the mental health of lesbian, gay, and bisexual people and found that they were more than twice as likely as heterosexual people to have attempted suicide. Lesbian, gay, and bisexual people were 1.5 times as likely to be anxious and depressed, to be overweight or obese, and to engage in substance abuse and smoke cigarettes. More recent research continues to support the finding of a disparity between the mental health of LGBTQ+ individuals and that of the general population (Abreu et al., 2022; Watson et al., 2018a, 2018b). For example, gay and bisexual men are more likely than heterosexual men to have eating disorders.

A survey of nearly 2,000 transgender adolescents in the United States found them to be at higher risk of depression and anxiety than their cisgender peers (Jardas et al., 2023). The researchers linked their poorer mental health to exposure to gender stress, such as exposure to prejudice, expectations of rejection, and their felt need to conceal their gender identity. Exposure to discrimination based on sexual orientation also places lesbian, gay, and bisexual (LGB) people at heightened risk of health problems (Huebner et al., 2021). Health researchers also recognize the need to take into account the intersectionality of race and ethnicity with sexual and gender identity, as by examining the particularly stressful effects of cultural biases faced by LGBT youth of color (Alegría & Cheng, 2023; Jackson et al., 2023).

There is also a connection between lifestyle and health—physical and psychological—among the LGBTQ+ population, just as there is among heterosexual people. Gay men and lesbians occupy all socioeconomic and vocational levels and follow a variety of lifestyles. It is worth mentioning the classic research of Alan P. Bell and Martin S. Weinberg (1978), who found variations in the mental health of LGBT individuals that seem to mirror the variations in the heterosexual community. Gay people who lived with partners in enduring relationships were about as healthy as married heterosexual couples.

Yet according to the Human Rights Campaign (2018), psychological well-being remains difficult for young LGBTQ+ people:

- Only 24% say they can definitely be themselves as LGBTQ at home.
- Only 25% have families that support them by getting involved in the larger LGBTQ community and its allies.
- 67% hear their families saying negative things about LGBTQ people.
- 78% have not disclosed their sexual orientations or gender identities to their parents because of the negative comments their parents make.

Because of the backdrop of social condemnation and discrimination, lesbians and gay males in our culture often struggle to come to terms with their sexual orientation (Savin-Williams, 2019, 2022). Lesbians and gay males speak of the process of accepting their sexual orientation as *coming out*. Coming out is a two-pronged process—coming out to oneself (recognizing one's own sexual orientation) and coming out to others (declaring one's orientation to the world).

Adolescents and young adults in big cities such as New York and Los Angeles may come out earlier than those in more remote areas (Hulko, 2018) due to a more accepting social atmosphere. Coming out to others occasionally means an open declaration to the world. Often, a person may inform only one or a few select people, perhaps friends rather than family members. Disclosure can be fraught with the risk of loss of jobs, friendships, and familial disapproval (Savin-Williams, 2019, 2022). If the organization at which an individual works is generally supportive of the LGBTQ+ community, however, coming out can be related to greater job satisfaction and less anxiety (Savin-Williams, 2019, 2022).

LGBTQ individuals experience many barriers when seeking health care. Their experiences with healthcare providers are frequently negative, resulting in hesitance to consult them (Baldwin et al., 2018). Just as healthcare providers too often attribute the health problems of people who are overweight to their weight, so do healthcare providers too often connect the health issues of LGBTQ people with their sexual or gender identity. An analysis of the healthcare experiences of 119 transgender and genderqueer individuals found that their experiences with providers were positive when the providers treated their identity disclosure as routine, did not show discomfort in treating them, and relied on their education and experience in working with them (Baldwin et al., 2019). According to Aleta Baldwin and her colleagues (2018), medical educators, administrators, and providers all share responsibility for improving the patient experiences of transgender people. Improved patient experiences lead to LGBTQ individuals being more likely to seek treatment when needed and to comply with treatment.

Homophobia and Transphobia

Homophobia and **transphobia** persist and account for the greatest challenge to the mental health of members of the LGBTQ community. They take many forms, including the following:

- Using derogatory names (such as "faggot" and "dyke")
- Telling disparaging jokes about LGBTQ individuals
- Barring gay people from housing, employment, or social opportunities
- Taunting (verbal abuse)
- Gay bashing (physical, sometimes deadly, abuse)

homophobia Fear of, hatred of, or discomfort with those attracted to members of the same sex.

transphobia Fear of, hatred of, or discomfort with people whose gender identity is inconsistent with their assigned sex.

biphobia Fear of, hatred of, or discomfort with people who are bisexual.

According to the FBI, about 1 in every 5 hate crimes in the United States is directed against gay men, lesbians, or transgender individuals (U.S. Department of Justice, 2023). Although some psychologists link homophobia to fears of gay men or lesbians within oneself, homophobic attitudes are more common among men who identify with a traditional tough male gender role and a conservative political orientation (Herek, 2016; Rosky, 2016). Men have more at stake in maintaining the tradition of male dominance, so perhaps it is not surprising that college men are more intolerant of gay men than college women are (Herek, 2016; Rosky, 2016).

Biphobia is fear of, hatred of, or discomfort with individuals who are sexually attracted to, and desire romantic relationships with, people of either sex. The ironic thing about biphobia is that it may be harbored by lesbians and gay males, themselves victims of prejudice and discrimination, who believe that biphobia represents lack of commitment to a lesbian or gay male sexual orientation (McConnell et al., 2018). Transphobia is the fear of, hatred of, or discomfort with transgender individuals. **Table 10.4** shows the relative health risk behaviors of cisgender male, cisgender female, and transgender high school students.

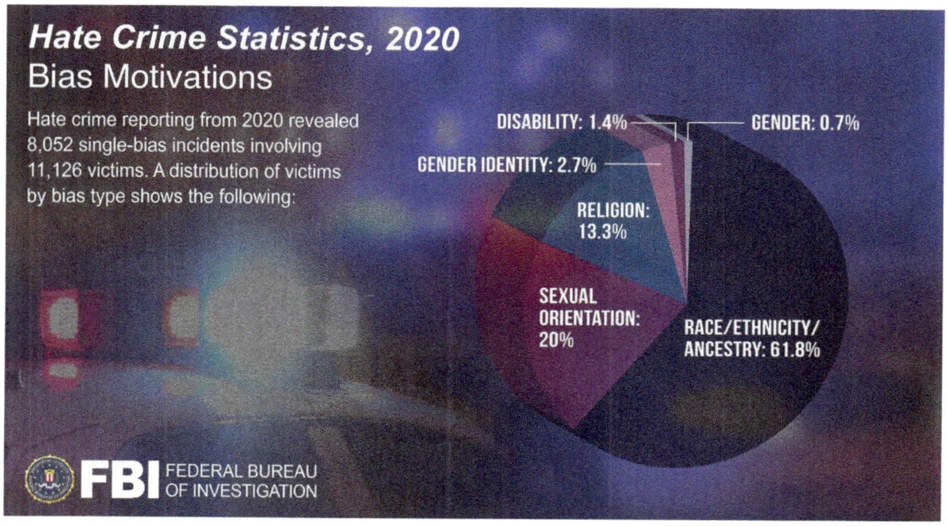

Federal Bureau of Investigation/Public Domain

Even in this climate of gradually increasing social acceptance, restrictive "bathroom laws" and policies in various locales prevent transgender youth from using facilities that are congruent with their gender identities. One youth says "I wait until I get home (from school) to use the bathroom, even when I'm at school for 10+ hours. . . . I wear my gym clothes over my normal clothes to avoid changing in locker rooms" (Human Rights Campaign, 2018). What in

TABLE 10.4 Health Risk Behaviors of Cisgender Male, Cisgender Female, and Transgender High School Students, in Percentages

Health Risk Behaviors or Experiences	Cisgender Males	Cisgender Females	Transgender Students
Felt unsafe at or traveling to/from school	4.6	7.1	26.9
Threatened or injured with a weapon at school	6.4	4.1	23.8
Bullied at school	14.7	20.7	34.6
Cocaine, lifetime use	4.3	2.6	27.2
Heroin, lifetime use	2.2	0.7	26.1
Attempted suicide	5.5	9.1	34.6
Did not use condom during last sexual intercourse	37.6	48.9	63.8
Drank alcohol or used drugs before last sexual intercourse	19.2	17.9	30.0

Source: Adapted from M. M. Johns, R. Lowry, J. Andrzejewski, L. C. Barrios, Z. Demissie, T. McManus, . . . & J. M. Underwood (2019). Transgender identity and experiences of violence victimization, substance use, suicide risk, and sexual risk behaviors among high school students—19 states and large urban school districts, 2017. *Morbidity and Mortality Weekly Report, 68*(3), 67–71.

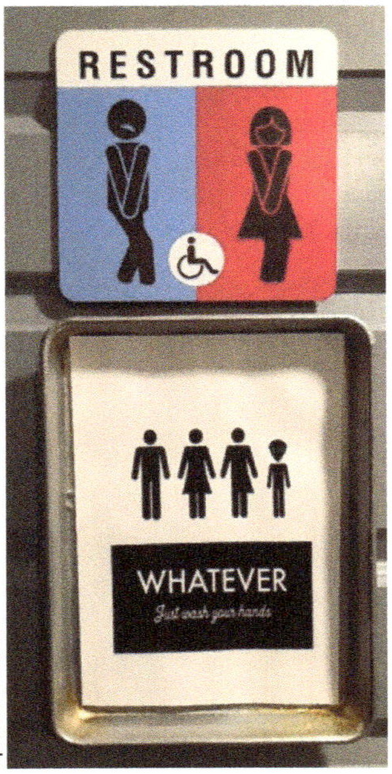

Spencer Rathus

general do trans youth who are unable to use the bathroom or locker room that is congruent with their gender identity do?

- 65% try not to use the bathroom at school.
- 65% use bathrooms and locker rooms that do not match their gender identity.
- 28% use facilities that are intended for only one person at a time.
- 25% try to avoid showing their bodies or changing their clothing.
- 19% do not shower or change their clothes "even when I should."

The health of LGBTQ+ individuals is intertwined with the attitudes they find in the families and communities in which they live, and in the ways in which health professionals welcome them and interact with them. Health psychologists emphasize the importance of the dignity of the individual. If society at large also focused on the dignity of LGBTQ+ individuals, the health of sexual and gender minorities would be enhanced.

Review 10.5

INTERACTIVE SELF-SCORING QUIZZES

Sentence Completion

1. The hormone __________ is essential to male sexual differentiation.
2. __________ is defined as fear of lesbians and gay males, although it could also be defined as hatred of lesbians and gay males.
3. According to the FBI, about 1 in every __________ hate crimes is directed against lesbians, gay males, and transgender individuals.
4. Our gender __________ is our psychological sense of being male, being female, or somewhere else along or outside the gender spectrum.
5. Sex __________ reflects the child's anatomy and typically occurs in the United States today with prenatal imaging or later, at birth.
6. People who are __________ have the gender identity of one sex but the sexual anatomy of the other sex.

Think About It

What kinds of comments about lesbians and gay males have you heard at home, in school, or among friends? How did the comments make you feel? Why? Do you know any lesbians or gay males? (Are you one?) How have they, or you, been treated by people you know? What can you do to improve the social climate for LGBTQ individuals?

Recite: An Active Summary

INTERACTIVE SELF-SCORING QUIZZES

Chapter 10 Practice Quiz

1. Identify and describe the female and male reproductive systems.

The external female reproductive organs are collectively called the vulva, which contains the urethral opening, clitoris, major and minor lips, and vagina. Internally, the ovaries produce ova and sex hormones that foster the development of female sex organs and regulate the menstrual cycle. In the male, the testes are the counterpart of the ovaries; they produce sperm and testosterone. Several glands, including the prostate, produce semen, the fluid that nourishes and transports sperm.

2. Discuss ways in which health psychologists help women with menstrual problems, postpartum depression, and menopause.

Premenstrual syndrome (PMS) refers to the biological and psychological symptoms during the 4- to 6-day interval that precedes menstruation. Most women who ovulate experience some mood-related problems associated with their menstrual cycles. The prevailing view of PMS is that it may be connected with biochemical changes during the menstrual cycle, but that negative attitudes toward menstruation can worsen menstrual problems. Women may develop the baby blues, postpartum depression, and—rarely—postpartum psychosis during the postpartum period. These problems are found around the world and mainly reflect hormonal changes following birth. Emotional and social support help women manage the baby blues; more serious cases of PPD are typically treated like other forms of clinical depression; postpartum psychosis, while rare, requires the attention of healthcare providers. Menopause is the cessation of menstruation. Perimenopause is the beginning of menopause and is characterized by irregular periods or amenorrhea. The climacteric is a multiyear process marked by declining levels of estrogen and ending in menopause. Menopause results from decreases in secretion of female sex hormones and is typically accompanied by symptoms such as hot flashes, hot flushes, decreased vaginal lubrication, and vaginal atrophy. Women's responses to menopause reflect physical changes and what the cessation of childbearing ability means to them.

3. Explain how theories of health behavior can help people make reproductive choices.

Theories of health behavior relate to weighing the benefits of and barriers to methods of contraception. Sterilization and hormonal methods (e.g., the pill) are the most reliable methods of contraception. A barrier concerning sterilization is that it should be considered reversible. The condom, used properly, provides protection against sexually transmitted infections as well as unwanted pregnancy; condoms also have the benefit of both members of the couple sharing responsibility for contraception. The withdrawal method has a high failure rate. Rhythm methods predict ovulation, which is the only phase of the menstrual cycle during which a woman can become pregnant.

4. Identify and discuss sexually transmitted infections, focusing on HIV/AIDS and how the Health Belief Model applies to people's decisions as to whether or not to use PrEP.

Most sexually transmitted infections (STIs) are bacterial or viral. Depending on the STI, it may be transmitted by vaginal, oral, or anal sex. Sometimes, as with chlamydia and genital herpes, there are no symptoms. Some infections clear by themselves, as do most cases of HPV in females; however, some cases that seem to clear may eventually lead to cancers and other serious health problems. Antibiotics are effective with nearly all bacterial STIs. HIV/AIDS is no longer lethal for most people if it is treated with antiretroviral drugs. PrEP can prevent the transmission of HIV, but there are barriers: Many people who would benefit from PrEP are inadequately educated about it, do not want to discuss it with healthcare providers, or cannot afford it. The Health Belief Model (HBM) focuses on key elements in the decision-making process regarding preventive health behaviors, such as PrEP, including perceived risk, barriers to use, and cues to actions.

5. Identify and discuss the origins of sexual dysfunctions and explain how psychologists help people overcome sexual dysfunctions.

Sexual problems include lack of desire, difficulty becoming sexually aroused (problems becoming lubricated in the female and erectile disorder in the male), difficulty reaching orgasm, premature ejaculation in the male, and painful sex. Persistent, recurrent problems may be called sexual dysfunctions. Premature ejaculation is most frequent among young males; other sexual problems in both females and males tend to increase in incidence with age. Fatigue and drugs such as alcohol can impede sexual response. Sexual problems can also reflect chronic health conditions or the side effects of medications prescribed to manage those very conditions. Performance anxiety about sex can be self-defeating and create a cycle of failure and then anxiety that leads to subsequent failures. Psychologists help clients reverse sexual dysfunctions by means of sex education, challenging irrational beliefs, reducing performance anxiety, and teaching sexual skills. The good-enough sex model helps older people maintain a vibrant sex life based on intimacy.

6. Define sexual orientation and gender identity and discuss the health challenges of LGBTQ individuals.

Sexual orientation involves the direction of one's erotic attractions. Most people are attracted to individuals of the other sex, but lesbians and gay males are attracted to people of their own sex. Bisexual people are attracted to both females and males. Gender minorities include people who are transgender or something else, such as feeling that they are both female and male or that they are gender neutral. Lesbians, gay males, bisexual people, and transgender individuals do not choose their orientation or identity any more than heterosexual people or cisgender people choose their sexual orientation or gender identity. Because of a history of misunderstanding and ostracism, sexual and gender minorities are exposed to threats, hate crimes, and other forms of bullying. As a result, they are more likely than heterosexual and cisgender people to be anxious and depressed and suicidal. They are also more likely to engage in substance abuse and risky sex. They may also feel uncomfortable with healthcare providers, feeling that they are not accepted.

Answers to Review Sections

10.1

1. progesterone
2. fallopian
3. menstrual
4. endometrium
5. Ovulation
6. dysmenorrhea
7. premenstrual
8. half
9. hormonal
10. Perimenopause
11. climacteric
12. blood
13. testosterone
14. prostate
15. blood
16. adrenal

10.2

1. 4 (27%)
2. condom
3. woman
4. pill (birth control pill)
5. Sterilization
6. sterilization

10.3

1. 26
2. herpes
3. papillomavirus
4. immunodeficiency
5. Chlamydia
6. semen (cum)
7. prophylaxis

10.4

1. Women
2. arousal
3. dysfunction
4. Performance
5. erectile disorder
6. premature ejaculation
7. Sex therapy

10.5

1. testosterone
2. Homophobia
3. 5
4. identity
5. assignment
6. transgender

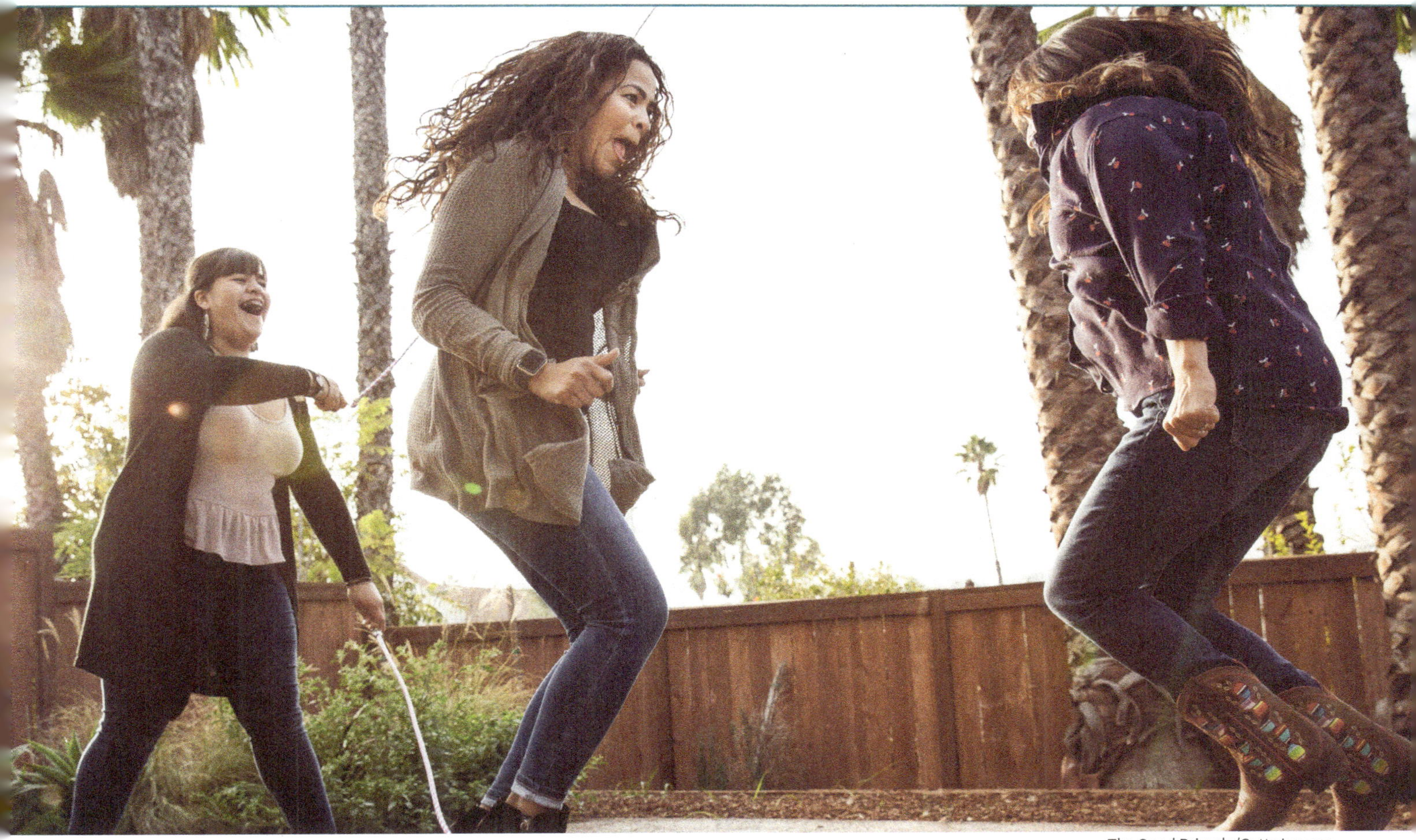

The Good Brigade/Getty Images

Psychological Health

LEARNING OBJECTIVES

After studying this chapter, you will be able to …

1. **Describe** the features of a healthy personality from the perspective of major theories of personality.
2. **Discuss** why we need adequate sleep to maintain our physical and psychological health.
3. **Discuss** the problem of insomnia and cognitive behavioral methods for managing it.
4. **Identify** criteria used to distinguish normal from abnormal behavior.
5. **Identify** and **describe** the major types of psychological disorders.
6. **Identify** and **describe** causal factors in psychological disorders.
7. **Identify** factors involved in suicide.

Did You Know That ...

- The Big Five is not the name of a new college basketball conference but a leading contemporary model of personality today?
- Extroverted students tend to have more Facebook friends than introverted students?
- A personality trait is linked to how long you are likely to live and how healthy you are likely to be?
- Some people can't fall asleep because they are trying too hard?
- Nearly 1 in 5 adults in the United States currently suffers from a serious psychological disorder?
- People may feel that they are having a heart attack when actually they are suffering a panic attack?
- Research evidence suggests that using Facebook can make us sadder?

Some 2,000 years ago the Roman poet Juvenal voiced his prescription for the good life: "*Pray for a sound mind in a sound body.*" He recognized the need to take care of both the body and the mind. In earlier chapters, we explored how health psychologists seek to understand the psychological or mental processes that affect physical health and adherence to medical treatment. In this chapter, we focus directly on our psychological health. Psychological health is essential for our well-being and our ability to cope with the challenges of life.

But what does it mean to be psychologically healthy? One yardstick of psychological health is the same as the minimal yardstick for physical health—the absence of a diagnosable health problem, in this case, the absence of a psychological or mental disorder. But just as psychologists focus on physical wellness, they also think of psychological wellness, which entails coping skills, regulation of our emotional states, and the possibilities of happiness and self-fulfillment.

Psychological health also incorporates conceptions of a healthy personality, the constellation of particular traits and behaviors that distinguishes each of us from everyone else. As we'll see, psychological theorists have differing conceptions of what constitutes a healthy personality.

VIDEO CONTENT

Understanding Personality

personality Distinctive patterns of behaviors and traits that make each of us unique and account for consistency of our behavior across situations and time.

trait perspective The view that reasonably stable internal characteristics determine behavior.

The Healthy Personality

The term **personality** refers to the unique constellation of psychological characteristics or behaviors that make each of us unique and account for consistency in behavior across situations and over time.

There is no one single theory or conceptualization of personality. Psychologists recognize that personality involves a complex web of factors that different theorists have approached from different perspectives. One prominent view, the *trait perspective*, looks at personality in terms of a constellation of underlying psychological traits. The **trait perspective** conforms to the view most people hold about personality, as when we say that someone has a "lively" personality or that someone else is "shy." Liveliness and shyness are examples of psychological traits that distinguish people based on their personalities and that may help us predict how people act in certain situations. Another theoretical approach, the *social cognitive perspective*, focuses on how personality is shaped by a combination of situational factors, such as learning experiences, and personal factors, such as individual expectancies and values. Those schooled in the *psychodynamic perspective* look at personality from a Freudian standpoint as consisting of underlying mental structures that continually jockey with each other in the unconscious depths of the mind that lie outside the range of ordinary awareness. From the *humanistic perspective*, personality is not something people possess but a way of interacting with the world and making choices that imbue our lives with a sense of meaning and purpose. None of these views offers a complete portrait of the person, but each can contribute something to our understanding.

We shall see what each of these theoretical perspectives has to say about the nature of personality and, importantly, what it means to have a healthy personality. We begin with the earliest psychological theory of personality, which is based on the work of the theorist Sigmund Freud.

VIDEO CONTENT

Psychodynamic Theories of Personality

psychodynamic perspective The view that drives and other forces within the person, some of which are unconscious, determine emotions and behavior.

The Psychodynamic Perspective

The **psychodynamic perspective**, which originated with Sigmund Freud (1856–1939), posits that personality is comprised of different elements or forces that clash with each other in a dynamic struggle within the personality.

Freud was trained as a physician specializing in neurological problems. Early in his practice he treated patients who, despite an absence of any medical disorder, experienced unexplained physical symptoms, such as loss of feeling in a hand or paralysis of the legs. He observed how these odd symptoms could sometimes disappear, at least for a time, when people were hypnotized or when, fully conscious, they recalled and expressed strong emotions. He became convinced that these symptoms were psychological in nature but that their causes were buried in the unconscious recesses of the mind. Based on his clinical work, he constructed the first psychological theory of personality.

Freud proposed that the human personality is composed of three mental or psychic structures—the *id*, the *ego*, and the *superego*. The **id**, the part of the personality present at birth, is a reservoir of instinctual drives, such as those that give rise to sexual and aggressive impulses. The guiding principle of the id is instant gratification of basic needs. It wants what it wants when it wants it, without regard to social niceties.

Although we are aware of what is in our conscious mind (what we are thinking, feeling, or sensing at any given time), the unconscious mind remains shrouded in mystery. Freud developed a type of mental detective work called **psychoanalysis**, which seeks clues to the workings of the unconscious mind by such means as interpreting dreams or slips of the tongue (so-called Freudian slips).

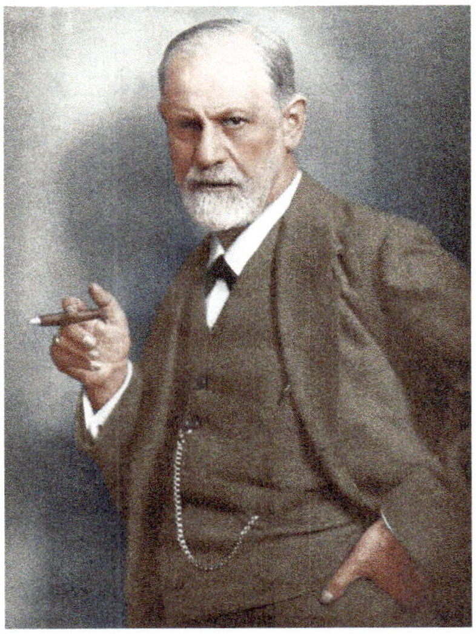

The Print Collector/Alamy Stock Photo

Sigmund Freud The founder of psychodynamic theory is shown here with his ever-present cigar. Even after he was operated on for cancer of the jaw, he returned to smoking.

The **ego**, which comes into being in the first year of life, stands for reason and good sense. The ego seeks ways to meet the demands of the id for satisfaction by means that are socially acceptable or fit social conventions. The ego takes into account what is practical along with what is urged by the id. The id may prompt you with hunger pangs, but it's the ego that directs you to order a sandwich at the cafeteria rather than rifling food off someone else's plate.

The ego operates consciously and unconsciously. At a conscious level, it constitutes the person's sense of self—the "I." The ego also constructs an *ideal self*, which represents an idealized sense of the self, or what the self strives to become. At the unconscious level, the ego acts as a censor that screens the impulses of the id and uses psychological defenses, such as repression, to prevent unacceptable sexual or aggressive urges from surfacing into conscious awareness (see **Table 5.1** for a list of defense mechanisms).

The **superego** develops during early childhood, as the child incorporates the moral standards and values of parents and others through a process called identification. The superego acts like a conscience, an internal moral guardian. Throughout life, the superego monitors the intentions of the ego and hands out judgments of right and wrong. It floods the ego with feelings of guilt and shame when the verdict is negative.

id Freud's concept of the mental structure that houses primitive or instinctual drives and impulses and which is fully unconscious (derived from a Latin word meaning "it").

psychoanalysis Freud's method of psychotherapy that focuses on providing insight into the workings of the unconscious mind.

ego Freud's concept of the mental structure that constitutes the sense of self and is responsible for satisfying instinctual impulses in a socially acceptable fashion (derived from a Latin word meaning "I").

superego Freud's concept of the mental structure that represents the moral conscience based on internalizing the standards and values of parents and important others.

social cognitive theory Albert Bandura's view, which emphasizes the interaction between people (personal factors), their behavior, and the environment (situational factors). Bandura's concept of reciprocal determinism holds that people are not only influenced by the environment but also influence the environment.

The Freudian View of the Healthy Personality

In Freud's view, the ego hasn't an easy time of it. It stands between the id and the superego, striving to satisfy the demands of the id and the moral sense of the superego. From this perspective, a healthy personality finds socially acceptable ways of gratifying most of the id's demands without seriously offending the superego. Most of the id's remaining demands are contained or repressed. If the ego is not a good problem solver or if the superego is too stern, psychological problems, such as fears, obsessions, or depression, may result.

Freud equated psychological health with the abilities *lieben und arbeiten*—that is, "to love and to work." Healthy people can care deeply for others. They can form intimate relationships and engage in sexual love and lead productive work lives. To accomplish these ends, Freud believed that sexual impulses must be allowed expression in the context of a committed heterosexual relationship—a view that might strike many contemporary readers as prudish, overly traditional, even small-minded and biased.

The Social Cognitive Perspective

Social cognitive theory embraces both mechanical classical and operant conditioning, and also social learning. Social cognitive theorists also focus on cognitive factors, such as the expectations we hold about the anticipated outcomes of events (outcome expectancies) and of our own abilities to accomplish what we set out to do (our self-efficacy). They also incorporate roles for social learning processes, such as modeling, or learning by observing the behavior of others in social situations. Social cognitive theorists believe that behavior reflects

VIDEO CONTENT

Social Cognitive Theories of Personality

the influences of both person variables (factors within the person, such as expectancies) and situational variables (e.g., rewards and punishments).

One goal of psychological theories is prediction of behavior. Social cognitive theorists believe we cannot predict behavior from knowledge of situational variables alone. Whether a person will behave in a certain way depends not only on situational variables but also on the person's expectancies about the outcomes of that behavior and perceived or subjective values of those outcomes—that is, the importance that the person attaches to them.

The Social Cognitive View of a Healthy Personality

To social cognitive theorists, a healthy personality is reflected by an active pursuit of learning and the development of personal variables, such as competencies, accurate interpretation of events, and the ability to regulate our emotional responses, enabling us to function effectively and pursue our goals. Let us briefly review these building blocks of a healthy personality.

- *Learning by observing others.* Because much human learning occurs by observation, we need to be exposed to a variety of models, such as teachers and parents. We also acquire skills vicariously, as by watching other people or instructional videos on YouTube.
- *Developing competencies.* Getting along and getting ahead require knowledge and skills, or competencies. We will be more effective if we learn the verbal, computational, and linguistic skills we need to adapt to the demands we face in a rapidly changing world. Competencies are acquired by means of learning opportunities. We require accurate, efficient models and the opportunities to practice and enhance our skills.
- *Accurate encoding of events.* Encoding is a process of bringing information into memory. The same event may mean very different things to different people depending on how they encode the information. We need to encode events accurately and productively. For example, we should not encode a disappointment or failure as a sign of total incompetence. A social provocation may be better encoded as a problem to be solved than an injury that must be avenged.
- *Accurate expectations.* Accurate expectancies enhance the probability that our efforts will pay off.
- *Developing self-efficacy.* To social cognitive theorists, psychologically healthy people believe in their ability to accomplish what they set out to do; that is, they have high levels of self-efficacy. Self-efficacious or self-confident people are more likely to face challenges in life than to shrink from them. They are more likely to make healthful changes in their behavior, such as quitting smoking, exercising regularly, and controlling their weight. They are also more likely to adhere to the pursuit of their desired changes, even when they face obstacles. People with higher self-efficacy about practicing COVID-19 protective behaviors were more likely to adhere to these protective measures (Shiloh, Peleg, & Nudelman, 2021). Yet self-efficacy is not a fixed trait; it can change for the better, and changes in self-efficacy can have healthful benefits. For example, evidence from a study of Latinas who participated in a culturally-tailored Web-based physical activity program showed that participating in the program boosted their self-efficacy and that changes in self-efficacy were associated with increased physical activity (Larsen et al., 2021).
- *Seeing the cup as half full rather than half empty.* Optimists are more likely than pessimists to make the most of every opportunity and to bounce back from disappointments. Optimism may add years to your life (Lee et al., 2019). We are more likely to pursue healthy changes in behavior when we are optimistic that the outcomes will be positive.
- *Developing efficient self-regulatory systems.* Our abilities to manage our emotions and plan out our behaviors shape our personal effectiveness. People who are capable of self-regulation may have thoughts such as "One step at a time" and "Don't get bent out of shape" that help them cope with difficulties.

VIDEO CONTENT

Humanistic Theories of Personality

self-theory The view that people are conscious and capable of choosing their behavior. People are healthiest when they make authentic choices—choices that reflect who they are as individuals and not choices that reflect the will of other people.

The Humanistic Perspective

Humanistic psychologists Carl Rogers (1902–1987) and Abraham Maslow (1908–1970) focused on the concept of the self, or "I," which they regarded as the sum total of our experience of being in the world. It's no surprise that Rogers dubbed his theory of personality **self-theory**.

Your self is your ongoing sense of who and what you are, of how you react to the environment, and, importantly, of how you choose what you do and how you act. To Rogers, the sense of self is an essential part of the experience of being human in the world and the guiding principle that underlies our behavior and our experience of ourselves in the world.

Sigmund Freud saw all motivation as stemming from the id, and he argued that the pursuit of creative expressions in the form of art and music are merely sublimated forms of basic sexual drives. By contrast, Maslow saw all levels of needs as real and legitimate in their own right. He believed that once we meet our lower-level needs, we strive to fulfill higher-order needs for personal growth (see **Figure 11.1**). We would not snooze away the hours until lower-order needs stirred us once more to act. In fact, some of us—as in the stereotype of the struggling artist—sacrifice basic comforts to devote ourselves to higher-level needs.

Maslow's hierarchy of needs includes the following:

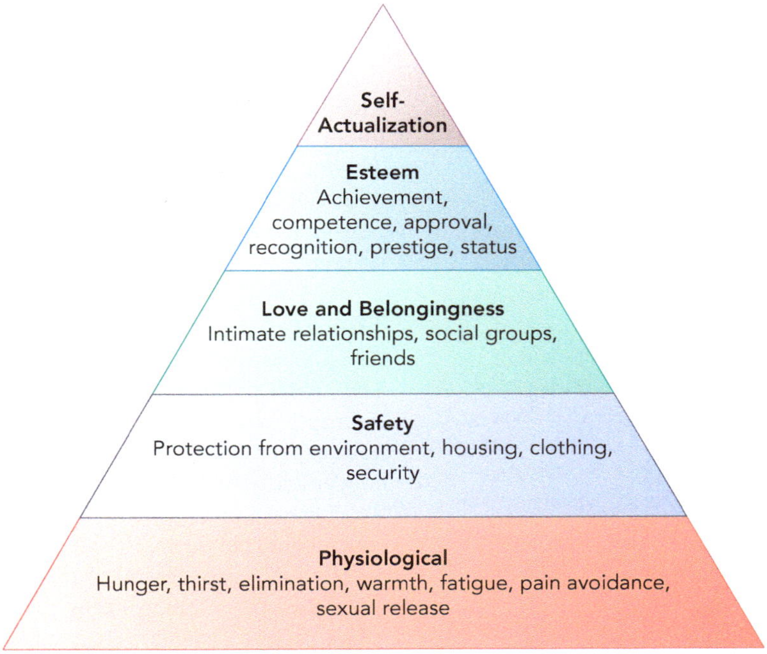

FIGURE 11.1 **Maslow's Hierarchy of Needs** Abraham Maslow believed that we progress toward higher social and psychological needs once we have met our basic needs for survival. Where do you fit into this picture? Where do you want to be?

INTERACTIVE FIGURES, CHARTS, & TABLES

1. *Biological needs.* Water, food, elimination, warmth, rest, avoidance of pain, sexual release, and so forth.
2. *Safety needs.* Protection from the physical and social environment by means of clothing, housing, and security from crime and financial hardship.
3. *Love and belongingness needs.* Love and acceptance through intimate relationships, social groups, and friends. Maslow believed that in a well-fed and well-housed society, a principal source of maladjustment lies in the frustration of needs for love and belongingness.
4. *Esteem needs.* Achievement, competence, approval, recognition, prestige, status.
5. *Self-actualization.* Personal growth, the development of our unique potentials. At the highest level are also needs for cognitive understanding (as found in novelty, understanding, exploration, and knowledge) and aesthetic experience (as found in order, music, poetry, and art).

Humanistic theorists place the "self" front and center in their concept of the healthy personality. People who are well adjusted are true to themselves—they know themselves and make authentic choices that are consistent with their individual needs, values, and goals. People with healthy personalities show the following qualities:

- *Experiencing life in the here and now.* They do not dwell excessively on the past or wish their days away as they strive toward future happiness.
- *Being open to new experience.* They do not turn away from ideas and ways of life that might challenge their own perceptions of the world or their own values.
- *Expressing their true feelings and beliefs.* They assert themselves in interpersonal relationships and are honest about their feelings. They believe in their own inner worth and are not afraid of their urges and impulses.
- *Seeking meaningful activities.* They strive to live up to their self-ideals, to enact fulfilling roles.
- *Being capable of making major changes in their lives.* They strive toward achieving new goals, act with freedom, and are open to change, including making changes in their health-related behavior.
- *Becoming their own persons.* They have developed their own values and their own beliefs, values, and goals, seeking to establish their individuality in the world.
- *Striving toward self-actualization.* They are in the process of striving to become self-actualized, to move toward fulfilling their own inner potential, whatever that might be. What inner potential might you seek to realize in your own life? Are you on the road toward self-actualization?

VIDEO CONTENT

Trait Theories of Personality

traits Relatively stable characteristics of personality used to explain a person's consistency in behavior and to distinguish one individual from another.

five-factor model A trait theory of personality based on factor analysis that finds five basic traits of personality: openness, conscientiousness, extraversion, agreeableness, and neuroticism. Also known as the Big Five model of personality.

Trait Theories of Personality

If you were asked to describe yourself, you would probably do so in terms of traits such as friendliness, outgoingness, and openness. (That *is* you, isn't it?). Trait theorists endeavor to understand the basic traits that comprise personality and to develop ways of measuring them. **Traits** are relatively stable characteristics of personality inferred from behavior. We don't directly observe "friendliness," but we infer friendliness from our observations of how the person acts in social situations. Traits are assumed to account for consistent behavior across situations. You probably expect your "shy" friend to be retiring in most social situations.

The Five-Factor Model The leading contemporary trait model of personality, the **five-factor model**, represents a consolidation of research on personality over many decades. The model posits five major traits of personality that investigators most consistently find in their research (Costa & McCrae, 2006; McCrae et al., 2004). The Big Five traits are openness to new experiences, conscientiousness, extraversion, agreeableness, and neuroticism, which conveniently spells out the acronym OCEAN (see Figure 11.2).

Big Five factors also relate to behavioral outcomes. One study showed a strong negative relationship between self-esteem and neuroticism (emotional instability)—that is, higher levels of neuroticism are linked to lower levels of life satisfaction (Olaru et al., 2023). Researchers also find a moderate to strong relationship between self-esteem and extraversion (i.e., higher scores on one variable were associated with higher scores on the other) (Watson et al., 2002).

People who are higher in neuroticism (emotional instability) also tend to achieve lower grades in school, to have lower levels of goal-oriented motivation, and to show poorer performance on the job (Soto, 2019; Vedel, 2014; Wilmot & Ones, 2021). We also have evidence from a Dutch study of more than 9,000 adults that found that neuroticism was the strongest of the Big Five traits in predicting poorer satisfaction in life, careers, and social relationships (Olaru et al., 2023).

People who report greater feelings of happiness and well-being are likely to score more highly than other people on emotional stability, agreeableness, conscientiousness, and extraversion (Roberts & Yoon, 2022; Soto, 2014). Extraverted people tend to participate more in enjoyable social interactions and activities (Anglim et al., 2020; Oerlemans & Bakker, 2014). They also tend to use the internet more for communicating with others (Mark & Ganzach, 2014). In addition, more conscientious people (no surprise here) and those who are more agreeable (friendlier) tend to be more successful in their jobs (Sackett & Walmsley, 2014).

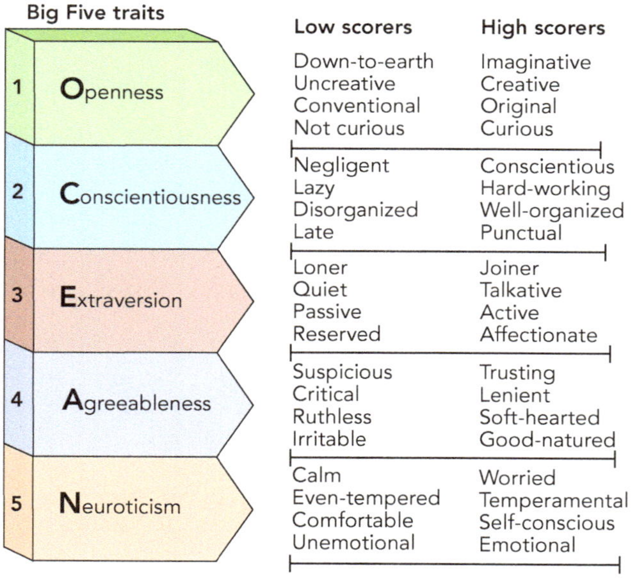

FIGURE 11.2 The Big Five Model of Personality Big Five traits are linked to health outcomes. Conscientiousness is linked to better health. Studies find that people who are highly conscientiousness adjust better to diabetes and multiple sclerosis. High neuroticism is associated with poorer health outcomes in general.

Links between Big Five Traits and Health Outcomes Big Five traits are linked to many aspects of our psychological and physical health. As shown in a *Health Psychology* article by Jason Strickhouser and his colleagues (2017), personality can predict physical health and well-being. The strongest links are between the resilience factors of conscientiousness and agreeableness and, conversely, the vulnerability factor of neuroticism (Strickhouser et al., 2017). Higher conscientiousness is associated with better adjustment in people with diabetes and multiple sclerosis, whereas higher neuroticism is associated with poorer adjustment in people with diabetes (Helgeson & Zajdel, 2017).

Benjamin Chapman and his colleagues (2019) drew data from 4,223 participants in studies on aging that included measurement of the Big Five personality traits. They found that neuroticism was connected with a greater mortality risk and that activity levels, an aspect of extraversion, were connected with a lower risk of mortality. Further supporting links between personality traits and health outcomes, researchers find that high neuroticism (low emotional stability) and low conscientious are associated with greater build-up of protein deposits in the brain associated with development of Alzheimer's disease (Terracciano et al., 2021). Findings along these lines suggest that personality traits may influence lifestyle behaviors in ways that predispose people to poorer health outcomes.

Catherine Rochefort and her colleagues (2019) studied Big Five personality traits among people with prostate or breast cancer and people without cancer. They found that higher conscientiousness and lower neuroticism were associated with more positive health behaviors and better health outcomes (Rochefort et al., 2019). Other researchers find links between emotional instability (high neuroticism) and poorer psychological adjustment and well-being and a greater risk of depression and substance abuse in college students (Rogers et al., 2018; Soto, 2019; Wilt & Revelle, 2018).

We would expect more conscientious students and workers to do better in school and on the job respectively. But did you know that conscientiousness is also linked to living longer and healthier lives (Jokela et al., 2013)? Research shows that conscientiousness is related to more positive health habits as well as work habits. Conscientious people are likely to control their weight, avoid smoking, avoid excess alcohol consumption, exercise more regularly, more closely follow medical advice, and avoid reckless behaviors that can shorten a person's life span, such as driving without seat belts (Bogg & Roberts, 2013; Israel et al., 2014; Shanahan et al., 2014).

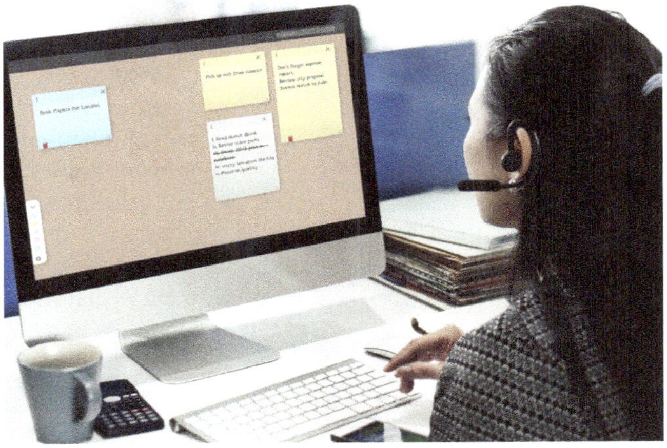

Rawpixel.com/Shutterstock.com

Conscientiousnes People who are conscientious are more likely to adhere to plans for maintaining or improving their health. When ill, they are more likely to adhere to medical advice.

Big Five traits also come into play in predicting other health behaviors, such as compliance with COVID-19 restrictions during the pandemic. Researchers found that people who were higher in agreeableness (friendliness) and lower in extraversion tended to be more compliant in adhering to health directives (Kleitman et al., 2021).

Translation of the Big Five Personality Traits into Health Behavior

The traits discussed in the trait perspective are seen as being largely heritable (Power & Pluess, 2015; South et al., 2018). But is biology destiny? Must introverted people remain reserved? Must disagreeable people remain stubborn and confrontational? We suggest that genetic tendencies toward these personality traits are just that: tendencies. Rather than thinking of biology as destiny, it might be more fruitful to look at things from a behavioral perspective and suggest that people can become what they do. The squanderer of time can focus (be conscientious) when need be. The "disagreeable person" can decide to be less argumentative and treat people more gently. The person who is reluctant to try new healthful foods can decide to be open to experiences and give them a whirl. People can choose to be more conscientious about their diets, exercise routines, and medical checkups. Once reinforcements start flowing for changing health behaviors, new, healthier habits can be formed. What began as a struggle—pushing yourself to jog and walk that first quarter mile—can become a pleasant feature of the day as you spin around the track or the neighborhood.

Review 11.1

INTERACTIVE SELF-SCORING QUIZZES

Sentence Completion

1. The __________ perspective conforms to the view most people hold about personality.
2. The __________ cognitive perspective focuses on how personality is shaped by a combination of situational factors and personal factors.
3. The three mental or psychic structures in Freud's theory of personality are id, ego, and __________.
4. In Freud's concept of defense mechanisms, the ejection of anxiety-evoking ideas from awareness is called __________.
5. Freud equated psychological health with the abilities to __________ and to work.
6. __________ is a process of bringing information into memory.
7. Evidence links optimism to living a (longer or shorter) life.
8. Psychologically healthy people have positive self-__________.
9. To become self-__________ is to move toward fulfilling one's own inner potential.
10. __________ are relatively stable characteristics of personality inferred from behavior.
11. The Big Five traits are openness to new experiences, conscientiousness, extraversion, __________, and neuroticism.
12. A study of people with cancer and healthy controls showed that both higher __________ and lower neuroticism were associated with more health-related behaviors and better health outcomes.

Think About It

How would you describe your own personality, looked at through the lens of the different perspectives discussed in this chapter?

VIDEO CONTENT

Sleep

Sleep

Sleep is essential to good psychological and physical health (Ramar, 2021). Persistent problems with getting enough sleep is linked to many health-related problems, including poorer immune system functioning.

You probably know from your own experience how important getting adequate sleep is to your psychological health and well-being. The National Sleep Foundation recommends that adults get at least 7 hours of sleep nightly, though many people say they need between 7 and 8 hours of sleep to function at their best (McMakin, 2021). It probably won't come as a surprise to learn that many Americans are not getting enough sleep. The CDC reports that about 1 in 3 adults in the United States are sleeping less than 7 hours a night (CDC, 2023b). **Table 11.1** shows the recommended levels of sleep according to the Centers for Disease Control, which are based on recommendations from the National Sleep Foundation.

Lack of sleep is associated with lower well-being for individuals but is also problematic for the U.S. economy because it increases the costs of health care and is linked to losses in productivity (McCarthy & Brown, 2015). Ninety percent of adults who report that they sleep well say they are able to get things accomplished each day; of adults who say they sleep poorly, only 46% report that they accomplish things well each day (National Sleep Foundation, 2018). These self-reports may be somewhat biased in that a positive response set could account for both reports of good sleeping and of good achievements, whereas a negative response set could account for both saying one doesn't get enough sleep and one doesn't get things done. But it would be foolhardy to dismiss the findings altogether; there is more than enough evidence that sleep is helpful—indeed, necessary.

More than 1 in 5 people polled by the National Sleep Foundation say they have fallen asleep at the wheel during the past year. Sleep deprivation is a serious problem for long-haul truck drivers (Soliani et al., 2024). It also contributes to many automobile accidents (Mahajan & Velaga, 2020).

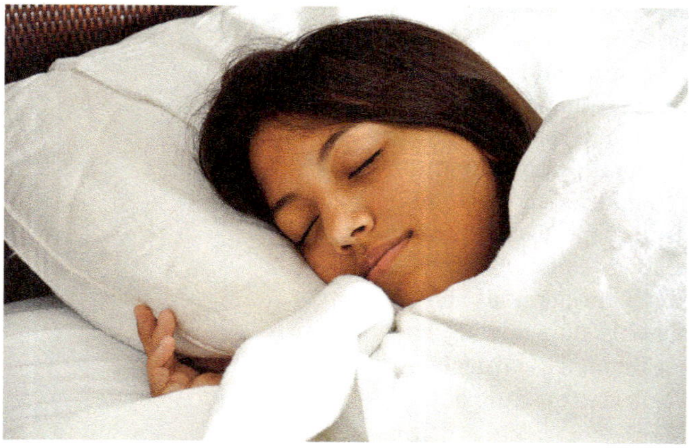

EMPPhotography/E+/Getty Images

Ah, She's Getting Her Z's "Beauty sleep" may be more than just a saying. Research suggests that when people have a good night's sleep, they look better the following day.

What about college students? How much do they sleep during an average night? Surveys of college students show that they average between 6 and 6.9 hours of sleep a night, which is less than the recommended level and may help explain why many feel groggy or drowsy while attending lectures or walking about campus during the day (Jalan et al., 2022). Only about 40% of American high school students obtain the recommended 8 to 10 hours of sleep they need (Basch et al., 2014).

Let us also note that Black and Hispanic people in the United States are far more likely than White people to report getting fewer than 6 hours of sleep a night (Ortega, 2021). The reasons underlying this health disparity remain unclear, but researchers suspect that one of the factors is that people of color are more likely to work nontraditional hours, including night shifts, that may interfere with normal sleep patterns. Exposure

TABLE 11.1 Table Showing Age Groups and Recommended Amount of Daily Sleep for Each Age Group

Age Group	Age	Recommended Hours of Sleep[1,2]
Infant	4–12 months	12–16 hours*
Toddler	1–2 years	11–14 hours per 24 hours*
Pre-School	3–5 years	10–13 hours per 24 hours*
School Age	6–12 years	9–12 hours per 24 hours
Teen	13–18 years	8–10 hours per 24 hours
Adult	18–64 years	7 or more hours per night
Older Adult	65+ years	7–9 hours per night

*Includes naps

Sources: CDC, 2022b; NIA, 2020

to discrimination, such as being treated unfairly because of one's race or ethnicity, may also be a source of stress that impacts sleep patterns of people of color. Whatever the cause, the need exists to find solutions to address this health disparity. We know we need an adequate amount of sleep to function at our best. But why do we need sleep? What functions does it serve?

Functions of Sleep

Researchers find that sleep serves multiple functions. One is a *restorative function*; sleep helps rejuvenate a tired brain and body. Sleep helps the brain restore itself and recover from daily wear and tear, performing basic housecleaning functions by flushing out cellular waste products from the brain (Delorme et al., 2021; Ghandour & Inokuchi, 2023; Helakari et al., 2022; Sterpenich et al., 2021). Sleep also helps refresh the mind and consolidate newly formed memories into more lasting ones (*memory consolidation function*). Sleep may also serve a *survival function*; by sleeping, animals, including human animals, keep from roaming about at night when nocturnal predators might be lurking.

Want to reduce your risk of coming down with a cold or other infection? Try getting more sleep. We've learned that sleep is good medicine, helping the body's immune system fight off disease-causing organisms (Dimitrov et al., 2019). And yes, it's true that when you have a good night's sleep, you tend to look better the next day (Raymond, 2013). People often need more sleep during times of stress, such as a change of job, an increase in workload, or an episode of depression. Sleep may help us recover from stress. Newborn babies tend to sleep about 16 hours a day, and teenagers seem to sleep around the clock. It is widely believed that older people need less sleep than younger adults do. However, sleep in older people is often interrupted by physical discomfort or the need to go to the bathroom. Older people often sleep more during the day—"nod off"—to make up for sleep lost at night.

Many people have so much difficulty falling asleep, remaining asleep, or falling back to sleep after a middle-of-the-night awakening that they cannot make up for lost sleep. They have chronic insomnia, a significant health problem that affects many of us at one time or another, sometimes for years.

Sleep and Social Support

Humans are social animals, and it is well established that social support helps people cope with stress. Health psychologists have also been investigating whether social support helps people get to sleep and have relatively stress-free sleep throughout the night. Social support in this case does not mean hand holding or warm telephone calls; it means the creation of an environment in which it is safe for the individual to let go of consciousness and vigilance when fatigued and to remain trustful during the night. From an evolutionary perspective, the effects of social support would reflect prehistoric days when the survival of the individual depended on the cohesiveness of the group.

Research by health psychologists concurs with the evolutionary perspective. One meta-analytic review of seven studies on the issue found that social support at work is associated with fewer sleep disturbances at night (Linton et al., 2015). A subsequent meta-analysis of 61 studies with more than 100,000 participants also found that social support was associated with better sleep outcomes.

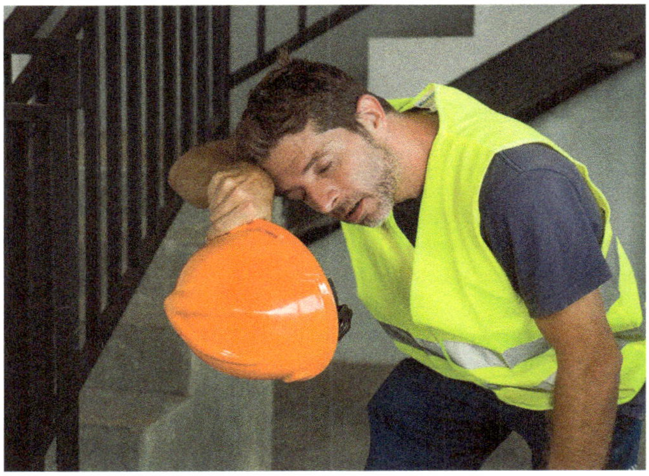
Marcos Calvo/Getty Images

Health Effects of Sleep Deprivation

If you miss a few hours of sleep or experience a sleepless night, you'll probably be able to muddle through the next day, although you may feel groggy. But pay attention to what you eat, as investigators find that missing even one night of sleep leads people to buy more high-calorie foods the next day (Benjamins et al., 2021; Okoli et al., 2021). As a result, sleep deprivation may lead people to reach for a doughnut rather than a healthful snack.

While occasional sleep deprivation is not linked to lasting health effects, persistent sleep deprivation is associated with greater risk of physical and psychological health problems,

insomnia A disorder characterized by persistent difficulty falling asleep or remaining asleep.

including increased risk of cardiovascular disease, infections, reduced immune system response, diabetes, poorer cognitive (thinking and memory) ability, and even premature death (Forthun et al., 2023; B.-H. Huang et al., 2023; S. Lee et al., 2022; Li et al., 2020). People who suffer chronic sleep deprivation, such as those with shifting work schedules, stand a greater chance of developing serious health problems, including cardiovascular disease, as well as psychological disorders and problems with mental alertness and concentration (S. Lee et al., 2022; Li et al., 2022; Meinhausen, Prather, Sumner, 2022; Sweeten et al., 2020). However, we shouldn't become alarmed if we occasionally miss a few hours of sleep; rather, we should restore our normal sleep pattern the following night.

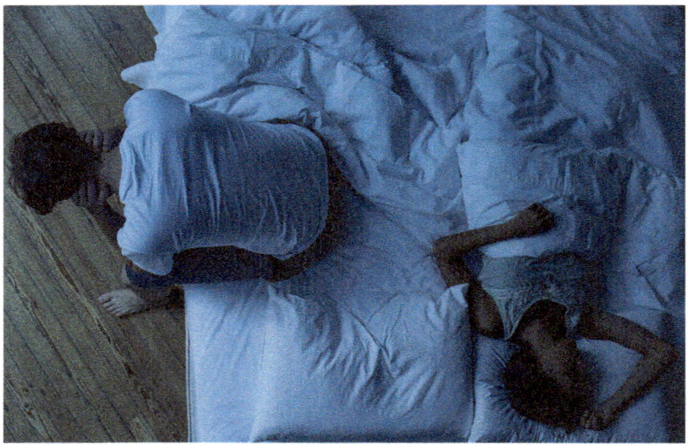

PhotoAlto/Alamy Stock Photo

Insomnia One of the contributors to insomnia is fear that we will not be able to get to sleep in time to be rested on the following day. The truth is that we can usually get by for a day or two with less than our optimal numbers of z's. But people with persistent difficulty getting to sleep might be well advised to try out the suggestions in the chapter, including challenging thoughts that are irrational and keeping them up at night.

Sleep deprivation has also been associated with inflammation in the brain, which can impair behavioral and cognitive performance (Atrooz & Salim, 2020).

If you are regularly deprived of sufficient sleep, it's likely to take a toll on your cognitive abilities, such as attention, learning, and memory—skills needed to succeed in school and on the job (McGuire & Lorenz, 2020). So we shouldn't be surprised that college students in a recent study who had more stable and consistent sleep patterns achieved better grades, averaging a 3.61 GPA as compared to a 3.1.21 among those with the most variable sleep patterns (Bono & Hill, 2022). People with erratic sleep schedules that play havoc with their internal body clock are also more likely to suffer from depression and anxiety than those with more regular sleep-wake schedules (O'Loughlin et al., 2021). Sleep deprivation can impair job performance even if workers themselves don't feel tired. Finally, persistent sleep deprivation is linked to an increased risk of obesity (Glaser & Styne, 2020).

Insomnia: When Sleep Eludes Us

Many people have difficulty falling asleep, remaining asleep, or falling back to sleep after a middle-of-the-night awakening. They may suffer from chronic insomnia, a significant health problem that affects many of us at one time or another, sometimes for years. Perhaps all of us have occasional trouble falling asleep, but about 10% to as many as 30% of adult Americans experience persistent or chronic **insomnia**, the most common type of sleep problem (National Sleep Foundation, 2021).

Insomnia is also common and persistent complaint among many adolescents and young adults. It affects about 20% of children and is highest in girls aged 11–12 years (31%) (Calhoun et al., 2014). Girls at these ages are in the throes of puberty, with floods of female sex hormones. Another study found that about one-third of adolescents overall report symptoms of insomnia during at least 2 weeks of the previous year, with Latino/Hispanic and Black adolescents reporting higher prevalences (42% and 41%, respectively) than White adolescents (30%) (Blank et al., 2015). During adolescence, a growing awareness of societal prejudices and discrimination mushrooms among people of color—more than enough to keep one awake at night.

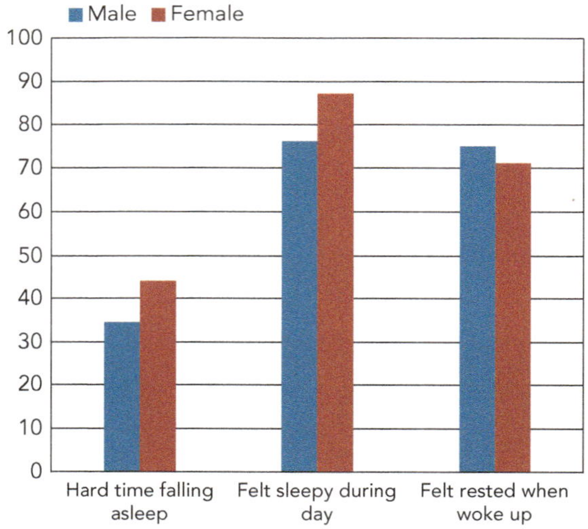

FIGURE 11.3 Sleeping (or Not!): Percentage of College Students Reporting These Experiences at Least 2 Days per Week During the Past Month

Source: Adapted from the American College Health Association, National College Health Assessment II, Fall 2017 Reference Group Data Report. American College Health Association, 2018. https://www.acha.org/documents/ncha/NCHA-II_FALL_2017_REFERENCE_GROUP_EXECUTIVE_SUMMARY.pdf

Insomnia also prevents achieving truly restorative sleep, the type of sleep that leaves us feeling refreshed and alert in the morning. Lack of sleep also takes a significant toll on the economy, resulting in lower productivity and increased sick days (Chalet et al., 2023). Psychologists find that a common theme among people with chronic insomnia is a pattern of poor sleep habits and intrusions of worrisome thoughts about not getting enough sleep. Staying up late at night staring at a cell phone is a major impediment to sleep among adolescents (de Sá et al., 2023; MacCarthaigh et al., 2020).

The American College Health Association found that approximately 35–45% of college men and women reported having a hard time getting to sleep at least 2 days a week (Figure 11.3). As a result, about 3 men in

Self-Assessment Are You Getting Your Z's?

INTERACTIVE SELF-ASSESSMENTS

Many people complain that they do not get enough sleep. How about you? This questionnaire will help you determine whether you are getting your Z's. If you answer several of these items in the affirmative, chances are that you are experiencing sleep deprivation or struggling with insomnia. If that's the case, the suggestions in the next *Applying Health Psychology* feature may be helpful. If the problem continues, it makes sense to consult your healthcare provider.

Directions: Read the following items and check whether each one is mostly true or mostly false for you. Try to work rapidly and answer every item.

TRUE	FALSE	
____	____	I have trouble staying awake when I do things in the evening.
____	____	I used to get more sleep than I do now.
____	____	I find myself hitting the snooze bar over and over again to grab a few more minutes of sleep.
____	____	I often have to fight to get out of bed in the morning.
____	____	Warm rooms can put me right to sleep.
____	____	I find myself nodding off during classes or at work.
____	____	I will suddenly realize that I haven't heard what someone is saying to me.
____	____	Sometimes it is almost impossible to keep my eyes open while I am driving.
____	____	I often fall asleep after I have had a drink or two.
____	____	I am one of those people who often falls asleep when my head hits the pillow.
____	____	I have bags, or dark circles, under my eyes.
____	____	I have to set the alarm clock loud in order to get up at the right time.
____	____	There are not enough hours in the day.
____	____	During the day I am often grumpy and worn out.
____	____	My eyes will sort of glaze over while I am working on something.
____	____	I need coffee or tea to get going in the morning.
____	____	I will be thinking about something, like solving a problem, and all of a sudden everything will go out of my mind.
____	____	I have trouble staying awake after eating a heavy meal.

4 and 8 to 9 women in 10 felt sleepy at least 2 days during a week. Ironically, about 7 in 10 men and women felt rested when they woke up in the morning. For many undergraduates, fatigue hits as the day wears on.

There are many causes of insomnia, including pain or physical disorders, psychological problems such as feelings of anxiety, depression, and substance abuse. Some factors are situational—intrusions from roommates or children; noise, light, and uncomfortable temperatures; even a partner's snoring. Insomnia often comes and goes with many people, increasing during periods of stress (National Sleep Foundation, 2018).

Applying Health Psychology

Sleep Habits for Getting to Sleep and Staying Asleep

No question about it—the most common medical method for fighting insomnia in the United States is taking sleeping pills. Pills (sleep medications) may work—for a while. They generally work by reducing arousal, which makes your brain more receptive to sleep. Positive expectations of success (the so-called placebo effect) may also contribute to their effectiveness. However, there are several concerns about using sleep meds on a regular basis.

If sleep meds help you fall asleep more easily, you are likely to attribute your success to the pills, not to yourself. As a result, you may come to depend on taking pills to fall asleep. Sleep medications also have significant drawbacks with respect to safety and efficacy (see Brooks, 2022). For one thing, people develop tolerance for many kinds of sleeping pills, so that with regular use they need higher doses to achieve the same effects. For another, there is a risk of overdose, especially if other drugs are mixed with alcohol. Regular use of sleep medications can also lead to physical or psychological dependence. Moreover, sleeping pills do not help you acquire healthier sleep habits. Thus, when you stop taking them, insomnia is likely to return. If these medications are to be used at all, they should be used only for a brief period of time, and only under a physician's care.

On the other hand, cognitive behavioral therapy (CBT), a psychological approach that focuses on changing problem sleep habits and disruptive thinking patterns, has emerged as the most effective (and safest) method for overcoming insomnia, even more effective than sleep meds (e.g., Felder et al., 2020; McCurry et al.. 2021; Simon et al., 2023; Zhou et al., 2022; among others). Although sleep medications may produce faster results, behavioral changes produce longer-lasting results—and good habits. Taking a sleeping pill doesn't help a person learn more adaptive sleep habits. Social-cognitive theory also points out that managing the problem without medication builds self-efficacy. Cognitive behavioral therapists use a combination of techniques to help people develop healthier sleep habits, including the following:

1. *Relax yourself.* Take a hot bath at bedtime or try meditating. Releasing muscle tension can reduce the amount of time needed to fall asleep and the incidence of waking up during the night.
2. *Challenge exaggerated fears.* You need not be a sleep expert to recognize that worrying that your next day will be ruined unless you get to sleep right now increases feelings of tension that interfere with natural sleep. People often exaggerate the problems they believe will befall them if they do not get a good night's rest. By thinking that it is absolutely necessary to get a full night's sleep, you bump up your anxiety to a level that makes sleep difficult if not impossible. Table 11.2 shows some beliefs that increase bedtime tension and some alternative beliefs.
3. *Don't ruminate in bed.* Worrying or ruminating about your daily concerns interferes with sleep, in part because it increases bodily arousal and makes the bed a cue for anxiety (Tutek et al., 2020). Don't plan or worry about the next day while lying in bed. When you lie down for sleep, you may organize your thoughts for the day for a few minutes, but then allow yourself to relax or engage in mental excursions or fantasy. If you don't doze after about 15 or 20 minutes, get out of bed and go to a quiet place and restore a state of relaxation for a few minutes by sitting quietly or reading under a dim light. Then return to bed.
4. *Establish a regular bedtime routine.* Sleeping late can make matters worse by altering your body's natural wake–sleep cycle. Set your alarm for the same time each morning and get up, regardless of how long you have slept. By establishing a regular time for going to bed and waking up, you allow your body to fall into a regular sleep–wake pattern. Give yourself a half hour or so before bedtime to wind down (reading may help). Turn off any electronic devices for at least an hour before going to bed. Avoid any caffeinated beverages for at least several hours prior to sleep and avoid or minimize exposure to bright lighting late at night (like bathroom lighting fixtures).
5. *Try a little fantasy.* Fantasies or daydreams are almost universal and may occur naturally as we fall asleep. You can allow yourself to go with fantasies that occur at bedtime or plan particular fantasies in nightly installments. You may be able to ease yourself to sleep by focusing on a sun-drenched beach with waves lapping on the shore or on a walk through a mountain meadow on a summer day. You can construct your own "mind trips" and paint in the details. With mind trips, you conserve fuel and avoid delays at airports.

Above all: Accept the idea that it's not the end of the world if you don't get a full night's sleep this night. You will survive. (You really will, you know.) In fact, you'll be just fine.

TABLE 11.2 Beliefs That Increase Nightly Tension and Calming Alternatives

Beliefs That Increase Nightly Tension	Calming Alternatives
If I don't get to sleep, I'll feel wrecked tomorrow.	Not necessarily. If I'm tired, I can go to bed early tomorrow night.
It's unhealthy for me not to get more sleep.	Not necessarily. Some people do very well on only a few hours of sleep.
I'll wreck my sleeping schedule for the whole week if I don't get to sleep right away.	Not at all. If I'm tired, I'll just go to bed a bit earlier. I'll get up about the same time with no problem.
If I don't get to sleep, I won't be able to concentrate on that big test/conference tomorrow.	Possibly, but my fears may be exaggerated. I may just as well relax or get up and do something enjoyable for a while.

Review 11.2

INTERACTIVE SELF-SCORING QUIZZES

Sentence Completion

1. Only about __________ in 5 high school students obtain(s) the recommended amount of sleep.
2. Missing a night of sleep leads people to eat (more or less) high-calorie foods the following day.
3. People need (more or less) sleep during times of stress.
4. Social support aids sleep by creating a safe __________ in which people can let go of consciousness.
5. Persistent difficulty falling asleep or remaining asleep is termed __________.
6. Cognitive behavioral therapists help people with insomnia get to sleep by challenging __________ fears.

Think About It

Do you have difficulty falling asleep? Does it happen now and then or persistently? If you have a recurrent problem, which of the suggestions offered in this section sound as if they could be of help to you?

Psychological Disorders

psychological disorders Patterns of abnormal behavior or mental processes that are connected with deep emotional distress or significant impairment in functioning. Also called *mental disorders* or *mental illnesses*.

Psychological disorders, which medical professionals call *mental disorders* or *mental illnesses*, are all too common. It is likely that you or someone close to you will experience a diagnosable psychological disorder at one time or another. Evidence from national surveys show that nearly half (46%) of adult Americans develop a diagnosable psychological disorder at some point in their lives (Kessler et al., 2005; Scott et al., 2018). Recent estimates put the number of people in the United States who are living with some type of diagnosable psychological or mental disorder at close to 60 million people, which works out to more than 1 in 5 adults (NIMH, 2023b). If we also consider the economic costs incurred in diagnosing and treating psychological disorders, as well as the lost productivity and wages of people affected by these health conditions, we could say that nearly all of us are affected by them in one way or another.

Many effective treatments are available to help people suffering from psychological disorders, including psychotherapy and various types of psychiatric medications. However, despite the range of available treatments, many people suffering from mental health problems, perhaps most, do not receive adequate mental health care (González et al., 2010; Olfson et al., 2016; Winerman, 2016). The underutilization of mental health care is in part explained by lack of access to qualified professionals or lack of insurance coverage for their services, but also because of the continued stigma associated with receiving psychological or psychiatric treatment. But it is also the case that many people with the most severe psychological disorders do not adhere to medical regimens (Dobber et al., 2020; Tessier et al., 2020). Health psychologists are investigating methods for helping people most in need adhere to the treatments that can make it possible for them to function in society.

What Are Psychological Disorders?

VIDEO CONTENT

Understanding Psychological Disorders

Psychological disorders are patterns of disturbed behavior or problems with mental processes such as thinking and perception that are associated with significant emotional distress or impaired functioning. In determining whether a person has a psychological disorder, a clinician needs to first rule out normative or expected responses to specific events. For example, some psychological disorders are characterized by anxiety, but many people are anxious now and then without having an anxiety disorder. It is appropriate to be anxious before an important date or on the eve of a midterm exam.

When, then, are feelings like anxiety deemed to be abnormal or signs of a psychological disorder? For one thing, anxiety may be a sign or feature of a psychological disorder when it is not appropriate to the situation. It is inappropriate to be anxious when boarding a well-maintained elevator or looking out of a fourth-story window. The magnitude of the problem may also suggest the presence of a definable disorder. Some anxiety is expected before or during a job interview. However, it is not customary to feel that your heart is pounding so intensely that it might leap out of your chest—and then avoiding the interview. Other factors

hallucinations Sensory experiences in the absence of sensory stimulation, as in hearing voices or seeing things that are not there.

delusions of persecution Fixed, false ideas of being persecuted or targeted by malicious forces or individuals.

in diagnosing psychological disorders include faulty perceptions or thinking, as in **hallucinations**—hearing or seeing things that are not there—and **delusions of persecution**—as in thinking that the mafia or the FBI are out to get you (unless, of course, they are truly out to get you). People with psychological disorders may also engage self-defeating and socially unacceptable behavior.

The Biopsychosocial Model: Examining the Mind–Body Interaction in Psychological Disorders

The biopsychosocial model, introduced in Chapter 1, is an explanatory framework for understanding health and wellness by considering biological, psychological, and social factors and their interactions. The biopsychosocial model is also the leading contemporary view of psychological disorders (Gandal et al., 2016).

diathesis-stress model A biopsychosocial model positing that disorders arise from a combination of a disposition to develop a particular disorder, called a diathesis, and life stress.

diathesis A proneness, vulnerability, or disposition to develop a particular disorder, usually genetic in nature.

A prominent example of the biopsychosocial model in mental health is the **diathesis-stress model**. According to this model, certain people have a vulnerability, called a **diathesis**, which increases their risk of developing a particular disorder. A diathesis is usually genetic in nature, but it can also involve psychological factors, such as maladaptive personality traits or self-defeating ways of thinking (Van Meter & Youngstrom, 2015). When a diathesis for a disorder is present, the likelihood of the disorder emerging may depend on the level of stress the person encounters. If the person encounters low levels of life stress or has effective skills for handling stress, the disorder may never emerge. However, the stronger the diathesis, the less stress is likely to be needed for the disorder to develop. In some cases, the diathesis may be so strong that the disorder develops even under the most benign life circumstances.

Classifying Psychological Disorders

The most widely used system of classification of psychological disorders (called mental disorders by the psychiatric profession) is the *DSM* system. The term *DSM* stands for *Diagnostic and Statistical Manual,* which is a compendium of diagnosable mental disorders published by the American Psychiatric Association. Now in a fifth, text-revised (TR) edition, the DSM-5-TR classifies disorders based on their particular features or symptoms (American Psychiatric Association, 2022). In our approach, we adapt the DSM classification to highlight several major categories of psychological or mental disorders—anxiety-related disorders, mood disorders, and schizophrenia.

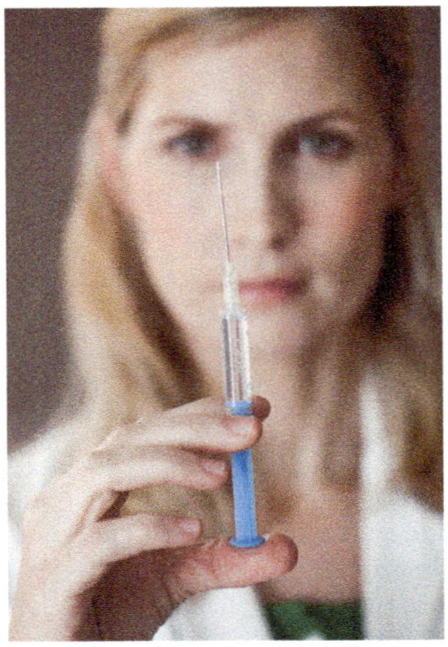

Emely/Cultura RM/Alamy Stock Photo

"Uh Oh, Do I Really Need That Injection"? Many people with a specific phobia for injections would gladly suffer greater pain than that caused by the needle, as long as it is caused by a pinch or a punch. Some people avoid important medical interventions, such as vaccinations, because of fear of needles.

Anxiety-Related Disorders

Anxiety is an emotional state that is accompanied by subjective, behavioral, and physical features. Subjective features include worrying, fear of something awful or terrible happening, fear of losing control, nervousness, and inability to relax. Physical features reflect arousal of the sympathetic branch of the autonomic nervous system. They include trembling, sweating, a pounding or racing heart, elevated blood pressure, and faintness. The behavioral features of anxiety are dominated by avoidance of situations or cues associated with the source of the anxiety. For example, dental anxiety is associated with avoidance or delay of dental examinations and treatment. Anxiety experienced in specific situations or in response to particular objects (like insects or large animals) or situations (enclosed spaces or heights) is called fear. Excessive or inappropriate fear is classified as a phobia, which is called clinically a phobic disorder.

Anxiety disorders involve excessive or unwarranted anxiety reactions and include phobic disorders, generalized anxiety disorder, social anxiety disorder, and panic disorder. These disorders are quite common, affecting an estimated 1 in 3 adults in the United States in their lifetimes and about 1 in 10 adults in any given year (Hudson, 2017; Smoller, 2020; Szuhany & Simon, 2022). Anxiety disorders usually develop during the teen years or early adulthood and may become chronic problems, although the severity of symptoms tends to decline with age

(Barry et al., 2023). In this section we also feature two related types of disorders in which problems with anxiety play a prominent role, obsessive-compulsive disorder and posttraumatic stress disorder (Hudson, 2017; Stein & Craske, 2017).

VIDEO CONTENT

Anxiety Disorders

Phobic Disorders The *DSM* classifies three major types of phobic disorder (phobias): *specific phobia, social phobia,* and *agoraphobia*. **Specific phobia** is an excessive, irrational fear of a specific object or situation, such as snakes or heights. One example of a specific phobia is fear of elevators. Some people will not board an elevator despite the hardships they incur as a result (such as walking up six flights of steps). Yes, the cable could break. The ventilation could fail. One could be stuck in midair waiting for repairs. These problems are uncommon, however, and it does not make sense to most people to walk up and down many flights of stairs to avoid the possibility that they might occur. Similarly, people with a specific phobia for hypodermic needles may refuse injections, even to treat severe illness. Injections can be painful, but most people with a phobia for needles would gladly suffer an even more painful pinch if it would help them combat illness. In other words, people with phobias may realize their fears are unreasonable or excessive, but nonetheless they feel they cannot control them.

specific phobia A type of phobic disorder involving excessive or inappropriate fear of a particular situation or object.

ANIMATION CONTENT

How Phobias are Created

Other specific phobias include **claustrophobia**; **acrophobia**; and fear of mice, snakes, and other creepy-crawlies. If there were a spider in the room, you can bet that a spider-phobic person will be the first to notice it and point it out to others (Purkis et al., 2011). Fear also affects the perception of environmental stimuli. The stronger a person's fear of spiders, the larger a spider may look to them (Vasey et al., 2012). Fears of animals and imaginary creatures are common among children.

claustrophobia A type of specific phobia involving a fear of enclosed spaces.

acrophobia A type of specific phobia involving a fear of heights.

Health Psychology in the Digital Age

Little Miss Muffet Confronts a Spider—Virtually

Little Miss Muffet,
She sat on her tuffet,
Eating her curds and whey.
Along came a spider
Who sat down beside her
And frightened Miss Muffet away.

This is a well-known nursery rhyme, and, no, we can't say that it is important to know what "curds" and "whey" are. (Or a "tuffet" for that matter.)[1]

The nursery rhyme is "make-believe," but there is a real woman who was playfully dubbed "Miss Muffet" by her psychologist. She did not sit on her tuffet but rather in her house, fearing that a spider might happen by if she ventured out. She suffered from a severe specific phobia for spiders. She recounted, "I washed my truck every night before I went to work in case there were webs. I put all my clothes in plastic bags and taped duct tape around my doors so spiders couldn't get in. I thought I was going to have a mental breakdown. I wasn't living." If she summoned up the courage to leave the house, she would check the cracks in the sidewalk for spiders. Finally, she almost became housebound, and, after years of anxiety, she sought help.

Her real name is Joanne Cartwright and, fortunately, she met with psychologist Hunter Hoffman at the Human Interface Technology Laboratory of the University of Washington. Hoffman was treating phobic clients with virtual therapy (Sears, 2016). He enabled his clients to reach out and touch spiders through the use of a toy spider and a device that tracked clients' hand movements to provide tactile sensations similar to those of touching a real spider (see **Figure 11.4**).

Twelve virtual therapy desensitization sessions later, Cartwright said that her life had changed profoundly. "I'm amazed," she reported, "because I am doing all this stuff I could never do," including camping and hiking. The point is that "Miss Muffet" was exposed to "virtual" spiders under circumstances that did not throw her into a fit of anxiety. Gradually she attained the ability to approach real spiders.

Now, if "along came a spider," she would be just fine.

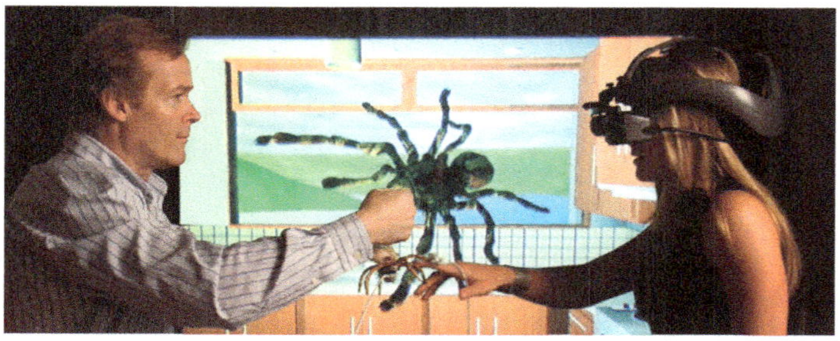

Courtesy of Dr. Hunter Hoffman

FIGURE 11.4 Dr. Hunter Hoffman of the University of Washington Uses Virtual Reality to Treat a Client's Phobia for Spiders Hoffman playfully dubbed her "Miss Muffet" after the nursery rhyme. She is wearing virtual reality headgear and sees the spider on the monitor in the background while she touches a toy spider.

[1]For the curious: curds are a white substance that derives from sour milk, used to make cheese. Whey: the watery part of milk, which remains after making curds. Tuffet: a footstool or low seat.

social anxiety disorder A type of phobic disorder characterized by intense fears and avoidance of social interactions.

Social anxiety disorder is a persistent fear of social interactions in which one might be scrutinized or judged negatively by others. Social anxiety disorder tends to develop early, by around age 15 on average (Stein & Stein, 2008). People with the disorder live in constant fear of doing something that will be humiliating or embarrassing. Fear of public speaking is a common social phobia. Social phobia can severely affect daily functioning, leading people to avoid socializing with others or accepting jobs or promotions that would bring them into closer contact with others.

agoraphobia A type of phobic disorder characterized by fear of venturing into open, public places.

Agoraphobia is fear of open or crowded places. The term "agoraphobia" is derived from the Greek root *agora*, meaning "marketplace." It is a fear of being out in open, busy areas, such as marketplaces, shopping malls, and the like. People with agoraphobia fear being in places from which it might be difficult to escape or in which help might not be available if they experience panicky symptoms. People who receive this diagnosis may even refuse to venture outside their homes, especially by themselves. They find it difficult to hold a job or maintain an ordinary social life.

gradual exposure A psychological technique for treating phobias involving the step-wise exposure to increasingly fearful objects or situations on a gradual basis.

In vivo ("in life") exposure to the fear-inducing stimulus is the gold standard of treatment for phobias (Wechsler et al., 2020). Exposure can be gradual, as by increasing a person's approach to the stimulus over time, or it can be all at once. (**Gradual exposure** is less unpleasant.) Exposure can also be virtual, in the form of viewing or hearing the stimulus through media, as in virtual reality. In a statistical analysis of nine experiments comparing the effectiveness of in vivo exposure versus virtual reality, Theresa Wechsler and her colleagues (2020) found a small advantage for in vivo therapy. However, the authors emphasize that virtual reality is also highly effective.

Panic Disorder

> *It happened while I was sitting in the car at a traffic light. I felt my heart beating furiously fast, like it was just going to explode. It just happened, for no reason. I started breathing really fast but couldn't get enough air. It was like I was suffocating and the car was closing in around me. I felt like I was going to die right then and there. I was trembling and sweating heavily. I felt this incredible urge to escape, to just get out of the car and get away. I somehow managed to pull the car over to the side of the road but just sat there waiting for the feelings to pass. I told myself if I was going to die, then I was going to die. I didn't know whether I'd survive long enough to get help. Somehow—I can't say how—it just passed and I sat there a long time, wondering what had just happened to me.*
>
> **—Authors' files**

panic disorder A psychological disorder characterized by episodes of sheer terror called panic attacks.

generalized anxiety disorder (GAD) A psychological disorder involving persistent feelings of worry accompanied by states of bodily tension and heightened levels of arousal.

In **panic disorder**, people experience abrupt attacks of acute, intense anxiety or sheer terror. At first panic attacks occur spontaneously, as if arising out of the blue. Over time they may become associated with situations in which they have previously occurred, such as boarding an elevator or airplane. Panic attacks are accompanied by strong physical symptoms of anxiety, such as shortness of breath, heavy sweating, tremors, and pounding of the heart. It is not unusual for people in a panic to think they are having a heart attack. Saliva levels of cortisol (a stress hormone) are elevated during attacks. Many people with panic disorder have difficulty breathing and may feel as though they are suffocating. During attacks, they may experience nausea, numbness or tingling, flushes or chills, and fear of dying, going crazy, or losing control. Afterward, they usually feel drained. Some people with panic attacks have accompanying agoraphobia, fearing venturing outside of home for fear of having an attack in public. About 5% of the population develops panic disorder at some point in their lives.

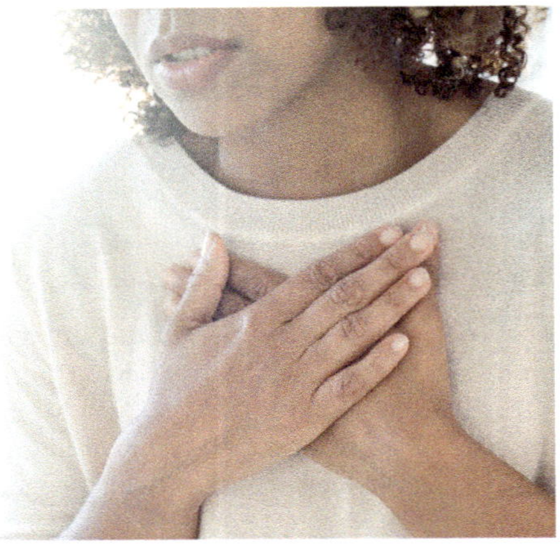

Science Photo Library/Getty Images

Panic Disorder Panic attacks are accompanied by strong physical symptoms of anxiety, such as shortness of breath, heavy sweating, tremors, and pounding of the heart. People with the disorder may think that they are having a heart attack.

Generalized Anxiety Disorder

The central feature of **generalized anxiety disorder (GAD)** is a general state of anxiety characterized by feelings of being on edge or tense most or much of the time and by persistent worrying

(Stefanopoulou et al., 2014). People with GAD experience persistent anxiety that is not tied to any specific object or situation. In such cases, the anxiety has a free-floating quality, as it seems to travel with the person from place to place. The hallmark feature of GAD is excessive worry. People with GAD are chronic worriers who tend to worry over just about everything. Symptoms may include motor tension (shakiness, inability to relax, furrowed brow, fidgeting), sympathetic overarousal (sweating, dry mouth, racing heart, light-headedness, frequent urination, diarrhea), feelings of dread and foreboding, and excessive worrying and vigilance. The disorder is estimated to affect about 9% of the general population.

Obsessive-Compulsive Disorder

VIDEO CONTENT

Obsessive-Compulsive Disorder

Jack, a successful chemical engineer, was urged by his wife, Mary, a pharmacist, to seek help for "his little behavioral quirks," which she had found increasingly annoying. Jack was a compulsive checker. When they left their apartment, he would insist on returning to check that the lights or gas jets were off, or that the refrigerator doors were shut. Sometimes he would apologize at the elevator and return to the apartment to carry out his rituals. Sometimes the compulsion to check struck him in the garage. He would return to the apartment, leaving Mary fuming. Going on vacation was especially difficult for Jack. The rituals occupied the better part of the morning of their departure. Even then, he remained plagued by doubts.

Mary had also tried to adjust to Jack's nightly routine of bolting out of bed to recheck the doors and windows. Her patience was running thin. Jack realized his behavior was impairing their relationship as well as causing himself distress. Yet he was reluctant to enter treatment. He gave lip service to wanting to be rid of his compulsive habits. However, he also feared that surrendering his compulsions would leave him defenseless against the anxieties they helped ease.

—Authors' files

People with obsessive-compulsive disorder (OCD) have recurring and troubling obsessions, compulsions, or both obsessions and compulsions. The obsessions or compulsions cause personal distress or impaired functioning. An obsession is a recurrent and intrusive anxiety-provoking thought or image that is beyond one's ability to control. Obsessions are so compelling and occur so often that they disrupt daily life. They may include doubts about whether one has locked the doors and shut the windows, or images such as one mother's repeated fantasy that her children had been run over on the way home from school. In another case, a woman became obsessed with the notion that she had contaminated her hands with a toilet cleanser and that the contamination was spreading to everything she touched.

A **compulsion** is a seemingly irresistible urge to perform a specific act, often repeatedly, such as elaborate washing after using the bathroom. The impulse is recurrent and forceful, interfering with daily life. The woman who felt contaminated by the toilet cleanser spent 3–4 hours at the sink each day and complained, "My hands look like lobster claws." Compulsions may temporarily reduce the anxiety connected with obsessions, but the obsessive thoughts typically return, leading to a vicious cycle of obsessive thoughts followed by compulsive behaviors, which are followed by more obsessive thoughts and compulsive behaviors, and so on. About 2–3% of American adults develop OCD at some point in their lives.

compulsion A seemingly irresistible urge to repeat an act or engage in ritualistic behavior, such as repetitive hand washing.

At her request, the woman with the obsession that she was contaminated by the toilet cleanser was treated with exposure and response prevention. She was asked to imagine that her hands were contaminated (exposure) and prevented from washing her hands. After a few sessions and an occasional booster session, she recognized that her fears were groundless and abandoned the compulsive hand washing.

Posttraumatic Stress Disorder Exposure to trauma in the form of physical attacks, combat, medical emergencies, witnessing a death or near death, accidents, and terrorist attacks can lead to the development of **posttraumatic stress disorder (PTSD)**. The disorder is a prolonged and maladaptive stress disorder that may not begin for months or years after exposure to trauma but can last for years afterward.

posttraumatic stress disorder (PTSD) A prolonged maladaptive reaction to a traumatic event characterized by intense fear and avoidance of stimuli associated with the trauma and by intrusive memories or images of the trauma.

PTSD is characterized by anxiety-related symptoms, such as a rapid heart rate and other symptoms of overarousal of the sympathetic nervous system, feelings of helplessness, intrusive thoughts, and flashbacks to the disturbing experience. The disorder frequently affects combat veterans, people whose homes and communities have been swept away by natural disasters,

Health Psychology in Action

Cognitive Behavioral Therapy Goes Digital in Treating Illness Anxiety Disorder

Imagine having an ache or pain in your side and fearing that it might be a sign of a serious illness, maybe cancer, so you consult a physician. After a physical exam and an X-ray, the doctor tells you it's a muscle strain that should heal relatively quickly. You walk out of the office, breathing a sigh of relief. Now imagine that you are someone with **illness anxiety disorder** facing the same situation, hearing the same report from the doctor. Despite medical assurance, you continue to be preoccupied with your symptoms, assuming that the doctor missed something or is incompetent. So perhaps you go from one doctor to another, looking for the one who might discover the condition that confirms your worst fears.

It's not the symptoms that people with illness anxiety disorder and related anxieties about their health find so disturbing—the passing feelings of tightness in the chest, the vague aches and pains—but rather what they believe the symptoms might mean. They tend to appraise relatively minor or mild physical symptoms as signs of serious illness, and their fears persist despite medical reassurance (Halldorsson & Salkovskis, 2017).

Cognitive behavioral therapy is often used to treat illness anxiety disorder and similar concerns about health. The method helps patients reappraise their responses to their physical symptoms and recognize that their fears are distorted or magnified out of proportion. Patients may be guided through behavioral experiments in which they break their habit of running from doctor to doctor for reassurance when a new symptom appears or compulsively checking the internet for the latest information about their symptoms—and then discover that they have survived (Fallon et al., 2017).

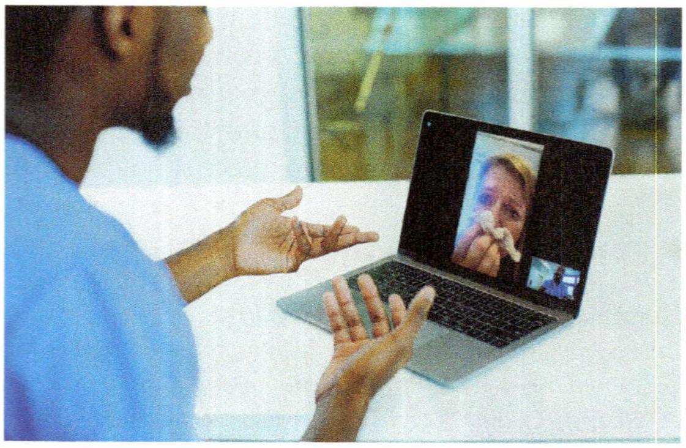

Carlos David/Alamy Stock Photo

Swedish researcher Elin Axelsson and his colleagues (2020) examined whether online cognitive behavioral therapy for illness anxiety disorder and related problems involving anxiety about health would work as well as treatment in a therapist's office. A sample of 204 people with illness anxiety disorder was randomized to receive cognitive behavioral therapy online or in person. People in both treatment conditions were encouraged to face their fears directly. For example, an otherwise healthy person who was preoccupied with unfounded fear of having a weak heart was encouraged to exercise without compulsively checking their pulse rate. The results showed that both treatments produced significant benefits in reducing health anxiety and did not differ in overall effectiveness. Although internet-delivered therapy may not replace in-person therapy (just as remote learning may not replace classroom teaching), it offers the advantage of reaching people who might not otherwise be able to consult a therapist, such as older people or people living in rural or remote areas.

illness anxiety disorder Unfounded, persistent fear that bodily symptoms or sensations represent serious health problems in the absence of medical findings.

epidemics, survivors of sexual assaults or childhood sexual abuse, and people directly exposed to terrorist attacks, including the terrorist attack on September 11, 2001.

Exposure to combat is closely associated with PTSD, yet the most commonly linked traumatic events are not combat experiences but rather motor vehicle accidents involving serious physical injury or death (Blanchard & Hickling, 2004). Exposure to violence, particularly acts of rape and assault, are more likely to lead to PTSD than are other forms of trauma (North, Oliver, & Pandya, 2012).

In PTSD, the traumatic event may be reexperienced in the form of intrusive memories, recurrent dreams, and flashbacks—the sudden feeling that the event is recurring. People with PTSD may try to avoid thoughts and activities connected to the traumatic event. They may find it difficult to enjoy life and may develop sleeping problems, irritable outbursts, difficulty concentrating, extreme vigilance, an exaggerated startle response to sudden noise, and suicidal thoughts or attempts.

Most people who experience trauma do not develop PTSD; in fact, most bounce back without professional assistance, with fewer than 1 in 10 eventually developing PTSD (Bonanno et al., 2010; Hu et al., 2020; Marin et al., 2019). Still, more than 10 million Americans experience PTSD at some point in their lives.

acute stress disorder A traumatic stress reaction in the days and weeks following a traumatic event, characterized by intrusive images or flashbacks of the trauma, high levels of anxiety, and feelings of detachment, as if walking around in a fog.

Vulnerability to PTSD depends on many factors, including the degree of exposure to the trauma, the perceived threat of the trauma, the availability of social support, and personal factors, such as a history of childhood sexual abuse, genetic vulnerability, and lack of coping responses (Hu et al., 2020; North et al., 2012). Investigators also find that people exposed to trauma who develop symptoms of **acute stress disorder** (a pattern of symptoms similar to those of PTSD that occur within a month of experiencing a trauma) are at greater risk of later developing PTSD (Marin et al., 2019). People with acute stress disorder may feel detached from their surroundings, as though they are walking around in a fog, and have high levels of anxiety and recurring intrusive thoughts, nightmares, and flashbacks relating to the traumatic event.

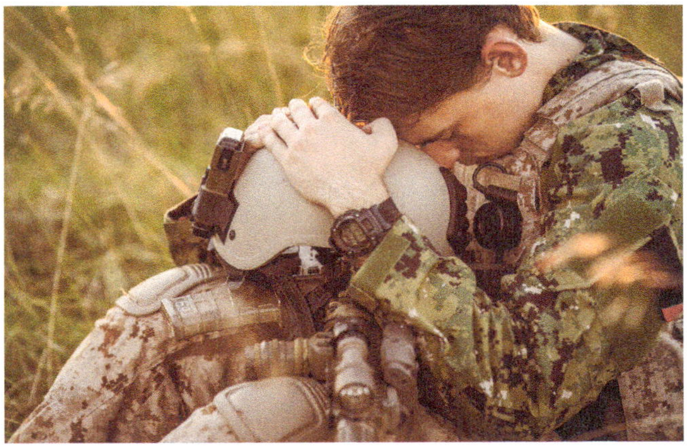

PRESSLAB/Shutterstock.com

PTSD PTSD can result from many traumatic experiences, including combat, sexual assault, earthquakes, stabbings, shootings, suicides, medical emergencies, accidents, explosions, and natural disasters, such as hurricanes and wildfires. Though people tend to associate PTSD most strongly with combat trauma and sexual assault, the most common traumatic events are serious motor vehicle accidents.

Exploring Mind–Body Interactions in Anxiety-Related Disorders Health psychologists focus on the psychological and biological factors involved in the development of anxiety-related disorders. Learning plays an important role in the development of such disorders. For example, phobias may be acquired on the basis of *classical conditioning*. A person who has been trapped in an elevator may develop a fear of riding on elevators. Some phobias may be conditioned fears acquired in early childhood so that the episodes are lost to memory. Other learning factors, such as observational learning, also play a role in the development of phobic behaviors. If parents squirm, grimace, and shudder at the sight of mice, insects, or blood, children might assume that these stimuli are threatening and learn to imitate their parents' behavior.

Another form of learning, *operant conditioning*, helps explain a pattern of avoiding a phobic stimulus. A person with an elevator phobia may opt to take the stairs rather than ride an elevator. Avoidance becomes reinforced (strengthened) by relief from anxiety and becomes a habitual way of coping with a phobic stimulus. By continually avoiding the stressful stimulus, the person is deprived of the opportunity to overcome the fear.

People who struggle with problems of anxiety may be prone to exaggerate or blow out of proportion the consequences of threatening situations, as when taking exams, meeting new people, or boarding an airplane. They also tend to have low self-efficacy, or lack of confidence in their ability to handle these threats or the anxiety they produce (Schultz & Heimberg, 2008).

The biological perspective on anxiety-related disorders considers genetics and the functioning of the brain (Goodman et al., 2021; Hu et al., 2020; Smoller, 2020). In OCD, for instance, researchers suspect the brain may be repeatedly sending messages that something is terribly wrong and needs immediate attention, which may then lead to the kinds of nagging obsessive thoughts we tend to see in people with OCD. The compulsive pattern in OCD may reflect a malfunction of the brain's ability to curb repetitive, ritualistic behaviors (Dougherty et al., 2018).

People who are prone to anxiety may possess a genetic tendency for greater sympathetic nervous system arousal in response to fearful stimuli, leading them to become unduly anxious in response to threats (Ullrich et al., 2017). Biochemical abnormalities in the brain may also be involved, such as irregularities in the functioning of neurotransmitters, perhaps involving the neurotransmitter **gamma-aminobutyric acid (GABA)**, a brain chemical that serves to calm excess sympathetic arousal. The class of antianxiety drugs called **benzodiazepines** (for example, *Xanax* and *Ativan*) works to calm anxiety by boosting the effects of GABA.

gamma-aminobutyric acid (GABA) An inhibitory neurotransmitter that curbs central nervous system activity and that is implicated in anxiety-related disorders.

benzodiazepines A class of antianxiety drugs that appear to work by increasing the sensitivity of receptor sites to GABA.

According to the Health Belief Model, people who face health threats, such as those posed by anxiety, weigh the perceived costs and benefits of treatment alternatives. In consultation with their healthcare providers, they evaluate whether the expected benefits (reduced anxiety, improved mood) outweigh the expected costs, such as the financial costs of medications and their potential side effects. They may also weigh the relative benefits and costs of taking medications against alternative treatment approaches, such as cognitive behavioral therapy.

According to an integrative model, cognitive factors such as catastrophic appraisal of changes in bodily sensations or physical symptoms can set into motion a chain of events that lead to a full-blown panic attack. In primary appraisal, momentary dizziness, rapid heartbeat, or light-headedness become blown out of proportion to the threat they pose (Ohst & Tuschen-Caffier, 2018). The person may think, "Oh, my God, I'm having a heart attack!" or "I've got to get out of here or I'll die," or "My heart is going to leap out of my chest." Primary appraisal intensifies the physical symptoms of anxiety, which in turn lead to more catastrophic thinking, producing yet more anxiety. The cycle may quickly spiral into a full-blown panic attack.

VIDEO CONTENT

Depressive and Bipolar Disorders

mood disorders A class of psychological disorders characterized by patterns of disturbed mood, as in major depression and bipolar disorder.

Mood Disorders

Mood disorders are characterized by severe or persistent disturbances of mood that may take the form of depression or extreme elation. Most of us feel joyful when fortune shines on us or deflated when we fail or encounter disappointments. If you have failed an important test, if you have lost money in business, or if your closest friend becomes ill, it is understandable to be sad about it. It would be odd, in fact, if you were not affected by adversity. But in mood disorders, the disturbance of moods may be extreme, persistent, or out of keeping with events. Here we consider two major types of mood disorders: major depressive disorder and bipolar disorder.

Major Depressive Disorder

> *What I had begun to discover is that, mysteriously and in ways that are totally remote from normal experience, the gray drizzle of horror induced by depression takes on the quality of physical pain. But it is not an immediately identifiable pain, like that of a broken limb. It may be more accurate to say that despair, owing to some evil trick played upon the sick brain by the inhabiting psyche, comes to resemble the diabolical discomfort of being imprisoned in a fiercely overheated room.*
>
> **—William Styron, *Darkness Visible: A Memoir of Madness***

> *Life is bloodless, pulseless, and yet present enough to allow a suffocating horror and pain. ... The body is bone-weary; there is no will; nothing is that is not an effort, and nothing at all seems worth it.*
>
> **—Kay Redfield Jamison, *Night Falls Fast***

major depressive disorder A severe type of mood disorder characterized by depressed mood, negative thinking, changes in appetite and sleep patterns, and lack of interest or pleasure in activities of daily life.

Major depressive disorder has been dubbed the "common cold" of psychological problems, affecting more than 1 in 5 adults (20.6%) in the United States at some point in their lives (Hasin et al., 2018). About 1 in 10 adults suffers from major depression in a given year. Worldwide, major depression is the most prevalent psychiatric disorder and the leading cause of disability, accounting for more years lost to disability than heart disease and cancer (Cipriani et al., 2018; Holingue, 2018; Scott et al., 2018). A major health challenge in the United States is addressing the unmet needs of people with major depression, as fewer than half of cases are identified by healthcare providers (Barry et al., 2023).

Largely because of the lingering stigma associated with seeking mental health care, or the belief that depressed people should be able to just "snap out of it," fewer than 30% of people diagnosed with depression in the United States receive professional help (Olfson et al., 2016). Latino/Hispanic Americans, Asian Americans, and non-Hispanic Black Americans are less likely than non-Hispanic Americans to receive professional care for depression (Barry et al., 2023; Waitzfelder et al., 2018).

In major depression, people may experience a downcast mood and lose interest or pleasure in activities they might otherwise enjoy, including the ordinary activities of daily life (Kalin, 2022; Pan et al., 2022). They may complain of feeling down in the dumps or have a sense of hopelessness about the future. They may have difficulty concentrating or summoning the energy to get going in the morning or even to get out of bed. They may experience changes in appetite (eating too much or too little) and sleep (sleeping either too much or too little). They may be tearful at times and contemplate or attempt suicide. In extreme cases, they may experience **psychotic** behaviors, including hallucinations and **delusions**, such as believing that their body is rotting away.

psychotic Referring to a break with reality, as in hallucinations and delusions.

delusions Fixed but patently false beliefs or ideas; characteristic of schizophrenia.

Major depression occurs in discrete episodes that can last months or a year or more, especially if untreated, and that have a high rate of recurrence (about 50% over the course of a lifetime) (Hamilton & Alloy, 2017; Judd et al., 2016). Women are about twice as likely as men to develop major depression in their lifetime—26.1% versus 14.7% (Barry et al., 2023; Hartung & Lefler, 2019; Landhuis, 2020). Although underlying hormonal or other biological differences between men and women may play a role in explaining this gender gap, we also need to consider the greater stress burden that many women carry in our society, as described in the Closer Look (Eagly et al., 2012).

A Closer Look

Why Are More Women Depressed Than Men?

Women are about twice as likely to suffer from major depression as men (Barry et al., 2023). But what explains this sex difference? As in other health issues, we need to consider biological, psychological, and social factors.

Although biological factors, such as hormonal influences relating to the menstrual cycle and childbirth, may contribute to the greater risk of depression in women, we also need to recognize the greater stress burdens many women carry (Eagly et al., 2012; Harkness et al., 2010; Hyde & Mezulis, 2020). Women often face a disproportionate level of stress, such as holding a job and bearing the bulk of housekeeping and childcare responsibilities at home. Women are also more likely than men to experience stresses such as physical and sexual abuse, poverty, single parenthood, and sexism. They are also more likely to assume caregiving responsibilities for aging family members who are sick or disabled. The sex difference found in rates of depression may also reflect different social expectations and social pressures. In our culture, for example, men are less likely than women to admit to depression or seek treatment for it. They may think that depression is a weakness and that they should just get over it.

Differences in coping styles between men and women also play a role. Psychologist Susan Nolen-Hoeksema (2008, 2012) believed that men are more likely to cope with depression by distracting themselves from their feelings, whereas women are more likely to ruminate, or dwell, on their problems. Distraction may help take one's mind off one's problems, whereas rumination may compound feelings of misery. Because men are more likely to distract themselves by turning to alcohol, they may expose themselves and their families to another set of problems. Frequent rumination can also increase emotional distress in men as well as women, setting the stage for depression (Connolly & Alloy, 2018; du Pont et al., 2018; Samtani, 2017).

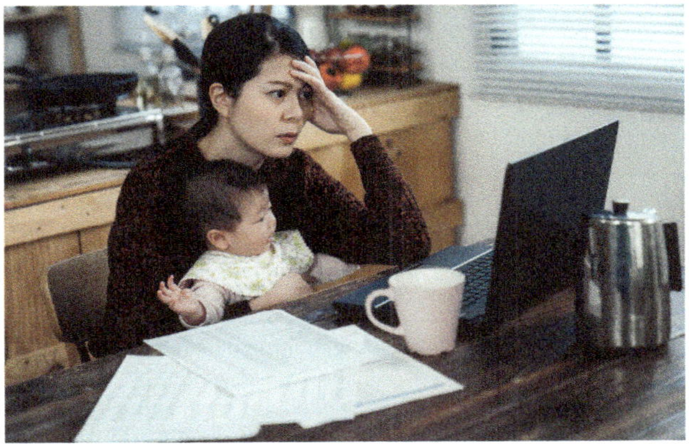

PRImageFactory/Getty Images

Why Is She Depressed? About twice as many women as men are diagnosed with major depressive disorvder. Is the difference due to biological factors? To differences in the tendency to ruminate about problems? To differences in the family and social demands placed on women as opposed to men?

Mind–Body Interactions in Mood Disorders The causes of mood disorders include biological, psychological, and social (environmental) factors. An important environmental factor is exposure to stress (Kendler & Gardner, 2010; Liu & Alloy, 2010). Many sources of stress are linked to increased risk of depression, including loss of loved ones, marital conflict, physical illness, low income, prolonged unemployment, work-related pressure, and maltreatment in childhood (Kõlves et al., 2010; Schultebraucks et al., 2021, among others).

In 2023, researchers linked various lifestyle behaviors to a lower risk of depression, making the case that healthy habits are associated with psychological as well as physical health (Zhao et al., 2023). The habits tied to a lower risk of depression were leading a more physically active and less sedentary lifestyle, following a healthy diet, never smoking, maintaining social connections, avoiding excess alcohol consumption, and the habit most strongly tied to lower risk of depression, healthy sleeping.

Psychological factors in mood disorders highlight the roles of learning, thinking patterns or cognitions, and behaviors. Learning theory teaches that a lack of reinforcement in a person's life may lead to depression by sapping motivation to engage in daily activities. Cognitive theorists such as Aaron Beck and psychologist Albert Ellis believe that the ways we interpret negative life events leads to emotional disorders such as depression. For example, Beck and his colleagues argue that people who are prone to depression tend to see the world through a dark mental filter that slants or biases their appraisal of life experiences (Beck, 2019; Beck & Bredemeier, 2016; Beck et al., 1979). Minor disappointments, such as getting a poor grade on a test, are appraised as catastrophic. People come to expect the worst and tend to focus only on the negative aspects of events. Beck calls these faulty thinking patterns "cognitive distortions" and believes that they pave the way for depression in the face of negative life events. Table 11.3 lists some examples of the cognitive distortions associated with depression.

Research conducted by learning theorists shows links between depression and the concept of **learned helplessness**. In classic research, psychologist Martin Seligman and his

learned helplessness A model for acquisition of depressive behavior, based on laboratory findings that animals and humans in aversive situations learn to become inactive when their attempts to escape are unreinforced.

TABLE 11.3 Cognitive Distortions Associated with Depression

INTERACTIVE FIGURES, CHARTS, & TABLES

Type of Cognitive Distortion	Description	Examples
All-or-nothing thinking	Viewing events in black-or-white terms, as either all good or all bad	• Do you view a relationship that ended as a total failure, or are you able to see some benefits in the relationship? • Do you consider any less-than-perfect performance as a failure?
Misplaced blame	Tendency to blame or criticize yourself for disappointments or setbacks while ignoring external circumstances	• When things don't go as planned, do you automatically assume that it's your fault?
Misfortune telling	Tendency to think that one disappointment will inevitably lead to another	• If your job application is rejected, do you assume that all the other applications you sent will meet the same fate?
Negative focusing	Focusing your attention only on the negative aspects of your experiences	• Do you tend to harp on the negative side of events and overlook the positive? • When you get a job evaluation, do you overlook the praise and focus only on the criticism?
Dismissing the positives	Snatching defeat from the jaws of victory by trivializing or denying your accomplishments; minimizing your strengths or assets	• Do you give yourself short shrift when sizing up your abilities? • When someone compliments you, do you find some way of dismissing it by saying something like "It's no big deal" or "Anyone could have done it"?
Jumping to conclusions	Drawing a conclusion that is not supported by the facts at hand	• If you meet someone new, do you naturally assume that they couldn't possibly like you? • If you feel a passing tightness in your chest, do you assume that it must be a sign of heart trouble?
Catastrophizing	Exaggerating the importance of negative events or personal flaws (making mountains out of molehills)	• Does your mind automatically run to the worst possible case? • Do you react to a disappointing grade in a course as though your life is ruined?
Emotion-based reasoning	Reasoning based on your emotions rather than on a clear-headed evaluation of the available evidence	• Do you think that things are really hopeless because it feels that way at the moment? • Do you believe that you must have done something really bad to feel so awful about yourself?
Shouldisms	Placing unrealistic demands on yourself that you "should" or "must" accomplish certain tasks or reach certain goals	• Do you think that you *should* be able to ace this course or else you're just a loser? • Do you feel that you *should* be further along in your life than you are now?
Name calling	Attaching negative labels to yourself or others as a way of explaining your own or someone else's behavior	• Do you think that people fail to meet your needs because they are *selfish*? • Do you label yourself *lazy* or *stupid* when you fall short of reaching your goals?
Mistaken responsibility	Assuming that you are the cause of other people's problems	• Do you automatically assume that your partner is depressed or upset because of something you said or did (or didn't say or do)?

colleagues (Maier & Seligman, 2016; Overmier & Seligman, 1967; Seligman & Maier, 1967) exposed dogs to inescapable electric shock. The dogs learned they were helpless to escape the shock. Later, a barrier to a safe compartment was removed, offering the animals a way out. But when the dogs were shocked again, they made no effort to escape. Their helplessness apparently prevented them from attempting to escape. The lethargy and lack of motivation they displayed resembled that seen in people who are depressed. In humans, the failure to garner reinforcements for one's efforts—to continually try but fail—may also produce the lethargy and sense of helplessness that Seligman observed in dogs. In the face of continued lack of

Self-Assessment: Are You Depressed?

INTERACTIVE SELF-ASSESSMENTS

Might you be struggling with depression? Although a diagnosis of a depressive disorder should be made only by a qualified mental health professional, such as a psychologist or psychiatrist, the National Institutes of Health offers some guidance to raise awareness about depressive symptoms. They offer this list of common symptoms of depression. Consider whether any of the following items apply to you.

	YES	NO
1. Persistent sad, anxious, or "empty" feelings	_____	_____
2. Feelings of hopelessness or pessimism	_____	_____
3. Feelings of guilt, worthlessness, or helplessness	_____	_____
4. Irritability, restlessness	_____	_____
5. Loss of interest in activities or hobbies once pleasurable, including sex	_____	_____
6. Fatigue and decreased energy	_____	_____
7. Difficulty concentrating, remembering details, and making decisions	_____	_____
8. Insomnia, early-morning wakefulness, or excessive sleeping	_____	_____
9. Overeating, or appetite loss	_____	_____
10. Thoughts of suicide, suicide attempts	_____	_____
11. Aches or pains, headaches, cramps, or digestive problems that do not ease even with treatment	_____	_____

Evaluating your responses: Depression may present in different ways from case to case with respect to particular symptoms, as well as their severity, frequency, and duration. However, if you have experienced two or more of these possible symptoms or signs of depression for a period of 2 or more weeks, it would be prudent to consult a mental health professional for a more complete evaluation. We recommend an immediate consultation if you have experienced thoughts of death or suicide (#10). If you're not sure whom to contact, speak with a counselor at your college counseling center, call a local mental health center or clinic in your neighborhood, or contact your healthcare provider.

Source: Adapted from National Institute of Mental Health, Depression. https://www.nimh.nih.gov/health/topics/depression/index.shtml

reinforcement for our efforts, we may begin to give up and resign ourselves to having a lack of control over potential reinforcements.

The concept of learned helplessness was expanded in the 1970s to include cognitive factors (Abramson et al., 1978). This revised theory, called *reformulated helplessness theory*, held that perception of lack of control over reinforcement alone did not explain the persistence and severity of depression. It was also necessary to consider cognitive factors, especially people's attributions about the causes of events—that is, how they explain to themselves their failures and disappointments (Haeffel et al., 2017; Liu et al., 2015).

attributional styles Tendencies to attribute one's behavior to internal or external factors, stable or unstable factors, and global or specific factors.

Let us explain. When things go wrong, we may think of the causes of failure along three dimensions—as internal or external, stable or unstable, and global or specific. These personal styles of explanation, or **attributional styles**, can be illustrated using the example of having a date that does not work out. An internal attribution involves self-blame (as in "I really loused it up"). An external attribution places the blame elsewhere (as in "Some couples just don't develop a liking for each other" or "She was the wrong sign for me"). A stable attribution ("It's my personality") suggests a problem that cannot be changed. An unstable attribution ("It was because I had a head cold") suggests a temporary condition. A global attribution of failure ("I have no idea what to do when I'm with other people") suggests that the problem is quite large. A specific attribution ("I have problems making small talk at the beginning of a relationship") chops the problem down to a manageable size.

Attributional style also has a bearing on adjusting to chronic disease. People who have a pessimistic attributional style—who appraise negative events as being internal, stable, and global while explaining positive events in terms of external, unstable, and specific causes—have a more difficult time adjusting to chronic illness (Helgeson & Zajdel, 2017). When things go wrong, they tend to hold themselves responsible and believe other bad things will follow, whereas they tend to attribute positive outcomes to blind luck or the actions of others. Consequently, they may not make the active coping efforts needed to adjust to the demands of living with a chronic health condition.

Evidence supports the value of these cognitive perspectives in understanding depression (Baer et al., 2012; Everaert et al., 2018). People who are depressed are more likely to attribute the causes of their failures to internal, stable, and global

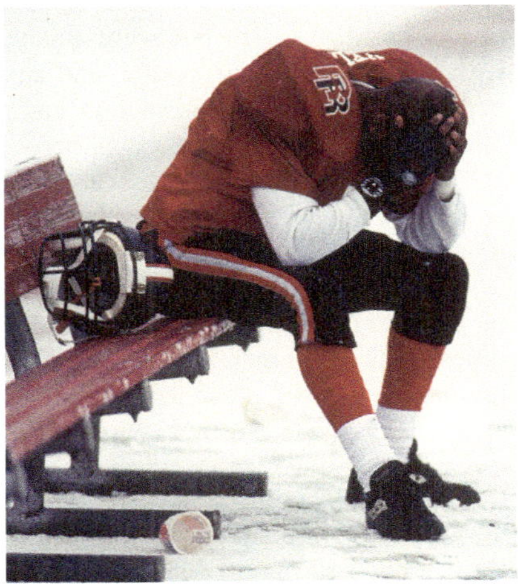

PCN Photography/Alamy Stock Photo

Why Did I Mess Up That Play? If he believes that he's just not skilled or talented enough and that he's likely to mess up again, he may be heading toward depression. But appraising the situation as a one-off—a single event that doesn't reflect his overall abilities—is likely to help him adjust to his disappointment.

factors—factors that they are relatively powerless to change (Hamilton et al., 2015). Consistent with Beck's cognitive theory, investigators find links between negative, distorted thinking and depression (e.g., Baer et al., 2012; Koster et al., 2011). That said, psychologists continue to debate whether attributional styles or distorted thinking cause depression or are themselves effects of depression. As this debate continues to play out, we may find that causal linkages work both ways—in other words, negative or distorted thinking patterns affect moods and moods affect how people think.

Evidence also points to genetic factors in the development of major depression and even more strongly in bipolar disorder (Carvalho, Firth, & Vieta, 2020; Kendler et al., 2020, 2023; Suran, 2022). For example, identical twins, who share 100% genetic overlap, are more likely to have bipolar disorder in common than are fraternal twins, who share 50% of their genes in common. There appear to be multiple genes involved in determining the risk of developing mood disorders (Musliner et al., 2019).

The links between depression and neurotransmitters are complex, but one thing is clear—depression is not caused by a chemical imbalance in the levels of these brain chemicals (Moncrieff et al., 2022). We know that antidepressant drugs increase levels of certain neurotransmitters in the brain within days or even a few hours of use, but the therapeutic effects of these drugs don't usually emerge until several weeks later. Current research in the field suggests that complex processes are involved that require more time to unfold, perhaps involving actions of

Health Psychology in the Digital Age

Is Social Media a Risk to the Nation's Psychological Health?

Does Facebook and other social media bring people down? Research at Utah Valley University showed that students who used Facebook longer and more frequently tended to see others as happier and leading better lives than they did (Chou & Edge, 2012). University of Michigan researchers found that greater Facebook use among students was associated with lower levels of happiness and life satisfaction (Kross et al., 2013).

Researchers suspect that an increase in depression among adolescent girls over the past decade or so may in part reflect increased use of social media sites such as Facebook (Twenge et al., 2018a, 2018b). Evidence is accumulating that greater use of social media sites in adolescents and young adults is associated with higher levels of depression and anxiety and lower levels of personal happiness, life satisfaction, and self-esteem (Bollen et al., 2017; Marino et al., 2018a, 2018b; Rozgonjuk et al., 2018). In 2023, the U.S. Surgeon General issued an alarm about social media use, pointing to a growing body of evidence linking use of social media to mental health problems in the nation's youth (Abbasi, 2023).

The average teen today spends about 3.5 hours a day on social media sites (Abbasi, 2023). It may not be the amount of screen time that is of concern as much as using social media as a basis for making unfavorable social comparisons with others (Ferguson et al., 2022; Spitzer, Crosby, & Witte, 2023; Stefana et al., 2022). The take-away message is that when we spend time comparing ourselves to others on social media sites like Facebook or Instagram, we may start thinking less of ourselves (Verduyn, Gugushvili, & Kross, 2021). To preserve self-esteem, it may be prudent to limit time spent online and to use social media time wisely to check in with friends, not to check out how other people's lives compare to your own. Also of concern to the mental health of the nation's youth is exposure to harmful content online, such as hateful messages, cyberbully, and sexual and violent content (Abbasi, 2023).

What might be at work here are the unintended consequences of social comparison (Joseph, 2020). Heavy users may

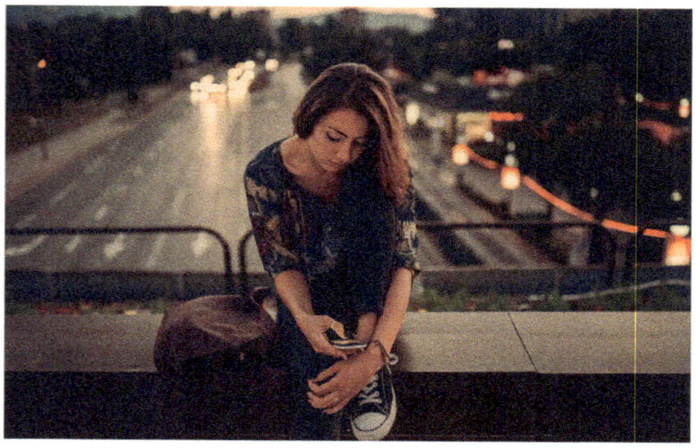

martin-dn/Getty Images

Alone and Depressed? Why is she on social media rather than interacting with her friends in person? Why does she care about who gets more likes? Researchers find that adolescents and emerging adults who spend more time on social media sites like Facebook are less happy and satisfied with their lives than those who are more likely to engage people in the flesh.

feel that they don't measure up in numbers of friends and likes. As a Michigan researcher said, "When you're on a site like Facebook, you get lots of posts about what people are doing. That sets up social comparison—you may feel your life is not as full and rich as those people you see on Facebook" (cited in Hu, 2013). Other researchers note that repeated exposure to idealized images of others leads adolescents to feel, again, that they "don't measure up" (Boers et al., 2019; Lee et al., 2020).

Links between social media use and psychological health are correlational, so we cannot say whether people who are unhappier become heavier users of social media, or whether heavier use of social media makes people unhappy. But even if cause and effect is somewhat clouded, heavy users of Facebook might be well advised to limit their time in the risk group.

these drugs on the sensitivity of receptors to which neurotransmitters bind or possibly changes in the numbers of these receptors (Chottekalapanda et al., 2020; Moriguchi et al., 2017).

We've come to understand that depression is a complex problem involving multiple causal factors. Other factors besides brain chemicals come into play, as we find in evidence from studies of brain scans of people with mood disorders that often show abnormalities in parts of the brain involved in processes that regulate thinking, memory, and emotional functioning (Roberts et al., 2022).

Applying Health Psychology

Coping with Depression

Be not afraid of life. Believe that life is worth living and your belief will help create the fact.

—William James

If you or someone close to you is struggling with depression, it makes sense to seek help from a professional. If emotional problems cause significant personal distress, if they persist for weeks or months, and if they impact the ability to function effectively in daily life—especially if there are intimations of suicide—then a professional evaluation is appropriate. But if you are confident that you can handle your feelings on your own, here are some ideas for lifting your mood—engaging in pleasant activities and practicing rational thinking.

Engaging in Pleasant Activities

Our emotions reflect our behavior. According to operant theory, maintaining our moods on an even keel depends on keeping reinforcement levels flowing. But a major contributor to depression is withdrawal from activities that we normally enjoy, leading to a vicious cycle of inactivity, lessened motivation, and continued inactivity. You may be able to lift your mood by increasing your participation in pleasant or pleasurable activities (Cujjpers et al., 2020; Hoyer et al., 2020).

List some 20 or 30 activities you have enjoyed, even if you have not engaged in them for some time. Examples might include attending a concert, going to a movie or a comedy club, bingeing on Netflix, watching a sunset, walking in a park, climbing a mountain, visiting friends, eating out, taking in a play or performance, reading for pleasure (not for work or school), and so on. Here is a list of activities that lift the mood for many people.

Why not set up a schedule in which you plan to engage in two or three activities each week? Afterward, jot down how you felt about the activity, from (1) "the pits" to (10) "totally great, wonderful." Repeat activities you enjoyed the most and experiment with new ones.

Rearranging a room
Dancing or singing
Helping a social or political group
Going to the park
Going to a museum or a concert
Reading a book or a magazine
Baking cookies or a cake
Visiting a sick person
Improving your diet
Hugging someone
Enjoying a sauna or a jacuzzi
Checking out old photos
People watching
Surfing the internet
Caring for houseplants
Riding a bike or jogging
Donating time to a charity
Playing an instrument
Flossing your teeth
Meditating

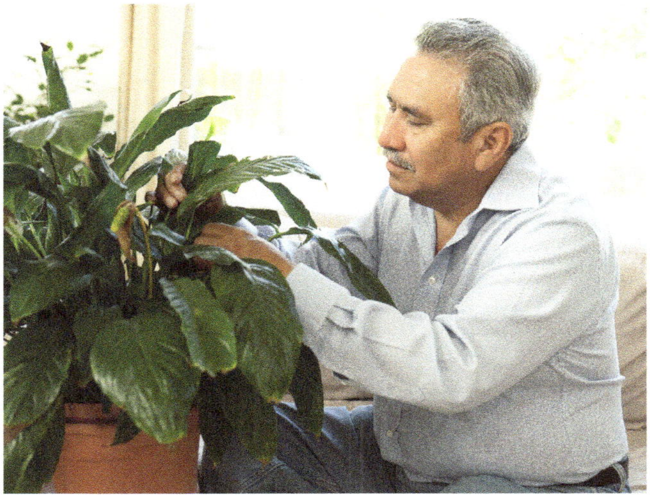

MBI/Alamy Stock Photo

A Pleasurable Activity A study conducted in the Twin Cities of Minnesota found that household gardening brings about as much happiness as eating out or going for a bicycle ride (Ambrose et al., 2020). Pleasurable activities help many people cope with depression and other psychological problems.

Thinking Rationally

Depressed people tend to appraise their failures and problems as stable (lasting) and global (pervasive)—as all but impossible to change. Depressed people also tend to appraise their problems as catastrophes and minimizing their accomplishments. Are you prone to these types of faulty patterns of thinking? Are your thoughts bringing you down? Might it be time to talk back to yourself?

Column 1 in **Table 11.4** shows examples of distorted, depressing thoughts. How many of these describe your own thinking patterns? Column 2 indicates the type of cognitive error (such as internalizing or catastrophizing), and Column 3 shows examples of rational alternatives for thoughts that bring you down.

You can pinpoint distorted thoughts by identifying the kinds of thoughts you have when you're feeling down. What thoughts pop in your head when things go wrong? Look for the fleeting thoughts that trigger mood changes. It may help to jot them down and examine them in the light of reality. Challenge their accuracy. Do you appraise difficult situations as impossible and hopeless? Do you set unrealistic expectations for yourself or minimize your achievements? Do you internalize more than your fair share of blame?

Challenge negative thoughts whenever and wherever they occur. When you catch a negative thought, stop and think again. Jot down the negative thought. Then challenge the thought by talking back to yourself, rationally. You can get the ball rolling by posing challenging countermands to your negative thoughts, as in the following examples:

- Why must it be so?
- Who says it must be so?
- Is there any evidence that it must be so?
- Is there an alternative way of appraising the situation?
- What rational thought can I substitute for this disturbing thought?

Put negative and irrational beliefs on trial. Challenge their validity and their hold over you.

Many of us create or compound feelings of depression because of cognitive errors such as those we see here. Do any of these distorted thoughts hit home with you? If so, it might be advisable to challenge them and substitute rational alternatives.

TABLE 11.4 Distorted, Depressing Thoughts and Rational Alternatives

Distorted Thoughts	Types of Distorted Thoughts	Rational Alternatives
"There's nothing I can do."	Catastrophizing, Jumping to Conclusions	"I can't think of anything to do right now, but if I work at it, I may."
"I'm no good."	Internalizing, Globalizing, Stabilizing	"I did something I regret, but that doesn't make me evil or worthless as a person."
"This is absolutely awful."	Catastrophizing	"This is pretty bad, but it's not the end of the world."
"I just don't have the brains for college."	Globalizing, Stabilizing	"I guess I really need to go back over the basics in that course."
"I just can't believe I did something so disgusting!"	Catastrophizing	"That was a bad experience. Well, I won't be likely to try that again soon."
"I can't imagine ever feeling right."	Jumping to Conclusions	"This is painful, but if I try to work it through step by step, I'll probably eventually see my way out of it."
"It's all my fault."	Internalizing	"I'm not blameless, but I wasn't the only one involved. It may have been my idea, but he went into it with his eyes open."
"I can't do anything right."	Internalizing, Globalizing, Stabilizing	"I sure screwed this up, but I've done a lot of things well, and I'll do other things well."
"I hurt everybody who gets close to me."	Internalizing, Globalizing, Stabilizing	"I'm not totally blameless, but I'm not responsible for the whole world. Others make their own decisions, and they have to live with the results too."
"If people knew the real me, they would have it in for me."	Dismissing the Positives, Jumping to Conclusions, All-or-Nothing Thinking	"I'm not perfect, but nobody's perfect. I have positive as well as negative features, and I am entitled to some self-interests."

Whatever roles biological factors may play in mood disorders, psychological factors, such as stress, availability of social support, and negative thinking patterns, are also important influences. Sorting out the interactions among psychological and biological factors leads researchers to zero in on interactions of mind and body.

microbiome The communities of microbial life, including bacteria and viruses, living within the body.

An intriguing line of inquiry into depression examines how stress interacts with underlying biological processes, such as the immune system and the human **microbiome**. Researchers recognize that our mental and physical health depends on maintaining a delicate balance between the body's stress response, immune system functioning, and the microbiome in the human gut or digestive track (Cruz-Pereira et al., 2020). Stressful life events may disrupt this fine balance, leading to dysregulation in brain physiology and behavior that contributes the development of major depression and other mood disorders. One possibility is that stressful life events trigger an immune system response, resulting in inflammation in neural pathways in the brain, thereby affecting mood states and leading to depression (Nie et al., 2018).

Inflammation results from the body's immune system response to various types of bodily threats, such as invading pathogens like bacteria and viruses, and to negative life events which the body may perceive as imminent threats (Cruz-Pereira et al., 2020). Increasing evidence points to brain inflammation playing a role in depression (Caneo et al., 2016; Fleshner et al., 2017). We are only beginning to learn about the role that gut bacteria may play in these pathways, but researchers suspect that changes in the microbial balance in the gut may affect the immune system, which in turn may affect brain functioning, leading to disturbed mood states (Cruz-Pereira et al., 2020). All things considered, mood disorders are complex problems reflecting the roles of many factors and their interactions (Dunn et al., 2015).

Bipolar Disorder

> *When you're high it's tremendous. The ideas and feelings are fast and frequent like shooting stars, and you follow them until you find better and brighter ones. Shyness goes, the right words and gestures are suddenly there, the power to captivate others a felt certainty ... Sensuality is pervasive and the desire to seduce and be seduced irresistible. Feelings of ease, intensity, power, well-being, financial omnipotence, and euphoria pervade one's marrow. But, somewhere, this changes. The fast ideas are far too fast, and there are far too many; overwhelming confusion replaces clarity. Memory goes. Humor and absorption on friends' faces are replaced by fear and concern.*
>
> —**Kay Redfield Jamison, *An Unquiet Mind***

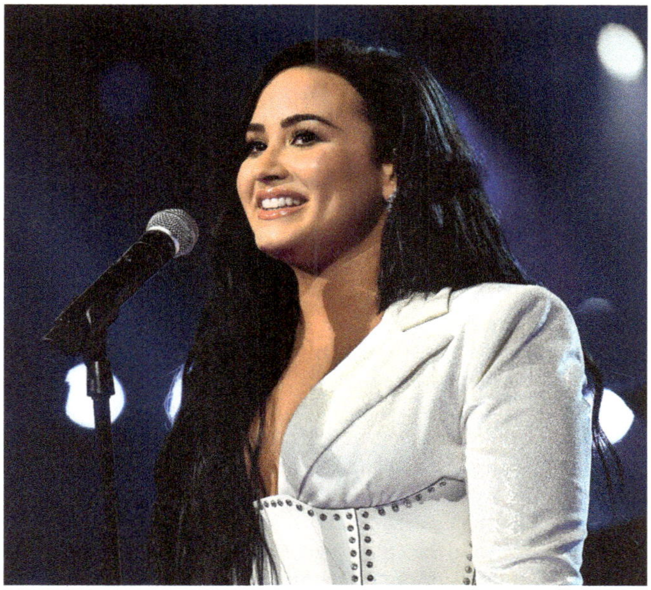

Emma McIntyre/Getty Images

Demi Lovato Singer Demi Lovato was reportedly diagnosed with bipolar disorder. She has been a strong mental health advocate, openly discussing her problems with alcohol and an eating disorder as well as bipolar disorder.

Bipolar disorder affects about 1% of adults at some point in their lives (Moreira et al., 2017). People with bipolar disorder, formerly known as *manic-depression*, have mood swings from great elation to deep depression. The cycles seem to be unrelated to external events. In the elated phase, or **mania**, the person may show excessive excitement or silliness, such as carrying jokes too far.

The person in a manic phase may be argumentative, destroy property, and show poor judgment, as by making huge contributions to charity they can ill afford or giving away expensive possessions. Others tend to find people in a manic phase to be abrasive and so they avoid them. In a manic phase, the person may be restless and unable to sit still or sleep restfully, may speak rapidly (showing "pressured speech"), and may jump from topic to topic (showing rapid flights of ideas). It can be hard to get a word in edgewise. **Table 11.5** shows differences in symptoms between manic and depressive episodes.

Depression is the other side of the proverbial coin. In the depressive phase of bipolar disorder, the person is likely to have a downcast mood, sleep more than usual, and feel unmotivated and lethargic. They may become socially withdrawn and irritable. Some people with bipolar disorder attempt suicide when the mood shifts from the elated phase toward depression. They will do almost anything to escape the depths of depression that lie ahead.

bipolar disorder A psychological disorder that is associated with unusual shifts in mood, energy, activity levels, concentration, and the ability to carry out day-to-day tasks.

mania A state of excessive elation and overactivity, characteristic of the manic phase of bipolar disorder.

TABLE 11.5 Comparing Symptoms of Manic and Depressive Episodes

INTERACTIVE FIGURES, CHARTS, & TABLES

Symptoms of a Manic Episode	Symptoms of a Depressive Episode
Feeling very up, high, elated, or extremely irritable or touchy	Feeling very down or sad, or anxious
Feeling jumpy or wired, more active than usual	Feeling slowed down or restless
Having a decreased need for sleep	Having trouble falling asleep, waking up too early, or sleeping too much
Talking fast about a lot of different things ("flight of ideas")	Talking very slowly, feeling unable to find anything to say, or forgetting a lot
Racing thoughts	Having trouble concentrating or making decisions
Feeling able to do many things at once without getting tired	Feeling unable to do even simple things
Having excessive appetite for food, drinking, sex, or other pleasurable activities	Having a lack of interest in almost all activities
Feeling unusually important, talented, or powerful	Feeling hopeless or worthless, or thinking about death or suicide

Source: NIMH (2023). https://www.nimh.nih.gov/health/topics/bipolar-disorder.

Health Psychology in Action

The Pandemic and Psychological Health: What Have We Learned?

The effects of the COVID-19 pandemic rippled across virtually every aspect of human life. Primary of course were the millions of lives lost worldwide, a staggering total of about 7 million deaths by the middle of 2023. Nearly 700 million people were confirmed infected, but the numbers of confirmed cases were but the tip of the proverbial iceberg. Virtually everyone in virtually every country on the planet was either infected or had a close friend or family member with the disease. COVID preyed upon the most vulnerable of us, the elderly and those with pre-existing medical conditions that put them at higher risk of serious and often fatal complications. But what about of the mental health effects of the pandemic? What have we learned of the emotional consequences of living through a deadly pandemic?

The mental health consequences are often thought of as the hidden costs of the pandemic. We might be able to measure the staggering economic costs of a global shutdown, but what of the costs that cannot be measured in dollars and cents? What of the loss of educational development and socialization of children schooled virtually rather than having engaging others in the classroom and playground? It's as if we were all part of a vast, unplanned experiment, the outcomes of which will be unfolding for years to come.

Health psychologists and other health researchers are actively involved in efforts to understand the psychological consequences of the disease and the disruptions the pandemic caused in our daily lives. We lived through a time in which we masked up, kept our distance from others, and used videoconferencing in place of direct human interactions. People got hitched in zoom weddings and families gathered in front of their laptops to "share" a Thanksgiving dinner or family celebration.

As researchers continue to explore the emotional consequences of the pandemic, certain trends have emerged. We've learned, not surprisingly, that there was a spike in rates of anxiety and depression early in the pandemic as our lives were turned upside down and we collectively faced a threat of disease for which there was no effective vaccine or treatment (Fitzpatrick et al., 2020; Haydon & Salvatore, 2021; McGinty et al., 2020; Stix, 2022). British researchers reported the greatest levels of emotional distress reported among people in their 50s and early 60s that had ever been reported since they had started keeping records some 40 years earlier, with women bearing more of the brunt of the emotional effects than men (Moreno-Agostino et al., 2023).

Coping with the disease itself and its aftermath also took an emotional toll, as evidence showed that about 20% of people who survived COVID-19 infection went on to develop a diagnosable psychiatric or psychological disorder within 90 days of infection (Taquet et al., 2021). The most common mental disorders involved problems relating to anxiety and insomnia, but there were also increased rates of dementia, suggesting that in some cases the virus may have directly invaded the brain.

Signs of Resilience

But there were some hopeful signs as well that speak to the resilience of people in the face of extreme stress. Despite the rise in levels of anxiety and depression, health researchers did not find any significant change in rates of suicide, or lower levels of life satisfaction, or, perhaps most surprisingly of all in light of the COVID restrictions, no significant increase in reported loneliness, at least through the first year of the pandemic (Aknin et al., 2022). Perhaps most remarkably, levels of emotional distress tended to bounce back, though not completely, to pre-pandemic levels within the first year of the pandemic (Aknin et al., 2022).

Who Was Most Affected?

Not everyone was affected in the same way. Health researchers have begun drilling down to study the effects of the pandemic on the most vulnerable groups. One population group which appears more vulnerable to the emotional toll of social isolation during lockdowns were young people. Researchers find that rates of eating disorders surged among teens during the pandemic, along with sharp increases in anxiety, as young people struggled with the isolating effects of the early lockdowns (Kwong et al., 2022; Morales et al., 2022).

The consequences of the pandemic were also more pronounced among groups with fewer economic resources and those lacking social and family support. A study of Black Americans in the rural south found that people showing the greatest emotional consequences of the pandemic—more depression and sleep problems—as well as greater physical health problems more often struggled with significant stressors before the pandemic, such as financial hardship (Adesogan et al., 2022).

Other research groups in different parts of the world showed that the groups of people most affected emotionally by the pandemic tended to be young women and parents of young children (Aknin et al., 2022). Here we see the close interdependence of emotional effects between people, especially between mothers and children. Researchers find that depression in mothers tracked to depression in their children. Although these connections need to be more fully mapped out, it's likely that the parent's emotional well-being affected their children and, vice-versa, that their children's mental health affected their own. To health psychologists, it's no surprise that emotional or psychological health reflects interdependency between people. For example, we know that people with strong social networks and supportive others whom they can depend upon are generally more resilient in the face of stress, even the stress of a global pandemic.

It's important to note that most people who were infected with COVID-19 recovered within a few weeks or months, but many others continue to suffer from long-term effects of the virus and its aftermath. One of the continuing challenges health investigators will need to address in the years and decades ahead is to better understand the physical and mental health impacts effects of long-term COVID infection and developing ways of helping people cope with these continuing challenges (Liu, 2022).

Schizophrenia

VIDEO CONTENT
Schizophrenia

Jennifer was 19. Her husband David brought her into the emergency room because she had cut her wrists. When she was interviewed, her attention wandered. She seemed distracted by things in the air or something she might be hearing. It was as if she had an invisible earphone. She explained that she had cut her wrists because the "hellsmen" had told her to. Then she seemed frightened. Later she said that the hellsmen had warned her not to reveal their existence. She had been afraid that they would punish her for talking about them. David and Jennifer had been married for about 1 year. At first they had been together in a small apartment in town. But Jennifer did not want to be near other people and had convinced him to rent a bungalow in the country. There she would make fantastic drawings of goblins and monsters during the day. Now and then she would become agitated and act as if invisible things were giving her instructions.

"I'm bad," Jennifer would mutter, "I'm bad." She would begin to jumble her words. David would then try to convince her to go to the hospital, but she would refuse. Then the wrist-cutting would begin. David thought he had made the cottage safe by removing knives and blades. But Jennifer would always find something. Then Jennifer would be brought to the hospital, have stitches put in, be kept under observation and medicated with antipsychotic drugs. She would explain that she cut herself because the hellsmen had told her that she was bad and must die. After a few days she would deny hearing the hellsmen, and she would insist on leaving the hospital. Once she was stabilized, she would be released, but the pattern would continue.

—Authors' files

schizophrenia A chronic psychological disorder that is characterized by illogical thinking, incoherent speech, inappropriate emotional responses, delusions, hallucinations, and bizarre behavior.

Schizophrenia is a chronic disorder that corresponds most closely to popular concepts of "madness" or "insanity." The disorder follows a chronic, lifelong course and typically develops in late adolescence or early adulthood, the very time in life when young people are beginning to make their way in the world (Kuo et al., 2022). The disorder is characterized by disturbances in thought, coherence of speech, perception, emotional responses, and interpersonal functioning. The primary feature is a break with reality that may take the form of bizarre, irrational behavior and by hallucinations (sensory experiences in the absence of external stimuli, such as hearing voices, or seeing things that are not physically there) and delusions, which are fixed but patently false beliefs or ideas. Recent estimates indicate that schizophrenia affects about 0.7% to 1% of the U.S. population (Goff, 2020; Keepers et al., 2020).

Delusions often involve paranoid themes, such as delusions of persecution or jealousy, that are disconnected from reality. Delusions tend to be unshakable even in the face of evidence that they are not true. People with delusions of persecution may believe that they are sought by the mafia, CIA, FBI, or some other group. A woman with delusions said that news stories contained coded information about her. A man with schizophrenia complained that neighbors had "bugged" his walls with "radios." Other people with schizophrenia have delusions that they have committed unpardonable sins, that they are rotting away from disease, or that they or the world doesn't exist. The onset of schizophrenia is typically during late adolescence or early adulthood, the time in life that young people are starting to make their way into the world (McGrath et al., 2016; NIMH, 2018b).

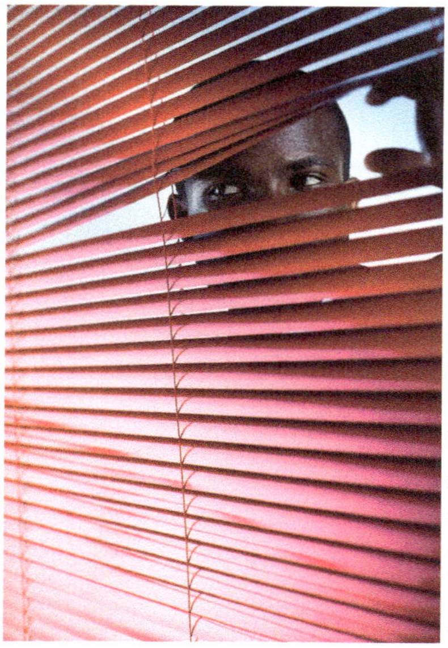

Classic Collection/Shotshop GmbH/Alamy Stock Photo

Paranoia People with schizophrenia often have delusions of persecution. They may also have delusions that their partners are cheating on them. They may believe that news stories refer to them in some sort of code. They also frequently have hallucinations, as in "hearing" voices in their heads.

Schizophrenia affects 0.79% to 1% of the general population in the United States, which is about 8 to 10 cases in 1,000 people (Goff, 2020; Keepers et al., 2020). Men are somewhat more likely to develop the disorder and to develop it earlier than women, as well as to have a more severe form of the disorder. Nearly 1 million people are treated for schizophrenia each year in the United States, with about one-third receiving care in a hospital.

People with schizophrenia tend to have problems in memory, attention, and communication. Their ability to think and process information becomes unraveled. Unless people without schizophrenia allow their thoughts to wander, their thinking is normally tightly knit. They start at a certain point, and thoughts that come to mind (their associations) tend to be logically connected. But people with schizophrenia often think illogically. Their speech becomes jumbled and their thoughts loosely associated. They may combine parts of words into new words or make meaningless rhymes. They may jump from topic to topic, conveying little useful information. They usually do not recognize that their thoughts and behavior are abnormal.

catatonic behavior Striking impairments in bodily movements and thinking processes, as in a state of stupor; sometimes seen in people with schizophrenia and other severe disorders.

Although uncommon, people with schizophrenia may show **catatonic behavior**, in which their movements slow down to a state of stupor and then suddenly change to an agitated phase. People in a catatonic state may maintain unusual, even difficult, postures for hours, even as their limbs grow swollen or stiff. A striking feature of catatonia is waxy flexibility, in which the person maintains positions into which he or she has been manipulated by others. These individuals may also be mute but afterward report that they heard what others were saying at the time. They may also make strange gestures and facial expressions.

Emotional responses of people with schizophrenia may be flat (nonexpressive) or inappropriate—as in giggling upon hearing bad news. People with schizophrenia may withdraw from others and become wrapped upon in their own thoughts and fantasies and have difficulty understanding other people's feelings.

Origins of Schizophrenia The origins of schizophrenia remain somewhat elusive, but most researchers believe that schizophrenia is a brain disorder that arises from a combination of psychosocial factors, such as stressful life experiences, and biological factors, such as genetics and neurotransmitter irregularities in the brain. A large body of evidence points to a strong role of genetics in the development of schizophrenia (e.g., Kahn, 2020; Kendler et al., 2023; Trubetskoy et al., 2022, among others). Also, the more closely two people are related, the more likely they are to share the diagnosis of schizophrenia.

Scientists are making headway pinpointing particular genes involved in the disorder (Thyme et al., 2019; Wilkinson et al., 2018). A landmark study published in 2016 linked certain genetic variations associated with schizophrenia to a thinning of the synapses (connections) between neurons in the prefrontal cortex of the brain, the so-called executive center where people plan and make decisions (Dhindsa & Goldstein, 2016; Sekar et al., 2016; Weidenauer et al., 2020). Also, the more closely two people are related, the more likely they are to share the diagnosis of schizophrenia.

concordance rate The rate of agreement, or co-occurrence, as in the percentage of twins who share a particular disorder with their twin.

Although genetics plays a key role in determining vulnerability to schizophrenia, it is not the only risk factor. If it were, we would expect a 100% **concordance rate** (percentage of agreement) between identical twins (who share all their genes), as opposed to the observed rate in the 40–50% range. Therefore, scientists are suggesting that genetic factors may be a *necessary* condition for the development of schizophrenia in that they create a vulnerability or predisposition to the disorder, but at least in many cases, genetic factors are not a *sufficient* cause of its development. Thus other environmental and biological factors may come into the picture.

For example, the mothers of many people who later developed schizophrenia had complications during pregnancy and birth (Murray et al., 2017). Many of these mothers came down with flu during the sixth or seventh month of pregnancy (Ersoy et al., 2017; Racicot & Mor, 2017). Birth complications, especially prolonged labor, may be connected with the development of brain abnormalities in people with schizophrenia (Eom et al., 2020; Kahn, 2020; Li et al., 2020). Poor maternal nutrition has also been implicated (Mackay et al., 2017). We also have evidence showing structural abnormalities in the brain in many people with schizophrenia that indicates a loss or thinning of brain tissue needed to think and perceive the world clearly (e.g., Cheng et al., 2021; Kuo et al., 2022; Zhao et al., 2022). These brain abnormalities may also be a product of genetic factors.

Problems in the nervous system may involve disturbances in brain chemistry as well as brain structures. Research along these lines has led to the *dopamine theory* of schizophrenia. The theory explains the breakdown in thinking and perception in schizophrenia in terms of the brain's oversensitivity to the neurotransmitter dopamine (Gallagher, 2021; Honer, 2021; Schmack et al., 2021). This explanation is bolstered by evidence that antipsychotic medications that help control the symptoms of schizophrenia reduce dopamine activity in the brain (Weidenauer et al., 2020). The chemicals in these medications fit into dopamine receptors in the brain, blocking out excess dopamine.

In sum, it seems clear that schizophrenia is a brain disorder. The parts of the brain most strongly implicated are those that enable us to organize our thoughts, keep information in working memory, develop and carry out plans, process emotional experiences, distinguish reality from mental imaginings, and maintain attention—the very functions that tend to be impaired in people with schizophrenia.

Treatment and Adherence Antipsychotic medications help quell the more flagrant symptoms of schizophrenia. They are typically administered orally, once a day. But the medications are effective only if people take them, and they are not a cure. Problems of adherence to medication, as discussed in Chapter 2, have special relevance to the treatment of schizophrenia, as evidence shows better symptom control and psychosocial functioning in people who take their medication reliably (Bernardo et al., 2017).

According to the Health Belief Model (HBM), people adhere to medical treatment when they perceive the benefits of doing so to outweigh the costs, or barriers. As schizophrenia typically involves disturbed thinking many patients with the disorder become paranoid and suspicious of medication, seeing it as a method that others are using to attempt to control them (Freudenreich, 2020a; Smart et al., 2019; Zink & Englisch, 2016).

Healthcare professionals have attempted to promote adherence in many ways. One method is the use of long-acting injectable antipsychotic medication (Freudenreich, 2020). The injections are given every 2 to 12 weeks, depending on the chosen medicine. To be fully effective, however, "oral overlap" is recommended for many of these injectable antipsychotics, at least for early doses. Therefore, there remains the problem of patients skipping oral medications. Moreover, patients must return to the clinic for injections as previous doses are wearing off. When doses begin to wear off, patients may become less likely to perceive the benefits of the medication and become reluctant to continue their use, or even become suspicious of the treatment or treatment providers.

Psychological treatments to encourage people with schizophrenia to adhere to treatment include motivational interviewing. A Dutch study using a structured form of interviewing that focuses on increasing motivation for treatment helped improve adherence in many but not all people with schizophrenia. The development of a trusting relationship and empathy were also of help (Dobber et al., 2020). Other studies support the importance of developing a good therapeutic relationship in boosting adherence (Dobber et al., 2020; Tessier et al., 2020).

Cognitive behavioral therapy has also been shown to be of help with many patients in reducing hallucinations, delusions, and bizarre behaviors while at the same time ameliorating social withdrawal (Rector & Beck, 2001; Rector et al., 2011). Many studies have shown that cognitive behavioral therapy is especially effective when used along with antipsychotic medication (e.g., Grant et al., 2012).

Adherence to treatment remains a problem with people with schizophrenia, but combinations of psychological and medical treatments hold much promise.

Review 11.3

INTERACTIVE SELF-SCORING QUIZZES

Sentence Completion

1. Nearly a (quarter or half) of adult Americans develop a diagnosable psychological disorder at some point in their lives.

2. More than 1 in (2 or 5) adults in the United States are currently affected by a diagnosable psychological or mental disorder.

3. Psychologists take the __________ context into account when making judgments about abnormal behavior.

4. A vulnerability or predisposition is called a __________.

5. Anxiety-related disorders affect an estimated 1 in (3 or 5) adults in the United States during their lifetimes.

6. Persistent anxiety that is not limited to particular situations is called __________ anxiety.

7. The stronger a person's fear of spiders, the (larger or smaller) the person is likely to perceive the size of a spider in a room.

8. An irresistible urge to perform a specific act is called a(n) __________.

9. An __________ is a recurrent, intrusive, anxiety-provoking thought or image.

10. About 1 in (2 or 10) adults suffers from major depression in any given year.

11. Genetic and __________ factors interact in a complex interplay that gives rise to abnormal behavior patterns.

12. The leading cause of disability worldwide is major __________.

13. Reasoning based on your emotions is called __________ based reasoning.

14. The large jump in depression among adolescent girls over the past decade may partly be the result of increased use of __________ sites.

15. Multiple genes, not any one single gene, appear to be involved in the development of __________.

16. The brains of people with schizophrenia often show (larger or smaller) ventricles (hollow spaces).

Think About It

Do you or someone close to you suffer from a diagnosable psychological disorder? Have you or they sought professional help? Why or why not?

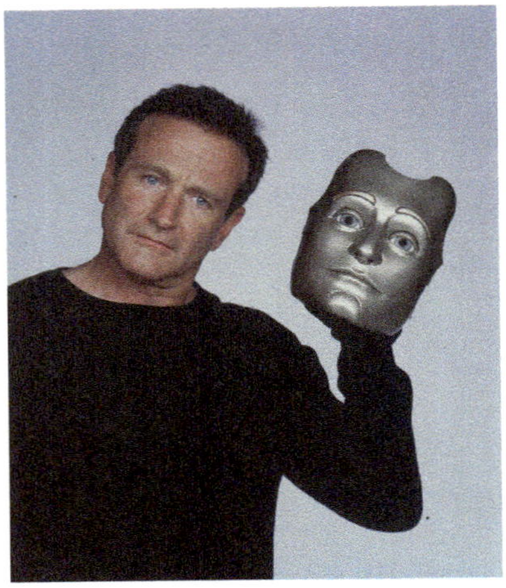

Granamour Weems Collection/Alamy Stock Photo

Comedian and Actor Robin Williams Fans were shocked when Williams committed suicide, because he was always—as far as they knew—so quick-witted, bubbly, and humorous. Only a few people knew that his final years were wracked with despair and pain due to illness.

Suicide: A Growing Public Health Crisis

After motor vehicle accidents, what would you say is the next leading cause of death among college students and among young people in general in the 10–24-year age range? Homicide? AIDS? Drugs? The answer is suicide (Curtin, 2020). Tragically, we lose more than 12,000 young people annually in the United States as the result of suicide, including more than 1,000 college students. Overall, approximately 47,000 Americans commit suicide each year. For the U.S. adult population, suicide is the 10th leading cause of death (Barry et al., 2023). The most common and most lethal method of suicide involves the use of firearms (Kuehn, 2021). Suicide attempts and completed suicides are rising in the United States, having jumped by more than 30% over the past twenty years or so (Bommersbach, Rosenheck, & Rhee, 2022; O'Connor et al., 2023).

Who's at Risk?

Consider some facts about suicide. More adolescents and young adults die from suicide than from cancer, heart disease, AIDS, birth defects, stroke, pneumonia and influenza, and chronic lung disease combined. The public's attention is focused on suicide among adolescents, which can border on sensationalism and may make it seem romantic in the minds of impressionable young people struggling with problems. However, older adults are actually much more likely to take their own lives. Table 11.6 shows some facts about suicide. Women are more likely to attempt suicide, but about three times more men complete the act, largely because men typically use more lethal means, especially firearms (Barry et al., 2023).

Suicide attempts are increasing, especially among adolescents and young adults (Miron et al., 2019). We can trace the rise in suicidal behavior in young people in large part to the greater prevalence of anxiety and depressive disorders and the meteoric rise in social networking use, which as we noted raises concerns about those who regularly compare themselves unfavorably to others on these sites.

Factors in Suicide

People with psychiatric disorders and those who have attempted suicide in the past are at heightened risk of suicidal behavior (Barry et al., 2023). The psychological disorders most commonly linked to suicide are major depression and bipolar disorder, especially when

TABLE 11.6 Some Facts About Suicide

- More than 47,000 Americans take their own lives each year—1 every 12 minutes. Every day, nearly 130 Americans take their own lives and more than 2,500 attempt to do so.
- Suicide is the 10th leading cause of death in the United States.
- About 2.5 times as many deaths result from suicide as from homicide.
- Native Americans (American Indians and Alaska Natives) have the highest suicide rates in the nation, followed by non-Hispanic White Americans.
- More than half of all suicides occur in adult men, aged 25–65 years.
- Many people who make suicide attempts do not seek professional care afterward.
- Among adolescents and young adults, more deaths result from suicide than from cancer, heart disease, AIDS, birth defects, stroke, pneumonia and influenza, and chronic lung disease combined.

Sources: Department of Health and Human Services (2001), CDC (2019), Kuehn (2018), NCHS (2023), Rey et al., 2023

Applying Health Psychology

Suicide Prevention

Imagine that you are having a heart-to-heart talk with Jamie, one of your best friends. Things haven't been going well. Jamie's grandmother died a month ago, and they were very close. Jamie's coursework has been suffering, and things have also been going downhill with the person Jamie has been seeing. But you are not prepared when Jamie looks you in the eye and says, "I've been thinking about this for days, and I've decided that the only way out is to kill myself."

If someone tells you that they are considering suicide, you may become frightened and flustered or feel that an enormous burden has been placed on you. You are right—it has. In such a case, your objective should be to encourage the person to consult a healthcare provider, or to consult one yourself, as soon as possible. But if the person refuses to talk to anyone else and you feel that you can't break free for a consultation, there are a number of things you can do:

1. *Keep talking.* Encourage the person to talk to you or to some other trusted person. Draw the person out with questions like "What's happening?," "Where do you hurt?," "What do you want to happen?" Questions like these may encourage the person to express frustrated needs and thereby provide some relief. They also give you time to think.
2. *Be a good listener.* Be supportive with people who express suicidal thoughts or feel depressed, hopeless, or worthless. They may believe their condition will never improve, but let them know that you are there for them and are willing to assist them to get help. Show that you understand how upset the person is. Do not say "Don't be silly."
3. *Suggest that something other than suicide might solve the problem, even if it is not evident at the time.* Many suicidal people see only two solutions—either death or a magical resolution of their problems. Therapists try to "remove the mental blinders" from suicidal people.
4. *Emphasize as concretely as possible how the person's suicide would be devastating to you and to other people who care.*
5. *Ask how the person intends to commit suicide.* People with concrete plans and a weapon are at greater risk. Ask if you might hold on to the weapon for a while. Sometimes the answer is yes.
6. *Do not tell people threatening suicide that they're acting stupid or crazy.*
7. *Do not insist on contact with specific people, such as parents or a spouse:* Conflict with these people may have led to the suicidal thinking in the first place.
8. *Suggest that the person go with you to obtain professional help now:* Call the local emergency department, suicide hotline, campus counseling center or infirmary, campus or local police station, or 911 for assistance. Explain that your friend is threatening suicide and you require immediate assistance. Offer to accompany the person to a healthcare provider or facility. If you cannot maintain contact with the suicidal person before the person can be brought to a healthcare professional, get professional assistance as soon as you separate.

You can also look into the following resources for assistance:

- The National Suicide Prevention Lifeline: 1-800-273-TALK (8255). The website of the American Association of Suicidology (www.suicidology.org) provides information on ways to prevent suicide. You will also find a list of crisis centers.
- American Foundation for Suicide Prevention: Its website (www.afsp.org) offers information about suicide and links to other suicide and mental health sites.
- American Psychological Association (APA): The APA website (www.apa.org) provides information about risk factors, warning signs, and prevention. Go to TOPICS, then Suicide.
- Suicide Awareness—Voices of Education (SA/VE): Its website (www.save.org) offers educational and practical information on suicide and depression. It highlights ways in which family members and friends can help suicidal people. The Canadian Centre for Suicide Prevention (www.siec.ca) offers a specialized library on suicide.

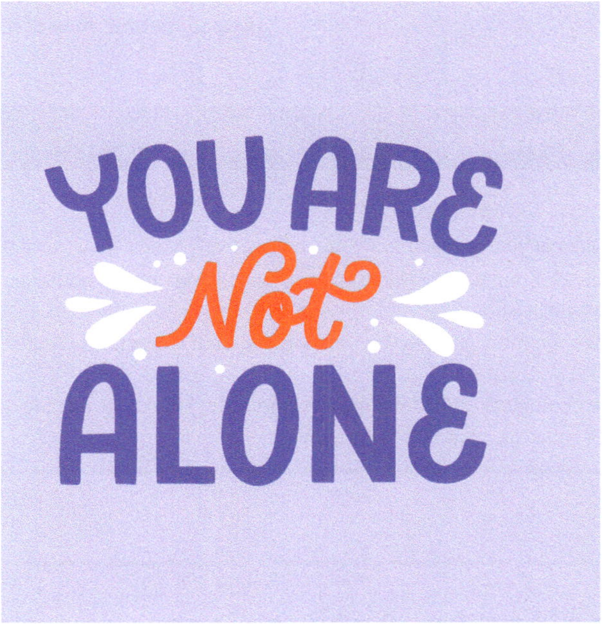

Камилла Хайруллина/Getty Images

compounded by deep feelings of hopelessness and helplessness in coping with life problems (Fazel & Runeson, 2020; Lannoy et al., 2023; Omary, 2021). Between 2% and 15% of people who are depressed eventually commit suicide, generally at a point in their lives when they feel utterly hopeless about their lives and helpless to change them.

Other factors implicated in suicide are problems in relationships (42%) and alcohol or other types of substance abuse (28%) (Fox, 2018). Other risk factors include persistent pain, severe chronic illness, financial problems, and a family history of suicide (Fazel & Runeson, 2020). Copycat suicides contribute to a so-called cluster effect among adolescents.

Stressful life events often serve as triggers for suicidal thoughts and behaviors, especially life events that entail loss of social support—as in the loss of a spouse, friend, or close relative (Liu & Miller, 2014). People under stress who have difficulty resolving problems, especially conflict with other people, may consider suicide. They may see no way of resolving their problems other than taking their own lives.

Biological factors are also implicated in suicide. Like depression, suicide may involve irregularities in the utilization of neurotransmitters in the brain (Petersen et al., 2014; Sullivan et al., 2015). Reduced availability in the brain of serotonin and norepinephrine are linked to depression, so the linkage between suicide and these neurotransmitters is not surprising (Santos & Miller, 2020). But serotonin's influence on curbing impulsive behavior, including impulses to harm oneself, may play a more direct role.

Myths About Suicide

You may have heard that individuals who threaten suicide are only seeking attention; those who are serious just "do it." Not so. Most people who commit suicide had earlier given warnings about their intentions, consulted a healthcare provider, or made earlier attempts (Luoma et al., 2002). One study showed that among adolescents who attempted suicide and were treated in hospital emergency departments, rates of later completed suicide were more than 10 times higher among females and more than 20 times higher among males than were the rates among the general adolescent population (Olfson et al., 2005). Recognize, too, that contrary to widespread belief, discussing suicide with a person who is depressed does not prompt the person to attempt suicide. Extracting a promise not to commit suicide before calling or visiting a healthcare provider may actually prevent some suicides.

Some people believe that you have to be "insane" to take your own life. However, suicidal thinking is not necessarily a sign of inability to perceive reality and organize one's thoughts. Instead, people may consider suicide when they think they have run out of options.

Review 11.4

INTERACTIVE SELF-SCORING QUIZZES

Sentence Completion

1. (Older or younger) adults are much more likely to take their own lives.
2. Suicide attempts are (increasing or decreasing) among adolescents and young adults.
3. Men are more likely to commit suicide than women by a factor of about __________ to 1.
4. Psychological disorders most commonly linked to suicide are severe __________ disorders.
5. It is not true that people who threaten suicide are only seeking __________.

Think About It

What would you say or do if a friend or loved one threatened suicide? Who might you turn to for help? What resources are available in your college or community to assist someone in a suicidal crisis?

Recite: An Active Summary

INTERACTIVE SELF-SCORING QUIZZES

Chapter 11 Practice Quiz

1. Describe the features of a healthy personality from the perspective of major theories of personality.

From a Freudian or psychodynamic perspective, a healthy personality balances the demands of id, ego, and superego, so that instinctual impulses can be gratified within the constraints of social reality and one's moral conscience. From a social cognitive perspective, a healthy personality incorporates personal variables that allow us to function effectively and pursue our goals, such as competencies, accurate encoding of events and expectancies, ability to regulate our emotional responses, and ability to learn by observing others in our social environment. Humanistic theorists propose that a healthy personality involves knowing oneself and making authentic choices consistent with one's needs, values, and goals. From a trait perspective, a healthy personality is one that possesses psychological traits associated with healthy outcomes, such as conscientiousness and emotional stability.

2. Discuss why we need adequate sleep to maintain our physical and psychological health.

Sleep restores the body and the psychological functions of attention, learning, memory, and executive planning and helps maintain healthy functioning of our immune systems. Seven hours a night is the recommended minimum for adults.

3. Discuss the problem of insomnia and cognitive behavioral methods for managing it.

Insomnia is persistent difficulty falling asleep or remaining asleep. People who are troubled by insomnia may benefit from developing healthier sleep habits and challenging irrational, exaggerated fears about what might happen if they do not get enough sleep.

4. Identify criteria used to distinguish normal from abnormal behavior.

Clinicians identify abnormal behavior based on multiple criteria that include unusualness, faulty perceptions or thinking, significant emotional distress, self-defeating behavior, dangerousness, and social unacceptability.

5. Identify the major types of psychological disorders.

Types of psychological disorders are organized in terms of patterns of abnormal behaviors or symptoms. Anxiety-related disorders typically involve anxiety that is excessive, self-defeating, or inappropriate to a person's situation. Mood disorders involve abnormal fluctuations in mood. Schizophrenia involves a break with reality and associated features involving disturbed thinking, speech, behavior, and emotions and difficulties in social or interpersonal functioning.

6. Identify causal factors in psychological disorders.

Biological causes of psychological disorders include genetic variants, brain abnormalities, and biochemical imbalances in the brain involving irregularities in neurotransmitter functioning. Psychological factors include learning influences, faulty thinking or cognition, and lack of reinforcement in daily life.

7. Identify factors involved in suicide.

Factors involved in suicide include psychological disorders, especially mood disorders, feelings of hopeless and helplessness, relationship problems, substance abuse, persistent physical pain or severe chronic illness, financial problems, social contagion (in adolescents, exposure to peer suicides), stressful life events, and possible biological influences.

Answers to Review Sections

11.1

1. trait
2. social
3. superego
4. repression
5. love
6. Encoding
7. longer
8. esteem
9. actualized
10. Traits
11. agreeableness
12. conscientiousness

11.2

1. 2
2. more
3. more
4. environment
5. insomnia
6. exaggerated, irrational, catastrophizing

11.3

1. half
2. 5
3. cultural
4. diathesis
5. 3
6. generalized
7. larger
8. compulsion
9. obsession
10. 10
11. environmental
12. depression
13. emotion
14. social media
15. schizophrenia
16. larger

11.4

1. Older
2. increasing
3. 3
4. mood
5. attention

CHAPTER 12

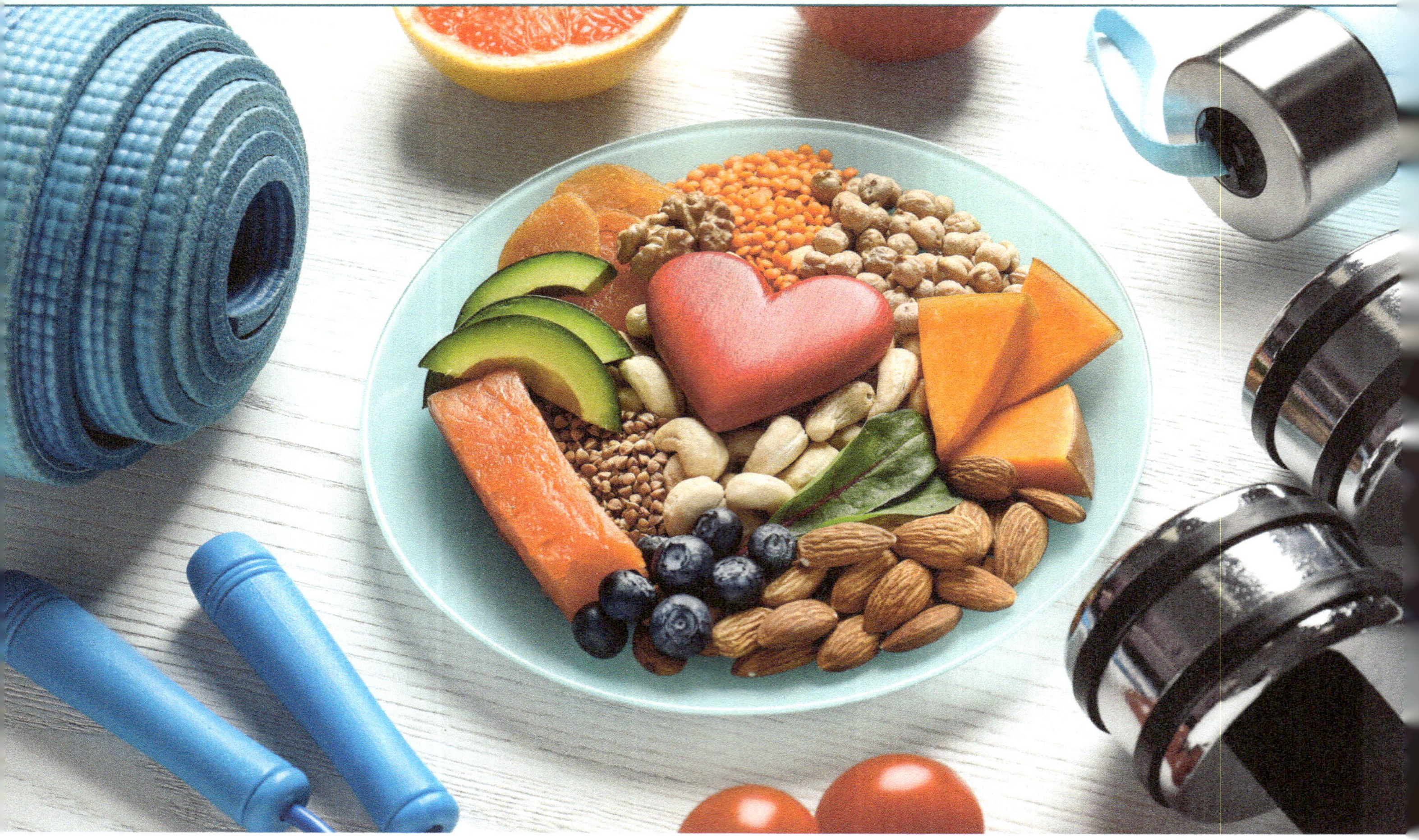

New Africa/Shutterstock.com

Cardiovascular Health

LEARNING OBJECTIVES

After studying this chapter, you will be able to …

1. **Describe** the parts of the circulatory system.
2. **Describe** the underlying disease process in coronary heart disease and stroke.
3. **Identify** risk factors for cardiovascular disease you cannot control.
4. **Identify** risk factors you can control.
5. **Describe** how psychological factors are related to risk of heart disease.
6. **Describe** ways of becoming heart healthy.

Did You Know That ...

- If you laid out all of an adult's blood vessels in a straight line, that line would be nearly 100,000 miles long?
- Despite the publicity given to infectious diseases such as HIV/AIDS and COVID-19 and to alcohol and drug overdoses, heart disease has been the perennial leading cause of death?
- Many of the risk factors for cardiovascular disease involve health behaviors that we can control?
- You can have a heart attack without feeling any chest pain?
- Aspirin is no longer used only for headaches and fever?
- You can have high blood pressure for years and not know it?
- A stroke is like a heart attack of the brain?
- Persistent anger and hostility can be dangerous for your heart?
- There is a type of cholesterol that decreases the risk of coronary heart disease?
- There may be some truth to the saying that you can die of a broken heart?

What is the single most important muscle in your body? If you said your biceps or triceps or your leg muscles, think again.

The most important muscle in your body is your heart. The heart is a muscular pump that moves blood through the circulatory system, bringing oxygen and nutrients to every cell in the body. It begins beating between the third and fourth weeks of prenatal development and will beat more than 3 billion times by the time you reach the age of 80. Like other muscles the heart profits from conditioning to function at its best, as by cardiovascular training in the form of vigorous physical activity or aerobic exercise. But the heart also needs its owner to care for its health in other ways—by following a healthful diet, managing body weight, avoiding smoking (of course), and controlling other risk factors, such as high blood pressure (HBP) and blood levels of cholesterol.

Most young people have healthy hearts and may not give much thought to their cardiovascular health. They may assume their hearts will continue to beat without any need to consider how their behavior might affect the health of their cardiovascular system. Yet over time, unhealthful behaviors can take a toll, leading to serious, life-threatening heart problems that could have been prevented by developing healthier habits earlier in life.

This chapter is about some unpleasant topics, including heart problems and strokes. In 2020 COVID-19 inserted itself among the leading causes of death. However, heart disease remains the nation's perennial leading cause of death, and strokes have been among the top five. The chapter is also about the steps that we can take to lower the probability of becoming yet another grim statistic of lives cut prematurely short by cardiovascular disease. We will see how heart-healthy behaviors can be incorporated within a healthful lifestyle and consider the roles that health psychologists play in treatment teams that work to prevent and treat cardiovascular disease.

The Cardiovascular System

The cardiovascular system is a network comprising your heart, blood, and blood vessels, which carries life-sustaining oxygen and nutrients throughout the body and carts away cellular wastes. Like other roadways there are accidents—many with fatalities—along this highway, accidents in the form of **cardiovascular disease (CVD)**.

cardiovascular disease (CVD) Disorders of the heart and circulatory system.

CVD affects the heart and circulatory system. CVD includes a host of diseases, such as *coronary heart disease* (CHD), *arrhythmias* (abnormal heart rhythms), *congenital* (inborn) *heart disease*, *stroke*, and diseases affecting blood vessels. CVD is the leading cause of death in the United States, claiming nearly 800,000 lives annually, which works out to about 1 in every 3 deaths, most often as the result of heart attacks or strokes (Heron, 2019). CVD leaves millions more people with disabilities or impairments. But road signs in the form of risk factors alert us to dangers lurking within our cardiovascular system. Many of these signs point to unhealthful choices, such as smoking, physical inactivity, and a poor diet. Health psychologists and other health professionals are involved in efforts to help people recognize these dangers and develop a heart-smart lifestyle to prevent them from becoming yet another casualty on the highway of life.

Might you be at risk of developing CVD in the next 10 years or so? The American College of Cardiology offers a risk estimator that health professionals use to evaluate a patient's relative risk of developing the major form of CVD over the next 10 years. You can use the risk calculator yourself to gauge your own personal risk (go to https://tools.acc.org/ascvd-risk-estimator-plus/#!/calculate/estimate/).

The risk estimator considers:

- Your age
- Your sex
- Your race
- Your blood pressure
- Your cholesterol levels
- Whether you have a history of diabetes
- Whether you are a smoker
- Whether you are being treated for high blood pressure
- Whether you are taking a statin (a medicine that lowers "bad" cholesterol)
- Whether you are on low-dose aspirin therapy (for people who have a certain risk profile for cardiovascular disease)

We will be looking at each of these factors throughout the chapter. If you have concerns about your own personal risk, why not consult a healthcare professional?

Let's take a tour of your cardiovascular system, starting with the remarkable pump that keeps the system humming, the heart. We then take a closer look at two major forms of CVD (CHD and stroke) and consider how we can protect ourselves from these serious threats to our health and longevity.

The Heart

heart The muscle that pumps blood through the circulatory system.

Weighing a mere 11 ounces, the **heart** is a muscular pump, a very powerful pump capable of pushing 5 or more quarts of blood through the circulatory system every minute of every day, day in and day out that amounts to some 2,000 gallons each day. Through the course of an 80-year lifetime, the heart will beat—contract and expand—more than 3 billion times. That works out to about 72 beats per minute while we are resting and faster when we exert ourselves. If you do the math, you'll see that the heart beats about 100,000 times per day. The main function of the heart is to supply oxygen and nutrients to the tissues of the body and to remove carbon dioxide and other waste products. Therefore, it should not be surprising that once it stops beating for longer than a few seconds, life comes to an end.

Places in the Heart

You might think that the heart resembles a Valentine, but it actually looks more like an upside-down pear (see **Figure 12.1**). The heart sits in the middle of the chest between the lungs, where it is protected by the rib cage.

atrium The upper chamber on each side of the heart.

ventricle The lower chamber on each side of the heart.

aorta The body's main artery, carrying blood from the heart into smaller blood vessels for delivery of oxygen-rich blood to all parts of the body.

Within the heart are four open spaces called chambers. The upper chamber on each side of the heart is called an **atrium**, and the lower chamber is called a **ventricle**. Unoxygenated blood enters the heart through the right atrium and then passes into the right ventricle, where it is pumped through the pulmonary artery into the lungs. In the lungs, oxygen passes into the blood and carbon dioxide is removed. Once it is oxygenated, blood enters the left atrium of the heart and is pumped into the left ventricle, which propels the blood into the body's main artery, the **aorta**. Blood vessels branching off from the aorta carry the oxygen-rich blood to every cell in the body.

The Circulatory System

If you were to place all blood vessels in a human adult end to end, they would be nearly 100,000 miles long, or more than a third of the distance to the moon. The circulatory system is a network of blood vessels that furnishes cellular tissues and organs with oxygen and

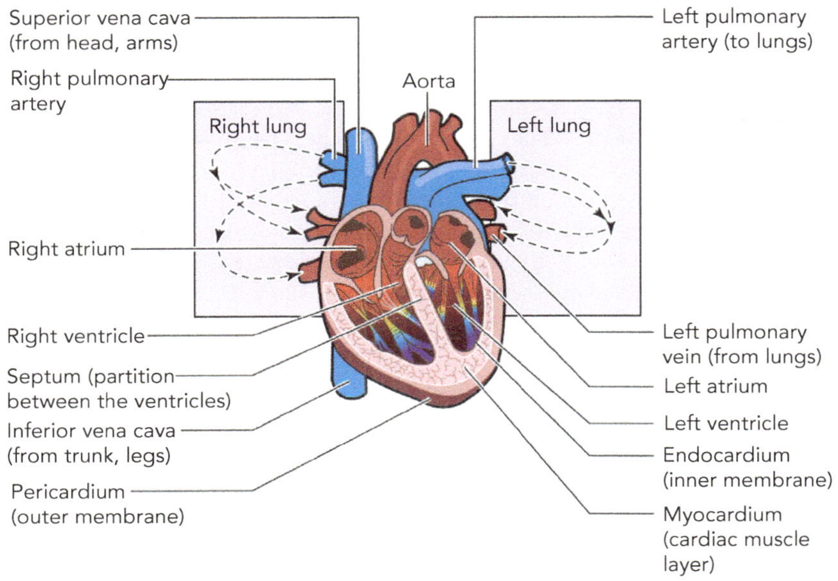

FIGURE 12.1 **Places in the Heart** The heart is composed of four chambers. The upper chambers are called atria and the lower chambers are called ventricles. Unoxygenated blood enters the right atrium. It then passes into the right ventricle, from where it is pumped through the pulmonary artery into the lungs. In the lungs, the blood releases carbon dioxide and picks up oxygen. The oxygenated blood then enters the left atrium and from there is pumped into the left ventricle, the heart's most powerful pump, which forces the blood into the aorta. Blood vessels branch off from the aorta, eventually reaching every cell in the body.

nutrients and carts away their waste products. Body cells need oxygen to metabolize nutrients, such as sugars and fats, converting them into energy. Resulting from this oxidative process is the gas carbon dioxide, which is a bodily waste product that is carried by the circulatory system to the lungs. From there it is expelled from the body through breathing.

And yet there's more—much more—to what the cardiovascular system does than deliver oxygen and nutrients and cart away waste products. It also carries hormones released by endocrine glands. Hormones are chemical secretions that exert effects on different organ systems in the body. In Chapter 4 you learned that the adrenal glands, which sit atop the kidneys, release stress hormones epinephrine and norepinephrine into the bloodstream, which transports them to the heart, causing it to beat faster and allowing your muscles to work harder to handle increased stressful demands (such as running to catch the bus). The circulatory system also transports armies of disease-fighting white blood cells and antibodies that comprise the immune system's defenses against invading microorganisms and rids the body of diseased and worn-out cells.

Blood

Blood is literally the liquid of life, ferrying oxygen, nutrients, hormones, and antibodies through the circulatory system to cells and carting away their waste products. The liquid part of the blood, which has a straw-colored or yellowish appearance, is **blood plasma**. Blood also contains several other components that perform specialized functions—erythrocytes, leukocytes, and platelets.

Erythrocytes, or red blood cells, are responsible for carrying oxygen to body cells. They contain red, iron-rich substance called **hemoglobin**, which gives blood its familiar reddish color. Hemoglobin binds to oxygen in the lungs and is carried in the bloodstream to body tissues. It then releases oxygen in the capillaries so that can pass into body cells.

Leukocytes, or white blood cells, form part of the body's immune system. Various types of leukocytes perform specialized functions in destroying invading organisms.

Platelets are small cell fragments in the blood that form clots to plug holes in the walls of injured blood vessels. They stop bleeding. They accumulate at a site of injury when the wall of a blood vessel is damaged or punctured. The process by which clots are formed (coagulation) is completed by specialized proteins called *clotting factors*, which are found in blood plasma. Without platelets we would bleed to death from the slightest wound.

blood plasma The liquid part of the blood.

erythrocytes Red blood cells that carry oxygen to cells.

hemoglobin An iron-rich protein in red blood cells that carries oxygen from the lungs to tissues and organs in the body and carries carbon dioxide back to the lungs.

leukocytes White blood cells that combat disease-causing organisms.

platelets Small cell fragments in the blood that allow blood to clot following a wound or injury.

Most blood cells are manufactured in the bone marrow, the soft material that fills the inner cavities of bones. Some leukocytes, called lymphocytes, are produced in lymph glands and other organs in the body's lymphatic system.

arteries Blood vessels that carry oxygenated blood from the heart to capillaries that deliver it to body tissues.

capillaries Small blood vessels that carry oxygenated blood from arteries directly to body cells and transport blood carrying carbon dioxide and cellular waste products from body cells to veins.

veins Blood vessels that carry blood back to the heart.

vena cava The largest vein, which carries blood directly into the heart.

Types of Blood Vessels The circulatory system is composed of three types of blood vessels—**arteries**, **capillaries**, and **veins**. Arteries carry oxygen-rich blood to the smallest blood vessels, the capillaries, which transport blood directly to body cells. Other capillaries take carbon dioxide and cellular waste products from body cells, transporting them in the blood and connecting to veins that carry the blood back to the heart. The veins widen as they approach the heart. The largest of the veins, called the **vena cava**, carries what is now oxygen-poor blood into the right atrium of the heart, from where it begins again to circulate (see **Figure 12.1**). There are two vena cava, the *superior vena cava*, which carries blood from the upper body, and the *inferior vena cava*, which carries blood from the lower body. Rounding out its journey on the way to the heart, the blood passes through the liver and kidneys, which remove cellular waste products for excretion in urine and through exhalation.

Cardiovascular diseases affect the health of the heart and circulatory system. We discuss two major types of CVD, CHD and stroke. These diseases are of particular interest to health psychologists because of the roles of health-related behaviors as risk factors. We also consider hypertension, or high blood pressure, a condition that can lead to both heart disease and stroke.

Self-Assessment

INTERACTIVE SELF-ASSESSMENTS

Are You Heart-Smart?

Test your cardiac IQ by answering the following questions. Then check your answers against the scoring key at the end of the chapter.

True	False	
___	___	1. A heart attack occurs when the heart stops beating.
___	___	2. You can have a heart murmur without actually having heart disease.
___	___	3. Cardiovascular disease does not begin until people reach middle age.
___	___	4. People can generally feel if their blood pressure is elevated.
___	___	5. People who are overweight or obese are not any more likely to have hypertension than people of normal weight.
___	___	6. People with cardiovascular disease should avoid physical exercise so that they do not put strain on their heart.
___	___	7. The pumping of the heart is controlled by the heart muscle.
___	___	8. Non-Hispanic White Americans are about as likely to die from coronary heart disease as non-Hispanic Black Americans.
___	___	9. Your risk of having a heart attack is in the cards—either you have a family history or you don't.
___	___	10. Cholesterol is harmful to the heart.

Review 12.1

INTERACTIVE SELF-SCORING QUIZZES

Sentence Completion

1. Cardiovascular diseases are conditions that affect the heart and __________ system.
2. The leading forms of CVD are CHD, abnormal heart rhythms or arrhythmias, and __________.
3. The heart has (two or four) open spaces called chambers.
4. The pumping action of the heart propels blood into the __________.
5. __________ stop bleeding by clumping and forming plugs in blood vessel injuries.

Think About It

Consider the factors assessed by the American College of Cardiology's risk estimator. Are you concerned about how the college would evaluate you if you complete the estimator? Why or why not? Do the factors in the calculator lead you to wonder about whether any family members or other people you know are at risk? Why or why not? If you have concern, what can you do about it?

Coronary Heart Disease: The Nation's Perennial Leading Cause of Death

The heart is made of muscle tissue, which like other bodily tissue requires oxygen and nutrients carried by the blood. In **coronary heart disease** (CHD), the flow of blood to the heart is insufficient to meet its needs, damaging the heart itself. (The word "coronary" is derived from the Latin *corona*, meaning "crown," which reflects the crown like manner in which the arteries encircle the heart.)

coronary heart disease The major type of heart disease, usually caused by insufficient blood supply to the heart as the result of a buildup of plaque in arteries serving the heart.

atherosclerosis A form of arteriosclerosis in which artery walls thicken and narrow due to the buildup of fatty deposits or plaque.

arteriosclerosis A condition in which the walls of arteries become thicker, harder, and lose elasticity.

thrombus A blood clot that impedes the flow of blood.

angina A type of chest pain that is a symptom of coronary heart disease; the pain may spread to the shoulders, arms, and neck and is caused by inadequate blood flow to the heart.

CHD is the major form of CVD and the leading cause of death for both men and women in the United States, accounting for nearly 700,000 deaths each year (CDC, 2023h). That approximates 1 in every 4 deaths (CDC, 2019c; Heron, 2019). Nearly half of men and one-third of women develop CHD. Yet according to a Cleveland Clinic survey, about 2 out of 3 Americans don't know that heart disease is the leading cause of death in women, with many assuming that it is breast cancer (Walters, 2020). Surveys also show that women tend to worry more about breast cancer than CHD, although CHD takes the lives of more than 6 times as many women (Harvard Health, 2017). But let us remain hopeful in our discussion of CHD, armed with the knowledge that we can take steps to reduce our personal risks of developing it.

Although most deaths from CHD result from heart attacks, the underlying cause is often years in the making, involving a disease process called **atherosclerosis**, or narrowing of arteries as the result of a buildup along artery walls of fatty deposits called plaque (see **Figure 12.2**). The word "atherosclerosis" is derived from the Greek *athero,* meaning "paste," and *sclerosis,* meaning "hardness." This is an apt description of the "hardening" of artery-clogging "paste" (plaque). When plaques form, arteries become narrower, which can reduce the flow of life-sustaining blood to the heart.

Atherosclerosis is the major form of **arteriosclerosis**, a condition commonly called hardening of the arteries, in which artery walls become thicker, harder, and less elastic. A blood clot (**thrombus**) is more likely to form in arteries narrowed by atherosclerosis. Affected arteries may no longer be able to provide an adequate supply of oxygenated blood that the heart needs to do its work, especially during physical exertion, leading to chest pain or **angina** (the technical term is *angina pectoris*). Angina is a symptom of CHD and the associated pain is similar to that of a heart attack, but less severe and prolonged. An angina attack typically lasts for a few minutes and doesn't leave enduring damage. Although many people with angina never experience a heart attack, angina should be taken seriously as a warning sign of a potential heart attack.

If a blood clot forms in a coronary artery and blocks or nearly blocks the flow of blood to a part of the heart, the result is a **myocardial infarction**, more commonly known as a heart attack. (The word "myocardial" is derived from Greek roots *myo* ["muscle"] and *kardia* ["heart"].) An area of dead or dying tissues is an *infarct*. When the heart does not receive enough oxygen, heart tissue in the affected area dies; therefore, a myocardial infarction is the death of heart tissue resulting from an insufficient blood supply, or **ischemia**. Survival from a heart attack depends on the extent of the damage to heart tissue and to the heart's electrical system, which controls the heart rhythm. Although CHD typically develops over a period of years, its first sign may be a heart attack. Someone in the United States has a heart attack on average every 30 seconds.

In a heart attack, minutes count—literally. During the attack, heart tissue begins to die within minutes of disruption of its blood supply. As the area of the infarct expands, the heart may no longer be able to pump enough blood to sustain life. Brain death can occur within minutes if the heart fails to pump enough blood.

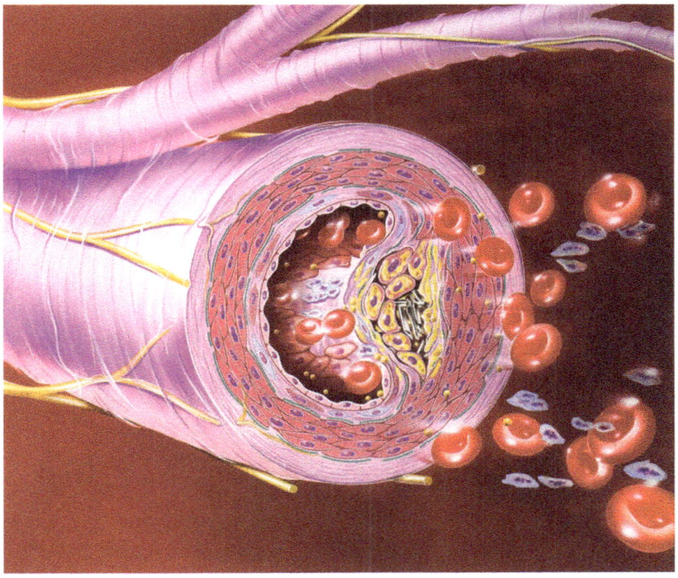

John Bavosi/Science Source

FIGURE 12.2 **Atherosclerosis of an Artery** An artery that has become narrowed due to atherosclerosis. A raised yellow plaque (atheroma) is seen in the wall of the artery. This plaque is made of lipids (yellow) and decaying muscle cells encasing crystals of calcium (white). At right are red blood cells, yellow lipid particles, and white blood cells (pink). Atheroma plaques are found in people who have a high concentration of cholesterol in their bloodstream. Narrowing of the arteries increases the risk of blood clots forming and is associated with coronary heart disease and stroke.

A Closer Look

Women and Coronary Heart Disease

Although we may hear more about CHD in men, CHD affects about one-third of women in the United States, and 1 woman in 4 dies from it. CHD is the leading cause of death of women as well as men. Unfortunately, the gender stereotype that heart disease primarily affects men may have contributed to an underrepresentation of women in clinical research trials. Progress has been made with respect to inclusion of women as participants in cardiovascular research, but female underrepresentation continues in some medication trials (Scott et al., 2018; Watson, 2018).

CHD usually develops more gradually in women than in men, about 7 to 10 years later (Maas & Appelman, 2010). Prior to the age of 65 years, a woman's risk of dying from a heart attack lags that of a man's by about 10 years. Thus, a 60-year-old woman has about the same chance of dying of a heart attack as a 50-year-old man. In part, these differences reflect the fact that men generally engage in unhealthier behaviors than women, behaviors that increase their risk of a heart attack, such as smoking and excessive drinking. Women may also be protected at younger ages by the secretion of female sex hormones (Schrager et al., 2020). Yet women are less likely to survive after heart surgery, and more likely to have a second heart attack than men (Wenger, 2020). These poorer outcomes may reflect the fact that women with CHD tend to be older than their male counterparts. Moreover, CHD is typically recognized sooner and treated more aggressively in men than in women (Wenger, 2020). Differences in aggressive treatment may stem from a long-standing misperception that heart disease is primarily a male problem. Women are also more likely than men to experience a "silent" heart attack, one without chest pain.

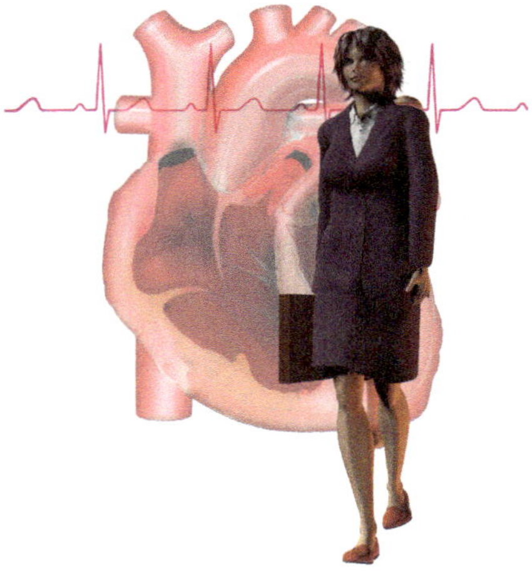

Carol and Mike Werner/Science Source

Women and CHD Heart disease is the leading killer of women, as it is of men.

myocardial infarction Damage or death of heart tissue due to insufficient blood flow to the heart, typically as the result of a blockage in a coronary artery; commonly referred to as a heart attack.

ischemia A restriction in the blood supply to bodily tissues, leading to a shortage of oxygen needed for cellular metabolism.

Inflammation

Medical researchers are zeroing in on inflammation in blood vessels as a contributing cause of heart disease. Inflammation can cause plaque along artery walls to burst, releasing particles of fatty deposits which then form blood clots. If these blood clots block the flow of blood to the heart, the result can be a heart attack. A particular marker of inflammation, produced by the liver and called *C-reactive protein* (CRP), is associated with increased risk of CVD. Medical researchers are studying whether people should be routinely screened for CRP and how best to treat people who present with high levels of the protein.

Signs of a Heart Attack

The first seconds and minutes after a heart attack are critical, as most deaths from a heart attack occur within 2 hours. Immediate medical attention is needed, yet about half of the people who suffer a heart attack wait 2 hours or longer to get medical help. Heart attacks are medical emergencies that require immediate attention. Why the delay? In many cases, symptoms of a heart attack are taken as signs of something less serious, like indigestion or heartburn. Public health officials recognize the need to raise public awareness of the signs of a heart attack so that people who are stricken can recognize it as a medical emergency and get the help they need. Would you recognize the signs of a heart attack? Here's a list of common symptoms—common, yes, but not every one of these symptoms is present in all cases (NIA, 2018; see **Figure 12.3**):

- Crushing chest pain or pressure and/or discomfort or pain elsewhere in the upper body, neck, or arms
- Nausea
- A cold sweat

A Closer Look

Aspirin—Not Just for Headaches?

The common aspirin tablet sitting in your medicine cabinet can reduce headache and bring fever down, but can it also be helpful in preventing heart attacks? Many people—1 in 4, according to a recent survey (Herman, 2019)—take a low dose of aspirin daily (a "baby" aspirin tablet) to help prevent heart attacks. But should they? Aspirin has legitimate medical uses in preventing blood clots in some cases. Blood clots are dangerous because of the risk that they might break free and travel to the heart, lungs, or brain, causing a heart attack, stroke, or serious respiratory problems. Aspirin may be a helpful part of a comprehensive treatment plan for preventing the recurrence of blood clots in people with established heart disease (Becattini et al., 2012; Yoo et al., 2023). But the question remains: Should healthy people without a history of a heart attack or stroke take a daily dose of aspirin to reduce their risk of a first heart attack or stroke? The answer, according to medical experts, is no (Baumgaertner, 2023; Croft, 2023).

Whatever slight benefit daily aspirin might offer in preventing heart attacks or strokes may not outweigh the risks, such as a greater potential of stomach problems and hemorrhaging (internal bleeding from a damaged blood vessel) (Cloud et al., 2023; Schwenk & Brett, 2019). Because of such risks, medical care providers do not routinely recommend taking a daily aspirin for prevention of heart disease or stroke. Yet the American Heart Association and American College of Cardiology does advise that low-dose aspirin therapy might be considered for middle-age adults at high risk of CVD who do not have an increased risk of bleeding problems (Herman, 2019; Peters & Mutharasan, 2020). Even then, people taking aspirin regularly should do so only under a physician's direction (Jain & Davis, 2019).

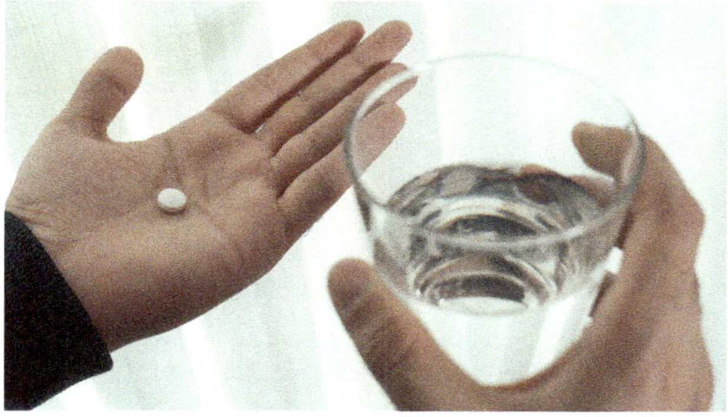
Sina Salehian/Getty Images

Is This Good for Your Heart? Should you be taking a small dose of aspirin daily to protect your heart? What do health authorities recommend?

- Fainting or light-headedness
- Shortness of breath

Crushing, intense, prolonged chest pain is present in many, but not all, heart attacks. In fact, some people have "silent" heart attacks; they experience little if any chest pain or shortness of breath. The possibility of a silent heart attack underscores the importance of seeking a medical evaluation if there is any suspicion that someone may be having a heart attack. If you or someone you know experiences the signs or symptoms of a heart attack, seek immediate medical attention by calling 911 and following the instructions given by an operator. The sooner the person can get to a hospital, the greater the chances for limiting the damage caused by a heart attack.

arrhythmia A type of cardiovascular disease involving abnormal heartbeat or rhythm.

tachycardia An abnormally fast heartbeat.

bradycardia An abnormally slow heartbeat.

Arrhythmias

An **arrhythmia** is an abnormal heartbeat or rhythm. Normally, the heart beats between 50 and 100 times a minute. One type of arrhythmia is **tachycardia**, or an abnormally fast heartbeat, whereas another is **bradycardia**, an abnormally slow beat. In other arrhythmias, the heart beats irregularly, which reduces the heart's efficiency in pumping blood.

Some arrhythmias are commonplace. It is not unusual for people to have occasional episodes of a racing heart (tachycardia), which they may experience as "palpitations," or fluttering sensations. Or the heart may occasionally skip a beat, which doesn't usually present a problem unless it becomes recurrent or persistent.

Arrhythmias resulting from underlying conditions, such as heart disease or congenital defects, can be dangerous or

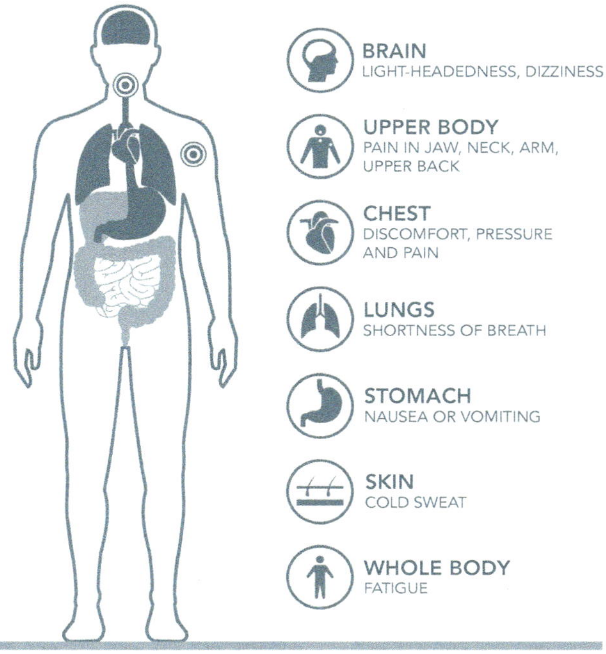

ElenaBs/Alamy Stock Photo

FIGURE 12.3 Common Symptoms of Heart Attack

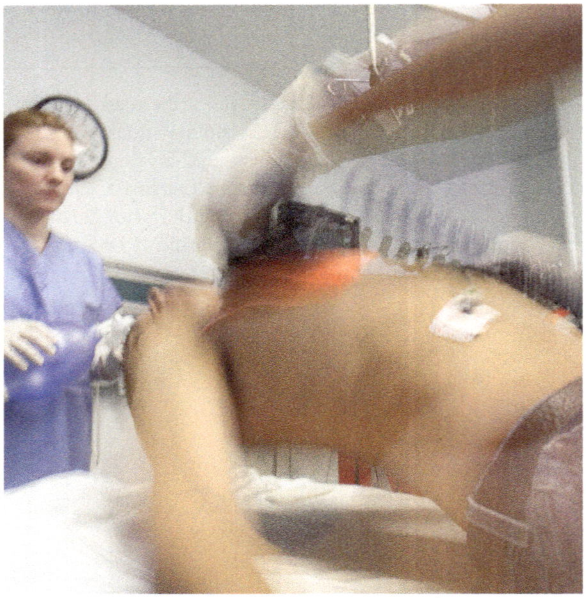

The Shock of Life A defibrillator is used to administer an electric shock to the chest to restore a normal heartbeat.

life-threatening. Severe bradycardia, for example, can result in loss of consciousness or even death. Damage to the heart muscle following a heart attack can lead to life-threatening arrhythmias, such as *ventricular fibrillation* in which a disruption in the electrical impulses regulating heartbeat causes the heart to beat erratically or quiver (fibrillate). Most heart attack deaths result from ventricular fibrillation in which the two ventricles (lower chambers of the heart) contract irregularly and are unable to pump effectively.

An electrical device called a *defibrillator* may be used to stop the heart from quivering and to restore a normal rhythm. Electrodes are placed on the chest to administer an electric shock to the heart to restore a normal heartbeat (a technique no doubt familiar to viewers of medical dramas on television). Ventricular fibrillation can trigger *cardiac arrest*, a condition in which the heart suddenly stops beating, resulting in loss of consciousness and the stoppage of breathing. Death occurs shortly after cardiac arrest, as the brain and other vital body organs fail to receive blood.

Other emergency techniques can also be lifesavers, such as *cardiopulmonary resuscitation (CPR)*, in which chest compressions or mouth-to-mouth breathing (administered by persons who have undergone training) is used to restore the heartbeat of someone in cardiac arrest. The CPR should be learned *before* a life-threatening emergency occurs. Classes that train laypeople in CPR techniques are available in most communities. Contact your local health department or hospital center for information.

stroke A type of cardiovascular disease in which a blockage of oxygen-rich blood to a part of the brain causes damage or death of brain tissue, or the sudden bleeding in the brain due to a rupture of a blood vessel in the brain.

ischemic stroke The most common type of stroke caused by a blockage in an artery supplying blood to a part of the brain.

cerebral hemorrhage A severe type of stroke in which a blood vessel in the brain ruptures and leaks blood into brain tissue; also called a *hemorrhagic stroke*.

Stroke

A **stroke** is like a heart attack of the brain. Like the heart, the brain requires an adequate supply of oxygen-rich and nutrient-rich blood. If an obstruction or blood clot in an artery blocks the flow of blood to the brain, the result can be a stroke (also called a *cerebrovascular accident*).

There are different kinds of strokes (see **Figure 12.4**). The most common type, accounting for 87% of all strokes, is an **ischemic stroke**, which is caused by a blockage in an artery that chokes off the blood supply to parts of the brain (CDC, 2023n). A much less common type of stroke, accounting for about 10% of strokes, is a **cerebral hemorrhage** (hemorrhagic stroke), a severe type of stroke that results in death about half the time. In a cerebral hemorrhage, a blood vessel in the brain ruptures, causing blood to seep into brain tissue, damaging or destroying it. Both types of strokes are linked to high blood pressure.

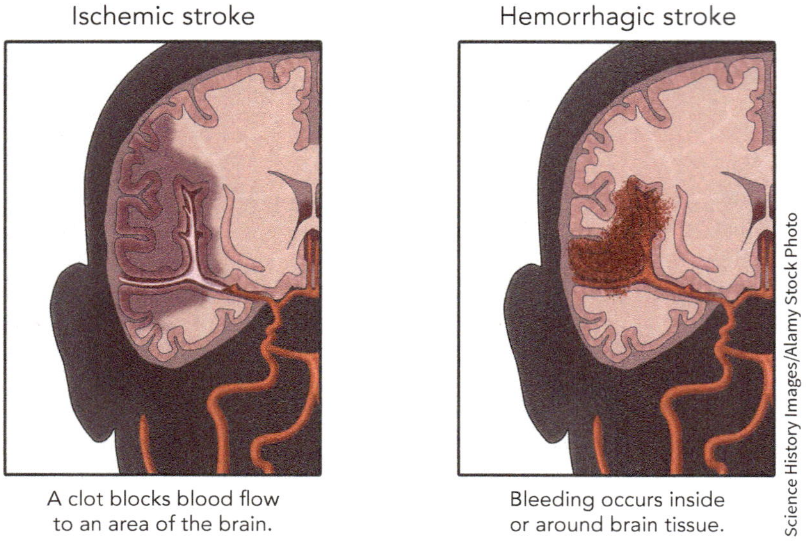

FIGURE 12.4 **Two Types of Stroke**

Brain tissue can be damaged or destroyed by a stroke within minutes after its blood supply is blocked. The functions controlled by areas of the brain affected by stroke may be lost or severely impaired—even the ability to speak or walk. In a massive stroke, death may result within minutes.

About 800,000 Americans have a stroke each year and 140,000 die of a stroke, accounting for about 1 in 20 deaths (CDC, 2020f). Stroke is the fifth leading cause of death among Americans overall, but it disproportionately affects non-Hispanic Black Americans, who have nearly twice the frequency of strokes as non-Hispanic White Americans and the highest rates of stroke among major racial/ethnic groups in the United States (CDC, 2020f). Reasons for this racial disparity is that Black Americans as a group have more risk factors for the condition, especially hypertension and smoking (CDC, 2020c).

Depending on the location and extent of damage, the effects of stroke can range from relatively minor to serious disability, even coma and death. The symptoms of stroke vary with the particular area of the brain that is damaged. There may be loss of speech or difficulty understanding speech, loss of feeling, numbness, weakness, or paralysis of a limb or of parts of the face. A person who has had a stroke may show significant declines in cognitive abilities, such as memory, reasoning, and judgment. The person may also experience severe headaches, have blurred or double vision, and experience dizziness or loss of balance or coordination. Typically, stroke affects only one side of the brain, so that loss of sensation or movement is limited to the opposite side of the body. (Each side of the body is regulated by the opposite side of the brain.)

Like a heart attack, a stroke is a medical emergency that requires immediate attention. Getting help as quickly as possible may mean the difference between life and death or may minimize the risk of permanent disability. If you or someone else experiences the following signs or symptoms, call 911 immediately (CDC, 2023o):

- Sudden numbness or weakness in the face, arm, or leg, especially on one side of the body
- Sudden confusion, trouble speaking, or difficulty understanding speech
- Sudden trouble seeing in one or both eyes
- Sudden trouble walking, dizziness, loss of balance, or lack of coordination
- Sudden severe headache with no known cause

If the symptoms subside after a few minutes, the person may have had a **transient ischemic attack (TIA)**. But the experience should not be ignored. Informing one's healthcare provider can save one's life.

The biopsychosocial model takes a broad view of health problems such as CVD by considering the roles of biological, psychological, and sociocultural factors.

transient ischemic attack (TIA) A brief episode of neurological dysfunction resulting from an interruption of the blood supply to the brain.

Heart Failure

Six to 7 million people in the United States are living with a chronic cardiovascular condition known as **heart failure**. Heart failure can result from inability of the heart to pump enough blood and oxygen to support other organs or fill adequately with sufficient blood that is returned to the heart. Although the "making" of heart failure typically proceeds for years, it can come on suddenly and may be initially indicated by shortness of breath (panting for air), rapid heart rate as the heart attempts to compensate for its weakness, and feelings of fatigue (CDC, 2019f). These symptoms are soon accompanied by weight gain as fluid swells the feet, ankles, legs, or abdomen (see **Figure 12.5**).

heart failure A chronic condition in which the heart cannot adequately pump blood or fill with blood, characterized by shortness of breath, rapid heartbeat, fatigue, and, typically, swelling of the legs.

The biological risk factors for heart failure mirror those that are associated with other cardiovascular disorders: buildup of plaque in the walls of arteries, hypertension, obesity, diabetes, and age. The behavioral risk factors include smoking tobacco; eating foods high in fat, cholesterol, and sodium; physical inactivity; and excessive drinking of alcohol.

Heart failure is not curable, but in many people it can be treated successfully by medications that enhance the flow of blood through the body, aid the heartbeat, and control high blood pressure; reducing dietary intake of sodium; drinking less liquids; using devices that purge the body of excess water and salt; and engaging in regular physical activity.

Adherence to medication is an issue with heart failure, as with other chronic conditions. One study examined the relationship between adherence to medication in more than 55,000 people with heart failure, as measured by the regularity of transactions at pharmacies and outcomes, including visits to emergency departments, hospitalizations, length of hospital stays, and mortality (Hood et al., 2018). For every 10% increase in the number of transactions at pharmacies, emergency department visits decreased by 11%; hospitalizations decreased by 6%, length of hospital stays decreased by 1%, and mortality decreased by 9%. Other studies support the conclusion that adherence to medication regimens reduces the rates of hospitalization and mortality among people with heart failure (e.g., Ruppar et al., 2016). Successful interventions to improve adherence included education about heart failure and about the medications used

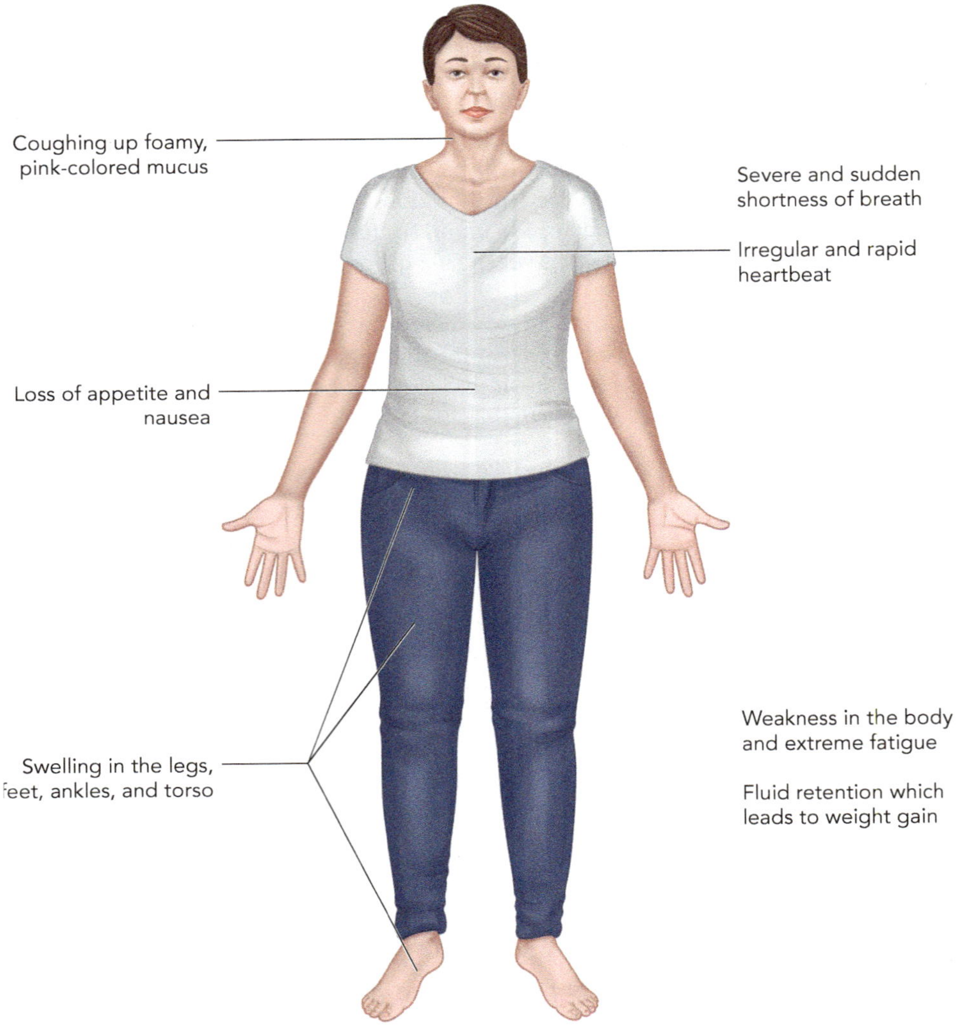

FIGURE 12.5 **Symptoms of Heart Failure**

to treat it. Face-to-face interventions are recommended, and various kinds of healthcare professionals, such as nurses, dieticians, pharmacists, physicians, social workers, and psychologists, may be involved (Ruppar et al., 2016).

Review 12.2

INTERACTIVE SELF-SCORING QUIZZES

Sentence Completion

1. One of every __________ men and 1 of every __________ women eventually develops CHD.
2. The underlying disease process in most cases of CHD is __________.
3. A myocardial infarction is more commonly known as a __________.
4. CHD usually develops (more gradually or more quickly) in women than in men.
5. Women are (less likely or more likely) as men to survive after heart surgery.
6. A marker of inflammation linked to CVD is __________ protein (CRP).
7. __________ include an abnormally fast heart rate, or __________, an abnormally slow heart rate, or __________, or irregular heart rates.
8. In an __________ stroke, a blood clot blocks blood flow to an area of the brain.

Think About It

Do you or someone close to you suffer from cardiovascular disease or hypertension? What are you (or they) doing about? Are you (or they) getting appropriate medical care and making heart-healthy lifestyle changes? *If not, why not?*

Risk Factors for Cardiovascular Disease

We've learned a great deal about the factors that increase a person's chances of developing CVD. Knowing these risk factors can raise your awareness of your own risk profile and what you can do to reduce your personal risk. These risk factors related to a number of risk include age (risk increases with age after about age 40), male gender (men are at greater risk until about age 65), life stress, family history (heredity), hypertension (high blood pressure), smoking, obesity, diabetes, lack of physical activity, and high levels of LDL cholesterol (low-density lipoproteins) in the bloodstream (Krist et al., 2020; Mangione et al., 2022; Shakhnoza & Asalya, 2022; Wang et al., 2021, and many others).

Some risk factors cannot be controlled: You cannot choose your parents or your gender of birth or stop aging. Health psychologists and other health professionals recognize that other factors, such as hypertension, smoking, obesity, diabetes, and high LDL cholesterol levels, can be controlled through behavioral changes (diet and exercise) or appropriate medical treatment. Adopting a healthier lifestyle, such as by exercising regularly, avoiding smoking and excess alcohol use, maintaining a healthy weight, and following a healthy diet, is linked with positive health outcomes, such as lower risks of hypertension, diabetes, and heart disease (Hill et al., 2023; Kelly et al., 2023; U.S. Preventive Services Task Force, 2020; among others).

Adoption of healthier lifestyles seems to be paying off, as deaths due to heart disease and stroke in the United States are on the decline. Even if you are young and healthy, and without any known risk factors, taking preventive measures now to protect your cardiovascular system may prevent CVD later on. Even if you are young and healthy, and without any known risk factors, taking preventive measures now to protect your cardiovascular system may prevent CVD later in life.

Three key risk factors are high blood pressure, high blood cholesterol, and smoking. Nearly 1 of 2 Americans (49%) have at least one of these risk factors (CDC, 2014). Health psychologists are keenly interested in CVD because many of the risk factors involve behaviors that we can change.

Risk Factors You Can't Control

There are a number of risk factors over which we have no control. Knowing where we stand on these factors can raise our awareness of our individual risks.

Age and Gender

The risk of CVD increases as we age, especially in late adulthood. CHD tends to develop at later ages in women than it does in men. Unfortunately, rates of CHD are rising among younger women, apparently because of unfavorable lifestyle changes, such as unhealthful diet and excess body weight (EUGenMed, 2016). In men, the risk of CHD rises sharply after about age 40. But among women, heart disease is uncommon until about menopause and then begins to rise sharply with increasing age. A first heart attack in women usually does not occur until about the age of 70 on average (Harvard Health, 2017). Like other forms of CVD, strokes most often affect people in late adulthood, typically after the age of 65 years.

Genetics and Family History

Genetics plays a role in the development of heart disease (CDC, 2019h). People are at higher risk if they have family members with heart disease. Of course, families share common environments (including meals) as well as genes, so it's difficult to separate environmental and genetic influences. But even if the genetic dice work against you, there is much you can do to lower your personal risk profile.

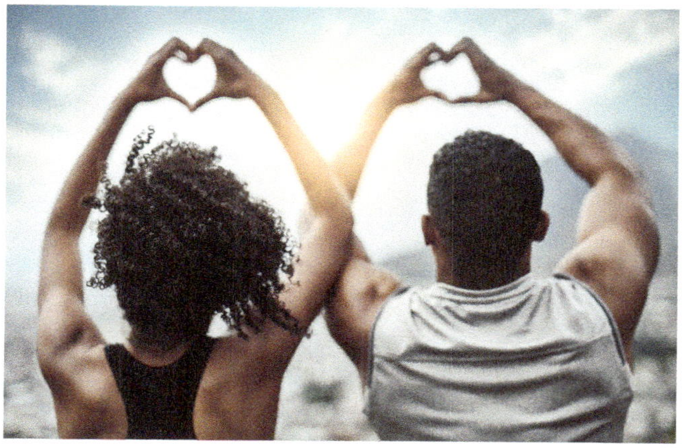

PeopleImages/Getty Images

Staying Heart Healthy What behavioral changes can you make in your daily life to protect yourself from heart disease?

Race and Ethnicity Heart disease is not an equal opportunity destroyer (Ruiz & Brondolo, 2016). **Figure 12.6** shows the mortality (death) rates for heart disease in relation to race or ethnicity. The good news is that death rates for heart disease have been falling for all racial and ethnic groups shown in the chart below. The not-so-good news is that disparities remain with respect to the death rates due to heart disease between non-Hispanic Black Americans and the other groups.

There are likely many reasons for the disparity between Black Americans and White Americans and other racial/ethnic groups with respect to deaths due to heart disease. One reason is that Black people with heart disease have more limited access to heart disease treatment services, often because they don't have adequate health insurance coverage (Office of Minority Health, 2022; NCHS, 2023). This dual standard of care results in health disparities that can have deadly consequences for people who lack equal access to medical services, including the more aggressive treatments that can save lives of people stricken with heart attacks and strokes.

Evidence shows that Black people with heart disease tend to not receive the same level of aggressive and potentially life-saving medical treatments, such as cardiac catheterization and coronary artery bypass surgery, even when they would benefit from them as much as White people (e.g., Mehta et al., 2016; Van Dyke et al., 2018). Moreover, when White patients and Black patients show up in the emergency department with heart attacks or other severe cardiac problems, physicians are more likely to misdiagnose these conditions in Black patients (Moy et al., 2015). Might it be that some emergency department physicians pay less attention to the health concerns of Black patients?

A dual standard of care, then, may reflect unequal access to quality healthcare services and discrimination by (some) healthcare providers. Black patients may also not be as aggressive as White patients in seeking health care for CVD, in part because of distrust of the healthcare system. The reluctance among some Black Americans to push the system for better treatment may limit their utilization of healthcare services, especially at earlier and more treatable stages of CVD. That said, let us note a hopeful sign, that racial disparities in measures of cardiovascular health have been narrowing somewhat in recent years (Mensah, 2018; Van Dyke, 2018).

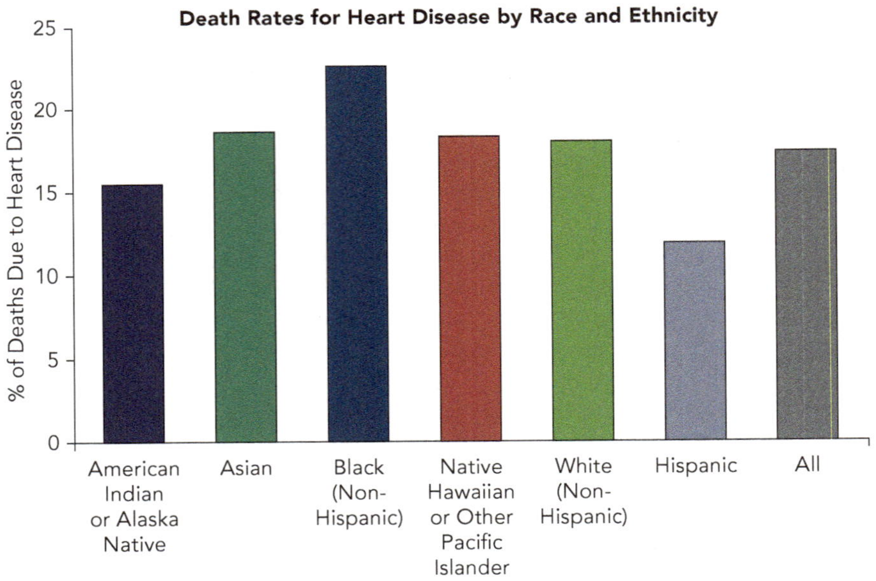

FIGURE 12.6 **Black Americans have the highest mortality rates due to heart disease of any major racial or ethnic group. The question is: Why?**

Source: CDC (2023q)

We should not overlook socioeconomic differences. As compared to non-Hispanic White Americans and Asian Americans, Black Americans more often live in neighborhoods that are lacking in accessible healthcare services, especially specialized services, such as cardiac care. Blacks and other minoritized groups in the United States tend to face greater economic hardships than Whites, and people on the low end of the socioeconomic spectrum tend to have higher rates of risk factors such as smoking, obesity, diets rich in fatty foods, physical inactivity, and stress, all of which can contribute to increased mortality rates (Chirinos et al., 2022; Qamar & Braunwald, 2018). Another contributing factor is that older residents of poorer neighborhoods also tend to show less improvement from medical care in the aftermath of a heart attack than those in more affluent areas (Krumholz et al., 2019; Watson, 2019b).

To address disparities in cardiovascular care, health psychologists and other health professionals recognize the need to harness community resources, such as by placing health-promotion flyers in neighborhood barbershops where they are more likely to reach Black men and enlisting barbers to help more directly by encouraging their customers to make lifestyle changes and schedule doctor's appointments (Chirinos et al., 2021; Wippold et al., 2023).

Risk Factors You Can Control

Adoption of healthier behaviors across the life span can substantially reduce the risk of CVD—behaviors such as following a healthy diet, exercising regularly, controlling excess body weight, and avoiding tobacco use (Arnett et al., 2019; Grundy et al., 2019). People can also reduce their risk of heart disease by having regular medical checkups and adhering to medical treatment for underlying conditions, such as high blood cholesterol levels and hypertension.

Taking stock of one's lifestyle choices in one's 20s or 30s can help prevent the development of CVD in later life. Even if your genetic profile increases your risk of heart disease, adopting a healthier lifestyle early in life can reduce this risk by up to 50% (Grundy et al., 2019; Khera et al., 2016).

Among people with heart disease, controlling behavioral risk factors increases the likelihood of long-term survival. The factors most strongly linked to survival in people with existing heart disease include not smoking, regular physical activity, controlling blood pressure, and following a healthful diet (Maron et al., 2018).

The lesson to be drawn for us all is that whether we currently have any signs of heart disease or not, it's important to take healthier living to heart (pun intended). We have some encouraging news to share, but it comes with a qualifier. Americans have begun to take better care of their cardiovascular health. Death rates from heart disease have declined steadily since the 1960s, in large part because fewer people are smoking and because of reduced intake of dietary fat, increased physical activity and exercise, and improved treatment of CHD (Jain & Davis, 2019; Joyner & Paneth, 2019).

Death rates from CHD continued to decline in the early 2000s for all major ethnic/racial groups. However, the qualifier is that the rate of decline has been slowing since 2016 and may actually have risen slightly in the past couple of years. This is a worrisome sign but can also serve as a call to action to expand public health efforts to get the nation back on track in taking better care of its cardiovascular health (CDC, 2019d; Joyner & Paneth, 2019). A likely culprit in this worrisome trend is the continuing rise in obesity among Americans (see Chapter 7), because obesity is a major contributing factor to CHD and other forms of CVD.

low-density lipoprotein (LDL) cholesterol A type of cholesterol that can stick to artery walls, forming fatty deposits that can impede blood flow, setting the stage for a heart attack or stroke; commonly referred to as "bad" cholesterol.

high-density lipoprotein (HDL) cholesterol A type of cholesterol that sweeps away plaque deposits from artery walls and thus lowers the risk of cardiovascular disease; commonly referred to as "good" cholesterol.

Blood Cholesterol Levels Elevated levels of a type of blood cholesterol, **low-density lipoprotein (LDL) cholesterol** (often called bad cholesterol), is a major contributor to atherosclerosis and the risk of CHD (Michos et al., 2019). LDL can cling to artery walls, leading to blockages that impair the flow of blood to the heart, brain, and other organs. Another type of blood cholesterol, **high-density lipoprotein (HDL) cholesterol**, is the good guy in our story. This "good" cholesterol helps lower the risk of CVD by sweeping away deposits of LDL cholesterol from artery walls for transport to

TABLE 12.1 Desirable Cholesterol Numbers for Adults

Total cholesterol	Less than 200 mg/dL*
LDL "bad" cholesterol	Less than 100 mg/dL
HDL "good" cholesterol	Greater than or equal to 60 mg/dL

**Cholesterol levels are measured in milligrams (mg) of cholesterol per deciliter (dL) of blood.*
Source: Cholesterol & Your Heart: What You Need to Know Fact Sheet, National Heart, Lung, and Blood Institute, 2022

the liver, where it is eliminated from the body. Consequently, a major focus of efforts to prevent CVD involves management of blood cholesterol levels with the aim of lowering LDL levels and boosting HDL to desirable levels.

How high is too high when it comes to LDL, or how low is too low for HDL? Healthy blood cholesterol levels vary with age, as shown in **Table 12.1**. Desirable blood cholesterol levels for men and women above age 20 are less than 200 mg/dL for total cholesterol, less than 100 mg/dL for LDL (bad cholesterol), and 40 mg/dL or higher in men and 50 mg/dL or higher in women for HDL (good cholesterol). A more comprehensive evaluation of blood cholesterol takes into account the ratio between HDL and total blood cholesterol. An optimal ratio is 3.5:1. For example, if HDL cholesterol is 36 mg/dL and total cholesterol is 200, the risk ratio is 200/36, or 5.55. A ratio of 5:1 or higher is associated with increased risk of CVD.

Blood cholesterol levels are influenced by genetic factors that you can't control but also by dietary factors, which you can control. Heredity influences how quickly LDL is produced in the body and how fast it is removed from the blood. Blood cholesterol levels also tend to rise with age. Healthy dietary changes that can have a positive impact on blood cholesterol levels include limiting consumption of foods that are high in saturated fat and cholesterol. Diet modification and exercise are generally recommended as the first steps in reducing blood cholesterol levels. If these lifestyle changes are insufficient, healthcare providers may recommend using cholesterol-lowering medications, such as *statins*. These medications are widely used because they have proven to be effective in lowering LDL levels and can also raise HDL levels. Statins slow the body's production of cholesterol and increase the liver's ability to remove LDL. However, some people who take statins develop abnormal liver function or muscle problems. Therefore, people on statins need to be regularly monitored to detect side effects. Health investigators recognize that, even when statins or other medications are used, lifestyle modifications also need to be part of the equation for controlling cholesterol levels (Arnett et al., 2019).

triglycerides The main type of fat carried in the blood and stored in fatty tissue.

Triglycerides

Triglycerides are the most common type of fat (lipid) found in the bloodstream and in fatty tissue throughout the body. The body converts excess calories in your diet into triglycerides. High level of triglycerides in the bloodstream contribute to arteriosclerosis, which in turn increases the risk of heart attacks and strokes (Mayo Clinic, 2018). High triglyceride levels are also associated with other risk factors, including obesity and high blood cholesterol. People with high triglyceride levels should ask their healthcare providers whether they would benefit from drugs or dietary changes to lower triglycerides in the blood.

Diet

Your dietary choices have an important bearing on your risk of CHD and other major forms of CVD. Foods that are high in saturated fat, such as red meat, processed meats, high-fat dairy products, and trans fats (found in many baked goods, snack foods, and fast food) increase levels of LDL cholesterol, which over time can lead to atherosclerosis. Foods high in sodium, such as snack foods and processed foods, can increase blood pressure, and foods high in sugar can add extra weight, which can increase blood pressure and blood cholesterol levels. Unfortunately, most Americans exceed recommended levels of sodium consumption. The average sodium intake among people in the United States is about 3,400 mg a day, which is about 50% higher than the recommended limit of 2300 mg a day in people 14 years of age and older (Mayne, McKinnon, & Woodcock, 2021).

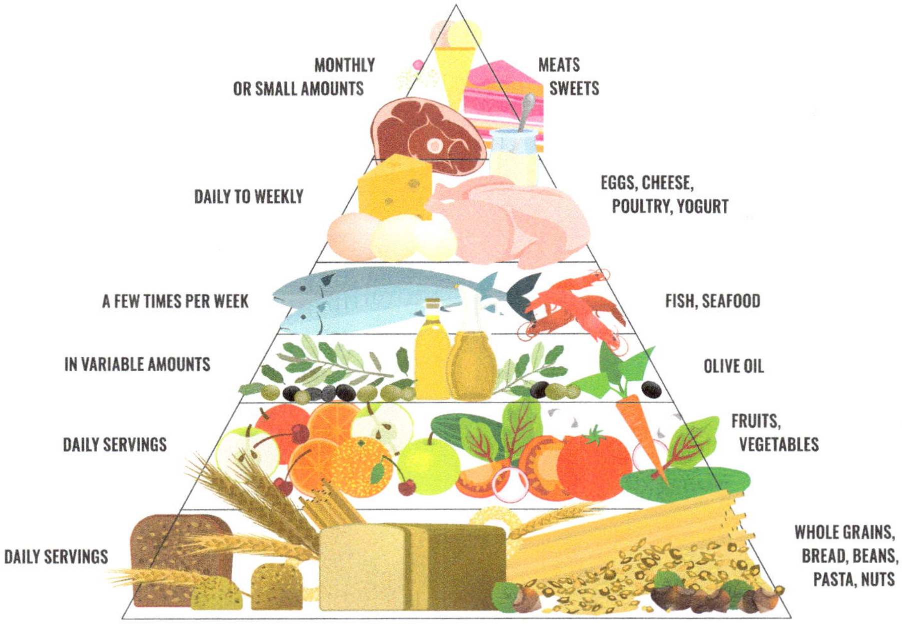

Double Brain/Shutterstock.com

From the Mediterranean to Your Plate The Mediterranean diet presents an ideal way to obtain the nutrients you need without "offending" the cardiovascular system.

Smoking

Smoking is linked to more than 1 in 5 deaths from heart disease (Duncan, 2019). It more than doubles the risk of heart attacks and doubles the risk of sudden cardiac death. Smokers are also less likely to survive a heart attack.

Smoking damages the heart and circulatory system in many ways. The constituents of cigarette smoke damage the lining of the blood vessels, making them more receptive to the formation of plaque. Tobacco smoke contains carbon monoxide, which reduces the supply of oxygen reaching vital body organs, including the heart. Smoking also increases the risk of dangerous blood clots by making platelets "stickier." In addition, smoking increases levels of LDL cholesterol and reduces levels of HDL cholesterol, and the nicotine in tobacco, a stimulant drug, directly increases heart rate and raises blood pressure (World Heart Foundation, 2024).

Obesity

Obesity is a significant risk factor for CHD as well as for hypertension, stroke, and diabetes (James et al., 2014; Massetti et al., 2017; U.S. Burden of Disease Collaborators, 2018). Obesity increases the risk of CVD in part because it is linked to high levels of LDL cholesterol. Although obesity is a complex health problem that involves genetic, metabolic, and lifestyle factors (see Chapter 7), developing healthy eating and exercise habits can help people lose excess weight and maintain a healthy weight.

Interestingly, it's not just excess weight that conveys added risk, but also how weight is distributed in the body. Carrying excess weight around the midsection (waist) is associated with greater risk of heart disease and diabetes than carrying excess fat in the hips, buttocks, and thighs. Put more simply, people with excess fat around their midsections ("apples") have a higher risk of CHD, diabetes, and hypertension than those with excess weight around the hips ("pears") (Pischon et al., 2008; Yusef et al., 2005) (see **Figure 12.7**)

The reason for differences in relative risk between "apples" and "pears" is that body fat accumulating around the pelvis (pear-shared) is linked to higher blood levels of good cholesterol, the HDL that helps remove fatty deposits in arteries. "Apples" tend to have lower levels of HDL. Men are more likely to be apple-shaped, which may in part explain their greater risk of CHD until late adulthood, when rates between men and women tend to even out.

Overweight and obesity is part of a complex of health problems referred to as **metabolic syndrome**. The syndrome is associated with increased risk of CVD and Type 2 (adult-onset) diabetes (see Chapter 14). Other risk factors for metabolic syndrome include high blood pressure, high blood sugar, high triglyceride and LDL levels, and low levels of HDL. Fifty million Americans are believed to have metabolic syndrome.

metabolic syndrome A cluster of risk factors for cardiovascular disease and other health conditions, such as diabetes.

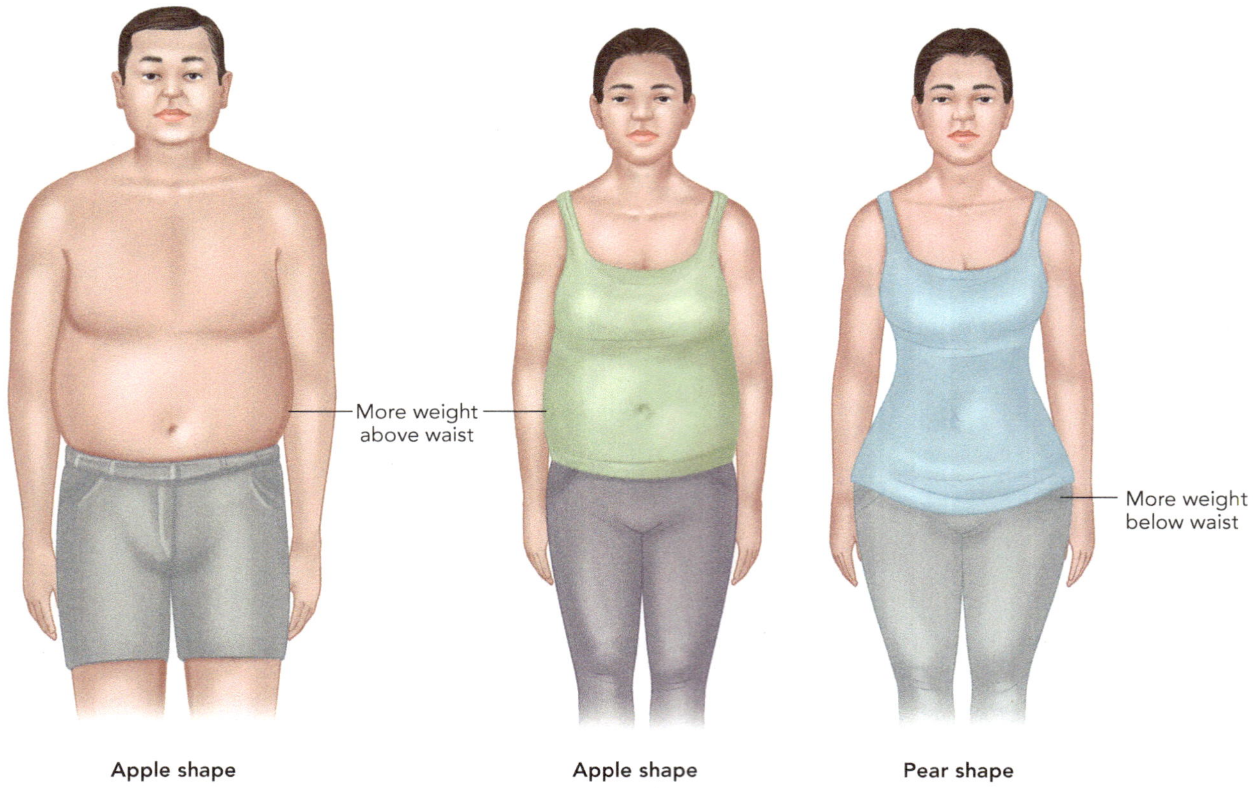

FIGURE 12.7 Distribution of Body Fat: Apples Versus Pears Fat distribution on the body is associated with relative risk of cardiovascular disease and diabetes. People who are apple-shaped are at greater risk than those who are pear-shaped.

Alcohol Use Evidence links higher levels of alcohol use to greater risk of CVD (and other health problems) (Piano, 2017). But evidence is less clear concerning moderate use of alcohol (one to two drinks per day for men, one drink for women). Ironically, a number of studies link low to moderate drinking to a lower risk of heart attacks and strokes and to lower death rates overall (e.g., see Bell et al., 2017; GBD 2016 Alcohol Collaborators, 2018; Naimi et al., 2019).

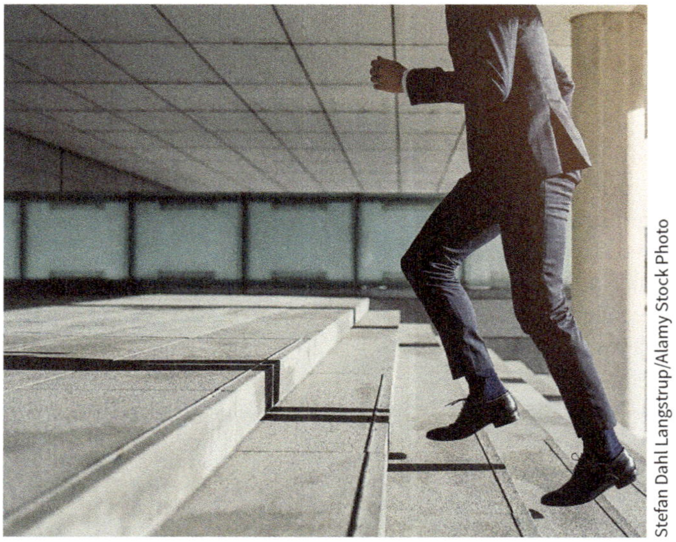

Steps! Taking the steps rather than an elevator is good for you, unless, perhaps, you work in a 60-story building. But there is no reason to believe that counting the steps you take per day has a magic effect—unless it motivates you to ... take the steps.

Low to moderate use of alcohol may have beneficial effects on blood levels of HDL (Huang et al., 2017). However, as noted in Chapter 9, other investigators question the possible health benefits of modest or moderate drinking, so we need further research to clarify these mixed findings (Biddinger et al., 2022; Millwood et al., 2019). Meanwhile, take note that no major health organization or federal health agency recommends that people begin to drink alcohol to control their cholesterol because of concerns that low levels of drinking may eventually develop into drinking problems (Piano, 2017).

Physical Inactivity Physical inactivity tends to add excess weight and increases the risk of CHD (McGowan et al., 2019). In fact, evidence shows that a sedentary lifestyle doubles the risk of developing CHD (Manson et al., 2004). A major culprit in a sedentary lifestyle is prolonged sitting, which is linked to a wide range of serious diseases, including CVD, cancer, diabetes, as well as overall mortality (Yang et al., 2019). We are spending about an hour more a day sitting than we did even 10 years ago (Yang et al., 2019). It turns out that the amount of time spent sitting while watching TV or videos is about the same as it was about 10 years ago, about 2 hours per day on average, but we are now spending about an hour more of leisure time on the computer.

Sitting for prolonged lengths of time is clearly hazardous to your health. The good news is that even seasoned couch potatoes can reduce their risk of CVD by becoming more physically active (Pasanen et al., 2017). Evidence shows that people who don't start leisure time physical activity until midlife still reap the benefits of reduced risk of CVD and premature death (Saint-Maurice et al., 2019).

The use of Fitbit-type electronic step counters has become popular in helping people keep track of the number of steps they take during the day. But it turns out that there is no magic number of steps for living longer, no set number such as 10,000 steps daily. Researchers find that walking just a little less than 4,000 steps a day is associated with lower death rates (Blum, 2023). Another study showed that older women who averaged 4,400 daily steps had lower mortality rates, on average, than those who took half as many steps (Abbasi, 2019). But there wasn't any further reduction in mortality beyond a level of about 7,500 steps daily. The health benefit comes from increasing physical activity, not from wearing a step-monitoring device. Nor has it been shown that using a wearable physical activity device has any advantages in boosting physical activity levels as compared with standard behavioral weight-loss programs (Jakicic et al., 2016).

Hypertension **Hypertension**, or high blood pressure, is a leading risk factor for CVD, contributing to the deaths of more than 400,000 Americans annually or more than 1,100 deaths each day (Yang et al., 2019). Most of these deaths are due to heart attacks or strokes, but hypertension can also lead to congestive heart failure, kidney damage, and even blindness. These grim statistics highlight the importance of having blood pressure checked regularly and getting high blood pressure under control.

hypertension High blood pressure.

Over time, high blood pressure damages the heart and circulatory system because of the greater force and friction it imposes on the sensitive tissues within arteries (AHA, 2019). In people with hypertension, the artery walls may develop slight tears that allow plaques to form from a buildup of LDL (bad) cholesterol, setting the stage for atherosclerosis. Arteries begin to narrow from the buildup of plaque, which, in a vicious cycle, raises blood pressure, which further damages the arteries, heart, and other parts of the cardiovascular system and ultimately leads to heart attacks, strokes, or other cardiovascular problems like heart arrhythmias.

systolic blood pressure (SBP) The maximum pressure in arteries when the heart contracts with each heartbeat.

diastolic blood pressure (DBP) The minimum pressure in arteries when the heart relaxes between beats.

About one-third of American adults—some 75 million people—have hypertension. Another third has prehypertension, or elevated blood pressure that is higher than normal but not in the hypertensive range—not yet, at least, but many people in this category go on to develop hypertension (CDC, 2020c). Hypertension does not usually have noticeable symptoms. People with hypertension may find out about the condition only during a routine medical exam, which is yet another reason for regular healthcare visits. No wonder hypertension is called a silent killer! Unfortunately, only about 1 in 4 people with hypertension have it under control (Kochanek et al., 2019).

Blood pressure (BP) is the force or pressure that circulating blood applies to the walls of blood vessels and is defined by two numbers:

- **Systolic blood pressure (SBP)** is a measure of the maximum pressures in arteries when the heart contracts or beats, pushing blood throughout the body.
- **Diastolic blood pressure (DBP)** is the minimum pressure that remains in the arteries when the heart relaxes between beats.

Both numbers are expressed in terms of a standard measure of blood pressure, which is given in millimeters of mercury (mm Hg). Health officials usually write these numbers

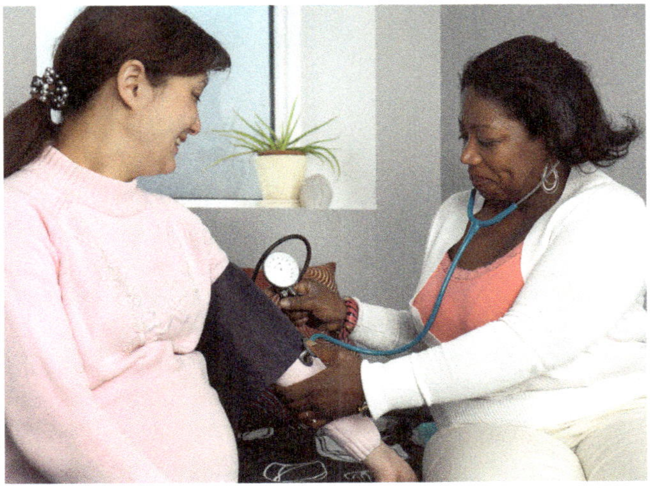

maximimages.com/Alamy Stock Photo

Do You Know Your Blood Pressure? Although it lacks telltale symptoms, high blood pressure can ultimately lead to heart attacks, strokes, and other serious health problems if left uncontrolled. When was the last time you had your blood pressure checked? You can take your blood pressure by yourself at home. Ask a pharmacist for a recommendation for a blood pressure monitor in your desired price range.

TABLE 12.2 Blood Pressure Categories: Are You Hypertensive?

Blood Pressure Category	Systolic Blood Pressure		Diastolic Blood Pressure
Normal	<120 mmHg	and	<80 mmHg
Elevated	120–129 mmHg	and	<80 mmHg
Hypertension			
Stage 1	130–139 mmHg	or	80–89 mmHg
Stage 2	≥140 mmHg	or	≥90 mmHg

Source: CDC (2024a)

in terms of an upper number (SBP) and a lower number (DBP), so that blood pressure of 120 SBP and 80 DBP is written in the form 120/80 mm Hg (read that as 120 over 80 millimeters of mercury).

Blood pressure readings of less than 120/80 mm Hg fall in a normal range. The ranges for elevated blood pressure (prehypertension) and hypertension are shown in **Table 12.2**, but note that different health organizations apply somewhat different standards. The risk of developing hypertension increases with age for both men and women. Men have a greater risk of developing HBP until about age 65, at which point the risk of developing HBP becomes greater among women (Mayo Clinic, 2019a).

Healthcare providers rely on both SBP and DBP in making diagnoses of high blood pressure. They can better appraise the risk of CVD by considering both systolic and diastolic pressures. However, health professionals generally place greater emphasis on systolic blood pressure for initiating antihypertensive medication for older people and on diastolic blood pressure for younger people.

Some cases of hypertension (HBP) can be traced to identifiable physical problems or defects, such as kidney malfunction. But in about 90% of cases, called essential hypertension or primary hypertension, the cause remains unclear, but many of the risk factors fall squarely on unhealthy behaviors, which is why it is a major focus in health psychology.

Behavioral Risk Factors in Hypertension Behavioral risk factors in hypertension mirror those for other forms of CVD, including unhealthful behaviors like these (CDC, 2020c; Mayo Clinic, 2019):

- *Using tobacco:* Smoking or chewing tobacco raises blood pressure.
- *Consuming foods high in sodium and low in potassium:* Sodium intake from foods and table salt causes the body to retain fluids, which increases blood pressure. High sodium intake is linked to higher rates of death due to CVD (Micha et al., 2017).
- *Physical inactivity:* Lack of physical activity or exercise is associated with increased heart rate, which increases the force applied by each heartbeat on the arteries and makes the heart work harder. Lack of exercise is also a risk factor for overweight and obesity.
- *Drinking too much alcohol:* Heavy consumption of alcohol, typically defined by regularly consuming more than one drink a day for women and more than two drinks a day for men, may increase blood pressure and can damage the heart over time.
- *Being overweight or obese:* With excess body weight, more blood is needed to supply bodily tissues. As blood volume increases, so too does pressure on artery walls, leading to higher blood pressure.
- *Stress:* Blood pressure can increase during times of stress and when stressful burdens become a feature of daily life.

There are steps each of us can take to lower our risk of developing hypertension by controlling modifiable risk factors (see **Table 12.3**). These healthy behaviors for reducing the risk of high

TABLE 12.3 Healthful Behaviors That Help Control Blood Pressure

- Adopt a diet that is rich in fresh fruit and vegetables and low in salt (sodium), total fat, saturated fat, and cholesterol.
- Avoid smoking. If you do smoke, quit as soon as possible.
- Maintain a healthy weight, keeping your body mass index (BMI) between 18 and 24.99.
- Keep physically active, at least 30 minutes a day of moderate intensity exercise, 5 days a week.
- Keep alcohol intake to a limit of one drink a day for women or two drinks a day for men.

Source: Adapted from Forman et al. (2009), NHLBI (2005)

blood pressure are all the more important because some risk factors, like age and family history, cannot be changed.

Differences in Hypertension

A greater percentage of men (47%) have hypertension than women (43%) (CDC, 2020c). Non-Hispanic Black adults have higher rates of hypertension than non-Hispanic White, Latino/Hispanic, or Asian American adults (CDC, 2020c) (see **Figure 12.8**). Black people also have higher rates of serious complications arising from high blood pressure, including heart attacks, strokes, and kidney failure (Schutte et al., 2020). Among people who have been prescribed blood pressure medication, control of blood pressure is higher among White American adults (32%) than among Black

Health Psychology in Action

Perceived Benefits and Barriers of Adhering to a Salt-Restricted Diet

According to the Health Belief Model, when people perceive a threat to their health, they function according to the perceived benefits and barriers concerning a course of action. In the case of hypertension, the perceived threats include heart attacks, heart failure, and strokes. People may see themselves as vulnerable to these cardiovascular disorders if there is a family history of CVD; if they are overweight, aging, and the like. A cue to action could be learning that someone they know, someone with a similar health profile, has died of a heart attack or stroke.

A study of 200 people with hypertension who were placed on salt-restricted diets (Zengin et al., 2018) reported perceived benefits and barriers to adhering to the diet.

Perceived benefits of adherence to a salt-restricted diet:

- "Eating a low-salt diet will keep me healthy."
- "Salty food is not good for me."
- "Eating a low-salt diet will keep my heart healthy."
- "Eating a low-salt diet will keep my swelling down."
- "Eating a low-salt diet will keep fluid from building up in my body."
- "When I follow my low-salt diet I feel better."
- "Eating a low-salt diet will help me breathe more easily."

Perceived barriers to adherence to a salt-restricted diet:

- "I can't eat in restaurants I like because of the low-salt diet."
- "Food does not taste good without salt."
- "Following a low-salt diet costs too much money."
- "Following a low-salt diet takes too much time."
- "It's too hard to understand exactly how to follow a low-salt diet."

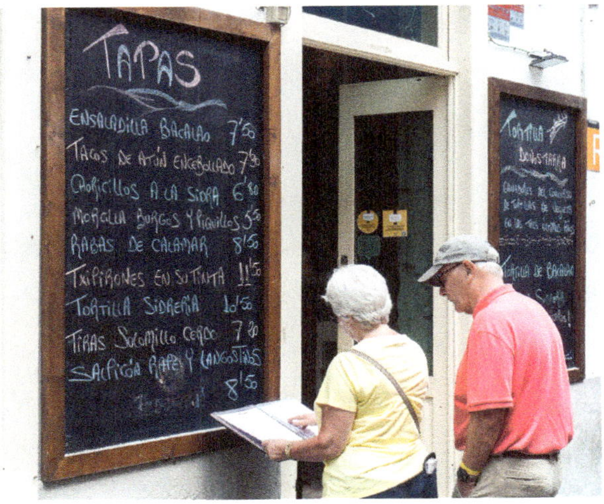

Islandstock/Alamy Stock Photo

Eating Out! Eating out is one of life's pleasures, and—for some of us—it can be one of life's health challenges. How can we control the amount of salt in the food we order?

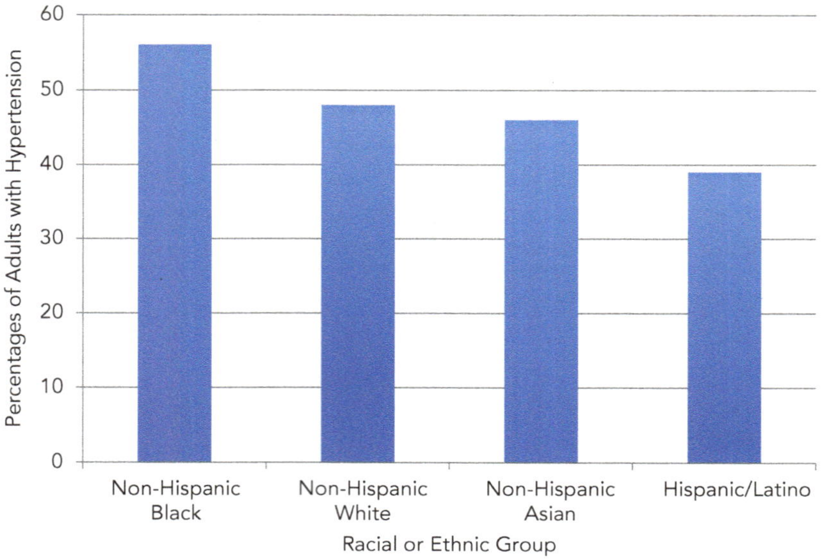

FIGURE 12.8 **Hypertension in Adults, United States, by Race/Ethnicity**
Source: CDC (2023i)

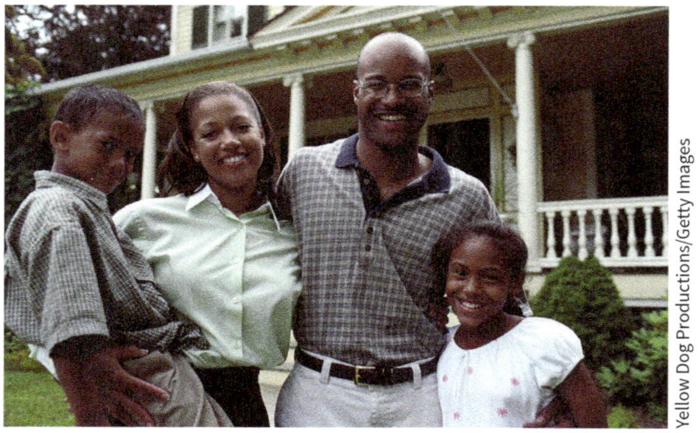

Discrimination and Social Class Middle-class Black Americans are more likely—not less likely—to encounter discrimination than lower SES Black Americans. Persistent active striving in the face of discrimination is associated with the secretion of stress hormones and hypertension.

American adults (25%), Asian American adults (19%), or Latino/Hispanic adults (25%) (CDC, 2020c).

Why are Black Americans at greater risk of hypertension? One reason is that they have higher rates of obesity and diabetes than the general population, and both of these factors are linked to an increased risk of high blood pressure (Lee, 2019). Another reason is that exposure to racial or ethnic discrimination is also linked to hypertension (Beatty Moody et al., 2016; Dolezsar et al., 2014). Black Americans also tend to develop high blood pressure earlier in life. We need to further explore mechanisms explaining links between blood pressure and discrimination, but a likely possibility is that discrimination is an important source of life stress, which can over time take a toll on the cardiovascular system.

Other factors also contribute to these health disparities. Black Americans may have a greater genetic sensitivity to sodium (salt) and a greater predisposition to retain sodium in the body (Jones & Rayner, 2020). Physical inactivity may also play a role, although activity levels may have more to do with socioeconomic status than race or ethnicity. Black Americans are disproportionately represented among the lower income strata, and people who are economically disadvantaged tend to exercise less, in part because they are less able than affluent people to pay for gym memberships, afford exercise classes or equipment, or have leisure time.

John Henryism, Hypertension, and Adherence to Medication The concept of "John Henryism" was developed to examine hypertension among Black Americans (Hudson et al., 2016). It is based on folklore concerning a Black American steel-driver,[1] John Henry, who reportedly raced a steam-powered steel-driving machine during the

[1] A railroad worker of the late 1800s who drove steel spikes into rock to make holes for explosives to clear the way for railroad tracks.

Health Psychology in Action

Should Salt Shakers Carry Tobacco-Style Health Warnings?

Cigarette packs are required to carry the explicit warning that smoking causes cancer. Should salt shakers and salt (sodium) packets carry a health warning as well? Most of us are aware of the health risks of smoking, thanks largely to the public health effort over the past 50 years to inform people of the dangers of tobacco products. But what about a health warning on salt?

The World Hypertension League and several other health and science organizations believe that countries should require a warning label (Campbell et al., 2019). Sodium intake is a recognized risk factor for hypertension, which contributes to the development of heart disease and stroke. A former president of the World Hypertension League, Dr. Norm Campbell, says that it is time to take action in the interests of public health: "Unhealthy diets are a leading cause of death globally and excess salt consumption is the biggest culprit, estimated to cause over 3 million deaths globally in [a year]" (cited in The George Institute for Global Health, 2019). No governmental authority in the world requires a warning label on salt, not yet at least. But we shouldn't be surprised if such a warning is in the offing, as governments and health authorities seek to address the devastating effects of CVD and ways of preventing it.

Though curbing use of table salt would certainly reduce sodium intake, we should note that only about 11% of daily salt intake comes from use of table salt or added salt when cooking at home (Mayne, McKinnon, & Woodcock, 2021). Most of the sodium we consume, more than 70%, comes from packaged foods or food we consume in restaurants or food service operations. More significant changes in reducing sodium intake will depend upon reducing the sodium content in the food supply and especially in processed foods, which are generally high in sodium. But at the individual level, each of us can directly monitor our sodium intake by checking product labels and avoiding prepared foods that are loaded with sodium (like Ramen noodles, sorry).

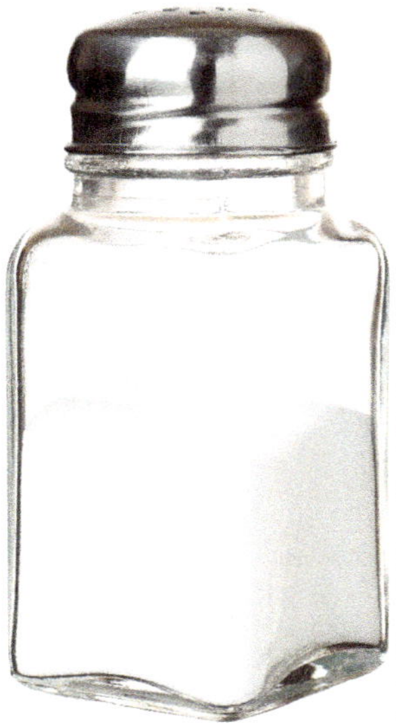

Andrei Kuzmik/Alamy Stock Photo

Should the Salt Shaker Carry a Health Warning? If cigarette packs must carry a health warning, why not salt shakers? High blood pressure is a major risk factor for CHD, and consumption of added salt may increase blood pressure. Do you think a warning label is warranted?

construction of the railroad. He won the race, but his heart gave out; he fell dead with a hammer in his hand. The point of the legend is that Black Americans must cope actively and strongly to surmount psychosocial and environmental stressors in a society that discriminates against them as they attempt to create an American identity characterized by hard work, self-reliance, and freedom.

The striving may gain Blacks of lower socioeconomic status a path to the middle class and beyond, but for many it comes at the cost of their physical health (DeAngelis, 2020). The stress associated with their striving to reach goals is associated with elevated levels of stress hormones and high blood pressure (DeAngelis, 2020). These bodily changes place goal-striving Black adults at risk of what stress researcher Hans Selye called diseases of adaptation and, given their greater risk of hypertension, particular vulnerability to cardiovascular disorders (DeAngelis, 2020).

There is also a connection between John Henryism and adherence to blood pressure medication. Black adults who are less prone to striving are also less likely to adhere to medication for hypertension (Cuffee et al., 2020). Those who strive are more likely to adhere to their medication, but they are also more suspicious of healthcare professionals, perhaps because they have come farther and are more likely to understand the kinds of discrimination shown by many—certainly not all—healthcare professionals.

Psychological Factors in Heart Disease

Might your personality, your emotions, and even your outlook on life put you at increased risk of CVD? As we shall see, research evidence from health psychology and other health disciplines points in this direction.

Stress and the Heart

Occasional stress is not likely to have adverse effects on the heart and circulatory system. But persistent or recurrent stress is a significant risk factor for CVD. As we noted, under stress, the body releases stress hormones, including epinephrine and norepinephrine, that speed up the heart and blood flow. Over time, excessive secretion of these stress hormones can damage the heart and blood vessels, increasing the potential for heart attacks and strokes. We also noted that high levels of stress that become a feature of daily life can contribute to hypertension, a major risk factor for CVD.

One of the major sources of daily stress is workplace stress from a demanding job. Stress on the job can contribute to increased CHD risk, especially for workers facing a combination of high-strain work (heavy demands) and little personal control over work (Aboa-Éboulé et al., 2007; Krantz et al., 1988). Occupational health psychologists are aware of the potentially toxic effects of a stressful workplace and work with managers to help reduce the stress levels workers face on the job.

Does Your Personality Place You at Risk of Heart Disease?

Type A behavior pattern A personality pattern characterized by a hurried pace to life, competitiveness, and proneness to hostility.

The **Type A behavior pattern** initially attracted attention in the medical community in the 1960s when medical reports appeared that linked this personality profile to increased risk of heart disease and heart attacks, especially in middle-age people. Although later investigations cast doubt on a link between the Type A personality and heart disease (Geipert, 2007), researchers revealed one element of the Type A behavior pattern that was a significant risk factor for heart disease and other serious health problems: hostility (Chida & Steptoe, 2009; Denollet & Pedersen, 2009).

Hostility and Anger: Getting Hot Under the Collar Can Be Dangerous to Your Health

Hostility is a psychological trait that describes people who have "short fuses" and are prone to anger. Their attitudes toward others are cynical and mistrustful. Investigators find that hostility, which is associated with proneness to anger, is the component of the Type A behavior pattern most strongly linked to the development of CHD. Whether other features of the Type A behavior pattern, such as a hurried pace of life, directly contribute to health problems remains open to further study.

Evidence shows that anger is closely associated with the risk of CHD (Andreeva & Gorbunov, 2022; Barefoot & Williams, 2022). Hostile people tend to be angry much of the time and persistent anger is linked to increased risk of both hypertension and CHD (Levine et al., 2021; Titova et al., 2022). To put the effects of anger in context, researchers statistically controlled for influences of high blood pressure and cholesterol levels, smoking, and obesity and found that people who become angered easily were about three times as likely as calmer people to experience heart attacks (J. E. Williams et al., 2000).

Underlying mechanisms explaining links between anger or hostility and cardiovascular problems remain to be determined, but the stress hormones epinephrine and norepinephrine appear to play roles. Anxiety and anger trigger the release of these stress hormones by the adrenal glands. These hormones increase heart rate, breathing rate, and blood pressure, which results in more oxygen-rich blood being pumped to the muscles to enable them to prepare for defensive action—to either fight or flee—in the face of a threatening stressor.

In people who frequently experience strong negative emotions such as anger or anxiety, the body may regularly pump out these stress hormones, eventually damaging the heart and blood vessels. The hormones speed up the heart rate and raise blood pressure, placing increased burdens on the cardiovascular system. Over time, this pattern of overarousal may eventually weaken the cardiovascular system, setting the stage for heart attacks, especially in genetically vulnerable people. An overproduction of stress hormones may also affect the stickiness of the clotting factors in the blood, which in turn may heighten the risk of potentially dangerous blood clots forming that can cause heart attacks or strokes.

Applying Health Psychology

Managing Hostility and Anger

Anger is an adaptive emotion when it motivates us to surmount obstacles in our paths or to defend ourselves. But anger is troublesome when it leads to excessive arousal and self-defeating aggression. Prolonged hostility is also stressful and may lead to diseases of adaptation, such as high blood pressure.

According to the cognitive theories of Albert Ellis and Aaron Beck, we become angry because we say infuriating things to ourselves under provocative circumstances. Something frustrating or annoying may have happened, but two people facing the same situation may respond quite differently—one remaining cool and the other getting hot under the collar. The difference may lie in what each person tells themselves about the situation.

We may be peeved when we mutter to ourselves how unfair it is to be treated like this and we can't stand for it. We may become irritated when our thinking is dominated by "musts" and "shoulds" about how other people should behave, perhaps that others *must* treat us fairly and *should* put our needs first. A world of mutual respect would be wonderful, but demanding that the world live up to these idealized expectations is a recipe for frustration and anger.

Thoughts that trigger anger may occur automatically, as in Table 12.4, but such thoughts may be irrational, and we need to tune in to them. Then we need to work to replace them with rational, calming alternatives. We can manage hostility and anger by identifying and correcting the kinds of thoughts that make us fume.

Here are the basics of managing hostility and anger:

- Tune into the thoughts that magnify frustrations and threats.
- Stop and think.
- Find rational alternatives and practice thinking them.
- Take a deep breath and relax; try relaxation breathing (see Chapter 5).
- Consider forgiving other people for their misdemeanors (really).
- Don't shout, scream, or curse.
- Stick up for your rights; explain why you feel as you do, but straightforwardly and assertively, not aggressively.
- Tell other people that you care about them.
- Pat yourself on the back for keeping your cool.
- Oh, yes: stop and think.

Preventing Road Rage

In road rage, anger caused by frustration with traffic spills over into violent confrontations between drivers. Drivers with low levels of tolerance for frustration have come to blows, chased cars, cut them off, and even taken potshots at them, sometimes over minor provocations, such as beeping the horn or being passed. Cases of road rage may start with beeping the horn but escalate into exchanges of obscene gestures, tailgating, or even bumping into the other vehicle. Here are some tips to avoid becoming a perpetrator or victim of road rage:

- Never use your vehicle as a weapon or as a means of threatening other drivers.
- Be aware of glare. Glaring at another driver is a hostile challenge.

TABLE 12.4 Irrational Thoughts That Intensify Feelings of Anger, and Rational Alternatives

INTERACTIVE FIGURES, CHARTS, & TABLES

Activating Event	Irrational Thoughts	Rational Alternatives
You are caught in traffic	"Who the hell are they to hold me up?" (Road-rage alert!)	"They're not doing it on purpose. They're probably just about as frustrated by it as I am."
	"I'll never get there! It'll be a disaster!"	"Don't catastrophize. It's not my fault, and the world won't come to an end."
Your partner says, "The baby's crying pretty hard."	"Are you blaming me for it?"	"Don't jump to conclusions." Your partner just made a statement of fact.
	"So do something about it!"	"Stop and think." Why not ask your partner to handle it this time?
Your roommate asks, "How's that paper of yours coming?"	Your roommate has nothing to do tonight!	"The paper is difficult, but that's not my roommate's fault."
	Your roommate is so competitive! Wouldn't your roommate love it if you failed!	"I shouldn't assume I can read my roommate's mind. Maybe it's a sincere question. And if it's not, why should I let my roommate get me upset?"
Your boss asks, "So how did the conference turn out?"	"I can handle conferences by myself!"	"Take it easy! Relax. Of course I can handle them. So why should I get bent out of shape?"
	"Always checking up on me!"	"Maybe my boss is just interested, and checking up is a part of a supervisor's job, after all is said and done."
	"Dammit, I'm an adult!"	"Of course I am an adult. So why should I get upset?"

- Control your anger. Ignore aggressive or inconsiderate drivers. You don't know them, so who cares? You need not teach them a lesson.
- Keep your distance. Maintain a safe distance from the car ahead of you on the road.
- Don't weave in and out without signaling. Aggressive driving can escalate into a dangerous confrontation.
- Don't lean on your horn. Use your horn only to prevent an accident, not to express frustration or anger.
- Do not respond to provocations. If a hostile driver provokes you, don't respond and don't make eye contact. Why should you care about it? Let it pass.
- Do not give another driver the finger or mouth curses.
- If your community has a witness tip line, report dangerous drivers, or dial 911.

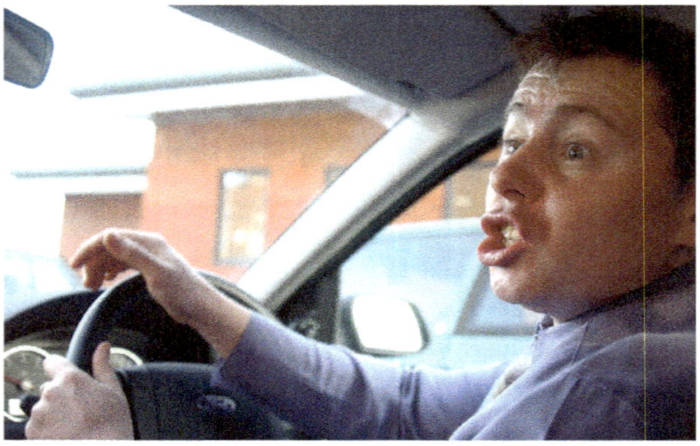

UK Stock Images Ltd/Alamy Stock Photo

Road Rage Control your anger on the road. Don't respond to aggressive or inconsiderate drivers. You need not.

Chronic hostility and the frequent episodes of anger it engenders can also lead to higher blood pressure and blood cholesterol levels, which are two of the major risk factors for CHD and early death. The results of this research on the risks posed by hostility and anger indicate the need to assist hostile and angry people to learn to remain calm in provocative situations.

Anxiety and Depression: Are Negative Emotions Dangerous to Your Heart? Much of the research linking negative emotions to heart disease has focused on the role of hostility and anger. But researchers have learned that other negative emotional states, such as anxiety and depression, also play a role in determining the risk of heart disease (Brugnera et al., 2022). Because of the close interaction of mind and body, prolonged emotional distress in the form of anxiety and depression may impair the cardiovascular system, raising the risk of both heart disease and stroke (Davidson, Pennells, & Di Angelantonio, 2021; Levine et al., 2021; Lee et al., 2022; Lu et al., 2021). Psychologists are developing ways of helping chronically angry or anxious people learn to control their emotional responses to reduce their risks of CHD and other serious health problems.

Depression is also linked to higher risk of cardiovascular disease, perhaps because of the burden on the cardiovascular system associated with increased life stress of people struggling with depression (Barry et al., 2023). Depression is also associated with more negative outcomes and higher death rates among people with established heart disease (Lichtman et al., 2014; Rajan et al., 2020). Even people without established heart disease who struggle with major depression may be at greater risk of dying from heart-related causes than people who are not depressed (Penninx, 2017).

Health psychologists help people struggling with negative emotions, such as anger, anxiety, and depression, learn to manage their emotional responses in order to reduce their risks of CHD and other serious health problems. All in all, taking care of our emotional health may yield benefits in physical as well as mental health. In the "Closer Look" on page 381, we examine intriguing evidence that considers whether there might be some truth to the belief that you can die from a broken heart.

A new personality type has entered the discussion of the role of negative emotions in CHD—the Type D personality. The D stands for "distressed." People with a Type D personality are typically unhappy, insecure, anxious, and irritable. However, they tend to keep their negative feelings bottled up out of fear of saying anything that could lead people to disapprove of them. Type D personality is found in about 1 in 4 people with CHD and is linked to an increased rate of death among CHD patients (Kupper & Denollet, 2018).

Optimism In Chapter 5 we asked what your general outlook on life is. Are you an optimist, someone who sees the proverbial cup as half full, or a pessimist who sees the cup as half empty? Optimism is an important health dimension, according to research showing that more optimistic people tend to have better cardiovascular health and immune system functioning and lower death (mortality) rates overall (Carver, 2014; Rozanski et al., 2019). One of the primary researchers in the field, cardiologist Alan Rozanski, said, "From teenagers to people in their 90's, all have better outcomes if they're optimistic" (cited in Brody, 2020). How does optimism translate into better health outcomes? Though more research is needed to identify the underlying mechanism, it may be that people who hold more hopeful expectancies about the future take better care of themselves and their health (Baumgartner et al., 2018). More optimistic people also practice more active coping strategies, such as problem-focused coping, and are less likely to rely on maladaptive ways of handling stress, such as avoidance (Carver et al., 2010; Helgeson & Zajdel, 2017).

A Closer Look

Can You Die of a Broken Heart?

You may be familiar with the expression "a broken heart" as applied to failed romantic relationships. It turns out, however, there is a recognized medical condition, called broken-heart syndrome, that can be deadly (Sancar, 2019). A part of the body's stress response (see Chapter 4) involves the release of stress hormones epinephrine and norepinephrine. Medical researchers suspect that in some individuals, an irregularity in the way the brain responds to stress may lead to excessive release of these stress hormones, which may "stun" the heart and prevent it from pumping normally (Sancar, 2019; Wittstein et al., 2005). The symptoms may be very similar to a true heart attack, including chest pains and difficulty breathing ("As Valentine's Day Approaches," 2012). Consider the following case report:

"Her heart was failing. She was only 45, but showed all the signs of having a heart attack. But it wasn't a heart attack. Were it a heart attack, there would have been blockage of blood flow through the arteries that service the heart. However, blood flowed freely to her heart. No, in this case, the woman's heart was failing because of the emotional shock of losing her husband in a car crash two days earlier. She had rushed to the crash site and collapsed next to his body, crying inconsolably and trying desperately, but unsuccessfully to wake him. Two days later, she was rushed to the hospital complaining of chest pain and difficulty breathing. This woman's heart was pumping only a fraction of the expected amount of blood. Fortunately, the woman survived, as the levels of stress hormones receded, and the heart returned to pumping at a nearly normal level. Later, she told a reporter, "If anyone had told me that you could die of a broken heart ... I'd never have believed it. But I almost did" (Sanders, 2006, p. 28).

The broken-heart syndrome acquired its name in cases where the source of significant stress that led to cardiac problems was intense grief after the loss of a loved one. However, other stressful events involving strong emotional reactions of anxiety, fear, or even sudden surprise may serve as triggers as well (Shams et al., 2015). Thankfully, the broken-heart syndrome is a rare condition, but it may explain some isolated cases of sudden death following emotional shock, such as the unexpected death of a spouse. In most cases, the symptoms are short-lived and the person survives without any permanent damage the heart ("As Valentine's Day Approaches," 2012). However, people with established heart disease may be especially susceptible to serious, even life-threatening coronary events in response to strong emotional stress (Strike et al., 2006).

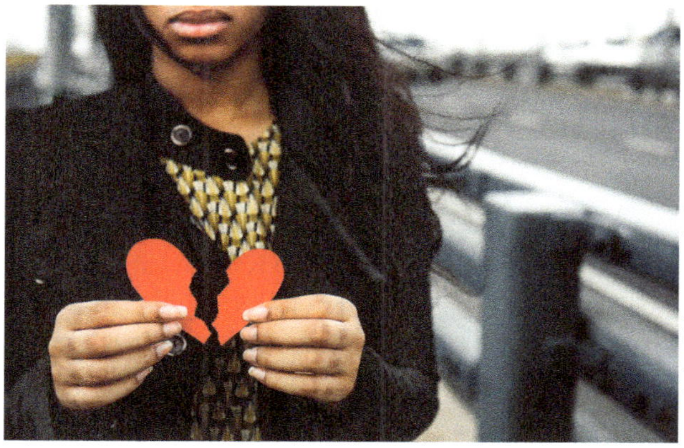

Rawpixel Ltd/Alamy Stock Photo

Can You Die of a Broken Heart? Not very likely, but ...

Review 12.3

INTERACTIVE SELF-SCORING QUIZZES

Sentence Completion

1. Low-density lipoprotein (LDL) cholesterol is often called (good or bad) cholesterol.

2. The most common types of blood fat are __________.

3. High-density lipoprotein (HDL) cholesterol is often called (good or bad) cholesterol.

4. Smoking is linked to more than one in (2 or 5) deaths from heart disease.

5. Heavy smokers (can or cannot) significantly reduce their risk of CVD by quitting.

6. Tobacco smoke contains __________ monoxide, which reduces the supply of oxygen reaching vital body organs, including the heart.

7. Carrying excess weight around the __________ is associated with greater risk of heart disease and diabetes than carrying excess fat in the hips, buttocks, and thighs.

8. __________ syndrome is associated with increased risk of Type 2 (adult-onset) diabetes.

9. Prolonged __________ is linked to a wide range of serious diseases.

10. Systolic blood pressure readings of less than __________ mm Hg fall in a normal range.

11. African Americans have (lower or higher) rates of obesity and diabetes than the general population.

12. The component of the Type A behavior pattern most closely linked to heart disease is __________.

13. The stress hormones __________ and norepinephrine appear to play significant roles in links between hostility and anger, on one hand, and cardiovascular problems, on the other.

14. Optimistic people tend to have (better or worse) cardiovascular health and immune system functioning.

Think About It

What are your personal risk factors for CVD? Which of these factors can you change? How would you go about changing them?

Prevention of Cardiovascular Disease

Health psychologists recognize that the best way to confront the challenge of cardiovascular disease lies in a biopsychosocial model that takes into account the roles of biological, psychological, and social factors (Gaffey et al., 2022). Let's be clear: Our daily behaviors and lifestyles play important roles in determining our risk of developing heart disease. Here's a number sure to garner attention: 94 million lives saved (Kontis et al., 2019; Rodriguez, 2019b). That's the number of lives investigators believe could be saved worldwide if public health interventions achieved the following objectives:

- Expanding treatment for hypertension—39.4 million lives saved
- Reducing sodium intake (sodium intake is a risk factor for CVD)—40.0 million lives saved
- Eliminating trans fats, which raise LDL and lower HDL—14.8 million lives saved

Here's another attention-grabbing number, this time in terms of a percentage—65%. That's an estimate from health researchers of the percentage of cases and deaths from CVD across 21 countries that were attributable to modifiable causes (Watson, 2019; Yusuf et al., 2019). The researchers identified more than 150,000 people who were free of CVD when the study began and then followed them for a period of nearly 10 years. Modifiable risk factors were broken down into two major categories, metabolic risk factors and behavioral risk factors (see **Table 12.5**). The take-away from this large-scale multinational study is that the great majority of cases of CVD and resulting deaths can be explained by factors that involve modifiable behaviors. That's good news for us all, because it demonstrates that reducing the risk of CVD is largely about developing healthier lifestyles.

Obesity, high blood cholesterol levels, and hypertension are among the major risk factors for CHD. The good news is that these factors are largely controllable. We can change our diet to make healthier food choices and start exercising regularly to keep fit and lose excess weight or prevent obesity from developing. We can avoid using tobacco, avoid or limit our use of alcohol, and watch our salt intake. We can have our cholesterol and blood pressure checked

TABLE 12.5 **Modifiable Risk Factors in CVD in 21 Countries**

Category	Individual Risk Factors	Percentage of CVD Disease (Morbidity) and Deaths (Mortality) Accounted For
Metabolic risk factors	Blood lipid (cholesterol) levels, blood pressure, diabetes, obesity, with blood pressure the strongest predictor	40%
Behavioral risk factors	Tobacco and alcohol use, diet, physical activity, and sodium intake, with tobacco use the strongest predictor	25%

Source: Adapted from Yusuf et al. (2019).

Health Psychology in Action

Practice Guidelines for Prevention Put the Emphasis on Healthful Behaviors

Two leading medical organizations, the American College of Cardiology and the American Heart Association, recently issued guidelines for the prevention of CVD (Arnett et al., 2019; Jain & Davis, 2019). The guideline endorses the idea that prevention of CVD takes a team effort that focuses on both medical interventions and behavior change strategies. Importantly, the guideline recognizes that the most important preventive measures involve adoption of a healthy lifestyle throughout the course of one's life.

Here we highlight recommendations from the guideline for promoting heart-healthy behaviors to prevent CVD (Arnett et al., 2019; Brett, 2019):

1. Targeting social determinants of health-related behaviors (see Table 12.6).
2. Promoting a healthful diet, such as a diet that is rich in vegetables, fruits, nuts, and whole grains; minimizes trans fats, red meat and processed red meats, refined carbohydrates such as sugary snacks and cereals, and sweetened beverages; and includes lean sources of protein from fish, plant, and animal sources.
3. Promoting calorie restriction to achieve and maintain weight loss in adults who are overweight or obese.
4. Promoting regular physical activity, consisting of at least 150 minutes per week in total of moderate-intensity physical activity or 75 minutes per week of vigorous-intensity physical activity.
5. Emphasizing the importance in adults with Type 2 diabetes mellitus of making healthy lifestyles changes in diet and exercise. (Diabetes is discussed further in Chapter 14.)
6. Regularly assessing tobacco use and assisting people to quit smoking.
7. Using lifestyle modifications (weight loss, healthful diet, regular exercise, quitting smoking) for adults with elevated blood pressure or hypertension.
8. Recommending lifestyle changes for people with Type 2 diabetes mellitus, including improving dietary habits and undertaking exercise.

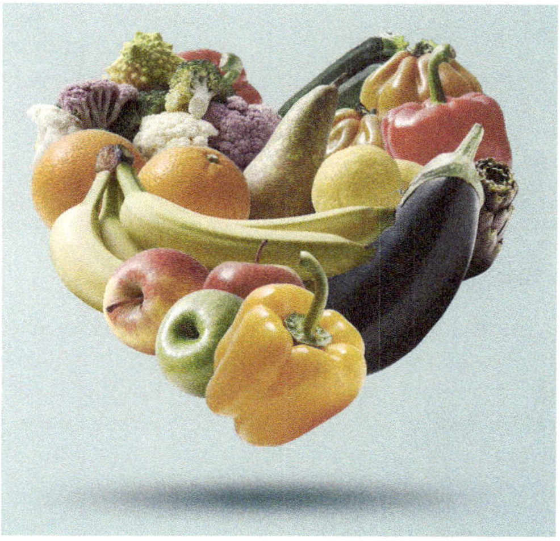

cyano66/Getty Images

TABLE 12.6 Strategies for Targeting Social Determinants to Prevent Cardiovascular Disease

Targets for Intervention	Strategies for Intervention
Cardiovascular risk	Assess presence of psychosocial stressors and provide counseling for coping with life stress.
Dietary factors	Examine social and cultural influences on diet and body size perception. Address any barriers to adopting a heart-healthy diet, such as access to healthful food, and socioeconomic factors affecting people from groups that are vulnerable or disadvantaged, such as those living in inner-city or rural environments, and those of advanced age.
Exercise and physical activity	Assess neighborhood access to physical activity centers, gyms, fitness centers, etc.
Obesity and weight loss	Examine barriers to weight management, such as psychosocial stressors, poor sleep habits, and other individual barriers. Promote weight management in persons unable to achieve recommended weight loss.
Diabetes mellitus	In addition to managing Type 2 diabetes mellitus, assess environmental and psychosocial factors that may affect adherence to treatment and ability to maintain glycemic control, such as depression, stress, self-efficacy, and social support.
High blood pressure	Assess short sleep duration (fewer than 6 hours nightly) and poor quality of sleep as well as other lifestyle habits, such as high salt intake and lack of physical activity, that may affect blood pressure management.
Tobacco treatment	Provide individual and group social support as part of counseling efforts to help patients become quit using tobacco.

Source: Adapted from Arnett et al. (2019). ACC/AHA Guideline on the Primary Prevention of Cardiovascular Disease.

regularly and control these risk factors through diet and regular exercise and, if necessary medication. All of these factors involve modifiable behaviors that reflect lifestyle choices and managing our healthcare needs.

We have yet more evidence that adopting a healthier lifestyle can prevent CVD. People who exercise regularly, avoid smoking and excess use of alcohol, maintain a healthy weight, and follow a healthful diet have more positive health outcomes overall, such as lower rates of hypertension, diabetes, and heart disease (Reusch & Manson, 2017; U.S. Preventive Services Task Force, 2017; Whelton & Carey, 2017). The message that healthier lifestyles pay off seems to be getting across, as the number of deaths from CVD has been declining over the past 50 years (Schwenk, 2017).

The challenge to health psychologists and other health professionals is to translate knowledge of health behavior into action. In far too many cases, modifiable risk factors, such as hypertension, remain poorly controlled. Obesity has become epidemic. Despite great progress in reducing smoking, more than one out of ten American adults still smoke. It's never too early to start thinking about cardiovascular health. Evidence links hypertension in young adults to a greater risk of CVD in later life (Vasan, 2018; Yano et al., 2018). Taking steps to reduce risk factors today can yield major payoffs in later years.

Applying Health Psychology

Becoming Heart Healthy

Unhealthful patterns of behavior linked to risk of CVD include heavy drinking, smoking, inactivity, overeating, and consuming a diet rich in saturated fat and cholesterol (Eckel et al., 2013; James et al., 2014; Yang et al., 2019). What changes can we make in our daily lives to adopt a heart-healthy lifestyle? The following are few suggestions.

Shed Extra Pounds

Obesity is a major risk factor for CHD and is associated with a greater likelihood of other risk factors, such as high LDL cholesterol levels and diabetes. As we discussed in Chapter 7, there are many causal factors in obesity, including genetics, metabolic factors, and dietary patterns. Whatever combination of factors may be involved, we can learn to manage our weight more effectively by adopting healthier dietary and exercise habits, such as by choosing healthier foods and substituting lower-calorie foods in place of high-calorie foods. For suggestions for reducing excess weight or body fat, see Chapter 7.

Limit or Avoid Alcohol

Evidence links higher levels of alcohol use to greater risk of CVD (and other health problems). An important component of a comprehensive cardiac care program is to help people curb excess alcohol intake. This may involve working with professional alcohol or drug or alcohol counselors or self-help groups to change problem drinking habits.

Avoid Smoking

Smoking alone more than doubles the risk of heart attacks and is linked to more than 1 in 5 deaths from heart disease. For current smokers, quitting smoking yields significant health benefits, including reduced risk of CVD. Even heavy smokers people who are heavy smokers can significantly reduce their risk of CVD within 5 years of quitting, although they still have an elevated risk relative to nonsmokers (Duncan et al., 2019). If you don't smoke, don't start. And if you do smoke, quit as soon as possible. (See Chapter 9 for a discussion of smoking cessation strategies.)

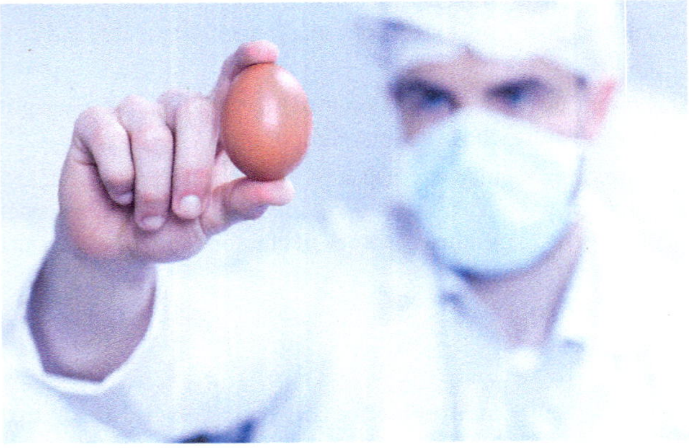

Wavebreak Media ltd/Alamy Stock Photo

To Eat or Not to Eat? It's just an egg! (Gulp.) Dare you eat it? Actually, research evidence suggests that it's safe to eat an egg a day, even for people with a history of cardiovascular disease. Of course, you can also choose to stick to egg whites, which are cholesterol-free.

Mind What You Eat

Health researchers estimate that nearly half of all deaths due to cardiovascular diseases and diabetes can be attributed to a set of dietary factors, including consumption of high levels of processed meats, high sodium intake, low levels of vegetable and fruit intake, and high levels of sugar-sweetened beverages (Micha et al., 2017).

The theory of planned behavior helps us better understand the factors that lead to healthful behavior changes, such as intentions to act and high levels of self-efficacy for carrying out one's plans. One of the challenges health psychologists and other helping professionals face in working with people with CVD is to assist them in developing healthier dietary habits. Recently investigators found that social support is an important intervening factor between intention to act and carrying through with planned actions. First they found, as the theory predicts, that self-efficacy (belief in one's ability to adopt a healthful diet) and outcome expectations (expecting that adopting a healthful diet will reap health benefits) jointly predicted intentions to act (Teleki et al., 2019). But second, the investigators also found that social support

TABLE 12.7 Making Healthier Food Choices to Reduce Blood Cholesterol

Your dietary choices are important determinants of blood cholesterol. These suggestions will help you make healthier, LDL-lowering choices that will also help you manage your weight. As a triple benefit, they are also consistent with dietary guidelines for reducing risks of cancer and other chronic diseases.

What to Buy More Often	What to Buy Less Often	How to Prepare Food	What to Snack On	What Not to Snack On
Lean cuts of meat, poultry, fish	Fatty cuts of meat, breaded poultry or fish	Trim the fat from meat before cooking.	Air-popped popcorn (no butter!); pretzels	Popcorn with butter
Skim or 1% milk	Whole milk, cream	Bake or broil meat. Do not fry.	Hard candy, jelly beans	Chocolate bars or other chocolate treats
Low-fat cottage cheese, low-fat yogurt	Cheese spreads and cheese (e.g., cheddar, American, Swiss)	Cook meat on a rack so the fat will drip off.	Bagels, raisin toast, or English muffins with margarine or jelly	Doughnuts, Danish pastry
Part-skim mild cheese (like part-skim mozzarella)	Lard, butter, fatback, salt pork, shortening	Use fat or oil sparingly.	Low-fat cookies	Cake, cookies, brownies
Vegetable oils low in saturated fats, squeezable margarine	Toppings (e.g., butter, cheese sauces, gravy, sour cream)	Take the skin off chicken and turkey.	Fruits, vegetables	Milkshakes, eggnogs, floats
Baking potatoes, rice, pasta	Vegetables in cream or cheese sauces	Pack fruits and low-fat cookies as ready-to-eat snacks.	Fruit juices and drinks	Ice cream (except low-fat ice cream or frozen desserts)
Plain fresh, frozen, or canned vegetables and fruit (without syrup)	French fries or hash browns		Frozen yogurt, sherbet, popsicles	
English muffins, bagels, breads, tortillas, pita; cold and hot cereals	Doughnuts, Danish pastry, desserts (e.g., cakes, cookies, and pies)			

Source: Adapted from National Heart Lung and Blood Institute, National Institutes of Health. (2011). National Cholesterol Education Program. http://www.nhlbi.nih.gov/about/ncep/index.htm

was an important intervening (mediating) factor in converting intentions into healthy actions. Having support from others may play a critical role in determining success in changing health behaviors.

Enlisting help from family members in making changes in family food purchases and meal planning may be a key factor in adopting a healthier diet. What we eat is largely determined by food choices we make in the market. Moreover, helping others make healthier choices may have a ripple effect in the family, leading other family members to adopt healthier eating habits.

Healthful eating starts with what you bring home from the grocery store, how you prepare food, and what you ultimately put into your mouth. It starts with buying healthier foods by comparing foods labels and avoiding unhealthful choices. Table 12.7 contrasts some heart-healthy food choices with less desirable choices. When you shop for groceries, arm yourself with a list of healthier food choices and stick to your list. Avoid walking down aisles containing rows of sugary snacks, processed foods, and other high-calorie, high-fat foods. There's any old adage that bears repeating: Out of sight is out of mind. If you don't bring it home from the store, you can't eat it.

Table 12.7 offers some tips on cutting cholesterol by making healthier food choices. By the way, the long-standing controversy about whether eggs are unhealthy (they are high in dietary cholesterol) may have been settled. In research reported in 2020, researchers found that moderate egg consumption, about 1 egg per day, is not associated with increased risk of CVD, even in people with a history of CVD (Dehghan et al., 2020). Also, the cholesterol in eggs is found in the yolk, so if you are concerned about limiting dietary cholesterol, eat egg whites. There are also cholesterol-free egg substitutes that are made from egg whites.

Manage Stress

Persistent stress is linked to increased blood pressure and may have more direct effects on the heart, so it makes sense to take stock of the sources of stress in our lives. Some stress may be unavoidable, such as dealing with traffic to get to work, balancing budgets or stretching paychecks, but other sources of stress can be more directly controlled, such as taking on more projects than we can handle or setting unrealistic deadlines. In Chapter 5 we reviewed cognitive behavioral methods for coping with stress. Even when faced with stress we can't avoid, we can learn emotion-focused coping skills to manage stress more effectively, such as listening to podcasts or comedy shows to manage the wait time while stuck in traffic rather than just stewing behind the wheel.

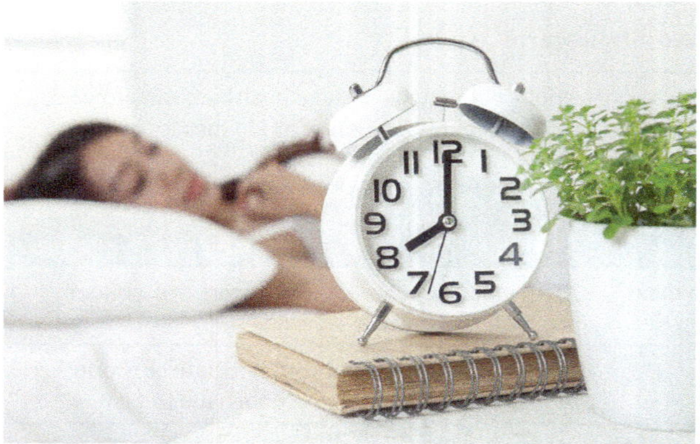

IMAGEMORE Co, Ltd./Getty Images

Uh Oh, What Will Happen to Her Cardiovascular System When That Alarm Goes Off? Why not select a pleasant-sounding alarm on your phone? One that will awaken you, but with less stress in the process?

Other sources of stress linked to cardiovascular risk may require professional assistance, such as couple or marital counseling for couples in distressed relationships. Researchers found that for women with established heart disease, marital stress tripled the risk of recurrent cardiac events, including heart and deaths due to CHD (Orth-Gomér et al., 2000).

Relaxation training and meditation can be a helpful antidote to stress and may even reduce high blood pressure. Investigators recently tested mindfulness meditation for people with high blood pressure and found that mindfulness significantly reduced blood pressure as well as perceived stress (Loucks et al., 2019).

Type A behavior can add stress to already stressful lives. Too often we jump out of bed to an abrasive alarm, hop into a shower, fight commuter crowds, and arrive at class or work with no time to spare. Then we become involved in our hectic day. For Type A people, the day begins urgently and never lets up. Following are some suggestions for combating time urgency:

1. Wake up to a pleasant alarm. Stretch.
2. Spend time socializing with friends and family.
3. Engage in enjoyable leisure and cultural activities. Read. Visit museums.
4. Enjoy snacks or relax at school or work before the day begins.
5. Slow down. Don't speed. Don't interrupt. Take the scenic route. Walk around the neighborhood, but leave the smartphone at home.
6. Don't multitask. Space chores. Why have the car repaired, shop, and drive a friend to the airport on the same day?
7. If rushed, postpone unessential work or chores to the next day.

Curb Hostility and Anger

Hostile people who anger easily and often are at greater risk of developing CHD. Occasional episodes of anger may not damage the cardiovascular system, but persistent or chronic hostility and proneness to anger may put your health and life at risk. Learning to calm down in provocative situations doesn't mean squelching your anger, as bottling up your feelings may also put stress on your cardiovascular system. It means channeling anger into healthy forms of assertive behavior.

Keep Blood Cholesterol Under Control

A prime goal in heart-healthy living is reducing LDL and boosting HDL. Making healthier dietary choices can help reduce LDL, and statin medications can help further when changes in diet aren't sufficient to reach desirable levels. Statins may also increase HDL, but another way within our direct control to give HDL a boost is through regular vigorous exercise.

Get Moving

Physical activity is associated with a range of health benefits, including a lower risk of death due to CVD, slowing the progression of established CVD, and reducing the risk of hypertension (USDHHS, 2018). Physically active adults have lower rates of heart disease and stroke and have lower blood pressure, better blood cholesterol profiles, and better physical fitness.

Evidence points to a dose-response relationship between physical activity levels and risk of CHD, meaning that higher levels of physical activity yield greater benefits (Arnett et al., 2019). Evidence shows that emphasizing the importance of exercise in primary healthcare settings translates into increased rates of physical activity among people (Jain & Davis, 2019). Also, better-educated people are more likely to modify unhealthy behavior patterns and reap the benefits of change. Is there a message here for you?

Review 12.4

INTERACTIVE SELF-SCORING QUIZZES

Sentence Completion

1. Health researchers estimate that __________ million lives could be saved worldwide if three key health objectives were achieved.

2. The two major categories of health risks accounting for 65% of CVD cases and deaths in a large multinational study were metabolic risk factors and __________ risk factors.

3. The number of deaths due to CVD has (increased or decreased) over the past 50 years.

4. The prevention of CVD is best achieved by both medical interventions and __________ change strategies.

5. Blood pressure targets for people in need of medication should be <__________ /80 mm Hg.

Think About It

Are you living a heart-healthy lifestyle? If not, what changes can you make to protect your heart and cardiovascular system?

Recite: An Active Summary

INTERACTIVE SELF-SCORING QUIZZES

Chapter 12 Practice Quiz

1. Describe the major parts of the circulatory system.

The circulatory system is the body's network of blood vessels, carrying oxygen, nutrients, and hormones to cells throughout the body, carrying away their waste products, and transporting disease-fighting white blood cells and antibodies to protect and defend the body against infectious organisms and rid the body of defective or cancerous cells. Blood consists of several components: erythrocytes, or red blood cells, that carry oxygen; leukocytes, or white blood cells, that fight disease-causing organisms; and platelets, or small cell fragments, needed for forming clots to plug holes in blood vessels due to injury. Three types of blood vessels make up the circulatory system: arteries, which carry blood to smaller blood vessels, called capillaries, and veins that carry blood back to the heart.

2. Describe the underlying disease process in coronary heart disease and stroke.

The major cause of coronary heart disease and stroke is atherosclerosis, the narrowing of arteries serving the heart and brain due to a buildup of fatty deposits or plaque along artery walls. When a blood clot blocks the flow of blood in these narrowed arteries, a heart attack or stroke may occur.

3. Identify risk factors for cardiovascular disease that you cannot control.

Some factors involved in CVD are beyond our direct control, including genetics or family history, age, and gender. But regardless of our individual risk profile, we can all take steps to reduce our personal risk by making healthy changes in behavior.

4. Identify risk factors you can control.

Many of the risk factors involve modifiable behaviors you can control, such as high blood levels of LDL and triglycerides, low blood levels of HDL, smoking, hypertension, obesity, alcohol use, inactivity, unhealthful diet, and hypertension. Some of these factors can be controlled by going for regular medical checkups and taking medication, while others can be controlled through lifestyle changes, such as losing weight, avoiding smoking and alcohol use, eating a healthful diet, and exercising regularly.

5. Describe how psychological factors are related to risk of heart disease.

Evidence links the personality factor of hostility to increased risk of heart disease. Negative emotions, such as anxiety and depression, also increase risk potential, while holding optimistic attitudes is tied to better cardiovascular and immune system health and lower mortality rates.

6. Describe ways of becoming heart healthy.

Leading a heart-healthy lifestyle involves adopting healthier behaviors, such as limiting or avoiding alcohol use, avoiding smoking, maintaining a healthy weight, following a healthy diet, managing stress and curbing anger, controlling hostility, exercising regularly, and controlling hypertension and blood cholesterol through regular medical treatment.

Answers to Review Sections

12.1

1. circulatory
2. stroke
3. four
4. aorta
5. Platelets

12.2

1. 2/3
2. atherosclerosis
3. heart attack
4. more gradually
5. less likely
6. C-reactive
7. Arrhythmias; tachycardia; bradycardia
8. ischemic

12.3

1. bad
2. triglycerides
3. good
4. 5
5. can
6. carbon
7. waist (or midsection)
8. Metabolic
9. sitting
10. 120
11. higher
12. hostility
13. epinephrine
14. better

12.4

1. 94
2. behavioral
3. decreased
4. behavior
5. 130

Scoring Key for Heart Smart Self-Assessment

1. False
2. True
3. False
4. False
5. False
6. False
7. False
8. False
9. False
10. False (HDL is actually good for your heart.)

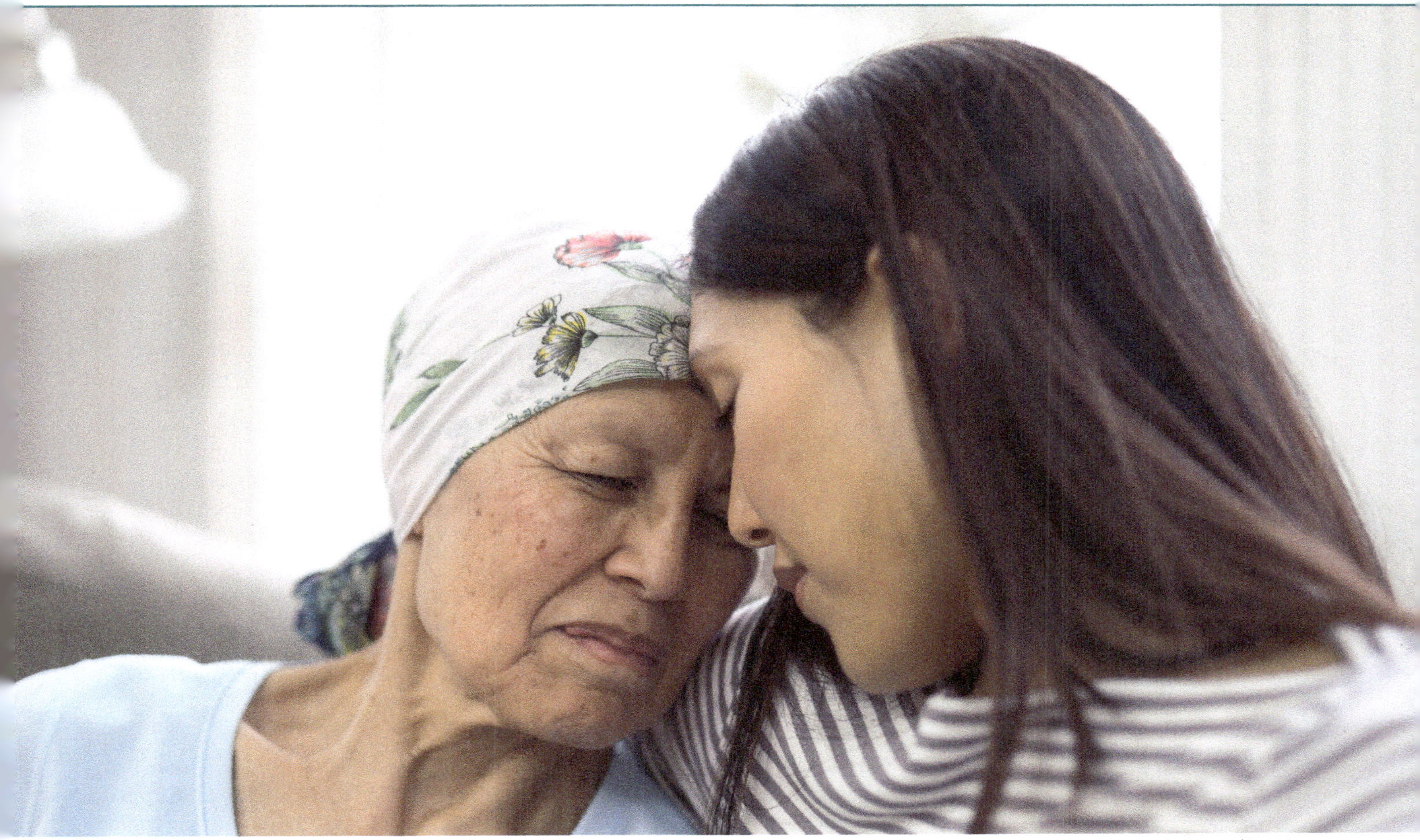

FatCamera/Getty Images

Cancer

LEARNING OBJECTIVES

After studying this chapter, you will be able to ...

1. **Define** cancer, and **explain** why we can think of *cancers* rather than a single disease called *cancer*.
2. **Identify** who is prone to developing cancer, focusing on gender and racial/ethnic disparities.
3. **Identify** 5-year survival rates for various kinds of cancer.
4. **Identify** the behavioral risk facts for cancer.
5. **Describe** psychological factors in living with cancer, focusing on the roles of health psychologists.

Did You Know That ...

- Cancer is not one disease but many?
- Cancer of the lung and bronchus takes the lives of more women than breast cancer?
- African American men are the racial/ethnic group most likely to develop and die from prostate cancer, and African American women are the racial/ethnic group most likely to die from breast cancer?
- Nearly 70% of people who receive a cancer diagnosis survive for at least 5 years?
- Tomatoes contain a plant chemical that may reduce the risks of certain types of cancer?
- Some viruses cause cancer?
- Smoking causes 1 in 3 cancer deaths?
- Some forms of cancer are curable?
- Many people who develop cancer are plagued by feelings of anxiety and depression?
- Some of the challenges of health psychologists include motivating people to adhere to screenings and treatment of cancer?

My gynecologist took on a somewhat professional attitude that felt different from her usual chumminess. She said that she and her partners had looked at the results of my test and that they saw cells that were consistent with endometrial cancer. She started talking about peripheral things, and after a while I got the courage to ask her directly: "Are you saying that I have endometrial cancer?" She took half a second that seemed like forever and then said "Yes."

—Shanice

My husband and I were at a meeting with everyone present: the oncologist, the neurologist, the rehab team, even a social worker. We understood what was going on but it didn't seem as if it could be real. There was an elephant in the room. After a while, the oncologist said, "I wish I could give you good news, but I can't." With it out in the open, my husband seemed to relax. He was always a take-charge kind of person and said, "Okay, what do we do next?"

—Sue

The very word elicits fear and dread—*cancer*. The fear is understandable. Each year more than 1.7 million Americans receive a diagnosis of cancer, and more than 600,000 people die from it, with about 1 death every minute (CDC, 2023j). More than 1 out of every 5 deaths in the United States is caused by cancer. **Figure 13.1** shows that cancer is the second leading cause of death in the United States. Cancer also takes a significant toll on mental health, as studies show that cancer patients face a higher risk of anxiety, depression, and even suicide (Deshields et al., 2022; Wapner, 2022).

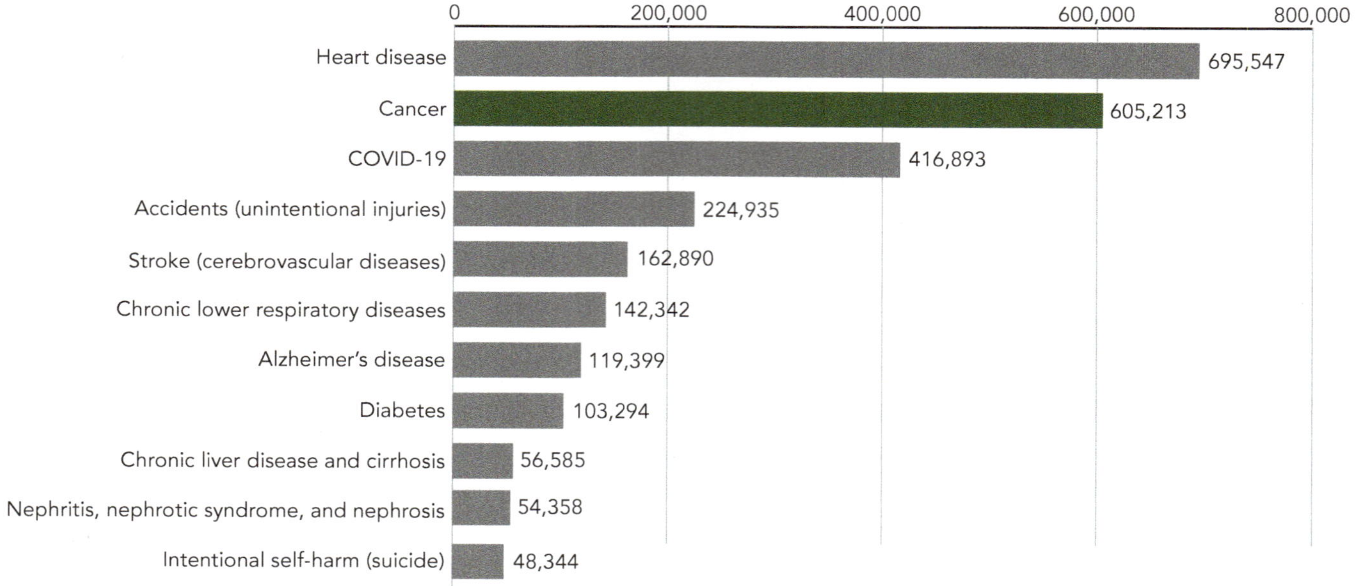

FIGURE 13.1 Leading Causes of Death in the United States Cancer is the second leading cause of death in the United States.

Source: Centers for Disease Control and Prevention (CDC) (2023p). Leading causes of death. https://www.cdc.gov/nchs/fastats/leading-causes-of-death.htm / Public Domain.

Yet we have good news to share as well, as cancer deaths in the United States have been on a steady decline for the past 30 years or so, resulting in all likelihood from reductions in smoking, increased cancer screenings (e.g., regular mammograms, Pap tests, and colonoscopies), and greater access to treatment at earlier stages of the disease and treatment at earlier stages of the disease (CDC, 2023j; U.S. Cancer Death Rates, 2023).

What Is Cancer?

Cancer is not one disease but many. Cancer is a group of more than 100 distinct diseases characterized by uncontrolled cell growth and spread of abnormal body cells (Stanton et al., 2019). Normally the body manufactures cells only when they are needed, replicating in an orderly fashion in a process directed by genes housed on chromosomes in the cell's nucleus. But in cancer, cells lose the ability to regulate their growth, multiplying even when they are not needed and forming growths of excess bodily tissue called **tumors**.

Tumors can be either benign (noncancerous) or malignant (cancerous). Cancerous tumors may *metastasize*—that is, spread by establishing colonies elsewhere in the body. Cancerous growths can form anywhere in the body—in the blood, bones, digestive tract, lungs, genital organs, and so on. Although the immune system destroys cancerous cells, a developing cancer may overwhelm the ability of the body to combat it. Malignant tumors invade and destroy surrounding tissue, damaging organs and bodily systems, which can lead to death.

There are many causes of cancer, including genetic factors, exposure to cancer-causing chemicals and certain viruses, and use of harmful substances, especially tobacco (Fruman et al., 2018). As with many other disorders, people can inherit a disposition toward developing certain types of cancer, such as breast cancer, prostate cancer, and colorectal cancer (cancer of the colon or rectum).

Cancer is primarily a genetic disease (Toker, 2019). It develops when changes occur in cellular **DNA** (deoxyribonucleic acid), the genetic material that makes up the chromosomes

cancer A group of more than 100 diseases characterized by development of malignant tumors, which may spread to other parts of the body.

tumors Abnormal growths of bodily tissue that may or may not be cancerous (malignant).

DNA Abbreviation of deoxyribonucleic acid, the basic chemical material in chromosomes that carries the individual's genetic code.

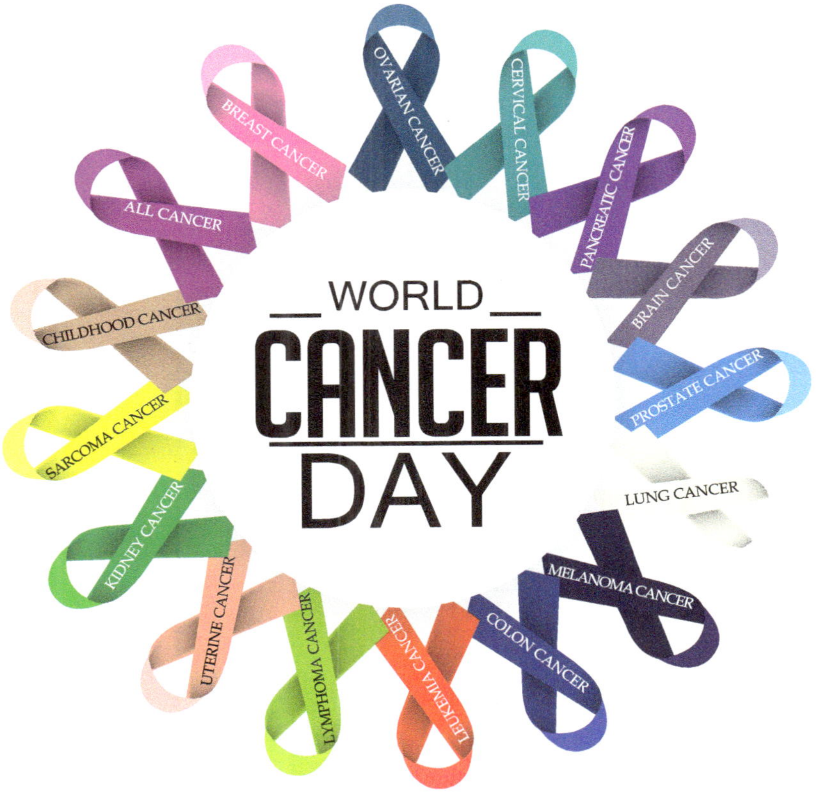

suns design/Shutterstock.com

The different-colored ribbons emphasize that "cancer" is actually a number of diseases.

and carries the genetic information encoded in genes. These changes result from mutations that cause the cell to begin dividing indefinitely. Mutations may arise from internal causes, such as genetic coding or immune system conditions, or from external causes, such as exposure to cancer-causing agents (*carcinogens*), including certain viruses, chemical compounds in tobacco, and ultraviolet (UV) radiation from the sun.

oncogenes Mutated genes that cause cancerous growths.

Oncogenes are cancer-causing genes that are mutated forms of normal genes that control cell replication and specialization (differentiation). Oncogenes remove the brakes from cell division, allowing cells to multiply wildly. In effect, oncogenes cause runaway cell replication. Scientists have identified more than 100 oncogenes and are working on ways to stop or inhibit them.

Who Develops Cancer?

The short answer is that cancer can affect anyone at any age; however, about three-quarters of cases of cancers develop in people aged 55 and older. Only about 1 in 10 cases occurs in people under 45 years of age. Nearly 40% of Americans develop cancer during their lifetime (NCI, 2020a). **Table 13.1** shows the relative lifetime risks for different types of cancers. **Figure 13.2** shows the leading cancer sites in men and women.

TABLE 13.1 Lifetime Risk of Developing and Dying from Cancer

Site	Men Developing/Dying From	Women Developing/ Dying From
All sites	1 in 2/1 in 5	1 in 3/1 in 5
Bladder	1 in 26/1 in 106	1 in 85/1 in 286
Brain	1 in 145/1 in 189	1 in 182/1 in 238
Breast	1 in 769/1 in 3,333	1 in 8/1 in 39
Cervix	---	1 in 159/1 in 455
Colon and rectum	1 in 23/1 in 55	1 in 25/1 in 60
Esophagus	1 in 125/1 in 132	1 in 417/1 in 500
Hodgkin's disease	1 in 417/1 in 2,500	1 in 500/1 in 3,333
Kidney and renal pelvis	1 in 46/1 in 167	1 in 81/1 in 303
Larynx	1 in 189/1 in 526	1 in 769/1 in 2,000
Leukemia	1 in 54/1 in 104	1 in 78/1 in 147
Liver and bile duct	1 in 69/1 in 98	1 in 161/1 in 185
Lung and bronchus	1 in 15/1 in 18	1 in 17/1 in 22
Melanoma of the skin	1 in 36/1 in 256	1 in 56/1 in 526
Multiple myeloma	1 in 108/1 in 213	1 in 141/1 in 263
Non-Hodgkin's lymphoma	1 in 41/1 in 123	1 in 52/1 in 156
Oral cavity and pharynx	1 in 60/1 in 238	1 in 141/1 in 526
Ovary	---	1 in 80/1 in 114
Pancreas	1 in 60/1 in 72	1 in 63/1 in 74
Prostate	1 in 9/1 in 41	---
Stomach	1 in 93/1 in 222	1 in 152/1 in 333
Testicles	1 in 250/1 in 5,000	---
Thyroid	1 in 143/1 in 1,667	1 in 52/1 in 1,429
Uterus	---	1 in 33/1 in 159

Source: Adapted from American Cancer Society (2020c). Lifetime risk of developing or dying from cancer. https://www.cancer.org/cancer/cancer-basics/lifetime-probability-of-developing-or-dying-from-cancer.html
Note: These numbers are average risks for the overall U.S. population. Your risk may be higher or lower than these numbers, depending on your particular risk factors.

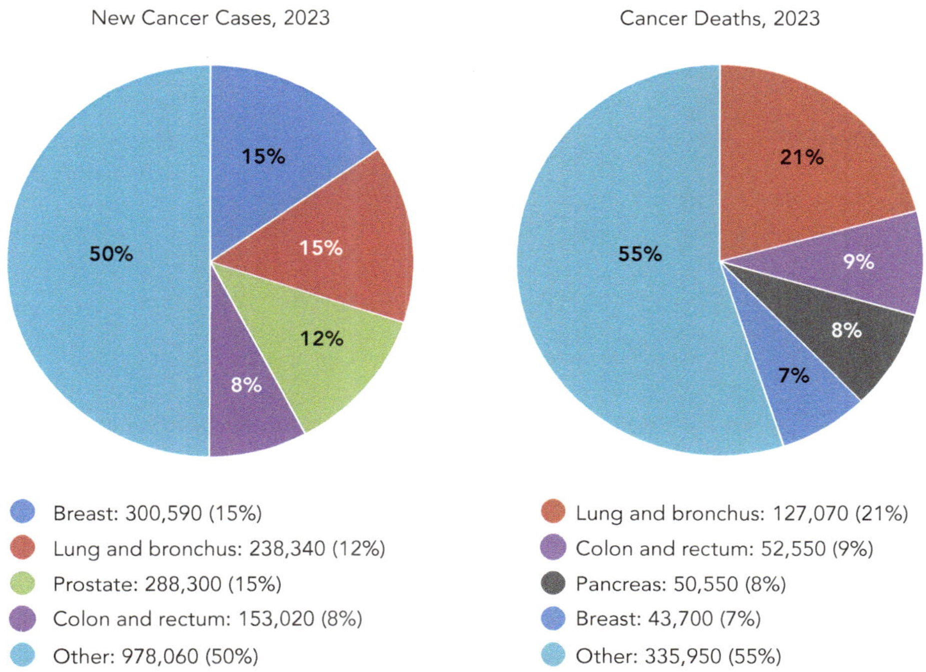

FIGURE 13.2 **Top Sites of Estimated New Cases of Cancer in Men and Women and Cancer Deaths**
Source: National Cancer Institute (NCI) (2023). Cancer stat facts: Common cancer sites. https://seer.cancer.gov/statfacts/html/common.html / Public Domain.

Racial and Ethnic Disparities in Cancer

Cancer rates and death rates from cancer vary widely across racial and ethnic groups in the United States (see **Figures 13.3** and **13.4**). The highest rates of new cases of cancer shown in Figure 13.3 are found among (non-Hispanic) Black Americans and (non-Hispanic) White Americans, although American Indian/Alaska Natives also have high rates of developing breast cancer and prostate cancer. The peak in the graph represents the fact that Black men are nearly twice as likely as White men to develop prostate cancer.

Cancer is not an equal opportunity destroyer. The death rates by race and ethnicity do not match the rates for developing cancer. As shown in Figure 13.4, death rates for all groups are highest for lung and bronchus cancer, followed, for most groups, by prostate cancer and breast cancer. For most types of cancer, (non-Hispanic) Black Americans have the highest mortality (death) rate and lowest survival rate of any racial/ethnic group in the United States (Mitchell et al., 2022). The

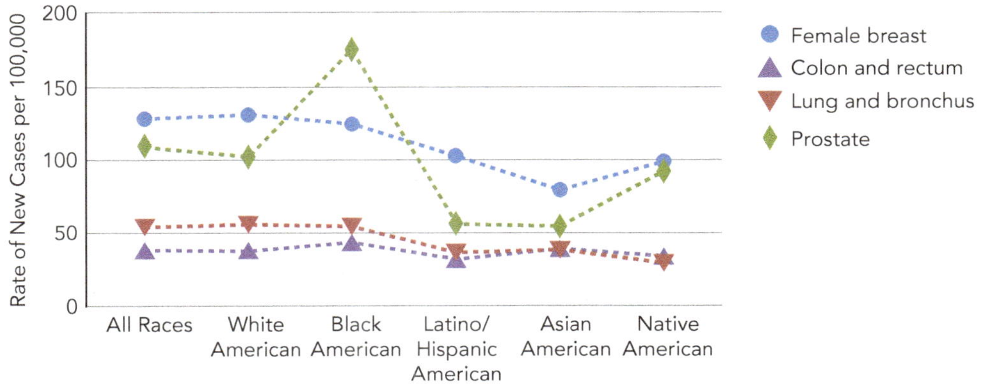

FIGURE 13.3 **Rates of New Cases of Common Kinds of Cancer by Race/Ethnicity**
Source: Adapted from National Cancer Institute (2023). Cancer stat facts: Cancer disparities. https://seer.cancer.gov/statfacts/html/disparities.html

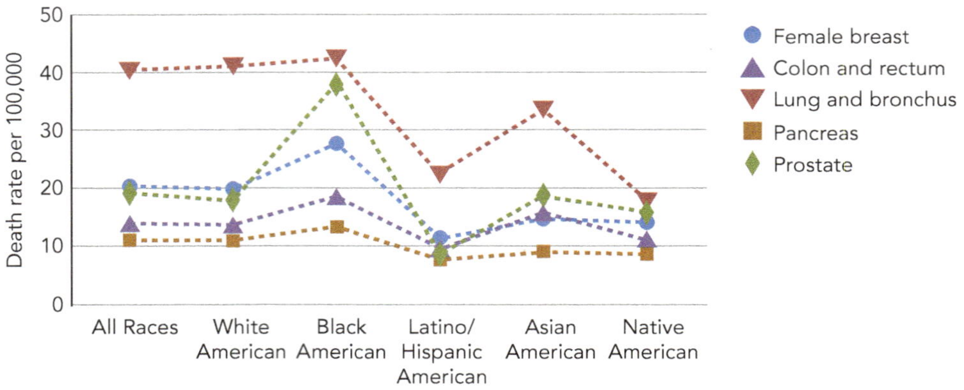

FIGURE 13.4 Mortality Rates of Common Kinds of Cancer by Race/Ethnicity
Source: Adapted from National Cancer Institute (2023). Cancer stat facts: Cancer disparities. https://seer.cancer.gov/statfacts/html/disparities.html

highest mortality rates are among Black men, who have a 19% higher rate of dying from cancer than White men (Islami et al., 2022). The death rate from cancer for Black women is 12% higher than White women, even though Black women have an 8% lower rate of cancer overall.

Let's look at disparities for different types of cancer. As you can see in Figure 13.4, Black men are significantly more likely to die of prostate cancer than all other groups. Black women are significantly more likely to die of breast cancer than all other groups. Black women also have significantly higher death rates and incident rates of cervical cancer than White women (Mitchell et al., 2022). For these reasons, Black men and women are advised to begin screening for these kinds of cancer at younger ages than members of other racial/ethnic groups.

Why are Black Americans more likely to die from cancer than any other population groups in this country? The reasons are complex, involving an array of factors. Black Americans are disproportionally represented in poorer communities, and people from economically distressed communities have higher cancer death rates than those from more affluent areas, in part because people from poorer areas tend to have more risk factors (physical inactivity, smoking, poor diet) and also because they often lack access to early detection (screening) programs and treatment services. Another factor is that poorer neighborhoods tend to have greater exposure to environmental factors that expose people to unhealthy contaminants, such as air pollution and water pollution (Mitchell et al., 2022).

Another factor in the mix is comorbidity—Black Americans are significantly more likely than White Americans to have diabetes, and adults with diabetes are approximately 30% more likely to die of cancer than people without diabetes (Harding et al., 2020). In addition, low-income communities with large minoritized populations can be described as "food deserts"—areas with limited access to healthy food choices, places with high concentrations of fast-food restaurants rather than supermarkets stocked with fresh produce and healthier food selections. We now have direct evidence showing that cancer survival is worse among people living in these food deserts (Fong et al., 2021).

Finally, another important factor is that differences in cancer care tend to favor White patients. A study of patients with gastrointestinal cancer showed that Black patients were more likely to be undertreated as compared to White patients (Bliton et al., 2021). Moreover, Black cancer patients have disproportionately low surgical rates for various forms of cancer, which may contribute to their lower survival rates as compared to White cancer patients.

There also appear to be genetic differences between (non-Hispanic) White Americans and Black Americans that play roles in developing and dying from cancer. Studies of DNA find that some—not all—Black American men may have alterations in genes that contribute to early-onset highly aggressive cases of prostate cancer (Ramakrishnan et al., 2018). Genetic factors may also be implicated in disparities in the development of lung cancer—White men in the United States smoke 30–40% more cigarettes than Black men, but Black men are approximately 34% more likely to develop lung cancer (Hall, 2020). Genetic factors also play roles in disparities in breast cancer in the United States (Murphy et al., 2017). As shown in Figure 13.3, White women are somewhat more likely than Black women to develop breast cancer, but as shown in Figure 13.4, Black women are more likely than any other U.S. racial or ethnic group to die from breast cancer. Breast cancer tends to be more aggressive in Black women in the United States (Saini et al., 2019). For genetic reasons, the onset of breast cancer also tends to be earlier in Black women (Bertrand et al., 2017).

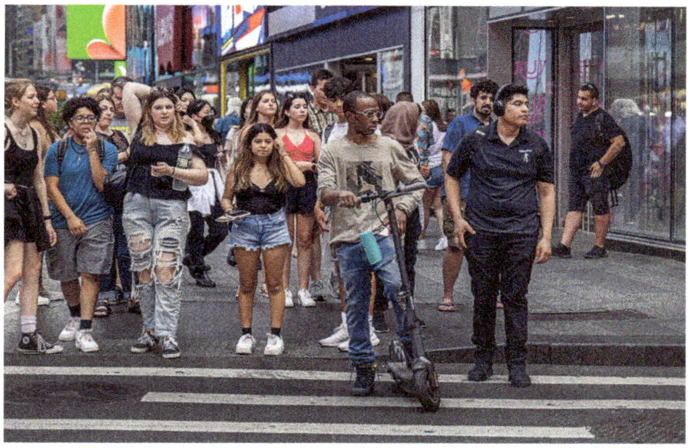

carstenbrandt/Getty Images

Is Your Neighborhood Toxic to Your Health? How might the neighborhood in which you live affect your chances of dying from cancer?

As we noted, the neighborhoods in which people live also make an important difference. Investigators find that mortality (death) rates from cancer are similar between (non-Hispanic) Black American and (non-Hispanic) White American women living in predominantly Black or African American neighborhoods. This finding points to the importance of neighborhood characteristics, such as poorer access to mammography and follow-up care in some neighborhoods (Smith & Madak-Erdogan, 2018). Other researchers note that adverse neighborhood conditions increase stress and inflammation (Saini et al., 2019). Stress and inflammation, in turn, heighten genetic vulnerability to the development of breast cancer (Saini et al., 2019).

Yet another important factor underlying higher cancer death rates among (non-Hispanic) Black Americans is that cancer is often detected at later and less treatable stages. Consider the experience of 59-year-old Cheryl King, a Black woman living on the South Side of Chicago, a predominantly African American area. King found a lump in her breast and consulted a healthcare professional in a local facility, who dismissed her concerns, saying that many Black women have lumps in their breasts. But King was not deterred, although it took her 3 months to get another medical appointment, at which time a diagnosis of breast cancer was confirmed. Unfortunately, by that time the lump had grown into a stage 2 tumor. King told a newspaper reporter, "I feel like if I lived on the [predominantly White American North Side and] I would have gone in for a diagnosis, I think they would have taken my concerns more seriously" (cited in Rockett, 2018).

Even after cancer is detected, there are racial disparities. An analysis by Hoppe et al. (2019) of more than half a million breast cancer patients whose cancer was detected at an early stage found that Black women experienced longer times than White women to:

- first treatment (36 days vs. 28 days),
- surgery (37 days vs. 29 days),
- chemotherapy (88 days vs. 75 days)
- radiation treatment (131 days vs. 99 days), and
- endocrine (hormonal) therapy (152 days vs. 127 days).

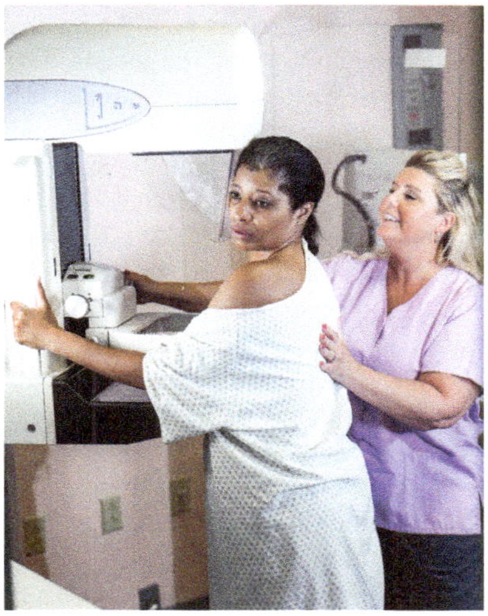

kali9/Getty Images

Screening for Breast Cancer by Mammography There are many reasons that Black American women are more likely to die from breast cancer than other racial/ethnic groups. Genetic factors may make Black women more susceptible to early-onset, highly aggressive forms of breast cancer. Another reason is that Black women are less likely than White women to be screened regularly for the development of tumors.

Racial and ethnic minority groups may also be underusers of healthcare services, including cancer care. For example, Latinos/Hispanics visit physicians less often than do (non-Hispanic) Black and Whites because of lack of health insurance, difficulty speaking English, misgivings about medical technology, and—for people who are in the country without documentation—concerns about deportation.

We also need to consider the role of acculturation among immigrants to better understand the adjustment of people who survive cancer. For example, a recent study of Chinese American and White American women who survived breast cancer showed a somewhat unexpected finding (Wang et al., 2019). As expected, poorly acculturated Chinese American women experienced higher levels of life stress than White American women did. But surprisingly, those same Chinese American women also showed better emotional adjustment—less anxiety and depression—than White American women did. Based on this pattern of results, the investigators speculate that adherence to traditional Chinese culture may have helped build resilience in coping with psychosocial stress.

So we've seen that marked disparities between ethnic and racial groups continue to exist in cancer outcomes in the United States. Addressing these disparities will require society marshaling its public health efforts to improve cancer screening, enhance treatment options, and tackling risk factors that increase the cancer burden and death rates in minoritized communities at the neighborhood level (e.g., improving food quality and reducing air and water pollution) and the individual level (e.g., reducing unhealthy behaviors such as smoking, poor diet, and physical inactivity).

Surviving Cancer

A century ago, few people survived cancer. Today, the chance of surviving cancer for at least 5 years after diagnosis is nearly 70% (Cherry et al., 2019; NCI, 2019a, 2019b). More than 15 million people in the United States have survived cancer (Stanton et al., 2019). Despite progress in fighting cancer, important challenges remain. We have made only limited progress in surviving certain forms of cancer, such as lung cancer, pancreatic cancer, and liver cancer (see Table 13.2). These cancers have poor survival rates even when they are diagnosed when the cancer is localized, before it has spread to other parts of the body.

Health Psychology in Action

Body Image After Mastectomy—Enter Tattoos

Women who undergo mastectomy for breast cancer lose more than their breasts. They also undergo a profound assault on their body images (Esplen et al., 2020; Hungr & Bober, 2020). One study interviewed 20 women in a traditional society who had undergone mastectomy and did not have reconstructive surgery (Koçan & Gürsoy, 2016). They found that most interviewees equated their breasts with femininity, beauty, and motherhood. They felt that they were missing "half of themselves." They chose clothing that hid the loss of the breasts and said that their relationships with their partners had changed. When women who choose not to have breast reconstruction surgery are experiencing adjustment problems, researchers have found that they tend to profit from education concerning the socialization messages internalized by women in Western society, how their body images and self-worth are caught up in these messages, and how they can boost their self-esteem by challenging them (Espen et al., 2020).

Results were somewhat different for a study of younger women aged 29–53 in a Western society (Grogran & Mechan, 2016). Responding to open-ended questions online, the women tended to report that aesthetics were much less important than survival. Impacts on their confidence about their postsurgical bodies varied. Some women rejected the dominant body shape ideals in the culture and wrote that they were proud of their scars. Authors of this study concluded that it was important for health psychologists to help women accept their changed bodies. Another study of younger women (30- and 40-year-old age group) found that some had rejected reconstruction because survival was their central concern (Holland et al., 2016). An Iranian study that included 71 women who had had mastectomies found that those women who accepted their changed appearances had a better body image than women who had poorer body images (Yamani Ardakani et al., 2020). The latter group spent more time attempting to fix their appearance. The researchers also reported that the support of their spouses helped women bear most of the complications and discomfort of the surgery and life thereafter.

Many women have breast reconstruction surgery, and it has been shown that who have the surgery generally report a better quality of life than those who do not (Archangelo et al., 2019; Zehra et al., 2020). Researchers surveyed 155 women considering postmastectomy breast reconstruction at Emory University Hospital (Duggal et al., 2013). Eighty-five of the women were Black (54.8%), and 64 were White (41.3%). The women generally agreed that their body image was the single most important motivating factor for breast reconstruction.

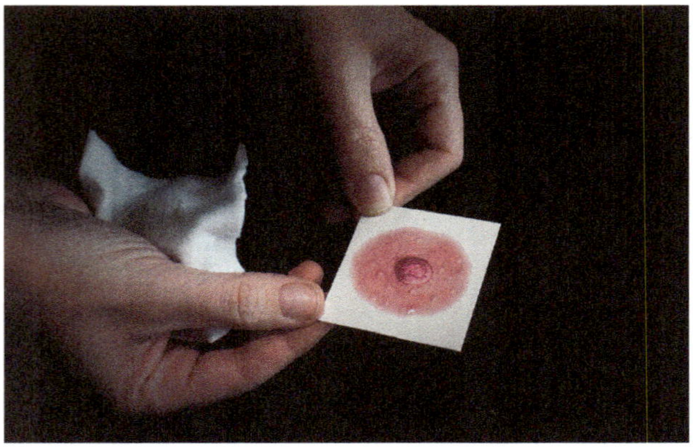

PHILIPPE LOPEZ/Getty Images

A Tattoo Made by Tattoo Artist Alexis Cassar Cassar is a former biologist who became a tattoo artist. She creates tattoos of nipples and areolas for women who have had mastectomies as a way of "giving back."

- 76% of the women desired to maintain a balanced appearance.
- 34% of the women said it was to continue to feel feminine.
- 7.7% said the purpose was to maintain sexual functioning.
- 51.6% said the surgery had been recommended by their referring physicians.

Enter tattoos. One of the challenges of breast reconstruction is the nipple. Surgery can be quite complex and additional corrective surgeries may be necessitated over the years (Jones & Erdmann, 2012). For this reason, efforts are made to spare the nipple during mastectomies, but it is not always possible to do so. Now tattoo artists as well as medical professionals are assisting women. A three-dimensional tattooing method is discussed in the journal *Plastic and Reconstructive Surgery* (Arouz et al., 2020). The height achieved by the tattoo is of value because the nipple protrudes from the areola.

TABLE 13.2 5-Year Survival Rates for Selected Sites (by Primary Cancer Sites)

Chance of 5-Year Survival	Selected Cancer Sites
Less than 10% chance	Pancreas
10–29% chance	Liver, esophagus, gallbladder, lung and bronchus
30–59% chance	Brain and nervous system, ovary, gum and oral cavity, floor of mouth, stomach, nose and middle ear, trachea and other respiratory organs, ovary, vagina, ureter, myeloma
60–89% chance	Leukemia (cancer of the blood and blood forming tissues of the body), tongue, salivary gland, small intestine, colon and rectum, anus and anal canal, larynx, bones and joints, soft tissue including heart, breast, bladder, kidney, cervix, uterus, lymphoma (cancer of the lymph system)
90% or better chance	Prostate, testis, thyroid, melanoma

Source: Adapted from SEER Cancer Statistics Review (2020). https://seer.cancer.gov/
Note: Percentages are rounded down to next nearest percent.

Review 13.1

INTERACTIVE SELF-SCORING QUIZZES

Sentence Completion

1. Approximately 1 out of every (2 or 5) deaths in the United States is caused by cancer.

2. Cancer is a group of more than __________ distinct diseases.

3. Tumors can be either benign (noncancerous) or __________ (cancerous).

4. Cancer is primarily a __________ disease.

5. __________ are cancer-causing genes that are mutated forms of normal genes.

6. About three-quarters of cases of cancers develop in people aged __________ years and older.

7. Nearly (20% or 40%) of Americans develop cancer during their lifetime.

8. Death (mortality) rates from cancer are highest among (Black or White) Americans.

9. The chances of surviving cancer for at least 5 years after diagnosis is nearly __________%.

Think About It

Almost all of us know people who have or have had cancer. Think of someone who had cancer. What type of cancer was it? Did the person survive?

Behavioral Risk Factors for Cancer

Like cardiovascular disease, certain risk factors for cancer cannot be controlled, such as age (risk of cancer increases with age) and family history (cancer tends to run in families because of shared genetic and home environments). We know that genes function abnormally in cancer. Genetic factors are involved in many forms of cancer, including some forms of colorectal cancer, skin cancer, prostate cancer, leukemia, ovarian cancer, and breast cancer (Gonzalez-Pons & Cruz-Correa, 2020; Marjaneh et al., 2020; Walsh et al., 2020). Our focus in this chapter is on risk factors we can control, especially modifiable behaviors.

The scientific study of the psychological, social, and behavioral aspects of cancer and its prevention and treatment is called *psycho-oncology, behavioral oncology*, or *psychosocial oncology* (Castelli et al., 2015; Piana, 2019). Health researchers believe we could prevent more than half of all cancers if people adopted a few healthier behaviors: avoiding smoking; adopting a sensible, low-fat diet; controlling excess body weight; limiting use of alcohol; exercising regularly; getting regular medical check-ups and vaccinations against human papilloma virus (HPV) and hepatitis B; and limiting their exposure to the sun (Brown et al., 2018; Colditz, Wolin, & Gehlert, 2012; Mayo Clinic, 2022). Hundreds of thousands of lives could be saved each year if all of us practiced these cancer-preventive behaviors.

An important step in saving lives is identifying cancer at its earliest and most treatable stage. A number of early signs and symptoms of cancer can serve as warning signals, but a diagnosis should be made only by a qualified medical care provider. A medical diagnosis of cancer is usually made upon physical examination and pathological analysis of a sample of suspicious tissue through a procedure called a **biopsy**. Medical treatment of cancer generally involves use of surgery (to remove cancerous tissue, especially before it spreads), chemotherapy (medications to kill cancerous cells), and radiation therapy.

biopsy A medical test involving surgical removal of a specimen of body tissue to detect cancerous cells.

Cancer can strike anyone; none of us is immune. But some of us are at greater risk than others. Your relative risk depends on many factors, especially your genetic inheritance and whether you engage in unhealthful behavior like smoking. Let us take a closer look at behavioral risk factors, beginning with the most dangerous of these: smoking. But first we need to become better aware of the early warning signs of cancer, such as those listed in Table 13.3, so that we might be able to identify cancer in its earliest and most treatable stages.

TABLE 13.3 Early Signs and Symptoms of Cancer

The chances of surviving cancer are greater if it is detected and treated early. The American Cancer Society identifies general and cancer-specific warning signs. But because these symptoms may result from other causes, they should be brought to the attention of a healthcare provider to arrive at a proper diagnosis.

General Signs and Symptoms	Signs and Symptoms of Specific Types of Cancer
Unexplained weight loss: Unexplained weight loss may be the first sign of cancer but can also occur due to many other causes. It is prudent to be aware of weight loss of about 10 pounds that cannot be explained by dieting or other obvious cause.	**Changes in bowel or bladder function:** Be alert to painful urination, blood in the urine, diarrhea, chronic constipation, or changes in the size of the stool or frequency of urination.
Fever: Fever is a very common symptom of cancer as well as other diseases. In cancer, it usually occurs after the cancer has metastasized.	**Sores that fail to heal:** Persistent sores that fail to heal over time may be signs of cancer, such as oral cancer and skin cancer. Also be alert to sores on the penis or vagina, which might be signs of infection or possibly early cancer.
Fatigue: Extreme fatigue that doesn't improve with rest may be an early sign of cancer.	**Unexplained bleeding or discharge:** Any unusual bodily discharge or bleeding should be evaluate medically—immediately! Blood in the stool is a common sign of colon or rectal cancer, whereas blood in the urine might indicate bladder or kidney cancer. Bleeding from a nipple may be a sign of breast cancer.
Pain: Be aware of any unexplained pain. Pain may stem from many causes, but it can be an early symptom of some forms of cancer, such as bone cancer and testicular cancer. Typically, pain occurs after cancer has spread (metastasized).	**A lump or thickening in the breasts or other areas in the body:** Be alert to any lumps or thickenings under the skin, especially when it involves the breasts, testicles, glands (lymph nodes), and soft tissues of the body. These can be signs of early or late cancer.
Changes in skin: Be alert to any skin changes, such as growths, yellowing, itching, darkening, or excessive hair growth or changes in the size or color of a mole. These types of changes can be symptoms of skin cancers as well as some internal forms of cancer.	**Indigestion or difficulty swallowing**: These symptoms may have many causes, including cancers of the esophagus, stomach, or pharynx (throat).
	Recent changes in warts or moles: Check your skin regularly for any changes in the size, color, or shape of warts or moles. Have a physician check them out to make sure they are not a sign of skin cancer.
	Nagging hoarseness or persistent cough: A persistent cough that won't go away may be a sign of lung cancer or serious respiratory disease. Persistent hoarseness may indicate cancer of the larynx (voice box) or thyroid.

Source: Adapted from American Cancer Society. (2014). Signs and symptoms of cancer. http://www.cancer.org/cancer/cancer-basics/signs-and-symptoms-of-cancer.html

Smoking

Smoking is responsible for at least 80–90% of deaths from lung cancer, a particularly virulent type of cancer. Although breast cancer occurs more frequently in women (affecting about 1 in 8 women) than lung and bronchus cancer (affecting about 1 in 17 women), lung and bronchus cancer is the leading cause of cancer deaths among women, as it is among men (ACS, 2018; NCI, 2019b).

Smoking also causes many other types of cancer, including bladder, kidney, pancreatic, and stomach cancers, as well as leukemia (cancer of the blood) and colorectal (colon and rectal) cancer. Smoking is also responsible for most cancers involving the mouth, larynx, pharynx, esophagus, and bladder.

Overall, cigarette smoking accounts for about 1 in 3 cancer deaths in the United States. It's not just cigarette smoking that causes cancer, but other means of using tobacco as well, including pipe and cigar smoking and chewing tobacco (dip or chew). It is also dangerous to inhale smoke from other people's cigarettes and cigars. Secondhand smoking contributes to several thousand cancer deaths per year.

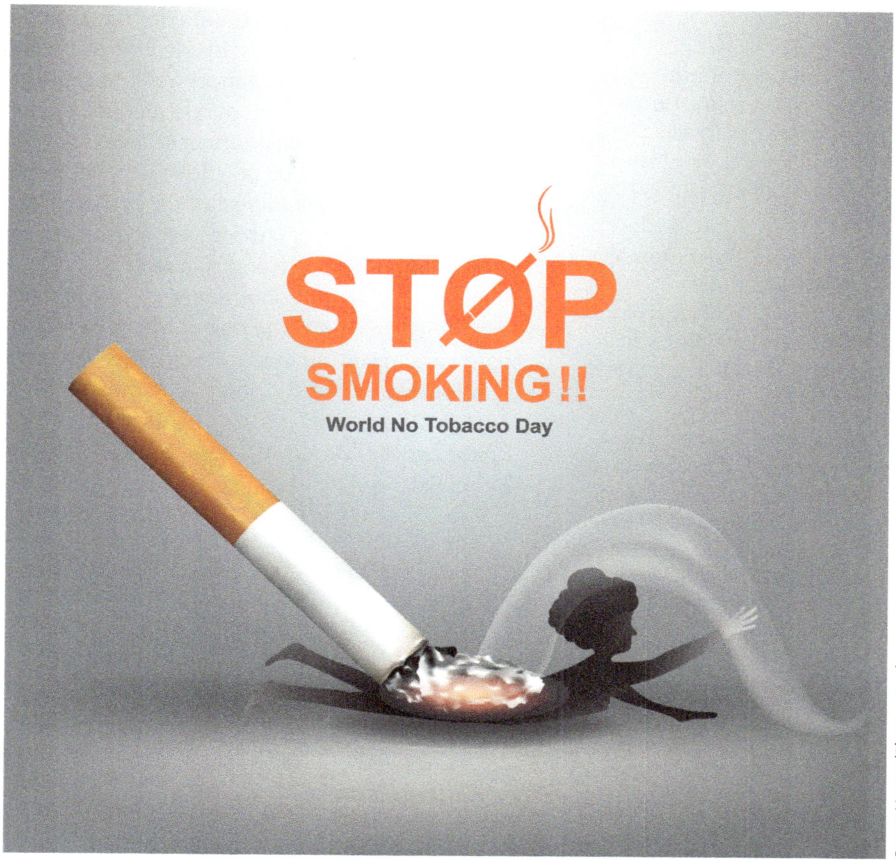

Space Vector/Shutterstock.com

Diet

Did you know that the food you consume may put you at greater risk of cancer? Saturated fat in our dietary intake is linked to two of the leading cancer killers, prostate cancer and colorectal cancer, and is believed to account for nearly 1 in 3 cancer deaths in the United States (Gorman, 2012; Taubes, 2012). Fortunately, we can modify our eating habits to make healthier dietary choices.

Because prostate cancer and colorectal cancer are linked to dietary factors, it makes sense to curb intake of high-fat foods—foods such as meat, dairy products, and cakes and cookies—and increase consumption of healthier food choices such as vegetables, fruits, and grains. Reducing fat intake may also reduce the risk of other health problems, such as cardiovascular disease and Type 2 (adult-onset) diabetes. Tomatoes may also help. *Yes, tomatoes.* Tomatoes contain plant chemicals called *lycopenes*, the substances that give them their red color.

Lycopenes may help prevent damage to DNA, which possibly could reduce the risk of prostate cancer and perhaps other cancers as well. Pink grapefruit and watermelon are also good sources of lycopenes.

Another possible preventive is antioxidant-rich green tea. Researchers across the globe are investigating whether the chemicals in tea—and especially green tea—have a preventive effect against forms of cancer, including esophageal cancer, to lung cancer and breast cancer (Wu et al., 2020; Xu et al., 2020b; Yi et al., 2020). The chemicals appear to have a small effect, and the investigators are planning to study the effects of greater concentrations of the chemicals.

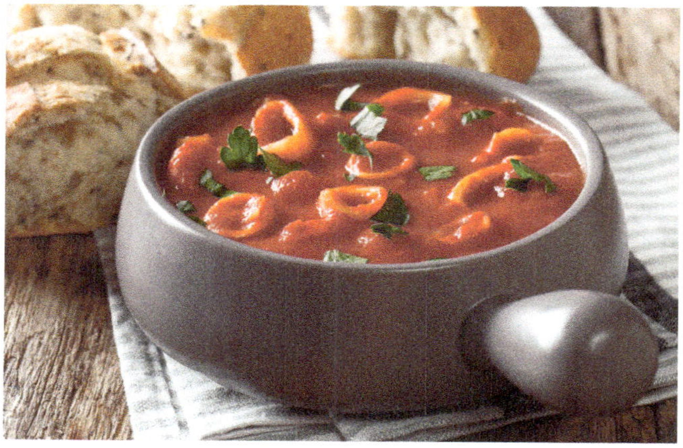

Sergii Koval/Alamy Stock Photo

Eating Red

Alcohol

Alcohol use is another preventable risk factor for cancer (Klein et al., 2020). An estimated 5.6% of cancers are associated with alcohol use (Islami et al., 2018). Heavier use of alcohol increases the risk, especially for cancers of the mouth, pharynx, larynx, and esophagus (Jayasekara et al., 2015). Yet even moderate alcohol intake is linked to increased rates of some forms of cancer, including breast cancer (Klein et al., 2020). A Japanese study evaluated drinking habits of more than 63,000 people with cancer, finding that moderate alcohol use daily was associated with a modest increase in the risk of cancer, while heavier drinking was associated with much higher rates of cancer as compared to nondrinkers (Zaitsu et al., 2020).

Modifiable behavioral risk factors account for nearly 1 in 4 (23%) cases of breast cancer, with obesity and alcohol being the two greatest risk factors (Sinclair et al., 2019). Alcohol consumption affects the risk of breast cancer by altering hormonal levels and their biological pathways, resulting in the development of carcinogens. By and large there is a dose–response relationship between drinking alcoholic beverages and breast cancer in women (Shield et al., 2016; Williams et al., 2016). That is, the more women drink, the more likely they are to develop breast cancer. Moreover, there is no guaranteed minimum safe amount of alcohol for women to imbibe.

basal cell carcinoma A form of skin cancer, characterized by appearance of translucent or pearly-looking tumors, which is easily curable if detected and treated early.

squamous cell carcinoma A form of skin cancer, characterized by reddish or pinkish raised nodules, which is easily curable if detected and treated early.

melanoma A potentially deadly form of cancer involving cancerous growths in melanin-forming cells in the body, which are most commonly found in the skin.

Body Weight

Obesity is a risk factor for many serious chronic diseases, including cardiovascular disease, diabetes, and some forms of cancer (Gorman, 2012; Key, 2020). Obesity is linked to colorectal cancer, breast cancer (in postmenopausal women), prostate cancer, cancer of the endometrium (the lining of the uterus), cancer of the kidney and esophagus, and possibly pancreatic cancer (e.g., Buzdar, 2006; Stolzenberg-Solomon et al., 2008). Obesity is determined by many factors, including biological factors like genetics and body metabolism that we can't control, but also by unhealthful patterns of food consumption and a sedentary lifestyle—factors that we can control.

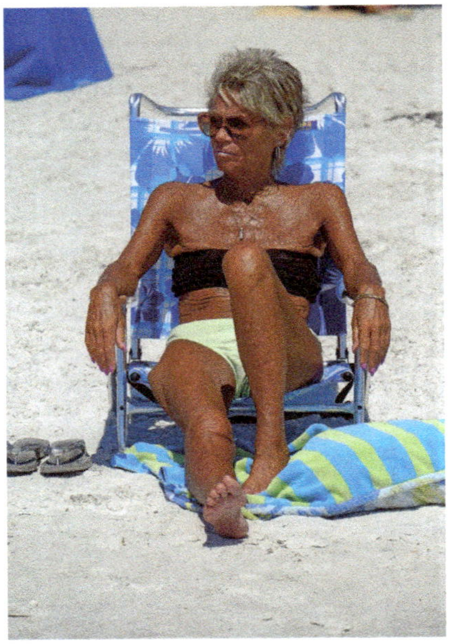

dmac/Alamy Stock Photo

OMG! You Mean That's What I'll Look Like! British investigators used morphing software to show people how their faces are likely to look at 72 years if they had limited sun exposure and used sun protection, and also if their faces were unprotected (Persson et al., 2018). Participants were shocked by the projected skin damage. A 40-year-old woman exclaimed, "Good grief, that's awful! I look like Yoda!" Another, a 47-year-old, told researchers, "The skin looks really wrinkled and leathery and ... much much older." The treatment increased the women's motivation to reduce their UV exposure or to continue to protect their skin if they were already doing so.

Exposure to the Sun

Prolonged exposure to ultraviolet radiation in the form of sunlight, especially if the skin is left unprotected, can lead to the two most common forms of skin cancer, **basal cell carcinoma** and **squamous cell carcinoma**. These are also the most easily treatable types of skin cancer. Basal cell carcinoma accounts for about 75% of cases of skin cancer. Cancerous growths may appear on the head, neck, and hands, the areas of the body most frequently exposed to direct sunlight. These types of skin cancer are relatively benign and readily curable if discovered at an early stage and surgically removed.

Melanoma, a type of cancer that forms in melanin-containing cells found most commonly in the skin, poses much more significant risks of mortality. Although melanoma accounts for only about 1% of skin cancers, it is responsible for a large majority of skin cancer deaths, claiming some 8,000 lives in the United States annually (ACS, 2023). Moreover, while new cases of cancers of the colon and rectum and cancers of the lung and bronchus have been declining, the incidence of melanoma has been on the rise in the United States (ACS, 2023; NCI, 2020b). Exposure to severe sunburns early in life increases the risk of later development of melanoma, which is a reminder that cancer-preventive behaviors need to start at an early age.

To protect ourselves from skin cancer, we need to limit our exposure to the sun and use sunscreen with SPF (sun protective factor) of 15 or more whenever we are exposed to the sun for longer than a few minutes. Evidence shows that it's difficult to get people to change their behavior to limit sun exposure. A recent meta-analysis showed only modest gains from health behavior interventions designed to

Applying Health Psychology

Recognizing the ABCs, D's, and E's of Melanoma

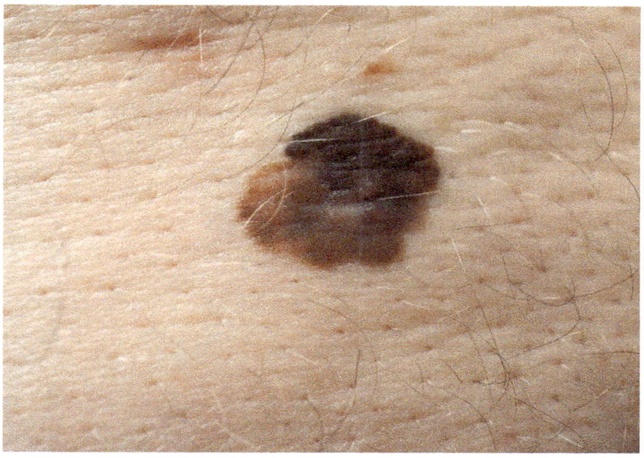
Barry Mason/Alamy Stock Photo

Can you identify the various moles and other spots, bumps, and growths on your body? Do you make it a regular practice to examine your skin from head to toe, front and back, or have a regular skin exam by a healthcare provider? Awareness of the various moles and areas of pigmentation on your skin provides a benchmark you can use to evaluate changes that might raise suspicions of cancerous growth. Look for warning signs and symptoms of skin cancer, such as unusual skin conditions, particularly changes in the size, shape, or pigmentation of moles or other dark areas of skin. Take note of any bleeding, ulceration, scaliness, or other changes in any nodule, growth, bump, or "beauty mark"; of changes in sensation (pain, tenderness, itchiness) of skin marks; or of a spreading of pigmentation. Contact your doctor or primary healthcare provider when you notice any changes or suspicious-looking moles or growths. Apply the following ABCDE rule to any moles on your body to detect warning signs of melanoma (Skin Cancer Foundation, 2019):

- *A is for asymmetry:* One half of the mole does not match the other half.
- *B is for border irregularity:* The edges are ragged, notched, or blurred.
- *C is for color:* The pigmentation is not uniform. Shades of brown, tan, and black are visible.
- *D is for diameter greater than 6 millimeters:* Any sudden or progressive increase in size should be of special concern.
- *E is for evolving:* "E" is to alert people to be aware of any evolving changes in the shape, size, color, or symptoms (itching, hurting, bleeding, etc.) of the mole.

Perform a full-body skin exam monthly and report any suspicious findings to your primary healthcare provider. Yes, it might just be a mole, but it is best to play it safe.

help people to reduce their exposure to dangerous UVR (Sheeran et al., 2020). The challenge awaits, as we need to find more effective ways of persuading people that when it comes to exposing skin to ultraviolet radiation, the sun is not their friend and can be a deadly nemesis. As we discuss in the nearby Health Psychology in Action feature, health psychologists recently applied the Common Sense Model to promoting sun protective behaviors to decrease the risk of skin cancer.

Environmental Factors

Many chemicals are identified as carcinogenic (cancer-causing) in humans including benzene, asbestos, vinyl chloride, coal tars, the hydrocarbons in tobacco smoke, and arsenic. Still others are classified as probable carcinogens. Sources of *ionizing radiation*—radiation that damages body cells—can also cause cancer, such as radiation from radon gas that can seep into homes from the ground below. The federal government maintains standards for limiting exposure to potentially dangerous chemicals in the environment and workplace as well as for protecting the quality of the air and water.

Infectious Agents

You can't "catch" cancer as you might an infectious disease like the flu. But you can contract infectious agents, especially viruses, that lead to the development of some forms of cancer. Viruses can insinuate themselves into the cell's DNA, where they can activate genes that lead to tumor growth or *de*activate those that suppress tumors. The bacterium *H. pylori,* when it proliferates in the stomach, can lead to stomach ulcers and is also linked to an increased risk of stomach cancer.

An example of a cancer-causing virus is *human papillomavirus* (HPV), the sexually transmitted virus that causes genital warts but is also responsible for the great majority of cases of cervical cancer. HIV, the virus that causes AIDS, can lead to a form of cancer called Kaposi's sarcoma, which is characterized by purplish spots on the body. Viruses like HIV can also weaken the immune system, making the body less capable of ridding itself of the cancerous cells. The hepatitis B and C viruses can cause liver cancer. Protecting ourselves from exposure to HIV and other sexually transmitted viruses (see Chapter 10) can reduce our risk of cancer.

Physical Inactivity

Physical inactivity is a risk factor not only for cardiovascular disease but also for some types of cancer (Campbell et al., 2019; Patel et al., 2019; Schmitz et al., 2019). A panel of health-care professionals issued a report stating that regular physical activity reduces the risks of many common cancers, including cancer of the colon, breast, kidney, endometrium, bladder, stomach, and esophagus (Collins, 2019). This panel also concluded that people with breast, colorectal, or prostate cancers who exercised more before receiving a cancer diagnosis or who started exercising after the cancer diagnosis had increased rates of survival. The mounting evidence of the risks posed by inactivity prompted the then Director of the National Institutes of Health, Dr. Francis Collins (2019), to write: "Every cancer survivor should, within reason, avoid inactivity."

Sedentary workers face a higher cancer risk than do physically active workers, which highlights the need for people who sit for long stretches of time to engage in physical activity during breaks and before or after their workdays. Reducing the time spent sitting may reduce the risks of some forms of cancer (Collins, 2019).

Health Psychology in Action

Using the CSM Model to Change Intentions to Practice Sun Protective Behaviors

You may recall from Chapter 3 the discussion of the Common Sense Model (CSM) of emotional regulation, the conceptual model that breaks down how people cope with illness in terms of their subjective appraisal of threats to their physical health (called *cognitive representations*) and their emotional reactions to physical health challenges (called *emotional representations*). Recently, health psychologists in Germany put this model to the test in the context of promoting sun protective behaviors (Vollmann, Engelhardt, & Salewski, 2021). The researchers targeted beliefs about skin cancer among a group of healthy individuals to see if they could increase intentions to practice conduct sun protective behaviors. The participants, 509 healthy volunteers with an average (mean) age of 39 years, were randomly assigned to either an intervention group or a control group. The online intervention included, in part, watching a video on skin protection and receiving information about skin cancer and the dangers of UV radiation. A control group received general information about skin cancer.

The intervention succeeded in increasing intentions of participants to engage in sun protective behaviors, such as use of UV protection and avoiding sun exposure. Supporting the common sense model, these changing intentions were at least partially accounted for by changes in cognitive representations of illness, such as development of a better understanding of skin cancer and changes in the beliefs that cancer can be prevented through one's own efforts. The investigators showed that illness representations are changeable and that by changing them, we can help people change their intentions to practice healthier behaviors. Future research is needed to see if changing intentions by means of altering illness representations leads to actual changes in sun protective behaviors.

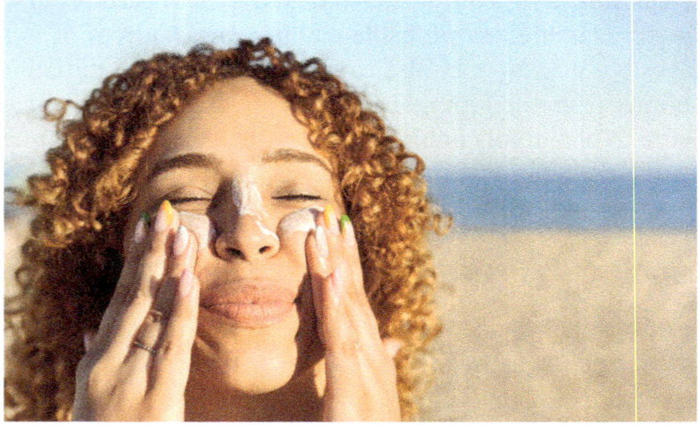

Javi Sanz/Getty Images

Protecting Your Skin To protect our skin, we should limit direct sun exposure as much as possible and apply sunscreen before any direct sun exposure.

Stress and Cancer: Is There a Link?

Is stress a risk factor for cancer? The immune system plays a critical role in ridding the body of diseased or defective cells, including the abnormal cells involved in cancer. If the immune system is weakened or compromised, it may be less capable of controlling abnormal cell growth, which may increase susceptibility to cancer. We know that psychological factors, such as stress, can adversely affect the immune system, so it is conceivable that life stress may increase the risk potential for cancer. Researchers who have explored links between stress and cancer have thus far reported inconclusive results, but it would be prudent to take reasonable steps to control the level of stress in our lives.

Although it has not been shown that stress is a cause of cancer, there is no doubt that cancer is stressful and that stress may affect patients' responses to cancer, including their survival. For example, Jessica Armer and her colleagues (2018) found that most women with ovarian cancer report increased anxiety at the time of diagnosis, which tends to diminish following treatment. However, some women report persistent anxiety, which can dysregulate the body's control of cortisol, leading to fatigue, a poorer quality of life, and, possible, shorter survival following treatment. A Brazilian study found that social support from family and healthcare providers lessens stress and improves the quality of life of patients undergoing chemotherapy for colorectal cancer (Costa et al., 2017). Anxiety and depression may also increase the risk of smoking-related cancers as people who struggle with negative emotions may develop unhealthy behaviors, like smoking, to ease negative emotional states (van Tuijl et al., 2023).

Self-Assessment

INTERACTIVE SELF-ASSESSMENTS

Assessing Personal Risk Factors for Cancer

Cancer can strike anyone, but some of us face a higher risk than others. Your relative risk depends on many factors, especially your family history and lifestyle. Examining your risk profile can help you identify risk factors you can change.

"Yes" answers to the following questions are associated with an increased cancer risk:

____ 1. Have you or someone in your immediate family suffered from cancer or precancerous growths (excluding basal and squamous skin cancers)?

____ 2. Are you 45 years of age or older?

____ 3. Do you currently smoke cigarettes or use other tobacco products, such as smokeless tobacco or snuff? If you are a former smoker, did you smoke regularly for at least a year or more?

____ 4. Are you overweight?

____ 5. Do you have more than 1 drink of alcohol daily?

____ 6. Do you have a history of severe sunburns, even in childhood? Do you fail to protect your skin when you are out in the sun?

"Yes" answers to the following questions are associated with a lower cancer risk:

____ 1. Are you mindful of the amount of fat in your diet, making sure not to consume more than 30% of your total caloric intake in the form of dietary fat?

____ 2. Have you adopted a diet rich in fruits, vegetables, and dietary fiber?

____ 3. Do you avoid foods that are smoked, nitrite- or salt-cured?

____ 4. Do you avoid using alcohol or limit use to 1 drink per day?

____ 5. Do you regularly use sunscreen protection (SPF value of 15 or higher) when you are in direct sunlight for longer than a few minutes? Do you wear protective clothing when exposed to direct sun?

____ 6. Do you avoid using tobacco products?

____ 7. Do you exercise regularly?

____ 8. Do you get regular health checkups and follow recommended cancer screening guidelines?

____ 9. Do you (women) regularly examine your breasts for lumps? Do you (men) regularly examine your testicles for lumps?

____ 10. Do you avoid exposure to environmental contaminants, such as asbestos, radiation, and toxic chemicals?

____ 11. Do you abstain from using tanning salons and home sunlamps?

____ 12. Do you follow a balanced, nutritional diet that is rich in food sources of essential vitamins and minerals?

Assessing your risk profile. No particular score represents a precise risk estimate. However, the more "Yes" answers to the first set of questions and fewer "Yes" answers to the second set, the greater your overall cancer risk. Look closely at these risk factors. Ask yourself which factors you can change to improve your chances of remaining healthy and cancer-free.

Review 13.2

INTERACTIVE SELF-SCORING QUIZZES

Sentence Completion

1. __________ weight loss may be the first sign of cancer.

2. __________ may have many causes, including cancers of the esophagus, stomach, or pharynx (throat).

3. Eating __________ fats is linked to prostate cancer and colorectal cancer.

4. Japanese researchers studied the drinking habits of more than 63,000 people with cancer; they found that __________ alcohol use daily was associated with a modest increase in the risk of cancer.

5. The two most common forms of skin cancer are __________ cell carcinoma and __________ cell carcinoma.

6. Although melanoma accounts for about 1% of skin cancers, it is responsible for much more than __________ of deaths due to skin cancer.

7. HPV is a sexually transmitted virus that causes genital warts but is also responsible for the great majority of cases of __________ cancer.

8. __________ workers face a higher cancer risk than do physically active workers.

9. Links between __________ and cancer are inconclusive.

Think About It

Consider your age and the behavioral risk factors for developing cancer. Do you see cancer as something far off in the future that affects a minority of people? Do you imagine that there will be cures for cancers 10, 20, or 30 years down the road? What do you perceive as your risk of developing cancer? Are you engaging in behaviors that increase your risk? Have you considered modifying them?

Psychological Factors in Living with Cancer

posttraumatic growth Positive changes in psychological functioning following traumatic life events.

Cancer takes a significant toll on mental health, as studies show that cancer patients have higher rates of anxiety and depressive disorders, and even suicide (Deshields et al., 2022; Wapner, 2022). Overall, nearly 1 in 3 people living with cancer has a mental health problem (Castelli et al., 2015). Prevalence rates of major depression and anxiety disorders among people living with cancer are estimated to be 16.3% and 10.3%, respectively (Stanton et al., 2019). Understandably, clinicians tend to focus on the negative emotional consequences of cancer and its treatment. But we should also recognize the potential for **posttraumatic growth**; that is, the trauma of cancer may lead to positive effects, such as renewal of connections with others or finding new meaning in life (Cormio et al., 2014).

Depression in cancer survivors is a threat not only to their mental health but also to their survival. Investigators find links between depression and reduced survival rates in people with cancer (Jansen et al., 2018; Satin et al., 2009). However, cancer patients who have a stronger sense of meaning in life tend to show less depression and to be better able to integrate living with cancer into their lives (Bamishigbin et al., 2020). We can't yet say why depression tends to lead to earlier death in people with cancer, but researchers suspect that adjusting to cancer leads to unhealthy lifestyle changes (increased smoking and alcohol consumption in people with depression) as well as increased risk of suicide (Jansen et al., 2019).

Another frequent emotional consequence of living with cancer is fear, including fear of cancer recurrence. In one study, researchers studied more than 2,000 people who had survived cancer over some 9 years (Séguin Leclair et al., 2019). They classified people according to three levels of fear of cancer recurrence (FCR). Those people with high levels of FCR were more often female, younger in age, Latino or Hispanic, and more likely to have advanced stages of cancer. The more fearful individuals also tended to show poorer adherence to recommendations for physical activity and increased intake of fruits and vegetables. Negative emotions such as fear can cripple efforts to increase healthful behaviors. Treatment providers need to address the specific needs of people at different levels of FCR to develop more targeted interventions.

Roles of Health Psychologists in Cancer Care

Health psychologists have become indispensable in the comprehensive treatment of people with cancer through their efforts to help the people make healthful behavior changes as well as assisting them in coping with the many emotional challenges of living with cancer. Health psychologists provide counseling and serve as group leaders in support programs where people with cancer share their struggles with others and benefit both from support they receive from other members and the support they provide others. They evaluate people with cancer for mental health problems, such as anxiety and depression, and provide treatment for these conditions. They develop and implement health promotion and cancer prevention programs focusing on helping people adopt healthier lifestyles to reduce the risks of cancer.

People who survive cancer face many challenges, from managing the physical symptoms of the illness itself and the side effects of treatment to the negative emotional consequences of having a life-threatening illness, as well as changes in body image after the removal of a breast or testicle, and disruptions in family relationships and responsibilities (Cherry et al., 2018; Ratcliff & Novy, 2018). Psychological interventions can help cancer patients develop skills for coping with their illness and managing stress, as well as combating depression and the sense of hopelessness that many experience (Antoni et al., 2023; Cillessen et al., 2019). Evidence strongly points to the benefits of psychological interventions, such as cognitive behavioral therapy and group support programs, in helping people with cancer manage stress and relieve depression, anger, anxiety, insomnia, and the feelings of helplessness that attend cancer (Murphy et al., 2020; Zhou et al., 2020).

A problem for people who must make repeated visits to treatment units for chemotherapy is that the stimuli associated with chemotherapy, such as visual cues and odors in the treatment unit, can become conditioned stimuli that elicit conditioned responses of nausea and vomiting, even before the chemotherapy is administered. To weaken the links between these conditioned stimuli and adverse reactions, health psychologists may educate people in ways of engaging in competing responses to the stimuli before they enter the treatment unit, such as a relaxation or meditation exercise.

Another challenge facing health psychologists is helping people with cancer cope with the persistent pain that often accompanies the disease (Ratcliff & Novy, 2018). Relaxation and mindfulness techniques, as well as distraction strategies (see Chapter 6), can help people who survive cancer develop coping skills for handling pain and anxiety (Ratcliff & Novy, 2018). Relaxation training also can help treat symptoms in people who survive cancer, such as anxiety and disturbed sleep patterns (Lazaridou & Edwards, 2019). As discussed in Chapter 6, cognitive behavioral therapists use various methods to combat chronic pain. These methods include helping people challenge and replace catastrophizing thoughts about pain and engage in rewarding daily activities in the *Health Psychology in Action* feature, "The Best Pickles Imaginable!," illustrates the importance of engaging life.

Cancer care psychologists also help people cope with another common feature of chemotherapy—"chemo brain" (Ahles & Root, 2020; Palmer, 2020). Chemo brain (sometimes called chemo fog) involves subtle changes in cognitive functioning resulting from the effects on the brain of chemotherapy or other treatments, such as surgery and anesthesia. These changes may include problems with memory, concentration, ability to organize tasks, or just a general slowing of the ability to process information. Cancer patients may also report feeling mentally slower than usual. These cognitive deficits are not as severe as those associated with disorders such as Alzheimer's disease, but they can affect daily functioning. Psychologists and other healthcare providers are using cognitive behavioral techniques to help people with cancer cope with cancer-related cognitive impairments, as by helping them focus their attention, handle distractions, and maintain journals and appointment calendars (Liou et al., 2020).

Health psychologists evaluate their intervention efforts to assess whether they yield benefits. An analysis of interventions designed to increase physical activity among people who survived cancer showed that they produced a significant effect, boosting physical activity by an average of some 1,100 additional steps per day (Sheeran et al., 2019). Greater increases in physical activity were generally found in supervised rather than in unsupervised programs. Even in supervised programs, larger effects were found in programs offering greater face-to-face time with participants. People profit when program developers provide direct supervision and spend time helping them achieve their physical activity goals.

It's not just the cancer patient who suffers, as evidence shows that caregivers of cancer patients also show higher than usual levels of anxiety and depression (Deshields et al., 2022). Health psychologists can be helpful in providing support and coping skills training to family members and others who care for the cancer patient. Finally, let's not overlook the important role that health psychologists play in conducting research on psychological factors in cancer

Health Psychology in Action

A Day in the Life of a Cancer Care Psychologist

Julie B. Schnur, Ph.D., is a licensed clinical psychologist at the Dubin Breast Center at Mount Sinai Medical Center in New York, an associate professor in the Department of Population Health Science and Policy, and a member of the Center for Behavioral Oncology, at the Icahn School of Medicine at Mount Sinai.

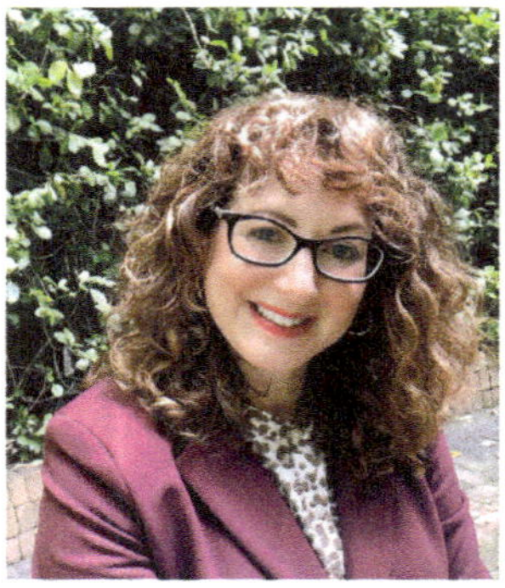

Source: Julie B. Schnur, Ph.D.

Julie B. Schnur, Ph.D.[1]

She writes:

My background is in clinical psychology, which traditionally focuses on evaluation and treatment of mental health concerns. My first full-time job was at a mental health clinic, where I primarily worked with patients with severe and persistent mental illness. But my career soon turned toward clinical health psychology when I had the opportunity to volunteer on a research study testing clinical hypnosis to help women undergoing breast cancer surgery. Hypnosis was being tested as a tool to help women reduce emotional distress before surgery and then to help alleviate pain, nausea, fatigue, and distress after surgery. I conducted hypnosis with breast cancer patients as they prepared for surgery, which typically involved either a lumpectomy or mastectomy, meeting with them in the pre-op area less than an hour before surgery. Perhaps you can imagine the anxiety the women felt as they prepared for major surgery on an intimate part of their body and faced an uncertain future. In my earlier work in mental health, I had helped patients work through long-standing emotional problems. But with breast cancer patients prepping for surgery, I was there to play a supportive role at one of the most stressful moments of their lives. In this setting, I had the opportunity to make a terrifying day a little bit less scary. There was something vital and profound about being able to listen, soothe, and shape a patient's experience of cancer care that connected with me, and I've been devoted to the field ever since, working to develop, test, and deliver psychotherapeutic and mind-body interventions at a large teaching hospital in New York.

So what do you call what I do? Some call it behavioral oncology, some psycho-oncology, some psychosocial oncology, and some health psychology or, more precisely, clinical health psychology. But what do I actually do on a day-to-day basis? I provide individual outpatient psychotherapy services to help improve the quality of life of women with breast cancer from the day they're diagnosed with cancer, through their course of treatment (which can include surgery, chemotherapy, radiotherapy, adjuvant hormonal therapy, and breast reconstruction), as they adjust to life after treatment (sometimes referred to as survivorship), and (in some cases) at the end of life.

What types of problems do I treat? Issues I see daily in my work with women with breast cancer include the following:

- Adjusting to a cancer diagnosis and threat of mortality (e.g., often going from one day thinking of yourself as healthy to the next day realizing you have a life-threatening disease)
- Body image concerns related to treatment (e.g., losing your hair and breasts, weight gain associated with steroids and hormone changes)
- Coping with physical changes (e.g., suffering with extreme cancer-related fatigue), cognitive changes (e.g., "chemo brain"), and changes in sexual function associated with treatment
- Learning how to communicate effectively with medical providers about treatment preferences and quality-of-life issues
- Learning how to communicate with family, friends, and colleagues about their cancer experience (e.g., how do you tell people about the diagnosis, how much information to share)
- Evaluating and adjusting priorities and goals (e.g., some patients choose to focus more on work-life balance when faced with concerns about their mortality)
- Fear of cancer recurrence (e.g., worry about cancer coming back or metastasizing) or in those cases where cancer metastasizes, helping the patient adjust to the end of life
- Traditional mental health issues such as depression and anxiety.

Also, given the mind–body connection and our understanding of how our thoughts and emotions are related to physical symptoms, I teach patients stress management and relaxation strategies to help them manage symptoms and side effects like pain, nausea, fatigue, and insomnia. My psychologist colleagues also treat caregivers, spouses, children, couples and families; help with weight management, smoking cessation, and treatment adherence; encourage patients to undergo recommended cancer screenings; conduct psychological and neuropsychological assessments; and counsel patients as they face acute crises throughout the course of their disease.

My time spent with patients can be as short as one session, as when a patient wants to talk to a psychologist about her fears of an upcoming medical procedure or to quickly learn a relaxation technique to prepare for an MRI. However, most typically I work with patients for longer periods of time, over the course of months, providing support and teaching skills as patients navigate their breast cancer journey.

Working at an academic cancer center means that in addition to conducting psychotherapy, I have the opportunity to teach, train, and mentor cancer care providers and colleagues and to conduct behavioral oncology research. In a given month I may use the interviewing skills I learned as a psychologist to train physicians how to conduct qualitative interviews with patients, teach radiation therapy students or breast surgery fellows about empathic communication, or conduct research to help improve patients' quality of life. For example, some clinical studies in which I've been involved include training cancer care providers how to work sensitively with sexual violence survivors, training psychosocial cancer care providers in how to deliver cognitive behavioral therapy plus hypnosis to reduce cancer-related fatigue, and testing whether hypnosis can reduce musculoskeletal pain in breast cancer survivors taking aromatase inhibitors (a type of hormonal therapy which is prescribed to reduce breast cancer risk). During my graduate career, I was trained to be a scientist and a practitioner, and my position in behavioral oncology affords me the opportunity to apply both aspects of my training to help patients feel less distressed and more comfortable during cancer care.

In sum, I strive to create a safe space for clients to share their emotions, to support them through the roller coaster that is cancer, to teach them skills and tools to endure the rigors of treatment, and to help them find their "new normal" past the disease. It is my honor and privilege to have the opportunity to do so."

care. Recently, investigators studied mindsets of 273 cancer survivors, breaking them down into maladaptive mindsets ("Cancer is a catastrophe") and adaptive mindsets ("Cancer is manageable" and "Cancer can be an opportunity") (Zeidman et al., 2022). The results showed that cancer survivors who endorsed adaptive mindsets reported better health-related quality of life than those with maladaptive mindsets ("Cancer is a catastrophe"). Findings like this underscore the need to address the psychological dimensions of living with cancer, a topic we explore further in the nearby *Health Psychology in Action*, "A Day in the Life of a Cancer Care Psychologist."

The need for integrated, multidisciplinary treatment of people with cancer may require new occupational roles. Some health psychologists have called for establishing a category of paraprofessionals devoted to helping people with cancer adopt healthier lifestyles (Spring et al., 2019). They proposed the category of *health promotionist*, essentially a lifestyle coach who could be routinely assigned to people with cancer to assist them in making healthful behavior changes, such as quitting smoking, losing excess weight, increasing physical activity, and adhering to treatment. Having a dedicated lifestyle coach would free up time for other healthcare professionals to focus on managing the medical and psychological needs of people with cancer.

Lack of Adherence to Recommendations for Screening and Treatment

Another problem concerning cancer is adherence, and it begins with screening for cancer. Screening is vital in battling cancer because the earlier cancer is detected, the better the treatment outcome. Consider screening for colorectal cancer. The major screening methods are stool tests (fecal occult blood tests and stool DNA tests) and colonoscopy. Fecal occult blood tests seek to detect and analyze small amounts of blood in the stool that are not visible to the naked eye but may be indicative of cancer. DNA stool tests seek to detect changes in genes that are indicative of cancer. In a colonoscopy, a thin, flexible tube with a light and video camera in the tip is inserted into the colon through the rectum to search for polyps—growths that can develop into cancer (Bretthauer et al.. 2023) (**Figure 13.5**). The physician removes any polyps that are found, and they are analyzed to see whether cancerous cells are present. Other tests include sigmoidoscopy and virtual colonoscopy.

These tests are potential lifesavers, but low screening rates remain a problem (Bretthauer et al., 2022; Tsipa et al., 2021). Unfortunately, only about two-thirds to three-quarters of people who are advised to have the tests actually do so (Daskalakis et al., 2020; Weiser et al., 2020). A few factors have been found to predict adherence to screening recommendations (Daskalakis et al., 2020):

- Offering people the option of having either a stool test or a colonoscopy,
- Older age, and
- Being married.

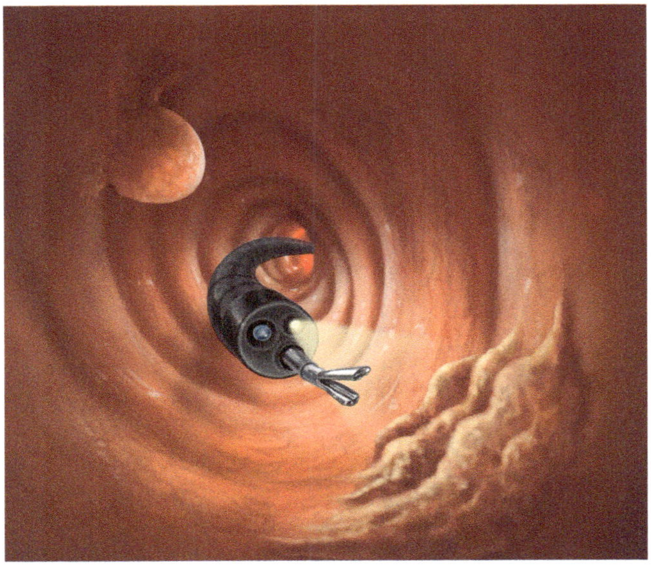

Jim Dowdalls/Science Source

FIGURE 13.5 **Colonoscopy** An illustration of discovery of cancer in the colon. A polyp is seen in the upper left of the image.

Health Psychology in Action

The Best Pickles Imaginable!

Jared was diagnosed with metastatic esophageal cancer when he was 60 years old. Before diagnosis, he retired after being an attorney for many years and moved to the Texas Hill country with his wife. This social and spiritual life in the new community had been very satisfying . ... [Although he] had a poor response to treatment with continued progression of disease, his desire to prolong his life remained strong ... [A] psychologist referred him to the pain center ... [where] he told us about his fear of dying and leaving his wife, and a strong desire to live. Since his diagnosis, he had shut out important people in his life and stopped doing things that gave meaning to his life. He was an avid gardener and loved growing his own food, but he now spent most of the day in bed feeling sad and worried about his prognosis ... [We] worked on pacing of activities and initiating some social and spiritual connections that were important to him. He started living a full life and became receptive to talk about how to live with hope and still be prepared for the end of life. Once he updated his will and included letters to those he loved, he felt less anxious because he was prepared for the unwanted possibility of his death. He was uplifted by important people in his life and once again had a garden full of cucumbers for pickling ... [He] became more active ... [and] tapered off his pain medications. For now, he's doing so much better and in our clinic staff members are enjoying the best pickles imaginable![1]

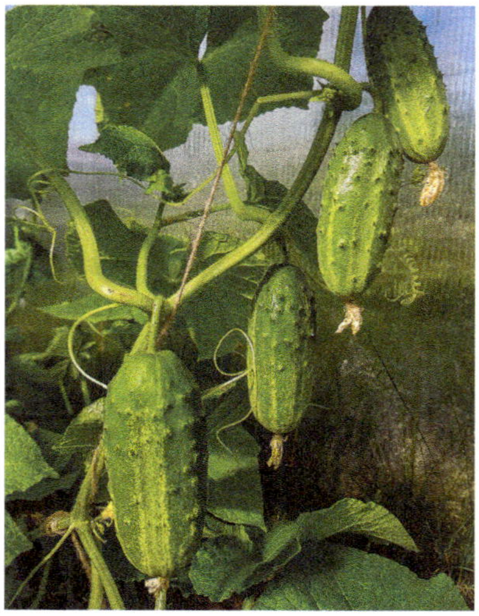

LARISA DUKA/Alamy Stock Photo

[1]Ratcliff, C., & Novy, D. (2018). Treating cancer patients with persistent pain. In D. C. Turk & R. J. Gatchel, *Psychological approaches to pain management: A practitioner's handbook* (3rd ed., pp. 485–514). Guilford Press.

A key concept in the Health Belief Model is perceived susceptibility to illness. This concept was recently put to the test as part of an effort to increase intentions to undergo mammography (Seitz et al., 2018). Investigators found that an intervention that focused on providing women with personalized risk assessments for breast cancer boosted their intentions to obtain a mammogram by increasing their perceived susceptibility.

Promoting Cancer Screening Despite the best of intentions, people may not follow through with mammography. A group of investigators compared the effectiveness of three interventions attempting to promote adherence to biennial screening mammograms for breast cancer (Costanza et al., 2020). The sample was more than 3,000 women in the 50–81-year age group. The interventions were a reminder letter only, a letter plus a reminder phone call, and two letters plus educational material and a counseling phone call. Three of 4 women (75%) who received the letter only had their mammograms as recommended. Nearly 4 out of 5 (79%) of women who received the letter and the reminder or two letters, educational material, and the counseling call adhered to their recommended mammography schedule. It would appear from this study that a letter and a phone call are the most cost-effective method used, but there remains the problem of the 21% who did not obtain their mammograms as recommended.

Another focus of health psychologists in treating people with cancer is lack of adherence to treatment recommendations. Despite the health benefits of physical activity and following a healthful diet, many people with cancer fail to follow through with these recommendations.

To address concerns of nonadherence, health psychologists evaluate barriers that impede progress toward making healthful behavior changes. Recently health researchers interviewed a group of people with cancer and reported that many of them did not intend to make healthful lifestyle changes (Corbett et al., 2018). Among the barriers they identified were uncertainty about how to put health behavior changes into practice and perceptions of a lack of support from healthcare providers. Some people also believed they didn't need to change their health behavior, as they thought that only nonmodifiable factors like genetics were involved in the development of cancer. Clearly, health psychologists need to assist people in removing these kinds of barriers to making healthful changes in order to increase their adherence to screening and treatment.

Health Psychology in the Digital Age

Colorectal Screening: Celebrate Life for Years to Come[1]

The Health Belief Model (HBM) was put into practice in a clinic waiting room where Black patients awaited appointments with their primary healthcare providers (Rawl et al., 2012). The challenge facing health researchers was to promote screening for colorectal cancer (CRC) using an intervention tailored to the user's health beliefs.

The participants first saw a video vignette in which friends are shown interacting at a 50th birthday party for a Black American man named Robert Gibson. The man had recently seen his doctor, who had recommended CRC screening. As the birthday cake is laid on the table, the narrator says, "Mr. Robert Gibson celebrates his 50th birthday today with his family and friends. Robert's in good health—he watches what he eats, stays active, and takes his blood pressure medicine. But there's something else he'll need to start doing to stay healthy in the years ahead. Colon testing is something everyone needs to think about when they get to be Robert's age. Some of his friends and family members have had their colon tested but others, like Robert, haven't even thought about it. Let's see what you think."

The people then completed the steps designed to measure their health beliefs about CRC. They were then instructed to use a video program on a computer that was tailored to address their particular health risks. People who were at low risk of colorectal cancer (a low susceptibility group) saw a health message on the screen emphasizing their own personal risk factors. Others with higher susceptibility by virtue of having a close relative who had been diagnosed with CRC saw a graph in which a bar representing the chances of developing CRC started at 0% and then increased to 18%, the risk level of someone having a close relative who developed CRC before age 60. The screen also showed a fixed marker at 6%, representing the risk of someone without any family history. As the bar inched upward, the person heard a narrator saying, "This picture shows how your chances of getting colon cancer go up when someone in your family has it." Those without a close relative affected by the disease received a health message highlighting general risk factors, such as age and race.

Other tailored messages emphasized factors relating to potential barriers to and benefits of CRC screening. Those who had earlier reported that they didn't want to know if anything was wrong with them saw a snippet of dialogue between two characters named James and Emmett:

James: "Why would I want to take a test to find something wrong? I don't go looking for trouble. If it ain't broke, don't fix it."

Emmett: "I used to think the same way. But then, I had the test. All I know is if I hadn't had the test they wouldn't have found those two polyps that may have turned into cancer."

Those who earlier reported that a colonoscopy would be painful or embarrassing saw a different dialogue between characters named Mary and Patricia:

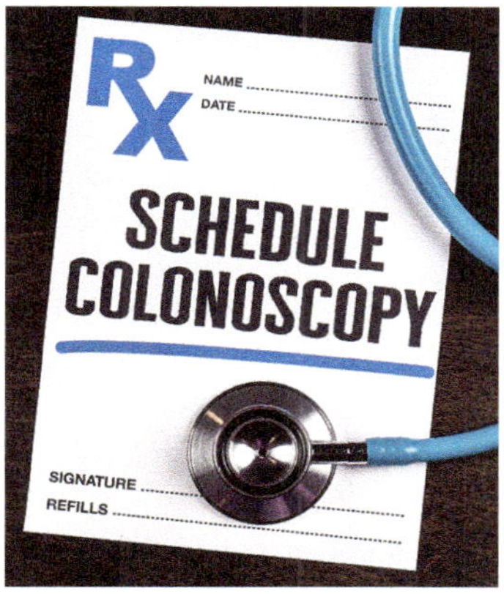

CatLane/Getty Images

Mary: "It sounds to me like a colonoscopy would just hurt, and I would just be too embarrassed."

Patricia: "Well, you know Mary, I thought the same thing. I went, they gave me some medicine, I dozed off, when I woke up it was over. I didn't have time to be embarrassed. I didn't even know what had happened."

In a randomized trial, participants who received the interactive computer program tailored to their susceptibility level showed greater increases in perceived susceptibility to CRC and greater benefits to CRC screening. They also perceived fewer barriers to screening than did control participants who received the general, nontailored material. Moreover, the tailored intervention participants were more likely to report they had discussed CRC screening with their healthcare providers and their healthcare providers were more likely to have documented in the electronic medical records a recommendation for CRC screening (Christy et al., 2013). Those receiving the tailored intervention were also likely to complete fecal occult blood testing, a commonly used screening procedure for colorectal cancer. The upshot of this intervention is that the use of tailored narratives can help change health beliefs (perceptions of susceptibility), which in turn may increase the likelihood of engaging in health-related behaviors.

Other health psychologists are experimenting with using culturally-tailored messages to promote CRC screening among Black adults, such as framing the message in terms of the need to overcome racial disparities in CRC (Lucas et al., 2023). As the field continues to develop, health psychologists are at the forefront of developing more nuanced ways of reaching traditionally underserved groups.

[1]Adapted from C. S. Skinner et al. (2015). The Health Belief Model. In K. Glanz et al. (Eds.), *Health behavior: Theory, research, and practice* (pp. 75–94). Wiley.

The concept of self-efficacy bears on translating intentions into actions. Health researchers find that higher levels of exercise behavior in people who survive cancer is associated with greater *exercise self-efficacy*—beliefs that one can successfully follow through with exercise plans (Basen-Engquist et al., 2013). This is a helpful reminder that interventions that focus on increasing activity levels in people who have survived cancer may first need to work on boosting their expectations of their ability to actually carry out their intentions. Another form of self-efficacy, called *coping self-efficacy*, or belief in one's ability to cope with the many challenges of living with cancer, predicts higher levels of life satisfaction in women with breast cancer (Raque-Bogdan et al., 2019).

Regular screening for colorectal cancer is associated with lower incidence of the disease and fewer deaths (Tsipa et al., 2021). Health psychologists play an important role in designing intervention programs to increase the use of colorectal cancer screening A recent scientific review examined the results of 102 studies based on nearly two million participants and found that intervention programs do indeed boost screening rates (Tsipa et al., 2021). When the researchers dug deeper into the data they discovered that interventions that focused on working to increase social support for screening and providing clear instructions or demonstrations of screening procedures produced stronger effects in getting people screened. Another key factor for improving screening outcomes is direct involvement of health professionals, which underscores the need to have primary healthcare providers directly involved in the screening effort.

Tailoring the content of the message to particular groups is also important. Recently, health psychologists showed that culturally targeted messages boosted screening rates for colorectal cancer among a group of Black Americans. The message focused on the need to overcome racial disparities in colorectal cancer through participating in cancer screening (Lucas et al., 2021). (See the nearby Health Psychology in Action feature focusing on a culturally tailored program to increase screening rates among Black Americans.)

A key concept in the Health Belief Model (HBM) is perceived susceptibility to illness. This concept was recently put to the test as part of an effort to increase intentions to undergo another important screening, mammography (Seitz et al., 2018). Investigators found that an intervention that focused on providing women with personalized risk assessments for breast cancer boosted their intentions to obtain a mammogram by increasing their perceived susceptibility to developing the disease.

Active Versus Passive Coping

People living with cancer cope in different ways (Serpentini & Errol, 2019). In coping with cancer, *active coping* involves direct engagement with the problem, such as making efforts to learn more about the cancer, seeking appropriate healthcare services, and reaching out for emotional support. By contrast, *passive coping* (also called *avoidant coping*) involves disengagement through denial, distancing, and detaching oneself from dealing with cancer.

Applying Health Psychology

Putting Cancer-Preventive Behaviors into Practice

Cancer is frightening, and for good reason, but we are not helpless in the face of it. We can assess our personal risks of cancer and take steps to reduce our risk potential. The Self-Assessment on page 403 can help you gauge your own personal risk factors. But whatever our individual risk profile may be, there are many health behaviors we can practice that can reduce our risk of developing cancer or detect it at its earliest and most treatable stages:

- *Avoid smoking and other tobacco products.* Note: Vaping may also have health hazards. Check with your healthcare provider.
- *Avoid using alcohol or limit its use.*
- *Modify diet by reducing intake of saturated fats and increasing intake of fruits and vegetables.* Plant foods contain many naturally occurring chemicals that may have cancer-preventive effects. (Yes, Grandma was right about veggies.)
- *Exercise regularly*. Regular vigorous exercise may help reduce the risk of some forms of cancer, such as colorectal cancer.
- *Get regular medical checkups so that cancer can be detected early.*
- *Minimize exposure to excess stress and learn to more effectively manage unavoidable stress.* (See Chapter 5 for suggestions for handling stress.)
- *Practice sun-safe behaviors.* Limit exposure to direct sun and use sunscreen (SPF or sun protection factors of 15 or higher) whenever you are in direct sun for more than a few minutes.
- *Maintain a sense of hope and take an active role in managing your health care.*
- *Check your skin regularly for signs of abnormal moles or growths.*
- *Follow recommended schedules for cancer screenings.* These include screenings for breast cancer (in women), prostate cancer (in men), and colorectal cancer (for both men and women). You can find out more information about cancer screening guidelines issued by the American Cancer Society at www.acs.org.
- *Perform regular self-care examinations*. Become familiar with performing breast self-exams and testicular self-exams. Online resources from the American Cancer Society can help you perform these behaviors.

Active coping is generally associated with lower levels of emotional distress in people with cancer (Langford et al., 2017). People with a more active or engaged style of coping tend to focus on the positives and seek out and use social support. Researchers find that people with cancer who rely on passive styles of coping, such as avoiding thinking about or dealing with the cancer, are more likely to become depressed than those who take a more active, engaged role (Stanton et al., 2018).

Health psychologists help people who survive cancer develop more positive attitudes and practice active coping skills, such as problem solving, seeking support from others, and finding ways of expressing their emotions rather than bottling them up. They may use cognitive behavioral therapy to help people develop more adaptive beliefs and behaviors. These methods include *behavioral activation* (e.g., encouraging engagement with life activities), *cognitive restructuring* (challenging and replacing cognition distortions, such as catastrophizing and focusing solely on the negatives), and *changing deeply held core beliefs* (as in correcting beliefs that one is unworthy, deserving of punishment, or doomed to fail) (Langford et al., 2017). Evidence shows that people with cancer who maintain a hopeful attitude and hold more positive expectancies tend to be better adjusted (Stanton et al., 2019).

Review 13.3

INTERACTIVE SELF-SCORING QUIZZES

Sentence Completion

1. Nearly 1 in __________ people living with cancer experiences mental health problems.

2. Two of the most common psychological problems affecting people with cancer are anxiety and __________.

3. Many "cured" people who have had cancer live in fear of cancer __________.

4. Health psychologists find that __________ support is of benefit to the psychological well-being of people with cancer.

5. Psychologists help people with __________ (also called chemo fog) focus their attention, handle distractions, and maintain journals and appointment calendars.

6. Higher levels of exercise in people who survive cancer is associated with greater exercise self-__________.

7. __________ is vital in battling cancer because the earlier cancer is detected, the better the treatment outcome.

8. Health psychologists research ways of motivating people at risk of cancer to __________ to recommended screening protocols.

9. Active, engagement-focused coping is generally associated with (lower or higher) levels of emotional distress in people with cancer.

Think About It

Does anyone you know go for recommended screening for cancer? What type of screening? Do you know anyone who might benefit from screening who does not go for screening? What types of interventions might help or motivate that person to be screened?

Recite: An Active Summary

INTERACTIVE SELF-SCORING QUIZZES

Chapter 13 Practice Quiz

1. Define cancer, and explain why we can think of cancers rather than a single disease called cancer.

The term "cancer" refers to more than 100 diseases characterized by uncontrolled proliferation of cells and the spread of abnormal cells throughout the body.

2. Identify who is prone to developing cancer, focusing on gender and racial/ethnic disparities.

Anybody can develop cancer at any age, but most new cases develop among people aged 55 years and older. Some cancers are limited to women (ovarian, cervical, uterine) or men (prostate, testicles). Women and men may both develop breast cancer, but it is much more common in women. Men are more likely to develop cancers of the bladder, larynx, esophagus, oral cavity, kidney, and stomach. The highest rates of new cancers are found among non-Hispanic Black Americans and White Americans. Black men are most likely to develop and die from prostate cancer. Black women are slightly less likely than White women to develop breast cancer, but they are more likely to die from it.

3. Identify 5-year survival rates for various kinds of cancer.

Fewer than 10% of people with pancreatic cancer survive for 5 years. Ten to 29% of people are likely to survive cancers of the liver and lungs. Sixty to 89% of women are likely to survive breast cancer and cancers of the reproductive system. Prostate, testicular, and thyroid cancer, along with melanoma, are most survivable.

4. Identify the behavioral risk factors for cancer.

General signs and symptoms of cancer include unexplained weight loss, fever, fatigue, pain, and changes in the skin. Other signs and symptoms include changes in bowel or bladder function. Foremost among the behavioral risk factors for cancer is smoking, which is connected with many cancers, including lung cancer. The saturated fats found in meats and dairy products are connected with colorectal cancer and prostate cancer. Alcohol intake is connected with breast cancer and cancers of the mouth, larynx, pharynx, and esophagus. Obesity is linked to several forms of cancer, including colorectal cancer. Exposure to sunlight is connected with skin cancers, including melanoma. Pollution, infectious agents, and physical inactivity are all connected with cancer.

5. Describe psychological factors in living with cancer, focusing on the roles of health psychologists.

About one person in three with cancer has a mental health problem, such as major depression or an anxiety disorder. Many people also have fear of recurrence, which can compromise adherence to recommendations for diet and exercise. Health psychologists evaluate and treat these problems. They often use cognitive behavior therapy and group support. They employ relaxation and mindfulness techniques to help people cope with pain and the side effects of chemotherapy. Psychologists use cognitive behavior therapy to help people with cancer cope with chemo brain by helping them focus their attention, handle distractions, and maintain journals and appointment calendars. Lack of adherence is a problem with recommendations for screening and treatment, and psychologists help people understand their vulnerability to cancer and the benefits of screening. Active coping with cancer is linked to lower levels of emotional distress than passive coping by denial or detaching oneself from dealing with the cancer.

Answers to Review Sections

13.1

1. 5
2. 100
3. malignant
4. genetic
5. Oncogenes
6. 55
7. 40%
8. Black
9. 70

13.2

1. Unexplained
2. Indigestion, Difficulty swallowing
3. saturated
4. moderate
5. basal cell carcinoma and squamous cell carcinoma
6. half
7. cervical
8. Sedentary
9. stress

13.3

1. 3
2. depression
3. recurrence
4. group, social, family
5. chemo brain
6. efficacy
7. Screening
8. adhere
9. lower

CHAPTER 14

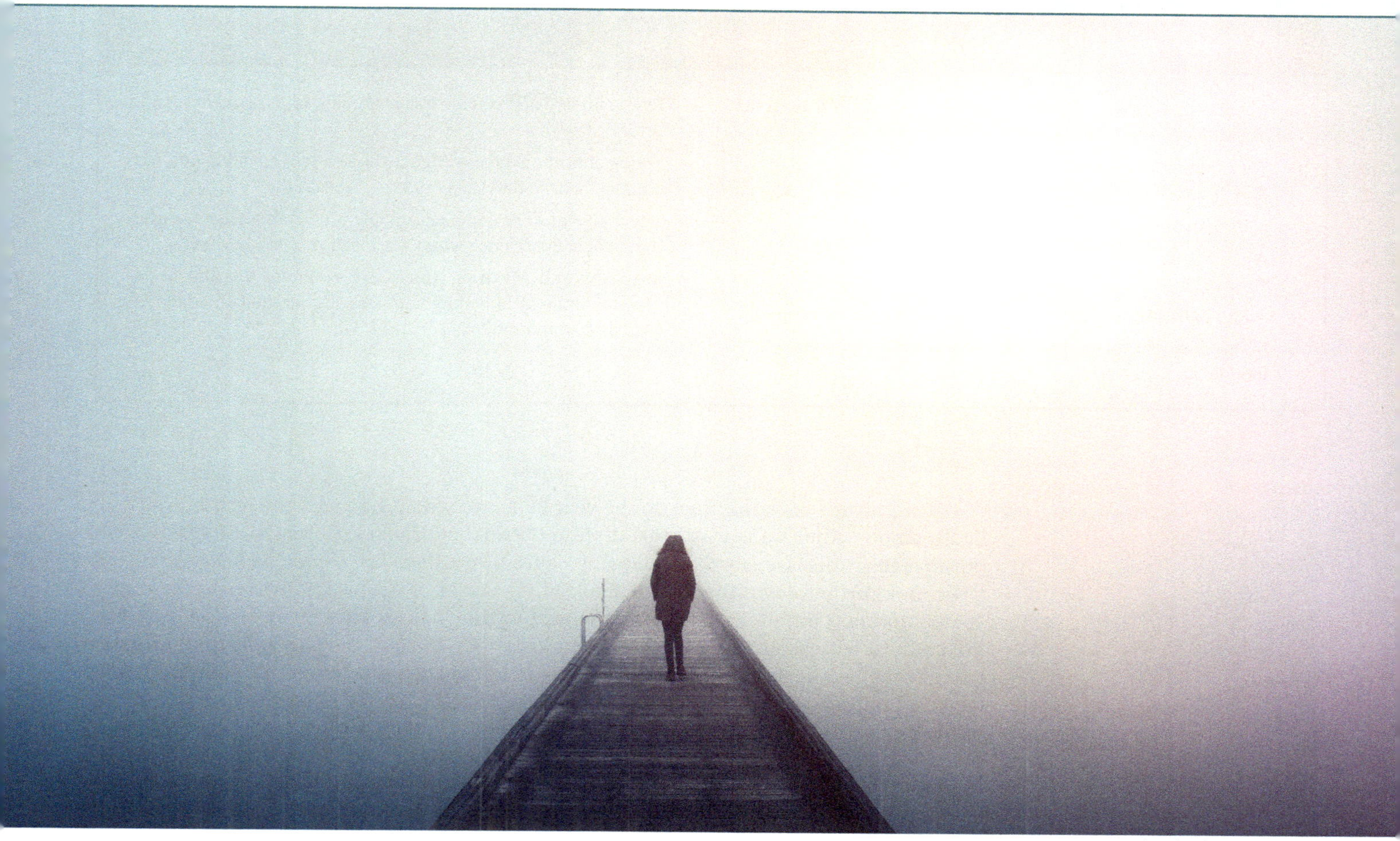

borchee/Getty Images

Chronic Diseases and End-of-Life Issues

LEARNING OBJECTIVES

After studying this chapter, you will be able to ...

1. **Identify** behavioral factors in the development and management of diabetes.
2. **Identify** behavioral factors in managing arthritis.
3. **Identify** behavioral factors in managing asthma.
4. **Describe** the major features of Alzheimer's disease and the challenges it poses to people with the disease and caregivers.
5. **Define** death, and **discuss** whether there are stages of dying.
6. **Identify** where people die, and **discuss** the challenges facing healthcare professionals, such as hospice workers.
7. **Identify** the various types of euthanasia, and **discuss** the legal and ethical issues associated with each one.
8. **Discuss** bereavement, focusing on bereavement over the life span and whether there are stages of grieving.

Did You Know That ...

- About 1 in 4 people with diabetes doesn't know they have the disease?
- There are more than 100 arthritic diseases?
- Alzheimer's and other dementias are not a normal consequence of aging?
- A person may stop breathing and have no heartbeat but still be alive?
- About half of the deaths in the United States occur in hospitals?
- Many hospice nurses find themselves battling "compassion fatigue"?
- Physician-assisted suicide for terminally ill patients is legal in several states?
- Young children who experience the death of a sibling or a parent may believe that the person will regain life?
- There appear to be some reasonably predictable stages of grief that people experience when a beloved person has died?
- Mexicans and Mexican Americans celebrate the *Dia de los Muertos* as a way of coping with loss and, in the United States, with discrimination?

If we turned back the clock to the year 1920, we would find that the leading cause of death among Americans was heart disease ("Principal Causes of Death," 1921). It turns out that heart disease is still the leading cause of death today, some 100 years later. But if we look further down the lists of the leading causes of death then and now, we notice some important differences. In 1920, the next leading causes after heart disease were two infectious diseases, pneumonia and tuberculosis (TB). In 2018, the only infectious diseases to make the list of leading causes of death were influenza and pneumonia, which together occupied 8th place (Xu et al., 2020a). In 2020, of course, COVID-19 added markedly to the number of deaths to infectious disease. On the other hand, TB has been nearly eradicated in the United States, with cases hitting an all-time low in 2018 (Talwar et al., 2019). However, TB remains one of the top 10 causes of death worldwide, underscoring the disparities in health care between Western countries like the United States and less developed countries.

Many people 100 years ago were stricken with life-threatening childhood illnesses and didn't survive to maturity. Others were felled in midlife by infectious diseases. Many infectious diseases that were scourges in the United States 100 years ago, like smallpox, TB, and childhood diseases such as mumps and measles, have been largely controlled or eliminated altogether as a result of public health efforts, widespread vaccination, and improved sanitation. With the exception of unpredictable pandemics, Americans today are more likely to die of noncommunicable diseases than from communicable diseases caused by infectious agents (Glanz et al., 2015a,b). Heart disease accounts for more than 10 times the numbers of deaths as pneumonia and influenza combined.

Among lifestyle and behavioral factors contributing to a reduced lifespan today, it is smoking, divorce, and alcohol abuse that top the list (Puterman et al., 2021). You can probably figure out why smoking and alcohol abuse are at the top of the list, as we know they contribute to serious chronic diseases such as cancer, but what about divorce? If you think about, it's not too surprising, as the psychological adjustment to a divorce is often a significant source of stress that may impact a person's long-term health, especially in cases in which financial hardship becomes a prominent issue as household funds and incomes are divided in the aftermath of the marital dissolution.

Differences in the leading causes of death between 1920 and 2020 are also explained by the greater life expectancy we enjoy today. The average baby born in 1920 could expect to live about 54 years. Today, the average life span is about 76 years. With people living longer today than their counterparts 100 years ago, they are more prone to develop noncommunicable (noninfectious) chronic diseases that tend to affect people as they age, such as heart disease, cancer, stroke, and Alzheimer's disease. The good news is that adopting healthier behaviors, such as being physically active, avoiding smoking, adopting a healthful diet, and drinking in moderation or not at all, can help protect us from many chronic diseases (Hagger et al., 2020). Medical checkups can help detect health problems when they are at their earliest and most treatable stages.

Now the bad news. Life expectancy in the United States declined from 2020 to 2021, from 77 years on the average to 76.4 years (Kuehn, 2023; Xu et al., 2023). The main reason for the decline, as you might guess, was COVID-19. By 2021, life expectancy in the United States, which had stagnated for some 30 years (Puterman et al., 2020), had reached the lowest level since 1996. Besides COVID-19, another major contribution to the decline are drug overdoses, a sad by-product of the opioid crisis we discussed in Chapter 9 and overdoses involving the very powerful opiate, *fentanyl.*

In Chapters 12 and 13 we discussed the chronic diseases of cardiovascular disorders and cancer. The focus of this chapter is on other chronic diseases that threaten our health, well-being, and survival, and the role of health psychology in helping people cope with living these major health challenges. We also discuss end-of-life issues that people may face as they approach life's final chapter.

Diabetes

Diabetes affects more than 37 million Americans, or about 1 in 10 people in the United States, and results in more than 100,000 deaths annually, making it the eighth leading cause of death in the country (CDC, 2023a, 2023b). It also contributes to more than 250,000 other deaths, mostly from heart disease. About 1.4 million new cases of diabetes occur annually in the United States (ADA, 2023). Because the symptoms of diabetes may not be obvious, about 1 in 4 people with the disease don't know they have it. But ignorance is far from bliss, as failure to control diabetes can lead to serious complications, even death.

diabetes A metabolic disease involving either insufficient production of insulin by the pancreas or failure of cells to properly use insulin, leading to the buildup of dangerously high sugar levels in the blood; properly called *diabetes mellitus*.

What Is Diabetes?

Diabetes (the proper medical term is *diabetes mellitus*) is a metabolic disorder in which the level of glucose (sugar) in the bloodstream is dangerously high. More than one in three Americans, which comes to more than 80 million people have *prediabetes*, a condition in which their blood sugar levels are higher than normal but not high enough to be diagnosed as diabetes (CDC, 2023a). About 1 in 5 adolescents and about 1 in 4 young adults are prediabetic (Andes et al., 2019). Obesity is a clear risk factor for both prediabetes and diabetes. People with prediabetes do not inevitably develop diabetes and in fact may be able to delay or prevent the development of the disease through a combination of weight loss, exercise, and possibly medication.

Glucose is a type of sugar and the major source of fuel the body uses for growth and energy. It is derived from the food we consume. Insulin, a hormone made by the pancreas, helps cells draw in glucose from the bloodstream. Most of the food we eat is converted into glucose by the liver, which then releases it into the bloodstream to be used by cells throughout the body.

Insulin works like a key in a lock, opening glucose receptors on cells so that glucose can be taken in. Normally, the pancreas regulates the appropriate amount of insulin the body needs. But in diabetes, the pancreas produces either too little insulin or none at all, or the insulin it does produce is not used efficiently by body cells. The result is that too much glucose accumulates in the blood, a condition called **hyperglycemia** (elevated blood sugar). Glucose in the bloodstream is ultimately excreted in urine, even as body cells remain starved for the glucose they need to function effectively. Cells then begin burning fat and even muscle as fuel. Excess glucose in the blood can also damage bodily organs, causing a range of serious health problems, such as heart disease, stroke, high blood pressure, kidney disease, dental disease, blindness, and lower-limb amputations (due to circulatory problems).

hyperglycemia A condition of elevated blood sugar.

Although we lack a cure for diabetes, people can practice self-management skills that help them manage the disease to avoid negative health outcomes (Fredrix et al., 2018). But effective self-management of diabetes is often difficult, complex, and challenging (Lee et al., 2019). Health psychologists work along with medical professionals to help people with diabetes make the lifestyle adjustments needed to manage the disease.

Types of Diabetes

There are three major types of diabetes: Type 1 diabetes, Type 2 diabetes, and gestational diabetes, which only affects pregnant women.

Type 1 diabetes A type of diabetes that usually develops in childhood or young adulthood, involving deficient production of insulin by the pancreas and need for daily doses of insulin. Previously labeled *juvenile diabetes* or *insulin-dependent diabetes mellitus*.

Type 1 Diabetes **Type 1 diabetes** typically develops in childhood or early adulthood. Formerly called *insulin-dependent diabetes mellitus* or *juvenile-onset diabetes*, it occurs when the body's own immune system attacks and destroys insulin-producing cells in the pancreas. Type 1 diabetes, which accounts for about 5–10% of cases of diabetes, is treated with daily injections of insulin (CDC, 2023a). If left untreated, it can induce a life-threatening coma.

Type 2 diabetes The most common type of diabetes, which typically develops in middle or later adulthood, in which body tissues develop a resistance to insulin. Previously labeled *adult-onset diabetes* or *non-insulin-dependent diabetes mellitus*.

Type 2 Diabetes **Type 2 diabetes** accounts for 90–95% of diabetes (CDC, 2023a). More than 200,000 new cases are reported each year. Formerly called *adult-onset diabetes* or *non-insulin-dependent diabetes mellitus*, Type 2 diabetes more commonly develops among overweight people in middle or late adulthood. In Type 2 diabetes there is either too much glucose in the blood or cells in the muscles, fat, and liver are not able to use insulin effectively, a condition called *insulin resistance*, which is the driving force behind the development of Type 2 diabetes. As the body places greater demands on the pancreas to produce more insulin, over time the ability of the pancreas to continue pumping out insulin declines, causing blood glucose levels to rise and leading to the development of diabetes.

Symptoms of Type 2 diabetes usually develop gradually and may go unnoticed. Common symptoms include increased thirst, hunger, and urination; tiring easily, blurred vision, and unexplained weight loss. Though Type 2 diabetes usually occurs after 45 years of age, incidence rates among younger adults are on the rise, an unfortunate consequence of the increasing prevalence of obesity in our society, even among younger adults (Nolt, 2018).

gestational diabetes A type of diabetes affecting pregnant women, characterized by insulin resistance.

Gestational Diabetes **Gestational diabetes**, which affects some women during pregnancy, is characterized by insulin resistance. Medical treatment is needed to ensure the blood glucose level remains within a normal level during pregnancy. Gestational diabetes generally disappears after childbirth but is associated with an increased risk of development of Type 2 diabetes later in life.

Risk Factors for Diabetes

Genetics plays a role in the development of diabetes, as it does in many chronic health conditions. Though we can't alter our genetic or family history, several factors that are potentially controllable increase our risk potential, especially excess body weight. Practicing healthier behaviors can reduce the risk of diabetes or delay its onset—behaviors such as adopting a healthful eating plan to lose excess weight, avoiding smoking, and exercising regularly (Diabetes Prevention Program Research Group, 2015; Nolt, 2018).

Health psychologists are at the vanguard of helping people with diabetes and those at high risk of developing the disease manage self-care behaviors, such as managing weight by adopting healthier dietary and exercise habits. As increasing numbers of young adults are affected by diabetes, even emerging adults in the 18–25-year age range, health psychologists are focusing on self-management of the disease in that age group. Guided by the biopsychosocial model, these self-management efforts include medical, social, and behavioral factors, as shown in **Figure 14.1**.

Ethnic and racial minority groups in the United States—non-Hispanic Black Americans, American Indian/Alaska Native Americans, and Latinos/Hispanics—have higher than average rates of diabetes (Helgeson, 2019; NIDDK, 2019; Ross et al., 2021). Although genetic factors may be involved, these population groups tend to have more risk factors for diabetes, including greater prevalence of overweight and obesity.

Managing Diabetes

Diabetes is a chronic disease that requires lifelong management. A comprehensive treatment approach incorporates control of blood glucose levels through continuous blood glucose

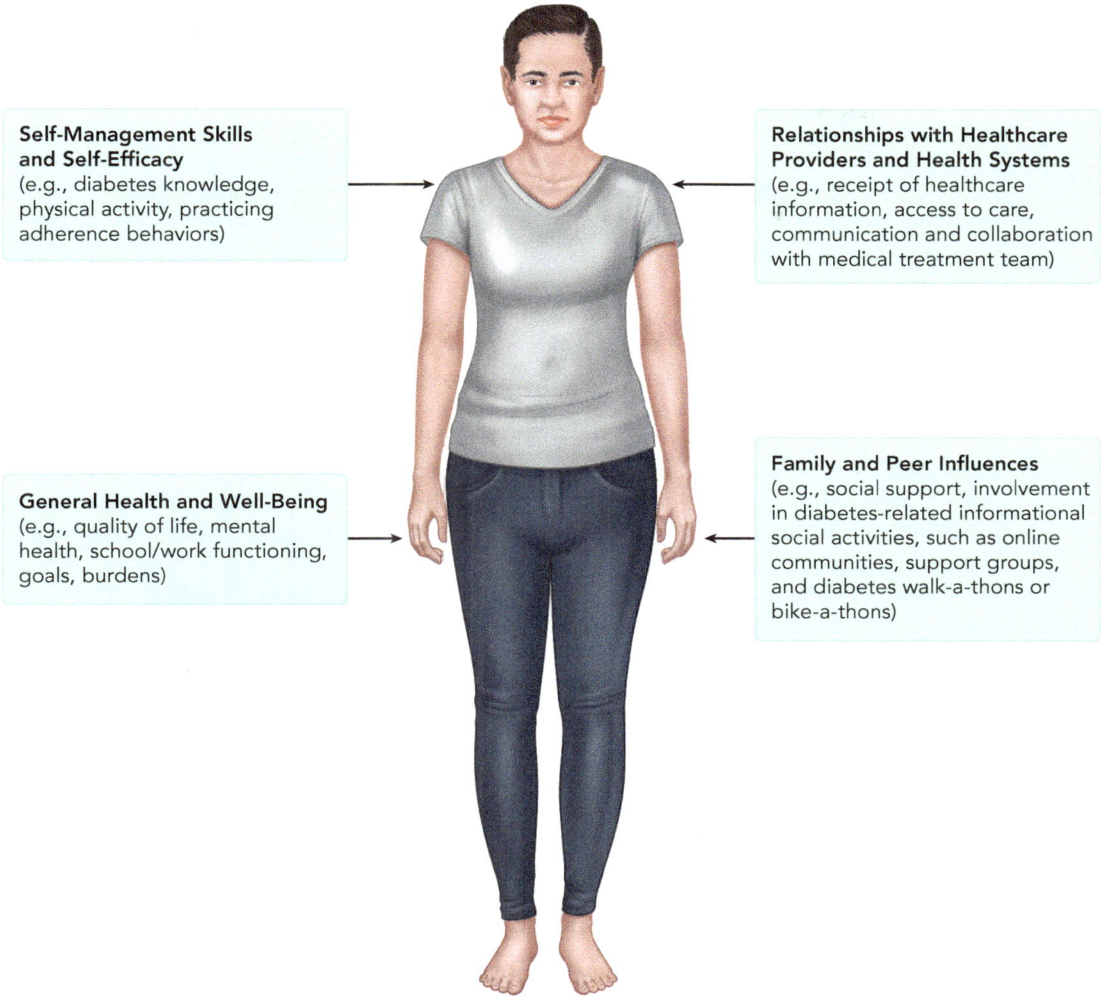

FIGURE 14.1 Modifiable Factors Associated with Positive Adaptations to the Demands of Managing Diabetes

Source: Adapted from Corathers et al. (2019). Depression screening of adolescents with diabetes: 5 years of implementation and outcomes. *Journal of the American Academy of Child and Adolescent Psychiatry*, *58*(6), 628–632.

monitoring (daily testing of blood sugar levels); following a healthful, low-sugar diet; increasing physical activity; and taking daily medication or daily insulin injections if needed to regulate blood sugar levels. Many people with Type 2 diabetes do not require daily insulin injections if they are able to control their blood sugar levels with diet, exercise, and oral medication.

Health psychologists have identified various psychological factors affecting diabetes self-management, including perceptions of personal effectiveness or self-efficacy for managing the day-to-day adjustments needed to maintain control of blood sugar (Helgeson, 2019). Not surprisingly, people who are depressed are less able to optimally manage their diabetes and as a result show poorer control of their blood sugar levels (glycemic control) (Schmitt et al., 2021).

Knowledge about how to manage the disease is not sufficient to ensure effective self-care. Knowledge must be translated into action. Health psychologists and other health professionals can be effective in helping people living with diabetes boost confidence in their ability to carry out appropriate self-management behaviors. They then help people follow through with making healthful changes in their daily behaviors. In addition, cognitive behavior therapy may be used to combat depression, which is a common mental health problem faced by people with diabetes (Kanapathy & Bogle, 2019). Evidence shows that psychological interventions are helpful in improving control of blood sugar and reducing psychological distress in people with Type 2 diabetes (Pouwer & Speight, 2019).

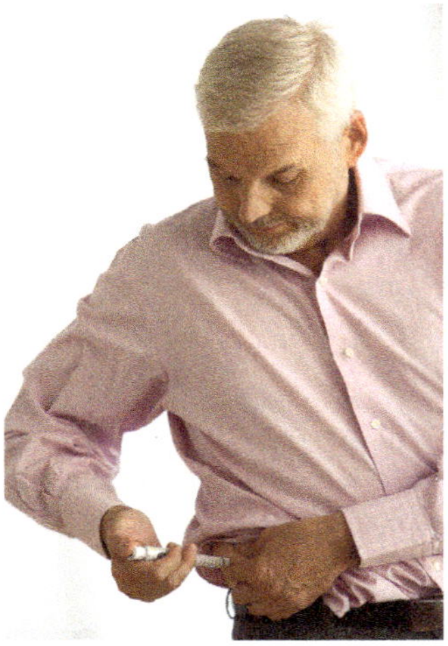

Philippe Garo/Science Source

Self-Injection with an Insulin Pen to Treat Diabetes

Recently health psychologists interviewed people who were successfully controlling their Type 1 diabetes in an attempt to determine common themes involved in successful self-management practices (Smith et al., 2018). The investigators found that people whose diabetes was well controlled were able to accept their condition and to learn to master it through developing self-management behaviors.

Family members and friends play pivotal roles in helping people manage diabetes effectively. We know that negative interactions, such as criticism, nagging, and arguing, are associated with poorer diabetes self-care and control of blood sugar levels (Lee et al., 2019). A primary focus of health psychologists is working with people with diabetes and their family members to build more positive interactions within the family. One relationship factor drawing interest among health psychologists is *autonomy support*, the kind of support seen in the willingness of a family member to just listen to the person with diabetes and to respect the person's health choices. A recent health psychology study identified the friend or family member who was most directly involved in the health care of the person with diabetes—the support person most likely to be there to remind them to take their medication or help motivate them to exercise. The researchers found that when the person with diabetes perceived there to be greater autonomy support from the support person, the person with diabetes had higher levels of self-efficacy for managing diabetes, lower distress about the disease, and more consistent self-monitoring of blood sugar levels (Lee et al., 2019).

Effective diabetes management requires a close coordination of treatment services, but people from ethnic minority and socially disadvantaged groups may face gaps in treatment owing to factors such as lack of insurance coverage, low utilization of services, and language barriers (Marquez et al., 2019). Comprehensive models of care need to take sociocultural factors into account to ensure that people with diabetes from all population groups receive the care they need to manage their disease.

Before moving on, let us note progress in the battle against diabetes. Newly diagnosed cases of diabetes have declined by about a third since 2009, driven in part, health officials believe, by changes in the nation's diet and exercise patterns (CDC, 2019a; Kuehn, 2019). This progress underscores the importance of addressing behavioral risk factors and what can be accomplished by helping people change their lifestyles. Much remains to be done, as the nation faces 1.43 million new cases of diabetes annually, and most of these cases involve Type 2 diabetes, a form of diabetes in which lifestyle factors play a prominent role. As CDC official Ann Albright described the recent decline in new cases, "The findings suggest that our work to stem the tide of Type 2 diabetes may be working—but we still have a very long way to go" (CDC, 2019a).

Health Psychology in the Digital Age

Texting to Manage Diabetes

Health psychologists recognize that management of chronic health conditions, like diabetes, requires lifestyle adjustments that include close monitoring of blood sugar levels and making adaptive behavioral changes in daily eating and exercise habits. Texting may be a useful tool for healthcare providers to keep in daily contact with people they are treating for diabetes. Recently researchers in New Zealand added text messaging to usual treatment to see if daily text prompts would improve clinical outcomes (Dobson et al., 2018; Mueller, 2018). One group of participants received individualized text messages that provided information, support and motivation, along with gentle reminders about the need to practice healthful behaviors and self-care. The texts also prompted the people with diabetes to text back their blood glucose test results. After a 9-month trial, people who received text messages showed modestly better improvements in blood sugar control than those who received usual care. Adding texting also improved other treatment outcomes relating to improvements in health. Most of the people in the texting condition were happy with the program and would recommend it to others. It turns out that texting health-related messages can be good medicine.

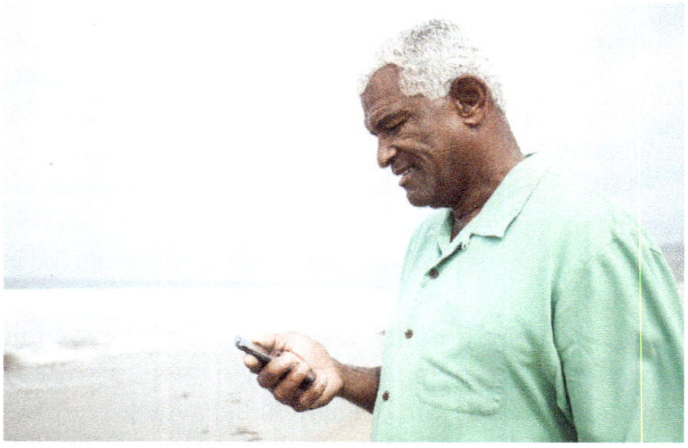

adamkaz/Getty Images

Texting for Self-Care Researchers find that adding text messaging to usual treatment can improve clinical outcomes in people with diabetes.

Review 14.1

INTERACTIVE SELF-SCORING QUIZZES

Sentence Completion

1. Diabetes affects nearly (1% or 10%) of the population.
2. __________ is a hormone that helps cells draw glucose from the bloodstream.
3. There are three major types of diabetes—type 1 diabetes, type 2 diabetes, and __________ diabetes.
4. Type (1 or 2) diabetes accounts for 90–95% of cases of diabetes.
5. Non-Hispanic Americans, American Indian/Alaska Native Americans, and Latino/Hispanic Americans have (higher than or lower than) average rates of diabetes.
6. Newly diagnosed cases of diabetes have (increased or decreased) by about a third since 2009.

Think About It

Do you or does someone you know have diabetes? What steps can you or they make to manage the disease more effectively? What can you do to reduce your risk factors for diabetes?

Arthritis

Arthritis is the commonly used term to refer to a group of more than 100 arthritic conditions or diseases that involve inflammation of the joints. Symptoms typically progress over time and include swelling, stiffness, and pain in the joints. The disease may progress to a loss of function and restricted mobility or movement. Though children can be affected by arthritis, it more commonly develops in middle or late adulthood. More than one in five American adults (22%), which amounts to more than 50 million people, have arthritis or a related condition (Eustice, 2022).

arthritis A general term for a group of diseases characterized by inflammation of one or more body joints and typically accompanied by pain, stiffness, and swelling of joints.

Types of Arthritis

Two of the most common arthritic diseases are *osteoarthritis* (OA), a painful, degenerative disease characterized by wear and tear on the joints, and *rheumatoid arthritis*, a chronic inflammation of the membranes lining the joints that causes joint pain that can lead to physical limitations due to joint damage if the disease is not controlled. In rheumatoid arthritis, the body's immune system attacks its own tissues, causing inflammation that can lead to severe disabilities as a result of joint damage (see Figure 14.2). About three times as many women as men suffer from rheumatoid arthritis. It most commonly affects joints in the knees, lower back, hips, neck, and fingers and hands.

Although specific symptoms of the disease depend upon the type of arthritis, all forms of the disease involve inflammation, pain, and stiffness in one or more joints (DeLongis et al., 2019). Fatigue is also a frequent complaint of people with arthritis, which may dampen their mood during the day (Hegarty et al., 2016). Reducing fatigue may have a side benefit with respect to improving daily moods.

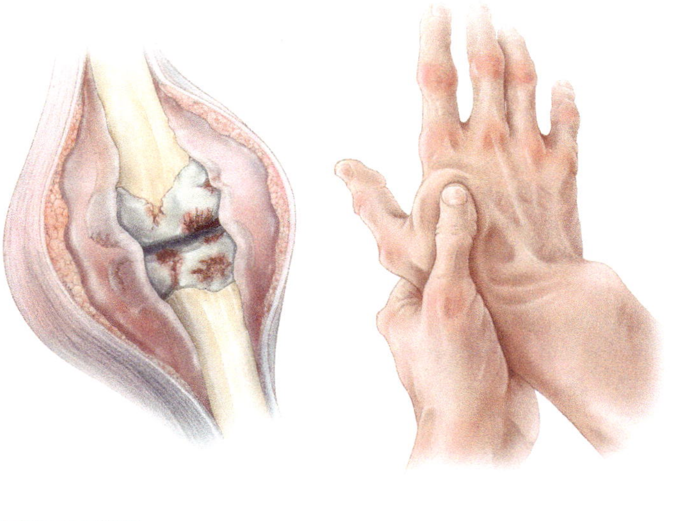

Evan Oto/Science Source

FIGURE 14.2 Rheumatoid Arthritis Rheumatoid arthritis is an autoimmune inflammatory disease that primarily affects joints but can spread to other areas of the body, such as the heart or lungs. Abnormal interactions between white blood cells initiate an autoimmune response against healthy tissue, promoting the inflammation of synovial joints. As a result, excess synovial fluid containing white blood cells, cytokines, and antibodies begins collecting in the joint cavity. As the disease progresses, the synovial membrane surrounding the joint begins to thicken as cartilage and bone are gradually eroded. This can eventually lead to pain, limited movement or deformity of the joint, as well as fever or fatigue. Rheumatoid arthritis is more common during middle age, and women and those with genetic susceptibility are more likely to be affected. Although rheumatoid arthritis is a chronic disease, medications or physical therapy can help slow its progression and damage to joints.

Treatment of Arthritis

People living with arthritis face many challenges coping with pain and stiffness and physical limitations, especially in more severe cases of joint damage. A class of anti-inflammatories called *NSAIDs* (nonsteroidal anti-inflammatory drugs), which includes the commonly used over-the-counter pain relievers aspirin, *ibuprofen* (brand names Advil and Motrin), and *naproxen* (brand name Aleve), is widely used to treat inflammation and pain of arthritis. More powerful NSAIDs available by prescription may be used if necessary, but when used routinely, all NSAIDs carry a risk of gastrointestinal problems. If anti-inflammatories aren't sufficient to control the pain and inflammation of arthritis, treatment providers may prescribe biologic drugs, such as *adalimumab* (brand name Humira), that block the source of inflammation but carry a risk of potentially serious side effects and complications. Physical therapy or occupational therapy may be recommended to help with joint mobility and to reduce pain. Evidence shows that both types of therapy can reduce pain in people with arthritis (Park & Shang, 2016).

Psychological interventions, especially cognitive behavior therapy, is often used alongside medication, especially when medication is not sufficient to control symptoms (DeLongis et al., 2019). Specific treatment techniques parallel those used in psychological treatment of other types of pain, such as helping people combat catastrophizing tendencies, challenge and correct negative and distorted thoughts, and increase adaptive behaviors. Psychological interventions may also be needed to treat depression that many people experience in the face of coping with arthritis. Arthritis is also associated with high rates of suicidal ideation (J. H. Park et al., 2019).

Coping with arthritis, like coping with other chronic diseases, may involve passive or avoidant efforts, which are characterized by disengagement or denial, or active coping efforts, which involve approach-oriented coping by directly dealing with the illness and its effects. Examples of active coping include keeping abreast of the latest medical developments and treatments, using medication and physical therapy as directed by healthcare providers, and making efforts to compensate for any loss of function. People with arthritis who use more active, approach-oriented styles of coping tend to be better adjusted and more effective in managing the disease (DeLongis et al., 2019).

Review 14.2

INTERACTIVE SELF-SCORING QUIZZES

Sentence Completion

1. Two of the most common arthritic diseases are __________, a painful, degenerative disease characterized by wear and tear on the joints, and rheumatoid arthritis.
2. Arthritis involves __________, pain, and stiffness in one or more joints.
3. A class of drugs called anti-__________ is widely used to treat inflammation and pain of arthritis.
4. __________ drugs block the source of inflammation in arthritis.
5. People with arthritis who use more active, __________-oriented styles of coping tend to be better adjusted.

Think About It

Do you or someone you know suffer from arthritis? If yes, what form of arthritis do you or they have? How is it affecting your or their life? What steps can you or they take to manage the disease more effectively?

Asthma

asthma A chronic lung disease involving temporary obstruction of the bronchial airways (bronchi), leading to attacks of wheezing and difficulty breathing.

Asthma is a chronic disease affecting about 25 million Americans, including about 6 million children (CDC, 2019i). Nearly 8% of children and adults in the United States have asthma. The disease is more common in boys than girls, but among teens and adults, more women are affected (NHLBI, 2019b). Although asthma can affect anyone at any age, it typically starts in childhood.

The prevalence of asthma has been rising rapidly, more than doubling in the past 30 years, which underscores the need for expansion of existing asthma control programs. Public health programs are of greatest need in poorer, inner-city neighborhoods, which are burdened by high rates of asthma and deaths due to the disease (Sullivan et al., 2019a; Sweenie et al., 2020). The clustering of cases of asthma in more distressed neighborhoods may reflect a range of factors, including poorer access to healthcare services, greater exposure to environmental pollution, and higher levels of psychosocial stress. Higher prevalence and mortality rates are also found among Black Americans and Puerto Ricans (NHLBI, 2019b; Wechsler et al., 2019). The COVID-19 pandemic increased racial disparities in health outcomes, and especially so with asthma, due to various complex factors (Willems, Castells, & Baptist, 2022). **Figure 14.3** shows the prevalence of asthma in relation to the major population groups in the United States.

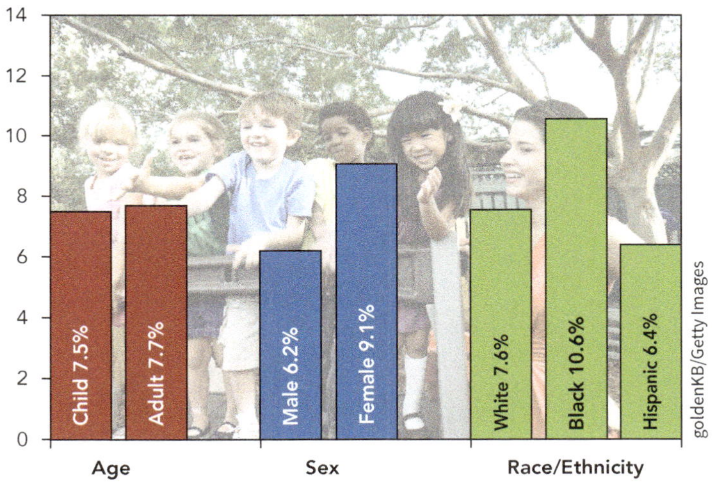

FIGURE 14.3 Current Asthma Prevalence, in Percentages, by Age, Sex, and Race/Ethnicity, United States

Source: National Center for Environmental Health (2020). Asthma surveillance data. https://www.cdc.gov/asthma/asthmadata.htm

Asthma Attacks

In asthma, the breathing passages in the lungs become narrow and swollen, which can lead to "attacks" (see **Figure 14.4**). Symptoms of an asthma attack include wheezing, coughing, and difficulty breathing, which in severe cases can cause death. Nearly 200 children and more than 3,000 adults die of asthmatic attacks each year in the United States (CDC, 2019i). Asthmatic attacks vary in intensity, lasting from minutes to hours. During an attack it may feel as if one is suffocating. Recurring attacks can damage the bronchial system, causing muscles involved in breathing to lose their elasticity and their capacity for movement.

Causal Factors in Asthma

Asthma involves an overreaction of the body's immune system to allergens in the environment, causing inflammation in the bronchial passages, which leads to a narrowing of the airways that can block the flow of air (CDC, 2019i). When symptoms become severe, an asthmatic attack may occur, which can be triggered by many factors, including allergens (e.g., pollen, ragweed, animal dander, and dust) in the air, environmental pollutants

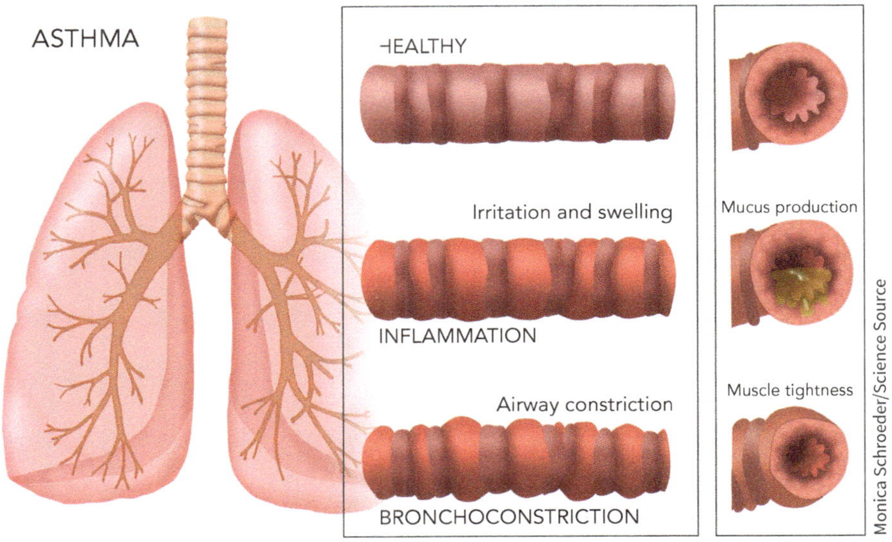

FIGURE 14.4 The Development of Constriction of Small Airways in the Lungs—Bronchioles, Resulting in Asthma At top right is a healthy bronchiole; the middle illustration shows some inflammation and mucus production; and in the bottom illustration, the bronchiole has narrowed and the airway is constricted.

that irritate the lungs (e.g., cigarette smoke and air pollution), strenuous exercise, and even intense anger or crying, which can cause hyperventilation and narrowing of the airways (NHLBI, 2019b). Even intense laughter can trigger an attack. Psychological factors, including stress, anxiety, and depression, also may increase the risk of asthmatic attacks (Meuret et al., 2020; Voelker, 2012).

Psychological factors play important roles in determining the severity of asthmatic attacks and the emotional consequences of living with asthma. Depression is more prevalent among people with asthma than it is in the general population and is linked to poorer control of the disease (Vargas, 2020). Another common feature of asthma is anxiety, which is also linked to poorer asthma control (González-Freire et al., 2019).

Treating Asthma

Although there is no cure for asthma, it can usually be controlled by avoiding exposure to allergens, undergoing desensitization therapy (allergy shots) to allow the body to become resistant to particular allergens, and using prescribed medications, such as *bronchodilators* that open blocked airways during asthma attacks and *anti-inflammatories* that help prevent asthma attacks from occurring by reducing swelling in the bronchial tubes, helping to keep them open. Biologic medicines, administered by injection every few weeks, may also be used to dampen the body's response to allergens (NHLBI, 2019).

Psychological interventions are often useful in helping people with asthma learn to cope with their symptoms (González-Freire et al., 2019). Cognitive behavior therapy focuses on changing negative thinking patterns that can trigger asthmatic attacks, such as perceptions of helplessness, and catastrophizing or assuming the worst. Behavioral techniques, such as relaxation training, sometimes used along with biofeedback, can help people with asthma learn to control stress and anxiety, which, in turn, can improve their respiratory function. Family therapy may also help control symptoms by changing dysfunctional family dynamics—another source of stress—in families of children with asthma.

Psychologists play important roles in the treatment process. They are often a part of an integrated treatment approach to help people with asthma develop active coping skills to

Health Psychology in Action

Addressing Health Disparities in Asthma Control

Children with asthma from minority, low-income families in inner-city areas face significant barriers in accessing health care, leading to higher rates of poorly controlled asthma. To make care more accessible, asthma specialists in Cincinnati, Ohio, teamed with a behavioral health psychologist to provide treatment to children with uncontrolled asthma in several inner-city, economically disadvantaged schools (Lin et al., 2020). The asthma specialists (pulmonologists and allergists) used a telehealth model in which they interacted with the children during the school day via video-conferencing software. They also used an electronic medication sensor to monitor the children's daily use of an inhaler and bronchodilator medication via a smartphone app or electronic hub. The health psychologist provided counseling sessions in the school focusing on asthma management skills. The results of the 6-month intervention showed improvements in asthma symptom control, demonstrating that a multicomponent treatment approach that provided medical and psychological services directly in a school-based setting can have a beneficial effect on the health of children who might otherwise lack access to healthcare services.

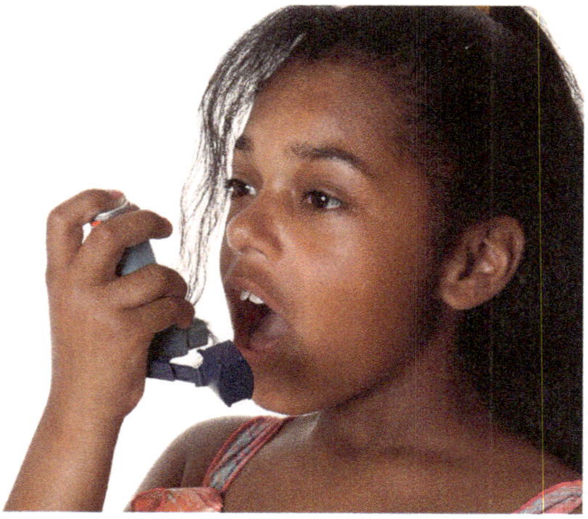

princessdlaf/Getty Images

A Girl with Asthma Using an Inhaler Use of a school-based care delivery model may help overcome barriers to access to healthcare services experienced by economically disadvantaged children with asthma.

manage stress, such as deep breathing exercises and relaxation skills. Self-management skills are especially important in helping people with asthma manage their medication and symptoms, as well as the psychological consequences of their illness. Behavioral research shows that people with asthma who rely on avoidant coping, such as tendencies to avoid thinking about asthma and not making efforts to control it, show less adherence to medical treatment and have poorer asthma control than people who adopt more active coping skills (González-Freire et al., 2019; Voorhees et al., 2020). In developing active coping skills, people with asthma come to accept the disease while maintaining an optimistic attitude about their ability to control it (Baiardini et al., 2015; Pappalardo & Martin, 2020). Coping skills training also increase people's sense of self-efficacy in handling the demands of living with asthma (Schreitmüller & Loerbroks, 2020).

Self-Management of Asthma

Learning to live with asthma involves making lifestyle adjustments to keep symptoms in check, including the following (NHLBI, 2019b; Voorhees et al., 2020):

- *Lose excess weight:* Obesity is implicated as a risk factor for asthma, so losing excess weight, even a 5–10% weight loss, can help reduce symptoms.
- *Become physically active:* Though strenuous exercise may trigger an asthmatic attack in susceptible individuals, health officials do not advise that asthma sufferers avoid physical activity. People living with asthma should discuss with their doctors what level of physical activity is appropriate for them.
- *Eat right:* Following a healthy diet rich in fruits and vegetables, and meeting recommended guidelines for vitamin D, can help with asthma control as well as contributing to other positive health outcomes.
- *Manage stress:* Stress can increase the risk of asthmatic attacks, so learning skills of turning down the body's alarm reaction, as by using relaxation and deep-breathing techniques, can help control symptoms.
- *Avoid exposure to tobacco smoke:* Tobacco smoke can induce an asthma attack, so it is important for asthma sufferers to avoid smoking (as it is for us all) and exposure to second-hand smoke.

Taking stock of our health behavior is important to us all, not just to people facing the challenge of living with a chronic condition. We noted at the end of the chapter on cardiovascular health (Chapter 12) that better-educated people—that means you—are more likely to alter unhealthy behavior patterns and to reap the benefits of change. College may not only help you prepare for a better job; it may save your life.

Review 14.3

INTERACTIVE SELF-SCORING QUIZZES

Sentence Completion

1. Asthma is a chronic disease affecting about (10 or 25) million Americans.

2. Asthma is more common in (boys or girls).

3. The prevalence of asthma has (risen or fallen) sharply in recent years.

4. __________ is more prevalent among people with asthma than it is in the general population.

5. __________ open blocked airways during asthma attacks and __________ reduce swelling in the bronchial tubes.

6. People with asthma who rely on __________ coping, such as not thinking about asthma or not making efforts to control it, show less adherence to medical treatment and poorer asthma control.

Think About It

Do you or does someone you know have asthma? If so, how does it affect your (or their) life? What lifestyle adjustments are you (or they) making to manage the disease more effectively?

Dementia and Alzheimer's Disease

dementia A syndrome comprising substantial deterioration of mental functioning.

Alzheimer's disease (AD) A progressive, deteriorative form of dementia caused by an underlying brain disorder.

Dementia is a syndrome characterized by a dramatic deterioration of mental abilities involved in thinking, memory, judgment, and reasoning. Dementia is more common among older people, but it is not considered to be a consequence of normal aging. It involves disease processes that damage brain tissue. Some of the causes of dementia are brain infections, such as meningitis, HIV, and encephalitis, as well as chronic alcoholism, infections, strokes, and tumors. But the most common cause of dementia, accounting for some 60–80% of cases, is **Alzheimer's disease (AD)** (Alzheimer's Association, 2019). AD is a chronic, progressive brain disease affecting nearly 6 million Americans. As the nation's population continues to age, the number of affected Americans is expected to reach nearly 14 million by the year 2050.

Though AD can affect people of different ages and different ethnic and racial backgrounds, it occurs more frequently among older adults, women, and Black people (Alty et al., 2022; Lennon et al., 2021; Suran et al., 2022). AD affects about 10% of people 65+ years of age and about a third of all adults over the age of 85 (Manly et al., 2022).

According to the most recent statistics, AD is the seventh leading cause of death in the United States, claiming nearly 120,000 lives annually (CDC, 2023f). The disease rarely affects people under 65 years. (**Figure 14.5**).

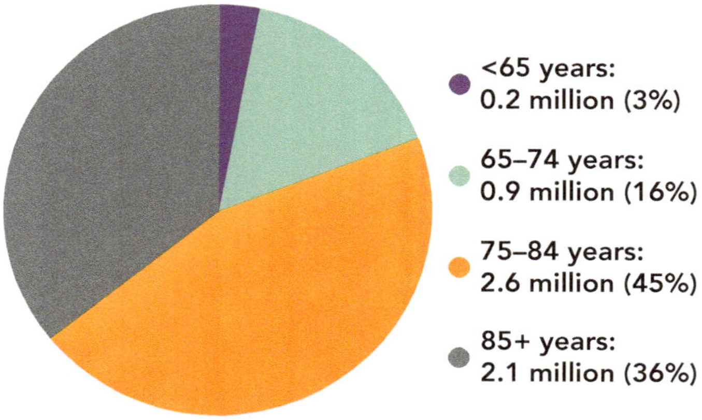

FIGURE 14.5 **Age Distribution of Cases of Alzheimer's Disease**

Source: 2019 Alzheimer's disease facts and figures, 2019. Reproduced with permission of ELSEVIER.

Features of Alzheimer's Disease

Although some forms of dementia may be reversible, such as those caused by treatable tumors or brain infections, dementia associated with AD is both irreversible and progressive. At first, the signs may be subtle or are confused with ordinary forgetfulness. Over time, however, the impairment becomes more apparent, as people with AD fail to remember names of family members (or even recognize them) and require help performing everyday activities, such as getting dressed, preparing meals, or maintaining personal hygiene. The person with AD may begin wandering off, become belligerent or overly suspicious or paranoid, and be unable to speak coherently. Although ordinary forgetfulness is common among older adults, AD involves significantly greater cognitive deficits. Think of it this way: You may occasionally forget where you left your keys, but forgetting what keys are for or how to use them is a sign of AD or other forms of dementia (IOM, 2015; Jacob et al., 2015). Though we lack a cure or effective treatment for AD, new drugs introduced in 2023 appear to modestly slow the cognitive decline we see in early stage Alzheimer's disease (Belluck, 2023; NIA, 2023; Reardon, 2023; Stern et al., 2023). These drugs target beta-amyloid build-up in the brain, which is suspected of playing an important role in the development of the disease.

A Closer Look

10 Warning Signs of Alzheimer's Disease

1. Memory loss that disrupts daily life
2. Challenges in planning or solving problems
3. Difficulty completing familiar tasks
4. Confusion with time or place
5. Trouble understanding visual images and spatial relationships
6. New problems with words in speaking or writing
7. Misplacing things and losing the ability to retrace steps
8. Decreased or poor judgment
9. Withdrawal from work or social activities
10. Changes in mood and personality

Source: Alzheimer's Association (2020). 10 early signs and symptoms of Alzheimer's. https://www.alz.org/alzheimers-dementia/10_signs

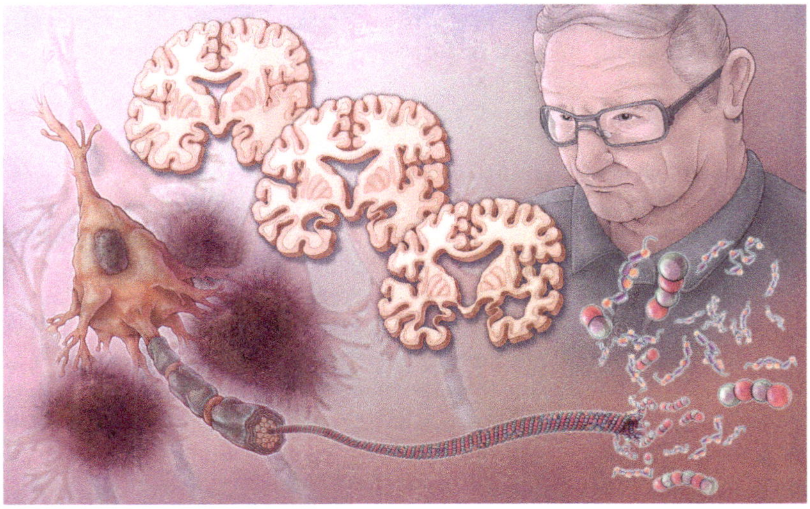

Evan Oto/Science Source

FIGURE 14.6 Alzheimer's Disease Alzheimer's disease is characterized by the progressive loss of neurons in the brain, leading to the degeneration of the cerebral cortex. Beta-amyloid peptides are proteins that can deposit outside the neuron and begin building up as amyloid plaque throughout the brain. Tau proteins normally hold microtubule subunits in the neuron together, which enables cell-to-cell communication. These tau proteins can destabilize and form neurofibrillary tangles, while the microtubules disintegrate and destroy the neuron. As plaque spreads and tangles accumulate, more neurons are destroyed or inhibited, leading to gradual atrophy of the brain and loss of cognitive function.

Causes of Alzheimer's Disease

The challenge of understanding AD highlights the delicate balance between mind and body and more specifically, how degenerative changes in the brain affect mental functioning. Although the cause or causes of AD remain unclear, researchers are focusing on two types of proteins that accumulate in the brains of people with AD, beta-amyloid and tau (Gouveia Roque et al., 2023; Paudel et al., 2024; Rajbanshi et al., 2023). These protein deposits form plaques and tangles of nerve fibers that may damage sensitive brain tissue involved in memory and other cognitive processes (see **Figure 14.6**).

One line of research raises the possibility that these abnormal protein deposits cause inflammation in the brain that damages sensitive networks of neurons involved in memory functioning and other cognitive processes (Lecca et al., 2022; Ralvenius et al., 2023). Genetic factors appear to play an important role in determining the risk of AD, just as they do in many other chronic diseases (e.g., Bourquard et al., 2023; Gao et al., 2023). Researchers also find that heart health is connected to brain health, as behavioral factors that protect the heart, such as physical activities and adoption of a heart-healthy diet, may also reduce the risk of AD (Alzheimer's Association, 2019).

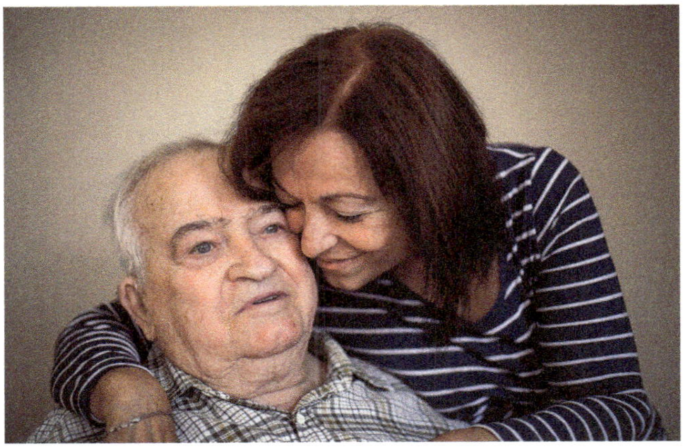

Gulcin Ragiboglu/Getty Images

Caring Takes a Toll Many caregivers suffer emotional and physical disorders from the stress of caring for a family member with Alzheimer's.

Living with Alzheimer's Disease

Alzheimer's has devastating effects on family members and caregivers as well as people with the disorder. People with AD may no longer be able to understand their situation or surroundings, becoming confused and frightened, even lashing out at family members. Caregiver burden and stress is compounded by the disturbing behaviors of the people with advanced AD, such as incontinence, screaming, wandering around the house at all hours, or wandering off by themselves. Family members may feel that they are living with a stranger who neither recognizes them nor appreciates their efforts and sacrifices. A family member of a person with AD described her life situation as a "funeral that never ends" (Aronson, 1988).

The stress of caring for a person with AD can exact a significant toll on the emotional health of family members, as about 1 in 4 suffers from clinical levels of anxiety and about 1 in 10 suffers from depression (Corrêa et al., 2019; Tentorio et al., 2020). Not surprisingly, serious physical disorders are also common among caregivers: They bear an increased risk of heart disease, cancer, and other health conditions (Russ et al., 2012). Typically, the burden of caregiving falls disproportionately on the adult daughters in the family, who may feel sandwiched between caring for the parent with AD and their own children and partners.

Many types of programs have been developed to help caregivers deal with the burdens they face. A review of evidence on interventions for caregivers of people with dementia showed that psychological help in the form of psychoeducation (teaching caregivers about the disease and how to manage problem behaviors) combined with cognitive behavior therapy (modifying dysfunctional thoughts, learning to regulate their own emotions, practicing self-care behaviors) can help reduce their distress (Cheng et al., 2019).

Review 14.4

INTERACTIVE SELF-SCORING QUIZZES

Sentence Completion

1. Dementia (is or is not) a normal consequence of aging.
2. The most common cause of dementia is __________.
3. Occasional forgetfulness (is or is not) a sign of Alzheimer's disease.
4. Alzheimer's presently affects nearly __________ million Americans.
5. Two types of abnormal protein deposits in the brain of Alzheimer's patients are beta-__________ and __________.

Think About It

Do you know someone who has Alzheimer's? How has the disease affected the person and their family members? How is the family coping? What adjustments might they make to deal better with problem behavior and their own self-care needs?

End-of-Life Issues

End-of-life issues have special poignancy as people age, in part because many of the diseases we discuss here and in Chapters 12 and 13—heart disease, cancer, diabetes, arthritis, and Alzheimer's disease—primarily affect older adults. However, death can occur at any age, a reality underscored during the COVID-19 pandemic. But even with COVID-19, the majority of deaths occurred among older adults and people affected by significant underlying health issues, such as heart disease, cancer, diabetes, and chronic respiratory disease.

In this section, we address some of the issues people and their families face during life's last passage, including stages of dying, palliative care, the living will, and bereavement. Although many of us prefer not to think about death, health issues relating to death are important to consider at whatever age we happen to be. Important questions to consider include: Should I donate my organs? Should I be buried or cremated when I die? Should I prepare a living will that gives clear directives to healthcare providers about my wishes regarding life-prolonging treatments if my medical condition is beyond hope?

Death and Dying

brain death Cessation of activity of the cerebral cortex.

How do we know that a person has died? Is it the stoppage of the heart? Of breathing? Of brain activity? Medical and legal professionals generally use **brain death** as the standard for determining that a person has died (Greer et al., 2020). The most widely used criteria for establishing brain death include absence of activity of the cerebral cortex, as shown by a flat recording of brain waves. When there is no activity in the cortex, consciousness—the sense of self and all psychological functioning—has ceased.

The broader concept of **whole-brain death** includes death of the brain stem, which is responsible for certain autonomic functions, such as reflexes like breathing (Lamb, 2020). Thus, a person who is "brain dead" can continue to breathe. In some cases people have been kept "alive," even though they were whole-brain dead, by life-support equipment that took over their breathing and circulation.

whole-brain death Cessation of activity of the cerebral cortex and of the brain stem.

Death is also a legal matter. In most states, a person is considered legally dead if there is an irreversible cessation of breathing and circulation or if there is an irreversible cessation of brain activity, including activity in the brain stem, which controls breathing (Greer et al., 2020).

Stages of Dying Death is not a part of life; it is the cessation of life. But the process of dying is a part of life that involves physical and psychological processes. From a biological standpoint, dying involves a deterioration in bodily processes needed to sustain life. Psychologically, dying involves a process of coming to terms with declining health and physical limitations and facing the prospect of imminent death. From her work with people who were terminally ill, psychiatrist Elisabeth Kübler-Ross (1969) identified five stages of dying that she believed characterized the final life passage:

1. *Denial:* In this stage people feel "Not me! It can't be me. The diagnosis must be wrong." Denial can be flat and absolute. It can fluctuate so that one minute the person accepts the medical verdict; the next, the person starts chatting animatedly about distant plans.
2. *Anger:* Denial usually gives way to anger and resentment toward the medical establishment, toward God, or toward the young and healthy ("Why me? It's so unfair. Why do I deserve this?).
3. *Bargaining:* Next, people may bargain with God to postpone death, promising, for example, to do good deeds if they are given another 6 months or another year, or just long enough to see their son or daughter graduate or get married.
4. *Depression:* A state of depression ensues with feelings of loss and hopelessness, along with grief of facing the loss of loved ones and of life itself.
5. *Final acceptance:* Ultimately, a sense of inner peace may come, a quiet acceptance of the inevitable. This "peace" is not contentment; it is nearly devoid of feeling.

Though Kübler-Ross's stages provide a useful framework for understanding how many people come to terms with dying, there are limitations to her theory. People facing impending death may not go through the same stages, or, if they do, they may not experience them in the same order. Many people facing death struggle with anxiety as well as depression. Moreover, Kübler-Ross's stages may be limited to people who receive a diagnosis of a terminal illness. Yet most people die without receiving a terminal diagnosis, so a stage model may not be of much value in understanding their adjustment. Overall, critics point to a lack of evidence supporting the validity of a stage model of dying (Corr, 2019).

Edwin Shneidman (2008), a psychologist who focused his research on suicide, recognized that people show various responses in the final stage of life, not any single sequence of responses. These responses can be fleeting or relatively stable, can ebb and flow, and can reflect pain and bewilderment. Some people become hopelessly depressed or suffer bouts of anxiety, while others show rapid changes in their mental states from day to day or hour to hour. How people respond to the end of life also reflects their own personalities and philosophies of life.

Where People Die In earlier times, most people died in their homes, surrounded by their families. Today only a minority of Americans die in their own homes. They tend to be of advanced old age or gravely or terminally ill. Many people who are terminally ill receive hospice care in their homes. According to the National Hospice and Palliative Care Organization (2020), two-thirds of people who receive hospice care die in their homes, a relative's home, a nursing home, or another residential facility. Many people, of course, die suddenly wherever they happen to be, either because of accidents, heart attacks, combat, homicide, or other unanticipated events. Overall, about half of the deaths in the United States occur in hospitals, and about 1 in 5 occur in nursing homes. Many people who are dying and their families find the hospital to be an impersonal setting in which to come to terms with impending death. Hospitals frequently do little to help prepare people who are dying and their families emotionally for impending death.

hospice An approach to caring for people who are dying using a palliative care approach in a more homelike and supportive treatment setting.

palliative care A form of medical care for terminally ill patients that focuses on support and pain relief rather than active treatment of the underlying condition.

The Hospice

A **hospice** is a treatment approach for people who are dying that provides a supportive, homelike atmosphere to make the individual's final days as meaningful and as free of pain as possible. Hospices provide **palliative care**, a form of treatment of people who are terminally ill that focuses on relief from pain and suffering rather than active treatment of disease. Historically, palliative care was developed in large part to meet the needs of people who were terminally ill with cancer. Today the increasing burdens posed by caring for people with Alzheimer's and other dementias has led to increased need for hospice services for this population. Nearly 1 in 5 hospice enrollees today are people with dementia (Hashimie et al., 2020). A hospice focuses on treating the person, not the disease, by expanding the scope of treatment to address the medical, emotional, psychological, and spiritual needs of the people who are dying as well as their families and friends. Some hospices are located in hospitals, while others are residential facilities located in the community. But most forms of hospice care are provided in the person's own home, so that final transition in life occurs in the most familiar and comfortable setting. Hospice workers enlist family and friends of the dying person to provide support through the final days. The person under hospice care is encouraged to take an active part in their own care, making decisions about their diet, activities, and pain-killing medications within the bounds set by their physical conditions. Once death occurs, hospice staff provide support to the deceased person's loved ones, helping them during their grief process.

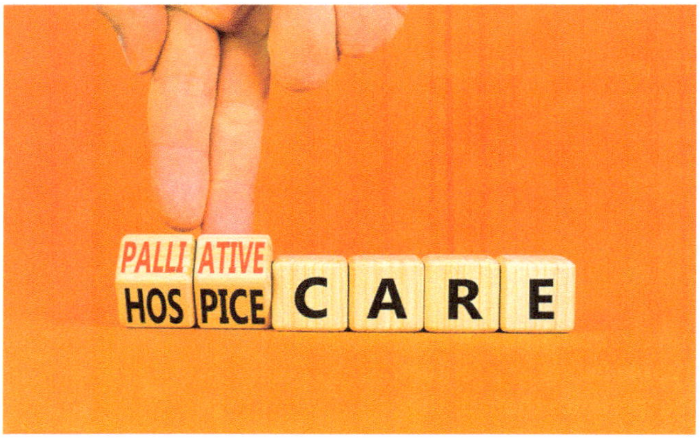

Dzmitry Dzemidovich/Getty Images

Like combat medics, hospice workers are literally surrounded by death, and they need to find the inner resources to continually provide social support to people in pain and grieving families. Perhaps it is reasonable to expect that many hospice workers experience burnout and something called *compassion fatigue* (Barnett et al., 2019; Portoghese et al., 2020). Hospice workers who develop compassion fatigue may show their emotions when it is preferable for them to be low key (Portoghese et al., 2020). It also appears that hospice volunteers vary a good deal in their resilience to being in settings with continual despair and death (Jo et al., 2020). Those who are less resilient are more likely to develop compassion fatigue, anxiety, and depression (Jo et al., 2020).

Euthanasia: Is There a Right to Die?

euthanasia The purposeful taking of life to relieve suffering.

The word **euthanasia** derived from Greek roots meaning "good" and "death." Also known as "mercy killing," euthanasia refers to the purposeful taking of a person's life through pain-free or gentle means in order to relieve pain or suffering.

Active Euthanasia: Mercy Killing or Murder?

In *active euthanasia,* a lethal treatment, usually a medication, is administered to cause a quick and pain-free death.

When euthanasia is conducted with the consent of the person it is referred to as *voluntary active euthanasia*. Voluntary active euthanasia is illegal throughout most of the United States, although there are legal challenges to the laws that prevent it. The practice is legal in many other countries, including Canada, the Netherlands, Belgium, Colombia, and parts of Australia.

Physician-assisted suicide is a form of voluntary active euthanasia in which physicians assist people with terminal or incapacitating illnesses who wish to die by providing them with lethal doses of medications or administering the medications themselves if the people are too ill to do it by themselves. Physician-assisted suicide is legal in Oregon, Washington, Montana, Vermont, and California.

Applying Health Psychology

Reflections of Hospice Patients on Wisdom and the Meaning of Life

Death is the greatest threat that humans face (Wong & Tomer, 2011). We may want to push away thoughts of our own demise or file away such thoughts in the back of our minds, along with other concerns about aging such as varicose veins, declining health and vitality, and potential dementia. But for people receiving hospice care, death is an impending reality and may evoke feelings of sheer terror and a range of negative emotions, including fear, anger, and depression, that were cataloged by Kübler-Ross. But Kübler-Ross's work also suggests that facing death can be an opportunity for personal growth and deeper reflection, not just suffering (Wong & Tomer, 2011). Psychologists recently interviewed a group of 15 dying hospice patients to learn about their perspectives on wisdom and the meaning of life (Wright et al., 2017). Their reflections, some of which are listed in the table, may be helpful to us all in thinking about the meaning of our own lives, whatever our age may be.

Theme	What They Said
On the Nature of Wisdom—Achieving Humility	"I think we should be humble. Because you know when you think you're doing really well and you're patting yourself on the back, that's probably not when you're at your best." "Wisdom is when we realize 'I don't really know much.'" "A lot of people think they have to have the answer. It is OK to say 'I don't know ...'"
On Facing Illness and Death—Changing Values and Priorities	"[Getting cancer] opens up your eyes to the possibilities of life can be cut short. I don't think people get that perspective very often ... I treat [my life] so much better as a beautiful journey and gift and don't take it lightly." "[Illness] has taught me to be a nicer person and not be in such a hurry ..." "I want to live until I die. I don't want to die until I die."
On Finding Personal Meaning—Connecting with Others	"The connection that you have with somebody else, whether it is man, woman or child ... [is what] we were put on Earth for, in my opinion ..." "... be the best I could possibly be and offer to others as much as I could possibly offer to others. Those are my goals. Nothing fancy. Very simple."

Source: Wright et al. (2017) / Reproduced with permission from Taylor & Francis Group.

The best-known cases of physician-assisted suicide were conducted by Dr. Jack Kevorkian, a retired pathologist who was dubbed "Dr. Death" by the press for having assisted in many publicized suicides. Following an assisted suicide that was aired on CBS's *60 Minutes* in 1998, Kevorkian was convicted of second-degree murder in Michigan and sentenced to 8 years in prison. Unlike Kevorkian, an activist for the legalization of euthanasia, most physicians who assist in suicides avoid public scrutiny for fear of legal prosecution and sanctions by medical societies (Yang & Curlin, 2016). In the United States, fewer than 20% of physicians report having received requests to assist people with suicide, and fewer than 5% have complied (Emanuel et al., 2016). About 70% of people who seek physician-assisted suicide have cancer.

In *involuntary active euthanasia,* a person terminates the life of another person without that person's informed consent. Involuntary active euthanasia usually involves people who are incapacitated or comatose and whose guardians believe that they would have wanted to die if they had been capable of making the decision. In the eyes of the law, involuntary active euthanasia is homicide.

Passive Euthanasia: Letting Go *Passive euthanasia* involves hastening the death of a person by withholding potentially life-saving treatments, such as not resuscitating a person who is terminally ill who has stopped breathing or withdrawing medicine, food, or life-support equipment, such as a respirator, from a person who is comatose. A form of passive euthanasia that is legal throughout the United States and Canada is the withdrawing or withholding of life-sustaining techniques or equipment from people who are terminally ill who have clearly specified that they would not wish to be kept alive by aggressive or heroic treatments. The declaration of these wishes may be in the form of a living will (discussed next), which specifies the conditions under which the person desires to have life-sustaining treatment withdrawn or withheld.

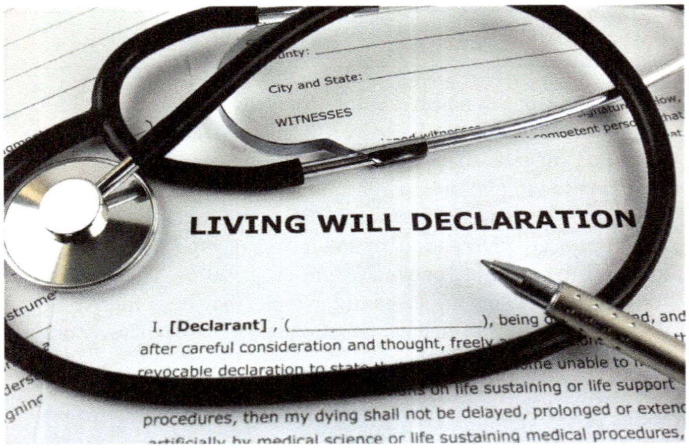

Ulf Wittrock/Shutterstock.com

The Living Will People in the United States are afforded legal protections to ensure that they—not their family members or doctors—decide when to end life-sustaining treatment if they become incapacitated or unable to communicate their wishes. A **living will** (also called an *advance directive*) is a legal document that directs healthcare providers to follow a person's wishes regarding end-of-life medical treatment. The document specifies the medical procedures or medications the person would like doctors to use or not use to prolong their life if they are unable to communicate directly. For example, people facing a terminal illness can have "Do Not Resuscitate" orders included in their medical charts, directing healthcare providers not to use cardiopulmonary resuscitation (CPR) in the event they suffer cardiac arrest. Without a living will, family members and healthcare providers must grapple with these difficult decisions, which can lead to conflicts or disputes or to use of procedures the person who is dying may not have wanted.

living will A legal document directing healthcare providers to terminate life-sustaining treatment under certain conditions in the event the person is incapacitated or unable to communicate directly.

bereavement The emotional state of adjusting to the death of a loved one, characterized by deep feelings of sadness, loneliness, and loss.

Bereavement

End-of-life health issues also affect those who are left behind. Grieving is not a disease but a normal reaction to the loss of loved ones. There is no one acceptable method of grieving or amount of time that it should take. The term **bereavement** refers to the emotional state of people who have experienced a loss; it typically involves feelings of sadness and loneliness as well as a process of mourning as survivors adjust to the loss of a loved one.

There are many aspects to bereavement—sorrow, emptiness and numbness, anger ("Why did he or she have to die?," "How could they let this happen?," "What do I do now?"), loneliness—even relief, as when the deceased person has been in pain over a prolonged period and we feel that we have reached the limits of our abilities to help sustain them. Another person's death also makes us mindful of our own mortality.

Children, Adolescents, and Bereavement Many young children lack the cognitive ability to understand the permanent nature of death (Fogarty, 2019; Rabenstein, 2018). Preschoolers may think that death is reversible or temporary, a belief reinforced by video games and cartoon characters that die and come back to life (Corr et al., 2018). Nevertheless, their thinking becomes increasingly realistic as they progress through the ages of 4 through 7 (Rabenstein, 2018). Loss is often most difficult to bear for children, especially when it involves the loss of a sibling or a parent (Corr et al., 2018; Koenig, 2018). Death of a parent strikes at the core of a child's sense of security and well-being. Older children may feel guilty because of the mistaken belief that they brought about the death by once wishing for the person to die. The loss of security may lead to anger, which may be directed toward surviving family or expressed in aggressive play. They also may show regressive or infantile behaviors, such as talking "baby talk" or becoming more demanding of food or attention. Some children may persist for several weeks in maintaining the belief that the deceased person is still alive. Though child psychiatrists believe this is normal, prolonged denial can be a harbinger of the development of more severe problems (Corr et al., 2018).

When children learn about death, it is normal for them to fear it. But children in various cultures are also taught that it is possible to survive death, either through reincarnation, as in some Eastern religions, or in the transcendence of the soul, as in Christianity (Gutiérrez et al., 2020; Yang & Park, 2017). Children in the United States are sometimes told things like "Your father is now in heaven and you will see him there again. Meanwhile, he is watching over you." The concept of surviving death renders death less permanent and less frightening to many children—and adults (Yang & Park, 2017).

Adolescents are "in between" in many ways. Teenagers understand that when life functions cease in a particular body, they cannot be restored, yet teens are not beyond constructing magical, spiritual, or pseudoscientific theories as to how some form of life or thought might survive (Corr et al., 2018).

As compared with young children, adolescents also are increasingly exposed to death among older family members, such as grandparents, and even among fellow adolescents, some of whom have died of illness but others from accidents, suicide, or foul play. Adolescents are more likely than young children to attend funerals, including funerals with open caskets. Even though adolescents come to recognize that the concept of death applies to them, they continue to engage in riskier behavior than adults do.

Although older children and adolescents may be prey to some cognitive distortions about death, they can also be remarkably insightful. When asked for advice on how to communicate with loved ones who are dying, a group of 49 children and adolescents suggested the following (Keeley & Generous, 2014):

- Confirm your deep relationship with the person who is dying.
- Try to remain as positive as possible.
- Seek support from external networks—people beyond the family.

Patterns of Grief and Mourning We can see parallels between stages of dying and patterns of grief and mourning that many bereaved people experience (although, as in the stages of dying, no single pattern fits everyone). There may be initial feelings of numbness or shock and difficulty accepting the reality of the loss. People who are mourning often say they expect the deceased person to walk through the door at any moment, or they may reach over in bed expecting to touch the departed person. Or they may feel the presence of the dead person around them. Once the reality sinks in, people who are mourning may develop a preoccupation with the dead person, or experience a deep ache or yearning for them. As feelings of loss deepen, they may experience depression, despair, and difficulty organizing their daily routines or meeting their usual responsibilities. Loss of appetite, insomnia, and forgetfulness are all normal reactions during the grieving process. It may take 2 or more years for the mourner to come to accept the loss and begin living life anew. Parental bereavement (loss of a child) may take longer or never be fully resolved. Usually the most intense grief may be experienced in the days after the funeral, after relatives and friends have left and the bereaved person is alone with their thoughts and feelings. Then they may need to come to grips with the reality of an empty house or an empty half of the bed. Mourning takes time. Social support is helpful throughout the process.

The majority of people who are bereaved come to deal with their loss, eventually resuming their usual lives or building new lives. They resume routines at work and in the home. They may continue to experience a deep sense of loss, even a gaping hole in their lives, but most resume functioning and live full and meaningful lives. Sometimes they grow in compassion because of their loss or gain a deeper appreciation of the value of life. People who

A Closer Look

Are There Stages of Grieving?

John Bowlby (1961), the psychology-of-attachment theorist, was the first to propose a stage theory of grief for coping with bereavement. It included four stages: shock-numbness, yearning-searching, disorganization-despair, and reorganization. Elisabeth Kübler-Ross (1969) adapted Bowlby's stage theory to describe her five-stage reaction of terminally ill patients to knowledge of their own impending death: denial-isolation, anger, bargaining, depression, and acceptance. The stage theory of grief has become generally accepted when applied to various kinds of losses, including children's responses to parental separation, adults' responses to marital separation (Gray et al., 1991), and hospital staffs' responses to the death of an inpatient. There is currently heavy emphasis in college textbooks and medical education on the Kübler-Ross model of grief (Corr, 2020; Maciejewski et al., 2007).

Jacobs (1993) modified the stage theory of grief to include the following stages: numbness-disbelief, separation distress (yearning-anger-anxiety), depression-mourning, and recovery. Jacobs's stage theory, like those that went before, is largely based on anecdotes and case studies.

In order to test Jacobs's theory, Paul Maciejewski and his colleagues (2007) administered five items measuring disbelief, yearning, anger, depression, and acceptance of death to 233 bereaved individuals from 1 to 24 months following their losses. A number of findings are clear. Disbelief was highest just after the loss and gradually waned over the course of 2 years. Acceptance of the loss shows the opposite course, being nonexistent at the outset, growing gradually throughout a couple of years. Yearning, anger, and depression rise suddenly in the predicted order and then each wanes gradually, reaching about half of its intensity a year afterward.

have personality traits of extraversion and conscientiousness tend to be more resilient during bereavement and less affected by depression; they may be better able to reach out to others for support and to reorganize their lives in the face of loss (Pai & Carr, 2010).

Perhaps unsurprisingly, another study applying the five-factor trait model to bereavement with 81 participants found that those who scored high on neuroticism were most likely to develop complicated, unrelenting grief (Goetter et al., 2019). How do we respond to this study? Do we say that these mourners are neurotic, so what can you do? Or do we say that they're undergoing an especially difficult period and need all the support we can give them?

Health Consequences of Bereavement Although most people adjust to loss without a need for professional help, many encounter significant psychological and medical problems. Most people experiencing bereavement rely on informal networks of support from friends and family (Rumbold et al., 2019). Others turn to medical or mental health professionals or to lay support groups who meet to share their grief and lend support and encouragement to each other. Though providing emotional support to bereaved family members is an essential part of end-of-life care, many health professionals feel inadequately trained to do so (Naef et al., 2020). Health psychologists, especially those working in cancer care, often help train medical staff members to develop more effective listening skills and ways of providing support and counseling to family members during bereavement.

Bereavement is among the most stressful experiences in life, so we shouldn't be surprised that people who are bereaved often experience emotional distress and have difficulties coping with changes in life circumstances. Evidence shows that bereaved people are at increased risk of poor physical health; emotional problems, such as anxiety, depression, suicide, and suicide attempts; and overall mortality (Molina et al., 2019; Shor et al., 2012). A study of family caregivers of people who had succumbed to cancer showed a suicide rate among caregivers of 12% before the death and 16.5% after the loss—rates many times higher than those in the general population (Abbott et al., 2014). Other researchers find that widowhood is associated with a 40% greater risk of early death (Moon et al., 2011).

One of the principal signs of stress is bodily inflammation. Research studies show evidence of increased inflammation following bereavement, which is suggestive of high levels of stress and proneness to stress-related disorders (Knowles et al., 2019). Inflammation may represent a physiological pathway that helps account for the poorer health of people during bereavement (O'Connor, 2019). Supporting bereaved people in coping with stress may help prevent adverse effects of bereavement on the body and mind.

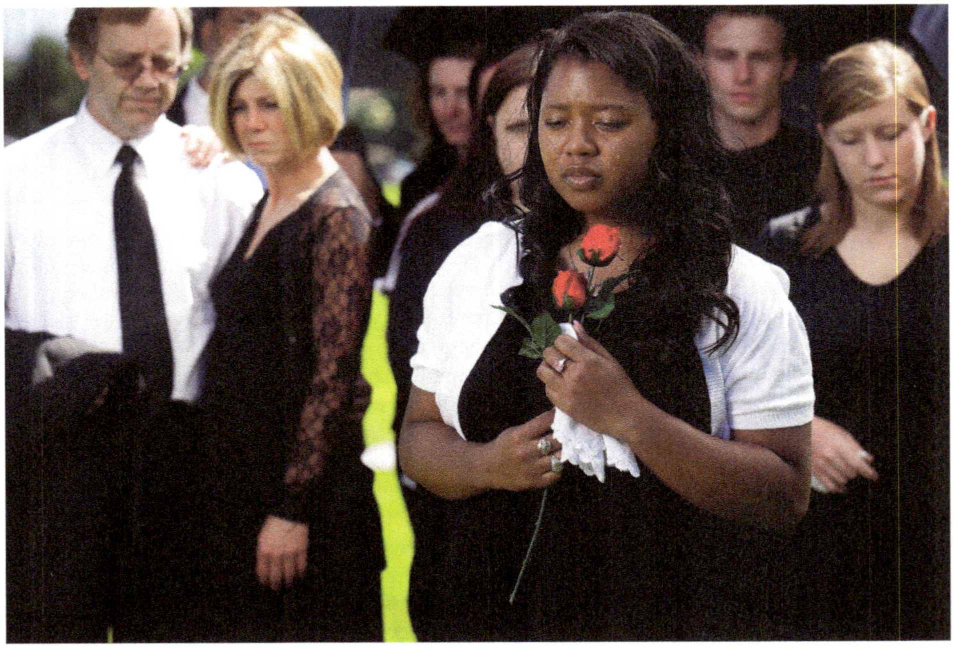

RichLegg/Getty Images

A Funeral The funeral is a social institution that provides an organized way for people to respond when they have lost someone.

Health Psychology in Action

Dia de los Muertos—Coping with Loss ... and with Discrimination

Around the world there are those who depart and those who are left behind to remember them and, often, to celebrate them. Many cultures have festivals or holidays during which they celebrate the dead. In many European countries, Roman Catholics take off from work on All Saints Day and All Souls Day, visit cemeteries with flowers and candles, and shower children with candy and toys. In Latin America, people build altars to the departed on the Day of the Dead (*Dia de los Muertos*), using skulls made of sugar, marigolds, and the favorite foods of the deceased.

The *Dia de los Muertos* celebrations in Mexico and among Mexican Americans can be traced back 2,500–3,000 years, to the cultures that dwelled in Mexico prior to European colonization. Aztecs and others kept the skulls of their ancestors and displayed them during rituals that symbolized life and death.

On the *Dia de los Muertos*, Mexicans and Mexican Americans visit cemeteries to communicate with the souls of the dead. They build altars and offer food, drink—tequila, mescal, pulque, and the like—along with photos of the departed to encourage the souls to visit. These are not somber occasions. Laughter can be heard as celebrants recount humorous stories about the departed. The *Dia de los Muertos* festivals provide comfort for the bereaved and enable them to channel their own concerns about the end of life into cultural festivals with joyous elements.

Psychologists find that the *Dia de los Muertos* also helps children and adults cope with death and loss. One study found that the festivals serve to shield children from death because adults fear that children are cognitively and emotionally incapable of coping with these matters (Gutiérrez et al., 2020). Another study found, however, that the *Dia de los Muertos* celebrations build children's coping skills by enabling them to observe what others are doing and to pitch in to help (Martinčeková et al., 2020). Other studies point out that these celebrations are times of high social support, buffering the celebrants from the stresses of life, including the stresses of acculturation in U.S. society (Rodriguez et al., 2019). The celebrations build and maintain harmonious relationships among Mexican Americans, reaffirming their cultural heritage and helping them cope with the discrimination many of them face in their daily lives.

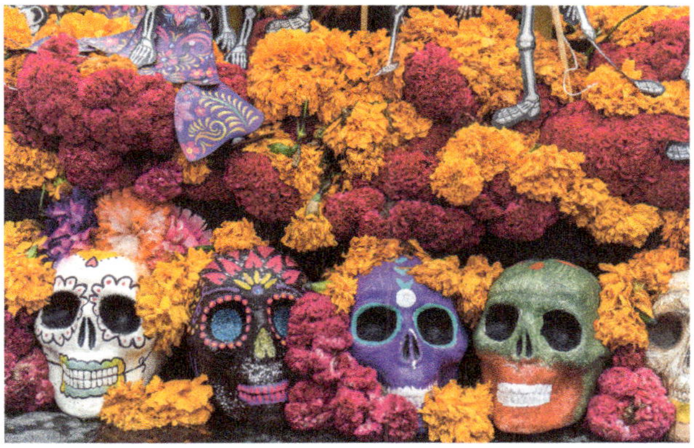

Sergio Mendoza Hochmann/Getty Images

Marigolds and Skulls—Traditional Accoutrements for the *Dia de los Muertos* These marigolds and skulls adorned an altar.

Review 14.5

INTERACTIVE SELF-SCORING QUIZZES

Sentence Completion

1. Elisabeth Kübler-Ross identified five stages of dying: denial, anger, ________, depression, and final acceptance.
2. A ________ creates a homelike environment in which terminally ill people can face death with physical and emotional supports that provide them with dignity.
3. Many hospice workers burn out and develop compassion ________.
4. In ________ active euthanasia, a lethal treatment is administered to cause a quick and pain-free death at the request of the individual who is dying.
5. ________ euthanasia involves hastening the death of a person who is terminally ill by withholding potentially life-saving treatments.
6. A ________ will is a legal document that directs healthcare providers to follow a person's wishes regarding end-of-life medical treatment, including passive euthanasia.
7. The term ________ refers to feelings of sadness and loneliness as well as a process of mourning as survivors adjust to the loss of a loved one.
8. Young children find the death of a ________ to be most devastating.
9. Research suggests that there might be five stages of grieving: disbelief, yearning, anger, depression, and ________.

Think About It

Have you or someone close to you suffered the loss of a parent, sibling, child, spouse, or partner? How did you (or they) cope with the loss? Did you (or they) receive social and emotional support? Was the support provided via informal networks of friends or other persons undergoing bereavement themselves? Or was it through a helping professional? Was the level of support adequate or could you (or they) have benefited from other types of support? If more support would have been beneficial, what type of support would have been helpful through the grieving process?

Recite: An Active Summary

INTERACTIVE SELF-SCORING QUIZZES

Chapter 14 Practice Quiz

1. Identify behavioral factors in the development and management of diabetes.

Obesity is a major contributor to the development of diabetes. People can reduce their risk of developing diabetes by losing excess weight, avoiding smoking, and exercising regularly. Self-management programs assist people with diabetes to manage the disease through continuous blood glucose monitoring, adopting a healthier diet and an exercise regimen, and adhering to medical treatment.

2. Identify behavioral factors in managing arthritis.

Psychological interventions, especially cognitive behavior therapy, may be a helpful adjunct to medical treatment in assisting patients with arthritis in managing pain, avoiding catastrophizing tendencies, challenging and correcting negative and distorted thoughts, increasing adaptive behaviors, and combating the depression that is a common feature in people with arthritis.

3. Identify behavioral factors in managing asthma.

Daily stress, as well as catastrophizing and exaggerating thinking, can trigger asthmatic attacks in people with asthma. People with asthma may benefit from behavioral techniques to help them manage anxiety and cope with stress more effectively, such as relaxation training and biofeedback training. Family therapy may be used to address family conflicts that contribute to the stress burden often faced by children with asthma.

4. Describe the major features of Alzheimer's disease and the challenges it poses to people with the disease and caregivers.

Alzheimer's disease is marked by a significant loss of mental abilities involved in memory, thinking, and judgment. As the disease progresses, the person becomes increasingly unable to manage their own personal needs and may show disruptive or disturbed behavior that cause undue stress on family caregivers.

5. Define death and discuss whether there are stages of dying.

Medical professionals usually use brain death as the standard for determining death, although people may be kept "alive" on life-support equipment. Kübler-Ross identified five stages of dying for terminally ill patients: denial, anger, bargaining, depression, and final acceptance. Shneidman argues that people who are terminally ill may experience feelings such as these, but not necessarily in stages.

6. Identify where people die, and discuss the challenges facing healthcare professionals, such as hospice workers.

About half of Americans die in hospitals. Many people who die use the hospice, which focuses on palliative care—that is, treatment of the person and not the disease—and social support of the family. Many hospice workers burn out due to being surrounded by despair and death, and some develop compassion fatigue.

7. Identify the various types of euthanasia, and discuss the legal and ethical issues associated with each one.

In active euthanasia, a lethal treatment, usually a medication, is administered to cause a quick and pain-free death. Physician-assisted suicide is a form of voluntary active euthanasia in which physicians assist people with terminal or incapacitating illnesses who wish to die by providing them with lethal doses of medications or administering the medications themselves if the people are too ill to do it by themselves. Passive euthanasia involves hastening the death of a person who is terminally ill by withholding potentially life-saving treatments, such as not resuscitating someone who has stopped breathing or withdrawing medicine, food, or life-support equipment, such as a respirator, from a person who is comatose. A living will is a legal document that directs healthcare providers to follow a person's wishes regarding end-of-life medical treatment, including passive euthanasia.

8. Discuss bereavement, focusing on bereavement over the life span and whether there are stages of grieving.

"Bereavement" refers to the emotional state of people who have suffered a loss; it typically involves feelings of sadness and loneliness as well as a process of mourning. Young children find the loss of a parent to be most devastating because it strikes at the core of the child's sense of security. Young children may also not understand that death is irreversible. Adolescents understand that death is permanent but may construct magical ways of surmounting death. Research suggests that there might be five stages of grieving: disbelief, yearning, anger, depression, and acceptance. Sociocultural factors influence our responses to death, such as whether we believe in an afterlife. The *Dia de los Muertos* helps Mexicans and Mexican Americans cope with loss and reaffirms their cultural heritage.

Answers to Review Sections

14.1

1. 10%
2. Insulin
3. gestational
4. 2
5. higher than
6. decreased

14.2

1. osteoarthritis
2. inflammation
3. inflammatory
4. Biologic
5. approach

14.3

1. 25
2. boys
3. risen
4. Depression
5. Bronchodilators/anti-inflammatories
6. avoidant

14.4

1. is not
2. Alzheimer's disease
3. is not
4. 6
5. amyloid; tau

14.5

1. bargaining
2. hospice
3. fatigue
4. voluntary
5. Passive
6. living
7. bereavement, grieving
8. parent
9. acceptance

CHAPTER 15

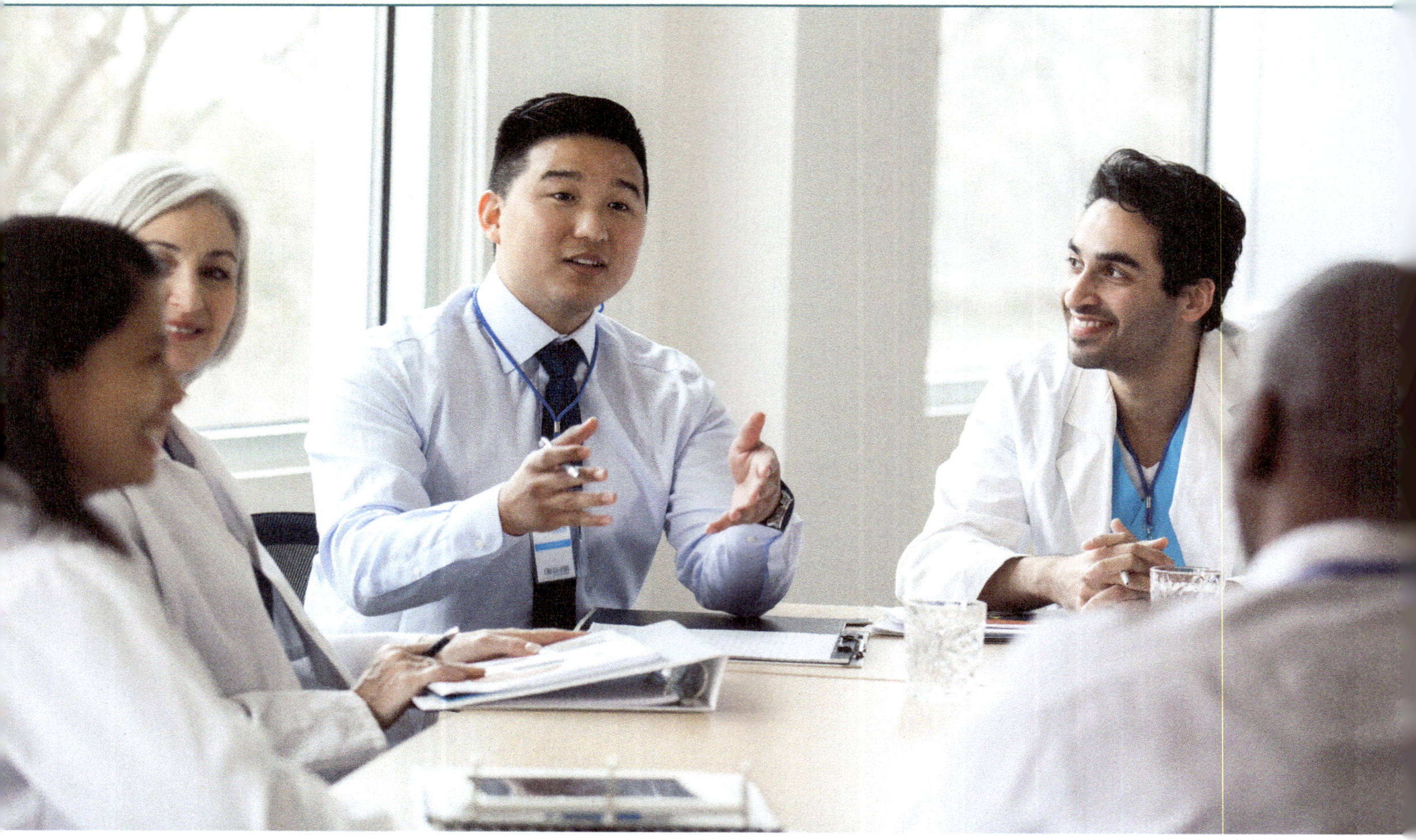

SDI Productions/Getty Images

New Directions in Health Psychology

LEARNING OBJECTIVES

After studying this chapter, you will be able to ...

1. **Evaluate** research evidence on the effectiveness of eHealth applications.
2. **Identify** the risks associated with using eHealth apps.
3. **Discuss** the uses of AI in promoting healthy behaviors.
4. **Identify** various types of eHealth wearable devices.
5. **Evaluate** the use of remote patient monitoring.
6. **Identify** health disparities associated with the digital divide.
7. **Describe** the Multiple Health Behavior Change (MHBC) Model.
8. **Identify** clusters of health risk behaviors found in surveys of college students and adults in the United States.
9. **Identify** two models of integrated primary care and describe how they differ.
10. **Identify** what is required to bring the HIV/AIDS epidemic to an end.

Did You Know That ...

- There are more than 400,000 health-related apps on the market today?
- Fewer than 2% of health claims made by eHealth apps have been validated in scientific studies?
- Researchers found that the first diagnosis offered by online symptom checkers ("Dr. Google") is incorrect about two-thirds of the time?
- There are apps that signal you when you've been sedentary for too long?
- Your smart watch might be able to tell you if your heart is in atrial fibrillation, an irregular heart rhythm that can be lethal?
- Having your blood pressure taken by a medical staff person who is wearing a white coat can elevate your readings?
- Only about 1 in 3 college students in a national survey fit a healthy profile in terms of health risk behaviors?
- Young people tend to have unhealthier risk behavior profiles than older people?
- The next time you go to your college health service for a physical health problem, you may also be asked to stop by for a talk with a behavioral health clinician?
- We already have the biological tools we need to end the HIV/AIDS epidemic?

The only constant in life is change.

—The ancient Greek philosopher Heraclitus

Is it true that the only unchanging fact of life is change? As the decade of the 2020s unfolded, the world faced the most significant health challenge since the influenza epidemic of 1918–1919, claiming more than 675,000 lives in the United States and more than 50 million worldwide—COVID-19. This virulent and deadly virus first appeared in China and soon engulfed the world in a pandemic. Contemporary transportation systems allow pathogens to be efficiently carried by infected passengers to all corners of Earth. Today a virus can spread its deadly tentacles worldwide in days or weeks. The first U.S. death from COVID-19 was reported in February 2020. Before year's end, nearly 20 million people in the United States had been infected, and there were several hundred thousand deaths.

The world was unprepared for the changes wrought by COVID-19. Whole regions of the world essentially closed down to curb the spread of the disease from person to person. Airplane travel virtually ceased. Rates of unemployment soared as businesses shut down and workers stayed at home. Businesses and educational institutions shifted seemingly overnight to online platforms, and new terms entered the vocabulary, such as Zooming and social distancing, as people adapted as best they could.

Change is also a touchpoint in our study of health psychology, as behavior change plays a central role in determining our health and longevity. In earlier chapters, we focused on models of behavior change and examined behavioral risk factors for various significant health threats, such as cardiovascular disease, cancer, and diabetes. We emphasized that many of the risk factors for these diseases involve modifiable behaviors, such as smoking, overeating, and physical inactivity. Health psychologists play important roles in conducting research on the behavioral aspects of health and illness and in developing effective behavior change interventions to help people live healthier and longer lives. As we look ahead to the 2030s, we expect that health psychologists will be in the forefront of efforts to curb the spread of infectious agents such as COVID by developing and promoting public health campaigns focused on changing health behaviors, as by practicing safe public distancing and frequent hand-washing.

In this concluding chapter, we look toward the future of health psychology by identifying four new directions in the field we expect will take center stage during the coming years. First, we focus on changes in technology that will continue to affect how people access health-related information and on the development of health applications (apps) that allow them to monitor their health status and help them adopt healthier behaviors. Second, we explore a growing movement within the field that focuses on changing combinations of health behaviors rather than individual health behaviors to foster healthier lifestyles. Third, we examine the integrated primary care model, a new model of delivering healthcare services in which behavioral health care is an integral part of primary care. Fourth, we consider the roles of health psychologists in bringing the HIV/AIDS epidemic to an end.

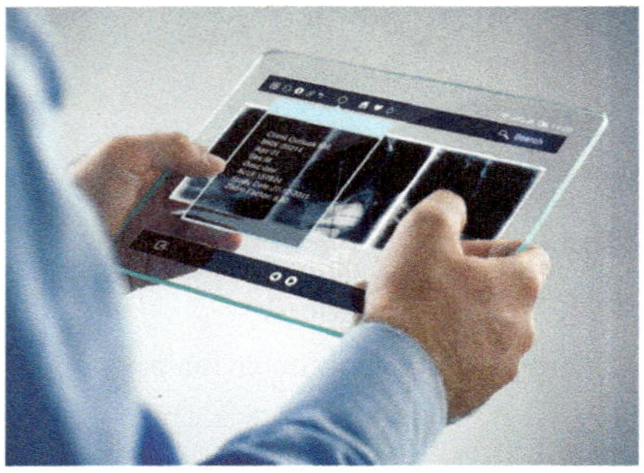

StudioThreeDots/Getty Images

eHealth and Wearables

Digital technology has transformed our lives in so many ways, including the ways in which we access health-related information and track health-related behaviors (Burton-Jones et al., 2020; Kwasnicka et al., 2022). The emerging subfield of *digital health psychology* focuses on development, effective utilization, and evaluation of digital devices to help empower people to take a more active role in managing their health needs. In earlier chapters, we recounted many of the ways in which technology has changed the field of health psychology. In Chapter 3, for example, we focused on the rise of telehealth services or telemedicine in which treatment providers, including physicians and psychologists, provide services to people seeking health care through telecommunications, such as video calling platforms. Healthcare providers can accomplish many things using telemedicine, even conducting a physical exam (Hollander & Sites, 2020). People can take their own pulse and report it remotely. Apps can also report their blood pressure. For people with psychological problems, telehealth is essentially as effective as face-to-face therapy, and retention rates are higher (Greenbaum, 2020). Why? Perhaps because it's easier for people to get online than get to an appointment that may be more than an hour away.

Throughout the text, we highlighted the development of smartphone apps and other uses of health-related technology. In this concluding chapter, we revisit the use of digital technology as we look ahead to future developments that will likely affect the field of health psychology and the lives that we live in the 2020s and beyond.

eHealth Apps: Yes, There's an App for That—Actually, There Are Many Apps

eHealth A shortened form of "electronic health"; it refers to the use of digital technology and telecommunications to improve access, efficiency, and quality of healthcare services.

mHealth A shortened form of "mobile health," referring to the ways in which we utilize mobile technologies, such as smartphones, tablets, and smart watches, to improve our health outcomes.

People today are asking "Dr. Google" and ChatGPT to explain their symptoms, or checking their blood pressure on portable devices, or tracking their steps as well as their sleep patterns using wearable devices with built-in sensors.

eHealth (sometimes written *e-Health*) is a broad term that applies to the use of electronic or digital technology, such as Internet-based services, to improve healthcare services and provide resources to people and healthcare providers to make health care and health-related information and services more efficient, accessible, and cost effective. **mHealth** comprises a subset of eHealth and refers to the specific ways in which we use mobile technologies, such as smartphones, to assess our health and transmit health-related information to data banks or health professionals.

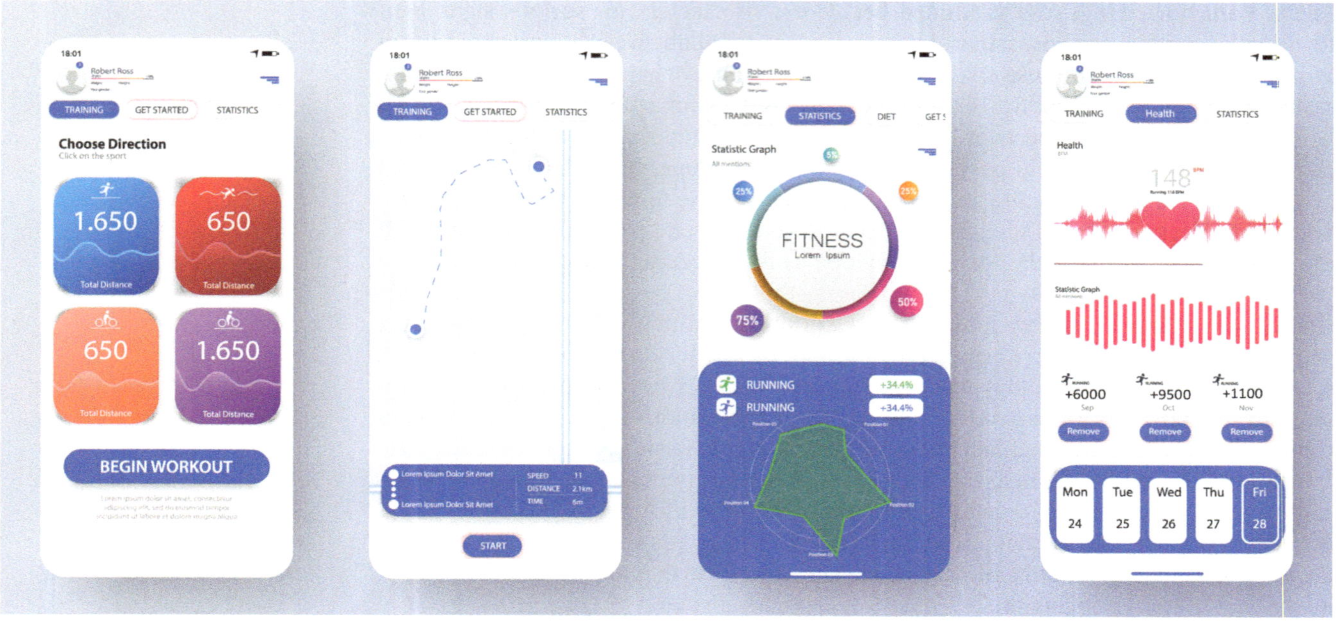

ZinetroN/Shutterstock.com

Included within the field of eHealth are health apps, health-related websites, telehealth and teletherapy services that allow providers and patients to communicate through phones, video calling platforms, and software-based health and wellness programs. eHealth applications allow people to take a more direct role in managing their healthcare needs and to communicate more effectively with their healthcare providers.

The growth of eHealth in recent years has been breathtaking. There are now more than 400,000 health-related apps (Statista, 2020). These apps help you monitor your health status, provide suggestions for making healthful behavior changes, and signal you when you reach certain health targets, such as walking 10,000 steps a day (although researchers question whether there is any special significance to this number).

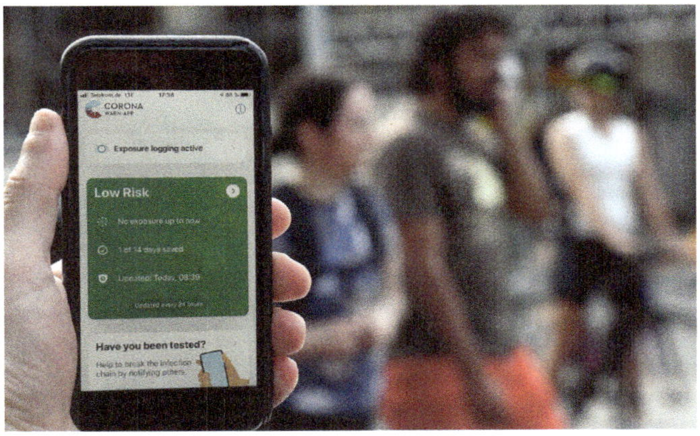

Adam Berry/Getty Images

The COVID-19 Tracking App In 2020 Germany launched its contact tracing smartphone app, which uses short-range Bluetooth to alert people who may have been exposed to an individual who has contracted the coronavirus, without relying on a centralized database.

Counting steps is only the start. eHealth apps allow users to count calories they consume and dietary choices they make, provide feedback about how much and well they sleep and how often they smoke, even allow them to adjust the volume of their hearing aids and monitor their mood states, along with other functions. Thousands of apps focus on mental health, including programs designed to help people relax, meditate, combat depression or anxiety, or battle addiction to alcohol and other substances, or quit smoking or lose excess weight (e.g., Berry et al., 2021; Miralles et al., 2020; Sala et al., 2021). One eHealth app called Sleepio features a cartoon therapist that offers behavioral suggestions to help people overcome insomnia (Singer, 2019).

Consumer interest in eHealth apps is on the rise, as people have become more aware of behavioral health risks and of the need to make behavioral changes to safeguard their health. Nearly 19% of Americans use a wearable fitness tracker, which is about the same percentage as those using any mobile health app (McCarthy, 2019). The digital health market overall is expected to grow to a $500 billion industry by 2025 (Hicks et al., 2019).

An advantage of mHealth applications, such as smartphone apps, is that they may reach population groups that have difficulty accessing quality healthcare services in person, such as low-income groups. Recently, health psychologists reported positive results from studies exploring the effectiveness of eHealth weight loss programs, and investigators reporting significant results tended to tailor their programs to meet the needs of low-income individuals (Clark et al., 2023). The programs studied included a variety of ways of providing guidance on weight loss strategies, including use of text messaging, social media, and access to websites hosting information about weight loss techniques and self-management tools.

Many health-related apps are popular with users and have high rates of adherence or utilization, but the question remains whether they help people succeed in achieving health-related goals, such as losing excess weight, reducing cardiovascular risk factors, and improving mental well-being. Some early studies show promising results in using eHealth apps for targeted behaviors, such as increasing step counts, reducing sedentary behaviors, and making healthful food choices (Milne-Ives et al., 2020). Many apps look promising, but a careful evaluation will need to be conducted app-by-app to ascertain which are helpful, which accomplish little to nothing, and which might actually be harmful.

The eHealth marketplace is in a nascent stage of development, and new or modified apps are coming into the marketplace virtually every day. The eHealth marketplace in the next 5 or 10 years will likely offer a wider range of health-related apps that pass scientific muster in terms of effectiveness. In the meantime, health consumers need to think carefully and critically about health claims made by app developers and marketers. Although more than half of eHealth apps make medical claims, closer scrutiny shows that fewer than 2% of these claims are validated in clinical studies (Larsen et al., 2021). Moreover, eHealth apps are not currently regulated by the Food and Drug Administration or other governmental watchdog agencies (Goz et al., 2019). As the regulatory landscape develops to accommodate new generations of eHealth apps, consumer protections may be enacted that will bolster confidence that these products actually accomplish the health benefits they claim they do.

Health Psychology in Action

An App for Quitting Smoking

In one research example of an eHealth application, health investigators used an interactive text messaging system to help people quit smoking. Called Text2Quit, the system relays text messages to keep participants engaged in the smoking cessation program, track their cigarette use, and complete survey instruments. Researchers randomly assigned participants to the Text2Quit program or to standard self-help programs and found that the Text2Quit program produced higher smoking cessation rates as compared to the self-help control. The researchers also found that the degree to which users engaged with the program predicted their success in quitting smoking (Abroms et al., 2014, 2020; Heminger et al., 2016).

Other research efforts have used text messaging in behavioral weight loss programs, allowing therapists to offer individualized feedback to participants as well as timely reminders and behavioral tips. Several studies support the effectiveness of text messaging in these types of programs (Cavero-Redondo et al., 2020). And in a study promoting physical activity for insufficiently active young adults, investigators sent upward of six text messages daily to the users' smartphones, prompting them to move more and sit less, and also providing them with inspirational quotes to help them keep going with their efforts (Hojjatinia et al., 2021).

In sum, do health apps work? Basically, it's too soon to tell. To date, too few apps and other digital health tools have been rigorously evaluated through clinical trials (Kwasnicka et al., 2022). Those that have been tested generally do not show results as successful as the Text2Quit approach (see *Health Psychology in Action* feature). Therefore, researchers conclude that it is too early to tell whether health-related apps in general produce reliable health benefits (McKay et al., 2019).

The "Dark Side" of eHealth

Acquiring health information from the internet (ask "Dr. Google") cuts both ways. On the positive side of the ledger, the information can help people become better informed about medical treatment, increasing their comprehension of medical advice they receive from healthcare professionals (Yardley et al., 2019). But the downside is that much of the information posted on the internet is incorrect or misleading. Using Dr. Google for self-diagnosis can lead to incorrect diagnoses and may increase anxiety, leading people to worry more about their symptoms (Jungmann et al., 2020). Australian health researchers recently assessed the accuracy of diagnostic advice given by symptom checkers on websites and mobile apps (Hill et al., 2020). Their findings showed that the first diagnosis listed by Dr. Google was incorrect about two-thirds of the time. Clearly, using Dr. Google is not a substitute for seeking an informed medical opinion.

Smartphone apps may also pose certain risks to users. For example, concerns have been raised about the privacy of the data collected by smartphone apps and wearable devices, including activity trackers, especially those with GPS-enabled tracking that can allow third parties to capture and market user location data (Puterman et al., 2021). Health data may not be protected once it is transmitted to cloud-based servers. Surveys of users of wearable devices indicate that there is a general lack of public awareness about security concerns and about whether data captured by these devices is protected (Cilliers, 2020; Zimmer et al., 2020).

Another concern is that self-directed health apps may convey to users a false sense of confidence that they are adequately addressing their health issues without assistance from healthcare professionals. Although many medical care providers encourage people to use health-related apps, they recognize that health needs are better served when technology is used in addition to regular healthcare services, not as a replacement for these services.

Going Remote

We all became familiar with remote means of interacting with others during the COVID-19 pandemic, whether it involved online course instruction or Zoom or FaceTime business meetings, birthday parties, and weddings. Well before COVID-19, medical care providers began making use of **remote patient monitoring (RPM)** to track important health data about their patients. RPM refers to the process of monitoring patients outside the hospital or doctor's office (Atreja et al., 2019). Many health-related apps provide a means of capturing biometric data from one location and transmitting it to healthcare providers in another location (Dunn & Hazzard, 2019). A University of Minnesota RPM program for more than 2,000 patients with COVID-19 resulted in over 2,000 alerts, more than 4,000 text messages, and a number of emergency department visits and hospital admission (Annis et al., 2020). All in all, the program provided an experience that was rated positively by patients and safe by healthcare providers. It also minimized exposure of healthcare workers to COVID-19. The growth of RPM was expected to more than double by the mid-2020s (Chau et al., 2019).

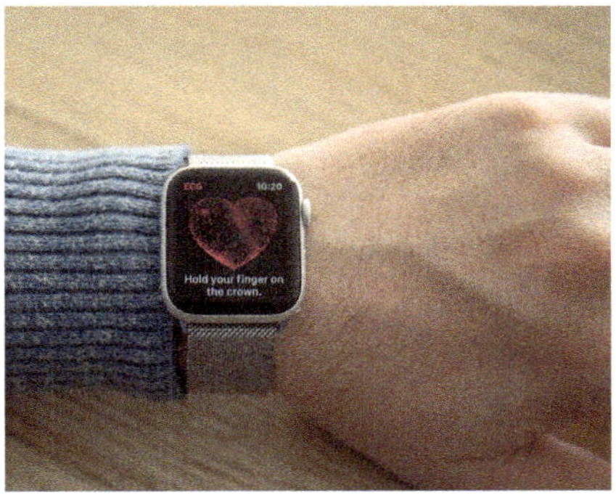

DenPhotos/Shutterstock.com

Telling Time or Saving a Life? Health sensors embedded in smart watches, such as the Apple Watch 4 Series shown here, can help us keep track of our steps and may even notify us of a potentially lethal abnormal heart rhythm.

remote patient monitoring (RPM) Assessing and tracking a person's health data outside the physician's office or healthcare facility.

Using a smartphone app, people can transmit data to their healthcare providers about their blood pressure and blood glucose levels, body weight, activity levels, smoking behavior, and other important health information that medical care providers can act upon to adjust treatment accordingly. People may also share information with clinicians about their symptoms and lifestyle information, such as dietary choices and exercise patterns. Some applications allow healthcare providers to push notifications to users to remind them to take their medication, exercise regularly, or check their blood pressure. Health psychologists can play an important role in helping medical practitioners increase people's adherence to using RPM consistently by leveraging behavior change principles, such as the ABCs of behavior change—for example, helping people avoid situations in which they may fall prey to the temptations of overeating, smoking, or excess drinking; encouraging healthful behaviors; and providing reinforcements, such as remote pats on the back for healthier behavior.

RPM is also used to capture patient data automatically from wearable devices equipped with biometric sensors (Chau et al., 2019). Wearable health technology is changing the ways in which we collect and use health-related data (Cilliers, 2020; Liao et al., 2019). Worn as accessories on the user's body, these devices can alert medical team members in real time to changes in the user's symptoms and medical condition, alerting them to a need to adjust a pacemaker or change medications (Dillard, 2020). Wearable devices with built-in sensors can automatically transmit a wide range of health data to treatment providers, such as heart rate, blood pressure, sleep patterns, number of steps taken, calories burned, and miles walked, and may even provide notifications when users have been sitting for too long (Glanz et al., 2015; Liao et al., 2019). The information may be directly accessed in real time by a healthcare provider, stored for review by a healthcare provider, or entered into a data bank with "electronic tripwires" that will inform healthcare providers, and patients, if a problem is sensed.

A wide range of biometric sensors are in use today, including implantable devices, ambulatory blood pressure cuffs, glucometers (devices that measure glucose levels from a test strip of blood taken from a finger prick), and pulse oximetry or Pulse Ox (a light-emitting probe that analyzes light passing through a finger or other body part to measure the level of oxygen in red blood cells) (American Heart Association, 2019).

Using specialized monitoring equipment, RPM has become a valuable tool for monitoring and transmitting data on heart rhythms in people with cardiac problems on a 24/7 basis. The American Heart Association (2019) finds that the RPM for atrial fibrillation (AF) appears to be about as effective as regular office evaluations with respect to reducing deaths due to heart disease or other causes and offers an advantage to people in remote areas who cannot readily attend in-office follow-up visits. In one study, people in pulmonary rehabilitation were able to learn to use remote pulse oximetry in their homes (Bonnevie et al., 2019).

Newer versions of fitness trackers are also equipped with special sensors to detect the heart's electrical signature and signal the wearer if an irregular heart rhythm occurs (Aschbacher et al., 2020; Semaan et al., 2020). Another example of a consumer device that measures heart rhythms is the Apple Watch, which is equipped with an electrocardiogram that can detect heart arrhythmias, such as AF, a potential cause of death. This information can be transmitted to a clinician.

A joint study by Apple, Inc., and researchers from Stanford University had some 419,000 people use the Apple Watch to detect incidents of AF over a period of several months (Perez et al., 2019). About 0.5 of the participants (about 1 in 200) received a pulse notification of an AF event and were instructed to contact a healthcare provider. More than 80% of the notifications were confirmed to be AF. Not surprisingly, rates of AF notifications were highest among people over age 65 and were least frequent among people under the age of 40.

RPM of blood pressure may provide more reliable measures than those taken during regular medical visits. Many patients are anxious about having their blood pressure taken in a medical office, a phenomenon described as *white coat hypertension* (named after the white coats that medical professionals typically wear), which can result in elevated blood pressure levels. Recording blood pressure at home may provide a more accurate measure of daily levels. Evidence shows that home blood pressure monitoring can help improve blood pressure control and increase adherence to taking blood pressure medications (Burke et al., 2015; Thomas et al., 2014; Tucker et al., 2017). However, some people may not take accurate readings of their blood pressure with do-it-yourself home devices. As an alternative, ambulatory blood pressure devices are also available. These small, lightweight monitoring devices are clipped to a belt and connected to a blood pressure cuff that can be worn comfortably under clothing. They automatically take blood pressure measures, typically every 15 or 30 minutes throughout the day, even while the user is sleeping.

Looking ahead, we expect tech companies to continue to expand their reach, and as they do, issues regarding privacy will increasingly come to the fore. Digital health companies are continually developing innovative technologies, including the use of voice data to detect early signs of Alzheimer's disease and face scanning technologies to reveal possible signs of mental health or neurological problems. These applications may improve health outcomes in users, but they also raise troubling concerns about protection of biometric data. Technology is advancing at a faster pace than regulatory agencies and legal safeguards can handle, so it is prudent for health consumers to question how their data will be collected and protected. Another issue facing the RPM industry is patient reimbursement for use of increasingly expensive medical devices, as questions remain about who—government, insurance companies, or users themselves—should foot the bill. We are encouraged to see that reimbursement systems have recently been introduced to cover RPM as legitimate medical expenses in recognition of the vital information that they can provide.

Health Disparities and the Digital Divide

A major challenge in eHealth is the digital divide that continues to separate people by social class, geography, and race. Although high-speed internet is nearly universal in many communities, more than 20 million Americans still lack broadband access, especially those living in rural areas and in disadvantaged urban communities (Anderson, 2019). These concerns were highlighted during the COVID-19 pandemic, as many underserved people with COVID-19 lacked digital devices needed to access eHealth apps (Yancy, 2020). In order to benefit from technological innovations, we need to ensure that the needs of diverse groups in our society are addressed in the implementation and dissemination of these applications. Closing the digital divide involves more than just providing access to digital devices and services; it also requires closing the digital literacy gap.

digital literacy The ability to find, access, and effectively use digital services and information.

Digital literacy refers to the ability to obtain, process, and understand digital services and information (Dunn & Hazzard, 2019). To use technology effectively, people need to know how to search and download relevant digital information, how to separate the wheat from the chaff (i.e., reliable vs. untrustworthy information), and how to use smartphone apps and web services effectively.

The Emergence of AI as a Tool to Promote Healthy Behavior Change

It's called the "next big thing" and it promises (or threatens?) to change the world as we know it. AI (artificial intelligence) is making inroads in virtually every aspect of our lives.

We make use of it when we "speak" to Siri or Alexa, which are AI chatbots, or when we ask questions of another AI chatbot, ChatGPT, which is built on a human language model that allows conversational interactions via text or voice between humans and a machine that is capable of drawing upon a vast storehouse of electronically stored information.

Introduced in late 2022, ChatGPT became the most widely adopted software application in history, quickly surpassing more than 100 million users, including your authors and most probably yourself and many of your friends. If you've had a "conversation" with ChatGPT, you begin to realize the vast potential it has for changing how we acquire and interact with information. With the meteoric rise in the use of AI-enabled devices, concerns have been raised about the need for guardrails to ensure that artificial intelligence works in the interests of humanity and not to its detriment or possibly becoming an existential threat to our very survival, as we see depicted in so many sci-fi scenarios.

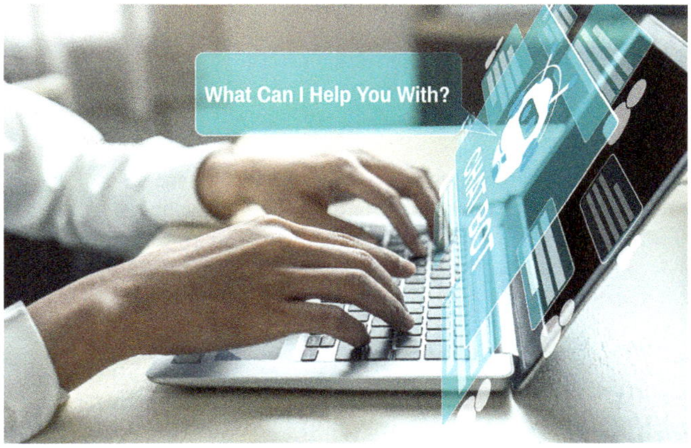

Blue Planet Studio/Getty Images

Can AI Promote Healthy Behaviors? What role might AI play in helping us live healthier lives? We decided to ask ChatGPT for its input.

Healthcare professionals are already focused on harnessing the potential benefits of AI. We see physicians and other healthcare professionals saving precious time by using AI to help them write case notes and keep up with their recordkeeping responsibilities, time they might better use in direct clinical service. We also find researchers gathering evidence supporting the effectiveness of AI chatbots in promoting various healthy behaviors, such as smoking cessation, adoption of healthy habits, adherence to treatment or medication regimens, and reducing misuse of psychoactive substances (Aggarwal et al., 2023).

In exploring current and potential uses of health-related AI applications, we thought it might be fitting to ask ChatGPT to list some examples of how AI can help promote healthy behavior changes. Here are seven applications of health-related AI programs that ChatGPT identified:

1. *Personalized health recommendations:* By analyzing an individual's health data from medical records and biometric information, AI can tailor personalized recommendations based on an individual's health profile, such as personalized exercise and dietary plans and stress management techniques.
2. *Behavior tracking and monitoring:* Using AI-equipped devices, it can track and monitor health information in real-time, such as exercise, food consumption, and sleep habits, helping people become more aware of their health habits and offering suggestions for making healthy changes in their daily routines.
3. *Virtual health coaches*: AI chatbots can serve as personal assistants, providing support and encouragement, answering questions, and offering reminders and motivational messages to encourage healthy behavior changes.
4. *Predictive analytics:* By using sophisticated algorithms, AI can detect behavioral patterns that predict health conditions or risk of developing certain diseases, while offering personalized preventive measures individuals can use to reduce their risk of disease.
5. *Gamification for healthy behaviors*: AI can create and run games that make following a healthy lifestyle more enjoyable and incentivize healthier behaviors, such as by creating challenges, leaderboards, and dispensing rewards for meeting behavioral goals.
6. *Personalized mental health support*: AI can adapt its conversational skills to provide personalized support to help people cope with stress, anxiety, and other mental health issues. It can draw upon cognitive behavior therapy techniques, mindfulness exercises, and other mental health tools at its disposal.
7. *Medication adherence*: As a personal assistant, AI can help people keep on track with their medication schedules, reminding them to take their medication as directed, tracking their medication use, and issuing alerts about drug interactions.

Self-Assessment

INTERACTIVE SELF-ASSESSMENTS

Using a Wearable—Is It for You?

How likely are you to use a wearable healthcare device, like a fitness tracker or heart rate monitor? Health psychologists recognize that your intention to purchase and use a wearable device depends on your beliefs about the device and about yourself (adapted from Chau et al., 2019).

Perceived Usefulness

1. Do you believe that using the device will improve your health or well-being? ____ yes ____ no
2. Do you believe the device is useful in your achieving your personal health goals? ____ yes ____ no

Perceived Convenience

3. Do you believe the device is easy to use and will fit into your lifestyle? ____ yes ____ no
4. Do you believe you have the time and opportunity to use the device? ____ yes ____ no

Perceived Irreplaceability

5. Do you believe the device is a "must have"? ____ yes ____ no
6. Do you believe that achieving your health goals depends on using the device? ____ yes ____ no

Perceived Credibility

7. Do you trust the device provides valid and reliable data? ____ yes ____ no
8. Do you believe the device is made by a trustworthy brand? ____ yes ____ no

Health Beliefs

9. Do you believe you can change unhealthful habits? ____ yes ____ no
10. Do you believe you can adopt a healthier lifestyle? ____ yes ____ no

The more of these questions you answered in the affirmative, the stronger your intention to use wearable health technology is likely to be. Of course, other factors also determine the likelihood of using these devices, such as affordability and social norms (whether you believe people in your reference groups are using these devices and what you think others might say about your use of the device).

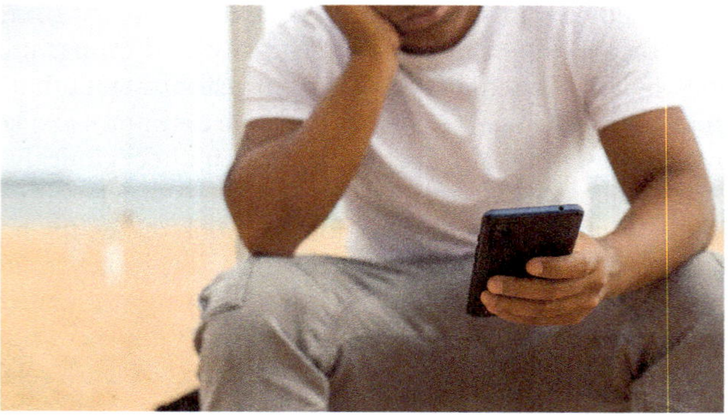

jorge mata/Getty Images

"Doctor AI Will See You Now" Mental health applications of AI allow people to interact with a virtual therapist on their smart devices. Perhaps by the time this text reaches your hands, you will have access to a personal AI therapist available 24/7 to provide emotional support and guidance.

Review 15.1

INTERACTIVE SELF-SCORING QUIZZES

Sentence Completion

1. The field of __________ involves the use of health-related digital apps, websites, communications, and electronic programs designed to improve healthcare services.
2. About __________% of Americans use wearable fitness trackers.
3. Health data (may or may not) be protected when it is transmitted to cloud-based servers.
4. __________ patient monitoring refers to the process of monitoring patients outside the hospital or doctor's office.
5. Devices that test a person's blood to measure glucose levels are called __________.
6. A large study of people using an electrocardiogram-enabled smart watch showed that about (1 in 50 or 1 in 200) received a pulse notification of an atrial fibrillation event.
7. Lack of broadband access is disproportionately found in __________ areas and __________ urban communities.
8. Digital health __________ involves the ability to obtain, process, and understand digital services and information.

Think About It

Do you use health apps? Why or why not? What factors would determine whether you would choose to use a health app? What questions should you ask before using a health app?

The Multiple Health Behavior Change Model

A developing area of interest in health psychology is helping people change multiple health-related behaviors, not just individual behaviors like smoking cessation or adopting a healthier diet. It is not that individual behaviors have lessened in importance. We know that the major causes of death in the United States and in many parts of the world are chronic noncommunicable diseases, such as cardiovascular disease, cancer, respiratory diseases, and diabetes. We also know that individual risk factors, such as smoking, consuming a high-fat diet, and physical inactivity, play important roles in the development of these diseases. But for many people, multiple risk factors cluster or co-occur, which further magnifies the risk of developing serious illnesses and shortening the life span (Rabel et al., 2019).

Most people report more than one behavioral health risk factor (Geller et al., 2016; Prochaska & Prochaska, 2011). They may smoke and also drink heavily. Or they may be sedentary and consume an unhealthful diet comprised of high levels of saturated fat, fat, and sugar (McSharry et al., 2015). Or they may smoke, consume too much alcohol, and make fast food a staple of their diet. It may be more difficult to change two or more unhealthful behavior patterns simultaneously, but it is possible, and health psychologists and many other health professionals address interventions that aim to improve lifestyles, not just individual behaviors (Geller et al., 2017).

It's a Matter of Unhealthful Lifestyles, Not Just Unhealthful Behaviors

Health professionals recognize that living a healthier life depends on making changes in lifestyles, not just individual behaviors. Millions of people receive similar advice from their healthcare providers to make these kinds of lifestyle adjustments: lose excess weight, follow a healthful diet, exercise regularly, don't smoke, and get adequate sleep (Kazi et al., 2019). The most common pattern of health risk factors among adults in the general population is a behavioral cluster of alcohol misuse and smoking (Meader et al., 2016, 2017). Another common thread in young adults is a cluster of sexual risk behavior and substance misuse.

The multiple health behavior change model targets multiple behaviors either within behavioral domains or across behavioral domains. For example, a person dealing with obesity might work within the same behavioral domain by reducing calorie consumption and changing the nutritional balance of their diet by increasing consumption of fruits and vegetables and high-fiber foods. A person with hypertension might make multiple choices across domains, such as reducing salt intake (a nutritional domain) and increasing the frequency of vigorous exercise (a physical activity domain). Concerning cardiovascular disease and cancer, we apparently have a long way to go. A review of research published in *Health Psychology* found that few if any healthcare facilities focus primarily on helping people who survive cancer modify the behaviors that make them susceptible to both cardiovascular disease and cancer (Spring et al., 2019).

A review of more than 220 studies of the multiple behavior change model showed that many of the interventions used to target multiple behaviors were highly successful (King et al., 2015). Most of these interventions targeted both dietary choices and physical activity. Health psychologists recognize that making effective behavior change strategies at the level of individual risk factors (e.g., behavioral treatment of excess body weight) may generalize to efforts to change other behavior risk factors, such as physical inactivity and smoking (Conner & Norman, 2017). But not always.

How Problem Health Behaviors Cluster

Health psychologists use the acronym SNAP to identify four unhealthful patterns of behavior commonly found among adults: smoking (S), poor nutrition (N), excess alcohol intake (A), and physical inactivity (P). Before making any snap judgments, we should recognize that people vary with respect to how many, if any, of this unholy quartet of health risk behaviors describes their own behavior risk profile. A review of international research on SNAP behaviors finds that many individuals fit a "healthy profile" in which none of the SNAP risk factors is present (Noble et al., 2015). Others show all four SNAP risk factors. The most frequent pairing of SNAP behaviors in this review was a clustering of smoking and excess alcohol use. The researchers also reported that clustering of two or more SNAP factors occurred more often among men and among people from socially or economically disadvantaged backgrounds.

Closer to home, other researchers culled data from a national health assessment survey of U.S. college students, which was the largest health survey of its kind, involving more than 100,000 college students (Jao et al., 2018). The researchers used the survey data to look for clusters of problem behaviors that could be used to classify particular groups of students. Their results revealed that students could be grouped into three classes or clusters based on their health risk behaviors. They then explored how these classes stacked up in terms of differences in mental health outcomes. Only about 1 in 3 students (35.3%) fit a healthy profile associated with low-risk health behaviors. About 4 in 10 (41.2%) students formed a cluster characterized chiefly by low levels of physical activity. A third definable cluster, comprising about 1 in 4 students (23.5%), reported high levels of use of alcohol and other drugs. This third cluster also had the greatest likelihood of reporting poor mental health outcomes, as indicated by higher rates of psychological disorders, self-harm, and psychological symptoms. Health surveys like this can help psychologists and other mental health professionals target particular groups of students who may be at greater risk of developing serious mental health problems.

All three clusters (classes) of college students had one health risk behavior in common. Can you guess what it might be? **Table 15.1** shows the percentages of students reporting health risk behaviors such as binge drinking, inactivity, and use of cigarettes, alcohol, and other drugs for each of the three clusters. The health risk they most shared in common, which was reported by greater than 90% of students in each of the three classes, was a low intake of fruits and vegetables. Adopting a healthful, nutritionally balanced diet—one with ample amounts of fruits, veggies, and foods with high fiber content—is an important element in leading a healthy lifestyle and reducing the risk of chronic diseases (see Chapter 7).

Another recent survey looked at clusters of health behavior patterns among U.S. adults. The data were drawn from a national epidemiological survey developed by the Centers for Disease Control and Prevention to assess unhealthful behaviors linked to disease and premature death (Fleary & Nigg, 2018). The researchers found three groupings or clusters of adults based

TABLE 15.1 **Health Risk Behaviors Overall and by Class**

	Overall	1 (high alcohol and drug use)	2 (low physical activity)	3 (low-risk behavior)
Number of students (% of group)	105,781	24,824 (23.5%)	43,507 (41.2%)	37350 (35.3%)
Insufficient fruit and vegetable consumption (%)	93.8	94.2	96.7	90.3
Binge drinking (%)	34.0	66.2	20.3	28.5
Insufficient physical activity (%)	53.7	54.5	100	0
Cigarette use (%)	15.1	62.3	0.8	0.4
Marijuana use (%)	15.7	66.1	0.3	0.2

Notes: Insufficient fruit and vegetable consumption—less than 5 servings of fruits/vegetables per day; binge drinking—number of times with 5 or more drinks of alcohol in a single sitting during the prior 2 weeks; and insufficient physical activity—less than 3 days of vigorous exercise for at least 20 minutes, or less than 5 days of moderate exercise for at least 30 minutes. Also, 0.4% in class 1, 41.3% in class 2, and 27.1% in class 3 do not drink alcohol.

Source: Jao et al., 2018. Reproduced with permission of Taylor and Francis.

on their health behavior patterns. As you look at the descriptions of three clusters described below, ask yourself which of the groups best describes your own health behavior profile.

1. *Healthy or physically active group:* 39% of the population, they tend to follow health guidelines for physical activity, have a low probability of smoking and drinking, and meet health recommendations for fruit and vegetable consumption.
2. *Apathetic group:* 48% of the population, they tend to have a low probability of smoking and drinking; however, they don't actively engage in preventive behaviors, such as consuming recommended levels of fruits and vegetables. Consequently, they stand an increased risk of developing serious chronic diseases later in life. They tend to be younger, more often male, and lower in income than the healthy, physically active group.
3. *Binge drinking group:* 13% of the population, they are described by a high probability of binge drinking. They tend to be younger, more often male, and have lower levels of education and income as compared to the healthy, physically active group.

It turns out that younger adults are more likely to be in the nonhealthy groups, which portends major health challenges as they enter later stages of life when chronic diseases begin to their toll. These findings that health behaviors of Americans can be used to group individuals into three relatively discrete categories support the value of using multiple health risk behaviors as an organizing principle for determining risk profiles. The investigators reported that these health behavior patterns seem to have been relatively stable in recent years, neither improving nor getting worse.

The challenge ahead for health psychologists and other health professionals going forward is to develop health promotion efforts to move the needle so that more adults develop healthier patterns of behavior or lifestyles that will increase their likelihood of living longer and healthier lives. The investigators point to the importance of taking multiple behaviors into account when developing behavior change interventions. They believe that targeting younger individuals with interventions focused on changing binge drinking, physical activity, and consumption of fruits and vegetables is likely to yield a greater payoff in terms of improved health outcomes than addressing individual unhealthy behaviors alone.

What is the payoff for leading a healthier lifestyle? Consider the results of a study by a group of Harvard University researchers who tracked health outcomes of more than 100,000 people from age 50 for as long as 34 years afterward (Li et al., 2020). The Harvard team repeatedly assessed the emergence of serious diseases in this sample, diseases that sap the quality of life and lead to early death. The primary outcome measure was the number of years that individuals lived free from chronic diseases, such as cardiovascular disease, diabetes, and cancer. The components of a healthful lifestyle were not ever smoking, maintaining a healthy weight, engaging in moderate to vigorous physical activity, avoiding excessive use of alcohol, and adopting a higher-quality diet. Men who met these healthful lifestyle standards had an average of 7.6 additional disease-free years as compared to men who met none of these standards. Women with healthful lifestyles had an additional 10.7 years of disease-free life. Though evidence from observational studies like this cannot pinpoint cause-and-effect relationships, the data point to a strong link between adoption of healthier lifestyles and living healthier for a greater number of years.

Closing the Gap in Health Disparities

One of the principal challenges facing health psychologists in the 2020s and beyond is to develop effective behavioral interventions that can help people change multiple behaviors linked to increased risk of serious illness and premature death. Yet it is important to note that health disparities remain a prominent obstacle in addressing these health challenges. Researchers find that socioeconomic status is the strongest predictor of the likelihood of engaging in multiple health risk behaviors (Meader et al., 2016). People at the lower end of the wealth and income spectrum suffer disproportionately from health risks associated with smoking, obesity, unhealthful diets, and physical inactivity, as we have noted throughout the book. Although psychologists and other health professionals continue to work with individuals to help them make healthier behavior changes, they also need to promote changes in social and environmental factors tied to unhealthful lifestyles, such as inadequate housing conditions, lack of job opportunities, and lack of access to health education and healthier

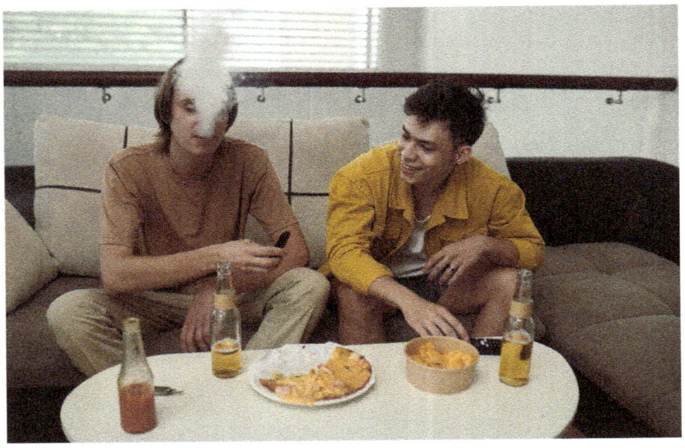

DragonImages/Getty Images

Where to Begin? One of the challenges facing health psychologists is whether to focus on helping people change multiple problem behaviors one at a time or all at once. How many behavioral risk factors are represented here?

food choices. Marshaling efforts to redress these social ills will likely contribute to improving the health and well-being of disadvantaged groups and reduce health disparities.

All Together Now—or One at a Time?

Should a person who is obese and smokes first try to quit smoking and then focus on losing excess weight? What about a sedentary person whose diet is packed with high-fat, high-sodium food choices? Should this person work on sitting less and exercising while also making healthier food choices, or should these goals be approached sequentially? Health psychologists face the challenge of deciding whether to help people address one problem at a time or tackle a combination of problem behaviors at the same time (Geller, 2017; King et al., 2015). The issue is far from settled, as research comparisons between treating multiple risk behaviors simultaneously or successively are sparse (Meader et al., 2017).

We recognize that health psychologists commonly target multiple behaviors within behavior domains simultaneously. For example, weight-loss programs typically include efforts to change both energy-balance factors simultaneously: diet and physical activity (Chevance et al., 2019). Less common are efforts that cross behavioral domains, such as health-promotion programs that target smoking cessation and weight loss simultaneously. In fact, preliminary evidence indicates that changing smoking behavior before tackling other health risk behaviors, such as changes in diet or food consumption, is more effective than trying to make these changes simultaneously (Meader et al., 2017). Most clinicians recognize the need to prioritize treatment goals and often put quitting smoking at the top of the list. It may turn out that certain combinations of behavioral goals may be best approached simultaneously (e.g., the energy-balance factors of diet and exercise) than other combinations.

Investigators undertook a study with 202 adults who showed a pattern of insufficient physical activity and excessive screen time, which is not atypical among many Americans today (Conroy et al., 2017). A 3-week intervention program designed to change these behavioral patterns resulted in some gains, as the frequency of daily moderate–vigorous intensity physical activity increased and leisure screen time decreased.

Building Sustainability for Lasting Behavior Changes

Another challenge facing the field of health psychology is the need for sustainable results of behavior change programs—that is, relapse prevention (Shahan, 2020). Much of the research emphasis among health researchers in past years has focused on immediate behavior changes following behavior change interventions and not on long-term maintenance of these changes (Connor & Norman, 2017).

Unfortunately, short-term gains may quickly evaporate. Investigators reviewed the effectiveness of eHealth programs used in school-based preventive programs targeting at least two unhealthful risk behaviors, such as smoking, physical inactivity, and sedentary behavior, as measured by screen time and sitting time (Champion et al., 2019). Overall, programs targeting multiple behaviors succeeded in reducing screen time and increased activity levels of students immediately after the intervention. However, these effects tended to be short-lived because unhealthful behaviors returned to earlier baseline levels.

Cancer researchers report similar problems with long-term adherence to health behavior change. An analysis of more than 3,000 studies showed low levels of adherence among people who survived cancer in sticking with recommended changes in physical activity and diet (Tollosa et al., 2019). Receiving a cancer diagnosis is considered a key period for making healthful behavior changes, but compliance tends to decrease over time. It would be helpful to develop programs that lead to more sustainable changes in health risk behaviors. Health psychologists face the hurdle of helping people to integrate healthful behavior changes into their lifestyles so that they can last a lifetime.

Review 15.2

INTERACTIVE SELF-SCORING QUIZZES

Sentence Completion

1. Multiple health risk factors tend to __________ or co-occur.
2. The most common cluster of health risk factors among adults in the general population involves alcohol misuse and __________.
3. SNAP identifies four unhealthy patterns of behavior commonly found among adults—smoking (S), poor __________ (N), excess __________ intake (A), and physical inactivity (P).
4. About (2 in 10 or 4 in 10) college students formed a cluster associated with low levels of physical activity.
5. A health risk shared in common by all health risk behavior clusters of college students in a national survey was a low level of intake of __________ and __________.
6. (Younger or older) adults are more likely to be clustered in the non-healthy groups.
7. The strongest predictor of engaging in multiple health risk behaviors is __________ __________.
8. Researchers report that successively changing smoking behavior before changing other health risk behaviors is (more effective or less effective) than trying to do both at the same time.

Think About It

Which cluster of college students best describes your own health risk behaviors? Does your health-related behavior fit a healthy profile? Why or why not? What changes can you make to join the healthy cluster?

Integrated Primary Care

Integrated primary care (IPC) is a transformative movement in health care today. It is changing the ways in which primary healthcare providers, such as family physicians and pediatricians, organize their practices and deliver health care to their patients. The traditional model of primary care is based on an independent or group practice model in which primary healthcare providers tend to the medical needs of their patients and families. The primary healthcare provider, typically a family physician, pediatrician, internist, or general practitioner, or a nurse practitioner or physician's assistant, treats the patient's medical problems, as needed, and makes referrals to behavioral health specialists, such as psychologists and psychiatrists. By contrast, IPC is a treatment model that directly incorporates behavioral health specialists as part of the healthcare team (De Paul & Caver, 2020).

integrated primary care (IPC) An approach to organizing primary medical care services that combines medical and behavioral care within the same outpatient treatment setting.

Many primary care providers (PCPs) continue to follow the standard treatment model, but times are changing. IPC has begun to dot the healthcare landscape, spurred in part by changes in healthcare policy, such as the advent of the Affordable Care Act, that encourage integration of behavioral health care as an essential part of primary care (Vogel et al., 2017). Another impetus for combining medical and behavioral care within the same treatment setting is the increasing recognition of the key role that unhealthful behaviors play in many serious medical conditions, from cancer to heart disease to asthma and diabetes. Health professionals recognize the need for more holistic treatment that is grounded within the biopsychosocial model of health and illness.

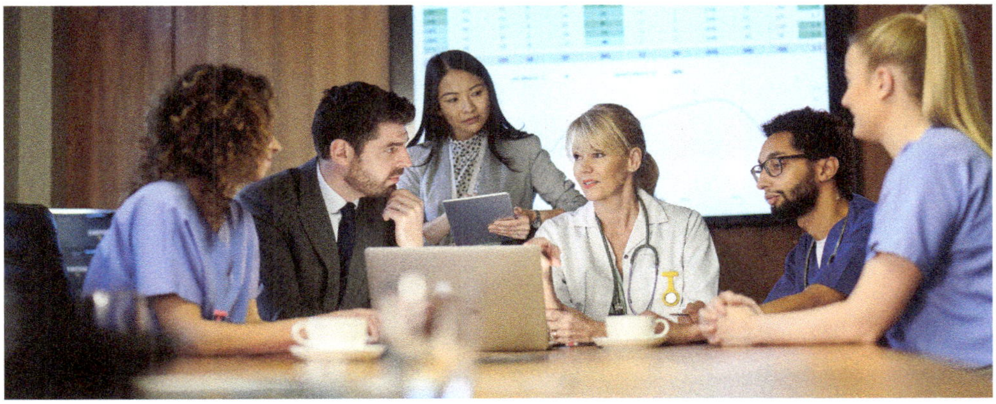

sturti/Getty Images

Integrated Primary Care In IPC, behavioral health specialists are incorporated as parts of healthcare teams.

Consider the case of a person with heart disease and hypertension who has several behavioral risk factors that increase the risk of life-threatening cardiovascular incidents, such as a heart attack or stroke. The behavioral risk factors in this case might include high stress levels as measured by stress hormones in the saliva, excess body weight, and physical inactivity. In the traditional healthcare model, a PCP, such as the person's family physician or internist, might refer the person to a heart specialist (cardiologist), who in turn might refer the person to a psychologist for stress management training and to a community-based weight-loss program, as well as advising the person to increase physical activity and cut back on high-fat foods. The person might access these additional services in different locations from a range of service providers who do not share medical records or have opportunities to coordinate care with one another as members of the same treatment team. Moreover, costs quickly mount as more outside services are added to the mix. In an IPC setting, medical and behavioral healthcare providers share case records and collaborate as members of the same treatment team that plans and coordinates the patient's treatment. This integration of services under the same roof can be delivered at a considerable cost advantage relative to the traditional referral-based system.

In IPC settings, behavioral healthcare specialists work closely with medical care providers in addressing people's medical and behavioral healthcare needs (Robinson & Reiter, 2016). IPC combines primary health care with behavioral health care in the same treatment setting. "Behavioral health care" is a generic term that applies to a wide range of behavioral health services, including the following:

- Behavioral weight control and smoking cessation programs
- Stress management programs
- Mental health treatment of emotional problems, such as depression and anxiety
- Behavioral treatment of chronic pain
- Behavioral treatment of substance use problems
- Behavioral problems in school-age children, such as attention-deficit/hyperactivity disorder (ADHD) and other disruptive behavior disorders, as well as anxiety and depression in childhood
- Behavioral treatment of insomnia and sleep-related problems
- Behavioral treatment of inactivity and other health risk behaviors

In traditional healthcare models, a person obtaining treatment might be referred to a psychologist or other behavioral healthcare provider. There would be separate billing, separate appointments, separate recordkeeping systems, and additional travel to meet with the behavioral healthcare specialist. By contrast, a treating physician in an IPC practice might escort the person down the hall to meet with a behavioral health specialist, such as a psychologist or mental health clinician, who would then evaluate the person's mental health concerns, all without the need for the person to leave the office. Afterward, the physician and behavioral health specialist would confer about the person's treatment plan.

Yet another advantage of incorporating behavioral health care in IPC settings is the fact, surprising as it may be, that most people who receive mental health services receive them within primary care settings. The family doctor is often the go-to resource for mental health problems people may encounter, such as anxiety, depression, and insomnia. At least 1 in 5 people in primary care has an anxiety or depressive disorder (De Paul & Caver, 2020). Many PCPs take a direct role in treating these problems, writing prescriptions for psychiatric and sleep medications and providing support to people during times of emotional stress. In IPC settings, medical care providers work directly with behavioral health specialists who provide more specialized care.

Models of Integrated Primary Care

There are different forms of integrated care, but two principal models have attracted the most attention among researchers in the field (Vogel et al., 2017):

1. *Care Manager Model:* This model designates a care manager who is responsible for coordinating people's care. The care manager typically conducts an initial interview

with the person, assesses the person's treatment needs, plans treatment options, and coordinates and communicates these treatment needs with other healthcare providers within the practice. The care manager may also participate in team meetings with the primary care team. In some cases, the care manager may be trained to use standardized manuals to provide structured behavioral health interventions. The training and experience of care managers varies widely, ranging from bachelor's-level mental health clinicians to nurses with psychiatric experience to master's or doctoral-level clinicians.

2. *Primary Care Behavioral Health (PCBH) Model:* Adopting a team-based approach, onsite behavioral health consultants (BHCs), typically psychologists or clinical social workers, work side-by-side with other members of the integrated care team, such as physicians and nurses (Hunter et al., 2017; Reiter et al., 2018; Robinson & Reiter, 2016; Vogel et al., 2017). The primary healthcare provider may refer people who have mental health issues to the BHC for evaluation. The BHC consults with the PCP to coordinate the person's care, perhaps bringing in other members of the primary care team to coordinate treatment services. The BHC regularly monitors the person's psychological health and may provide first-line treatment within the practice's standard of care, which typically involves a limited number of brief therapy sessions.

The behavioral consultants may have specialized training in short-term treatment methods, such as those used in crisis intervention, stress management, and treatment of depression or anxiety. Behavioral consultants may also refer people needing longer or more intensive psychological treatment to mental health professionals or facilities outside the IPC practice.

An analysis of 30 randomized controlled trials supported the effectiveness of psychological treatment of depression in primary care settings (Linde et al., 2015). Although there is no single PCBH model, University of Arizona health psychologists developed a comprehensive PCBH model that involves six key components that can be represented by the acronym GATHER, as shown in **Table 15.2** (Hunter et al., 2017).

IPC is still in an early stage of development, but evidence has already accrued showing it can help curb healthcare costs (Vogel et al., 2017). Cost savings typically result from reducing the need for costly emergency room visits and unnecessary diagnostic imaging tests. The IPC may also reduce additional expenses incurred by relying on outside providers for mental health services. Moreover, further significant cost savings can be reaped by providing effective behavioral health interventions that reduce risk factors for chronic diseases, including such unhealthy behavior patterns as poor diet, inactivity, smoking, and excessive alcohol use.

One of the major challenges faced by clinical health psychologists in busy primary care settings is to adapt their treatment models to treat large numbers of people. The typical 45- or 50-minute therapy hour limits the numbers of people that can be treated at any given time, especially when long-term treatment approaches are used. Typically, specialized treatment protocols developed for use in primary care settings last perhaps 12–18 sessions, but even this limited treatment model might not be feasible for implementation in many settings. Psychologists working in a Veterans Health Administration primary care clinic developed a 5-session mental health treatment protocol (De Paul & Caver, 2020). Preliminary results of this treatment protocol look promising, but further efforts are needed to develop treatment manuals that can be easily transported across IPC settings. Teletherapy is yet another treatment alternative that might be used within an IPC practice to increase access and efficiency of behavioral health services (Waugh et al., 2019).

One treatment setting in which integrated care has taken root may only be a short distance away from you—your college health center. A survey of student health centers on college campuses showed that nearly half (46%) were integrated health/counseling centers and the other (54%) were nonintegrated centers (Readdean et al., 2019). This means that if you walk into an integrated healthcare center on campus for a physical health problem, your care provider might also ask you about your emotional health and have you meet with a behavioral health clinician if you are having problems with anxiety or depression or difficulty coping with stress.

TABLE 15.2 The GATHER Model for Primary Care Behavioral Health

INTERACTIVE FIGURES, CHARTS, & TABLES

Key Components	Description	Comments
"G" is for Generalist	The BHC is a generalist who evaluates people seeking care across a range of conditions.	In some cases, the BHC may refer to specialty mental health providers to oversee the person's mental health needs.
"A" is for Accessibility	The BHC responds immediately to requests from the PCP when mental health or psychosocial needs are identified.	Typically, the PCP would brief the BHC about the referral issues and introduce the BHC to the person in the exam room. The BHC may attend the meeting with person on the same day to begin addressing these concerns.
"T" is for Team-based	The BHC uses the same electronic medical record system as the PCP so that all components of the patient's treatment are available to the different treatment providers and may meet with the PCP and other team members to coordinate the person's care.	Team-based sharing may also apply to clinic facilities, as BHCs may use exam rooms for visits, depending on availability, as well as having people wait for appointments in a common reception area.
"H" is for High productivity	The IPC functions as a high-volume treatment setting by limiting the length of appointments in order to serve a larger number of people.	The BHC may be expected to treat 10–14 people a day as compared to the 5–7 people that constitutes a typical caseload in a specialty mental health clinic.
"E" is for Educator	The BHC helps improve the skills of the treatment team by educating the PCP and other team members about mental health issues.	The BHC may consult with other treatment providers during team meetings or make formal presentations on selected topics during lunchtime or staff meetings. The BHC may leave education handouts on display in the waiting room or ask the PCP to distribute them during office visits.
"R" is for Routine	The BHC is a regular member of the treatment team who provides input across a range of cases.	Unlike a specialty mental healthcare provider, such as an off-site psychologist or psychiatrist, who may maintain client confidentiality by keeping their work separate from the primary care setting, the ICP functions within a team model that encourages sharing of information among team members in the interests of providing integrative care.

Source: Adapted from Hunter et al. (2017).

Review 15.3

INTERACTIVE SELF-SCORING QUIZZES

Sentence Completion

1. __________ primary care is a healthcare model that incorporates behavioral health specialists into primary care.

2. In an IPC setting, medical and behavioral healthcare providers (do or do not) share patient case records.

3. Upward of (1 in 2 or 1 in 5) people in primary care have anxiety or depressive disorders.

4. The two major types of integrated care models are the __________ __________ Model and the Primary Care __________ __________ (PCBH) Model.

5. In the GATHER model of IPC, "T" is for __________ -based approaches.

6. Nearly (one-quarter or one-half) of college health services operate on the basis of an integrated care model.

Think About It

How (if at all) does the IPC model differ from the health care you have experienced over the years? What advantages or disadvantages might it have in meeting your own healthcare needs?

Ending the HIV/AIDS Epidemic

We have come a long way in managing the HIV/AIDS epidemic. When the disease burst upon the scene in the 1980s, it was literally a death sentence. The immune system and HIV (human immunodeficiency virus) might wage a war with shifting fronts for a decade or more, but

HIV would eventually emerge as the victor, giving rise to the condition known as AIDS (acquired immunodeficiency syndrome), setting the stage for lethal "opportunistic" diseases to administer the *coup de grace*.

For decades, no treatment could be found that would change the eventual outcome. Today the outlook is very different. Combinations of antiretroviral drugs (drug "cocktails" referred to as antiretroviral therapy, or ART) can reduce the viral "load" in the bloodstream to undetectable levels, levels so low that the virus can no longer be transmitted to other people, levels so low that the infected individual can live long enough so that the "usual" lethal diseases—for example, cardiovascular disease and cancers unrelated to the HIV virus—cause death later in life. Moreover, the partners of people infected with HIV can also take drug cocktails known as PrEP (pre-exposure prophylaxis), which prevent them from becoming infected with HIV.

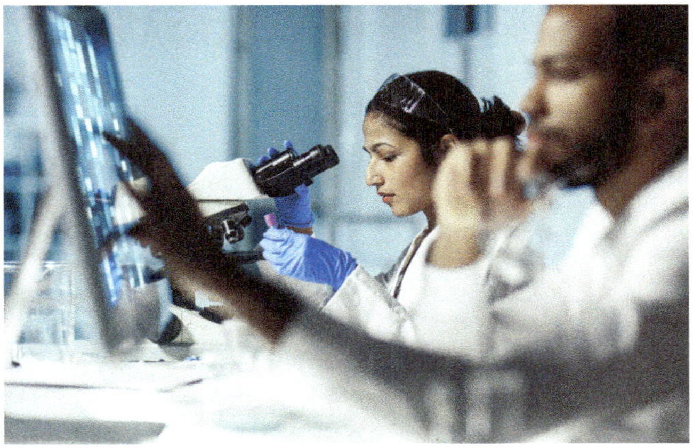
poba/E+/Getty Images

Ending the HIV Epidemic We have the tools in place—antiretroviral therapy (ART) that suppresses the viral load of HIV such that people living with HIV are highly unlikely to infect partners. We also have pre-exposure prophylaxis (PrEP) which makes it highly unlikely that sero-negative individuals will be infected with HIV by sex partners. People living with HIV need to obtain treatment, and people vulnerable to being infected with HIV should obtain prophylaxis. The benefits are clear; what are the barriers to doing so?

Despite all this progress, there is no vaccine for HIV, and there is no cure for AIDS. More than 1.2 million Americans are currently living with HIV and some 38,000 Americans are newly infected each year. Worldwide, the numbers remain staggering. It is estimated that more than 38 million people are living with HIV (World Health Organization, 2020b). Worldwide, there are about 1.3 million new infections each year and 630,000 deaths (WHO, 2023). ART has averted the deaths of millions of people worldwide (Kemnic & Gulick, 2022), but of the people living with HIV worldwide, only some 23 million, or some 62% of that total, are receiving ART, and many of these people do not adhere to the treatment (World Health Organization, 2023). Approximately 30% of people living with HIV do not know that they have the virus. These are some of the reasons that the global death rate remains so high.

In the United States, ART has been shown to virtually eliminate the risk of transmitting HIV to a sex partner, and PrEP, when used conscientiously (see Chapter 10), has the potential of reducing the rate of new infections by about 90% by 2030 (Bedimo & Jodlowski, 2023; Kemnic & Gulick, 2022). Use of PrEP also helps prevent female sex partners of men with HIV from being infected with HIV, as it does those who might be infected by sharing needles when injecting drugs (Kemnic & Gulick, 2022). However, it is estimated that only a minority, about 1 in 10 people, who could benefit by taking PrEP are currently doing so. Moreover, many do not reliably use condoms, which, used consistently, would also decrease the spread of the virus. That is one of the reasons that we still have AIDS-related deaths in the United States.

The Plan for America

President Barack Obama created the nation's first national HIV/AIDS strategy in 2010. His administration updated the strategy in 2015 and scheduled it to run until 2020. It was structured around four aims: reducing new infections with HIV, increasing access to care for people living with HIV, reducing HIV-related racial and ethnic disparities, and creating a coordinated national response to the HIV epidemic (Avert, 2019). The Trump administration also released a plan for ending the HIV/AIDS epidemic. The goals were to reduce the rate of new HIV infections by 75% within 5 years and by 90% within 10 years. The plan contains the elements shown in **Figure 15.1**.

The plan includes these elements:

1. Diagnosing people living with HIV as soon as possible so that they can receive treatment that will prevent them from transmitting the infection to others
2. Treating people with HIV to achieve sustained viral suppression. ART can reduce the viral load of HIV so that it becomes undetectable in the bloodstream; however, it would reproduce rapidly if ART were discontinued

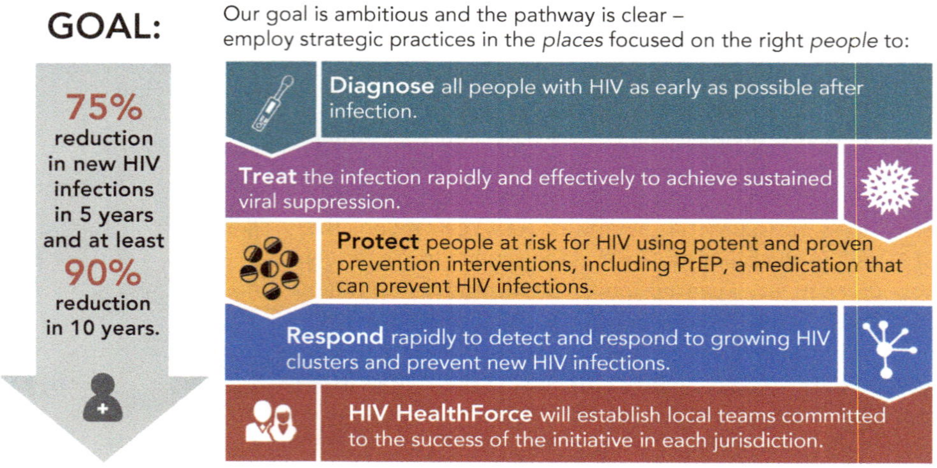

FIGURE 15.1 **Ending the HIV Epidemic—A Plan for America** ART and PrEP provide biological tools for ending the epidemic. However, it lies within the province of health psychologists to create interventions for managing the mental health and "health illiteracy" barriers to implementing the plan with all people who are living with HIV and those who are vulnerable to being infected.

3. Protecting people who are vulnerable to being infected with HIV through use of PrEP, education, and, as appropriate, treatment for mental health and substance abuse problems
4. Identifying areas of the nation that are developing new clusters of HIV infections as early as possible so that teams of federal healthcare professionals can work with local officials and healthcare professionals to diagnose and treat those who are living with HIV and those who are vulnerable to being infected with HIV
5. Establishing local teams of healthcare professionals to carry out the goals of the program

Barriers to Ending the HIV/AIDS Epidemic

The lowest rates of use of PrEP are among men who have sex with men, members of racial and ethnic minority groups, and people who live in the South and Southeast. For example, Black Americans, who comprise 13% of the U.S. population, account for 40% of people living with HIV (CDC, 2022). Despite comprising 18.5% of the U.S. population, Hispanic people account for 24.7% of new HIV diagnoses (Impact, 2023). Many Black Americans mistrust the healthcare system and are therefore less likely than White Americans to adhere to PrEP or to ART for lowering their viral loads (Mgbako et al., 2023). Let us consider the barriers to using PrEP and ART from a health psychology perspective (Padilla et al., 2020; Pleuhs et al., 2020):

- Many people living with HIV or vulnerable to being infected lack basic health literacy, which could possibly be reversed by means of education in their communities.
- Many people avoid being tested for HIV because they fear learning of the results.
- People are frequently reluctant to discuss their sexual behavior, particularly risky sexual behavior, such as unprotected anal intercourse, with their PCPs for fear that disclosing this information will meet with disapproval and lead to bias in their health care.
- PCPs themselves may not be familiar with the availability and proper use of PrEP.
- Mental health and substance abuse problems prevent many who would profit from PrEP from using it due to issues with impulse control or lack of clear understanding of the issues at stake and the availability of PrEP.
- The expense can be prohibitive, more than $20,000 a year.

Managing Barriers Concerning Mental Health It is essential that health clinics work to provide health literacy skills to people who would benefit from using PrEP or adhering to prescriptions to use ART in order to lower their viral loads (Pleuhs et al., 2020).

For some people, adherence to medication is connected to wider health issues such as diet and physical activity. In addition, unhealthy older people living with HIV are less likely to be able to effectively manage ART than are healthy older people living with HIV (Cooley et al., 2020). There is also a greater prevalence of mental health problems among people who are living with HIV and people who are vulnerable to being infected than we find in the general population (Remien et al., 2019; Waldron et al., 2021). In many cases we have the appropriate screening tools to assess mental health needs and can offer effective treatments for them. However, adequate resources need to be provided to address gaps in screening and treatment in the United States and elsewhere (Pleuhs et al., 2020; Vavani et al., 2020).

Managing Barriers Concerning Costs Even people who are insured for the cost may find that they are subjecting their physicians to many hurdles concerning preauthorization of the use of the drug cocktail, not only when they are first prescribed PrEP, but even when prescriptions are being renewed. California has undertaken some steps to make PrEP more available (Kazi et al., 2019). People living with HIV can receive the cocktail from their pharmacists without a prescription, insurance companies must shoulder the cost of at least one month's supply, and then the costs are buffered by the state's Medi-Cal program. California has found that pharmacists can be trained to safely dispense PrEP. In order for supports like these to be in place, state governments must desire to help people who will benefit from using PrEP, and they must be willing to discuss it in their legislatures. Pharmacists in California may dispense only a 60-day supply without prescription every two years, but PrEP users may feel more comfortable approaching their PCPs for renewals once they can show that they are using the drug conscientiously. But make no mistake: The wider use of PrEP would help prevent transmission of HIV.

The U.S. Department of Health and Human Services (USDHHS, 2020) states that its *Ready, Set, PrEP* program will make PrEP available at no cost for recipients who qualify. In order to qualify, recipients must

- Lack insurance coverage for prescription drugs,
- Be tested for HIV and have a negative result (be sero-negative), and
- Have a prescription for PrEP.

It remains to be seen how many people who would benefit from taking PrEP will qualify for the program and actually make use of it. The webpage www.getyourprep.com has links to assist individuals and healthcare professionals to enroll in the program.

The Plan for America is ambitious and will only succeed if the federal government and state and local governments provide the necessary resources. Some of the resources are financial. Others involve health psychology: the assistance of people who have expertise in creating interventions that can overcome psychological, social, and cultural barriers to participating in efforts to end the epidemic.

Review 15.4

INTERACTIVE SELF-SCORING QUIZZES

Sentence Completion

1. Some _____ thousand Americans are infected with HIV each year.
2. Approximately _____ % of people who are infected with HIV do not know that they have the virus.
3. The first step in the Plan for America to eradicate HIV/AIDS is __________ of people with HIV or considered to be vulnerable to being infected with HIV.
4. The two biological tools for ending the HIV epidemic are ART and __________.
5. Mental health problems are (more or less) prevalent among people living with HIV than in the general population.
6. The USDHHS states that its *Ready, Set, PrEP* program will make PrEP available at no cost for recipients who are sero-__________ for HIV.

Think About It

The biological tools for eradicating HIV/AIDS are in place. What are the barriers to making proper use of those tools? How can health psychologists help people overcome those barriers?

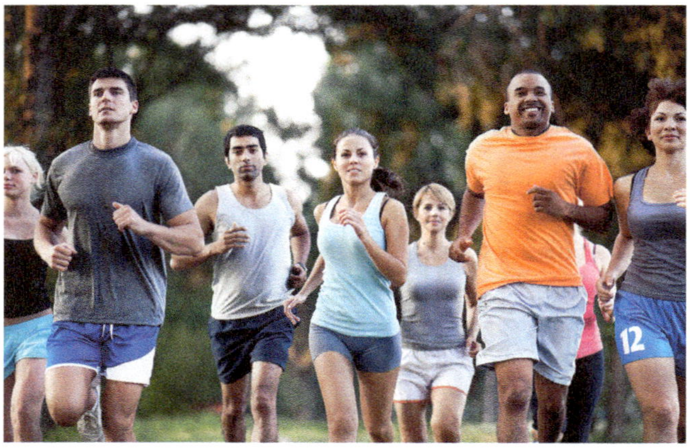

skyneshe r/Getty Images

Living Healthier, Living Longer What knowledge and skills from this course can you apply to living a healthier and longer life?

Health Psychology and *Your* Future

We have spoken about the Plan for America. What about the plan for you?

Return to the findings of the Harvard University study of more than 100,000 people (Li et al., 2020). The Harvard team considered the lifestyle factors of diet, overweight and obesity, physical activity, smoking, and alcohol. Women with healthful lifestyles lived 10.7 years longer than women who engaged in unhealthful behaviors. Men who led a healthful lifestyle lived 7.6 years longer. Yes, the study was correlational. It could be that the same factors—perhaps factors related to personality or genetics—that led to longer lives also led to adopting and maintaining healthful lifestyles. Even if cause-and-effect relationships are not crystal clear, to which group do you want to belong?

Do you see yourself as being vulnerable to any of the chronic diseases discussed throughout the book—cardiovascular disorders, cancer, diabetes, and so forth? Do you see benefits to avoiding smoking, eating more fruits and vegetables, eating foods with fewer calories and saturated fats, boosting your level of physical activity, controlling your use of alcohol, and, did we mention, avoiding smoking? Might we suggest that the information presented in the text can serve as a cue to action for you?

Assuming that you perceive benefits in adopting a healthful lifestyle, what are the barriers? Consider diet. The pleasures of eating high-calorie foods stuffed with fats and sugars are *now*, and they can be intense. Can you think of ways to bring the long-term negative health outcomes into the forefront? What types of things can you learn to say to yourself as you stop and think before giving in to temptation?

Consider smoking. If you smoke, do you want that drag now, because it miraculously provides relaxation and pleasure at once, and because it enables you to avoid the unpleasant sensations of withdrawal from nicotine? And do you tell yourself that health consequences of smoking may be 20, 30, or 40 years off in the future? What can you do to think more about that future now? Can you live with a week or so of withdrawal symptoms in order to live many years longer? Years without coughing and shortness of breath and the eventuality of the devastating health consequences of cancer and other smoking-related diseases? In Chapter 9 we noted that most people who successfully quit smoking did so without professional help. How did they do it? Is there a lesson in what they did that applies to you?

Are you spending too much time sitting and surfing the internet or watching television? What can you do to get a move on? Can you join (or create) a group so that you receive social support while you're engaging in physical activity? Can you inform others about your change of lifestyle—people who will approve of and encourage your changes? (Sadly, some people who are jealous and have no intention of changing their own sedentary lifestyles may not be encouraging.) Choose your social reinforcers carefully! Stimulus control also enters the picture. If you're having difficulty motivating yourself to exercise, perhaps you can plunk yourself in the gym or on a track for half an hour and see what happens. And treat yourself to that fantastic running gear!

Another barrier to losing weight and building stamina and muscle is that it takes time, which can be frustrating. Changing your lifestyle can be hard work, and it can take weeks or a few months before you begin to see changes in the mirror and feel better. The same is true of college, of course. You enter college with hopes for the future, but it will take many years of hard work to accomplish the goals you set for yourself. It has been said that if you have your health, you have everything. Are you ready to make the commitment to adopting a healthier lifestyle? Who is the only person who can truly answer that question?

Recite: An Active Summary

INTERACTIVE SELF-SCORING QUIZZES

Chapter 15 Practice Quiz

1. Evaluate research evidence on the effectiveness of eHealth apps.

There remains insufficient evidence to document the effectiveness of eHealth apps in producing significant health benefits. Early evidence shows positive effects on some targeted health behaviors. Future refinements to existing apps and development of new apps may yield significant health benefits in the future.

2. Identify risks associated with using eHealth apps.

These include privacy concerns, as collection of user health-related data may not be protected once it is transmitted to external servers, use of untested apps that might not yield measurable health benefits, and reliance on using health apps in place of standard medical treatment.

3. Identify several types of eHealth apps and devices.

eHealth apps range from devices that measure steps and activity levels, to others that monitor mood states, sleep patterns, smoking behavior, sedentary behavior, and calories consumed and dietary choices, among other functions.

4. Evaluate the use of remote patient monitoring.

Remote patient monitoring devices provide important tools used to track a person's health status outside the hospital or doctor's office. RPM can alert treatment providers to changes in a person's symptoms and medical condition, permitting them to make adjustments in medical treatment based on data provided in real time. Evidence shows that wearable RPM devices embedded in smart watches can detect abnormal heart rhythms, which may be a lifesaver for people who experience incidents of atrial fibrillation.

5. Identify health disparities associated with the digital divide.

Significant differences in access to digital health services exist with respect to social class, geography, and race. Disparities also affect broadband access, with people from rural areas and disadvantaged urban areas most likely to lack high-speed internet services. Disparities also exist in digital literacy, which prevents people from using technology effectively.

6. Describe the multiple health behavior change (MHBC) model.

The MHBC model proposes that behavior change efforts should focus on changing multiple health behavior risk behaviors rather individual behaviors alone. It is based on evidence showing clusters of unhealthful behaviors, such as those represented in the SNAP model, and recognizes that lifestyle adjustments are needed to make significant changes in health-related behaviors.

7. Identify clusters of health risk behaviors found in a national survey of college students and U.S. adults.

A national survey of health risk behaviors in college students showed that students clustered into three groups—(1) a healthy profile (35.3% of students) characterized by healthful behavior patterns; (2) a low physical activity cluster (41.2% of students); and (3) an alcohol/drug cluster (23.5% of students). This third cluster showed the poorest mental health outcomes. A CDC survey of U.S. adults identified three health risk behavior clusters—(1) a healthy or physically active group (39% of the population); (2) an apathetic group (48% of the population) who tended not to smoke or use alcohol but didn't engage in preventive behaviors; and (3) a binge drinking group (13% of the population) who had a high probability of binge drinking.

8. Identify two models of integrated primary care and describe how they differ.

Two major models of integrated primary care are (1) the Care Manager Model, in which a designated care manager coordinates patient care within the IPC practice and may provide some direct behavioral care consistent with the scope of practice of the IPC setting, and (2) the Primary Care Behavioral Health (PCBH) Model, in which behavioral health specialists are members of the treatment team and monitor the behavioral care needs of patients and consult with the primary health provider to coordinate and plan the patient's treatment needs.

9. Identify what is required to bring the HIV/AIDS epidemic to an end.

Bringing the HIV/AIDS epidemic to an end requires the use of medication (ART) that suppresses the viral load of the person living with HIV to undetectable levels so that (1) the person will survive, and (2) the person will not transmit the virus to others. It also requires the use of medication (PrEP) to prevent vulnerable people from contracting HIV. Barriers to obtaining the medicines include gaps in screening and diagnosis, lack of health literacy on the part of some people living with HIV, mistrust of the healthcare system by others, problems with mental health and substance abuse, and the cost of the medications.

Answers to Review Sections

15.1

1. eHealth
2. 19
3. may not
4. Remote
5. glucometers
6. 1 in 200
7. rural; disadvantaged
8. literacy

15.2

1. cluster
2. smoking
3. nutrition; alcohol
4. 4 in 10
5. fruits; vegetables
6. Younger
7. socioeconomic status
8. more effective

15.3

1. Integrated
2. do
3. 1 in 5
4. Care Manager; Behavioral Health
5. team
6. one-half

15.4

1. 38
2. 30
3. diagnosis
4. PrEP
5. more
6. negative

References

Abavi, R., Branston, A., Mason, R., & Du Mont, J. (2020). An exploration of sexual assault survivors' discourse online on help-seeking. *Violence and Victims*, 35(1), 126–140.

Abbasi, J. (2019). For mortality, busting the myth of 10,000 steps per day. *Journal of the American Medical Association*, 322, 492–493.

Abbasi, J. (2020). The American Heart Association takes on vaping. *Journal of the American Medical Association*, 323(3), 205–206.

Abbasi, J. (2023). Surgeon General sounds the alarm on social media use and youth mental health crisis. *JAMA*. https://doi.org/10.1001/jama.2023.10262

Abbott, C. H., Prigerson, H. G., & Maciejewski, P. K. (2014). The influence of patients' quality of life at the end of life on bereaved caregivers' suicidal ideation. *Journal of Pain and Symptom Management*, 48, 459–464.

Abdollahi, A., Abu Talib, M., Carlbring, P., Harvey, R., Yaacob, S. N., & Ismail, Z. (2018). Problem-solving skills and perceived stress among undergraduate students: The moderating role of hardiness. *Journal of Health Psychology*, 23(10), 1321–1331.

Aboa-Éboulé, C., Brisson, C., Maunsell, E., Mâsse, B., Bourbonnais, R., Vézina, M., ... Dagenais, G. R. (2007). Job strain and risk of acute recurrent coronary heart disease events. *Journal of the American Medical Association*, 298, 1652–1660.

Abraham, J. M. (2019). Employer wellness programs—A work in progress. *Journal of the American Medical Association*, 321, 1462–1463.

Abraído-Lanza, A. F., Mendoza, S., & Armbrister, A. N. (2019). Latino health. In T. E. Revenson & R. A. R. Gurung (Eds.), *Handbook of health psychology* (pp. 342–354). Routledge.

Abramson, L. T., Seligman, M. E. P., & Teasdale, J. D. (1978). Learned helplessness in humans: Critique and reformulation. *Journal of Abnormal Psychology*, 87, 49–74.

Abreu, R. L., Lefevor, G. T., Gonzalez, K. A., Teran, M., & Watson, R. J. (2022). Parental Support, Depressive Symptoms, and LGBTQ Adolescents: Main and Moderation Effects in a Diverse Sample. *Journal of Clinical Child & Adolescent Psychology*, 1–16. https://doi.org/10.1080/15374416.2022.2096047

Abroms, L. C., Boal, A. L., Simmens, S. J., Mendel, J. A., & Windsor, R. A. (2014). A randomized trial of Text2Quit. *American Journal of Preventive Medicine*, 47, 242–250.

Abroms, L. C., Heminger, C. L., Boal, A. L., Van Alstyne, J. M., & Krishnan, N. (2020). Text2Quit: An analysis of user experiences with a mobile smoking cessation program. *Journal of Smoking Cessation*, 15(1), 23–28. https://doi.org/10.1017/jsc.2019.22

Achstetter, L. I., Schultz, K., Faller, H., & Schuler, M. (2019). Leventhal's common-sense model and asthma control: Do illness representations predict success of an asthma rehabilitation? *Journal of Health Psychology*, 24(3), 327–336.

ACIP (Advisory Committee on Immunization Practices). (2019). Evidence to recommendations for HPV vaccination of adults, ages 27 through 45 years. https://www.cdc.gov/vaccines/acip/recs/grade/HPV-adults-etr.html

Adachi, T., Fujino, H., Nakae, A., Mashimo, T., & Sasaki, J. (2014). A meta-analysis of hypnosis for chronic pain problems: A comparison between hypnosis, standard care, and other psychological interventions. *International Journal of Clinical & Experimental Hypnosis*, 62, 1–28.

Adakai, M., Sandoval-Rosario, M., Xu, F., Aseret-Manygoats, T., Allison, M., Greenlund, K. J., & Barbour, K. E. (2018). Health disparities among American Indians/Alaska Natives—Arizona, 2017. *MMWR. Morbidity and Mortality Weekly Report*, 67(47), 1314–1318. https://doi.org/10.15585/mmwr.mm6747a4

Adam, M. B., McGuire, J. K., Walsh, M., Basta, J., & LeCroy, C. (2005). Acculturation as a predictor of the onset of sexual intercourse among Hispanic and white teens. *Archives of Pediatrics & Adolescent Medicine*, 159, 261–265.

Adesogan O., Lavner J. A., Carter S. E., Beach S. R. H. (2022). COVID-19 stress and the health of Black Americans in the rural south. *Clinical Psychological Science*, 10(6), 1111–1128. https://doi.org/10.1177/21677026211049379

Adsett, J. A., Morris, N. R., Kuys, S. S., Paratz, J. D., & Mudge, A. M. (2019). Motivators and barriers for participation in aquatic and land-based exercise training programs for people with stable heart failure: A mixed methods approach. *Heart & Lung*, 48(4), 287–293.

Adult Obesity Prevalence Maps. (2019). Prevalence of self-reported obesity among U.S. adults by state and territory (2018). https://www.cdc.gov/obesity/data/prevalence-maps.html#overall

Agency for Healthcare Research and Quality (AHRQ). (2019, October). *2018 National Healthcare Quality and Disparities Report*. Content last reviewed October 2019. Agency for Healthcare Research and Quality, Rockville, MD. https://www.ahrq.gov/research/findings/nhqrdr/nhqdr18/index.html

Aggarwal, A., Tam, C. C., Wu, D., Li, X., & Qiao, S. (2023). Artificial intelligence–based chatbots for promoting health behavioral changes: Systematic review. *Journal of Medical Internet Research*, 25, e40789. https://doi.org/10.2196/40789

Agras, W. S. & Bohon, C. (2021). Cognitive behavioral therapy for eating disorders. *Annual Review of Clinical Psychology*, 17, 417–438.

Ahles, T. A., & Root, J. C. (2018). Cognitive effects of cancer and cancer treatments. *Annual Review of Clinical Psychology*, 14, 425–445.

Ahmadi, M., Zaree, K., Leily, A. K., & Hoseini, A. S. S. (2019). Efficacy of a written prayer technique on the anxiety of mothers of children with cancer. *Palliative & Supportive Care*, 17(1), 54–59. https://doi.org/10.1017/S1478951518000743

Ahn, J., Lee, J. H., & Jung, Y. C. (2018). Predictors of suicide attempts in individuals with eating disorders. *Suicide and Life-Threatening Behavior*. https://doi.org/10.1111/sltb.12477

Aiyer, R., Johnson, E., & Poli, J. J. (2022). Transcutaneous electrical nerve stimulation. In R. K. Banik (Ed.), *Anesthesiology in-training exam review*. Springer. https://doi.org/10.1007/978-3-030-87266-3_66347–350

Aizenman, N. (2018, November 9). Deaths from gun violence: How the US compares with the rest of the world. *National Public Radio*. https://www.npr.org/sections/goatsandsoda/2018/11/09/666209430/deaths-from-gun-violence-how-the-u-s-compares-with-the-rest-of-the-world

Ajzen, I. (1991). The theory of planned behavior. *Organizational Behavior and Human Decision Processes*, 50, 179–211.

Ajzen, I. (2002). Perceived behavioral control, self-efficacy, locus of control, and the theory of planned behavior. *Journal of Applied Social Psychology*, 32(4), 665–683.

Ajzen, I. (2005, December). Constructing a Theory of Planned Behavior questionnaire. https://www.researchgate.net/publication/235913732_Constructing_a_Theory_of_Planned_Behavior_Questionnaire

Akbari, M., Lankarani, K., Tabrizi, R., Vali, M., Heydari, S., Motevalian, S., & Sullman, M. (2021). The effect of motorcycle safety campaign on helmet use: A systematic review and meta-analysis. *IATSS Research,* 45(4), 513–520. https://doi.org/10.1016/j.iatssr.2021.06.001

Aknin, L. B., De Neve, J.-E., Dunn, E. W., Fancourt, D. E., Goldberg, E., Helliwell, J. F., ... Ben Amor, Y. (2022). Mental health during the first year of the COVID-19 pandemic: A review and recommendations for moving forward. *Perspectives on Psychological Science,* 17(4), 915–936. https://doi.org/10.1177/17456916211029964

Akther, T., & Nur, T. (2022). A model of factors influencing COVID-19 vaccine acceptance: A synthesis of the theory of reasoned action, conspiracy theory belief, awareness, perceived usefulness, and perceived ease of use. *PLoS One*, 17(1), e0261869. https://doi.org/10.1371/journal.pone.0261869

Alashoor, T., & Han, S. (2021). The smoking paradox: exploring why attitudes toward cigarette smoking are a weak predictor of cigarette smoking. *Psychology & Health*, 36(7), 847–861. https://doi.org/10.1080/08870446.2020.1798958

Alcántara, C., Diaz, S. V., Cosenzo, L. G., Loucks, E. B., Penedo, F. J., & Williams, N. J. (2020). Social determinants as moderators of the effectiveness of health behavior change interventions: Scientific gaps and opportunities. *Health Psychology Review*, 14(1), 132–144.

Alegría, M., & Cheng, M. (2023). Intersectional approaches are essential to identify the multiple sources of oppression. *Journal of Psychopathology and Clinical Science,* 132(5), 590–593. https://doi.org/10.1037/abn0000842

Allan, J. L., Johnston, M., & Campbell, N. (2015). Snack purchasing is healthier when the cognitive demands of choice are reduced: A randomized controlled trial. *Health Psychology,* 34(7), 750–755. https://doi.org/10.1037/hea0000173

Allen, J. G., Flanigan, S. S., LeBlanc, M., Vallarino, J., MacNaughton, P., Stewart, J. H., & Christiani, D. C. (2016). Flavoring chemicals in e-cigarettes: Diacetyl, 2,3-pentanedione, and acetoin in a sample of 51 products, including fruit-, candy-, and cocktail-flavored e-cigarettes. *Environmental Health Perspectives*, 124(6), 733–739.

Almazan, A. N., & Keuroghlian, A. S. (2021). Association between gender-affirming surgeries and mental health outcomes. *JAMA Surgery,* 156(7), 611. https://doi.org/10.1001/jamasurg.2021.0952

Almosawi, S., Baksh, H., Qareeballa, A., Falamarzi, F., Alsaleh, B., Alrabaani, M., ... Kamal, A. (2018). Acute administration of caffeine: The effect on motor coordination, higher brain cognitive functions, and the social behavior of BLC57 mice. *Behavioral Sciences*, 8(8), 65. https://doi.org/10.3390/bs8080065

Al-Noumani, H., Wu, J.-R., Barksdale, D., Sherwood, G., AlKhasawneh, E., & Knafl, G. (2019). Health beliefs and medication adherence in patients with hypertension: A systematic review of quantitative studies. *Patient Education & Counseling*, 102(6), 1045–1056. https://doi.org/10.1016/j.pec.2019.02.022

Alonso-Castro, A. J., Ruiz-Padilla, A. J., Ramírez-Morales, M. A., Alcocer-García, S. G., Ruiz-Noa, Y., Ibarra-Reynoso, L. D. R., ... Alba-Betancourt, C. (2019). Self-treatment with herbal products for weight-loss among overweight and obese subjects from central Mexico. *Journal of Ethnopharmacology*, 234, 21–26.

Alsan, M., Garrick, O., & Graziani, G. C. (2018). Does diversity matter for health? Experimental evidence from Oakland. National Bureau of Economic Research Working Paper No. 24787.

Altekruse, S. F., Kosary, C. L., Krapcho, M., Neyman, N., Aminou, R., Waldron, W., ... Mariotto, A. (2010). *SEER Cancer Statistics Review, 1975–2007*. National Cancer Institute.

Alty, J. E., Bindoff, A. D., Stuart, K. E., Roccati, E., Collins, J. M., King, A. E., ... Vickers, J. C. (2022). Sex-specific protective effects of cognitive reserve on age-related cognitive decline. *Neurology,* 100(2), e211–e219. https://doi.org/10.1212/wnl.0000000000201369

Alzheimer's Association. (2019). 2019 Alzheimer's disease facts and figures. *Alzheimer's and Dementia*, 15(3), 321–387.

Ambrose, G., Das, K., Fan, Y., & Ramaswami, A. (2020). Is gardening associated with greater happiness of urban residents? A multi-activity, dynamic assessment in the Twin-Cities region, USA. *Landscape and Urban Planning*, 198.

American Cancer Society. (2014). Signs and symptoms of cancer. http://www.cancer.org/cancer/cancer-basics/signs-andsymptoms-of-cancer.html

American Cancer Society (ACS). (2018). Cancer facts & figures 2018.

American Cancer Society (ACS). (2020c). Lifetime risk of developing or dying from cancer. https://www.cancer.org/cancer/cancer-basics/lifetime-probability-of-developingor-dying-from-cancer.html

American Cancer Society (ACS). (2023). Melanoma skin cancer statistics. https://www.cancer.org/cancer/types/melanoma-skin-cancer/about/key-statistics.html

American College Health Association. (2018). *American College Health Association-National College Health Assessment II: Reference Group Executive Summary Fall 2018*. American College Health Association.

American College Health Association (2022). *Publications and reports*. https://www.acha.org/ACHA/Resources/Survey_Data/NCHA/NCHA/Data/Publications_and_Reports.aspx?hkey=42461a35-897f-4644-bde7-f2410d487ca5

American College Health Association. (2023). *Publications and reports*. https://www.acha.org/ACHA/Resources/Survey_Data/NCHA/NCHA/Data/Publications_and_Reports.aspx?hkey=42461a35-897f-4644-bde7-f2410d487ca5

American Diabetes Association (ADA). (2023). Statistics about diabetes. https://diabetes.org/about-us/statistics/about-diabetes#:~:text=Prevalence%20in%20seniors%3A%20The%20percentage,diagnosed%20with%20diabetes%20every%20year.

American Family Physician. (2022). Family planning and contraception. https://www.aafp.org/pubs/afp/topics/by-topic.html

American Heart Association. (2018a). Understand your risks to prevent a heart attack. http://www.heart.org/en/health-topics/heart-attack/understand-your-risks-to-prevent-a-heart-attack

American Heart Association. (2018). Understand your risks to prevent a heart attack. http://www.heart.org/en/health-topics/heart-attack/understand-your-risks-to-prevent-a-heart-attack

American Heart Association (AHA). (2009). Heart disease and stroke statistics 2009 update: A report from the American Heart Association Statistics Committee and Stroke Statistics Subcommittee. *Circulation*, 119, e121–e181.

American Heart Association (AHA). (2019). Understanding blood pressure readings. https://www.heart.org/en/health-topics/high-blood-pressure/understanding-blood-pressure-readings

American Lung Association. (2020). Lung cancer fact sheet. https://www.lung.org/lung-health-diseases/lung-disease-lookup/lung-cancer/resource-library/lung-cancer-fact-sheet

American Medical Association. (2020, March 16). Caring for our care givers during COVID-19. https://www.ama-assn.org/delivering-care/public-health/caring-our-caregivers-during-covid-19

American Pain Society. (2018). *Pediatric chronic pain programs by state/province*. Author.

American Psychiatric Association. (2013). *Diagnostic and statistical manual of mental disorders* (5th ed.). Author.

American Psychiatric Association. (2022). *Diagnostic and statistical manual of mental disorders,* (5th Ed., Text Revision). American Psychiatric Association.

American Psychological Association. (2015). Stress in America: Paying with our health. https://www.apa.org/news/press/releases/stress/2014/stress-report.pdf

American Psychological Association. (2017). Stress in America: The state of our nation. Stress in America Survey.

American Psychological Association. (2018b). Stress in America: Generation Z. *Stress in America Survey*. https://www.apa.org/news/press/releases/2018/10/generation-z-stressed

American Psychological Association. (2019). Stress in America 2019. Americans feeling stressed about presidential election, health care and mass shootings. https://www.apa.org/news/press/releases/stress/2019/stress-america-2019.pdf

American Psychological Association. (2020). Stress in the time of COVID-19. http://www.apa.org/covid-19.

Anderson, M. (2019). Mobile technology and home broadband 2019. Pew Research Center. https://www.pewresearch.org/internet/2019/06/13/mobile-technology-and-home-broadband-2019/

Anderson, M., & Karasz, A. (2017). Are vaginal symptoms ever normal? In M. A. Farage & H. I. Maibach (Eds.), *The vulva: Physiology and clinical management*. CRC Press.

Anderson, R. M., Heesterbeek, H., Kilnkenberg, D., & Hollingsworth, T. D. (2020). How will country-based mitigation measures influence the course of the COVID-19 epidemic? *The Lancet*, 395(10228), 931–934.

Andes, L. J., Cheng, Y. J., Rolka, D. B., Gregg, E. W., & Imperatore, G. (2019). Prevalence of prediabetes among adolescents and young adults in the United States, 2005–2016. *JAMA Pediatrics*. https://doi.org/10.1001/jamapediatrics.2019.4498

Andreeva, G. F., & Gorbunov, V. M. (2022). Hostility, anger, psychoemotional factors and cardiovascular disease. *Rational Pharmacotherapy in Cardiology*, 18(2), 191–199. https://doi.org/10.20996/1819-6446-2022-04-09

Andres-Rodriguez, L., Borras, X., Feliu-Soler, A., Perez-Aranda, A., Rozadilla-Sacanell, A., Montero-Marin, J., ... Luciano, J. V. (2019). Immune-inflammatory pathways and clinical changes in fibromyalgia patients treated with mindfulness-based stress Reduction (MBSR): A randomized, controlled clinical trial. *Brain, Behavior, and Immunity*, 80, 109–119.

Anglim, J., Horwood, S., Smillie, L. D., Marrero, R. J., & Wood, J. K. (2020). Predicting psychological and subjective well-being from personality: A meta-analysis. *Psychological Bulletin*, 146, 279–323.

Annis, T., Pleasants, S., Hultman, G., Lindemann, E., Thompson, J. A., Billecke, S., ... Melton, G. B. (2020). Rapid implementation of a COVID-19 remote patient monitoring Program. *Journal of the American Medical Informatics Association*. https://doi.org/10.1093/jamia.ocaa097

Antoni, M. H., Moreno, P. I., & Penedo, F. J. (2023). Stress management interventions to facilitate psychological and physiological adaptation and optimal health outcomes in cancer patients and survivors. *Annual Review of Psychology*, 74(1), 423–455. https://doi.org/10.1146/annurev-psych-030122-124119

Aquino, M., DiMenna, F. J., Petrizzo, J., Otto, R. M., & Wygand, J. (2020). Power training improves bone mineral density and fall risk for a postmenopausal woman with a history of osteoporosis and increased risk of falling. *Journal of Bodywork and Movement Therapies*, 24(3), 44–49.

Archangelo, S. D. C. V., Sabino Neto, M., Veiga, D. F., Garcia, E. B., & Ferreira, L. M. (2019). Sexuality, depression and body image after breast reconstruction. *Clinics*, 74. https://doi.org/10.6061/clinics/2019/e883

Arena, J. G., & Tankersley, J. D. (2018). Introduction to biofeedback training for chronic pain disorders. In D. C. Turk & R. J. Gatchel (Eds.), *Psychological approaches to pain management: A practitioner's handbook* (3rd ed., pp. 138–159). The Guilford Press.

Arias, E., Kochanek, K. D., & Anderson, R. N. (2015). How does cause of death contribute to the Hispanic mortality advantage in the United States? NCHS Data Brief, No. 221. National Center for Health Statistics.

Arias, E., Kochanek, K., Xu, J., & Tejada-Vera, B. (2023). Vital statistics rapid release provisional life expectancy estimates for 2022. https://www.cdc.gov/nchs/data/vsrr/vsrr031.pdf

Arias, E., & Xu, J. (2019). United States life tables, 2017. *National Vital Statistics Reports*, 68(7).

Armeli, S., Carney, M. A., Tennen, H., Affleck, G., & O'Neil, T. P. (2000). Stress and alcohol use: A daily process examination of the stressor vulnerability model. *Journal of Personality and Social Psychology*, 78, 979–994.

Armer, J. S., Clevenger, L., Davis, L. Z., Cuneo, M., Thaker, P. H., Goodheart, M. J., ... Slavich, G. M. (2018). Life stress as a risk factor for sustained anxiety and cortisol dysregulation during the first year of survivorship in ovarian cancer. *Cancer*, 124(16), 3401–3408. https://doi.org/10.1002/cncr.31570

Arnett, D. K., Blumenthal, R. S., Albert, M. A., Buroker, A. B., Goldberger, Z. D., Hahn, E. J., ... Ziaeian, B. (2019). 2019 ACC/AHA guideline on the primary prevention of cardiovascular disease: Executive summary: A report of the American College of Cardiology/American Heart Association Task Force on Clinical Practice Guidelines. *Journal of the American College of Cardiology*, 74, 1376–1414.

Arnold, L. M., Choy, E., Clauw, D. J., Goldenberg, D. L., Harris, R. E., Helfenstein Jr., M., ... Wang, G. (2016). Fibromyalgia and chronic pain syndromes: A white paper detailing current challenges in the field. *The Clinical Journal of Pain*, 32, 737–746.

Aronson, M. K. (1988). Patients and families: Impact and long-term-management implications. In M. K. Aronson (Ed.), Understanding Alzheimer's disease (pp. 74–78). New York: Charles Scribners and Sons.

Arsenović, S., Trajković, G., Pekmezović, T., & Gazibara, T. (2022). Beliefs about influenza and avoidance of free influenza immunization among people with chronic diseases. *Health Psychology*, 41(7), 455–462. https://doi.org/10.1037/hea0001176

Artiga, S., & Orgera, K. (2019, November 12). Key facts on health and health care by race and ethnicity. Kaiser Family Foundation.

Asare, M. (2015). Using the theory of planned behavior to determine the condom use behavior among college students. *American Journal of Health Studies*, 30(1), 43–50. PMID: 26512197.

Aschbacher, K., Yilmaz, D., Kerem, Y., Crawford, S., Benaron, D., Liu, J., ... Marcus, G. M. (2020). Atrial fibrillation detection from raw photoplethysmography waveforms: A deep learning application. *Heart Rhythm O2*, 1(1), 3–9.

Ashford, R. D., Giorgi, S., Mann, B., Pesce, C., Sherritt, L., Ungar, L., & Curtis, B. (2020). Digital recovery networks: Characterizing user participation, engagement, and outcomes of a novel recovery social network smartphone application. *Journal of Substance Abuse Treatment*, 109, 50–55.

As Valentine's Day Approaches. (2012, February). *ScienceDaily*. https://www.sciencedaily.com/releases/2012/02/120207121928.htm

Atreja, A., Francis, S., Kurra, S., & Kabra, R. (2019). Digital medicine and evolution of remote patient monitoring in cardiac electrophysiology: A state-of-the-art perspective. *Current Treatment Options in Cardiovascular Medicine*, 21(12). https://doi.org/10.1007/s11936-019-0787-3

Atrooz, F., & Salim, S. (2020). Sleep deprivation, oxidative stress and inflammation. In R. Doney (Ed.), *Advances in protein chemistry and structural biology* (Vol. 119, pp. 309–336). Academic Press.

Attia, E., & Guarda, A. S. (2022). Prevention and early identification of eating disorders. *JAMA*, 327(11), 1029. https://doi.org/10.1001/jama.2022.2458

Aubrey, A. (2020, April 18). Who's hit hardest by COVID-19? NPR.org. https://www.npr.org/sections/health-shots/2020/04/18/835563340/

whos-hit-hardest-by-covid-19-why-obesity-stress-and-race-all-matter

Avert. (2019). HIV and AIDS in the United States of America. https://www.avert.org/professionals/hiv-around-world/western-central-europe-north-america/usa

Avery, J. (2022). Naltrexone and alcohol use. *American Journal of Psychiatry,* 179(12), 886–887. https://doi.org/10.1176/appi.ajp.20220821

Axelsson, E., Andersson, E., Ljótsson, B., Björkander, D., Hedman-Lagerlöf, M., & Hedman-Lagerlöf, E. (2020). Effect of Internet vs face-to-face cognitive behavior therapy for health anxiety. *JAMA Psychiatry*. https://doi.org/10.1001/jamapsychiatry.2020.0940

Aydogan, U., Doganer, Y. C., Haymana, C., Kaplan, U., Aydogdu, A., Demirci, I., ... Sonmez, Y. A. (2023). Evaluation of sexual functional status and consistency of scales in patients with hypogonadotropic hypogonadism before and after testosterone replacement therapy: A single-center experience. *Archives of Endocrinology and Metabolism,* 67(2), 179–188. https://doi.org/10.20945/2359-3997000000539

Azouz, S., Swanson, M., Omarkhil, M., & Rebecca, A. (2020). A nipple-areola stencil for three-dimensional tattooing: Nipple by number. *Plastic and Reconstructive Surgery*, 145(1), 38–42.

Bach, D. S. (2023). Exercise benefits in CVD: Key points. American College of Cardiology.

Bäckström, T., Andreen, L., Birzniece, V., Björn, I., Johansson, I.-M., Nordenstam-Haghjo, M., ... Zhu, D. (2003). The role of hormones and hormonal treatments in premenstrual syndrome. *CNS Drugs,* 17(5), 325–342. https://doi.org/10.2165/00023210-200317050-00003

Baer, H. J., Rozenblum, R., De La Cruz, B. A., Orav, E. J., Wien, M., Nolido, N. V., ... Bates, D. W. (2020). Effect of an online weight management program integrated with population health management on weight change. *JAMA,* 324(17), 1737. https://doi.org/10.1001/jama.2020.18977

Baer, R. A., Peters, J. R., Eisenlohr-Moula, T. A., Geiger, P. J., & Sauer, S. E. (2012). Emotion-related cognitive processes in borderline personality disorder: A review of the empirical literature. *Clinical Psychology Review*, 32, 359–369.

Bahlburg, H. F. L. (2015). Gender identity and role: Clinical-psychological aspects. *The international encyclopedia of human sexuality*, 427–500.

Baiardini, I., Sicuro, F., Balbi, F., Canonica, G. W., & Braido, F. (2015). Psychological aspects in asthma: Do psychological factors affect asthma management? *Asthma Research and Practice*, 1, 7. https://doi.org/10.1186/s40733-015-0007-1

Bakalar, N. (2020, January 20). Drinking tea tied to better heart health. *New York Times*. https://www.nytimes.com/2020/01/13/well/eat/drinking-tea-tied-to-better-heart-health.html

Balderson, B. H., Pruitt, S. D., & Von Korff, M. (2018). Strengthening self-management of low back pain in primary care: An evolving paradigm. In D. C. Turk & R. J. Gatchel (Eds.), *Psychological approaches to pain management: A practitioner's handbook* (3rd ed., pp. 319–339). The Guilford Press.

Baldwin, A., Dodge, B., Schick, V. R., Light, B., Scharrs, P. W., Herbenick, D., & Fortenberry, J. D. (2018). Transgender and genderqueer individuals' experiences with health care providers: What's working, what's not, and where do we go from here? *Journal of Health Care for the Poor and Underserved*, 29(4), 1300–1318.

Baldwin, A., Fu, T. C., Reece, M., Herbenick, D., Dodge, B., Sanders, S. A., ... Fortenberry, J. D. (2019). Condom use completeness, perceptions, and sexual quality at most recent sexual event: Results from a US nationally representative probability sample. *International Journal of Sexual Health*, 31(4), 414–425.

Balkıs, M., & Duru, E. (2018). The protective role of rational beliefs on the relationship between irrational beliefs, emotional states of stress, depression and anxiety. *Journal of Rational-Emotive & Cognitive-Behavior Therapy*, 37(1), 96–112.

Balter, L. J., Raymond, J. E., Aldred, S., Drayson, M. T., van Zanten, J. J. V., Higgs, S., & Bosch, J. A. (2020). Loneliness in healthy young adults predicts inflammatory responsiveness to a mild immune challenge in vivo. *Brain, Behavior, and Immunity*, 82, 298–301.

Bamishigbin, O. N., Jr., Stein, K. D., Leach, C. R., & Stanton, A. L. (2020). Spirituality and depressive symptoms in a multiethnic sample of cancer survivors. *Health Psychology,* 39(7), 589–599. https://doi.org/10.1037/hea0000878

Bamonti, P. M., Moye, J., & Naik, A. D. (2018). Pain is associated with continuing depression in cancer survivors. *Psychology, Health & Medicine*, 23, 1182–1195.

Bandura, A. (1986). The explanatory and predictive scope of self-efficacy theory. *Journal of Social and Clinical Psychology*, 4(3), 359–373. https://doi.org/10.1521/jscp.1986.4.3.359

Bandura, A. (2010). Self-efficacy. *The Corsini Encyclopedia of Psychology*, 1–3. https://doi.org/10.1002/9780470479216.corpsy0836

Bansal, K., Rajput, S., & Mathur, V. S. (2019). Exploring reasons for medication non-adherence in hypertension patients. *International Journal of Pharmacy & Life Sciences*, 10(16), 16–16.

Barabási, A.-L. (2007). Network medicine—From obesity to the "diseasome." *New England Journal of Medicine*, 357, 404–407.

Barbeau, A. M., Burda, J., & Siegel, M. (2013). Perceived efficacy of e-cigarettes versus nicotine replacement therapy among successful e-cigarette users: A qualitative approach. *Addiction Science & Clinical Practice*, 8(1), 5.

Barcelos, T. M. R., Ferreira, C. H. J., Lerri, M. R., Brito, L. G. O., de Sá, M. F. S., de Sá, A. C. S., ... da Silva Lara, L. A. (2022). Sexual function of transgender women after gender affirming surgery: A mini review. *Clinical Anatomy,* 35(5), 560–570. https://doi.org/10.1002/ca.23863

Barefoot, J. C., & Williams, R. B. (2022). Hostility and health. In S. R. Waldstein, W. J. Willem, J. Kop, E. C. Suarez, W. R. Lovallo, & L. I. Katzel (Eds.), *Handbook of cardiovascular behavioral medicine* (pp. 503–524). Springer. https://doi.org/10.1007/978-0-387-85960-6_20

Barley, E., & Lawson, V. (2016). Using health psychology to help patients: Theories of behaviour change. *British Journal of Nursing*, 25, 923–927.

Barnes, B. (2020, February 18). Ben Affleck tried to drink away the pain. Now he's trying honesty. https://www.nytimes.com/2020/02/18/movies/ben-affleck.html?searchResultPosition=1

Barnett, M. D., Hale, T. M., & Sligar, K. B. (2017). Masculinity, femininity, sexual dysfunctional beliefs, and rape myth acceptance among heterosexual college men and women. *Sexuality & Culture*, 21(3), 741–753.

Barnett, M. D., Hays, K. N., & Cantu, C. (2019). Compassion fatigue, emotional labor, and emotional display among hospice nurses. *Death Studies*. https://doi.org/10.1080/07481187.2019.1699201

Barquissau, V., Léger, B., Beuzelin, D., Martins, F., Amri, E. Z., Pisani, D. F., ... Déjean, S. (2018). Caloric restriction and diet-induced weight loss do not induce browning of human subcutaneous white adipose tissue in women and men with obesity. *Cell Reports*, 22(4), 1079–1089.

Barreiro-de Acosta, M., Marín-Jiménez, I., Panadero, A., Guardiola, J., Cañas, M., Montoya, M. G., ... Casellas, F. (2018). Recomendaciones del Grupo Español de Trabajo en Enfermedad de Crohn y Colitis Ulcerosa (GETECCU) y de la Confederación de Asociaciones de Enfermedad de Crohn y Colitis Ulcerosa (ACCU) para el manejo de los aspectos psicológicos en la enfermedad inflamatoria intestinal. *Gastroenterología y Hepatología*, 41(2), 118–127.

Barry, M. J., Nicholson, W. K., Silverstein, M., Chelmow, D., Coker, T. R., Davidson, ... Wong, J. B. (2023). Screening for depression and suicide risk in adults. *JAMA*, 329(23), 2057. https://doi.org/10.1001/jama.2023.9297

Barry, M. J., Nicholson, W. K., Silverstein, M., Coker, T. R., Davidson, K. W., Davis, E. M., ... Wong, J. B. (2023). Screening for anxiety disorders in adults. *JAMA*. https://doi.org/10.1001/jama.2023.9301

Barton, B. K., Kologi, S. M., & Siron, A. (2016). Distracted pedestrians in crosswalks: An application of the Theory of Planned Behavior. *Transportation Research Part F: Traffic Psychology and Behaviour*, 37, 129–137.

Bartone, P. T., Valdes, J. J., & Sandvik, A. (2016). Psychological hardiness predicts cardiovascular health. *Psychology, Health & Medicine*, 21(6), 743–749.

Basch, C. E., Basch, C. H., Ruggles, K. V., & Rajan, S. (2014). Prevalence of sleep duration on an average school night among 4 nationally representative successive samples of American high school students, 2007–2013. *Preventing Chronic Disease*, 11. https://doi.org/10.5888/pcd11.140383

Basen-Engquist, K., Carmack, C. L., Li, Y., Brown, J., Jhingran, A., Hughes, D. C., ... Waters, A. (2013). Social-cognitive theory predictors of exercise behavior in endometrial cancer survivors. *Health Psychology*, 32, 1137–1148.

Basso, J. C., McHale, A., Ende, V., Oberlin, D. J., & Suzuki, W. A. (2019). Brief, daily meditation enhances attention, memory, mood, and emotional regulation in non-experienced meditators. *Behavioural Brain Research*, 356, 208–220. https://doi.org/10.1016/j.bbr.2018.08.023

Basten-Günther, J., Peters, M., & Lautenbacher, S. (2019). Optimism and the experience of pain: A systematic review. *Behavioral Medicine*, 45(4), 323–339.

Battalio, S. L., Huffman, S. E., & Jensen, M. P. (2020). Longitudinal associations between physical activity, anxiety, and depression in adults with long-term physical disabilities. *Health Psychology*, 39(6), 529–538.

Bauer, U., & Thompson, B. L. (2018). Mission possible: Addressing health disparities in heart disease and stroke outcomes. https://blogs.cdc.gov/healthequity/2018/02/26/heart-disease-and-stroke/

Baumeister, R. F., & Alghamdi, N. G. (2015). Role of self-control failure in immoral and unethical actions. *Current Opinion in Psychology*, 6, 66–69.

Baumgaertner, E. (2023, July 26). For healthy older people, aspirin could cause more bleeding. *New York Times*. https://www.nytimes.com/2023/07/26/health/aspirin-bleeding-stroke-heart-attack.html?utm_campacroft ign=KHN:%20First%20Edition&utm_medium=email&_hsmi=267980575&_hsenc=p2ANqtz-8Dtvyn6t542r5LzOaXIcCv3pg5TTF40aZ3q2J1blYWX4ZoTZyNQ-tZWmsKwPcq9RHsAEwM_EA2mJRzxFNQsi98XsYjzg&utm_con

Baumgartner, J. N., Schneider, T. R., & Capiola, A. (2018). Investigating the relationship between optimism and stress responses: A biopsychosocial perspective. *Personality and Individual Differences*, 129, 114–118.

Baum, M. J., & Bakker, J. (2017). Reconsidering prenatal hormonal influences on human sexual orientation: Lessons from animal research. *Archives of Sexual Behavior*, 46(6), 1601–1605.

Beatty Moody, D. L., Waldstein, S. R., Tobin, J. N., Cassells, A., Schwartz, J. C., & Brondolo, E. (2016). Lifetime racial/ethnic discrimination and ambulatory blood pressure: The moderating effect of age. *Health Psychology*, 35, 333–342.

Becattini, C., Agnelli, G., Schenone, A., Eichinger, S., Bucherini, E., Silingardi, M., ... WARFASA Investigators. (2012). Aspirin for preventing the recurrence of venous thromboembolism. *New England Journal of Medicine*, 366, 1959–1967.

Bechara, A., Berridge, K. C., Bickel, W. K., Morón, J. A., Williams, S. B., & Stein, J. S. (2019). A neurobehavioral approach to addiction: Implications for the opioid epidemic and the psychology of addiction. *Psychological Science in the Public Interest*, 20, 96–127.

Beck, A. T. (1993). Cognitive therapy: Past, present, and future. *Journal of Consulting and Clinical Psychology*, 61(2), 194–198. https://doi.org/10.1037/0022-006X.61.2.194

Beck, A. T. (2019). A 60-year evolution of cognitive theory and therapy. *Perspectives on Psychological Science*, 14, 16–20. https://doi.org/10.1177/1745691618804187

Beck, A. T., & Bredemeier, K. (2016). A unified model of depression: Integrating clinical, cognitive, biological, and evolutionary perspectives. *Clinical Psychological Science*, 4(4), 596–619.

Beck, A. T., Rush, A. J., Shaw, B. F., & Emery, G. (1979). *Cognitive therapy of depression*. Guilford Press.

Beck, M., & Schatz, A. (2014, January 17). American eating habits take a healthier turn. *The Wall Street Journal*, A1, A8.

Bedimo, R. J., & Jodlowski, T. (2023). PrEParing for the end of the HIV epidemic-A public health imperative. *JAMA Network Open*, 6(8), e2330195. https://doi.org/10.1001/jamanetworkopen.2023.30195

Bell, A. P., & Weinberg, M. S. (1978). *Homosexualities: A study of diversity among men and women*. Simon & Schuster.

Bell, B. T., & Dittmar, H. (2011). Does media type matter? The role of identification in adolescent girls' media consumption and the impact of different thin-ideal media on body image. *Sex Roles*, 65, 478–490.

Bellocco, R., Marrone, G., Ye, W., Nyrén, O., Adami, H. O., Mariosa, D., & Lagerros, Y. T. (2016). A prospective cohort study of the combined effects of physical activity and anthropometric measures on the risk of post-menopausal breast cancer. *European Journal of Epidemiology*, 31(4), 395–404.

Bell, S., Daskalopoulou, M., Rapsomaniki, E., George, J., Britton, A., Bobak, M., ... Hemingway, H. (2017). Association between clinically recorded alcohol consumption and initial presentation of 12 cardiovascular diseases: Population based cohort study using linked health records. *British Medical Journal*, 356, j909. https://doi.org/10.1136/bmj.j909

Belluck, P. (2023, January 6). F.D.A. approves new treatment for early Alzheimer's. (2023). *New York Times*. https://www.nytimes.com/2023/01/06/health/alzheimers-drug-leqembi-lecanemab.html?searchResultPosition=1

Benedetti, F. (2021). Placebos and movies: What do they have in common? *Current Directions in Psychological Science*. https://journals.sagepub.com/doi/10.1177/09637214211003892

Benedict, M. O. A., Steinberg, W. J., Claassen, F. M., Mofolo, N., & Van Rooyen, C. (2023). Knowledge, attitude and practice on screening and early diagnosis of prostate cancer of primary health care providers in the Free State. *African Journal of Primary Health Care & Family Medicine*, 15(1), e1–e12. https://doi.org/10.4102/phcfm.v15i1.3688

Benight, C. C., & Bandura, A. (2004). Social cognitive theory of posttraumatic recovery: The role of perceived self-efficacy. *Behaviour Research and Therapy*, 10, 1129–1148.

Benjamins, J. S., Hooge, I. T. C., Benedict, C., Smeets, P. A. M., & van der Laan, L. N. (2021). The influence of acute partial sleep deprivation on liking, choosing and consuming high- and low-energy foods. *Food Quality and Preference*, 88(104074), 104074. https://doi.org/10.1016/j.foodqual.2020.104074

Benner, A. D., Wang, Y., Shen, Y., Boyle, A. E., Polk, R., & Cheng, Y.-P. (2018). Racial/ethnic discrimination and well-being during adolescence: A meta-analytic review. *American Psychologist*, 73(7), 855–883. https://doi.org/10.1037/amp0000204

Bennie, J. A., Teychenne, M. J., De Cocker, K., & Biddle, S. J. (2019). Associations between aerobic and muscle-strengthening exercise with depressive symptom severity among 17,839 US adults. *Preventive Medicine*, 121, 121–127.

Benson, H. (1977). Systemic hypertension and the relaxation response. *The New England Journal of Medicine*, 296, 1152–1156.

Benyamini, Y., & Leventhal, H. (2019). Beliefs and perceptions of health and illness. In C. Llewellyn, S. Ayers, C. McManus, S. Newman, K. J. Petrie, T. A. Revenson, & J. Weinman (Eds.), *Cambridge handbook of psychology, health and medicine* (3rd ed., pp. 106–109). Cambridge University Press.

Bergman, B. C., & Goodpaster, B. H. (2020). Exercise and muscle lipid content, composition, and localization: Influence on muscle insulin sensitivity. *Diabetes*, 69(5), 848–858.

Bergström, G., Lohela-Karlsson, M., Kwak, L., Bodin, L., Jensen, I., Torgén, M., & Nybergh, L. (2017). Preventing sickness absenteeism among employees with common mental disorders or stress-related symptoms at work: Design of a cluster randomized controlled trial of a problem-solving based intervention versus care-as-usual conducted at the Occupational Health Services. *BMC Public Health*, 17(1), 436. https://doi.org/10.1186/s12889-017-4329-1

Bernardo, M., Cañas, F., Herrera, B., & Dorado, G. (2017). Adherence predicts symptomatic and psychosocial remission in schizophrenia: Naturalistic study of patient integration in the community. *Revista de Psiquiatría y Salud Mental*, 10, 149–159.

Bernstein, E. E., & McNally, R. J. (2018). Exercise as a buffer against difficulties with emotion regulation: A pathway to emotional well-being. *Behaviour Research and Therapy*, 109, 29–36. https://doi.org/10.1016/j.brat.2018.07.010

Berry, K. M., Fetterman, J. L., Benjamin, E. J., Bhatnagar, A., Barrington-Trimis, J. L., Leventhal, A. M., & Stokes, A. (2019). Association of electronic cigarette use with subsequent initiation of tobacco cigarettes in US youths. *JAMA Network Open*, 2(2), e187794–e187794.

Berry, M. P., Sala, M., Abber, S. R., & Forman, E. M. (2021). Incorporating automated digital interventions into coach-delivered weight loss treatment: A meta-analysis. *Health Psychology*, 40(8), 534–545. https://doi.org/10.1037/hea0001106

Bertrand, K. A., Bethea, T. N., Adams-Campbell, L. L., Rosenberg, L., & Palmer, J. R. (2017). Differential patterns of risk factors for early-onset breast cancer by ER status in African American women. *Cancer Epidemiology, Biomarkers & Prevention*, 26(2), 270–277.

Bethune, S. (2020). Americans are stressed about the presidential election. *Monitor on Psychology*, 51(1), 20.

Bhuptani, P. H., & Messman-Moore, T. L. (2019). Blame and shame in sexual assault. In W. T. O'Donohue & P. A. Schewe (Eds.), *Handbook of sexual assault and sexual assault prevention* (pp. 309–322). Springer.

Bianchi, R., Schonfeld, I. S., & Verkuilen, J. (2020). A five-sample confirmatory factor analytic study of burnout-depression overlap. *Journal of Clinical Psychology*, 76(4), 801–821.

Biddinger, K. J., Emdin, C. A., Haas, M. E., Wang, M., Hindy, G., Ellinor, P. T., Kathiresan, S., Khera, A. V., & Aragam, K. G. (2022). Association of habitual alcohol intake with risk of cardiovascular disease. *JAMA Network Open*, 5(3), e223849. https://doi.org/10.1001/jamanetworkopen.2022.3849

Biggs, A., Brough, P., & Drummond, S. (2017). Lazarus and Folkman's psychological stress and coping theory. In C. L. Cooper & J. C. Quick (Eds.), *The handbook of stress and health: A guide to research and practice* (pp. 351–364). John Wiley & Sons.

Bikdeli, B., Wayda, B., Bao, H., Ross, J. S., Xu, X., Chaudhry, S. I., ... Krumholz, H. M. (2014). Place of residence and outcomes of patients with heart failure: Analysis from the telemonitoring to improve heart failure outcomes trial. *Circulation: Cardiovascular Quality and Outcomes*, 7, 749–756.

Binny, J., Wong, N. L. J., Garga, S., Lin, C. W. C., Maher, C. G., McLachlan, A. J., ... Shaheed, C. A. (2019). Transcutaneous electric nerve stimulation (TENS) for acute low back pain: Systematic review. *Scandinavian Journal of Pain*, 19, 225–233.

Bishop, F. M. (2018). Self-guided change: The most common form of long-term, maintained health behavior change. *Health Psychology Open* (January–June), 1–14. https://doi.org/10.1177/2055102917751576

Bishop, K. C., Ketcham, J. D., & Kuminoff, N. V. (2018). Hazed and confused: The effect of air pollution on dementia. National Bureau of Economic Research, Working Paper No. 24970. http://www.nber.org/papers/w24970

Blanchard, E. B., & Hickling, E. J. (2004). *After the crash: Psychological assessment and treatment of survivors of motor vehicle accidents* (2nd ed.). American Psychological Association.

Blanco, C., Secades-Villa, R., Garcia-Rodriguez, O., Labrador-Mendez, M., Wang, S., & Schwartz, R. P. (2013). Probability and predictors of remission from life-time prescription drug use disorders: Results from the National Epidemiologic Survey on Alcohol and Related Conditions. *Journal of Psychiatric Research*, 47(1), 42–49.

Blank, M., Zhang, J., Lamers, F., Taylor, A. D., Hickie, I. B., & Merikangas, K. R. (2015). Health correlates of insomnia symptoms and comorbid mental disorders in a nationally representative sample of US adolescents. *Sleep*, 38(2), 197–204.

Bliton, J. N. Parides, M., Muscarella, P., & Papalezova, K. T. (2021). Understanding racial disparities in gastrointestinal cancer outcomes: Lack of surgery contributes to lower survival in African American patients. *Cancer Epidemiology, Biomarkers & Prevention*, 30(3), 529–538. https://doi.org/10.1158/1055-9965.EPI-20-0950.

Blum, D. (2023, August 9). Even 4,000 steps a day can have big health benefits. *The New York Times*. https://www.nytimes.com/2023/08/09/well/move/steps-walking-health-benefits.html

Bodell, L. P., Cheng, Y., & Wildes, J. E. (2018). Psychological impairment as a predictor of suicide ideation in individuals with anorexia nervosa. *Suicide and Life-Threatening Behavior*. https://doi.org/10.1111/sltb.12459

Boersma, P., & Black, L. I. (2020). Human papillomavirus vaccination among adults aged 18–26, 2013–2018. *NCHS Data Brief*, 354. https://www.cdc.gov/nchs/data/databriefs/db354-h.pdf

Bogg, T., & Roberts, B. W. (2013). The case for conscientiousness: Evidence and implications for a personality trait marker of health and longevity. *Annals of Behavioral Medicine*, 45, 278–288.

Bohm, M. K., Liu, Y., Esser, M. B., Mesnick, J. B., Lu, H., Pan, Y., & Greenlund, K. J. (2021). Binge drinking among adults, by select characteristics and State—United States, 2018. *Morbidity and Mortality Weekly Report*, 70(41), 1441–1446.

Bolívar, H. A., Klemperer, E. M., Coleman, S. R., DeSarno, M. J., Skelly, J. M., & Higgins, S. T. (2021). Contingency management for patients receiving medication for opioid use disorder. *JAMA Psychiatry*, 78(10), 1092. https://doi.org/10.1001/jamapsychiatry.2021.1969

Bollen, J., Gonçalves, B., van de Leemput, I., & Ruan, G. (2017). The happiness paradox: Your friends are happier than you. *EPJ Data Science*, 6(1), 4. https://doi.org/10.1140/epjds/s13688-017-0100-1

Bommersbach, T. J., Rosenheck, R. A., & Rhee, T. G. (2022). National trends of mental health care among US adults who attempted suicide in the past 12 months. *JAMA Psychiatry*. https://doi.org/10.1001/jamapsychiatry.2021.3958

Bonanni, R., Cariati, I., Tancredi, V., Iundusi, R., Gasbarra, E., & Tarantino, U. (2022). Chronic pain in musculoskeletal diseases: Do you know your enemy? *Journal of Clinical Medicine*, 11(9), 2609–2609. https://doi.org/10.3390/jcm11092609

Bonanno, G. A., Brewin, C. R., Kaniasty, K., & La Greca, A. M. (2010). Weighing the costs of disaster: Consequences, risks, and resilience in individuals, families, and communities. *Psychological Science in the Public Interest*, 11, 1–49.

Bonnevie, T., Gravier, F. E., Elkins, M., Dupuis, J., Prieur, G., Combret, Y., ... Lamia, B. (2019). People undertaking pulmonary rehabilitation are willing and able to provide accurate data via a remote pulse oximetry system: A multicentre observational study. *Journal of Physiotherapy*, 65(1), 28–36.

Bonomi, A., Nichols, E., Kammes, R., Chugani, C. D., De Genna, N. M., Jones, K., & Miller, E. (2018). Alcohol use, mental health disability, and violence victimization in college women: Exploring connections. *Violence Against Women*, 24(11), 1314–1326.

Bookwala, J., & Gaugler, T. (2020). Relationship quality and 5-year mortality risk. *Health Psychology*, 39(8), 633–641. https://doi.org/10.1037/hea0000883

Boskind-White, M., & White, W. C. (1983). *Bulimarexia: The binge/purge cycle*. W. W. Norton.

Bouchard, J., & Wong, J. S. (2020). Disparate approaches to intimate partner violence intervention: A preliminary investigation of participant outcomes across two community-based programs. *Deviant Behavior*, 1–20. https://doi.org/10.1080/01639625.2020.1750569

Bourquard, T., Lee, K., Al-Ramahi, I., Pham, M., Shapiro, D., Lagisetty, Y., ... Lichtarge, O. (2023). Functional variants identify sex-specific genes and pathways in Alzheimer's disease. *Nature Communications*, 14(1). https://doi.org/10.1038/s41467-023-38374-z

Bower, J. E., & Irwin, M. R. (2016). Mind–body therapies and control of inflammatory biology: A descriptive review. *Brain, Behavior, and Immunity*, 51, 1–11.

Bowlby, J. (1961). Processes of mourning. *International Journal of Psychoanalysis*, 42, 317–339.

Boyatzis, R. E. (1974). The effect of alcohol consumption on the aggressive behavior of men. *Quarterly Journal of Studies on Alcohol*, 35, 929–972.

Boylan, J. M., Tompkins, J. L., & Krueger, P. M. (2022). Psychological well-being, education, and mortality. *Health Psychology*, 41(3), 225–234. https://psycnet.apa.org/doi/10.1037/hea0001159

Bradley, R. H. (2019). Home life and health among Native American, African American, and Latino adolescents. *Health Psychology*, 38, 738–747.

Brady, D., Kohler, U., & Zheng, H. (2023). Novel estimates of mortality associated with poverty in the US. *JAMA Internal Medicine*, 183(6), 618–619.

Brady, S., D'Ambrosio, L. A., Felts, A., Rula, E. Y., Kell, K. P., & Coughlin, J. F. (2020). Reducing isolation and loneliness through membership in a fitness program for older adults: Implications for health. *Journal of Applied Gerontology*, 39(3), 301–310.

Branscombe, N. R., & Baron, R. A. (2017). *Social psychology* (14th ed.). Pearson.

Bray, G. A., & Bouchard, C. (2014). *Handbook of obesity—Epidemiology, etiology, & physiopathology*. CRC Press.

Breland, J. Y., Wong, J. J., & McAndrew, L. M. (2020). Are Common Sense Model constructs and self-efficacy simultaneously correlated with self-management behaviors and health outcomes: A systematic review. *Health Psychology Open*, 7(1). https://doi.org/10.1177/2055102919898846

Brett, A. S. (2019). Primary prevention of cardiovascular disease: New guideline. *New England Journal of Medicine Journal Watch*. https://www.jwatch.org/na48885/2019/04/10/us-outcomes-acute-myocardial-infarction-have-improved-last

Bretthauer, M., Løberg, M., Wieszczy, P., Kalager, M., Emilsson, L., Garborg, K., ... Kaminski, M. F. (2022). Effect of colonoscopy screening on risks of colorectal cancer and related death. *The New England Journal of Medicine*, 387(17), 1547–1556. https://doi.org/10.1056/nejmoa2208375

Bretthauer, M., Wieszczy, P., Løberg, M., Kaminski, M. F., Werner, T. F., Helsingen, L. M., . . . Kalager, M. (2023). Estimated lifetime gained with cancer screening tests: A meta-analysis of randomized clinical trials: A meta-analysis of randomized clinical trials. *JAMA Internal Medicine*, 183(11), 1196–1203. https://doi.org/10.1001/jamainternmed.2023.3798

Breuner, C. C., Mattson, G., & Committee on Psychosocial Aspects of Child and Family Health. (2016). Sexuality education for children and adolescents. *Pediatrics*, 138(2), e20161348.

Breuninger, M. M., Grosso, J. A., Hunter, W., & Dolan, S. L. (2020). Treatment of alcohol use disorder: Integration of Alcoholics Anonymous and cognitive behavioral therapy. *Training and Education in Professional Psychology*, 14(1), 19–26. https://doi.org/10.1037/tep0000265

Brewis, A., SturtzSreetharan, C., & Wutich, A. (2018). Obesity stigma as a globalizing health challenge. *Globalization and Health*, 14(1), 20.

Brody, J. E. (2020, January 28). To find better health, look on the bright side. *New York Times*, D5.

Bromet, E. J., Atwoli, L., Kawakami, N., Navarro-Mateu, F., Piotrowski, P., King, A. J., ... Florescu, S. (2017). Post-traumatic stress disorder associated with natural and human-made disasters in the World Mental Health Surveys. *Psychological Medicine*, 47(2), 227–241.

Brook, M. J., Christian, L. M., Hade, E. M., & Ruffin, M. T. (2017). The effect of perceived stress on Epstein-Barr virus antibody titers in Appalachian Ohio women. *Neuroimmunomodulation*, 24(2), 67–73.

Brooks, M. (2022, July 15). Best meds for insomnia identified? *Medscape*. https://www.medscape.com/viewarticle/977318

Brooks, M., Graham-Kevan, N., Lowe, M., & Robinson, S. (2017). Rumination, event centrality, and perceived control as predictors of post-traumatic growth and distress: The Cognitive Growth and Stress Model. *British Journal of Clinical Psychology*, 56(3), 286–302.

Brooks, S. K., Webster, R. K., Smith, L. E., Woodland, L., Wessely, S., Greenberg, N., & Rubin, G. J. (2020). The psychological impact of quarantine and how to reduce it: Rapid review of the evidence. *The Lancet*, 395, 912–920.

Brotons, M., & Bruni, L. (2020). Population-level impact of human papillomavirus vaccination. *Lancet*, 395(10221), 411–412.

Brown, E. G., Gallagher, S., & Creaven, A. M. (2018). Loneliness and acute stress reactivity: A systematic review of psychophysiological studies. *Psychophysiology*, 55(5), e13031.

Brownell, K. D., & Walsh, B. T. (2017). *Eating disorders and obesity: A comprehensive handbook* (3rd ed.). Guilford Press.

Brugnera, A., Compare, A., Omboni, S., Greco, A., Carrara, S., Tasca, G. A., ... Parati, G. (2022). Psychological covariates of blood pressure among patients with hypertension and metabolic syndrome. *Health Psychology*, 41(12), 946–954. https://doi.org/10.1037/hea0001205

Buchanan, A., Sint, K., Swanson, J., & Rosenheck, R. (2019). Correlates of future violence in people being treated for schizophrenia. *The American Journal of Psychiatry*, 176(9), 694–701. https://doi.org/10.1176/appi.ajp.2019.18080909

Buchholz, K. (2023, October 13). U.S. homicide rate comes Down from pandemic peak. Statista Daily Data. Retrieved March 27, 2024, from https://www.statista.com/chart/31062/us-homicide-rate

Burgoon, J. K. (2016). Expectancy violations theory. In C. R. Berger & M. E. Roloff (Eds.), *The international encyclopedia of interpersonal communication* (p. 1).

Burke, L. E., Ma, J., Azar, K. M. J., Bennett, G. G., Peterson, E. D., Zheng, Y., ... Quinn, C. C. (2015). Current science on consumer use of mobile health for cardiovascular disease prevention. *Circulation*, 132(12), 1157–1213.

Burns, J. A., Jensen, M. P., Thorn, B. E., Lillis, T. A., Carmody, J., Newman, A. K., & Keefe, F. J. (2022). Cognitive therapy, mindfulness-based stress reduction, and behavior therapy for the treatment of chronic pain: randomized controlled trial. *Pain*, 163(2), 376–389. https://doi.org/10.1097/j.pain.0000000000002357

Burrell, A., Tilchin, C., Ruhs, S., Schumacher, C., Fields, E., Wagner, J., ... Jennings, J. (2019). P450 Prep use, STD acquisition and sexual risk behavior. *British Medical Journal*, 95(Suppl. 1). https://doi.org/10.1136/sextrans-2019-sti.534

Burston, J. J., Valdes, A. M., Woodhams, S. G., Mapp, P. I., Stocks, J., Watson, D., ... Chapman, V. (2019). The impact of anxiety on chronic musculoskeletal pain and the role of astrocyte activation. *Pain*, 160(3), 658–669.

Burton-Jones, A., Akhlaghpour, S., Ayre, S., Barde, P., Staib, A., & Sullivan, C. (2020). Changing the conversation on evaluating digital transformation in healthcare: Insights from an institutional analysis. *Information and Organization*, 30(1). https://doi.org/10.1016/j.infoandorg.2019.100255

Buschmann, T., Horn, R. A., Blankenship, V. R., Garcia, Y. E., & Bohan, K. B. (2018). The relationship between automatic thoughts and irrational beliefs predicting anxiety and depression. *Journal of Rational-Emotive & Cognitive-Behavior Therapy*, 36(2), 137–162.

Bush, B. (2017, December 3). Yes, Donald Trump, you said that. *New York Times*, p. A21.

Bushman, B. J., Wang, M. C., & Anderson, C. A. (2005). Is the curve relating temperature to aggression linear or curvilinear? Assaults and temperature in Minneapolis reexamined. *Journal of Personality and Social Psychology*, 89, 62–66.

Butryn, M. L., Godfrey, K. M., Call, C. C., Forman, E. M., Zhang, F., & Volpe, S. L. (2021). Promotion of physical activity during weight loss maintenance: A randomized controlled trial. *Health Psychology*, 40(3), 178–187. https://doi.org/10.1037/hea0001043

Buzdar, A. U. (2006). Dietary modification and risk of breast cancer. *Journal of the American Medical Association*, 295, 691–692.

Cain, P., Donaghue, N., & Ditchburn, G. (2017). Concerns, culprits, counsel, and conflict: A thematic analysis of "obesity" and fat discourse in digital news media. *Fat Studies*, 6(2), 170–188.

Calhoun, S. L., Fernandez-Mendoza, J., Vgontzas, A. N., Liao, D., & Bixler, E. O. (2014). Prevalence of insomnia symptoms in a general population sample of young children and preadolescents: Gender effects. *Sleep Medicine*, 15(1), 91–95.

Campbell, K. L., Winters-Stone, K. M., Wiskemann, J., May, A. M., Schwartz, A. L., Courneya, K. L., ... Schmitz, K. H. (2019). Exercise guidelines for cancer survivors: Consensus statement from international multidisciplinary roundtable. *Medicine & Science in Sports & Exercise*, 51, 2375–2390.

Campbell, N. R. C., Webster, J., Blanco-Metzler, A., He, F. J., Tan, M., MacGregor, G. A., ... Whelton, P. K. (2019). Packages of sodium (Salt) sold for consumption and salt dispensers should be required to have a front of package health warning label: A position statement of the World Hypertension League, national and international health and scientific organization. *The Journal of Clinical Hypertension*, 21(11), 1623–1625.

Candeias, A. A., Calisto, I. P., Borralho, L., & Portelada, A. (2019). Burnout in teaching: The importance of personal and professional variables. In J. G. Pereira, J. Gonçalves, & V. Bizzari (Eds.), *The neurobiology-psychotherapy-pharmacology intervention triangle: The need for common sense in 21st century mental health* (pp. 221–234). Vernon Press.

Caneo, C., Marston, L., Bellón, J., & King, M. (2016). Examining the relationship between physical illness and depression: Is there a difference between inflammatory and non-inflammatory diseases? A cohort study. *General Hospital Psychiatry*, 43, 71–77.

Capps, K. P., Updegraff, J. A., Foust, J. L., O'Brien, A. G., & Taber, J. M. (2022). Field experiment of signs promoting hand hygiene during the COVID-19 pandemic. *Health Psychology*, 41(11), 826–832. https://doi.org/10.1037/hea0001211

Caraballo, C., Massey, D. S., Ndumele, C. D., Haywood, T., Kaleem, S., King, T., ... Krumholz, H. M. (2023). Excess mortality and years of potential life lost among the Black Population in the US, 1999–2020. *JAMA*, 329(19), 1662–1670. https://doi.org/10.1001/jama.2023.7022

Carnethon, M. R., Kershaw, K. N., & Kandula, N. R. (2020). Disparities research, disparities researchers, and health equity. *Journal of the American Medical Association*, 323, 211–212.

Carpenter, J., Murray, B. P., Atti, S., Moran, T. P., Yancey, A., & Morgan, B. (2019). Naloxone dosing after opioid overdose in the era of illicitly manufactured fentanyl. *A Journal of Medical Toxicology*, 1–8. https://doi.org/10.1007/s13181-019-00735-w

Carroll, D. J. (2016). Civil War veterans and opiate addiction in the Gilded Age. https://www.journalofthecivilwarera.org/2016/11/civil-war-veterans-opiate-addiction-gilded-age/

Carter, S. E., Ong, M. L., Simons, R. L., Gibbons, F. X., Lei, M. K., & Beach, S. R. H. (2019). The effect of early discrimination on accelerated aging among African Americans. *Health Psychology*, 38, 1010–1013.

Carvalho, A. F., Firth, J., & Vieta, E. (2020). Bipolar disorder. *New England Journal of Medicine*, 383(1), 58–66. https://doi.org/10.1056/nejmra1906193

Carver, C. S. (1997). You want to measure coping but your protocol's too long: Consider the Brief COPE. *International Journal of Behavioral Medicine*, 4, 92–100.

Carver, C. S. (2014). Dispositional optimism. *Trends in Cognitive Sciences*, 18, 293–299.

Carver, C. S. (2019). Coping. In D. Polsky, et al. (Eds.), *Cambridge handbook of psychology, health and medicine* (pp. 114–119). Cambridge University Press.

Carver, C. S., & Scheier, M. F. (2017). Optimism, coping, and well-being. In C. L. Cooper & J. C. Quick (Eds.), *The handbook of stress and health: A guide to research and practice* (pp. 400–414). Wiley.

Carver, C. S., Scheier, M. F., & Segerstrom, S. C. (2010). Optimism. *Clinical Psychology Review*, 30, 879–899.

Castelli, L., Castelnuovo, G., & Torta, R. (2015). Editorial: PsychOncology. *Frontiers in Psychology*, 6, 947. https://doi.org/10.3389/fpsyg.2015.00947

Castelnuovo, G., & Schreurs, K. M. G. (2019). Editorial: Pain management in clinical and health psychology. *Frontiers in Psychology*, 10, 1285.

Cavero-Redondo, I., Martinez-Vizcaino, V., Fernandez-Rodriguez, R., Saz-Lara, A., Pascual-Morena, C., & Álvarez-Bueno, C. (2020). Effect of behavioral weight management interventions using lifestyle mhealth self-monitoring on weight loss: A systematic review and meta-analysis. *Nutrients*, 12(7). https://doi.org/10.3390/nu12071977

Centers for Disease Control and Prevention (CDC). (2014). Controlling blood pressure.

Centers for Disease Control and Prevention (CDC). (2015). Vaccines do not cause autism. https://www.cdc.gov/vaccinesafety/concerns/autism.html

Centers for Disease Control and Prevention (CDC). (2017b). Leading causes of death. https://www.cdc.gov/nchs/fastats/leading-causes-of-death.htm

Centers for Disease Control and Prevention (CDC). (2017c). Accidents or unintentional injuries. https://www.cdc.gov/nchs/fastats/accidental-injury.htm

Centers for Disease Control and Prevention (CDC). (2017d). Stroke facts. https://www.cdc.gov/stroke/facts.htm

Centers for Disease Control and Prevention. (CDC). (2018). Opioid overdoses treated in emergency departments. https://www.cdc.gov/vitalsigns/opioid-overdoses/infographic.html

Centers for Disease Control and Prevention (CDC). (2019). Intimate partner violence. https://www.cdc.gov/violenceprevention/intimatepartnerviolence/index.html

Centers for Disease Control and Prevention (CDC). (2019a, May 28). 35% drop in new diabetes diagnoses—And no increase in total cases. *CDC Newsroom*.

Centers for Disease Control and Prevention (CDC). (2019b). CDC releases first national estimates on diabetes within Hispanic and Asian Populations in the US. https://www.cdc.gov/media/releases/2019/p1220-diabetes-estimate.html

Centers for Disease Control and Prevention (CDC). (2019c). Heart disease facts. https://www.cdc.gov/heartdisease/facts.htm

Centers for Disease Control and Prevention (CDC). (2019d, April). Health, United States spotlight: Racial and ethnic disparities in heart disease. https://www.cdc.gov/nchs/hus/spotlight/2019-heart-disease-disparities.htm

Centers for Disease Control and Prevention (CDC). (2019e). Intimate partner violence. https://www.cdc.gov/violenceprevention/intimatepartnerviolence/index.html

Centers for Disease Control and Prevention (CDC). (2019f). Heart failure. https://www.cdc.gov/heartdisease/heart_failure.htm

Centers for Disease Control and Prevention (CDC). (2019g). HPV (human papillomavirus) VIS. Vaccine Information Statements (VISs). https://www.cdc.gov/vaccines/hcp/vis/vis-statements/hpv.html

Centers for Disease Control and Prevention (CDC). (2019h). Know your risk for heart disease. https://www.cdc.gov/heartdisease/risk_factors.htm

Centers for Disease Control and Prevention (CDC). (2019i). Most recent national asthma data. https://www.cdc.gov/asthma/most_recent_national_asthma_data.htm

Centers for Disease Control and Prevention (CDC). (2019j). Show me the science—When & how to use hand sanitizer in community settings.

Centers for Disease Control and Prevention (CDC). (2020a). Trends in meeting the 2008 Physical Activity Guidelines, 2008–2018.

Centers for Disease Control and Prevention (CDC). (2020b). Coronavirus disease 2019 (COVID-19). Manage anxiety and stress. Stress and coping.

Centers for Disease Control and Prevention (CDC). (2020c). Facts about hypertension.

Centers for Disease Control and Prevention (CDC). (2020d). Handwashing: Clean hands save lives. https://www.cdc.gov/handwashing/

Centers for Disease Control and Prevention (CDC). (2020e). Measles, mumps, rubella (MMR) vaccine. https://www.cdc.gov/vaccinesafety/vaccines/mmr-vaccine.html

Centers for Disease Control and Prevention. CDC. (2020f). Stroke facts. Centers for Disease Control and Prevention. https://www.cdc.gov/stroke/facts.htm

Centers for Disease Control and Prevention (CDC) (2021a). Get the facts: Added sugars.

Centers for Disease Control and Prevention (CDC). (2021b). CDC estimates 1 in 5 people in the U.S. have a sexually transmitted infection.

Centers for Disease Control and Prevention (CDC). (2022a). HIV and Black/African American people in the U.S. (https://www.cdc.gov/nchhstp/newsroom/fact-sheets/hiv/black-african-american-fact-sheet.html

Centers for Disease Control and Prevention (CDC). (2022b). Preliminary 2021 STD surveillance data.

Centers for Disease Control and Prevention (CDC). (2022c). STDs and infertility. https://www.cdc.gov/std/infertility/default.htm

Centers for Disease Control and Prevention (CDC). (2023a). Diabetes fast facts.

Centers for Disease Control and Prevention (CDC). (2023b). Diseases and death. https://www.cdc.gov/tobacco/data_statistics/fact_sheets/fast_facts/diseases-and-death.html

Centers for Disease Control and Prevention (CDC) (2023c). Injuries and violence are leading causes of death.

Centers for Disease Control and Prevention (CDC). (2023d). FastStats. Homicide. https://www.cdc.gov/nchs/fastats/homicide.htm

Centers for Disease Control and Prevention (CDC) (2023e). *Fast facts:* Preventing sexual violence.

Centers for Disease Control and Prevention (CDC). (2023f). FastStats: Alzheimer Disease.

Centers for Disease Control and Prevention (CDC). (2023g). Tobacco-related mortality.

Centers for Disease Control and Prevention (CDC). (2023h). Heart disease facts. https://www.cdc.gov/heartdisease/facts.htm

Centers for Disease Control and Prevention (CDC). (2023i). Estimated hypertension prevalence, treatment, and control among U.S. adults. https://millionhearts.hhs.gov/data-reports/hypertension-prevalence.html

Centers for Disease Control and Prevention (CDC), National Center for Health Statistics. (2023j). National Vital Statistics System, Mortality 2018–2021. http://wonder.cdc.gov/ucd-icd10-expanded.html

Centers for Disease Control and Prevention (CDC) (2023k). Measles cases and outbreaks. https://www.cdc.gov/measles/cases-outbreaks.html

Centers for Disease Control and Prevention (CDC). (2023l). More than a quarter of U.S. adults and children have at least one allergy. https://www.cdc.gov/nchs/pressroom/nchs_press_releases/2022/20220126.htm

Centers for Disease Control and Prevention (CDC) (2023m). Heart disease deaths - Health, United States. https://www.cdc.gov/nchs/hus/topics/heart-disease-deaths.htm

Centers for Disease Control and Prevention (CDC). (2023n). Stroke facts. https://www.cdc.gov/stroke/facts.htm

Centers for Disease Control and Prevention (CDC). (2023o). Stroke signs and symptoms.

Centers for Disease Control and Prevention (CDC) (2023p). Leading causes of death. https://www.cdc.gov/nchs/fastats/leading-causes-of-death.htm/Public Domain.

Centers for Disease Control and Prevention (CDC). (2023q). Cancer deaths-Health,UnitedStates.https://www.cdc.gov/nchs/hus/topics/cancer-deaths.htm

Centers for Disease Control and Prevention (CDC). (2023r), 1918 Pandemic Influenza: Three Waves.

Centers for Disease Control and Prevention (CDC) (2024). Tuberculosis (TB).

Centers for Disease Control and Prevention (CDC). (2024a). Facts about hypertension. https://www.cdc.gov/bloodpressure/facts.htm

Cha, A. E., & Cohen, R. A. (2020). Problems paying medical bills, 2018. NCHS Data Brief, No. 357. National Center for Health Statistics.

Chaiton, M., Diemert, L., Cohen, J. E., Bondy, S. J., Selby, P., Philipneri, A., & Schwartz, R. (2016). Estimating the number of quit attempts it takes to quit smoking successfully in a longitudinal cohort of smokers. *BMJ Open*, 6(6), e011045.

Chakhtoura, M., Nassar, A., Arabi, A., Cooper, C., Harvey, N., Mahfoud, Z., . . . Nabulsi, M., El-Hajj Fuleihan, G. (2016). Effect of vitamin D replacement on maternal and neonatal outcomes: a randomised controlled trial in pregnant women with hypovitaminosis D. A protocol. *BMJ Open*, 6(3), e010818. https://doi.org/10.1136/bmjopen-2015-010818

Chalet, F.-X., Luyet, P.-P., Rabasa, C., Vaillant, C., Saskin, P., Ahuja, A., & Citrome, L. (2023). 0350 Daridorexant in patients with insomnia disorder: number needed to treat, number needed to harm & likelihood to be helped or harmed. *Sleep,* 46(Supplement 1), A155–A155. https://doi.org/10.1093/sleep/zsad077.0350

Chamie, J. (2023). America's high homicide rate. *Neodemos*. https://www.neodemos.info/2023/02/28/americas-high-homicide-rate/

Champion, K. E., Parmenter, B., McGowan, C., Spring, B., Wafford, Q. E., Gardner, L. A., ... Newton, N. C. (2019). Effectiveness of school-based eHealth interventions to prevent multiple lifestyle risk behaviours among adolescents: A systematic review and meta-analysis. *The Lancet Digital Health*, 1(5), e206–e221. https://doi.org/10.1016/S2589-7500(19)30088-3

Chang, C., Tsai, G., & Hsieh, C. J. (2013). Psychological, immunological and physiological effects of a laughing qigong program (LQP) on adolescents. *Complementary Therapies in Medicine*, 21(6), 660–668.

Chang, E. C., Tian, W., Jiang, X., Yi, S., Liu, J., Bai, Y., ... Li, M. (2020). Beyond the role of loneliness in psychological ill-being and well-being in females: Do social problem-solving processes still matter? *Personality and Individual Differences*, 155. https://doi.org/10.1016/j.paid.2019.109729

Chang, S. H., Freeman, N. L. B., Lee, J. A., Stoll, C. R. T., Calhoun, A. J., Eagon, J. C., & Colditz, G. A. (2018). Early major complications after bariatric surgery in the USA, 2003–2014: A systematic review and meta-analysis. *Obesity Reviews*, 19(4), 529–537.

Chang, Y., Cho, J., Cho, Y. K., Cho, A., Hong, Y. S., Zhao, D., ... Ryu, S. (2020). Alcoholic and nonalcoholic fatty liver disease and incident hospitalization for liver and cardiovascular diseases. *Clinical Gastroenterology and Hepatology*, 18(1), 205–215.

Chapman, B. P., & Elliot, A. J. (2019). How short is too short? An ultra-brief measure of the big-five personality domains implicates "agreeableness" as a risk for all-cause mortality. *Journal of Health Psychology*, 24, 1568–1573.

Chaudry, A., Jackson, A., & Glied, S. A. (2019). Did the Affordable Care Act reduce racial and ethnic disparities in health insurance coverage? *The Commonwealth Fund*. https://www.commonwealthfund.org/publications/issue-briefs/2019/aug/did-ACA-reduce-racial-ethnic-disparities-coverage

Chauhan, R. G., & Sharma, A. (2017). Effectiveness of Jacobson's progressive muscle relaxation therapy to reduce blood pressure among hypertensive patients: A literature review. *International Journal of Nursing Care*, 5(1), 26–29.

Chau, K. Y., Lam, M. H. S., Cheung, M. L., Tso, E. K. H., Flint, S. W., Broom, D. R., ... Lee, K. Y. (2019). Smart technology for healthcare: Exploring the antecedents of adoption intention of healthcare wearable technology. *Health Psychology Research*, 7(1).

Cheng, S., Au, A., & Losada, A. (2019). Psychological interventions for dementia caregivers: What we have achieved, what we have learned. *Current Psychiatry Reports*, 21, 59. https://doi.org/10.1007/s11920-019-1045-9

Cheng, W., Frei, O., van der Meer, D., Wang, Y., O'Connell, K. S., Chu, Y., ... Andreassen, O. A. (2021). Genetic association between schizophrenia and cortical brain surface area and thickness. *JAMA Psychiatry,* 78(9), 1020. https://doi.org/10.1001/jamapsychiatry.2021.1435

Chen, J., Li, J., Cao, B., Wang, F., Luo, L., & Xu, J. (2020). Mediating effects of self-efficacy, coping, burnout, and social support between job stress and mental health among young Chinese nurses. *Journal of Advanced Nursing*, 76(1), 163–173.

Chen, Y. F., Huang, X. Y., Chien, C. H., & Cheng, J. F. (2017). The effectiveness of diaphragmatic breathing relaxation training for reducing anxiety. *Perspectives in Psychiatric Care*, 53(4), 329–336.

Chen, Y., & VanderWeele, T. J. (2019). Associations of religious upbringing with subsequent health and well-being from adolescence to young adulthood: An outcome-wide analysis. *American Journal of Epidemiology*. https://doi.org/10.1093/aje/kwy142

Cherry, M. G., Salmon, P., Byrne, A., Ullmer, H., Abbey, G., & Fisher, P. L. (2019). Qualitative evaluation of cancer survivors' experiences of metacognitive therapy: A new perspective on psychotherapy in cancer care. *Frontiers in Psychology*, 10, 949. https://doi.org/10.3389/fpsyg.2019.00949

Chetty, R., Stepner, M., Abraham, S., Lin, S., Scuderi, B., Turner, N., ... Cutler, D. (2016). The association between income and life expectancy in the United States, 2001–2014. *Journal of the American Medical Association*, 315, 1750–1766.

Chevance, G., Golaszewski, N., Baretta, D., Hekler, E. B., Larsen, B., Patrick, K., & Godino, J. (2019, September 5). Modelling multiple health behavior change with network analyses: Results from a one-year study conducted among overweight and obese adults. *Journal of Behavioral Medicine*.

Chiang, J. J., Chen, E., Leigh, A. K. K., Hoffer, L. C., Lam, P. H., & Miller, G. E. (2019). Familism and inflammatory processes in African American, Latino, and White youth. *Health Psychology*, 38(4), 306–317.

Chida, Y., & Steptoe, A. (2009). The association of anger and hostility with future coronary heart disease: A meta-analytic review of prospective evidence. *Journal of the American College of Cardiology*, 53, 936–946.

Chinh, K., Mosher, C. E., Brown, L. F., Beck-Coon, K. A., Kroenke, K., & Johns, S. A. (2020). Psychological processes and symptom outcomes in mindfulness-based stress reduction for cancer survivors: A pilot study. *Mindfulness*, 11, 905–916.

Chirinos, D. A., Vargas, E., Kamsickas, L., & Carnethon, M. (2022). The role of behavioral science in addressing cardiovascular health disparities: A narrative review of efforts, challenges, and future directions. *Health Psychology: Official Journal of the Division of Health Psychology, American Psychological Association*, 41(10), 740–754. https://doi.org/10.1037/hea0001191

Chlamydia. (2019). Chlamydia—CDC fact sheet. https://www.cdc.gov/std/chlamydia/Chlamydia-FS.pdf

Choi, A., Marcus, K., Pohl, D., Eyck, P. T., Balfour Jr., H., & Jackson, J. B. (2020). Epstein-Barr virus infection status among first year undergraduate university students. *A Journal of American College Health*, 1–4. https://doi.org/10.1080/07448481.2020.1726927

Choi, N. G., Hegel, M. T., Sirrianni, L., Marinucci, M. L., & Bruce, M. L. (2012). Passive coping response to depressive symptoms among low-income homebound older adults: Does it affect depression severity and treatment outcome? *Behaviour Research and Therapy*, 50(11), 668–674. https://doi.org/10.1016/j.brat.2012.07.003

Cho, L., Kaunitz, A. M., Faubion, S. S., Hayes, S. N., Lau, E. S., Pristera, N., ... Lindley, K. J., & for the ACC CVD in Women Committee. (2023). Rethinking menopausal hormone therapy: For whom, what, when, and how long? *Circulation,* 147(7), 597–610. https://doi.org/10.1161/circulationaha.122.061559

Chottekalapanda, R. U., Kalik, S., Gresack, J., Ayala, A., Gao, M., Wang, W., ... Greengard, P. (2020). AP-1 controls the p11-dependent antidepressant response. *Molecular Psychiatry,* 25(7), 1364–1381. https://doi.org/10.1038/s41380-020-0767-8

Choudhary, V., Hatila, S., & Mehta, S. (2020). Post-partum depression—Treatment update. *International Journal of Medical and Biomedical Studies*, 4(1). https://doi.org/10.32553/ijmbs.v4i1.843

Chou, H. T.-G., & Edge, N. (2012). "They are happier and having better lives than I am": The impact of using Facebook on perceptions of others' lives. *Cyberpsychology, Behavior, and Social Networking*, 15, 117–121. https://doi.org/10.1089/cyber.2011.0324

Chou, R., Deyo, R., Friedly, J., Skelly, A., Hashimoto, R., Weimer, M., Fu, R., ... Brodt, E. D. (2017). Nonpharmacologic therapies for low back pain: A systematic review for an American College of Physicians Clinical Practice Guideline. *Annals of Internal Medicine*, 166(7), 493–505.

Chowdhury, K. P. (2020). Health benefits of green tea and herbal teas: A comparative review. *Our Heritage*, 68(30), 4703–4717.

Chowkwanyun, M., & Reed, A. L. (2020). Racial Health Disparities and Covid-19—Caution and context. *New England Journal of Medicine*. https://doi.org/10.1056/nejmp2012910

Christy, S. M., Perkins, S. M., Tong, Y., Krier, C., Champion, V. L., Skinner, C. S., ... Rawl, S. M. (2013). Promoting colorectal cancer screening discussion: A randomized controlled trial. *American Journal of Preventive Medicine*, 44(4), 325–329.

Cifu, A. S., Lembo, A., & Davis, A. M. (2020). Can an evidence-based approach improve the patient–physician relationship? *Journal of the American Medical Association*, 323, 31–32. https://doi.org/10.1001/jama.2019.19427

Cillessen, L., Johannsen, M., Speckens, A. E. M., & Zachariae, R. (2019). Mindfulness-based interventions for psychological and physical health outcomes in cancer patients and survivors: A systematic review and meta-analysis of randomized controlled trials. *Psycho-Oncology*, 28(12), 2257–2269. https://doi.org/10.1002/pon.5214

Cilliers, L. (2020). Wearable devices in healthcare: Privacy and information security issues. *Health Information Management Journal*, 49(2–3), 150–156.

Cipriani, A., Furukawa, T. A., Salanti, G., Chaimani, A., Atkinson, L. Z., Ogawa, Y., ... Geddes, J. R. (2018). Comparative efficacy and acceptability of 21 antidepressant drugs for the acute treatment of adults with major depressive disorder: A systematic review and network meta-analysis. *The Lancet*, 391, 1357–1366.

Clarke, N., Pechey, E., Kosīte, D., König, L. M., Mantzari, E., Blackwell, A., ... Hollands, G. J. (2020). Impact of health warning labels on selection and consumption of food and alcohol products: Systematic review with meta-analysis. *Health Psychology Review*, 15(3), 430–453. https://doi.org/10.1080/17437199.2020.1780147

Clarke, P. B., Lewis, T. F., Myers, J. E., Henson, R. A., & Hill, B. (2020). Wellness, emotion regulation, and relapse during substance use disorder treatment. *Journal of Counseling & Development*, 98(1), 17–28. https://doi.org/10.1002/jcad.12296

Clark, T. L., Savin, K. L., Perez-Ramirez, P., Valdez, T., Toba, G., & Gallo, L. C. (2023). eHealth weight loss interventions for adults with low income: A systematic review. *Health Psychology*, 42(6), 353–367. https://doi.org/10.1037/hea0001278

Cludius, B., Stevens, S., Bantin, T., Gerlach, A. L., & Hermann, C. (2013). The motive to drink due to social anxiety and its relation to hazardous alcohol use. *Psychology of Addictive Behaviors*, 27, 806–813.

Cobb, C. L., Meca, A., Branscombe, N. R., Schwartz, S. J., Xie, D., Zea, M. C., ... Sanders, G. L. (2019). Perceived discrimination and well-being among unauthorized Hispanic immigrants: The moderating role of ethnic/racial group identity centrality. *Cultural Diversity and Ethnic Minority Psychology*, 25, 280–287. http://dx.doi.org/10.1037/cdp0000227

Coderre, T. J., Mogil, J. S., & Bushnell, M. C. (2003). The biological psychology of pain. In M. Gallagher & R. J. Nelson (Eds.), *Handbook of psychology: Vol. 3. Biological psychology* (Vol. 3, pp. 237–268). John Wiley & Sons.

Cohen-Kettenis, P. T., & Klink, D. (2015). Adolescents with gender dysphoria. *Best Practice & Research Clinical Endocrinology & Metabolism*, 29(3), 485–495. https://doi.org/10.1016/j.beem.2015.01.004

Cohen, R. A., Terlizzi, E. P., & Martinez, M. E. (2019). *Health insurance coverage: Early release of estimates from the National Health Interview Survey, 2018*. National Center for Health Statistics.

Cohen, S. (2016). Psychological stress, immunity, and physical disease. In R. J. Sternberg, S. T. Fiske, & D. J. Foss (Eds.), *Scientists making a difference: The greatest living behavioral and brain scientists talk about their most important contributions*. Cambridge University Press.

Cohen, S., Frank, E., Doyle, W. J., Skoner, D. P., Rabin, B. S., & Gwaltney, J. M. (1998). Types of stressors that increase susceptibility to the common cold in healthy adults. *Health Psychology*, 17, 214–223.

Cohen, S., Gianaros, P. J., & Manuck, S. B. (2016). A stage model of stress and disease. *Perspectives on Psychological Science*, 11(4), 456–463.

Cohen, S., Murphy, M. L., & Prather, A. A. (2019). Ten surprising facts about stressful life events and disease risk. *Annual Review of Psychology*, 70, 577–597. https://doi.org/10.1146/annurev-psych-010418-102857

Cohn, D. (2016). 10 demographic trends that are shaping the U.S. and the world. *Pew Research Center*.

Colditz, G. A., Wolin, K. Y., & Gehlert, S. (2012). Applying what we know to accelerate cancer prevention. *A Science Translational Medicine*, 4(127), 127rv4.

Coleman, J. A., & Gouaux, E. (2018). Structural basis for recognition of diverse antidepressants by the human serotonin transporter. *Nature Structural & Molecular Biology*, 25(2), 170–175.

Collins, F. C. (2019, October 16). Panel finds exercise may lower cancer risk, improve outcomes. *NIH Director's Blog*.

Colloca, L. (2019). The placebo effect in pain therapies. *Annual Review of Pharmacology and Toxicology*, 59(1), 191–211. https://doi.org/10.1146/annurev-pharmtox-010818-021542

Colloca, L., & Barsky, A. J. (2020). Placebo and nocebo effects. *New England Journal of Medicine*, 382(6), 554–561. https://doi.org/10.1056/nejmra1907805

Comas-Díaz, L., Hall, G. N., & Neville, H. A. (2019). Racial trauma: Theory, research, and healing: Introduction to the special issue. *American Psychologist*, 74(1), 1–5. https://doi.org/10.1037/amp0000442

Conner, M. (2015). Health behaviors. In G. Wright (Ed.), *International encyclopedia of the social & behavioral sciences* (2nd ed.). Elsevier.

Conner, M., & Norman, P. (2017). Health behaviour: Current issues and challenges. *Psychology & Health*, 32, 895–906.

Conner, M., & Sparks, P. (2005). The theory of planned behavior. In M. Conner & P. Norman (Eds.), *Predicting health behaviour: Research and practice with social cognition models* (pp. 121–162). Open University Press.

Connolly, S. L., & Alloy, L. B. (2018). Negative event recall as a vulnerability for depression: Relationship between momentary stress-reactive rumination and memory for daily life stress. *Clinical Psychological Science*, 6, 32–47. https://doi.org/10.1177/2167702617729487

Connor, J. P., Stjepanović, D., Budney, A. J., Le Foll, B., & Hall, W. D. (2022). Clinical management of cannabis withdrawal. *Addiction (Abingdon, England)*, 117(7), 2075–2095. https://doi.org/10.1111/add.15743

Connor, M. T., & Norman, P. D. (2017). Health behaviour: Current issues and challenges. *Psychology and Health*, 32(8), 895–906. https://doi.org/10.1080/08870446.2017.1336240

Conroy, D. E., Hedeker, D., McFadden, H. G., Pellegrini, C. A., Pfammatter, A. F., Phillips, S. M., ... Spring, B. (2017). Lifestyle intervention effects on the frequency and duration of daily moderate–vigorous physical activity and leisure screen time. *Health Psychology*, 36(4), 299–308.

Cooley, S. A., Paul, R. H., & Ances, B. M. (2020). Medication management abilities are reduced in older persons living with HIV compared with healthy older HIV-controls. *Journal of NeuroVirology*, 264–269.

Cooney, G. M., Dwan, K., Greig, C. A., Lawlor, D. A., Rimer, J., Waugh, F. R., ... Mead, G. E. (2013). Exercise for depression. *The Cochrane Database of Systematic Reviews*, 9, CD004366.

Cope, L. M., Munier, E. C., Trucco, E. M., Hardee, J. E., Burmeister, M., Zucker, R. A., & Heitzeg, M. M. (2017). Effects of the serotonin transporter gene, sensitivity of response to alcohol, and parental monitoring on risk for problem alcohol use. *Alcohol*, 59, 7–16.

Corathers, S., Mara, C. A., Chundi, P. K., & Kichler, J. C. (2019). Depression screening of adolescents with diabetes: 5-years of implementation and outcomes. *Journal of the American Academy of Child and Adolescent Psychiatry*, 58(6), 628–632. https://doi.org/10.1016/j.jaac.2019.01.013

Corbett, T., Cheetham, T., Müller, A. M., Slodkowska-Barabasz, J., Wilde, L., Krusche, A., ... Bradbury, K. (2018). Exploring cancer survivors' views of health behaviour change: "Where do you start, where do you stop with everything?" *Psychooncology*, 27, 1816–1824.

Cormio, C., Romito, F., Viscanti, G., Turaccio, M., Lorusso, V., & Mattioli, V. (2014). Psychological well-being and post-traumatic growth in caregivers of cancer patients. *Frontiers of Psychology*, 5, 1342. https://doi.org/10.3389/fpsyg.2014.01342

Cornally, N., & McCarthy, G. (2011). Help-seeking behaviour for the treatment of chronic pain. *British Journal of Community Nursing*, 16, 90–98.

Corr, C. A. (2019). "The five stages" in coping with dying and bereavement: Strengths, weaknesses and some alternatives. *Mortality*, 24, 405–417.

Corr, C. A. (2020). Elisabeth Kübler-Ross and the "five stages" model in a sampling of recent American textbooks. *OMEGA-Journal of Death and Dying*, 82(2), 294–322. https://doi.org/10.1177/0030222818809766

Corr, C. A., Corr, D. M., & Doka, K. J. (2018). Death & dying, life & living. *Cengage Learning*. https://doi.org/10.1097/NJH.0000000000000640

Corrêa, M. S., de Lima, D. B., Giacobbo, B. L., Vedovelli, K., de Lima Argimon, I. I., & Bromberg, E. (2019). Mental health in familial caregivers of Alzheimer's disease patients: Are the effects of chronic stress on cognition inevitable? *Stress*, 22, 83–92.

Costa, A. L. S., Heitkemper, M. M., Alencar, G. P., Damiani, L. P., da Silva, R. M., & Jarrett, M. E. (2017). Social support is a predictor of lower stress and higher quality of life and resilience in Brazilian patients with colorectal cancer. *Cancer Nursing*, 40(5), 352–360. https://doi.org/10.1097/NCC.0000000000000388

Costanza, M. E., Luckmann, R., Frisard, C., White, M. J., & Cranos, C. (2020). Comparing telephone counseling with reminding to promote on-time repeated mammography: A randomized trial in a cohort with 4 years follow-up. *Health Education & Behavior*, 47, 37–46.

Costa, P. T., & McCrae, R. R. (2006). Changes in personality and their origins: Comment on Roberts, Walton, and Viechtbauer (2006). *Psychological Bulletin*, 132, 26–28.

Craig, M., Hales, M. D., Carroll, M. D., Fryarr, C. D., & Ogden, C. L. (2020). Prevalence of obesity and severe obesity among adults: United States, 2017–2018. NCHS Data Brief, No. 360. https://www.cdc.gov/nchs/data/databriefs/db360-h.pdf

Crandall, C. J., Mehta, J. M., & Manson, J. E. (2023). Management of menopausal symptoms: A review. *JAMA*, 329(5), 405–420.

Croft, J. (2023, July 27). Research casts doubt on value of daily aspirin for healthy adults. *Medscape*. https://www.medscape.com/s/viewarticle/994925

Crosby, C. L., Durkee, P. K., Meston, C. M., & Buss, D. M. (2020). Six dimensions of sexual disgust. *Personality and Individual Differences*, 156. https://doi.org/10.1016/j.paid.2019.109714

Crossman, A. (2018). *Sociology definition: Sick role*. thoughtco.com/sick-role-definition-3976325

Crucian, B., & Choukér, A. (2020). Immune system in space: General introduction and observations on stress-sensitive regulations. In A. Choukèr (Ed.), *Stress challenges and immunity in space* (pp. 205–220). Springer.

Cruz, D., Rodriguez, Y., & Mastropaolo, C. (2019). Perceived microaggressions in health care: A measurement study. *PLoS One*, 14(2), e0211620. https://doi.org/10.1371/journal.pone.0211620

Cruz-Pereira, J. S., Rea, K., Nolan, Y. M., O'Leary, O. F., Dinan, T. G., & Cryan, J. F. (2020). Depression's unholy trinity: Dysregulated stress, immunity, and the microbiome. *Annual Review of Psychology*, 71, 49–78.

Cuevas, A. G., & O'Brien, K. (2019). Racial centrality may be linked to mistrust in healthcare institutions for African Americans. *Journal of Health Psychology*, 24, 2022–2030.

Cuevas, A. G., O'Brien, K., & Saha, S. (2016). African American experiences in healthcare: "I always feel like I'm getting skipped over". *Health Psychology*, 35, 987–995.

Cuffee, Y. L., Hargraves, L., Rosal, M., Briesacher, B. A., Allison, J. J., & Hullett, S. (2020). An examination of John Henryism, trust, and medication adherence among African Americans with Hypertension. *Health Education & Behavior*, 47(1), 162–169.

Cuijpers, P., Noma, H., Karyotaki, E., Vinkers, C. H., Cipriani, A., & Furukawa, T. A. (2020). A network meta-analysis of the effects of psychotherapies, pharmacotherapies and their combination in the treatment of adult depression. *World Psychiatry: Official Journal of the World Psychiatric Association (WPA)*, 19(1), 92–107. https://doi.org/10.1002/wps.20701

Cummings, M., Hróbjartsson, A., & Ernst, E. (2018). Should doctors recommend acupuncture for pain? *BMJ (Clinical Research Ed.)*, 360, k970. https://doi.org/10.1136/bmj.k970

Cunningham, T. J., Croft, J. B., Liu, Y., Lu, H., Eke, P. I., & Giles, W. H. (2017). Vital signs: Racial disparities in age-specific mortality among Blacks or African Americans—United States, 1999–2015. *Morbidity and Mortality Weekly Report*, 66, 444–456. https://doi.org/10.15585/mmwr.mm6617e1

Curci, S. G., Hernández, J. C., Winstone, L. K., Perez, M., & Luecken, L. J. (2023). Discrimination and depressive symptoms among Mexican American women: Exploring multilevel sociocultural moderators. *Clinical Psychological Science*, 11(3), 444–457. https://doi.org/10.1177/21677026221129628

Currier, J. S. (2020). Monthly injectable antiretroviral therapy—Version 1.0 of a new treatment approach. *The New England Journal of Medicine*. https://doi.org/10.1056/NEJMe2002199

Curtin, S. C. (2020). State suicide rates among adolescents and young adults aged 10–24: United States, 2000–2018. *National Vital Statistics Reports*, 69(11). National Center for Health Statistics.

Curtin, S., & Garnett, M. (2023). *Suicide and homicide death rates among youth and young adults aged 10–24: United States, 2001–2021*. National Center for Health Statistics.

Curtin, S., Tejada-Vera, B. & Bastian, B. (2023). National Vital Statistics Reports. Deaths: Leading causes for 2020. https://www.cdc.gov/nchs/data/nvsr/nvsr72/nvsr72-13.pdf

Cystic Fibrosis Foundation. (2020). http://www.cff.org/AboutCF/

Dahlhamer, J., Lucas, J., Zelaya, C., Nahin, R., Mackey, S., DeBar, L., ... Helmick, C. (2018). Prevalence of chronic pain and high-impact chronic pain among adults—United States, 2016. *MMWR*

Morbidity and Mortality Weekly Report, 67(36), 1001–1006. https://doi.org/10.15585/mmwr.mm6736a2

Dahl, M. (2013, July 4). Heat waves lead to hot tempers—And here's why. *NBC News*. http://www.today.com/health/heat-waves-lead-hot-tempers-heres-why-6C10436073

Dakkak, M. (2023). Fat shame—Inside and out. *JAMA*, 329(21), 1827. doi: 10.1001/jama.2023.7784

Dalen, K., Ellertsen, B., Espelid, I., & Grønningsaeter, A. G. (2009). EMG feedback in the treatment of myofascial pain dysfunction syndrome. *Acta Odontologica Scandinavica*, 44, 279–284.

Danaei, G., Ding, E. L., Mozaffarian, D., Taylor, B., Rehm, J., Murray, C. J. L., ... Ezzati, M. (2011). The preventable causes of death in the United States: Comparative risk assessment of dietary, lifestyle, and metabolic risk factors. *PLoS Medicine*, 8(1). https://doi.org/10.1371/annotation/0ef47acd-9dcc-4296-a897-872d182cde57

Daniels, K., & Abma, J. C. (2018). Contraceptive status among women aged 15–49: United States, 2015–2017. NCHS Data Brief, No. 327. https://www.cdc.gov/nchs/data/databriefs/db327-h.pdf

Dardis, C. M., Ullman, S. E., & Brecklin, L. R. (2018). "It's worth the fight!": Women resisting rape. In L. M. Orchowski & C. A. Gidycz (Eds.), *Sexual assault risk reduction and resistance* (pp. 111–133). Elsevier.

Darnall, B. D. (2019). *Psychological treatment for patients with chronic pain*. American Psychological Association. https://doi.org/10.1037/0000104-000

Dascal, J., Reid, M., Ishak, W. W., Spiegel, B., Recacho, J., Rosen, B., & Danovitch, I. (2017). Virtual reality and medical inpatients: A systematic review of randomized, controlled trials. *Innovations in Clinical Neuroscience*, 14(1–2), 14.

Daskalakis, C., DiCarlo, M., Hegarty, S., Gudur, A., Vernon, S. W., & Myers, R. E. (2020). Predictors of overall and test-specific colorectal Cancer screening adherence. *Preventive Medicine*, 133(106022), 106022. https://doi.org/10.1016/j.ypmed.2020.106022

Dassah, E., Aldersey, H., McColl, M. A., & Davison, C. (2018). Factors affecting access to primary health care services for persons with disabilities in rural areas: A "best-fit" framework synthesis. *Health Research Policy*, 3, 36. https://doi.org/10.1186/s41256-018-0091-x

Datar, A., Mahler, A., & Nicosia, N. (2020). Association of exposure to communities with high obesity with body type norms and obesity risk among teenagers. *JAMA Network Open*, 3(3), e200846–e200846.

Davidson, K. W., Pennells, L., & Di Angelantonio, E. (2021). Depression and incident cardiovascular disease—Reply. *JAMA*, 325(16), 1680. https://doi.org/10.1001/jama.2021.2032

Davis, A. C. (2020). Resolving the tension between feminism and evolutionary psychology: An epistemological critique. *Evolutionary Behavioral Sciences*. https://doi.org/10.1037/ebs0000193

Davis, A., Kim, R., & Crifasi, C. K. (2023). A year in review: 2021 Gun deaths in the U.S. Johns Hopkins Center for Gun Violence Solutions. Johns Hopkins Bloomberg School of Public Health.

Davison, J., McLaughlin, M., & Giles, M. (2019). Factors influencing children's tooth brushing intention: An application of the theory of planned behaviour. *Health Psychology Bulletin*, 3(1), 8–66. https://doi.org/10.5334/hpb.8

Dawson, L. A. (2019). What factors affect adherence to medicines? *Archives of Disease in Childhood—Education and Practice*, 104, 49–52. https://doi.org/10.1136/archdischild-2017-312820

Deak, J. D., & Johnson, E. C. (2021). Genetics of substance use disorders: A review. *Psychological Medicine*, 51(13), 2189–2200. https://doi.org/10.1017/s0033291721000969

Dean, A. C., Morales, A. M., Hellemann, G., & London, E. D. (2018). Cognitive deficit in methamphetamine users relative to childhood academic performance: Link to cortical thickness. *Neuropsychopharmacology*, 43, 1745–1752.

DeAngelis, R. T. (2020). Striving while Black: Race and the psychophysiology of goal pursuit. *Journal of Health and Social Behavior*, 61(1), 24–42. https://doi.org/10.1177/0022146520901695

DeAngelis, T. (2021). Mental illness and violence: Debunking myths, addressing realities. *Monitor on Psychology*. https://www.apa.org/monitor/2021/04/ce-mental-illnes

Deas, S., Power, K., Collin, P., Yellowlees, A., & Grierson, D. (2011). The relationship between disordered eating, perceived parenting, and perfectionistic schemas. *Cognitive Therapy and Research*, 35, 414–424.

de-Graft Aikins, A., Awuah, R. B., & Pera, T. (2015). Explanatory models of diabetes in poor urban Ghanaian communities. *Ethnicity & Health*, 20, 391–408.

Dehghan, M., Mente, A., Rangarajan, S., Mohan, V., Lear, S., Swaminathan, S., ... Yusuf, S. (2020). Association of egg intake with blood lipids, cardiovascular disease, and mortality in 177,000 people in 50 countries. *The American Journal of Clinical Nutrition*. https://doi.org/10.1093/ajcn/nqz348

DeLongis, A., Levere, D., & Stephenson, D. (2019). Arthritis and musculoskeletal disease. In T. E. Revenson & R. A. R. Gurung (Eds.), *Handbook of health psychology* (pp. 436–449). Routledge.

Delorme, J., Wang, L., Kuhn, F. R., Kodoth, V., Ma, J., Martinez, J. D., ... Aton, S. J. (2021). Sleep loss drives acetylcholine- and somatostatin interneuron–mediated gating of hippocampal activity to inhibit memory consolidation. *Proceedings of the National Academy of Sciences*, 118(32). https://doi.org/10.1073/pnas.2019318118

Dempsey, A. F., & O'Leary, S. T. (2018). Human papillomavirus vaccination: Narrative review of studies on how providers' vaccine communication affects attitudes and uptake. *Academic Pediatrics*, 18(2), S23–S27. https://doi.org/10.1016/j.acap.2017.09.001

Dempster, M., Howell, D., & McCorry, N. K. (2015). Illness perceptions and coping in physical health conditions: A meta-analysis. *Journal of Psychosomatic Research*, 79(6), 506–513. https://doi.org/10.1016/j.jpsychores.2015.10.006

Denollet, J., & Pedersen, S. S. (2009). Anger, depression, and anxiety in cardiac patients: The complexity of individual differences in psychological risk. *Journal of the American College of Cardiology*, 53, 947–949.

Denys, D., Graat, I., Mocking, R., de Koning, P., Vulink, N., Figee, M., ... Schuurman, R. (2020). Efficacy of deep brain stimulation of the ventral anterior limb of the internal capsule for refractory obsessive–compulsive disorder: A clinical cohort of 70 patients. *American Journal of Psychiatry*. https://doi.org/10.1176/appi.ajp.2019.19060656

de Oliveira, C. C., Nicoletti, C. F., de Souza Pinhel, M. A., de Oliveira, B. A. P., Quinhoneiro, D. C. G., Noronha, N. Y., ... Nonino, C. B. (2017). Influence of expression of UCP3, PLIN1 and PPARG 2 on the oxidation of substrates after hypocaloric dietary intervention. *Clinical Nutrition*, 37(4), 1383–1388.

De Paul, N. F., & Caver, K. A. (2020). A pilot study of a brief group adaptation of the Unified Protocol in integrated primary care. *Psychological Services*. https://doi.org/10.1037/ser0000406

de Sá, S., Baião, A., Marques, H., Marques, M. do C., Reis, M. J., Dias, S., & Catarino, M. (2023). The influence of smartphones on adolescent sleep: A systematic literature review. *Nursing Reports*, 13(2), 612–621. https://doi.org/10.3390/nursrep13020054

Desbordes, G., Gard, T., Hoge, E. A., Hölzel, B. K., Kerr, C., Lazar, S. W., ... Vago, D. R. (2015). Moving beyond mindfulness: Defining equanimity as an outcome measure in meditation and contemplative research. *Mindfulness*, 6(2), 356–372.

Deshields, T. L., Asvat, Y., Tippey, A. R., & Vanderlan, J. R. (2022). Distress, depression, anxiety, and resilience in patients with cancer and caregivers. *Health Psychology*, 41(4), 246–255. https://doi.org/10.1037/hea0001170

De Sousa, A. (2019a). Disulfiram: The history behind the molecule. In *Disulfiram* (pp. 1–8). Springer.

De Sousa, A. (2019b). *Disulfirum*. Springer.

Deter, H.-C., Kruse, J., & Zipfel, S. (2018). History, aims and present structure of psychosomatic medicine in Germany. *Biopsychosocial Medicine*, 12, 1. https://doi.org/10.1186/s13030-017-0120-x

De Visser, R. (2019). Gender and health. In C. D. Llewellyn, S. Ayers, C. McManus, S. Newman, K. J. Petrie, T. A. Revenson, & J. Weinman (Eds.), *Cambridge handbook of psychology, health and medicine* (3rd ed., pp. 20–24). Cambridge University Press.

Dhindsa, R. S., &. Goldstein, D. B. (2016). Schizophrenia: From genetics to physiology at last. *Nature*, 530, 162–163. https://doi.org/10.1038/nature16874

Diabetes Prevention Program Research Group. (2015). Long-term effects of lifestyle intervention or metformin on diabetes development and microvascular complications over 15-year follow-up: The Diabetes Prevention Program Outcomes Study. *The Lancet Diabetes & Endocrinology*, 3, 866–875.

Diaz, C. D., Carroll, B. J., & Hemyari, A. (2020). Pulmonary illness related to e-cigarette use. *The New England Journal of Medicine*, 382, 384–386.

Diaz, T., & Bui, N. H. (2017). Subjective well-being in Mexican and Mexican American women: The role of acculturation, ethnic identity, gender roles, and perceived social support. *Journal of Happiness Studies*, 18(2), 607–624.

Dickie, R., Rasmussen, S., Cain, R., Williams, L., & MacKay, W. (2018). The effects of perceived social norms on handwashing behaviour in students. *Psychology, Health & Medicine*, 23, 154–159.

Dickman, S. L., Gaffney, A., McGregor, A., Himmelstein, D. U., McCormick, D., Bor, D. H., ... Woolhandler, S. (2022). Trends in health care use among Black and White persons in the US, 1963–2019. *JAMA Network Open*, 5(6), e2217383-e2217383.

Diefenbach, M. A., & Leventhal, H. (1996). The common-sense model of illness representation: Theoretical and practical considerations. *Journal of Social Distress & The Homeless*, 5(1), 11–38. https://doi.org/10.1007/BF02090456

Di Iorio, C. R., Watkins, T. J., Dietrich, M. S., Cao, A., Blackford, J. U., Rogers, B., ... Cowan, R. L. (2011). Evidence for chronically altered serotonin function in the cerebral cortex of female 3,4-methylenedioxymethamphetamine polydrug users. *Archives of General Psychiatry*, 69, 399–409.

Dillard, R. (2020, February 28). Every step you take: What is the future of remote patient monitoring? *Docwirenews*. https://www.docwirenews.com/blog/what-is-the-future-of-remote-patient-monitoring-rpm/

Dillon, K., Rollo, S., & Prapavessis, H. (2022). A combined health action process approach and mHealth intervention to reduce sedentary behaviour in university students - a randomized controlled trial. *Psychology & Health*, 37(6), 692–711. https://doi.org/10.1080/08870446.2021.1900574

Dimitrov, S., Lange, T., Gouttefangeas, C., Jensen, A. T. R., Szczepanski, M., Lehnnolz, J., ... Besedovsky, L. (2019). Gαs-coupled receptor signaling and sleep regulate integrin activation of human antigen-specific T cells. *The Journal of Experimental Medicine*, 216(3), 517–526. https://doi.org/10.1084/jem.20181169

Dion, J., Hains, J., Vachon, P., Plouffe, J., Laberge, L., Perron, M., ... Leone, M. (2016). Correlates of body dissatisfaction in children. *The Journal of Pediatrics*, 171, 202–207.

Distracted Driving. (2019). Centers for Disease Control and Prevention. National Center for Injury Prevention and Control.

Dittmar, H., Halliwell, E., & Ive, S. (2006). Does Barbie make girls want to be thin? The effect of experimental exposure to images of dolls on the body image of 5- to 8-year-old girls. *Developmental Psychology*, 42, 283–292.

Dobber, J., Latour, C., Van Meijel, B., Ter Riet, G., Barkhof, E., Peters, R., ... DeHaan, L. (2020). Active ingredients and mechanisms of change in motivational interviewing for medication adherence. A mixed methods study of patient-therapist interaction in patients with schizophrenia. *Frontiers in Psychiatry*, 11.

Dobson, K. S., Poole, J. C., & Beck, J. S. (2018). The fundamental cognitive model. In R. L. Leahy (Ed.), *Science and practice in cognitive therapy: Foundations, mechanisms, and applications* (pp. 29–47). Guilford.

Dobson, R., Whittaker, R., Jiang, Y., Maddison, R., Shepherd, M., McNamara, C., ... Murphy, R. (2018). Effectiveness of text message based, diabetes self management support programme (SMS4BG): Two arm, parallel randomised controlled trial. *British Medical Journal*, 361, k1959. https://doi.org/10.1136/bmj.k1959

Dolezsar, C. M., McGrath, J. J., Herzig, A. J. M., & Miller, S. B. (2014). Perceived racial discrimination and hypertension: A comprehensive systematic review. *Health Psychology*, 33, 20–34.

Donnelly, G. E., Guge, P. M., Howell, R. T., & John, L. K. (2021). A salient sugar tax decreases sugary-drink buying. *Psychological Science*, 32(11), 1830–1841. https://doi.org/10.1177/09567976211017022

Doran, N., Schweizer, C. A., & Myers, M. G. (2011). Do expectancies for reinforcement from smoking change after smoking initiation? *Psychology of Addictive Behaviors*, 25, 101–107.

Dossett, M. L., Fricchione, G. L., & Benson, H. (2020). A new era for mind–body medicine. *The New England Journal of Medicine*, 382, 1390–1391.

Dougherty, D. D., Brennan, B. P., Stewart, E., Wilhelm, S., Widge, A. S., & Rauch, S. L. (2018). Neuroscientifically informed formulation and treatment planning for patients with obsessive–compulsive disorder: A review. *JAMA Psychiatry*, 75, 1081–1087.

Dowell, D., Haegerich, T. M., & Chou, R. (2016). CDC guideline for prescribing opioids for chronic pain—United States, 2016. *Journal of the American Medical Association*, 315, 1624–1645.

Drazen, J. M., Morrissey, S., & Campion, E. W. (2019). The dangerous flavors of e-cigarettes. *NEJM*, 380(7), 679–680. https://doi.org/10.1056/NEJMe1900484.

Drolet, M., Bénard, É., Pérez, N., Brisson, M., Ali, H., Boily, M. C., ... Checchi, M. (2019). Population-level impact and herd effects following the introduction of human papillomavirus vaccination programmes: Updated systematic review and meta-analysis. *Lancet*, 394, 497–509.

Duggal, C. S., Metcalfe, D., Sackeyfio, R., Carlson, G. W., & Losken, A. (2013). Patient motivations for choosing postmastectomy breast reconstruction. *Annals of Plastic Surgery*, 70(5), 574–580.

Duncan, M. S., Freiberg, M. S., Greevy, R. A., Jr, Kundu, S., Ramachandran, S., Vasa, M. D., ... Tindle, H. A. (2019). Association of smoking cessation with subsequent risk of cardiovascular disease. *Journal of the American Medical Association*, 322(7), 642–650. https://doi.org/10.1001/jama.2019.10298

Dunn, E. C., Brown, R. C., Dai, Y., Rosand, J., Nugent, N. R., Amstadter, A. B., & Smoller, J. W. (2015). Genetic determinants of depression. *Harvard Review of Psychiatry*, 23, 1. https://doi.org/10.1097/HRP.0000000000000054

Dunn, E. C., Wang, M. J., & Perlis, R. H. (2020). A summary of recent updates on the genetic determinants of depression. In R. S. McIntyre (Ed.), *Major depressive disorder* (pp. 1–27). Elsevier.

Dunn, K. E., Weerts, E. M., Huhn, A. S., Schroeder, J. R., Tompkins, D. A., Bigelow, G. E., & Strain, E. C. (2020). Preliminary evidence of different and clinically meaningful opioid withdrawal phenotypes. *Addiction Biology*, 25(1). https://doi.org/10.1111/adb.12680

Dunn, P., & Hazzard, E. (2019). Technology approaches to digital health literacy. *International Journal of Cardiology*, 293, 294–296.

Dunski, S. (2015). Yes, my teenage son is transgender. No, you may not ask about his genitals. *Washington Post*.

du Pont, A., Rhee, S. H., Corley, R. P., Hewitt, J. K., & Friedman, N. P. (2018). Rumination and psychopathology: Are anger and depressive rumination differentially associated with internalizing and externalizing psychopathology? *Clinical Psychological Science*, 6, 18–31.

Eagly, A. H., Eaton, A., Rose, S. M., Riger, S., & McHugh, M. C. (2012). Feminism and psychology: Analysis of a half-century of research on women and gender. *American Psychologist*, 67, 211–230.

Eccleston, C., Tabor, A., & Keogh, E. (2018). Using advanced technologies to improve access to treatment, to improve treatment, and to directly alter experience. In D. C. Turk & R. J. Gatchel (Eds.), *Psychological approaches to pain management: A practitioner's handbook* (3rd ed., pp. 289–300). The Guilford Press.

Eckel, R. H., et al. (2013). AHA/ACC guideline on lifestyle management to reduce cardiovascular risk: A report of the American College of Cardiology/American Heart Association Task Force on Practice Guidelines. *Journal of the American College of Cardiology*, 129(25 Suppl. 2), S76–99. https://doi.org/10.1161/01.cir.0000437740.48606.d1

Edwards, R. R., Campbell, C., Jamison, R. N., & Wiech, K. (2009). The neurobiological underpinnings of coping with pain. *Current Directions in Psychological Science*, 18, 237–241. https://doi.org/10.1111/j.1467-8721.2009.01643.x

Egan, S. J., Watson, H. J., Kane, R. T., McEvoy, P., Fursland, A., & Nathan, P. R. (2013). Anxiety as a mediator between perfectionism and eating disorders. *Cognitive Therapy and Research*, 37, 905–913.

Egede, L. E., Walker, R. J., Garacci, E., & Raymond Sr, J. R. (2020). Racial/ethnic differences In COVID-19 screening, hospitalization, and mortality in southeast Wisconsin. *Health Affairs*, 39(11), 1926–1934.

Ellegaard, M., Bieler, T., Beyer, N., Kjaer, M., & Jørgensen, N. R. (2020). The effect of 4 months exercise training on systemic biomarkers of cartilage and bone turnover in hip osteoarthritis patients. *Translational Sports Medicine*, 3(1), 16–25.

Ellingson, J. M., Ross, J. M., Winiger, E., Stallings, M. C., Corley, R. P., Friedman, N. P., ... Hopfer, C. J. (2020). Familial factors may not explain the effect of moderate-to-heavy cannabis use on cognitive functioning in adolescents: A sibling-comparison study. *Addiction*, 116(4), 833–844. https://doi.org/10.1111/add.15207

Ellis, A. (2008). Rational emotive behavior therapy. In R. J. Corsini & D. Wedding (Eds.), *Current psychotherapies* (8th ed., pp. 187–222). Thomson Higher Education.

Elmaleh-Sachs, A., Schwartz, J. L., Bramante, C. T., Nicklas, J. M., Gudzune, K. A., & Jay, M. (2023). Obesity management in adults: A review. *JAMA: The Journal of the American Medical Association*, 330(20), 2000. https://doi.org/10.1001/jama.2023.19897

Emanuel, E. J., Onwuteaka-Philipsen, B. D., Urwin, J. W., & Cohen, J. (2016). Attitudes and practices of euthanasia and physician-assisted suicide in the United States, Canada, and Europe. *Journal of the American Medical Association*, 316(1), 79–90. https://doi.org/10.1001/jama.2016.8499

Eom, T.-Y., Han, S. B., Kim, J., Blundon, J. A., Wang, Y.-D., Yu, J., ... Zakharenko, S. S. (2020). Schizophrenia-related microdeletion causes defective ciliary motility and brain ventricle enlargement via microRNA-dependent mechanisms in mice. *Nature Communications*, 11(1). https://doi.org/10.1038/s41467-020-14628-y

Equity (Hope) Initiative, E., Siddiqui, N., Faria, A., Andrulis, D. P., Chapman, D. A., Christopher, G. C., ... Wilson, K. (2020). Mapping racial and ethnic inequities in health and opportunity. *The New England Journal of Medicine*, 383(23), e124. https://doi.org/10.1056/nejmp2029139

Ersoy, A. O., Unlu, S., Oztas, E., Ozler, S., Uygur, D., & Yucel, A. (2017). Influenza infections in the 2014–2015 season and pregnancy outcomes. *The Journal of Infection in Developing Countries*, 11(10), 766–771.

Esplen, M. J., Warner, E., Boquiren, V., Wong, J., & Toner, B. (2020). Restoring body image after cancer (ReBIC): A group therapy intervention. *Psycho-Oncology*, 29(4), 671–680. https://doi.org/10.1002/pon.5304

Eugenicos, M., & Ferreira, N. G. (2021). Psychological factors associated with inflammatory bowel disease. *British Medical Bulletin*, 138(1), 16–28. https://doi.org/10.1093/bmb/ldab010

Eustice, C. (2022). Arthritis prevalence and statistics. *Verywell Health Year: 2022*. https://www.verywellhealth.com/arthritis-prevalence-and-statistics-189356#:~:text=More%20than%2022%25%20of%20American,men%20have%20doctor%2Ddiagnosed%20arthritis

Everaert, J., Bronstein, M. V., Cannon, T. D., & Joormann, J. (2018). Looking through tinted glasses: Depression and social anxiety are related to both interpretation biases and inflexible negative interpretations. *Clinical Psychological Science*, 6, 517–528. https://doi.org/10.1177/2167702617747968

Ezenwa, M., Yao, Y., Nguyen, M., Mandernach, M., Hunter, C., Yoon, S., ... Wilkie, D. (2018). The effects of relaxation intervention on pain, stress, and autonomic responses among adults with sickle cell pain in the outpatient setting. *The Journal of Pain*, 19(3), S32–S33.

Fallon, B. A., Ahern, D. K., Pavlicova, M., Slavov, I., Skritskya, N., & Barsky, A. J. (2017). A randomized controlled trial of medication and cognitive-behavioral therapy for hypochondriasis. *American Journal of Psychiatry*, 174, 756–764.

Fan, H., Li, T.-F., Gong, N., & Wang, Y.-X. (2016). Shanzhiside methylester, the principle effective iridoid glycoside from the analgesic herb *Lamiophlomis rotata*, reduces neuropathic pain by stimulating spinal microglial β-endorphin expression. *Neuropharmacology*, 101, 98–109.

Farrell, A. K., & Sarah, C. E. (2019). Toward a mechanistic understanding of links between close relationships and physical health. *Current Directions in Psychological Science*, 28, 483–489.

Fattoracci, E. S. M., & King, D. D. (2023). The need for understanding and addressing microaggressions in the workplace. *Perspectives on Psychological Science*, 18(4), 738–742. https://doi.org/10.1177/17456916221133825

Fazel, S., & Runeson, B. (2020). Suicide. *New England Journal of Medicine*, 382, 266–274. https://doi.org/10.1056/NEJMra1902944

Feagin, J., & Bennefield, Z. (2014). Systemic racism and US health care. *Social Science & Medicine*, 103, 7–14.

Federal Bureau of Investigation (FBI). (2019). Crime in the U.S. 2019. https://ucr.fbi.gov/crime-in-the-u.s/2019/crime-in-the-u.s.-2019/topic-pages/expanded-offense

Federal Bureau of Investigation (FBI). (2023). FBI releases supplemental 2021 hate crime statistics. U.S. Department of Justice. https://www.fbi.gov/news/press-releases/fbi-releases-supplemental-2021-hate-crime-statistics

Fehr, F. S., & Stern, J. A. (1965). Heart rate conditioning in the rat. *Journal of Psychosomatic Research*, 8(4), 441–453.

Felder, J. N., Epel, E. S., Neuhaus, J., Krystal, A. D., & Prather, A. A. (2020). Efficacy of digital cognitive behavioral therapy for the treatment of insomnia symptoms among pregnant women. *JAMA Psychiatry*, 77(5), 484–492. https://doi.org/10.1001/jamapsychiatry.2019.4491

Feldstein Ewing, S. W., & Bryan, A. D. (2020). Have we missed the boat? The current preventable surge of sexually transmitted infections (STIs) in the United States. *Health Psychology*, 39(3), 169–171.

Felt, J. M., Russell, M. A., Ruiz, J. M., Johnson, J. A., Uchino, B. N., Allison, M., ... Smyth, J. (2020). A multimethod approach examining the relative contributions of optimism and pessimism to cardiovascular disease risk markers. *Journal of Behavioral Medicine*. https://doi.org/10.1007/s10865-020-00133-6

Ferguson, C. J., Kaye, L. K., Branley-Bell, D., Markey, P., Ivory, J. D., Klisanin, D., ... Wilson, J. (2022). Like this meta-analysis: Screen media and mental health. *Professional Psychology: Research and Practice*, 53(2), 205–214. https://doi.org/10.1037/pro0000426

Fernandes, J., Fialho, M., Santos, R., Peixoto-Plácido, C., Madeira, T., Sousa-Santos, N., ... Carneiro, A. V. (2020). Is olive oil good for you? A systematic review and meta-analysis on anti-inflammatory benefits from regular dietary intake. *Nutrition*, 69, 110559. https://doi.org/10.1016/j.nut.2019.110559

Fernández-Ruiz, I. (2020). Exercise protects against cardiovascular disease by modulating immune cell supply. *Nature Reviews Cardiology*, 17(5). https://doi.org/10.1038/s41569-019-0311-1

Ferrer, R. A., & Klein, W. M. (2015). Risk perceptions and health behavior. *Current Opinion in Psychology*, 5, 85–89. https://doi.org/10.1016/j.copsyc.2015.03.012

Ferrer, R. A., & Mendes, W. B. (2018). Emotion, health decision making, and health behaviour. *Psychology & Health*, 33(1), 1–16. https://doi.org/10.1080/08870446.2017.1385787

Fervaha, G., Izard, J. P., Tripp, D. A., Aghel, N., Shayegan, B., Klotz, L., ... Siemens, D. R. (2020). Psychological morbidity associated with prostate cancer: Rates and predictors of depression in the RADICAL PC study. *Canadian Urological Association Journal*, 15(6). https://doi.org/10.5489/cuaj.6912

Field-Springer, K., Randall-Griffiths, D., & Reece, C. (2018). From menarche to menopause: Understanding multigenerational reproductive health milestones. *Health Communication*, 33, 733–742.

Figueira, M. E. (2019). Tea extracts. In S. M. Nabavi & A. S. Silva (Eds.), *Nonvitamin and nonmineral nutritional supplements* (pp. 433–436). Academic Press.

Figueroa, W. S., Zoccola, P. M., Manigault, A. W., Hamilton, K. R., Scanlin, M. C., & Johnson, R. C. (2021). Daily stressors and diurnal cortisol among sexual and gender minority young adults. *Health Psychology: Official Journal of the Division of Health Psychology, American Psychological Association*, 40(2), 145–154. https://doi.org/10.1037/hea0001054

Filippi, V., Chou, D., Ronsmans, C., Graham, W., & Say, L. (2016). Levels and causes of maternal mortality and morbidity. *Disease control priorities: Reproductive, maternal, newborn, and child health* (3rd ed., Vol. 2, pp. 51–70). https://doi.org/10.1596/978-1-4648-0348-2_ch3

Fink, E. (2019). Central pain syndromes. In A. Abd-Elsayed (Ed.), *Pain* (pp. 927–929). Springer.

Finkelstein, A. (2020). A strategy for improving U.S. health care delivery—Conducting more randomized, controlled trials. *The New England Journal of Medicine*, 382, 1485–1488.

Finkelstein, A., Zhou, A., Taubman, S., & Doyle, J. (2020). Health care hotspotting—A randomized, controlled trial. *New England Journal of Medicine*, 382, 152–162.

Fishbein, M., & Ajzen, I. (1975). *Belief, attitude, intention and behavior: An introduction to theory and research*. Addison-Wesley.

Fishel, J., Thomas, E., & Lantry, L. (2020, March 16). Fact check: Trump's coronavirus response plagued with misstatements. https://abcnews.go.com/Politics/fact-check-friday-trumps-coronavirus-response-plagued-misstatements/story?id=69590582

Fitzpatrick, K. M., Harris, C., & Drawve, G. (2020). How bad is it? Suicidality in the middle of the COVID-19 pandemic. *Suicide and Life-Threatening Behavior.* https://doi.org/10.1111/sltb.12655

Flagel, S. B., Clark, J. J., Robinson, T. E., Mayo, L., Czuj, A., Willuhn, I., ... Akil, H. (2011). A selective role for dopamine in stimulus–reward learning. *Nature*, 469, 53–57.

Fleary, S. A., & Nigg, C. R. (2018). Trends in health behavior patterns among U.S. adults, 2003–2015. *Annals of Behavioral Medicine*, 53, 1–15.

Fleshner, M., Frank, M., & Maier, S. F. (2017). Danger signals and inflammasomes: Stress-evoked sterile inflammation in mood disorders. *Neuropsychopharmacology*, 42, 36–45.

Flowers, K. M., Patton, M. E., Hruschak, V. J., Fields, K. G., Schwartz, E., Zeballos, J., ... Schreiber, K. L. (2021). Conditioned open-label placebo for opioid reduction following spine surgery: A randomized, controlled trial. *Pain,* 162(6), 1828–1839. https://doi.org/10.1097/j.pain.0000000000002185

Fogarty, J. A. (2019). *The magical thoughts of grieving children: Treating children with complicated mourning and advice for parents*. Routledge.

Folkman, S. (Ed.). (2011). *The Oxford handbook of stress, health and coping*. Oxford University Press.

Fong, A., Lafaro, K. J., Ituarte, P. H. G., & Fong, Y. (2021). Association of living in urban food deserts with mortality from breast and colorectal cancer. *Annals of Surgical Oncology,* 28(3). https://doi.org/10.1245/s10434-020-09049-6

Foreman, A. (2022, February 18). Anorexia's ancient roots and present toll. *The Wall Street Journal*. https://www.wsj.com/articles/anorexias-ancient-roots-and-present-toll-11645215947?mod=Searchresults_pos1&page=

Forsyth, J. K., & Asarnow, R. F. (2020). Genetics of childhood-onset schizophrenia 2019 update. *Child and Adolescent Psychiatric Clinics*, 29(1), 157–170.

Forthun, I., Eliassen, K. E. R., Emberland, K. E., & Bjorvatn, B. (2023). The association between self-reported sleep problems, infection, and antibiotic use in patients in general practice. *Frontiers in Psychiatry,* 14. https://doi.org/10.3389/fpsyt.2023.1033034

Foster, S. J., Carvallo, M., Wenske, M., & Lee, J. (2021). Damaged masculinity: How honor endorsement can influence prostate cancer screening decision-making and prostate cancer mortality rates. *Personality and Social Psychology Bulletin,* 49(2), 296–308. https://doi.org/10.1177/01461672211065293

Foti, S. A., Khambaty, T., Birnbaum-Weitzman, O., Arguelles, W., Penedo, F., Giacinto, R. A. E., ... Llabre, M. M. (2020). Loneliness, cardiovascular disease, and diabetes prevalence in the Hispanic community health study/study of Latinos sociocultural ancillary study. *Journal of Immigrant and Minority Health*, 22(2), 345–352.

Fox, M. (2018, June 7). Suicide rates are up 30 percent since 1999, CDC says. *NBCnews.com*. https://www.nbcnews.com/health/health-news/suicide-ratesare-30-percent-1999-cdc-says-n880926

Frajerman, A., Morvan, Y., Krebs, M. O., Gorwood, P., & Chaumette, B. (2019). Burnout in medical students before residency: A systematic review and meta-analysis. *European Psychiatry*, 55, 36–42.

Franczyk, B., Gluba-Brzózka, A., Aleksandra Ciałkowska-Rysz, Janusz Ławiński, & Rysz, J. (2023). The impact of aerobic exercise on HDL quantity and quality: A narrative review. *International Journal of Molecular Sciences,* 24(5), 4653–4653. https://doi.org/10.3390/ijms24054653

Franko, D. L., Keshaviah, A., Eddy, K. T., Krishna, M., Davis, M. C., Keel, P. K., ... Herzog, D. B. (2013). A longitudinal investigation of mortality in anorexia nervosa and bulimia nervosa. *The American Journal of Psychiatry,* 170(8), 917–925. https://doi.org/10.1176/appi.ajp.2013.12070868

Fredrix, M., McSharry, J., Flannery, C., Dinneen, S., & Byrne, M. (2018). Goal-setting in diabetes self-management: A systematic review and meta-analysis examining content and effectiveness of goal-setting interventions. *Psychology & Health*, 33, 955–977.

Freedland, K. E. (2022). Progress in health-related behavioral intervention research: Making it, measuring it, and meaning it. *Health Psychology,* 41(1), 1–12. https://doi.org/10.1037/hea0001160

Freedman, A., & Nicolle, J. (2020). Social isolation and loneliness: The new geriatric giants: Approach for primary care. *Canadian Family Physician*, 66(3), 176–182.

Free, J. L. (2020). "We're brokers": How youth violence prevention workers intervene in the lives of at-risk youth to reduce violence. *Criminal Justice Review*. https://doi.org/10.1177/0734016820907663

Freudenreich, O. (2020). *Psychotic disorders: A practical guide*. Springer International Publishing.

Friedman, R. A. (2014, May 28). Why can't doctors identify killers. *The New York Times*. https://www.nytimes.com/2014/05/28/opinion/why-cant-doctors-identify-killers.html

Friedman, R. A. (2018, February 8). Opinion. *The New York Times*. https://www.nytimes.com/2018/02/08/opinion/marijuana-opiates-jeff-sessions.html

Frizon, L. A., Yamamoto, E. A., Nagel, S. J., Simonson, M. T., Hogue, O., & Machado, A. G. (2020). Deep brain stimulation for pain in the modern era: A systematic review. *Neurosurgery*, 86(2), 191–202. https://doi.org/10.1093/neuros/nyy552

Fruman, D. A., Chiu, H., Hopkins, B. D., Bagrodia, S., Cantley, L. C., & Abraham, R. T. (2018). The PI3K pathway in human disease. *Cell*, 170, 605–635.

Gabriel, E. H., Hoch, M. C., & Cramer, R. J. (2019). The development of the theory of planned behavior and health belief model scales: Assessing behavioral determinants of exercise-related injury prevention program participation. *Athletic Training & Sports Health Care*, 11(3), 113–123.

Gaffey, A. E., Harris, K. M., Mena-Hurtado, C., Sinha, R., Jacoby, D. L., & Smolderen, K. G. (2022). The Yale roadmap for health psychology and integrated cardiovascular care. *Health Psychology,* 41(10), 779–791. https://doi.org/10.1037/hea0001152

Galante, J., Friedrich, C., Dalgleish, T., Jones, P. B., & White, I. R. (2023). Systematic review and individual participant data meta-analysis of randomized controlled trials assessing mindfulness-based programs for mental health promotion. *Nature Mental Health*, 1(7). https://doi.org/10.1038/s44220-023-00081-5

Gallagher, N. (2021, April). Dopamine levels predict hallucination-like experiences in mice. *Academictimes.com*. https://academictimes.com/dopamine-levels-predict-hallucination-like-experiences-in-mice/

Gall, T. L., & Bilodeau, C. (2020). The role of positive and negative religious/spiritual coping in women's adjustment to breast cancer: A longitudinal study. *Journal of Psychosocial Oncology*, 38(1), 103–117. https://doi.org/10.1080/07347332.2019.1641581

Galsworthy-Francis, L. (2014). Cognitive behavioral therapy for anorexia nervosa: A systematic review. *Clinical Psychology Review*, 34, 54–72.

Gandal, M. J., Leppa, V., Won, H., Parikshak, N. N., & Geschwind, D. H. (2016). The road to precision psychiatry: Translating genetics into disease mechanisms. *Nature Neuroscience*, 19, 1397–1407.

Gandal, M. J., Zhang, P., Hadjimichael, E., Walker, R. L., Chen, C., Liu, A., ... Geschwind, D. H. (2018). Transcriptome-wide isoform-level dysregulation in ASD, schizophrenia, and bipolar disorder. *Science*, 362(6420), 8127. https://doi.org/10.1126/science.aat8127

Gandy, M., Karin, E., Jones, M. P., McDonald, S., Sharpe, L., Titov, N., & Dear, B. F. (2018). Exploring psychological mechanisms of clinical response to an internet-delivered psychological pain management program. *European Journal of Pain (London, England),* 22(8), 1502–1516. https://doi.org/10.1002/ejp.1239

Gandy, M., Pang, S. T., Scott, A. J., Heriseanu, A. I., Bisby, M. A., Dudeney, J., ... Dear, B. F. (2022). Internet-delivered cognitive and behavioural based interventions for adults with chronic pain: A systematic review and meta-analysis of randomized controlled trials. *Pain*, 163(10), e1041–e1053.

Gao, X. R., Chiariglione, M., Qin, K., Nuytemans, K., Scharre, D. W., Li, Y.-J., & Martin, E. R. (2023). Explainable machine learning aggregates polygenic risk scores and electronic health records for Alzheimer's disease prediction. *Scientific Reports,* 13(1). https://doi.org/10.1038/s41598-023-27551-1

Garcia-Silva, J., Navarrete, N. N., Peralta-Ramírez, M. I., García-Sánchez, A., Ferrer-González, M. Á., & Caballo, V. E. (2018). Efficacy of cognitive behavioral therapy in adherence to the Mediterranean Diet in metabolic syndrome patients: A randomized controlled trial. *Journal of Nutrition Education and Behavior*, 50(9), 896–904.

Garcia, T. A., Hultgren, B. A., Canning, J. R., Gilson, M. S., & Larimer, M. E. (2022). "On a night like this": A mixed-methods approach to understanding high-risk drinking events in college students. Alcoholism: *Clinical and Experimental Research,* 46(6), 1121–1132. https://doi.org/10.1111/acer.14844

Garland, E. L., Brintz, C. E., Hanley, A. W., Roseen, E. J., Atchley, R. M., Gaylord, S. A., ... Keefe, F. J. (2019). Mind–body therapies for opioid-treated pain: A systematic review and meta-analysis. *JAMA Internal Medicine*. https://doi.org/10.1001/jamainternmed.2019.4917

Gast, A., & Mathes, T. (2019). Medication adherence influencing factors—An (updated) overview of systematic reviews. *Systematic Reviews.*

Gatchel, R. J., Neblett, R., Kishino, N., & Ray, C. T. (2016). Fear-avoidance beliefs and chronic pain. *Journal of Orthopaedic and Sports Physical Therapy*, 46(2), 38–43.

Gatchel, R. J., & Noe, C. (2019). Biofeedback. In C. D. Llewellyn, S. Ayers, C. McManus, S. Newman, K. J. Petrie, T. A. Revenson, & J. Weinman (Eds.), *Cambridge handbook of psychology, health and medicine* (3rd ed., pp. 242–245). Cambridge University Press.

Gauntlett-Gilbert, J., & Brook, P. (2018). Living well with chronic pain: the role of pain-management programmes. *BJA Education*, 18(1), 3–7. https://doi.org/10.1016/j.bjae.2017.09.001

GBD 2016 Alcohol Collaborators. (2018). Alcohol use and burden for 195 countries and territories, 1990–2016: A systematic analysis for the Global Burden of Disease study. *Lancet*, 39, 1015. https://doi.org/10.1016/S0140-6736(18)31310-2

Gehlert, S., & Browne, T. (2019). *Handbook of health social work* (3rd ed.). Jossey-Bass Wiley.

Gehlert, S., & Ward, T. S. (2019). Theories of health behavior. In S. Gehlert & T. Browne (Eds.), *Handbook of health social work* (3rd ed., pp. 143–162). Jossey-Bass Wiley.

Geipert, N. (2007, January). Don't be mad: More research links hostility to coronary risk. *Monitor on Psychology*, 38, 50–51.

Geller, K., Lippke, S., & Nigg, C. R. (2016). Future directions of multiple behavior change research. *Journal of Behavioral Medicine*, 40(1), 194–202. https://doi.org/10.1007/s10865-016-9809-8

Ge, L., Sadeghirad, B., Ball, G. D. C., da Costa, B. R., Hitchcock, C. L., Svendrovski, A., ... Johnston, B. C. (2020). Comparison of dietary macronutrient patterns of 14 popular named dietary programmes for weight and cardiovascular risk factor reduction in adults:

Systematic review and network meta-analysis of randomised trials. *British Medical Journal, m696*. https://doi.org/10.1136/bmj.m696

Geniole, S. N., Bird, B. M., McVittie, J. S., Purcell, R. B., Archer, J., & Carré, J. M. (2020). Is testosterone linked to human aggression? A meta-analytic examination of the relationship between baseline, dynamic, and manipulated testosterone on human aggression. *Hormones and Behavior*, 123(104644), 104644. https://doi.org/10.1016/j.yhbeh.2019.104644

Genital Herpes. (2019). Genital herpes—CDC fact sheet.

George Institute for Global Health. (2019, September 27). Salt shakers should carry tobacco-style health warning, say experts.

George, J. C. (2015). Mind, metabolism, and melatonin: Time's arrow towards the future. *Journal of Science Technology and Humanities*, 1(2), 195–216.

Gerber, M., Schilling, R., Colledge, F., Ludyga, S., Pühse, U., & Brand, S. (2020). More than a simple pastime? The potential of physical activity to moderate the relationship between occupational stress and burnout symptoms. *International Journal of Stress Management*, 27(1), 53–64.

Gerend, M. A., Patel, S., Ott, N., Wetzel, K., Sutin, A.R., Terracciano, A., ... Maneret, J. K. (2022) A qualitative analysis of people's experiences with weight-based discrimination. *Psychology & Health*, 37(9), 1093–1110. doi: 10.1080/08870446.2021.192117

Gerhardt, U. (2022). Parsons, role theory, and health interaction. In G. Scrambler (Eds.), *Sociological theory and medical sociology* (e-book). Routledge.

Geuter, S., & Büchel, C. (2013). Facilitation of pain in the human spinal cord by nocebo treatment. *Journal of Neuroscience*, 33, 3784–13790.

Ghandour, K., & Inokuchi, K. (2023). Memory reactivations during sleep. *Neuroscience Research*, 189, 60–65. https://doi.org/10.1016/j.neures.2022.12.018

Ghomrawi, H. M., Funk, R. J., Parks, M. L., Owen-Smith, J., & Hollingsworth, J. M. (2018). Physician referral patterns and racial disparities in total hip replacement: A network analysis approach. *PLoS One*, 13(2), e0193014.

Ginley, M. K., Pfund, R. A., Rash, C. J., & Zajac, K. (2021). Long-term efficacy of contingency management treatment based on objective indicators of abstinence from illicit substance use up to 1 year following treatment: A meta-analysis. *Journal of Consulting and Clinical Psychology*, 89(1), 58–71. https://doi.org/10.1037/ccp0000552

Gladden, P. R., & Cleator, A. M. (2018). Sexual assault and Intimate partner violence. In T. K. Shakelford & V. A. Weekes-Shakelford (Eds.), *Encyclopedia of evolutionary psychological science*. Springer International Publishing. https://doi.org/10.1007/978-3-319-16999-6_1722-1

Glanz, K., & Bishop, D. B. (2010). The role of behavioral science theory in the development and implementation of public health interventions. *Annual Review of Public Health*, 31, 399–418. https://doi.org/10.1146/annurev.publhealth.012809.103604

Glanz, K. B., Rimer, B. K., & Viswanath, K. (2015a). Theory, research, and practice: Interrelationships. In K. B. Glanz, B. K. Rimer, & K. Viswanath (Eds.), *Health behavior: Theory, research, and practice* (5th ed., pp. 23–42). Jossey-Bass.

Glanz, K. B., Rimer, B. K., & Viswanath, K. (2015). *Health behavior: theory, research, and practice* (5th ed.). San Francisco: Jossey-Bass.

Glanz, K., Rimer, B. K., & Viswanath, K. (2015). The scope of health behavior. In K. B. Glanz, B. K. Rimer, & K. Viswanath (Eds.), *Health behavior: Theory, research, and practice* (5th ed., pp. 3–22). Jossey-Bass.

Glaser, N., & Styne, D. (2020). Thoughts on the association between sleep and obesity. *Pediatrics*, 145(3). https://doi.org/10.1542/peds.2019-3676

Glogan, E., Liu, P., & Meulders, A. (2023). Generalization of costly pain-related avoidance based on real-life categorical knowledge. *Psychological Science*, 34(7), 809–821. https://doi.org/10.1177/09567976231170878

Goetter, E., Bui, E., Horenstein, A., Baker, A. W., Hoeppner, S., Charney, M., & Simon, N. M. (2019). Five-factor model in bereaved adults with and without complicated grief. *Death Studies*, 43(3), 204–209. https://doi.org/10.1080/07481187.2018.1446059

Goff, D. C. (2020). The pharmacologic treatment of schizophrenia—2021. *JAMA*. https://doi.org/10.1001/jama.2020.19048

Goffman, E. (1963). *Stigma; notes on the management of spoiled identity*. Prentice-Hall.

Goldberg, S. B., Riordan, K. M., Sun, S., & Davidson, R. J. (2021). The empirical status of mindfulness-based interventions: A systematic review of 44 meta-analyses of randomized controlled trials. *Perspectives on Psychological Science*, 17(1), 108–130. https://doi.org/10.1177/1745691620968771

Gold, J. M., Carr, L. J., Thomas, J. G., Burrus, J., O'Leary, K. C., Wing, R., ... Bond, D. S. (2020). Conscientiousness in weight loss maintainers and regainers. *Health Psychology*, 39(5), 421–429. https://doi.org/10.1037/hea0000846

Goldstein, I., Kim, N. N., Clayton, A. H., DeRogatis, L. R., Giraldi, A., Parish, S. J., ... Stahl, S. M. (2017, January). Hypoactive sexual desire disorder: International Society for the Study of Women's Sexual Health (ISSWSH) expert consensus panel review. *Mayo Clinic Proceedings*, 92(1), 114–128.

Goldstein, P., Weissman-Fogel, I., Dumas, G., & Shamay-Tsoory, S. G. (2018). Brain-to-brain coupling during handholding is associated with pain reduction. *PNAS*, 115(11), E2528–E2537. https://doi.org/10.1073/pnas.1703643115

González-Freire, B., Vázquez, D., & Pértega-Díaz, S. (2019). The relationship of psychological factors and asthma control to health-related quality of life. *The Journal of Allergy and Clinical Immunology: In Practice*, 8, 197–207. https://doi.org/10.1016/j.jaip.2019.07.009

González, H. J., Vega, W. A., Williams, D. R., Tarraf, W., West, B. T., & Neighbors, H. W. (2010). Depression care in the United States: Too little for too few. *Archives of General Psychiatry*, 67, 37–46.

Gonzalez-Pons, M., & Cruz-Correa, M. (2020). Colorectal cancer disparities in Latinos: Genes vs. environment. In A. G. Ramirez & E. J. Trapido (Eds.), *Advancing the science of cancer in Latinos* (pp. 35–41). Springer.

Goodman, W. K., Storch, E. A., & Sheth, S. A. (2021). Harmonizing the neurobiology and treatment of obsessive-compulsive disorder. *American Journal of Psychiatry*, 178(1), 17–29. https://doi.org/10.1176/appi.ajp.2020.20111601

Goodnough, A. (2019, May 19). Heroin is vanishing as fentanyl swamps streets. *New York Times*, pp. A1, A24.

Gordon, D., Moos, M., Amborski, D., & Taylor, Z. (2018). The future of the suburbs: Policy challenges and opportunities in Canada. *The School of Public Policy Publications*, 11. https://doi.org/10.11575/sppp.v11i0.53000

Gordon, J. S. (2024). Poverty, human rights, and just distribution check for updates. *International Public Health Policy and Ethics*, 106, 147–158

Gorman, C. (2012, January). Five hidden dangers of obesity: Excess weight can harm health in ways that may come as a surprise. *Scientific American*. www.scientificamerican.com/article.cfm?id=five-hidden-dangers-of-obesity

Gosling, S. D., & Mason, W. (2015). Internet research in psychology. *Annual Review of Psychology*, 66, 877–902. https://doi.org/10.1146/annurev-psych-010814-015321

Gostin, L. O., Ratzan, S. C., & Bloom, B. R. (2019). Safe vaccinations for a healthy nation: Increasing us vaccine coverage through law, science, and communication. *Journal of the American Medical Association*, 321, 1969–1970.

Gouveia Roque, C., Chung, K. M., McCurdy, E. P., Jagannathan, R., Randolph, L. K., Herline-Killian, K., Baleriola, J., & Hengst, U. (2023). CREB3L2-ATF4 heterodimerization defines a transcriptional hub of Alzheimer's disease gene expression linked to neuropathology. *Science Advances*, 9(9), eadd2671. https://doi.org/10.1126/sciadv.add2671

Goz, V., Spiker, W. R., & Brodke, D. (2019). Mobile messaging and smartphone apps for patient communication and engagement in spine surgery. *Annals of Translational Medicine*, 7(Suppl. 5), S163. https://doi.org/10.21037/atm.2019.08.10

Graf, N., Brown, A., & Patten, E. (2019). The narrowing but persistent gender gap in pay. *Pew Research Center*.

Grandgenett, H. M., Steel, A. L., Brock, R. L., & DiLillo, D. (2020). Responding to disclosure of sexual assault: The potential impact of victimization history and rape myth acceptance. *Journal of Interpersonal Violence*. https://doi.org/10.1177/0886260519898429

Grant, J. E., Lust, K., & Chamberlain, S. R. (2019). Hallucinogen use is associated with mental health and addictive problems and impulsivity in university students. *Addictive Behaviors Reports*, 10. https://doi.org/10.1016/j.abrep.2019.100228

Grant, P. M., Huh, G. A., Perivoliotis, D., Stolar, N. M., & Beck, A. T. (2012). Randomized trial to evaluate the efficacy of cognitive therapy for low-functioning patients with schizophrenia. *Archives of General Psychiatry*, 69(2), 121–127.

Gravel, J., Allison, B., West-Fagan, J., McBride, M., & Tita, G. E. (2018). Birds of a feather fight together: Status-enhancing violence, social distance and the emergence of homogenous gangs. *Journal of Quantitative Criminology*, 34(1), 189–219.

Gray, C., Koopman, E., & Hunt, J. (1991). The emotional phases of marital separation: an empirical investigation. *American Journal of Orthopsychiatry*, 61, 138–143.

Greenbaum, Z. (2020). How well is telehealth working? *Monitor on Psychology*, 51(5), 46.

Greenhalgh, S. (2015). *Fat-talk nation: The human costs of America's war on fat*. Cornell University Press.

Greer, D. M., Shemie, S. D., Lewis, A., Torrance, S., Varelas, P., Goldenberg, F. D., ... Baldisseri, M. (2020). Determination of brain death/death by neurologic criteria: The World Brain Death Project. *Journal of the American Medical Association*, 324(11). 1078–1097. https://doi.org/10.1001/jama.2020.11586

Griffin, S. C., Williams, A. B., Ravyts, S. G., Mladen, S. N., & Rybarczyk, B. D. (2020). Loneliness and sleep: A systematic review and meta-analysis. *Health Psychology Open*, 7(1). https://doi.org/10.1177/20551029209132352055102920913235

Griffith, K., Evans, L., & Bor, J. (2017). The Affordable Care Act reduced socioeconomic disparities in health care access. *Health Affairs*. https://doi.org/10.1377/hlthaff.2017.0083.

Grogan, S., & Mechan, J. (2017). Body image after mastectomy: A thematic analysis of younger women's written accounts. *Journal of Health Psychology*, 22(11), 1480–1490. https://doi.org/10.1177/1359105316630137

Groves, C. L., & Anderson, C. A. (2018). Aversive events and aggression. *Current Opinion in Psychology*, 19, 144–148.

Grundy, S. M., Stone, N. J., Bailey, A. L., Beam, C., Birtcher, K. K., Blumenthal, R. S., ... Yeboahet, J. (2019). AHA/ACC/AACVPR/AAPA/ABC/ACPM/ADA/AGS/APhA/ASPC/NLA/PCNA guideline on the management of blood cholesterol: Executive summary: A report of the American College of Cardiology/American Heart Association Task Force on Clinical Practice Guidelines. *Journal of the American College of Cardiology*, 73, 3168–3209.

Guardino, C., & Dunkel Schetter, C. (2022). Subjective social status and allostatic load in mothers 1 year after birth. *Health Psychology*, 41(3), 235–241. https://doi.org/10.1037/hea0001148

Guasch-Ferré, M., Liu, G., Li, Y., Sampson, L., Manson, J. E., Salas-Salvadó, J., ... Hu, F. B. (2020). Olive oil consumption and cardiovascular risk in US adults. *Journal of the American College of Cardiology*, 75(15), 1729–1739. https://doi.org/10.1016/j.jacc.2020.02.036

Guevarra, D. A., Moser, J. S., Wager, T. D., & Kross, E. (2020). Placebos without deception reduce self-report and neural measures of emotional distress. *Nature Communications*, 11(1). https://doi.org/10.1038/s41467-020-17654-y

Gunstad, J., Sanborn, V., & Hawkins, M. (2020). Cognitive dysfunction is a risk factor for overeating and obesity. *American Psychologist*, 75(2), 219–234.

Guo, F., Xu, Q., Salem, H. M. A., Yao, Y., Lou, J., & Huang, X. (2016). The neuronal correlates of mirror therapy: A functional magnetic resonance imaging study on mirror-induced visual illusions of ankle movements. *Brain Research*, 1639, 186–193.

Gustavson, D. E., Franz, C. E., Kremen, W. S., Carver, C. S., Corley, R. P., Hewitt, J. K., & Friedman, N. P. (2019). Common genetic influences on impulsivity facets are related to goal management, psychopathology, and personality. *Journal of Research in Personality*, 79, 161–175.

Gutiérrez, I. T., Menendez, D., Jiang, M. J., Hernandez, I. G., Miller, P., & Rosengren, K. S. (2020). Embracing death: Mexican parent and child perspectives on death. *Child Development*, 91(2), e491–e511.

Gyatso, T. (2003, April 26). The monk in the lab. *New York Times*, p. A29.

Hachem, A., & Brennan, L. (2016). Quality of life outcomes of bariatric surgery: A systematic review. *Obesity Surgery*, 26(2), 395–409.

Haddad, N., Allen, R. H., Szkwarko, D., Forcier, M., & Paquette, C. (2018). Eliminating parental consent for adolescents receiving human papillomavirus vaccination. *Rhode Island Medical Journal*, 101(7), 12–14.

Hadi, S., Momenan, M., Cheraghpour, K., Hafizi, N., Pourjavidi, N., Malekahmadi, M., ... Alipour, M. (2020). Abdominal volume index: A predictive measure in relationship between depression/anxiety and obesity. *African Health Sciences*, 20(1), 257–265.

Haeffel, G. J., Hershenberg, R., Goodson, J. T., Hein, S., Square, A., Grigorenko, E. L., & Chapman, J. (2017). The hopelessness theory of depression: Clinical utility and generalizability. *Cognitive Therapy and Research*, 41(4), 543–555.

HaGani, N., Yagil, D., & Cohen, M. (2022). Burnout among oncologists and oncology nurses: A systematic review and meta-analysis. *Health Psychology*, 41(1), 53–64. https://doi.org/10.1037/hea0001155

Hagger, M. S., Cheung, M. W. -L., Ajzen, I., & Hamilton, K. (2022). Perceived behavioral control moderating effects in the theory of planned behavior: A meta-analysis. *Health Psychology*, 41(2), 155–167. https://doi.org/10.1037/hea0001153

Hagger, M. S., Moyers, S., McAnally, K., & McKinley, L. E. (2020). Known knowns and known unknowns on behavior change interventions and mechanisms of action. *Health Psychology Review*, 14(1), 199–212.

Hagger, M. S., & Orbell, S. (2003). A meta-analytic review of the common-sense model of illness representations. *Psychological Health*, 18, 141–184.

Hagger, M. S., & Orbell, S. (2022). The common sense model of illness self-regulation: A conceptual review and proposed extended model. *Health Psychology Review,* 16(3), 347–377. https://doi.org/10.1080/17437199.2021.1878050

Hahn, C. K., Hahn, A. M., Gaster, S., & Quevillon, R. (2020). Predictors of college students' likelihood to report hypothetical rape: Rape myth acceptance, perceived barriers to reporting, and self-efficacy. *Ethics & Behavior*, 30(1), 45–62.

Hajek, P., Phillips-Waller, A., Przulj, D., Pesola, F., Myers Smith, K., Bisal, N., ... McRobbie, H. J. (2019). A randomized trial of e-cigarettes versus nicotine-replacement therapy. *New England Journal of Medicine,* 380(7), 629–637.

Hales, C. M., Carroll, M.D., Fryar, C. D., & Ogden, C. L. (2020). *Prevalence of obesity and severe obesity among adults: United States, 2017–2018.* NCHS Data Brief, No. 360. National Center for Health Statistics.

Haley, J. (1987). *Problem-solving therapy* (2nd ed.). Jossey-Bass.

Halldorsson, B., & Salkovskis, P. M. (2017). Why do people with OCD and health anxiety seek reassurance excessively? An investigation of differences and similarities in function. *Cognitive Therapy and Research*, 41(4), 619–631.

Hall, G. L. (2020). Important differences in cancer care. In G. Hall (Ed.), *Patient-centered clinical care for African Americans* (pp. 69–84). Springer.

Hamed, S., Bradby, H., Ahlberg, B. M., & Thapar-Björkert, S. (2022). Racism in healthcare: A scoping review. *BMC Public Health,* 22(1), 988.

Hamel, J. (2020). Explaining symmetry across sex in intimate partner violence: Evolution, gender roles, and the will to harm. In J. Hamel (Ed.), *Partner abuse.* Springer. http://dx.doi.org/10.1891/PA-2020-0014

Hamilton, B. E., & Chong, L. L. (2015). U.S. and state trends on teen births, 1990–2013. National Center for Health Statistics. http://blogs.cdc.gov/nchs-data-visualization/2015/08/14/us-and-state-trends-on-teen-births-1990-2013/

Hamilton, J. C., Hedge, K. A., & Feldman, C. D. (2015). Excessive illness behavior: Psychiatric care of the medical patient. https://oxfordmedicine.com/mobile/view/10.1093/med/9780199731855.001.0001/med-9780199731855-chapter-37

Hamilton, J. L., & Alloy, L. B. (2017). Physiological markers of interpersonal stress generation in depression. *Clinical Psychological Science*, 5, 911–929.

Hamilton, K., Cornish, S., Kirkpatrick, A., Kroon, J., & Schwarzer, R. (2018). Parental supervision for their children's toothbrushing: Mediating effects of planning, self-efficacy, and action control. *British Journal of Health Psychology*, 23, 387–406.

Hamzelou, J. (2020). World in lockdown. *NewScientist*, 245(3275). https://doi.org/10.1016/S0262-4079(20)30611-4

Han, B., Compton, W. M., Blanco, C., Crane, E., Lee, J., & Jones, C. M. (2017). Prescription opioid use, misuse, and use disorders in US adults: 2015 national survey on drug use and health. *Annals of Internal Medicine*, 167(5), 293–301.

Han, B., Compton, W. M., Jones, C. M., Einstein, E. B., & Volkow, N. D. (2021). Methamphetamine use, methamphetamine use disorder, and associated overdose deaths among US. *JAMA Psychiatry*, 78(12), 1329. https://doi.org/10.1001/jamapsychiatry.2021.2588

Han, M., & Lee, E. (2018). Effectiveness of mobile health application use to improve health behavior changes: A systematic review of randomized controlled trials. *Healthcare Informatics Research*, 24(3), 207–226. http://dx.doi.org/10.1177/1833358319851684

Hanscom, B., Janes, H. E., Guarino, P. D., Huang, Y., Brown, E. R., Chen, Y. Q., ... Donnell, D. J. (2016). Preventing HIV-1 infection in women using oral pre-exposure prophylaxis: A meta-analysis of current evidence. *Journal of Acquired Immune Deficiency Syndromes*, 73(5), 606–608.

Harding, J. L., Andes, L. J., Gregg, E. W., Cheng, Y. J., Weir, H. K., Bullard, K. M., ... Imperatore, G. (2020). Trends in cancer mortality among people with vs without diabetes in the USA, 1988–2015. *Diabetologia*, 63(1), 75–84.

Harkness, K. L., Alavi, N., Monroe, S. M., Slavich, G. M., Gotlib, I. H., & Bagby, R. M. (2010). Gender differences in life events prior to onset of major depressive disorder: The moderating effect of age. *Journal of Abnormal Psychology*, 119, 791–803.

Harlow, B. L., Kunitz, C. G., Nguyen, R. H., Rydell, S. A., Turner, R. M., & MacLehose, R. F. (2014). Sexual pain prevalence of symptoms consistent with a diagnosis of vulvodynia: Population-based estimates from 2 geographic reasons. *American Journal of Obstetrics & Gynecology*, 210(1), 40.e1–40.e8.

Harlow, H. F. (1958). The nature of love. *American Psychologist*, 13(12), 673–685.

Harris, E. (2023a). Study: No more than 6 teaspoons of added sugar per day. *JAMA*, 329(18), 1543. https://doi.org/10.1001/jama.2023.6285

Harris, E. (2023b). Gun violence affects more than half of US adults. *JAMA*, 329(18), 1543. https://doi.org/10.1001/jama.2023.6289

Hart, R. J. (2016). Physiological aspects of female fertility: Role of the environment, modern lifestyle, and genetics. *Physiological Reviews*, 96, 873–909.

Hartung, C. M., & Lefler, E. K. (2019). Sex and gender in psychopathology: DSM–5 and beyond. *Psychological Bulletin*, 145, 390–409. https://doi.org/10.1037/bul0000183

Harvard Health, Harvard Medical School. (2017). Gender matters: Heart disease risk in women. https://www.health.harvard.edu/heart-health/gender-matters-heart-disease-risk-in-women

Harvard Health Letter. (2014). Eat more fiber-rich foods to foster heart health. Harvard Medical School. https://www.health.harvard.edu/heart-health/eat-more-fiber-rich-foods-to-foster-heart-health

Hashimie, J., Schultz, S. K., & Stewart, J. T. (2020). Palliative care for dementia: 2020 update. *Clinical Geriatric Medicine*, 36, 329–339.

Hasin, D. S., Sarvet, A. L., Meyers, J. L., Saha, T. D., Ruan, W. J., Stohl, M., ... Grant, B. F. (2018). Epidemiology of adult DSM-5 major depressive disorder and its specifiers in the United States. *JAMA Psychiatry*, 75, 336–346.

Hatcher, R. A., Nelson, A. L., Trussell, J., Cwiak, C., Cason, P., Policar, M. S., ... Aiken, A. R. A. (2018). *Contraceptive technology* (21st ed). *Managing Contraception LLC.*

Haught, H. M., Rose, J. P., & Brown, J. A. (2015). Social-class indicators differentially predict engagement in prevention vs. detection behaviours. *Psychology & Health*, 31(1), 21–39. https://doi.org/10.1080/08870446.2015.1068313

Haydon, K. C., & Salvatore, J. E. (2021). A prospective study of mental health, well-being, and substance use during the initial COVID-19 pandemic surge. *Clinical Psychological Science,* 10(1), 58–73. https://doi.org/10.1177/21677026211013499

Heap, M. (2019). Hypnosis. In C. D. Llewellyn, S. Ayers, C. McManus, S. Newman, K. J. Petrie, T. A. Revenson, & J. Weinman (Eds.), *Cambridge handbook of psychology, health and medicine* (3rd ed., pp. 278–283). Cambridge University Press.

Heath, A. C., Madden, P. A. F., Bucholz, K. K., Dinwiddie, S. H., Slutske, W. S., Bierut, L. J., ... Martin, N. G. (1999). Genetic differences in alcohol sensitivity and the inheritance of alcoholism risk. *Psychological Medicine*, 29(5), 1069–1081.

Hedegaard, H., Minino, A. M., & Warner, M. (2020). Drug overdose deaths in the United States, 1999–2018. NCHS Data Brief, No. 356. https://www.cdc.gov/nchs/data/databriefs/db356-h.pdf

Heeren, G. A., Jemmott III, J. B., Marange, C., Rumosa Gwaze, A., Batidzirai, J. M., Ngwane, Z., ... Tyler, J. C. (2018). Health-promotion intervention increases self-reported physical activity in sub-Saharan African university students: A randomized controlled pilot study. *Behavioral Medicine*, 44, 297–305.

Hegarty, R. S. M., Treharne, G. J., Stebbings, S., & Conner, T. S. (2016). Fatigue and mood among people with arthritis: Carry-over across the day. *Health Psychology*, 35, 492–499.

He, J., Zhu, Z., Bundy, J. D., Dorans, K. S., Chen, J., & Hamm, L. L. (2021). Trends in cardiovascular risk factors in US adults by race and ethnicity and socioeconomic status, 1999–2018. *JAMA*, 326(13), 1286. https://doi.org/10.1001/jama.2021.15187

Helakari, H., Korhonen, V., Holst, S. C., Piispala, J., Kallio, M., ... Väyrynen, T. (2022). Human NREM sleep promotes brain-wide vasomotor and respiratory pulsations. *The Journal of Neuroscience*. https://doi.org/10.1523/jneurosci.0934-21.2022

Helgeson, V. S., Naqvi, J. B., Van Vleet, M., & Zajdel, M. (2019). Diabetes. In T. E. Revenson & R. A. R. Gurung (Eds.), *Handbook of health psychology* (pp. 423–435). Routledge.

Helgeson, V. S., & Zajdel, M. (2017). Adjusting to chronic health conditions. *Annual Review of Psychology*, 68, 545–571.

Heminger, C. L., Boal, A. L., Zumer, M., & Abroms, L. C. (2016). Text2Quit: An analysis of participant engagement in the mobile smoking cessation program. *The American Journal of Drug and Alcohol Abuse*, 42, 450–458.

Hendershot, C. S., Witkiewitz, K., George, W. H., & Marlatt, G. A. (2011). Relapse prevention for addictive behaviors. *Substance Abuse Treatment, Prevention, and Policy*, 6(1), 17. https://doi.org/10.1186/1747-597X-6-17

Hennessy, E. A., Johnson, B. T., Acabchuk, R. L., McCloskey, K., & Stewart-James, J. (2019). Self-regulation mechanisms in health behaviour change: A systematic meta-review of meta-analyses, 2006–2017. *Health Psychology Review*, 14, 1–14.

Hennessy, M., Bleakley, A., & Ellithorpe, M. (2018). Prototypes reflect normative perceptions: Implications for the development of reasoned action theory. *Psychology, Health & Medicine*, 23(3), 245–258.

Henriksson, M., Wall, A., Nyberg, J., Adiels, M., Lundin, K., Bergh, Y., ... Åberg, M. (2022). Effects of exercise on symptoms of anxiety in primary care patients: A randomized controlled trial. *Journal of Affective Disorders*, 297, 26–34. https://doi.org/10.1016/j.jad.2021.10.006

Hensley, R. D. (2018). Primary care management of obesity: Individualized treatment strategies. *The Nurse Practitioner*, 43(7), 41–48.

Herbenick, D., Fu, T. C., Arter, J., Sanders, S. A., & Dodge, B. (2018). Women's experiences with genital touching, sexual pleasure, and orgasm: Results from a US probability sample of women ages 18 to 94. *Journal of Sex & Marital Therapy*, 44(2), 201–212.

Herek, G. M. (2016). A nuanced view of stigma for understanding and addressing sexual and gender minority health disparities. *LGBT Health*, 3(6). https://doi.org/10.1089/lgbt.2016.0154

Herman, A. O. (2019). 1 in 4 U.S. adults uses aspirin to prevent heart disease. https://www.jwatch.org/fw115634/2019/07/23/1-4-us-adults-uses-aspirin-prevent-heart-disease

Hernandez, R., Kershaw, K. N., Siddique, J., Boehm, J. K., Kubzansky, L. D., Diez-Roux, A., ... Lloyd-Jones, D. M. (2015). Optimism and cardiovascular health: Multi-ethnic study of atherosclerosis (MESA). *Health Behavior and Policy Review*, 2, 62–73.

Heron, M. (2019). *Deaths: Leading causes for 2017*. National Vital Statistics Reports, 68(6). Accessed November 19, 2019.

Heron, M. (2019). Deaths: Leading causes for 2017. *National Vital Statistics Reports*, 68(6). National Center for Health Statistics.

Hicks, A., Siwik, C., Phillips, K., Zimmaro, L. A., Salmon, P., Burke, N., ... Sephton, S. E. (2019). Dispositional mindfulness is associated with lower basal sympathetic arousal and less psychological stress. *International Journal of Stress Management*, 21(1), 88–92.

Hildebrandt, T., Alfano, L., Tricamo, M., & Pfaff, D. W. (2010). Conceptualizing the role of estrogens and serotonin in the development and maintenance of bulimia nervosa. *Clinical Psychology Review*, 30, 655–668.

Hill, E. B., Cubellis, L. T., Wexler, R. K., Taylor, C. A., & Spees, C. K. (2023). Differences in adherence to American Heart Association's life's Essential 8, diet quality, and weight loss strategies between those with and without recent clinically significant weight loss in a nationally representative sample of us adults. *Journal of the American Heart Association*, 12(8). https://doi.org/10.1161/jaha.122.026777

Hill, M. G., Sim, M., & Mills, B. (2020). The quality of diagnosis and triage advice provided by free online symptom checkers and apps in Australia. *Medical Journal of Australia*. https://doi.org/10.5694/mja2.50600

Hines, M., Constantinescu, M., & Spencer, D. (2015). Early androgen exposure and human gender development. *Biology of Sex Differences*, 6(3), https://doi.org/10.1186/s13293-015-0022-1

Hinman, R. S., McCrory, P., Pirotta, M., Relf, I., Forbes, A., Crossley, K. M., ... Bennell, K. L. (2014). Acupuncture for chronic knee pain: A randomized clinical trial. *Journal of the American Medical Association*, 312, 1313–1322.

Hirschey, R., Bryant, A. L., Macek, C., Battaglini, C., Santacroce, S., Courneya, K. S., ... Sheeran, P. (2020). Predicting physical activity among cancer survivors: Meta-analytic path modeling of longitudinal studies. *Health Psychology*, 39, 269–280.

Hjalmarsson, E., Fernandez-Gonzalo, R., Lidbeck, C., Palmcrantz, A., Jia, A., Kvist, O., ... von Walden, F. (2020). RaceRunning training improves stamina and promotes skeletal muscle hypertrophy in young individuals with cerebral palsy. *BMC Musculoskeletal Disorders*, 21, 1–9.

Hochbaum, G. M. (1958). Public participation in medical screening programs: A socio-psychological study. US Department of Health, Education, and Welfare, Public Health Service, Bureau of State Services, Division of Special Health Services, Tuberculosis Program.

Hodson, R. (2023a). Smoking: An avoidable health disaster explained. *Nature*, 618(7964), S2–S3. https://doi.org/10.1038/d41586-023-01837-w

Ho, E. K., Chen, L., Simic, M., Ashton-James, C. E., Comachio, J., Hayden, D., ... Ferreira, P. H. (2022). Psychological interventions for chronic, non-specific low back pain: Systematic review with network meta-analysis. *The British Medical Journal*, 376, e067718–e067718.

Hogarth, L., Hardy, L., Mathew, A. R., & Hitsman, B. (2018). Negative mood-induced alcohol-seeking is greater in young adults who report depression symptoms, drinking to cope, and subjective reactivity. *Experimental and Clinical Psychopharmacology*, 26(2), 138–146.

Hojjatinia, S., Hojjatinia, S., Lagoa, C. M., Brunke-Reese, D., & Conroy, D. E. (2021). Person-specific dose-finding for a digital messaging intervention to promote physical activity. *Health Psychology*, 40(8), 502–512. https://doi.org/10.1037/hea0001117

Holingue, C. (2018). Mental disorders around the world: Facts and figures from the WHO World Mental Health Surveys. *American Journal of Psychiatry*. https://doi.org/10.1176/appi.ajp.2018.18050506

Hollander, J. E., & Carr, B. G. (2020). Virtually perfect? Telemedicine for Covid-19. *New England Journal of Medicine*. https://doi.org/10.1056/NEJMp2003539

Holland, F., Archer, S., & Montague, J. (2016). Younger women's experiences of deciding against delayed breast reconstruction post-mastectomy following breast cancer: An interpretative phenomenological analysis. *Journal of Health Psychology*, 21(8), 1688–1699.

Holman, R. J. (2016). Potentially preventable deaths in the United States. Society of Actuaries. https://www.soa.org/research-reports/2016/potentially-preventable-deaths/

Holt-Lunstad, J. (2018). Why social relationships are important for physical health: A systems approach to understanding and modifying risk and protection. *Annual Review of Psychology*, 69, 437–458.

Honer, W. G. (2021) Better evidence for pharmacological maintenance treatment in nonaffective psychoses: Implications for relapse prevention. *American Journal of Psychiatry.* https://ajp-psychiatryonline-org.jerome.stjohns.edu/doi/10.1176/appi.ajp.2021.21030281

Hood, S. R., Giazzon, A. J., Seamon, G., Lane, K. A., Wang, J., Eckert, G. J., ... Murray, M. D. (2018). Association between medication adherence and the outcomes of heart failure. *Pharmacotherapy: The Journal of Human Pharmacology and Drug Therapy*, 38(5), 539–545.

Hope, H. F., Binkley, G. M., Fenton, S., Kitas, G. D., Verstappen, S. M. M., & Symmons, D. P. M. (2019). Systematic review of the predictors of statin adherence for the primary prevention of cardiovascular disease. *PLoS One*, 14(1). https://doi.org/10.1371/journal.pone.0201196.

Hoppe, E. J., Hussain, L. R., Grannan, K. J., Dunki-Jacobs, E. M., Lee, D. Y., & Wexelman, B. A. (2019). Racial disparities in breast cancer persist despite early detection: Analysis of treatment of stage 1 breast cancer and effect of insurance status on disparities. *Breast Cancer Research and Treatment*, 173(3), 597–602.

Horne, R., Chan, A., & Wileman, V. (2019). Adherence to treatment. In T. E. Revenson & R. A. R. Gurung (Eds.), *Handbook of health psychology* (pp. 148–161). Routledge.

Hou, J., Yu, L., Fang, X., & Epstein, N. B. (2016). The intergenerational transmission of domestic violence: The role that gender plays in attribution and consequent intimate partner violence. *Journal of Family Studies*, 22(2), 121–139.

Hourani, L. L., Davila, M. I., Morgan, J., Meleth, S., Ramirez, D., Lewis, G., ... Lane, M. (2020). Mental health, stress, and resilience correlates of heart rate variability among military reservists, guardsmen, and first responders. *Physiology & Behavior*, 214. https://doi.org/10.1016/j.physbeh.2019.112734

Hoyer, J., Hoefler, M., & Wuellhorst, V. (2020). Activity and subsequent depression levels: A causal analysis of behavioural activation group treatment with weekly assessments over 8 weeks. *Clinical Psychology & Psychotherapy*. https://doi.org/10.1002/cpp.2430

Hruschaka, V., & Cochran, G. (2018). Psychosocial predictors in the transition from acute to chronic pain: A systematic review. *Psychology, Health & Medicine*, 23, 1151–1167.

Hsu, T., & Raposa, E. B. (2021). Effects of stress on eating behaviours in adolescents: A daily diary investigation. *Psychology & Health*, 36(2), 236–251. https://doi.org/10.1080/08870446.2020.1766041

Huang, B.-H., del Pozo Cruz, B., Teixeira-Pinto, A., Cistulli, P. A., & Stamatakis, E. (2023). Influence of poor sleep on cardiovascular disease-free life expectancy: A multi-resource-based population cohort study. *BMC Medicine*, 21(1). https://doi.org/10.1186/s12916-023-02732-x

Huang, C., Fan, Y., & Hu, S. (2023). The prevalence and influencing factors of postpartum depression between primiparous and secundiparous. *Journal of Nervous & Mental Disease,* 211(3), 190–194. https://doi.org/10.1097/nmd.0000000000001591

Huang, L., Fu, M. X., & Liu, H. R. (2020). Emotional responses and coping strategies of nurses and nursing college students during COVID-19 outbreak. *medRxiv*. https://doi.org/10.1101/2020.03.05.20031898

Huang, S., Li, J., Shearer, G. C., Li, J., Shearer, G. C., Lichtenstein, A. H., Zheng, X., ... Gao, X. (2017). Longitudinal study of alcohol consumption and HDL concentrations: A community-based study. *American Journal of Clinical Nutrition*, 105, 905–912.

Hudson, D. L., Neighbors, H. W., Geronimus, A. T., & Jackson, J. S. (2018). Racial discrimination, John Henryism, and depression among African Americans. *Journal of Black Psychology*, 42(3), 221–243. https://doi.org/10.1177/0095798414567757

Hudson, J. L. (2017). Prevention of anxiety disorders across the lifespan. *JAMA Psychiatry*, 74, 1029–1030.

Hu, E. A., Lazo, M., Rosenberg, S. D., Grams, M. E., Steffen, L. M., Coresh, J., & Rebholz, C. M. (2020). Alcohol consumption and incident kidney disease: Results from the atherosclerosis risk in communities study. *Journal of Renal Nutrition*, 30(1), 22–30.

Huebner, D. M., McGarrity, L. A., Perry, N. S., Spivey, L. A., & Smith, T. W. (2021). Cardiovascular and cortisol responses to experimentally-induced minority stress. *Health Psychology*, 40(5), 316–325. https://doi.org/10.1037/hea0001067

Huecker, M. R., King, K. C., Jordan, G. A., & Smock, W. (2023). Domestic violence. *StatPearls.* https://www.ncbi.nlm.nih.gov/books/NBK499891/)

Hughto, J. W., Reisner, S., Cahill, S., Santostefano, C., McMahon, J., Pletta, D., & Mimiaga, M. (2019, November). Understanding facilitators and barriers to PrEP use among PrEP naïve and PrEP experienced transgender adults. In APHA's 2019 Annual Meeting and Expo (November 2–6). American Public Health Association.

Hulko, W. (2018). Being queer in the small city. Power and possibility in the small city. In C. Walmsley & T. Kading (Eds.), *Small cities big issues* (pp. 105–124). AU Press.

Human Papillomavirus. (2019). https://www.cdc.gov/vaccines/pubs/pinkbook/hpv.html

Human Rights Campaign. (2018). A national epidemic: Fatal anti-transgender violence in America in 2018.

Hungr, C., & Bober, S. (2020). Sexual health and body image after breast cancer. In O. Gentilini, A. H. Partridge, & O. Pagani (Eds.), *Breast cancer in young women* (pp. 155–166). Springer.

Hunleth, J. M., Steinmetz, E. K., McQueen, A., & James, A. S. (2016). Beyond adherence: Health care disparities and the struggle to get screened for colon cancer. *Qualitative Health Research*, 26(1), 17–31.

Hunter, C. L., Funderburk, J. S., Polaha, J., Bauman, D., Goodie, J. L., & Hunter, C. M. (2017). Primary Care Behavioral Health model (PCBH) research: Current state of the science and a call to action. *Journal of Clinical Psychology in Medical Settings*, 25, 127–156.

Huppin, M., & Malamuth, N. M. (2017). Aggression for sexual access. In T. K. Shakelford & V. A. Weekes-Shakelford (Eds.), *Encyclopedia of evolutionary psychological science*. Springer International Publishing. https://doi.org/10.1007/978-3-319-16999-6_1681-1

Hyde, J. S., & Mezulis, A. H. (2020). Gender differences in depression: Biological, affective, cognitive, and sociocultural factors. *Harvard Review of Psychiatry*, 28(1), 4–13.

Hystad, S. W., Eid, J., & Brevik, J. I. (2011). Effects of psychological hardiness, job demands, and job control on sickness absence: A prospective study. *Journal of Occupational Health Psychology*, 16(3), 265–278.

IARC Working Group on the Evaluation of Carcinogenic Risk to Humans. (2004). Tobacco smoke and involuntary smoking. International Agency for Research on Cancer. IARC Monographs on the Evaluation of Carcinogenic Risks to Humans, No. 83.

Iglesias, A. H. (2020). Transcranial magnetic stimulation as treatment in multiple neurologic conditions. *Current Neurology and Neuroscience Reports*, 20, 1. https://doi.org/10.1007/s11910-020-1021-0

Imeri, H., Toth, J., Arnold, A., & Barnard, M. (2022). Use of the transtheoretical model in medication adherence: A systematic review. *Research in Social and Administrative Pharmacy,* 18(5), 2778–2785. doi: 10.1016/j.sapharm.2021.07.008.

Institute of Medicine (IOM). (2015). Cognitive aging: Progress in understanding and opportunities for action. Report Brief. http://www/"http://www. iom.edu/~/media/Files/Report%20Files/2015/Cognitive_aging/Cognitive%20Aging%20report%20brief.pdf

Islami, F., Goding, S. A., Miller, K. D., Siegel, R. L., Fedewa, S. A., Jacobs, E. J., ... Jemal, A. (2018). Proportion and number of cancer cases and deaths attributable to potentially modifiable risk factors in the United States. *CA: A Cancer Journal for Clinicians*, 68, 31–54.

Islami, F., Guerra, C. E., Minihan, A., Yabroff, K. R., et al. (2022). American Cancer Society's report on the status of cancer disparities in the United States, 2021. *CA: A Cancer Journal for Clinicians,* 72(2), 112–143. https://doi.org/10.3322/caac.21703

Ismail, L. M. N., Selim, M. A.-A., & El-Khashab, S. O. (2017). Factors affecting medication adherence among patients with rheumatic disorders. *Journal of Nursing Education and Practice*, 7(8). https://doi.org/10.5430/jnep.v7n8p7

Israel, S., Moffitt, T. E., Belsky, D. W., Hancox, R. J., Poulton, R., Roberts, B., ... Caspi, A. (2014). Translating personality psychology to help personalize preventive medicine for young adult patients. *Journal of Personality and Social Psychology*, 106, 484–498.

Itriyeva, K. (2022). Premenstrual syndrome and premenstrual dysphoric disorder in adolescents. *Current Problems in Pediatric and Adolescent Health Care,* 52(5). https://doi.org/10.1016/j.cppeds.2022.101187

Jackson, S. D., Harvey, T. D., Watson, R. J., Pereira, K., & Clark, K. A. (2023). Multilevel stigma and depression among a national sample of Black and Latinx LGBTQ+ adolescents in the United States. *Journal of Psychopathology and Clinical Science,* 132(5), 577–589. https://doi.org/10.1037/abn0000841

Jacob, R. G., Hugo, J. A., & Dunbar-Jacob, J. (2015). History of psychosomatic medicine and consultation-liaison psychiatry. https://doi.org/10.1093/med/9780199329311.003.0001

Jacobs, S. (1993). *Pathologic grief: Maladaptation to loss.* American Psychiatric Press.

Jafar, T. H., Gandhi, M., de Silva, H. A., Jehan, I., Naheed, A., Finkelstein, E. A., ... Shah Ebrahim, D. M., for the COBRA-BPS Study Group. (2020). A community-based intervention for managing hypertension in rural South Asia. *New England Journal of Medicine*, 382, 717–726.

Jain, A., & Davis, A. M. (2019). Primary prevention of cardiovascular disease. *Journal of the American Medical Association*, 322, 1817–1818.

Jain, A., & Yilanli, M. (2023, July 31). Bulimia nervosa. StatPearls–NCBI Bookshelf. https://www.ncbi.nlm.nih.gov/books/NBK562178/

Jakicic, J. M., Davis, K. K., Rogers, R. J., King, W. C., Marcus, M. D., Helsel, D., ... Belle, S. H. (2016). Effect of wearable technology combined with a lifestyle intervention on long-term weight loss: The IDEA Randomized Clinical Trial. *Journal of the American Medical Association*, 316, 1161–1171.

Jakubiak, B. K., & Feeney, B. C. (2017). Affectionate touch to promote relational, psychological, and physical well-being in adulthood: A theoretical model and review of the research. *Personality and Social Psychology Review*, 21(3), 228–252.

Jalan, S., Vishnu, P. V., & Gayathri, R. (2022). Awareness on effects of sleep deprivation among college students - A questionnaire based survey. *Journal for Educators, Teachers and Trainers,* 13(6), 11–19. https://doi.org/10.47750/jett.2022.13.06.002

James, P. A., Oparil, S., Carter, B. L., Cushman, W. C., Dennison-Himmelfarb, C., Handler, J., ... Ortiz, E. (2014). 2014 evidence-based guideline for the management of high blood pressure in adults: Report from the panel members appointed to the Eighth Joint National Committee (JNC 8). *Journal of the American Medical Association*, 311, 507–520.

Jansen, F., Verdonck-de Leeuw, I. M., Cuijpers, P., Leemans, C. R., Waterboer, T., Pawlita, M., ... Ness, A. R., (2018). Depressive symptoms in relation to overall survival in people with head and neck cancer: A longitudinal cohort study. *Psychooncology,* 27, 2245–2256. https://doi.org/10.1002/pon.4816.

Jao, N. C., Robinson, L. D., Kelly, P. J., Ciecierski, C. C., & Hitsman, B. (2018). Unhealthy behavior clustering and mental health status in United States college students. *Journal of American College Health*, 67(8), 790–800.

Jarab, A. S., Alefishat, E. A., Bani Nasur, R., & Mukattash, T. L. (2018). Investigation of variables associated with medication nonadherence in patients with hypertension. *Journal of Pharmaceutical Health Services Research*, 9(4), 341–346.

Jardas, E. J., Ladd, B. A., Maheux, A. J., Choukas-Bradley, S., Salk, R. H., & Thoma, B. C. (2023). Testing the minority stress model across gender identity, race, and ethnicity among U.S. gender minority adolescents. *Journal of Psychopathology and Clinical Science,* 132(5), 542–554. https://doi.org/10.1037/abn0000834

Jarman, A. F., MacLean, J. V., Barron, R. J., Wightman, R. S., & McGregor, A. J. (2020). Brexanolone for postpartum depression: A novel approach and a call for comprehensive postpartum care. *Clinical Therapeutics.* https://doi.org/10.1016/j.clinthera.2019.11.005

Jayasekara, H., MacInnis, R. J., Room, R., & English, D. R. (2016). Long-term alcohol consumption and breast, upper Aero-digestive tract and colorectal cancer risk: A systematic review and meta-analysis. *Alcohol and Alcoholism (Oxford, Oxfordshire)*, 51(3), 315–330. https://doi.org/10.1093/alcalc/agv110

Jensen, M. P. (2018). Enhancing motivation to change in pain treatment. In D. C. Turk & R. J. Gatchel (Eds.), *Psychological approaches to pain management: A practitioner's handbook* (3rd ed., pp. 71–95). New York: The Guilford Press.

Jensen, T. S. (2008). Pathophysiology of pain: from theory to clinical evidence. *European Journal of Pain Supplements*, 2(S1), 13–17. https://doi.org/10.1016/s1754-3207(08)70058-0

Jewett, A., Beck, L. F., Taylor, C., & Baldwin, G. (2016). Bicycle helmet use among persons 5 years and older in the United States, 2012. *Journal of Safety Research,* 59, 1–7. https://doi.org/10.1016/j.jsr.2016.09.001

Jha, P., Ramasundarahettige, C., Landsman, V., Rostron, B., Thun, M., Anderson, R. N., ... Peto, R. (2013). 21st-century hazards of smoking and benefits of cessation in the United States. *New England Journal of Medicine*, 368(4), 341–350.

Jiang, C., Cifu, A. S., & Sam, S. (2022). Obesity and weight management for prevention and treatment of Type 2 diabetes. *JAMA,* 328(4), 389. https://doi.org/10.1001/jama.2022.10338

Jin, J. (2022). Screening for eating disorders in adolescents and adults. *JAMA,* 327(11), 1100. https://doi.org/10.1001/jama.2022.2428

Johns Hopkins Medicine. (2018). Nutrition. *Health Library.* https://www.hopkinsmedicine.org/healthlibrary/conditions/adult/pediatrics/malnutrition_22

Johns, M. M., Lowry, R., Andrzejewski, J., Barrios, L. C., Demissie, Z., McManus, T., ... Underwood, J. M. (2019). Transgender identity and experiences of violence victimization, substance use, suicide risk, and sexual risk behaviors among high school students—19 states and large urban school districts, 2017. *Morbidity and Mortality Weekly Report*, 68(3), 67–71.

Johnson, C. O., Boon-Dooley, A. S., DeCleene, N. K., Henny, K. F., Blacker, B. F., Anderson, J. A., ... Roth, G. A. (2022). Life expectancy for White, Black, and Hispanic race/ethnicity in US states: Trends and disparities, 1990 to 2019. *Annals of Internal Medicine,* 175(8), 1057–1064.

Johnson, L. E., Robins, R. W., Guyer, A. E., & Hastings, P. D. (2023). Ethnic pride and cultural values promote positive youth development in a conceptual replication of the Five Cs model. *Developmental Psychology,* 59(9), 1543–1558. https://doi.org/10.1037/dev0001570

Johnston, J., Shu, C. Y., Hoiles, K. J., Clarke, P. J., Watson, H. J., Dunlop, P. D., & Egan, S. J. (2018). Perfectionism is associated with higher eating disorder symptoms and lower remission in children and adolescents diagnosed with eating disorders. *Eating Behaviors*, 30, 55–60.

Johnston, L. D., Miech, R. A., O'Malley, P. M., Bachman, J. G., Schulenberg, J. E., & Patrick, M. E. (2018). *Monitoring the Future national survey results on drug use: 1975–2017: Overview, key findings on adolescent drug use.* Institute for Social Research, The University of Michigan.

Jokela, M., Batty, G. D., Nyberg, S. T., Virtanen, M., Nabi, H., Singh-Manoux, A., ... Kivimäki, M. (2013). Personality and all-cause mortality: Individual-participant meta-analysis of 3,947 deaths in 76,150 adults. *American Journal of Epidemiology*, 178, 667–675.

Jo, M., Na, H., & Jung, Y. E. (2020). Mediation effects of compassion satisfaction and compassion fatigue in the relationships between resilience and anxiety or depression among hospice volunteers. *Journal of Hospice & Palliative Nursing*, 22(3), 246–253.

Jones, A. P., & Erdmann, M. (2012). Projection and patient satisfaction using the "Hamburger" nipple reconstruction technique. *Journal of Plastic, Reconstructive & Aesthetic Surgery*, 65(2), 207–212.

Jones, D. W., Chambless, L. E., Folsom, A. R., Heiss, G., Hutchinson, R. G., Sharrett, A. R., ... Taylor, H. A., Jr. (2002). Risk factors for coronary heart disease in African Americans: The Atherosclerosis Risk in Communities Study, 1987–1997. *Archives of Internal Medicine*, 162, 2565–2571.

Jones, E., & Rayner, B. (2020). The importance of the epithelial sodium channel in determining salt sensitivity in people of African origin. *Pediatric Nephrology*, 1–7. https://doi.org/10.1007/s00467-019-04427-z

Joshi, P. K., Pirastu, N., Kentistou, K. A., Fischer, K., Hofer, E., Schraut, K. E., ... Wilson, J. F. (2017). Genome-wide meta-analysis associates HLA-DQA1/DRB1 and LPA and lifestyle factors with human longevity. *Nature Communications*, 8(1). https://doi.org/10.1038/s41467-017-00934-5

Joyner, M. J., & Paneth, N. (2019). Cardiovascular disease prevention at a crossroads: Precision medicine or polypill? *Journal of the American Medical Association*, 322, 2281–2282.

Judd, L. L., Schettler, P. J., & Rush, A. J. (2016). A brief clinical tool to estimate individual patients' risk of depressive relapse following remission: Proof of concept. *American Journal of Psychiatry*, 173, 1140–1146.

Jungmann, S. M., Brand, S., Kolb, J., & Witthöft, M. (2020). Do Dr. Google and health apps have (comparable) side effects? An experimental study. *Clinical Psychological Science*, 8, 306–317.

Kahn, R. S. (2020). On the origins of schizophrenia. *American Journal of Psychiatry,* 177(4), 291–297. https://doi.org/10.1176/appi.ajp.2020.20020147

Kaiser Family Foundation. (2018). Employer health benefits 2018 annual survey. http://files.kff.org/attachment/Report-Employer-Health-Benefits-Annual-Survey-2018.

Kaiser Family Foundation (KFF). (2022). Five key findings on mental health and substance use disorders by race/ethnicity. https://www.kff.org/racial-equity-and-health-policy/issue-brief/five-key-findings-on-mental-health-and-substance-use-disorders-by-race-ethnicity/#:~:text=Just%20over%20a%20quarter%20of,nonelderly%20adults%20(Figure%204)

Kalin, N. H. (2020). Substance use disorders and addiction: Mechanisms, trends, and treatment implications. *The American Journal of Psychiatry,* 177(11), 1015–1018. https://doi.org/10.1176/appi.ajp.2020.20091382

Kalin, N. H. (2022). Neuroscientific advances supporting new treatments for major depression. *American Journal of Psychiatry,* 179(7), 441–444. https://doi.org/10.1176/appi.ajp.20220445

Kam-Hansen, S., Jakubowski, M., Kelley, J. M., Kirsch, I., Hoaglin, D. C., Kaptchuk, T. J., ... Burstein, R. (2014). Altered placebo and drug labeling changes the outcome of episodic migraine attacks. *Science Translational Medicine*, 8, 218ra5.

Kanapathy, J., & Bogle, V. (2019). The effectiveness of cognitive behavioural therapy for depressed patients with diabetes: A systematic review. *Journal of Health Psychology*, 1, 137–149.

Kandola, A., Ashdown-Franks, G., Hendrikse, J., Sabiston, C. M., & Stubbs, B. (2019). Physical activity and depression: Towards understanding the antidepressant mechanisms of physical activity. *Neuroscience & Biobehavioral Reviews*, 107, 525–539.

Kanny, D., Naimi, T. S., Liu, Y., & Brewer, R. D. (2020). Trends in total binge drinks per adult who reported binge drinking—United States, 2011–2017. *Morbidity and Mortality Weekly Report*, 69(2), 30–34. https://doi.org/10.15585/mmwr.mm6902a2

Kanny, D., Naimi, T. S., Liu, Y., Lu, H., & Brewer, R. D. (2018). Annual total binge drinks consumed by US adults, 2015. *American Journal of Preventive Medicine*, 54(4), 486–496. https://doi.org/10.1016/j.amepre.2017.12.021

Kaplan, S., & Hoffman, J. (2018, September 12). F.D.A. cracks down on Juul and e-cigarette retailers. *New York Times*. https://www.nytimes.com/2018/09/12/health/juul-fda-vaping-ecigarettes.html?action=click&module=Top%20Stories&pgtype=Homepage

Karasek, R., Baker, D., Marxer, F., Ahlbom, A., & Theorell, T. (1981). Job decision latitude, job demands, and cardiovascular disease: A prospective study of Swedish men. *American Journal of Public Health*, 71, 694–705.

Karlsson Linnér, Richard, Mallard, T. T., Barr, P. B., Sanchez-Roige, S., Madole, J. W., Driver, M. N., ... Vrieze, S. (2021). Multivariate analysis of 1.5 million people identifies genetic associations with traits related to self-regulation and addiction. *Nature Neuroscience*, 24(10), 1–10. https://doi.org/10.1038/s41593-021-00908-3

Kasardo, A. E., & McHugh, M. C. (2015). From fat shaming to size acceptance: Challenging the medical management of fat women. In M. C. McHugh & J. C. Chrisler (Eds.), *The wrong prescription for women: How medicine and media create a "need" for treatments, drugs, and surgery* (pp. 179–201). ABC-Clio, LLC.

Kaster, T. S., Downar, J., Vila-Rodriguez, F., Thorpe, K. E., Feffer, K., Noda, Y., ... Blumberger, D. M. (2019). Trajectories of response to dorsolateral prefrontal rTMS in major depression: A THREE-D study. *American Journal of Psychiatry*, 176(5), 367–375. https://doi.org/10.1176/appi.ajp.2018.18091096

Katzmarzyk, P. T., Powell, K. E., Jakicic, J. M., Troiano, R. P., Piercy, K., Tennant, B., & 2018 Physical Activity Guidelines Advisory Committee. (2019). Sedentary behavior and health: Update from the 2018 physical activity guidelines advisory committee. *Medicine and Science in Sports and Exercise*, 51(6), 1227–1241. https://doi.org/10.1249/MSS.0000000000001935

Kazi, D. S., Katz, I. T., & Jha, A. K. (2019). Preparing to end the HIV epidemic—California's route as a road map for the United States. *The New England Journal of Medicine*. https://doi.org/10.1056/NEJMp1912293

Kearney, D. J., & Simpson, T. L. (2020). *Mindfulness-based interventions for trauma and its consequences.* American Psychological Association.

Keeley, M. P., & Generous, M. A. (2014). Advice from children and adolescents on final conversations with dying loved ones. *Death Studies*, 38(5), 308–314. https://doi.org/10.1080/07481187.2012.753556

Keenan, G. S., Childs, L., Rogers, P. J., Hetherington, M. M., & Brunstrom, J. M. (2018). The portion size effect: Women demonstrate an awareness of eating more than intended when served larger than normal portions. *Appetite*, 126, 54–60.

Keepers, G. A., Fochtmann, L. J., Anzia, J. M., Benjamin, S., Lyness, J. M., Mojtabai, R., ... Hong, S.-H. (2020). The American Psychiatric Association Practice Guideline for the treatment of patients with schizophrenia. *American Journal of Psychiatry*, 177(9), 868–872. https://doi.org/10.1176/appi.ajp.2020.177901

Keer, R., Ullrich, S., Destavola, B. L., & Coid, J. W. (2013). Association of violence with emergence of persecutory delusions in untreated schizophrenia. *American Journal of Psychiatry*, 171, 332–339. doi:10.1176/appi.ajp.2013.13010134.2013

Keller, K. L., English, L. K., Fearnbach, S. N., Lasschuijt, M., Anderson, K., Bermudez, M., ... Wilson, S. J. (2018). Brain response to food cues varying in portion size is associated with individual differences in the portion size effect in children. *Appetite*, 125, 139–151.

Kelly, R. K., Tong, T. Y. N., Watling, C. Z., Reynolds, A., Piernas, C., Schmidt, J. A., ... Perez-Cornago, A. (2023). Associations between types and sources of dietary carbohydrates and cardiovascular disease risk: A prospective cohort study of UK Biobank participants. *BMC Medicine*, 21(1). https://doi.org/10.1186/s12916-022-02712-7

Kemnic, T. R., & Gulick, P. G. (2022). *HIV antiretroviral therapy*. StatPearls Publishing. https://www.ncbi.nlm.nih.gov/books/NBK513308/

Kendler, K. S., & Gardner, C. O. (2010). Dependent stressful life events and prior depressive episodes in the prediction of major depression: The problem of causal inference in psychiatric epidemiology. *Archives of General Psychiatry*, 67, 1120–1127.

Kendler, K. S., Ohlsson, H., Sundquist, J., & Sundquist, K. (2020). An extended Swedish national adoption study of bipolar disorder illness and cross-generational familial association with schizophrenia and major depression. *JAMA Psychiatry*, 77(8), 814. https://doi.org/10.1001/jamapsychiatry.2020.0223

Kendler, K. S., Ohlsson, H., Sundquist, J., & Sundquist, K. (2023). Relationship of family genetic risk score with diagnostic trajectory in a Swedish national sample of incident cases of major depression, bipolar disorder, other nonaffective psychosis, and schizophrenia. *JAMA Psychiatry*, 80(3), 241. https://doi.org/10.1001/jamapsychiatry.2022.4676

Kennedy, J., Roll, J. M., Schraudner, T., Murphy, S., & McPherson, S. (2014). Prevalence of persistent pain in the U.S. adult population. *Journal of Pain*, 10, 979–984.

Kent, P., Haines, T., O'Sullivan, P., Smith, A., Campbell, A., Schutze, R., ... Hancock, M. (2023). Cognitive functional therapy with or without movement sensor biofeedback versus usual care for chronic, disabling low back pain (RESTORE): A randomised, controlled, three-arm, parallel group, phase 3, clinical trial. *The Lancet*, 401(10391), 1866–1877. https://doi.org/10.1016/s0140-6736(23)00441-5

Kerns, J., Itriyeva, K., & Fisher, M. (2022). Etiology and management of amenorrhea in adolescent and young adult women. *Current Problems in Pediatric and Adolescent Health Care*. https://doi.org/10.1016/j.cppeds.2022.101184

Kessler, R. C., Berglund, P. A., Demler, O., Jin, R., & Walters, E. E. (2005). Lifetime prevalence and age-of-onset distributions of DSM-IV disorders in the National Comorbidity Survey Replication (NCS-R). *Archives of General Psychiatry*, 62, 593–602.

Keum, S., & Shin, H. S. (2019). Genetic factors associated with empathy in humans and mice. *Neuropharmacology*, 159. https://doi.org/10.1016/j.neuropharm.2019.01.029

Key, T. J., Bradbury, K. E., Perez-Cornago, A., Sinha, R., Tsilidis, K. K., . . .Tsugane, S. (2020). Diet, nutrition, and cancer risk: What do we know and what is the way forward? *British Medical JournalJ*, m511. https://doi.org/10.1136/bmj.m511

Khan, S. U., Lone, A. N., Yedlapati, S. H., Dani, S. S., Khan, M. Z., Watson, K. E., ... Michos, E. D. (2022). Cardiovascular disease mortality among Hispanic versus non-Hispanic white adults in the United States, 1999 to 2018. *Journal of the American Heart Association*, 11(7), e022857.

Khera, A. V., Emdin, C. A., Drake, I., Connor, A., Natarajan, P., Bick, A. G., ... Boerwinkle, E. (2016). Genetic risk, adherence to a healthy lifestyle, and coronary disease. *New England Journal of Medicine*, 375, 2349–2358.

Kidd, D. G., & Singer, J. (2019). Consumer acceptance of enhanced seat belt reminders, a gearshift interlock, or different speed-limiting interlocks to encourage seat belt use following a brief hands-on experience. *Safety Science*, 120(1), 617–624. https://doi.org/10.1016/j.ssci.2019.07.039

Kiecolt-Glaser, J. K., Renna, M. E., Shrout, M. R., & Madison, A. A. (2020). Stress reactivity: What pushes us higher, faster, and longer—and why it matters. *Current Directions in Psychological Science*, 29(5), 492–498. https://doi.org/10.1177/0963721420949521

Kiecolt-Glaser, J. K., Speicher, C. E., Holliday, J. E., & Glaser, R. (1984). Stress and the transformation of lymphocytes by Epstein-Barr virus. *Journal of Behavioral Medicine*, 7(1), 1–12.

Kim, S. C., Namkoong, K., Fung, T., Heo, K., & Gunther, A. (2018). Understanding public opinion change of HPV vaccination controversy: Effects of exemplification and the mediating role of projection. *Health Education*, 118(5), 402–412.

King, D., Vlaev, I., Everett-Thomas, R., Fitzpatrick, M., Darzi, A., & Birnbach, D. J. (2016). "Priming" hand hygiene compliance in clinical environments. *Health Psychology*, 35, 96–101.

King, K., Meader, N., Wright, K., Graham, H., Power, C., Petticrew, M. ... Sowden, A. J. (2015). Characteristics of interventions targeting multiple lifestyle risk behaviours in adult populations: A systematic scoping review. *PLoS One*, 10(1). https://doi.org/10.1371/journal.pone.0117015

King, M., Semlyen, J., Tai, S. S., Killaspy, H., Osborn, D., Popelyuk,D.,...Nazareth,I.(2008).Asystematicreviewofmentaldisorder, suicide, and deliberate self harm in lesbian, gay and bisexual people. *BMC Psychiatry*, 8(1). https://doi.org/10.1186/1471-244x-8-70

Kinzel, J. (2018, August 22). Fat shaming is not an individual problem, it's a cultural one. http://www.lesleykinzel.com/fat-shaming-is-not-an-individual-problem-its-a-cultural-one/

Kirsten, H., Seib-Pfeifer, L. E., & Gibbons, H. (2022). Helpless against food cues: The influence of pro- and anti-sugar videos on instrumental food-seeking behaviour in a Pavlovian-to-instrumental transfer paradigm. *Psychology & Health*, 37(5), 633–657. https://doi-org.jerome.stjohns.edu/10.1080/08870446.2021.1907388

Kiviniemi, M. T., Klasko-Foster, L. B., Erwin, D. O., & Jandorf, L. (2018). Decision-making and socioeconomic disparities in colonoscopy screening in African Americans. *Health Psychology*, 37(5), 481–490. https://doi.org/10.1037/hea0000603

Klein, W. M. P., Jacobsen, P. B., & Helzlsouer, K. J. (2020). Alcohol and cancer risk: Clinical and research implications. *Journal of the American Medical Association*, 323, 23–24.

Kleitman, S., Fullerton, D. J., Zhang, L. M., Blanchard, M. D., Lee, J., Stankov, L., ... Thompson, V. (2021). To comply or not comply? A latent profile analysis of behaviours and attitudes during the COVID-19 pandemic. *PLoS One*, 16(7), e0255268. https://doi.org/10.1371/journal.pone.0255268

Klenofsky, B., Pace, A., Natbony, L. R., & Sheikh, H. U. (2019). Episodic migraine comorbidities: Avoiding pitfalls and taking therapeutic opportunities. *Current Pain and Headache Reports*, 23(1). https://doi.org/10.1007/s11916-019-0742-8

Klopack, E. T., Crimmins, E. M., Cole, S. W., Seeman, T. E., & Carroll, J. E. (2022). Social stressors associated with age-related T lymphocyte percentages in older US adults: Evidence from the US Health and Retirement Study. *Proceedings of the National Academy of Sciences*, 119(25). https://doi.org/10.1073/pnas.2202780119

Knowles, L. M., Ruiz, J. M. F., & O'Connor, F. (2019). A systematic review of the association between bereavement and biomarkers of immune function. *Psychosomatic Medicine*, 81, 415–433.

Koban, L., Kross, E., Woo, C.-W., Ruzic, L., & Wager, T. D. (2017). Frontal-brainstem pathways mediating placebo effects on social rejection. *The Journal of Neuroscience*, 37, 3621. https://doi.org/10.1523/JNEUROSCI.2658-16.2017

Kobasa, S. C. O., Maddi, S. R., Puccetti, M. C., & Zola, M. A. (1994). Effectiveness of hardiness, exercise, and social support as resources against illness. In A. Steptoe & J. Wardle (Eds.), *Psychosocial processes and health* (pp. 247–260). Cambridge University Press.

Koçan, S., & Gürsoy, A. (2016). Body image of women with breast cancer after mastectomy: A qualitative research. *The Journal of Breast Health*, 12(4), 145–150.

Kochanek, K. D., Murphy, S. L., Xu, J., & Arias, E. (2019). Deaths: Final data for 2017. *National Vital Statistics Reports*, 68(9). National Center for Health Statistics.

Koenig, A. (2018). A lifetime loss: Death of a sibling. In C. Arnold (Ed.), *Understanding child and adolescent grief: Supporting loss and facilitating growth* (pp. 62–77). Routledge/Taylor & Francis Group.

Koga, H. K., Trudel-Fitzgerald, C., Lee, L. O., James, P., Kroenke, C., & Kubzansky, L. D. (2022). Optimism, lifestyle, and longevity in a racially diverse cohort of women. *Journal of the American Geriatrics Society*. https://doi.org/10.1111/jgs.17897

Kokkinos, P. F., Holland, J. C., Narayan, P., Colleran, J. A., Dotson, C. O., & Papademetriou, V. (1995). Miles run per week and high-density lipoprotein cholesterol levels in healthy, middle-aged men: A dose–response relationship. *Archives of Internal Medicine*, 155(4), 415–420.

Koliaki, C., Liatis, S., Dalamaga, M., & Kokkinos, A. (2020). The implication of gut hormones in the regulation of energy homeostasis and their role in the pathophysiology of obesity. *Current Obesity Reports*, 9, 255–271. https://doi.org/10.1007/s13679-020-00396-9

Kolker, R. (2022, July 26). Why was Joshua Held for more than two years for someone else's crimes? *The New York Times*. https://www.nytimes.com/2022/07/26/magazine/joshua-spriestersbach-wrongful-incarceration.html#:~:text=Because%20he%20had%20a%20mental,and%20couldn't%20be%20released

Kõlves, K., Ide, N., & De Leo, D. (2010). Suicidal ideation and behaviour in the aftermath of marital separation: Gender differences. *Journal of Affective Disorders*, 120, 48–53.

Kondo, K., Noonan, K. M., Freeman, M., Ayers, C., Morasco, B. J., & Kansagara, D. (2019). Efficacy of biofeedback for medical conditions: An evidence map. *Journal of General Internal Medicine*. https://doi.org/10.1007/s11606-019-05215-z

Kontis, V., Cobb, L. K., Mathers, C. D., Frieden, T. R., Ezzati, M., & Danaei, G. (2019). Three public health interventions could save 94 million lives in 25 years: Global impact assessment analysis. *Circulation*, 140, 715–725.

Kosinski, M., Matz, S. C., Gosling, S. D., Popov, V., & Stillwell, D. (2016, March). Facebook as a research tool. *Monitor on Psychology*, 47, 70–75.

Koskela, T. H., Ryynanen, O. P., & Soini, E. J. (2010). Risk factors for persistent frequent use of the primary health care services among frequent attenders: A Bayesian approach. *Scandinavian Journal of Primary Health Care*, 28, 55–61.

Koss, M. P. (2018). Hidden rape: Sexual aggression and victimization in a national sample of students in higher education. In P. Searles & R. J. Berger (Eds.), *Rape and society* (pp. 35–49). Routledge.

Koster, E. H. W., De Lissnyder, E., Derakshan, N., & De Raedt, R. (2011). Understanding depressive rumination from a cognitive science perspective: The impaired disengagement hypothesis. *Clinical Psychology Review*, 31, 138–145. https://doi.org/10.1016/j.cpr.2010.08.005

Kovich, H. (2020). Rural matters—Coronavirus and the Navajo Nation. *New England Journal of Medicine*.

Krantz, D. S., Contrada, R. J., Hill, D. R., & Friedler, E. (1988). Environmental stress and biobehavioral antecedents of coronary heart disease. *Journal of Consulting and Clinical Psychology*, 56, 333–341.

Kranzler, H. R. (2023). Overview of alcohol use disorder. *American Journal of Psychiatry*. https://ajp.psychiatryonline.org/doi/10.1176/appi.ajp.20230488

Krist, A. H., Davidson, K. W., Mangione, C. M., Barry, M. J., Cabana, M., Caughey, A. B., . . . Wong, J. B. (2020). Behavioral counseling interventions to promote a healthy diet and physical activity for cardiovascular disease prevention in adults with cardiovascular risk factors: US Preventive Services Task Force Recommendation Statement. *JAMA: The Journal of the American Medical Association*, 324(20), 2069. https://doi.org/10.1001/jama.2020.21749

Krivoshchekov, V., Gulevich, O., & Blagov, I. (2023). Traditional masculinities and men's sexism: A meta-analysis. *Psychology of Men & Masculinity*, 24(4), 365–380. https://doi.org/10.1037/men0000444

Kross, E., Verduyn, P., Demiralp, E., Park, J., Lee, D. S., Lin, N., ... Ybarra, O. (2013). Facebook use predicts declines in subjective well-being in young adults. *PLoS One*, 8, e69841.

Krumholz, H. M., Normand, S. L. T., & Wang, Y. (2019). Twenty-year trends in outcomes for older adults with acute myocardial infarction in the United States. *JAMA Network Open*, 2, e191938. https://doi.org/10.1001/jamanetworkopen.2019.1938

Kübler-Ross, E. (1969). *On death and dying*. Macmillan.

Kuehn, B. (2018). Suicide: The leading cause of violent death. *Journal of the American Medical Association*, 319(10), 973. https://doi.org/10.1001/jama.2018.1699

Kuehn, B. (2019). Diabetes incidence decreases. *Journal of the American Medical Association*, 322, 108. https://doi.org/10.1001/jama.2019.8668

Kuehn, B. M. (2021). Disparities in suicide persist despite overall dip in US rate. *The Journal of the American Medical Association*, 325(14), 1386. doi:10.1001/jama.2021.4131

Kuehn, B. M. (2023). US life expectancy in 2021 lowest since 1996. *JAMA*, 329(4), 280. https://doi.org/10.1001/jama.2022.23562

Kühn, S., Mascherek, A., Filevich, E., Lisofsky, N., Becker, M., Butler, O., & Gallinat, J. (2021). Spend time outdoors for your brain – An in-depth longitudinal MRI study. *The World Journal of Biological Psychiatry*, 23(3), 201–207. https://doi.org/10.1080/15622975.2021.1938670

Kuo, S. S., Roalf, D. R., Prasad, K. M., Musket, C. W., Rupert, P. E., Wood, J., ... Pogue-Geile, M. F. (2022). Age-dependent effects of schizophrenia genetic risk on cortical thickness and cortical surface area: Evaluating evidence for neurodevelopmental and neurodegenerative models of schizophrenia. *Journal of Psychopathology and Clinical Science,* 131(6), 674–688. https://doi.org/10.1037/abn0000765

Kupper, N., & Denollet, J. (2018). Type D personality as a risk factor in coronary heart disease: A review of current evidence. *Current Cardiology Reports*, 20, 104. https://doi.org/10.1007/s11886-018-1048-x

Kutner, B. A., Simoni, J. M., Aunon, F. M., Creegan, E., & Balán, I. C. (2020). How stigma toward anal sexuality promotes concealment and impedes health-seeking behavior in the US among cisgender men who have sex with men. *Archives of Sexual Behavior*. https://doi.org/10.1007/s10508-019-01595-9

Kuypers, K. P. C., Verkes, R. J., Van Den Brink, W., Van Amsterdam, J. G. C., & Ramaekers, J. G. (2020). Intoxicated aggression: Do alcohol and stimulants cause dose-related aggression? A review. *European Neuropsychopharmacology*, 30, 114–147.

Kwasnicka, D., Keller, J., Perski, O., Potthoff, S., ten Hoor, G. A., Ainsworth, B., ... Sanderman, R. (2022). White paper: Open digital health—accelerating transparent and scalable health promotion and treatment. *Health Psychology Review,* 16(4), 475–491. https://doi.org/10.1080/17437199.2022.2046482

Kwong, A. S. F., Northstone, K., Pearson, R. M., McIntosh, A. M., & Timpson, N. J. (2022). Tracking population mental health before and across stages of the COVID-19 pandemic in young adults. https://doi.org/10.1101/2022.03.24.22272899

Kwong, W., Tomlinson, G., & Feig, D. S. (2018). Maternal and neonatal outcomes after bariatric surgery; a systematic review and meta-analysis: Do the benefits outweigh the risks? *American Journal of Obstetrics and Gynecology*, 218(6), 573–580.

Labbott, S. M. (2018). *Health psychology consultation in the inpatient medical setting*. Washington, D. C.: American Psychological Association. https://www.apa.org/pubs/books/4317499

Lacey, R. J., Belcher, J., Rathod, T., Wilkie, R., Thomas, E., & McBeth, J. (2014). Pain at multiple body sites and health-related quality of life in older adults: Results from the North Staffordshire Osteoarthritis Project. *Rheumatology*, 53, 2071–2079.

Lamb, D. (2020). *Death, brain death and ethics*. Routledge.

Lambiase, M. J., Kubzansky, L. D., & Thurston, R. C. (2014). Prospective study of anxiety and incident stroke. *Stroke*, 45, 438–443.

Lami, M. J., Martínez, M. P., & Miró, E. (2018). Efficacy of combined cognitive-behavioral therapy for insomnia and pain in patients with fibromyalgia: A randomized controlled trial. *Cognitive Therapy and Research*, 42, 63–79.

Lamuela-Raventos, R. M., Estruch, R., & Kirwan, R. (2020). Genetic individuality and alcohol consumption. In R. Caterina, J. Martinez, & M. Kohlmeier (Eds.), *Principles of nutrigenetics and nutrigenomics* (pp. 231–235). Academic Press.

Landhuis, E. (2020, April 14). Why women may be more susceptible to mood disorders. *Scientific American*. https://www.scientificamerican.com/article/why-women-may-be-more-susceptible-to-mood-disorders/

Langford, D. J., Cooper, B., Paul, S., & Humphreys, J. (2017). Evaluation of coping as a mediator of the relationship between stressful life events and cancer-related distress. *Health Psychology*, 36, 1147–1160.

Lannoy, S., Ohlsson, H., Kendler, K. S., Sundquist, J., Sundquist, K., & Edwards, A. C. (2023). Examining common and distinct contributions to the etiology of suicide attempt and reattempt. *Journal of Psychopathology and Clinical Science,* 132(2), 165–172. https://doi.org/10.1037/abn0000802

Lapowsky, I. (2014, September 5). This app is a 21st century rape whistle. *Wired Magazine*. http://www.wired.com/2014/09/circle-of-6/

Lara, B., Ruiz-Moreno, C., Salinero, J. J., & Del Coso, J. (2019). Time course of tolerance to the performance benefits of caffeine. *PLoS One*, 14(1), e0210275.

Larimer, M. E., & Marlatt, G. A. (2004). Relapse prevention: An overview of Marlatt's cognitive-behavioral model. In E. McCance-Katz & H. W. Clark (Eds.), *Psychosocial treatments* (pp. 11–28). Routledge.

Larkin, H. D. (2023). Substance use, mental health challenges widespread in 2021. *JAMA*, 329(5), 363. https://doi.org/10.1001/jama.2022.24491

Larrick, R. P., Timmerman, T. A., Carton, A. M., & Abrevay, J. (2011). Temper, temperature, and temptation: Heat-related retaliation in baseball. *Psychological Science*, 22, 423–428.

Larsen, B., Dunsiger, S. I., Pekmezi, D., Linke, S., Hartman, S. J., & Marcus, B. H. (2021). Psychosocial mediators of physical activity change in a web-based intervention for Latinas. *Health Psychology,* 40(1), 21–29. https://doi.org/10.1037/hea0001041

Lauricella, S. K., Phillips, R. E., & Dubow, E. F. (2017). Religious coping with sexual stigma in young adults with same-sex attractions. *Journal of Religion and Health*, 56(4), 1436–1449.

Lawson, A., & Vaganay-Miller, M. (2019). The effectiveness of a poster intervention on hand hygiene practice and compliance when using public restrooms in a university setting. *International Journal of Environmental Research and Public Health*, 16(24), 5036.

Lazaridou, A., & Edwards, R. R. (2019). Relaxation techniques and biofeedback for cancer pain management. In A. Gulati, V. Puttanniah, B. Bruel, W. Rosenberg, & J. Hung (Eds.), *Essentials of interventional cancer pain management*. Springer.

Lazarus, R. S., & Folkman, S. (1984). *Stress, appraisal and coping*. New York: Springer.

Lecca, D., Jung, Y. J., Scerba, M. T., Hwang, I., Kim, Y. K., Kim, S., ... Greig, N. H. (2022). Role of chronic neuroinflammation in neuroplasticity and cognitive function: A hypothesis. *Alzheimer's & Dementia*. https://doi.org/10.1002/alz.12610

Lee, A. A., Piette, J. D., Heisler, M., Janevic, M. R., & Rosland, A. M. (2019). Diabetes self-management and glycemic control: The role of autonomy support from informal health supporters. *Health Psychology*, 38, 122–132.

Leech, T. G., Jacobs, S., & Watson, D. (2020). Factors associated with binge drinking during the transition into adulthood: Exploring associations within two distinct young adult age ranges. *Substance Abuse: Research and Treatment*, 14. https://doi.org/10.1177/1178221820951781

Lee, H. S., & O'Malley, D. (2018). Abstinence-only: Are you not working the program or is the program not working for you? *Journal of Social Work Practice in the Addictions*, 18(3), 289–304.

Lee, I. M., Shiroma, E. J., Kamada, M., Bassett, D. R., Matthews, C. E., & Buring, J. E. (2019). Association of step volume and intensity with all-cause mortality in older women. *JAMA Internal Medicine*, 79, 1105–1112.

Lee, J. H., Gamarel, K. E., Bryant, K. J., Zaller, N. D., & Operario, D. (2016). Discrimination, mental health, and substance use disorders among sexual minority populations. *LGBT Health*, 3(4), 258–265.

Lee, J. S., & Lee, S. K. (2020). The Effects of Laughter Therapy for the relief of employment-stress in Korean student nurses by assessing psychological stress salivary cortisol and subjective happiness. *Osong Public Health and Research Perspectives*, 11(1), 44–52. https://doi.org/10.24171/j.phrp.2020.11.1.07

Lee, L. K., Flaherty, M. P., Blanchard, A., & Agarwal, M. (2022). Helmet use in preventing head injuries in bicycling, snow sports, and other recreational activities and sports. *Pediatrics*. https://doi.org/10.1542/peds.2022-058878

Lee, L. O., Grodstein, F., Trudel-Fitzgerald, C., James, P., Okuzono, S. S., Koga, H. K., ... Kubzansky, L. D. (2022). Optimism, daily stressors, and emotional well-being over two decades in a cohort of aging men. *The Journals of Gerontology: Series B*. https://doi.org/10.1093/geronb/gbac025

Lee, L. O., James, P., Zevon, E. S., Kim, E. S., Trudel-Fitzgerald, C., Spiro, A., ... Kubzansky, L. D. (2019). Optimism is associated with exceptional longevity in 2 epidemiologic cohorts of men and women. *Proceedings of the National Academy of Sciences*, 116(37), 18357–18362. https://doi.org/10.1073/pnas.1900712116

Lee, S., Mu, C. X., Wallace, M. L., Andel, R., Almeida, D. M., Buxton, O. M., & Patel, S. R. (2022). Sleep health composites are associated with the risk of heart disease across sex and race. *Scientific Reports,* 12(1). https://doi.org/10.1038/s41598-022-05203-0

Legrand, L. N., Iacono, W. G., & McGue, M. (2005). Predicting addiction: Behavioral genetics uses twins and time to decipher the origins of addiction and learn who is most vulnerable. *American Scientist*, 93(2), 140–147.

Leigh-Hunt, N., Bagguley, D., Bash, K., Turner, V., Turnbull, S., Valtorta, N., & Caan, W. (2017). An overview of systematic reviews on the public health consequences of social isolation and loneliness. *Public Health*, 152, 157–171.

Lembo, A., Kelley, J. M., Nee, J., Ballou, S., Iturrino, J., Cheng, V., ... Kaptchuk, T. J. (2021). Open-label placebo vs double-blind placebo for irritable bowel syndrome: A randomized clinical trial. *Pain,* 162(9), 2428–2435.

Lennon, J. C., Aita, S. L., Bene, V. A. D., Rhoads, T., Resch, Z. J., Eloi, J. M., & Walker, K. A. (2021). Black and White individuals differ in dementia prevalence, risk factors, and symptomatic presentation. *Alzheimer's & Dementia.*

Leplus, A., Lanteri-Minet, M., Donnet, A., Darmon, N., Régis, J., & Fontaine, D. (2022). Treatment of chronic refractory pain by combined deep brain stimulation of the anterior cingulum and sensory thalamus (EMOPAIN study): Rationale and protocol of a feasibility and safety study. *Brain Science,* 12(9), 1116–1116. https://doi.org/10.3390/brainsci12091116

Leventhal, H., Phillips, L. A., & Burns, E. (2016). The Common-Sense Model of Self-Regulation (CSM): A dynamic framework for understanding illness self-management. *Journal of Behavioral Medicine*, 39, 935–946.

Leventhal, H., Yu, J., & Leventhal, E. A. (2015). Illness behavior and care-seeking. *International encyclopedia of the social & behavioral sciences* (2nd ed., pp. 596–602). Elsevier.

Levine, G. N., Cohen, B. E., Commodore-Mensah, Y., Fleury, J., Huffman, J. C., Khalid, U., ... Kubzansky, L. D. (2021). Psychological health, well-being, and the mind-heart-body connection: A scientific statement from the American Heart Association. *Circulation,* 143(10). https://doi.org/10.1161/cir.0000000000000947

Levinson, C. A. (2017). The core symptoms of bulimia nervosa, anxiety, and depression: A network analysis. *Journal of Abnormal Psychology*, 26(3), 340–354.

Lezin, N. (2019). Theory of reasoned action (TRA). http://recapp.etr.org/recapp/

Liao, Y., Thompson, C., Peterson, S., Mandrola, J., & Beg, M. S. (2019). The future of wearable technologies and remote monitoring in health care. *American Society of Clinical Oncology Educational Book*, 39, 115–121.

Li, A., Zalesky, A., Yue, W., Howes, O., Yan, H., Liu, Y., ... Liu, B. (2020). A neuroimaging biomarker for striatal dysfunction in schizophrenia. *Nature Medicine.* https://doi.org/10.1038/s41591-020-0793-8

Lichtman, J. H., Froelicher, E. S., Blumenthal, J. A., Carney, R. M., Doering, L. V., Frasure-Smith, N., ... Vaccarino, V. (2014). Depression as a risk factor for poor prognosis among patients with acute coronary syndrome: Systematic review and recommendations: A scientific statement from the American Heart Association. *Circulation*, 129(12), 1350–1369. https://doi.org/10.1161/CIR.0000000000000019

Liddon, L., Kingerlee, R., & Barry, J. A. (2018). Gender differences in preferences for psychological treatment, coping strategies, and triggers to help-seeking. *British Journal of Clinical Psychology*, 57(1), 42–58.

Li, D. H., Newcomb, M., Macapagal, K., Remble, T., & Mustanski, B. (2020). Condom-associated erectile function, but not other domains of sexual functioning, predicts condomless insertive anal sex among young men who have sex with men. *Archives of Sexual Behavior*, 49(1), 161–174.

Lilley, C., Willmott, D., Mojtahedi, D., & Labhardt, D. (2023). Intimate partner rape: A review of six core myths surrounding women's conduct and the consequences of intimate partner rape. *Social Sciences,* 12(1), 34. https://doi.org/10.3390/socsci12010034

Limakatso, K., Bedwell, G. J., Madden, V. J., & Parker, R. (2019). The prevalence of phantom limb pain and associated risk factors in people with amputations: A systematic review protocol. *Systematic Reviews*, 8(1), 17. https://doi.org/10.1186/s13643-018-0938-8

Limbu, Y. B., Gautam, R. K., & Pham, L. (2022). The Health Belief Model applied to COVID-19 vaccine hesitancy: A systematic review. *Vaccines,* 10(6), 973. https://doi.org/10.3390/vaccines10060973 10(6), 973–973.

Lim, J. S., & Noh, G. Y. (2017). Effects of gain-versus loss-framed performance feedback on the use of fitness apps: Mediating role of exercise self-efficacy and outcome expectations of exercise. *Computers in Human Behavior*, 77, 249–257.

Lindberg, L., Hagman, E., Danielsson, P., Marcus, C., & Persson, M. (2020). Anxiety and depression in children and adolescents with obesity: A nationwide study in Sweden. *BMC Medicine*, 18(1), 1–9. https://doi.org/10.1186/s12916-020-1498-z

Linde, K., Sigterman, K., Kriston, L., Rücker, G., Jamil, S., Meissner, K., & Schneider, A. (2015). Effectiveness of psychological treatments for depressive disorders in primary care: Systematic review and meta-analysis. *Annals of Family Medicine*, 13(1), 56–68. https://doi.org/10.1370/afm.1719

Lin, N. Y., Ramsey, R. R., Miller, J. L., McDowell, K. M., Zhang, N., Hommel, K., & Guilbert, T. W. (2020). Telehealth delivery of adherence and medication management system improves outcomes in inner-city children with asthma. *Pediatric Pulmonology*, 55(4), 858–865. https://doi.org/10.1002/ppul.24623

Linton, S. J. (2018). The cognitive-behavioral approach to early interventions to prevent chronic pain-related disability. In D. C. Turk & R. J. Gatchel (Eds.), *Psychological approaches to pain management: A practitioner's handbook* (3rd ed., pp. 340–356). The Guilford Press.

Linton, S. J., Kecklund, G., Franklin, K. A., Leissner, L. C., Sivertsen, B., Lindberg, E., ... Hall, C. (2015). The effect of the work environment on future sleep disturbances: A systematic review. *Sleep Medicine Reviews*, 23, 10–19.

Liou, K. T., Root, J. C., Garland, S. N., Green, J., Li, Y., Li, Q. S., ... Mao, J. J. (2020). Effects of acupuncture versus cognitive behavioral therapy on cognitive function in cancer survivors with insomnia: A secondary analysis of a randomized clinical trial. *Cancer.* https://doi.org/10.1002/cncr.32847

Lipari, R. N., Park-Lee, E., & Van Horn, S. (2016). *America's need for and receipt of substance use treatment in 2015.* Center for Behavioral Health Statistics and Quality, Substance Abuse and Mental Health Services Administration.

Lipsitt, D. R. (2006). Psychosomatic medicine: History of a "new" specialty. In M. Blumenfield & J. J. Strain (Eds.), *Psychosomatic medicine.* Lippincott Williams & Wilkins.

Liu, R. T., & Alloy, L. B. (2010). Stress generation in depression: A systematic review of the empirical literature and recommendations for future study. *Clinical Psychology Review*, 30, 582–593.

Liu, R. T., Kleiman, E. M., Nestor, B. A., & Cheek, S. M. (2015). The hopelessness theory of depression: A quarter-century in review. *Clinical Psychology: Science and Practice*, 22(4), 345–365.

Liu, R. T., & Miller, I. (2014). Life events and suicidal ideation and behavior: A systematic review. *Clinical Psychology Review*, 34(3), 181–192. https://doi.org/10.1016/j.cpr.2014.01.006

Liu, T. (2021). Placebo effects: A new theory. *Clinical Psychological Science*, 10(1), 27–40. https://doi.org/10.1177/21677026211009799

Liu, Y., Hu, X., Xiong, M., Li, J., Jiang, X., Wan, Y., ... Zhang, X. (2023). Association of BMI with erectile dysfunction: A cross-sectional study of men from an andrology clinic. *Frontiers in Endocrinology*, 14, 1135024. https://doi.org/10.3389/fendo.2023.1135024

Liu, Y., Yang, Y., Bai, X., Chen, Y., & Mo, L. (2022). Do immediate external rewards really enhance intrinsic motivation? *Frontiers in Psychology*, 13. doi: 10.3389/fpsyg.2022.853879

Li, X., Xue, Q., Wang, M., Zhou, T., Ma, H., Heianza, Y., & Qi, L. (2020). Adherence to a healthy sleep pattern and incident heart failure: A prospective study of 408802 UK biobank participants. *Circulation*. https://doi.org/10.1161/circulationaha.120.050792

Li, Z., & Heber, D. (2020). Ketogenic diets. *Journal of the American Medical Association*, 323(4), 386. https://doi.org/10.1001/jama.2019.18408

Lloyd, J., Bond, F. W., & Flaxman, P. E. (2017). Work-related self-efficacy as a moderator of the impact of a worksite stress management training intervention: Intrinsic work motivation as a higher order condition of effect. *Journal of Occupational Health Psychology*, 22(1), 115–127.

Lobel, M., & Ibrahim, S. M. (2018). Emotions and mental health during pregnancy and postpartum. *Women's Reproductive Health*, 5(1), 13–19.

Lock, M., Post, D., Dollman, J., & Parfitt, G. (2020). Efficacy of theory-informed workplace physical activity interventions: A systematic literature review with meta-analyses. *Health Psychology Review*. https://doi.org/10.1080/17437199.2020.1718528

Lo Coco, G., Maiorana, A., Mirisola, A., Salerno, L., Boca, S., & Profita, G. (2018). Empirically-derived subgroups of Facebook users and their association with personality characteristics: A latent class analysis. *Computers in Human Behavior*, 86, 190–198.

Loeb, C., Miller, J. A., Schneider, D., Grimaud, L., Moukhtar Hammad, M. A., & Yafi, F. A. (2023). Testosterone replacement therapy is associated with high satisfaction rates: Results of a survey study. *International Journal of Impotence Research*. https://doi.org/10.1038/s41443-023-00724-2

Lofland, L. H. (2017). *The public realm: Exploring the city's quintessential social territory*. Routledge.

Lopes, A. R., & Nihei, O. K. (2020). Burnout among nursing students: Predictors and association with empathy and self-efficacy. *Revista Brasileira de Enfermagem*, 73(1). https://doi.org/10.1590/0034-7167-2018-0280

Lopez-Quintero, C., Hasin, D. S., De Los Cobos, J. P., Pines, A., Wang, S., Grant, B. F., & Blanco, C. (2011). Probability and predictors of remission from life-time nicotine, alcohol, cannabis or cocaine dependence: Results from the national epidemiologic survey on alcohol and related conditions. *Addiction*, 106(3), 657–669.

Loprinzi, P. D., Wolfe, C. D., & Walker, J. F. (2015). Exercise facilitates smoking cessation indirectly via improvements in smoking-specific self-efficacy: Prospective cohort study among a national sample of young smokers. *Preventive Medicine*, 81, 63–66.

Losina, E., Yang, H. Y., Deshpande, B. R., Katz, J. N., & Collins, J. E. (2017). Physical activity and unplanned illness-related work absenteeism: Data from an employee wellness program. *PLoS One*, 12(5). https://doi.org/10.1371/journal.pone.0176872

Loucks, E. B., Nardi, W. R., Gutman, R., Kronish, I. M., Saadeh, F. B., ... Li, Y. (2019). Mindfulness-based blood pressure reduction (MB-BP): Stage 1 single-arm clinical trial. *PLoS One*, 14(11). https://doi.org/10.1371/journal.pone.0223095

Lovelace, B., Jr. (2023, August 21). Guns are leading cause of death for kids, teens in U.S., CDC says. NBC News. https://www.nbcnews.com/health/kids-health/gun-deaths-us-children-rose-2021-cdc-data-shows-rcna100601

Lozano-Blasco, R., Latorre-Martínez, M., & Cortés-Pascual, A. (2022). Screen addicts: A meta-analysis of internet addiction in adolescence. *Children and Youth Services Review*, 135, 106373.

Lucas, J. W., Ho, H.-Y., & Kerns, K. (2018). Power, status, and stigma: Their implications for health. In B. Major, J. F. Dovidio, & B. G. Link (Eds.), *The Oxford handbook of stigma, discrimination, and health* (pp. 69–84). Oxford University Press.

Lucas, M. W., Versluis, J. M., Rozeman, E. A., & Blank, C. U. (2023). Personalizing neoadjuvant immune-checkpoint inhibition in patients with melanoma. *Nature Reviews. Clinical Oncology*, 20(6), 408–422. https://doi.org/10.1038/s41571-023-00760-3

Lucas, T., Thompson, H. S., Blessman, J., Dawadi, A., Drolet, C. E., Hirko, K. A., ... Penner, L. A. (2021). Effects of culturally targeted message framing on colorectal cancer screening among African Americans. *Health Psychology*, 40(5), 305–315. https://doi.org/10.1037/hea0001073

Ludwick-Rosenthal, R., & Neufeld, R. W. J. (1993). Preparation for undergoing an invasive medical procedure. *Journal of Consulting and Clinical Psychology*, 61, 156–164.

Ludyga, S., Gerber, M., Pühse, U., Looser, V. N., & Kamijo, K. (2020). Systematic review and meta-analysis investigating moderators of long-term effects of exercise on cognition in healthy individuals. *Nature Human Behaviour*.

Lumley, M. A., & Schubiner, H. (2019). Psychological therapy for centralized pain: An Integrative assessment and treatment model. *Psychosomatic Medicine*, 81, 114–124.

Luoma, J. B., Martin, C. E., & Pearson, J. L. (2002). Contact with mental health and primary care providers before suicide: A review of the evidence. *American Journal of Psychiatry*, 159, 909–916.

Lupton, D. (2017). Digital media and body weight, shape, and size: An introduction and review. *Fat Studies*, 6(2), 119–134.

Lu, S. (2015, April). Great expectations. *Monitor on Psychology*, 46(4), 50.

Lutz, J., Mashal, N., Kramer, A., Suresh, M., Gould, C., Jordan, J. T., ... Beaudreau, S. A. (2020). A case report of problem solving therapy for reducing suicide risk in older adults with anxiety disorders. *Clinical Gerontologist*, 43(1), 110–117.

Lu, X., Juon, H. S., He, X., Dallal, C. M., Wang, M. Q., & Lee, S. (2019). The association between perceived stress and hypertension among Asian Americans: Does social support and social network make a difference? *Journal of Community Health*, 44(3), 451–462.

Lu, Y., Wang, Z., Georgakis, M. K., Lin, H., & Zheng, L. (2021). Genetic liability to depression and risk of coronary artery disease, myocardial infarction, and other cardiovascular outcomes. *Journal of the American Heart Association*, 10(1). https://doi.org/10.1161/jaha.120.017986

Lynch, J., Prihodova, L., Dunne, P. J., McMahon, G., Carroll, A., Walsh, C., & White, B. (2018). Impact of mantra meditation on health and wellbeing: A systematic review protocol. *European Journal of Integrative Medicine*, 18, 30–33.

Maas, A. H., & Appelman, Y. E. (2010). Gender differences in coronary heart disease. *Netherlands Heart Journal*, 18, 598–602.

Mabe, A. G., Forney, K. J., &. Keel, P. K. (2014). Do you "like" my photo? Facebook use maintains eating disorder risk. *International Journal of Eating Disorders*, 47, 516–523.

MacCárthaigh, S., Griffin, C., & Perry, J. (2020). The relationship between sleep and problematic smartphone use among adolescents:

A systematic review. *Developmental Review: DR*, 55(100897), 100897. https://doi.org/10.1016/j.dr.2020.100897

Maciejewski, P. K., Zhang, B., Block, S. D., & Prigerson H. G. (2007). An empirical examination of the stage theory of grief. *Journal of the American Medical Association*, 297, 716–723. https://doi.org/10.1001/jama.297.7.716

Mackay, E., Dalman, C., Karlsson, H., & Gardner, R. M. (2017). Association of gestational weight gain and maternal body mass index in early pregnancy with risk for nonaffective psychosis in offspring. *JAMA Psychiatry*, 74(4), 339–349.

MacLean, P. S., Higgins, J. A., Giles, E. D., Sherk, V. D., & Jackman, M. R. (2015). The role for adipose tissue in weight regain after weight loss. *Obesity Reviews*, 16, 45–54.

Macready, A. L., Fallaize, R., Butler, L. T., Ellis, J. A., Kuznesof, S., Frewer, L. J. ... Stewart-Knox, B. J. (2018). Application of behavior change techniques in a personalized nutrition electronic health intervention study: Protocol for the web-based Food4Me randomized controlled trial. *JMIR Research Protocols*, 7(4), e87.

Maddi, S. R. (2007). Relevance of hardiness assessment and training to the military context. *Military Psychology*, 19(1), 61–70.

Maddi, S. R. (2016). Hardiness as a pathway to resilience under stress. In U. Kumar (Ed.), *The Routledge international handbook of psychosocial resilience* (pp. 104–110). Routledge.

Mahajan, K., & Velaga, N. R. (2020). Effects of partial sleep deprivation on braking response of drivers in hazard scenarios. *Accident Analysis & Prevention*, 142. https://doi.org/10.1016/j.aap.2020.105545

Maier, S. F., & Seligman, M. E. P. (2016). Learned helplessness at fifty: Insights from neuroscience. *Psychological Review*, 123, 349–367. https://doi.org/10.1037/rev0000033

Maisto, S. A., & Simons, J. S. (2016). Research on the effects of alcohol and sexual arousal on sexual risk in men who have sex with men: Implications for HIV prevention interventions. *AIDS and Behavior*, 20(1), 158–172.

Major, B., Dovidio, J. F., Link, B. G., & Calabre, S. K. (2018). Stigma and its implications for health: Introduction and overview. In B. Major, J. F. Dovidio, & B. G. Link (Eds.), *The Oxford handbook of stigma, discrimination, and health* (pp. 3–28). Oxford University Press.

Major, B., & Schmader, T. (2018). Stigma, social identity threat, and health. In B. Major, J. F. Dovidio, & B. G. Link (Eds.), *The Oxford handbook of stigma, discrimination, and health* (pp. 85–103). Oxford University Press.

Mangione, C. M., Barry, M. J., Nicholson, W. K., Cabana, M., Chelmow, D., Coker, T. R., ... Wong, J. B. (2022). Statin use for the primary prevention of cardiovascular disease in adults. *JAMA*, 328(8), 746. https://doi.org/10.1001/jama.2022.13044

Manly, J. J., Jones, R. N., Langa, K. M., Ryan, L. H., Levine, D. A., McCammon, R. J., ... Weir, D. (2022). Estimating the prevalence of dementia and mild cognitive impairment in the US. *JAMA Neurology*, 79(12), 1242. https://doi.org/10.1001/jamaneurol.2022.3543

Mannes, Z. L., Ferguson, E. G., Perlstein, W. M., Waxenberg, L. B., Cottler, L. B., & Ennis, N. (2020). Negative health consequences of pain catastrophizing among retired National Football League athletes. *Health Psychology: Official Journal of the Division of Health Psychology, American Psychological Association*, 39(5), 452–462. https://doi.org/10.1037/hea0000847

Manson, J. E., Skerrett, P. J., Greenland, P., & VanItallie, T. B. (2004). The escalating pandemics of obesity and sedentary lifestyle a call to action for clinicians. *Archives of Internal Medicine*, 164, 249–258.

Mansoor, N., Vinknes, K. J., Veierød, M. B., & Retterstøl, K. (2016). Effects of low-carbohydrate diets v. low-fat diets on body weight and cardiovascular risk factors: A meta-analysis of randomised controlled trials. *British Journal of Nutrition*, 115(3), 466–479.

Manworren, R. C., Anderson, M. N., Girard, E. D., Ruscher, K. A., Verissimo, A. M., Palac, H., ... Hight, D. (2018). Postoperative pain outcomes after Nuss Procedures: Comparison of epidural analgesia, continuous infusion of local anesthetic, and preoperative self-hypnosis training. *Journal of Laparoendoscopic & Advanced Surgical Techniques*. https://www.liebertpub.com/doi/abs/10.1089/lap.2017.0699?journalCode=lap

Marcus, A. (2023, August 4). FDA approves first pill for postpartum depression. *Medscape Psychiatry*. https://www.medscape.com/viewarticle/995204?src=FYE

Marín-Jiménez, I., Gobbo Montoya, M., Panadero, A., Cañas, M., Modino, Y., Romero de Santos, C., ... GETECCU Study Group and ACCU. (2017). Management of the psychological impact of inflammatory bowel disease: Perspective of doctors and patients—The ENMENTE Project. *Inflammatory Bowel Diseases*, 23(9), 1492–1498.

Marin, M.-F., Geoffrion, S., Juster, R.-P., Giguèrea, C.-E., Marchand, A., Lupien, S. J., & Guay, S. A. (2019). High cortisol awakening response in the aftermath of workplace violence exposure moderates the association between acute stress disorder symptoms and PTSD symptoms. *Psychoneuroendocrinology*, 104, 238–242.

Marino, C., Gini, G., Vieno, A., & Spada, M. M. (2018a). A comprehensive meta-analysis on problematic Facebook use. *Computers in Human Behavior* 83, 262–277. https://doi.org/10.1016/j.chb.2018.02.009

Marino, C., Gini, G., Vieno, A., & Spada, M. M. (2018b). The associations between problematic Facebook use, psychological distress and well-being among adolescents and young adults: A systematic review and meta-analysis. *Journal of Affective Disorders*, 226, 274–281. https://doi.org/10.1016/j.jad.2017.10.007

Mariotto, A. B., Zou, Z., Johnson, C. J., Scoppa, S., Weir, H. K., & Huang, B. (2018). Geographical, racial and socio-economic variation in life expectancy in the US and their impact on cancer relative survival. *PLoS One*, 13(7), e0201034.

Marjaneh, M. M., Beesley, J., O'Mara, T. A., Mukhopadhyay, P., Koufariotis, L. T., Kazakoff, S., ... Kaufmann, S. (2020). Non-coding RNAs underlie genetic predisposition to breast cancer. *Genome Biology*, 21(1), 1–14.

Markel, H. (2020). Was Freud a Freudian? Not in your dreams. *Washington Post*. https://www.washingtonpost.com/wp-srv/special/opinions/outlook/whats-in-a-name/freud.html

Markfelder, T., & Pauli, P. (2020). Fear of pain and pain intensity: Meta-analysis and systematic review. *Psychological Bulletin*, 146(5), 411–450. https://doi.org/10.1037/bul0000228

Mark, G., & Ganzach, Y. (2014). Personality and Internet usage: A large-scale representative study of young adults. *Computers in Human Behavior*, 36, 274–281.

Marks, L., Nesteruk, O., Swanson, M., Garrison, B., & Davis, T. (2005). Religion and health among African Americans: A qualitative examination. *Research on Aging*, 27(4), 447–474.

Maron, D. J., Mancini, G. B., Hartigan, P. M., Spertus, J. A., Sedlis, S. P., Kostuk, W. J., ... COURAGE Trial Group. (2018). Healthy behavior, risk factor control, and survival in the Courage trial. *Journal of the American College of Cardiology*, 72, 2297–2305.

Marquez, I., Calman, N., & Crump, C. (2019). A framework for addressing diabetes-related disparities in US Latino populations. *Journal of Community Health*, 44, 412–422.

Martinčeková, L., Jiang, M. J., Adams, J. D., Menendez, D., Hernandez, I. G., Barber, G., & Rosengren, K. S. (2020). Do you remember being told what happened to grandma? The role of early socialization on later coping with death. *Death Studies*, 44(2), 78–88.

Martin, M. J. (1978). Psychosomatic medicine: A brief history. *Psychosomatics*, 19, 697–700.

Martin, P. R., Reece, J., MacKenzie, S., Bandarian-Balooch, S., Brunelli, A., & Goadsby, P. J. (2021). Integrating headache trigger management strategies into cognitive-behavioral therapy: A randomized controlled trial. *Health Psychology,* 40(10), 674–685. https://doi.org/10.1037/hea0001115

Massaro, M., Scoditti, E., Carluccio, M. A., Calabriso, N., Santarpino, G., Verri, T., & De Caterina, R. (2020). Effects of olive oil on blood pressure: Epidemiological, clinical, and mechanistic evidence. *Nutrients*, 12(6), 1548. https://doi.org/10.3390/nu12061548

Massetti, G. M., Dietz, W. H., & Richardson, L. C. (2017). Excessive weight gain, obesity, and cancer. *Journal of the American Medical Association*, 318(20), 1975–1976.

Masters, W. H., & Johnson, V. E. (1970). *Human sexual inadequacy*. Little, Brown.

Matsushita, S., & Higuchi, S. (2017). Use of Asian samples in genetic research of alcohol use disorders: Genetic variation of alcohol metabolizing enzymes and the effects of acetaldehyde. *The American Journal on Addictions*, 26(5), 469–476.

Matta, J., Wiernik, E., Robineau, O., Carrat, F., Touvier, M., Severi, G., ... De Lamballerie, X. (2022). Association of self-reported COVID-19 Infection and SARS-CoV-2 serology test results with persistent physical symptoms among French adults during the COVID-19 pandemic. *JAMA Internal Medicine,* 182(1), 19. https://doi.org/10.1001/jamainternmed.2021.645

Matthews, K. A. (1982). Psychological perspectives on the type A behavior pattern. *Psychological Bulletin*, 91(2), 293–323.

Maxwell, J. A., & McNulty, J. K. (2019). No longer in a dry spell: The developing understanding of how sex influences romantic relationships. *Current Directions in Psychological Science*, 28(1), 102–107. https://doi.org/10.1177/0963721418806690

Maya, J., & Misra, M. (2022). The female athlete triad: Review of current literature. *Current Opinion in Endocrinology & Diabetes and Obesity,* 29(1), 44–51.

Mayne, S. T., McKinnon, R. A., & Woodcock, J. (2021). Reducing sodium intake in the US. *JAMA,* 326(17), 1675. https://doi.org/10.1001/jama.2021.18611

Mayo Clinic. (2018). Triglycerides: Why do they matter? https://www.mayoclinic.org/diseases-conditions/high-blood-cholesterol/in-depth/triglycerides/art-20048186

Mayo Clinic. (2019a). High blood pressure (hypertension). https://www.mayoclinic.org/diseases-conditions/high-blood-pressure/symptoms-causes/syc-20373410

Mayo Clinic. (2019b, January 26). Mediterranean diet: A heart-health eating plan. https://www.mayoclinic.org/healthy-lifestyle/nutrition-and-healthy-eating/in-depth/mediterranean-diet/art-20047801

Mayo Clinic. (2019). *High blood pressure (hypertension).* https://www.mayoclinic.org/diseases-conditions/high-blood-pressure/symptoms-causes/syc-20373410

Mayo Clinic. (2022). 7 healthy habits that can reduce your risk of cancer. https://www.mayoclinic.org/healthy-lifestyle/adult-health/in-depth/cancer-prevention/art-20044816

McCarthy, J. (2019). One in FIVE U.S. adults use health apps, wearable trackers. https://news.gallup.com/poll/269096/one-five-adults-health-apps-wearable-trackers.aspx

McCarthy, J. (2023, June 5). *U.S. same-sex marriage support holds at 71%.* https://news.gallup.com/poll/506636/sex-marriage-support-holds-high.aspx

McCarthy, J., & Brown, A. (2015). Getting more sleep linked to higher well-being. The Gallup Organization. https://news.gallup.com/poll/181583/getting-sleep-linked-higher.aspx

McCaul, M. E., Hutton, H. E., Stephens, M. A. C., Xu, X., & Wand, G. S. (2017). Anxiety, anxiety sensitivity, and perceived stress as predictors of recent drinking, alcohol craving, and social stress response in heavy drinkers. *Alcoholism: Clinical and Experimental Research*, 41(4), 836–845.

McClintock, A. S., Brown, R., Coe, C. L., Zgierska, A., & Barrett, B. (2019). Mindfulness practice and stress following mindfulness-based stress reduction: Examining within-person and between-person associations with latent curve modeling. *Mindfulness*, 10(9), 1905–1914.

McConnell, E. A., Janulis, P., Phillips, I. I., Truong, R., & Birkett, M. (2018). Multiple minority stress and LGBT community resilience among sexual minority men. *Psychology of Sexual Orientation and Gender Diversity*, 5(1), 1–12.

McCormack, S., Dunn, D. T., Desai, M., Dolling, D. I., Gafos, M., Gilson, R., ... Mackie, N. (2016). Pre-exposure prophylaxis to prevent the acquisition of HIV-1 infection (PROUD): Effectiveness results from the pilot phase of a pragmatic open-label randomised trial. *The Lancet*, 387(10013), 53–60. https://doi.org/10.1016/S0140-6736(15)00056-2

McCracken, L. M., Yu, L., & Vowles, K. E. (2022). New generation psychological treatments in chronic pain. *British Medical Journal,* 376, e057212–e057212. https://doi.org/10.1136/bmj-2021-057212

McCrae, R. R., Costa, P. T., Jr., Martin, T. A., Oryol, E., Rukavishnikov, A. A., Senin, I. G., ... Urbánek, T. (2004). Consensual validation of personality traits across cultures. *Journal of Research in Personality*, 38, 17–20.

McCurry, S. M., Zhu, W., Von Korff, M., Wellman, R., Morin, C. M., Thakral, M., ... Vitiello, M. V. (2021). Effect of telephone cognitive behavioral therapy for insomnia in older adults with osteoarthritis pain. JAMA Internal Medicine. https://doi.org/10.1001/jamainternmed.2020.9049

McCutcheon, V. V., Agrawal, A., Kuo, S. I. C., Su, J., Dick, D. M., Meyers, J. L., ... Schuckit, M. A. (2018). Associations of parental alcohol use disorders and parental separation with offspring initiation of alcohol, cigarette and cannabis use and sexual debut in high-risk families. *Addiction*, 113(2), 336–345.

McEvoy, K. (2020). Clinical phenotypes of postpartum psychosis. In J. L. Payne & L. M. Osborne (Eds.), *Biomarkers of postpartum psychiatric disorders* (pp. 137–147). Academic Press.

McGinty, E. E., Presskreischer, R., Han, H., & Barry, C. L. (2020). Psychological distress and loneliness reported by US Adults in 2018 and April 2020. *JAMA,* 324(1), 93. https://doi.org/10.1001/jama.2020.9740

McGowan, L., Devereux-Fitzgerald, A., Powell, R., & French, D. P. (2019). Physical activity and health. In C. D. Llewellyn, S. Ayers, C. McManus, S. Newman, K. J. Petrie, T. A. Revenson, & J. Weinman (Eds.), *Cambridge handbook of psychology, health and medicine* (3rd ed., pp. 61–64). Cambridge University Press.

McGrath, J. J., Saha, S., Al-Hamzawi, A. O., Alonso, J., Andrade, L., Borges, G., ... Fayyad, J. (2016). Age of onset and lifetime projected risk of psychotic experiences: Cross-national data from the World Mental Health Survey. *Schizophrenia Bulletin*, 42, 933–941.

McGuire, K., & Lorenz, R. (2020). Exploring the relationships between sleep, stress, and performance in simulation-based learning. *Sleep*, 43(Suppl. 1), A88–A89.

McHugh, R. K., Votaw, V. R., Sugarman, D. E., & Greenfield, S. F. (2017). Sex and gender differences in substance use disorders. *Clinical Psychology Review*. https://doi.org/10.1016/j.cpr.2017.10.012

McKay, F. H., Wright, A., Shill, J., Stephens, H., & Uccellini, M. (2019). Using health and well-being apps for behavior change: A systematic search and rating of apps. *JMIR mHealth and uHealth*, 7(7). https://doi.org/10.2196/11926

McKernan, L. C., Nash, M. R., & Patterson, D. R. (2018). Clinical hypnosis in the treatment of chronic and acute pain. In D. C. Turk &

R. J. Gatchel (Eds.), *Psychological approaches to pain management: A practitioner's handbook* (3rd ed., pp. 162–176). The Guilford Press.

McMakin, D. (2021). How much sleep do you really need? *The Conversation*. https://theconversation.com/how-much-sleep-do-you-really-need-156819

McPhillips, D. (2023, April 17). As gun violence reaches record levels in the US, an underlying trauma may be building up. *CNN*. https://www.cnn.com/2023/04/17/health/mass-shootings-mental-health/index.html

McSharry, J., Olander, E. K., & French, D. P. (2015). Do single and multiple behavior change interventions contain different behavior change techniques? A comparison of interventions targeting physical activity in obese populations. *Health Psychology*, 34(9), 960–965.

Meade, L. B., Bearne, L. M., Sweeney, L. H., Alageel, S. H., & Godfrey, E. L. (2019). Behaviour change techniques associated with adherence to prescribed exercise in patients with persistent musculoskeletal pain: Systematic review. *British Journal of Health Psychology*, 24, 10–30.

Meader, N., King, K., Moe-Byrne, T., Wright, K., Graham, H., Petticrew, M., ... Sowden, A. J. (2016). A systematic review on the clustering and co-occurrence of multiple risk behaviours. *BMC Public Health*, 16(1), 657. https://doi.org/10.1186/s12889-016-3373-6

Meader, N., King, K., Wright, K., Graham, H. M., Petticrew, M., Power, C., ... Sowden, A. J. (2017). Multiple risk behavior interventions: Meta-analyses of RCTs. *American Journal of Preventive Medicine*, 53(1), e19–e30.

Mechanic, D., & Volkart, E. H. (1960). Illness behavior and medical diagnoses. *Journal of Health and Human Behavior*, 1(2), 86–94. https://doi.org/10.2307/2949006

Meeusen, R., Van Cutsem, J., & Roelands, B. (2020). Endurance exercise-induced and mental fatigue and the brain. *Experimental Physiology*. https://doi.org/10.1113/EP088186

Mehta, R. H., Shahian, D. M., Sheng, S., O'brien, S. M., Edwards, F. H., Jacobs, J. P., & Peterson, E. D. (2016). Association of hospital and physician characteristics and care processes with racial disparities in procedural outcomes among contemporary patients undergoing coronary artery bypass grafting surgery. *Circulation*, 133(2), 124–130.

Meichenbaum, D. (2017). *The evolution of cognitive behavior therapy*. Routledge.

Meinhausen, C., Prather, A. A., & Sumner, J. A. (2022). Posttraumatic stress disorder (PTSD), sleep, and cardiovascular disease risk: A mechanism-focused narrative review. *Health Psychology*, 41(10), 663–673. https://doi.org/10.1037/hea0001143

Mekawi, Y., Hyatt, C. S., Maples-Keller, J., Carter, S., Michopoulos, V., & Powers, A. (2021). Racial discrimination predicts mental health outcomes beyond the role of personality traits in a community sample of African Americans. *Clinical Psychological Science*, 9(2), 183–196. https://doi.org/10.1177/2167702620957318

Melo, B. P., Guariglia, D. A., Pedro, R. E., Bertolini, D. A., de Paula Ramos, S., Peres, S. B., & de Moraes, S. M. F. (2019). Combined exercise modulates cortisol, testosterone, and immunoglobulin a levels in individuals living with HIV/AIDS. *Journal of Physical Activity and Health*, 16(11), 993–999.

Melzack, R. (1999a). From the gate to the neuromatrix. *Pain* (Suppl. 6), S121–S126.

Melzack, R., & Wall, P. D. (1965). Pain mechanisms: A new theory. *Science*, 150, 971–979.

Melzack, R., & Wall, P. D. (1983). *The challenge of pain*. Basic Books.

Menatti, A. R., Weeks, J. W., Levinson, C. A., & McGowan, M. M. (2013). Exploring the relationship between social anxiety and bulimic symptoms: Mediational effects of perfectionism among females. *Cognitive Therapy and Research*, 37, 914–922.

Mendez Colmenares, A., Voss, M. W., Fanning, J., Salerno, E. A., Gothe, N. P., Thomas, M. L., ... Burzynska, A. Z. (2021). White matter plasticity in healthy older adults: The effects of aerobic exercise. *NeuroImage*, 239, 118305. https://doi.org/10.1016/j.neuroimage.2021.118305

Mensah, G. A. (2018). The black–white cardiovascular health disparity is narrowing, but not for the reason you think. *Annals of Internal Medicine*, 168, 590–591. https://doi.org/10.7326/M18-0349

Merchant, J. (2016, January 26). How meditation, placebos and virtual reality help power 'mind over body.' http://www.npr.org

Meredith, G. R., Rakow, D. A., Eldermire, E. R., Madsen, C. G., Shelley, S. P., & Sachs, N. A. (2020). Minimum time dose in nature to positively impact the mental health of college-aged students, and how to measure it: A scoping review. *Frontiers in Psychology*, 10. https://doi.org/10.3389/fpsyg.2019.02942

Mescouto, K., Olson, R. E., Hodges, P. W., & Setchell, J. (2022). A critical review of the biopsychosocial model of low back pain care: Time for a new approach? *Disability and Rehabilitation*, 44(13), 3270–3284. https://www.tandfonline.com/doi/full/10.1080/09638288.2020.1851783

Meshe, O. F., Bungay, H., & Claydon, L. S. (2020). Participants' experiences of the benefits, barriers and facilitators of attending a community-based exercise programme for people with chronic obstructive pulmonary disease. *Health & Social Care in the Community*, 28(3), 969–978.

Meston, C. M., & Stanton, A. M. (2017). Evaluation of female sexual interest/arousal disorder. In W. W. IsHak (Ed.), *The textbook of clinical sexual medicine* (pp. 155–163). Springer.

Metrebian, N., Weaver, T., Pilling, S., Goldsmith, K., Carr, E., Shearer, J., ... van der Waal, R. (2020). Telephone delivered incentives for encouraging adherence to supervised methadone consumption (TIES): Study protocol for a feasibility study for an RCT of clinical and cost effectiveness. *Contemporary Clinical Trials Communications*, 17.

Metz, M. E., & McCarthy, B. W. (2007). The "Good-Enough Sex" model for couple sexual satisfaction. *Sexual and Relationship Therapy*, 22(3), 351–362.

Meuret, A. E., Tunnell, N., & Roque, A. (2020). Anxiety disorders and medical comorbidity: Treatment implications. In Y.-K. Kim (Ed.), *Anxiety disorders* (pp. 237–261). Springer.

Mgbako, O., Loughran, C., Mathu, R., Castor, D., McLean, J., Sobieszczyk, M. E., ... Remien, R. H. (2023). Rapid or immediate ART, HIV stigma, medical mistrust, and retention in care: An exploratory mixed methods pilot study. *AIDS and Behavior*, 27(10), 3430–3446.

Micha, R., Peñalvo, J. L., Cudhea, F., Imamura, F., Rehm, C. D., & Mozaffarian, D. (2017). Association between dietary factors and mortality from heart disease, stroke, and type 2 diabetes in the United States. *Journal of the American Medical Association*, 317, 912–924.

Michielsen, C. C., Hangelbroek, R. W., Feskens, E. J., & Afman, L. A. (2019). Disentangling the effects of monounsaturated fat from other components of a Mediterranean Diet on serum metabolite profiles: A randomized fully controlled dietary intervention in healthy subjects at risk of the metabolic syndrome. *Molecular Nutrition & Food Research*, 1801095. https://onlinelibrary.wiley.com/doi/full/10.1002/mnfr.201801095

Michie, S., Marques, M. M., Norris, E., & Johnston, M. (2019). Theories and interventions in health behavior change. In T. E. Revenson & R. A. R. Gurung (Eds.), *Handbook of health psychology* (pp. 69–88). Routledge.

Michos, E. D., McEvoy, J. W., & Blumenthal, R. S. (2019). Lipid management for the prevention of atherosclerotic cardiovascular disease. *New England Journal of Medicine*, 17(381), 1557–1567.

Miech, R. A., Johnston, L. D., O'Malley, P. M., Bachman, J. G., Schulenberg, J. E., & Patrick, M. E. (2019). *Monitoring the future national survey results on drug use, 1975–2018: Volume I, Secondary school students*. Institute for Social Research, The University of Michigan.

Miech, R. A., Johnston, L. D., Patrick, M. E., O'Malley, P. M., Bachman, J. G., & Schulenberg, J. E., (2023). Monitoring the Future national survey results on drug use, 1975–2022: Secondary school students. Monitoring the Future Monograph Series. Ann Arbor, MI: Institute for Social Research, University of Michigan. Available at https://monitoringthefuture.org/results/publications/ monographs/

Mikolajczak, M., Gross, J. J., Stinglhamber, F., Norberg, A. L., & Roskam, I. (2020). Is parental burnout distinct from job burnout and depressive symptomatology? *Clinical Psychological Science*. http://doi.org/10.1177/2167702620917447

Milesi, P., Süssenbach, P., Bohner, G., & Megías, J. L. (2020). The interplay of modern myths about sexual aggression and moral foundations in the blaming of rape victims. *European Journal of Social Psychology*, 50(1), 111–123.

Miller, A. L., Lo, S. L., Bauer, K. W., & Fredericks, E. M. (2020) Developmentally informed behaviour change techniques to enhance self-regulation in a health promotion context: A conceptual review. *Health Psychology Review*, 14(1), 16–31.

Millwood, I. Y., Walters, R. G., Mei, X. W., Guo, Y., Yang, L., Bian, Z., ... Zhou, G. (2019). Conventional and genetic evidence on alcohol and vascular disease aetiology: A prospective study of 500 000 men and women in China. *The Lancet*, 393(10183), 1831–1842. https://doi.org/10.1016/S0140-6736(18)31772-0

Milne-Ives, M., Lam, C., De Cock, C., Van Velthoven, M. H., & Meinert, E. (2020). Mobile apps for health behavior change in physical activity, diet, drug and alcohol use, and mental health: Systematic review. *JMIR MHealth and UHealth,* 8(3), e17046.

Milner, A. N., & Baker, E. H. (2017). Athletic participation and intimate partner violence victimization: Investigating sport involvement, self-esteem, and abuse patterns for women and men. *Journal of Interpersonal Violence*, 32(2), 268–289.

Miralles, I., Granell, C., Díaz-Sanahuja, L., Van Woensel, W., Bretón-López, J., Mira, A., ... Casteleyn, S. (2020). Smartphone apps for the treatment of mental disorders: Systematic review. *JMIR mHealth and uHealth,* 8(4), e14897. https://doi.org/10.2196/14897

Miron, O., Yu, K.-H., Wilf-Miron, R., & Kohane, I. S. (2019). Suicide rates among adolescents and young adults in the United States, 2000–2017. *Journal of the American Medical Association*, 321, 2362–2364. https://doi.org/10.1001/jama.2019.5054

Mitchell, E., Alese, O. B., Yates, C., Rivers, B. M., Blackstock, W., Newman, L., ... Harris, A. E. (2022). Cancer healthcare disparities among African Americans in the United States. *Journal of the National Medical Association,* 114(3), 236–250. https://doi.org/10.1016/j.jnma.2022.01.004

Mitchell, J. E., & Peterson, C. B. (2020). Anorexia nervosa. *The New England Journal of Medicine*, 382, 1343–1351.

Mitchell, J. E., Roerig, J., & Steffen, K. (2013). Biological therapies for eating disorders. *International Journal of Eating Disorders*, 46, 470–477.

Miya, N., Uratani, A., Chikamoto, K., Naito, Y., Terao, K., Yoshikawa, Y., & Yasui, H. (2020). Effects of exercise on biological trace element concentrations and selenoprotein P expression in rats with fructose-induced glucose intolerance. *Journal of Clinical Biochemistry and Nutrition*, 66(2), 124–131.

Modzelewska, D., Bellocco, R., Elfvin, A., Brantsæter, A. L., Meltzer, H. M., Jacobsson, B., & Sengpiel, V. (2019). Caffeine exposure during pregnancy, small for gestational age birth and neonatal outcome – Results from the Norwegian Mother and Child Cohort Study. *BMC Pregnancy and Childbirth*, 19(1), 80. https://doi.org/10.1186/s12884-019-2215-9

Moeller, R. W., Seehuus, M., Wahl, L., & Gratch, I. (2020). Use of PrEP, sexual behaviors and mental health correlates in a sample of gay, bisexual and other men who have sex with men. *Journal of Gay & Lesbian Mental Health*, 24(1), 94–111.

Molina, N., Viola, M., Rogers, M., Ouyang, D., Gang, J., Derry, H., & Prigerson, H. G. (2019). Suicidal ideation in bereavement: A systematic review. *Behavioral Sciences*, 9, 53.

Moncrieff, J., Cooper, R. E., Stockmann, T., Amendola, S., Hengartner, M. P., & Horowitz, M. A. (2022). The serotonin theory of depression: A systematic umbrella review of the evidence. *Molecular Psychiatry*. https://doi.org/10.1038/s41380-022-01661-0

Montanaro, D. (2020, March 17). Poll: Americans don't trust what they're hearing from Trump on coronavirus. https://www.npr.org/2020/03/17/816680033/poll-americans-dont-trust-what-they-re-hearing-from-trump-on-coronavirus

Montanaro, E. A., Kershaw, T. S., & Bryan, A. D. (2018). Dismantling the theory of planned behavior: Evaluating the relative effectiveness of attempts to uniquely change attitudes, norms, and perceived behavioral control. *Journal of Behavioral Medicine,* 41(6), 757–770. https://doi.org/10.1007/s10865-018-9923-x

Montano, D. E., & Kasprzyk, D. (2015). Theory of reasoned action, theory of planned behavior, and the integrated behavioral model. In K. Glanz, B. K. Rimer, & K. Viswanath (Eds.), *Health behavior: Theory, research and practice* (pp. 95–124). Jossey-Bass.

Monteiro, F. C., Schuch, F. B., Deslandes, A. C., Vancampfort, D., Mosqueiro, B. P., Messinger, M. F., ... de Almeida Fleck, M. P. (2020). Perceived barriers, benefits and correlates of physical activity in outpatients with major depressive disorder: A study from Brazil. *Psychiatry Research*, 112751.

Moon, J. R., Kondo, N., Glymour, M. M., & Subramanian, S. V. (2011). Widowhood and mortality: A meta-analysis. *PLoS One*, 6(8), e23465.

Moon, Z., Moss-Morris, R., Hunter, M. S., Norton, S., & Hughes, L. D. (2019). Nonadherence to tamoxifen in breast cancer survivors: A 12-month longitudinal analysis. *Health Psychology*, 38, 888–899.

Moore, A. S. (2014, November 2). This is your brain on drugs. *New York Times*, Education Life Section, p. 17.

Moos, R. H., & Moos, B. S. (2004). Long-term influence of duration and frequency of participation in alcoholics anonymous on individuals with alcohol use disorders. *Journal of Consulting and Clinical Psychology*, 72, 81–90.

Morales S., Zeytinoglu S., Lorenzo N. E., Chronis-Tuscano A., Degnan K. A., Almas A. N., ... Fox N. A. (2022). Which anxious adolescents were most affected by the COVID-19 pandemic? *Clinical Psychological Science,* 10(6), 1044–1059. https://doi.org/10.1177/21677026211059524

Moreira, A. L. R., Van Meter, A., Genzlinger, J., & Youngstrom, E. A. (2017). Review and meta-analysis of epidemiologic studies of adult bipolar disorder. *The Journal of Clinical Psychiatry*, 78, e1259–e1269. https://doi.org/10.4088/JCP.16r11165

Moreno-Agostino, D., Fisher, H. L., Goodman, A., Hatch, S. L., Morgan, C., Richards, M., ... Ploubidis, G. B. (2023). Long-term psychological distress trajectories and the COVID-19 pandemic in three British birth cohorts: A multi-cohort study. *PLoS Medicine,* 20(4), e1004145. https://doi.org/10.1371/journal.pmed.1004145

Moreno-Rius, J. (2019). The cerebellum, THC, and cannabis addiction: Findings from animal and human studies. *The Cerebellum*, 18(3), 593–604.

Morgan, N., Irwin, M. R., Chung, M., & Wang, C. (2014). The effects of mind-body therapies on the immune system: Meta-analysis. *PLoS One*, 9(7), E100903.

Moriguchi, S., Yamada, M., Takano, H., Nagashima, T., Takahata, K., ... Suhara, T. (2017). Norepinephrine transporter in major depressive disorder: A PET study. *American Journal of Psychiatry*, 174, 36–41.

Mouilso, E. R., & Wilson, L. F. (2019). Alcohol and sexual assault. In W. T. O'Donohue & P. A. Schewe (Eds.), *Handbook of sexual assault and sexual assault prevention* (pp. 195–209). Springer.

Moy, E., Barrett, M., Coffey, R., Hines, A. L., & Newman-Toker, D. E. (2015). Missed diagnoses of acute myocardial infarction in the emergency department: Variation by patient and facility characteristics. *Diagnosis*, 2(1), 29–40.

Mueller, P. S. (2018, July 3). Can text messages improve glycemic control? *NEJM Journal Watch*. https://www.jwatch.org/na46803/2018/07/03/can-text-messages-improve-glycemic-control

Mueller, P. S. (2023, November 22). Gender gap in U.S. life expectancy continues to widen. *Journal Watch*. www.jwatch.org. https://doi.org/10.1056/nejm-jw.NA56830

Mulhall, J. P., Giraldi, A., Hackett, G., Hellstrom, W. J., Jannini, E. A., Rubio-Aurioles, E., ... Hassan, T. A. (2018). The 2018 revision to the process of care model for management of erectile dysfunction. *The Journal of Sexual Medicine*, 15(10), 1434–1445.

Mulugeta, A., Zhou, A., King, C., & Hyppönen, E. (2019). Association between major depressive disorder and multiple disease outcomes: A phenome-wide Mendelian randomisation study in the UK Biobank. *Molecular Psychiatry*. https://doi.org/10.1038/s41380-019-0486-1

Mundle, R., Afenya, E. & Agarwal, N. (2021). The effectiveness of psychological intervention for depression, anxiety, and distress in prostate cancer: A systematic review of literature. *Prostate Cancer Prostatic Disease,* 24, 674–687 (2021). https://doi.org/10.1038/s41391-021-00342-3

Murphy, M. E., Liu, S., Yao, S., Huo, D., Liu, Q., Dolfi, S. C., ... Ogundiran, T. O. (2017). A functionally significant SNP in TP53 and breast cancer risk in African-American women. *NPJ Breast Cancer*, 3(1), 1–4.

Murphy, M. J., Newby, J. M., Butow, P., Loughnan, S. A., Joubert, A. E., Kirsten, L., ... Andrews, G. (2020). Randomised controlled trial of internet-delivered cognitive behaviour therapy for clinical depression and/or anxiety in cancer survivors (iCanADAPT Early). *Psycho-Oncology*, 29(1), 76–85.

Murphy, M. Z., Jackson, T. P., & Mishra, P. (2022). Chronic pain. In D. A. Edwards, P. Gulur, & C. M. Sobey (Eds.), *Hospitalized chronic pain patient* (pp. 11–14). Springer, Cham.

Murray, R. M., Bhavsar, V., Tripoli, G., & Howes, O. (2017). 30 Years on: How the neurodevelopmental hypothesis of schizophrenia morphed into the developmental risk factor model of psychosis. *Schizophrenia Bulletin*, 43(6), 1190–1196.

Murray, S. B., Brown, T. A., Lavender, J. M., Nagata, J. M., & Keel, P. K. (2020). The evolving nature of weight dissatisfaction and eating behaviors among men: Secular trends among college men across four decades. *Journal of Abnormal Psychology,* 129(8), 824–830. https://doi.org/10.1037/abn0000587

Mursa, R., Patterson, C., & Halcomb, E. (2022). Men's help-seeking and engagement with general practice: An integrative review. *Journal of Advanced Nursing,* 78(7), 1938–1953. https://doi.org/10.1111/jan.15240

Musliner, K. L., Mortensen, P. B., McGrath, J. J., Suppli, N. P., Hougaard, D. M., Bybjerg-Grauholm, J., ... Agerbo, E. (2019). Association of polygenic liabilities for major depression, bipolar disorder, and schizophrenia with risk for depression in the Danish population. *JAMA Psychiatry*.

Mustaquium, D., Jones, C M., & Compton, W. M. (2021). Trends and correlates of cocaine use among adults in the United States, 2006-2019 | SAMHDA. (2021, April 1). https://www.datafiles.samhsa.gov/publication/trends-and-correlates-cocaine-use-among-adults-united-states-2006-2019

Naar, S., Czajkowski, S. M., & Spring, B. (2018). Innovative study designs and methods for optimizing and implementing behavioral interventions to improve health. *Health Psychology*, 37, 1081–1091.

Nabalamba, A., & Millar, W. J. (2007). Going to the doctor. *Rapports Sur La Sante [Health Reports]*, 18(1), 23–35. https://pubmed.ncbi.nlm.nih.gov/17441441/

Nabalamba, A., & Millar, W. J. (2020). Going to the doctor. *Health Reports*, 18(1). https://pubmed.ncbi.nlm.nih.gov/17441441/

Nadimpalli, S. B., Cleland, C. M., Hutchinson, M. K., Islam, N., Barnes, L. L., & Van Devanter, N. (2016). The association between discrimination and the health of Sikh Asian Indians. *Health Psychology*, 35, 351–355.

Naef, R., Peng-Keller, S., Rettke, H., Rufer, M., & Petry, H. (2020). Hospital-based bereavement care provision: A cross-sectional survey with health professionals. *Palliative Medicine*, 34, 547–552.

Naimi, T. S., Stadtmueller, L. A., Chikritzhs, T., Stockwell, T., Zhao, J., Britton, A., ... Sherk, A. (2019). Alcohol, age, and mortality: Estimating selection bias due to premature death. *Journal of Studies on Alcohol & Drugs*, 80(1). https://doi.org/10.15288/jsad.2019.80.63

Nappi, R. E., Chedraui, P., Lambrinoudaki, I., & Simoncini, T. (2022). Menopause: a cardiometabolic transition. *The Lancet. Diabetes & Endocrinology*, 10(6), 442–456. https://doi.org/10.1016/s2213-8587(22)00076-6

Narayanan, M. V., & Shimozaki, K. K. (2016, August 31). Months after first outbreak, campus rid of mumps. Thecrimson.Com. https://www.thecrimson.com/article/2016/9/1/mumps-gone-not-forgotten/

Nashin, R. L. (2015). Estimates of pain severity in adults. *Journal of Pain*, 8, 969–780.

National Cancer Institute (NCI). (2019a). Annual report to the nation: Overall cancer mortality continues to decline; Special section on adults ages 20 to 49 shows higher cancer incidence and mortality for women than men. https://www.cancer.gov/news-events/press-releases/2019/annual-report-nation-2019

National Cancer Institute (NCI). (2019b). Annual Report to the Nation on the Status of Cancer. https://seer.cancer.gov/report_to_nation/

National Cancer Institute (NCI). (2020a). Cancer stat facts: Common cancer sites. https://seer.cancer.gov/statfacts/html/common.html

National Cancer Institute (NCI). (2020b). Melanoma of the Skin-Cancer Stat Facts. https://seer.cancer.gov/statfacts/html/melan.html

National Cancer Institute (NCI). (2023). Cancer stat facts: Common cancer sites. https://seer.cancer.gov/statfacts/html/common.html

National Center for Complementary and Integrative Health (NCCIH). (2015). Complementary and alternative medicine: What people aged 50 and older discuss with their health care providers.

National Center for Complementary and Integrative Health (NCCIH). (2017). Complementary and alternative medicine. Introduction.

National Center for Complementary and Integrative Health (NCCIH). (2018a). Complementary, alternative, or integrative health: What's in a name? NCCIH Pub No. D347.

National Center for Education Statistics (NCES). (2023). Criminal incidents at postsecondary institutions. Condition of education. U.S. Department of Education, Institute of Education Sciences. https://nces.ed.gov/programs/coe/indicator/a21.

National Center for Environmental Health. (2020). Asthma surveillance data. https://www.cdc.gov/asthma/asthmadata.htm

National Center for Health Statistics (NCHS). (2023). National Health Interview Survey. Interactive summary health statistics for adults. NHIS-Detailed Race and Ethnicity Summary Health Statistics. https://wwwn.cdc.gov/NHISDataQueryTool/SHS_adult3yr/index.html

National Heart, Lung, and Blood Institute, National Institutes of Health (NHLBI). (2005a). Your guide to lowering high blood pressure. www.nhlbi.nih.gov/hbp/index.html

National Heart Lung and Blood Institute, National Institutes of Health. (2011). *National Cholesterol Education Program*. http://www.nhlbi.nih.gov/about/ncep/index.htm

National Heart, Lung, and Blood Institute, National Institutes of Health (NHLBI). (2019b). Asthma. https://www.nhlbi.nih.gov/health-topics/asthma

National Highway Traffic Safety Administration. (2020). Seat belts. https://www.nhtsa.gov/risky-driving/seat-belts

National Highway Traffic Safety Administration (NHTSA). (2023a, April 20). NHTSA estimates for 2022 show roadway fatalities remain flat after two years of dramatic increases. https://www.nhtsa.gov/press-releases/traffic-crash-death-estimates-2022#:~:text=NHTSA%20Estimates%20for%202022%20Show,Two%20Years%20of%20Dramatic%20Increases&text=The%20National%20Highway%20Traffic%20Safety,in%20motor%20vehicle%20traffic%20crashes.

National Highway Traffic Safety Administration (NHTSA). (2023b). Drowsy driving. https://www.nhtsa.gov/risky-driving/drowsy-driving

National Institute of Diabetes and Digestive and Kidney Diseases (NIDDK). (2019). Changing your habits for better health. hniddk.nih.gov/health-information/diet-nutrition/changing-habits-better-health

National Institute of Mental Health (NIMH) (2023). Mental illness. https://www.nimh.nih.gov/health/statistics/mental-illness

National Institute of Mental Health (NIMH). (2023b). Warning signs of suicide. https://www.nimh.nih.gov/sites/default/files/documents/health/publications/warning-signs-of-suicide/Warning_Signs_of_Suicide.pdf

National Institute of Neurological Disorders and Stroke, National Institutes of Health. (2018). Chronic pain: In depth. U.S. Department of Health & Human Services, National Institutes of Health, USA.gov. https://nccih.nih.gov/health/pain/chronic.htm

National Institute on Aging, National Institutes of Health (NIA). (2018). What is a heart attack? https://www.nia.nih.gov/health/what-heart-attack

National Institute on Aging (NIA). (2023, January 6). NIA statement on report of lecanemab reducing cognitive decline in Alzheimer's clinical trial. https://www.nia.nih.gov/news/nia-statement-report-lecanemab-reducing-cognitive-decline-alzheimers-clinical-trial

National Institute on Alcohol Abuse and Alcoholism (NIAAA). (2018). Alcohol facts and statistics.

National Institute on Alcohol Abuse and Alcoholism (NIAAA). (2020). Alcohol facts and statistics. https://www.niaaa.nih.gov/publications/brochures-and-fact-sheets/alcohol-facts-and-statistics

National Institute on Alcohol Abuse and Alcoholism (NIAAA). (2023, April). Understanding alcohol use disorder. https://www.niaaa.nih.gov/publications/brochures-and-fact-sheets/understanding-alcohol-use-disorder

National Institute on Drug Abuse. (2020). Methamphetamine. https://www.drugabuse.gov/drugs-abuse/methamphetamine

National Institute on Drug Abuse (NIDA). (2023). Drug overdose death rates. https://nida.nih.gov/research-topics/trends-statistics/overdose-death-rates

National Institutes of Health. (2014). Cold, flu, or allergy? *News in Health*. https://newsinhealth.nih.gov/2014/10/cold-flu-or-allergy

National Institutes of Health (NIH) (2022). Stress and cancer. https://www.cancer.gov/about-cancer/coping/feelings/stress-fact-sheet

National Institutes of Health (NIH) News Release. (2020, January 16). Patients with newly diagnosed musculoskeletal pain are prescribed opioids more often than recommended.

National Safety Council. (2023a). Seat belts - data details. https://injuryfacts.nsc.org/motor-vehicle/occupant-protection/seat-belts/data-details/

National Safety Council. (2023b). Gun deaths in America, 2022. https://injuryfacts.nsc.org/home-and-community/safety-topics/guns/

National Sexual Violence Resource Center. (2018). Sexual assault in the United States. https://www.nsvrc.org/statistics

National Sleep Foundation. (2018). National Sleep Foundation's 2018 Sleep in America poll.

National Sleep Foundation (2021). *Sleep in America® Polls*. https://www.thensf.org/sleep-in-america-polls/

Naumova, I., & Castelo-Branco, C. (2018). Current treatment options for postmenopausal vaginal atrophy. *International Journal of Women's Health*, 10, 387–395.

Neff, H. A., Kellar-Guenther, Y., Jankowski, C. M., Worthington, C., McCandless, S. A., Jones, J., & Erlandson, K. M. (2019). Turning disability into ability: Barriers and facilitators to initiating and maintaining exercise among older men living with HIV. *AIDS Care*, 31(2), 260–264.

Neumann, M. S., Plant, A., Margolis, A. D., Borkowf, C. B., Malotte, C. K., Rietmeijer, C. A., ... Klausner, J. D. (2018). Effects of a brief video intervention on treatment initiation and adherence among patients attending human immunodeficiency virus treatment clinics. *PLoS One*, 13(10), 1–16.

Neumer, A., Schweizer T, Bogdanić, V., Boecker, L., & Loschelder, D. D. (2022). How health message framing and targets affect distancing during the COVID-19 pandemic. *Health Psychology: Official Journal of the Division of Health Psychology, American Psychological Association*, 41(9). https://doi.org/10.1037/hea0001203

Newport, F. (2018). In U.S., estimate of LGBT population rises to 4.5%. Gallup Organization. https://news.gallup.com/poll/234863/estimate-lgbt-population-rises.aspx

Nezu, A. M., Nezu, C. M., & D'Zurilla, T. (2013). *Problem-solving therapy: A treatment manual*. Springer Publishing Company.

Nicholas, M. K. (2022). The biopsychosocial model of pain 40 years on: Time for a reappraisal? *Pain*, 163(S1), S3–S14. https://doi.org/10.1097/j.pain.0000000000002654

Nie, X., Kitaoka, S., Tanaka, L., Segi-Nishida, E., Imoto, Y., Ogawa, A., ... Narumiya, S. (2018). The innate immune receptors TLR2/4 mediate repeated social defeat stress-induced social avoidance through prefrontal microglial activation. *Neuron*, 99, 464–479.

Nigg, C. R., & Harmon, B. (2018). The sedentariness epidemic—Demographic considerations. In S. Razon & M. L. Sachs (Eds.), *Applied exercise psychology: The challenging journey from motivation to adherence* (pp. 5–14). Routledge.

Nigol, S. H., & Di Benedetto, M. (2020). The relationship between mindfulness facets, depression, pain severity and pain interference. *Psychology, Health & Medicine*, 25(1), 53–63.

Niknejad, B., Boiler, R., Henderson, C. R., Jr., Delgado, D., Kozlov, E., Löckenhoff, C. E., & Reid, M. D. (2018). Association between psychological interventions and chronic pain outcomes in older adults: A systematic review and meta-analysis. *JAMA Internal Medicine*, 178, 830–839.

Niloy, N., Hediyal, T. A., Vichitra, C., Sonali, S., Chidambaram, S. B., Gorantla, V. R., & Mahalakshmi, A. M. (2023). Effect of cannabis on memory consolidation, learning and retrieval and its current legal status in India: *A review. Biomolecules*, 13(1), 162. https://doi.org/10.3390/biom13010162

Noble, N., Paul, C., Turon, H., & Oldmeadow, C. (2015). Which modifiable health risk behaviours are related? A systematic review of the clustering of smoking, nutrition, alcohol and physical activity ('SNAP') health risk factors. *Preventive Medicine*, 81, 16–41.

Nokia, M. S., Lensu, S., Ahtiainen, J. P., Johansson, P. P., Koch, L. G., Britton, S. L., & Kainulainen, H. (2016). Physical exercise increases adult hippocampal neurogenesis in male rats provided it is aerobic and sustained. *The Journal of Physiology*, 594(7), 1855–1873.

Nolen-Hoeksema, S. (2008). It is not what you have; it is what you do with it: Support for Addis's gendered responding framework. *Clinical Psychology: Science and Practice*, 15, 178–181.

Nolen-Hoeksema, S. (2012). Emotion regulation and psychopathology: The role of gender. *Annual Review of Clinical Psychology*, 8, 161–187.

Nolt, K. L. (2018). Persons with medical conditions. In S. Razon & M. L. Sachs (Eds.), *Applied exercise psychology: The challenging journey from motivation to adherence* (pp. 432–444). Routledge.

North American Menopause Society. (2013). Management of symptomatic vulvovaginal atrophy: 2013 position statement of the North American Menopause Society. *Menopause: The Journal of the North American Menopause Society*, 20(9), 888–902.

North, C. S., Oliver, J. and Pandya, A. (2012) Examining a comprehensive model of disaster-related posttraumatic stress disorder in systematically studied survivors of 10 disasters. *American Journal of Public Health*, 102, e40–e48. http://dx.doi.org/10.2105/ajph.2012.300689

Norton, L. H., Norton, K. I., & Lewis, N. R. (2015). Adherence, compliance, and health risk factor changes following short-term physical activity interventions. *BioMed Research International*, 12, 1-9604-15. https://doi.org/10.1155/2015/929782

Novaco, R. W. (2017). Cognitive-behavioral factors and anger in the occurrence of aggression and violence. In P. Sturmey (Ed.), *The Wiley handbook of violence and aggression*. Wiley.

Nova, E., San Mauro-Martín, I., Díaz-Prieto, L. E., & Marcos, A. (2019). Wine and beer within a moderate alcohol intake is associated with higher levels of HDL-c and adiponectin. *Nutrition Research*, 63, 42–50.

Nyamayaro, P., Bere, T., Magidson, J. F., Simms, V., O'Cleirigh, C., Chibanda, D., & Abas, M. (2020). A task-shifting problem-solving therapy intervention for depression and barriers to antiretroviral therapy adherence for people living with HIV in Zimbabwe: Case series. *Cognitive and Behavioral Practice*, 27(1), 84–92.

O'Carroll, R. E. O. (2020). Self-regulation interventions – What do we know and where should we go? *Health Psychology Review*, 14(1), 159–164.

O'Connor, D. B., Thayer, J. F., & Vedhara, K. (2021). Stress and health: A review of psychobiological processes. *Annual Review of Psychology*, 72(1), 663–688.

O'Connor, E. A., Perdue, L. A., Coppola, E. L., Henninger, M. L., Thomas, R. G., & Gaynes, B. N. (2023). Depression and suicide risk screening. *The Journal of the American Medical Association*, 329(23), 2068. https://doi.org/10.1001/jama.2023.7787

O'Connor, M. F. (2019). Grief: A brief history of research on how body, mind, and brain adapt. *Psychosomatic Medicine*, 81, 731–738.

O'Connor, P. J., Pronk, N. P., Tan, A., & Whitebird, R. R. (2005). Characteristics of adults who use prayer as an alternative therapy. *American Journal of Health Promotion*, 19(5), 369–375.

O'Dea, C. J., Rapp, S., Brand, O. R., & Greco-Henderson, D. (2022). "Act like a real man!" A novel examination of how socializing others to masculine honor-based norms bolsters men's reputations. *Psychology of Men & Masculinities*, 23(3), 299–308.

Odedina, F. T., Dagne, G. A., Pressey, S., Odedina, O., Emanuel, F., Scrivens, J., ... Larose-Pierre, M. (2011). Prostate cancer health and cultural beliefs of black men: The Florida Prostate Cancer Disparity Project. *Infectious Agents and Cancer*, 6(S2). https://doi.org/10.1186/1750-9378-6-s2-s10

O'Donohue, W. T. (2019). Reporting sexual assault: Process and barriers victims experience. In W. T. O'Donohue & P. A. Schewe (Eds.), *Handbook of sexual assault and sexual assault prevention* (pp. 591–608). Springer.

O'Dwyer, M. C. T., Dune, T., Bidewell, J., & Liamputtong, P. (2019). Critiquing the Health Belief Model and sexual risk behaviours among adolescents: A narrative review of familial and peer influence. *International Journal of Social Science Studies*, 7(6), 62–70.

Oerlemans, W. G. M., & Bakker, A. B. (2014). Why extraverts are happier: A day reconstruction study. *Journal of Research in Personality*, 50, 11–22.

Office of Minority Health. (2022). *Heart disease and African Americans*. The Office of Minority Health. U.S. Department of Health and Human Services. https://minorityhealth.hhs.gov/omh/browse.aspx?lvl=4&lvlid=19

Ogden, C. L., Fryar, C. D., Martin, C. B., Freedman, D. S., Carroll, M. D., Gu, Q., ... Hales, C. M. (2020). Trends in obesity prevalence by race and Hispanic origin—1999–2000 to 2017–2018. *JAMA*, 324(12), 1208. https://doi.org/10.1001/jama.2020.14590

Ohst, B., & Tuschen-Caffier, B. (2018). Catastrophic misinterpretation of bodily sensations and external events in panic disorder, other anxiety disorders, and healthy subjects: A systematic review and meta-analysis. *PLoS One*, 13, e0194493.

Okoli, A., Hanlon, E. C., & Brady, M. J. (2021). The relationship between sleep, obesity, and metabolic health in adolescents–A review. *Current Opinion in Endocrine and Metabolic Research*, 17, 15–19. https://doi.org/10.1016/j.coemr.2020.10.007

Okubo, H., Miyake, Y., Tanaka, K., Sasaki, S., & Hirota, Y. (2015). Maternal total caffeine intake, mainly from Japanese and Chinese tea, during pregnancy was associated with risk of preterm birth: The Osaka Maternal and Child Health Study. *Nutrition Research*, 35(4), 309–316.

Olaru, G., Laukka, E. J., Dekhtyar, S., Sarwary, A., & Brehmer, Y. (2023). Association between personality traits, leisure activities, and cognitive levels and decline across 12 years in older adults. *Psychology and Aging*, 38(4), 277–290. https://doi.org/10.1037/pag0000743

O'Leary, D., Suri, G., & Gross, J. J. (2018). Reducing behavioural risk factors for cancer: An affect regulation perspective. *Psychology & Health*, 33, 17–39.

Olfson, M., Blanco, C., & Marcus, S. C. (2016). Treatment of adult depression in the United States. *Journal of the American Medical Association Internal Medicine*, 176, 1482–1491.

Olfson, M., Gameroff, M. J., Marcus, S. C., Greenberg, T., & Shaffer, D. (2005). Emergency treatment of young people following deliberate self-harm. *Archives of General Psychiatry*, 62, 1122–1128.

O'Loughlin, J., Casanova, F., Jones, S. E., Hagenaars, S. P., Beaumont, R. N., Freathy, R. M., ... Tyrrell, J. (2021). Using Mendelian randomisation methods to understand whether diurnal preference is causally related to mental health. *Molecular Psychiatry*. https://doi.org/10.1038/s41380-021-01157-3

Omary, A. (2021). National prevalence rates of suicidal ideation and suicide attempts among adults with and without depression. *Journal of Nervous & Mental Disease*, 209(5), 378–385. https://doi.org/10.1097/nmd.0000000000001309

Onyeador, I. N., Wittlin, N. M., Burke, S. E., Dovidio, J. F., Perry, S. P., Hardeman, R. R., ... van Ryn, M. (2020). The value of interracial contact for reducing anti-black bias among non-black physicians: A Cognitive Habits and Growth Evaluation (CHANGE) Study report. *Psychological Science*, 31, 18–30.

Opel, N., Martin, S., Meinert, S., Redlich, R., Enneking, V., Richter, M., ... Repple, J. (2019). White matter microstructure mediates the association between physical fitness and cognition in healthy, young adults. *Scientific Reports*, 9(1), 1–9.

Ordaz, D. L., Schaefer, L. M., Choquette, E., Schueler, J., Wallace, L., & Thompson, J. K. (2018). Thinness pressures in ethnically diverse college women in the United States. *Body Image*, 24, 1–4.

Orrow, G., Kinmonth, A. L., Sanderson, S., & Sutton, S. (2012). Effectiveness of physical activity promotion based in primary care. *British Medical Journal*, 344, e1389.

Ortega, R. P. (2021, October 28). Poor sleep takes a heavy toll on communities of color. Can scientists help? Science.org. https://www.science.org/content/article/poor-sleep-takes-heavy-toll-communities-color-can-scientists-help

Orth-Gomér, K., Wamala, S. P., Horsten, M., Schenck-Gustafsson, K., Schneiderman, N., & Mittleman, M. A. K. (2000). Marital stress worsens prognosis in women with coronary heart disease: The Stockholm Female Coronary Risk Study. *Journal of the American Medical Association*, 284, 3008–3014.

Oshri, A., Cui, Z., Carvalho, C., & Liu, S. (2022a). Is perceived stress linked to enhanced cognitive functioning and reduced risk for psychopathology? Testing the hormesis hypothesis. *Psychiatry Research*, 314, 114644. https://doi.org/10.1016/j.psychres.2022.114644

Oshri, A., Cui, Z., Owens, M. M., Carvalho, C. A., & Sweet, L. (2022b). Low-to-moderate level of perceived stress strengthens working memory: Testing the hormesis hypothesis through neural activation. *Neuropsychologia*, 176,

Ouimette, P. C., Finney, J. W., & Moos, R. H. (1997). Twelve-step and cognitive-behavioral treatment for substance abuse. *Journal of Consulting and Clinical Psychology*, 65, 230–240.

Overmier, J. B., & Seligman, M. E. P. (1967). Effects of inescapable shock upon subsequent escape and avoidance learning. *Journal of Comparative and Physiological Psychology*, 63, 23–33.

Overstreet, N. M., Quinn, D. M., & Agocha, V. B. (2010). Beyond thinness: The influence of a curvaceous body ideal on body dissatisfaction in black and white women. *Sex Roles*, 63, 91–103.

Padilla, M., Frazier, E. L., Carree, T., Luke Shouse, R., & Fagan, J. (2020). Mental health, substance use and HIV risk behaviors among HIV-positive adults who experienced homelessness in the United States–Medical Monitoring Project, 2009–2015. *AIDS Care*, 32(5), 594–599.

Padovano, H. T., Janssen, T., Sokolovsky, A., & Jackson, K. M. (2020). The altered course of learning: How alcohol outcome expectancies are shaped by first drinking experiences. *Psychological Science*, 31(12), 1573–1584. https://doi.org/10.1177/0956797620959006

Padovano, H. T., Janssen, T., Sokolovsky, A., & Jackson, K. M. (2020). The altered course of learning: How alcohol outcome expectancies are shaped by first drinking experiences. *Psychological Science*, 31(12), 1573–1584. https://doi.org/10.1177/0956797620959006

Pai, M., & Carr, D. (2010). Do personality traits moderate the effect of late life spousal loss on psychological distress? *Journal of Health and Social Behavior*, 51, 183–199.

Palmer, A., Tomko, R. L., Squeglia, L. M., Gray, K. M., Carpenter, M. J., Smith, T. T., ... McClure, E. A. (2022). A pilot feasibility study of a behavioral intervention for nicotine vaping cessation among young adults delivered via telehealth. *Drug and Alcohol Dependence*, 232, 109311. https://doi.org/10.1016/j.drugalcdep.2022.109311

Palmer, C. (2020, March). Cognition and cancer treatment. *Monitor on Psychology*, 51(2), 42.

Palmer, T., Wallace, L., Pollock, K. G., Cuschieri, K., Robertson, C., Kavanagh, K., & Cruickshank, M. (2019). Prevalence of cervical disease at age 20 after immunization with bivalent HPV vaccine at age 12–13 in Scotland: Retrospective population study. *British Medical Journal*, 365, I1161.

Pan, P. M., Sato, J. R., Martinot, M.-L. P., Martinot, J.-L., Artiges, E., Penttilä, J., ... Ernst, T. M. (2022). Longitudinal trajectory of the link between ventral striatum and depression in adolescence. *American Journal of Psychiatry*, 179, 470–481

Panter-Brick, C., Wiley, K., Sancilio, A., Dajani, R., & Hadfield, K. (2019). C-reactive protein, Epstein-Barr virus, and cortisol trajectories in refugee and non-refugee youth: Links with stress, mental health, and cognitive function during a randomized controlled trial. *Brain, Behavior, and Immunity*. https://doi.org/10.1016/j.bbi.2019.02.015

Papadimitriou, N., Dimou, N., Tsilidis, K. K., Banbury, B., Martin, R. M., Lewis, S. J., ... Berndt, S. I. (2020). Physical activity and risks of breast and colorectal cancer: A Mendelian randomisation analysis. *Nature Communications*, 11(1), 1–10.

Pappalardo, A. A., & Martin, M. A. (2020). Asthma health disparities. In *Health disparities in allergic diseases* (pp. 145–179). Springer.

Paradis, V., Cossette, S., Frasure-Smith, N., Heppell, S., & Guertin, M.-C. (2010). The efficacy of a motivational nursing intervention based on the stages of change on self-care in heart failure patients. *Journal of Cardiovascular Nursing*, 25(2), 130–141. https://doi.org/10.1097/JCN.0b013e3181c52497

Parandeh, A., Ashtari, S., Rahimi-Bashar, F., Gohari-Moghadam, K., & Vahedian-Azimi, A. (2022). Prevalence of burnout among health care workers during coronavirus disease (COVID-19) pandemic: A systematic review and meta-analysis. *Professional Psychology: Research and Practice*, 53(6), 564–573. https://doi.org/10.1037/pro0000483

Pargament K. I. (1997). The psychology of religion and coping. *Theory, research, practice*. New York: Guilford Press, s. 21–33, 163–197.

Park, I., Díaz, J., Matsumoto, S., Iwayama, K., Nabekura, Y., Ogata, H., & Vogt, K. E. (2021). Exercise improves the quality of slow-wave sleep by increasing slow-wave stability. *Scientific Reports*, 11(1). https://doi.org/10.1038/s41598-021-83817-6

Park, J. H., Kim, D. J., & Kim, S. J. (2019). Is arthritis associated with suicidal ideation and quality of life? *Psychology, Health, & Medicine*, 24, 144–154.

Park, J. W., Howe, C. J., Dionne, L. A., Scarpaci, M. M., Needham, B. L., Sims, M., . . . Dulin, A. J. (2022). Social support, psychosocial risks, and cardiovascular health: Using harmonized data from the Jackson Heart Study, Mediators of Atherosclerosis in South Asians Living in America Study, and Multi-Ethnic Study of Atherosclerosis. *SSM - Population Health*, 20(101284), 101284. https://doi.org/10.1016/j.ssmph.2022.101284

Park, Y., & Shang, M. (2016). Effects of rehabilitation for pain relief in patients with rheumatoid arthritis: A systematic review. *Journal of Physical Therapy Science*, 28, 304–308.

Pasanen, T., Tolvanen, S., Heinonen, A., & Kujala, U. M. (2017). Exercise therapy for functional capacity in chronic diseases: An overview of meta-analyses of randomised controlled trials. *British Journal of Sports Medicine*, 51, 1459–1465.

Pascoe, E. A., Lattanner, M. R., & Richman, L. S. (2022). Meta-analysis of interpersonal discrimination and health-related behaviors. *Health Psychology*, 41(5), 319–331. https://doi.org/10.1037/hea0001147

Patel, A. V., Friedenreich, C. M., Moore, S. C., Hayes, S. C., Silver, J. K., Campbell, K. L., ... Matthews, C. E. (2019). American College of Sports Medicine roundtable report on physical activity, sedentary behavior, and cancer prevention and control. *Medicine & Science in Sports & Exercise*, 51, 2391–2402.

Pathak, V., Jena, B., & Kalra, S. (2013). Qualitative research. *Perspectives in Clinical Research*, 4(3), 192. https://doi.org/10.4103/2229-3485.115389

Patrick, M. E., Evans-Polce, R., Kloska, D. D., Maggs, J. L., & Lanza, S. T. (2017). Age-related changes in associations between reasons for alcohol use and high-intensity drinking across young adulthood. *Journal of Studies on Alcohol and Drugs*, 78(4), 558–570.

Paudel, B., Jeong, S.-Y., Martinez, C. P., Rickman, A., Haluck-Kangas, A., Bartom, E. T., ... Peter, M. E. (2024). Death induced by survival gene elimination (DISE) correlates with neurotoxicity in Alzheimer's disease and aging. *Nature Communications*, 15(1), 1–19. https://doi.org/10.1038/s41467-023-44465-8

Paulus, G. F., de Vaan, L. E., Verdam, F. J., Bouvy, N. D., Ambergen, T. A., & van Heurn, L. E. (2015). Bariatric surgery in morbidly obese adolescents: A systematic review and meta-analysis. *Obesity Surgery*, 25(5), 860–878.

Payne, J. L. (2021). The search for postpartum depression biomarkers. *The Psychiatric Times*. https://www.psychiatrictimes.com/view/postpartum-depression-biomarkers?utm_source=sfmc&utm_medium=email&utm_campaign=08142021_PT_NEU-21-PSV0105_eNL_Case%20Based%20TD%20Promo&eKey=amVmZm5ldmlkQGdtYWlsLmNvbQ==

Pearce, M., Garcia, L., Abbas, A., Strain, T., Schuch, F. B., Golubic, R., ... Woodcock, J. (2022). Association between physical activity and risk of depression. *JAMA Psychiatry*, 79(6), 550. https://doi.org/10.1001/jamapsychiatry.2022.0609

Pears, S., & Sutton, S. (2020). Effectiveness of acceptance and commitment therapy (ACT) interventions for promoting physical activity: A systematic review and meta-analysis. *Health Psychology Review*, 1–26. https://doi.org/10.1080/17437199.2020.1727759

Peltz, G., & Südhof, T. C. (2018). The neurobiology of opioid addiction and the potential for prevention strategies. *JAMA: The Journal of the American Medical Association*, 319(20), 2071–2072. https://doi.org/10.1001/jama.2018.3394

Penlington, C., Urbanek, M., & Barker, S. L. (2022). Psychological theories of pain. In T. Renton, T. (Ed.), Optimal pain management for the dental team. *BDJ clinician's guides*. Springer.

Pennebaker, J. W. (2018). Expressive writing in psychological science. *Perspectives on Psychological Science*, 13, 226–229.

Pennington, M. L., Carpenter, T. P., Synett, S. J., & Torres, V. A. (2018). The influence of exposure to natural disasters on depression and PTSD symptoms among firefighters. *Prehospital Disaster Medicine*, 33(1), 102–108.

Penninx, B. W. (2017). Depression and cardiovascular disease: Epidemiological evidence on their linking mechanisms. *Neuroscience & Biobehavioral Reviews*, 74, 277–286. https://doi.org/10.1016/j.neubiorev.2016.07.003

Percy, J. (2023, August 22). What people misunderstand about rape. *The New York Times*. https://www.nytimes.com/2023/08/22/magazine/immobility-rape-trauma-freeze.html

Perez, M. V., Mahaffey, K. W., Hedlin, H., Rumsfeld, J. S., Garcia, A., Ferris, T., ... Turakhia, M. P. (2019). Large-scale assessment of a smartwatch to identify atrial fibrillation. *New England Journal of Medicine*, 381(20), 1909–1917.

Perez-Tejada, J., Garmendia, L., Labaka, A., Vegas, O., Gómez-Lazaro, E., & Arregi, A. (2019). Active and passive coping strategies: Comparing psychological distress, cortisol, and proinflammatory cytokine levels in breast cancer survivors. *Clinical Journal of Oncology Nursing*, 23, 583–590.

Perkins, K. M., Munguia, N., Angulo, A., Anaya, C., Rios, R., & Velazquez, L. (2020). Evaluation of aquafitness exercise on the physical and mental health of older women: A pilot study. *Journal of Women & Aging*. https://doi.org/10.1080/08952841.2020.1730681

Perlis, R. H., Ostacher, M., Fava, M., Nierenberg, A. A., Sachs, G. S., & Rosenbaum, J. F. (2010). Assuring that double-blind is blind. *American Journal of Psychiatry*, 167, 2502–2552. https://doi.org/10.1176/appi.ajp.2009.09060820

Persson, S., Grogan, S., Dhingra, K., & Benn, Y. (2018). "It's bit of an eye opener"—A qualitative study of women's attitudes towards tanning, sun protection and a facial morphing intervention. *Psychology & Health*, 33, 381–397.

Peter G. Peterson Foundation (PGPF). (2019, July 22). How does the U.S. healthcare system compare to other countries? https://www.pgpf.org/blog/2019/07/how-does-the-us-healthcare-system-compare-to-other-countries

Peters, A. T., & Mutharasan, R. K. (2020). Aspirin for prevention of cardiovascular disease. *Journal of the American Medical Association*, 323, 676. https://doi.org/10.1001/jama.2019.18425

Petersen, L., Sørensen, T. I. A., Andersen, P. K., Mortensen, P. B., & Hawton, K. (2014). Genetic and familial environmental effects on suicide attempts: A study of Danish adoptees and their biological and adoptive siblings. *Journal of Affective Disorders*, 155, 273–277.

Petersen, R. C., Joyner, M. J., & Jack, C. R. (2020). Cardiorespiratory fitness and brain volumes. *Mayo Clinic Proceedings*, 95(1), 6–8.

Peterson Jr., A. V., & Marek, P. M. (2017). Late smoking relapse among adolescent quitters. *Addictive Behaviors*, 65, 171–173.

Petrosino, J. M., DiSilvestro, D., & Ziouzenkova, O. (2014). Aldehyde dehydrogenase 1A1: Friend or foe to female metabolism? *Nutrients*, 6(3), 950–973.

Petrosky, E., Bocchini Jr, J. A., Hariri, S., Chesson, H., Curtis, C. R., Saraiya, M., ... Markowitz, L. E. (2015). Use of 9-valent human papillomavirus (HPV) vaccine: Updated HPV vaccination recommendations of the advisory committee on immunization practices. *MMWR. Morbidity and Mortality Weekly Report*, 64(11), 300–304.

Petrosky, E., Harpaz, R., Fowler, K. A., Bohm, M. K., Helmick, C. G., Yuan, K., & Betz, C. J. (2018). Chronic pain among suicide decedents, 2003 to 2014: Findings from the National Violent Death Reporting System. *Annals of Internal Medicine*, 169, 448–455.

Pette, D. (2019). Sex-education and safe-sex compliance for gay men prescribed Truvada: An integrative literature review. *The Grace Peterson Nursing Research Colloquium*. https://via.library.depaul.edu/nursing-colloquium/2019/summer/6/

Pew Research Center. (2002, September 20). American psyche reeling from terror attacks. www.people-press.org/terrorist01rpt.htm

Phillips, L. A., & Gardner, B. (2016). Habitual exercise instigation (vs. execution) predicts healthy adults' exercise frequency. *Health Psychology*, 35(1), 69–77.

Piadeh Zavardehi, Z., Faramarzi, M., & Mirzaeian, B. (2018). Quality of mother–infant attachment after physiological birth. *International Journal of Pediatrics*, 6(7), 7929–7936.

Piana, R. (2019, July). Looking into the future of psychosocial oncology: A conversation with Jana Bolduan Lomax, PsyD. https://www.ascopost.com/issues/july-25-2019/looking-into-the-future-of-psychosocial-oncology/

Piano, M. R. (2017). Alcohol's effects on the cardiovascular system. *Alcohol Research*, 38, 219–241.

Picheta, R. (2020, January 15). Rich people are staying healthy for almost a decade longer than poor people. *CNN.com*.

Picker-Roesch, C., Schweiker, M., Kraus, T., & Lang, J. (2024). Psychosocial job characteristics comparison between work from home and work in the office: a study from the pandemic onwards. *Frontiers in Organizational Psychology*, 2, 1352526. https://doi.org/10.3389/forgp.2024.1352526

Pillai, K. G., Liang, Y. S., Thwaites, D., Sharma, P., & Goldsmith, R. (2019). Regulatory focus, nutrition involvement, and nutrition knowledge. *Appetite*, 137, 267–273.

Pinto, P. R., McIntyre, T., Almeida, A., & Araújo-Soares, V. (2011). The mediating role of pain catastrophizing in the relationship between pre-surgical anxiety and acute postsurgical pain after hysterectomy. *Pain*, 153, 218–226.

Pischon, T., Boeing, H., Hoffmann, K., Bergmann, M., Schulze, M. B., Overvad, K., ... Riboli, E. (2008). General and abdominal adiposity and risk of death in Europe. *New England Journal of Medicine*, 359, 2105–2120.

Plackett, R., Kaushal, A., Kassianos, A. P., Cross, A., Lewins, D., Sheringham, J., ... Von Wagner, C. (2020). Use of social media to promote cancer screening and early diagnosis: Scoping review. *Journal of Medical Internet Research,* 22(11), e21582. https://doi.org/10.2196/21582

Pleuhs, B., Quinn, K. G., Walsh, J. L., Petroll, A. E., & John, S. A. (2020). Health care provider barriers to HIV pre-exposure prophylaxis in the United States: A systematic review. *AIDS Patient Care and STDs,* 34(3), 111–123. https://doi.org/10.1089/apc.2019.0189

Plomin, B. (2018). *Blueprint: How DNA makes us who we are.* MIT Press.

Poh, M. Z., Loddenkemper, T., Reinsberger, C., Swenson, N. C., Goyal, S., Madsen, J. R., ... Picard, R. W. (2012). Autonomic changes with seizures correlate with postictal EEG suppression. *Neurology*, 78, 1868–1876.

Portenoy, R. K., & Dhingra, K. K. (2017). Overview of cancer pain syndromes. *UpToDate.* https://www.uptodate.com/contents/overview-of-cancer-pain-syndromes.

Portoghese, I., Galletta, M., Larkin, P., Sardo, S., Campagna, M., Finco, G., & D'Aloja, E. (2020). Compassion fatigue, watching patients suffering and emotional display rules among hospice professionals: A daily diary study. *BMC Palliative Care*, 19(1). https://doi.org/10.1186/s12904-020-0531-5

Pouget, E. R., Fong, C., & Rosenblum, A. (2018). Racial/ethnic differences in prevalence trends for heroin use and non-medical use of prescription opioids among entrants to opioid treatment programs, 2005–2016. *Substance Use & Misuse*, 53(2), 290–300.

Poulsen, S., Lunn, S., Daniel, S. I. F., Folke, S., Mathiesen, B. B., Katznelson, H., ... Fairburn, C. G. (2014). A randomized controlled trial of psychoanalytic psychotherapy or cognitive-behavioral therapy for bulimia nervosa. *American Journal of Psychiatry*, 171, 109–113.

Poulter, N. (2020). Lower blood pressure in South Asia? Trial evidence. *New England Journal of Medicine*, 382, 758–760.

Pouwer, F., & Speight, J. (2019). Diabetes mellitus, Type 2. In C. D. Llewellyn, S. Ayers, C. McManus, S. Newman, K. J. Petrie, T. A. Revenson, & J. Weinman (Eds.), *Cambridge handbook of psychology, health and medicine* (3rd ed., pp. 481–483). Cambridge University Press.

Powell, A. (2023, January 25). A laugh a day keeps the doctor away? *Harvard Gazette.* https://news.harvard.edu/gazette/story/2023/01/a-laugh-a-day-keeps-the-doctor-away/

Powell, D., Pacula, R. L., & Taylor, E. (2020). How increasing medical access to opioids contributes to the opioid epidemic: Evidence from medicare part D. *Journal of Health Economics.*

Power, R. A., & Pluess, M. (2015). Heritability estimates of the Big Five personality traits based on common genetic variants. *Translational Psychiatry*, 5(7), e604. https://doi.org/10.1038/tp.2015.96

Pradhan, D. S., Solomon-Lane, T. K., & Grober, M. S. (2015). Contextual modulation of social and endocrine correlates of fitness: Insights from the life history of a sex changing fish. *Frontiers in Neuroscience*, 9(8), https://doi.org/10.3389/fnins.2015.00008

Prichard, I., Kavanagh, E., Mulgrew, K. E., Lim, M. S. C., & Tiggemann, M. (2020). The effect of Instagram #fitspiration images on young women's mood, body image, and exercise behaviour. *Body Image,* 33, 1–6. https://doi.org/10.1016/j.bodyim.2020.02.002

Principal Causes of Death in the United States Registration Area, 1920: Census Bureau's Summary of Mortality Statistics. (1921). *Public Health Reports (1896–1970)*, 36(44), 2723–2725.

Prochaska, J. J., & Prochaska, J. O. (2011). A review of multiple health behavior change interventions for primary prevention. *American Journal of Lifestyle Medicine*, 5(3), 208–221. https://doi.org/10.1177/1559827610391883

Proctor, R. N. (2012). The history of the discovery of the cigarette–lung cancer link: Evidentiary traditions, corporate denial, global toll: Table 1. *Tobacco Control*, 21(2), 87–91. https://doi.org/10.1136/tobaccocontrol-2011-050338

Puhlmann, L. M. C., Vrtička, P., Linz, R., Stalder, T., Kirschbaum, C., Engert, V., & Singer, T. (2021). Contemplative mental training reduces hair glucocorticoid levels in a randomized clinical trial. *Psychosomatic Medicine,* 83(8), 894–905. https://doi.org/10.1097/psy.0000000000000970

Purkis, H. M., Lester, K. J., & Field, A. P. (2011). But what about the Empress of Racnoss? The allocation of attention to spiders and doctor who in a visual search task is predicted by fear and expertise. *Emotion*, 11, 1484–1488.

Puterman, E., Pauly, T., Ruissen, G., Nelson, B., & Faulkner, G. (2021). Move more, move better: A narrative review of wearable technologies and their application to precision health. *Health Psychology*, 40(11), 803–810. https://doi.org/10.1037/hea0001125

Puterman, E., Weiss, J., Hives, B. A., Gemmill, A., Karasek, D., Mendes, W. B., . . . Rehkopf, D. H. (2020). Predicting mortality from 57 economic, behavioral, social, and psychological factors. *Proceedings of the National Academy of Sciences of the United States of America*, 117(28), 16273–16282. https://doi.org/10.1073/pnas.1918455117

Qamar, A., & Braunwald, E. (2018). Treatment of hypertension: Addressing a global health problem. *Journal of the American Medical Association*, 320, 1751–1752. https://doi.org/10.1001/jama.2018.16579

Qasim, A., Turcotte, M., Souza, R. J., Samaan, M. C., Champredon, D., Dushoff, J., ... Meyre, D. (2018). On the origin of obesity: Identifying the biological, environmental and cultural drivers of genetic risk among human populations. *Obesity Reviews*, 19(2), 121–149.

Qin, W., Hamler, T. C., & Miller, D. B. (2022). Self-efficacy and importance of participation reasons as predictors for prostate cancer screening intention in African American men. *Ethnicity & Health,* 27(2), 316–328, https://doi.org/10.1080/13557858.2020.1724269

Quick, J. C. (2018). Cited in B. L. Smith, What it really takes to stop sexual harassment. *Monitor on Psychology*, 49(2), 36–42.

Quinn, S. C. (2018). African American adults and seasonal influenza vaccination: Changing our approach can move the needle. *Human Vaccines & Immunotherapeutics*, 14(3), 719–723.

Rabel, M., Laxy, M., Thorand, B., Peters, A., Schwettmann, L., & Mess, F. (2019). Clustering of health-related behavior patterns and demographics: Results from the population-based KORA S4/F4 Cohort Study. *Frontiers in Public Health*, 6. https://doi.org/10.3389/fpubh.2018.00387

Rabenstein, S. (2018). Assessing grief and loss in children and adolescents. In C. Arnold (Ed.), *Understanding child and adolescent grief: Supporting loss and facilitating growth* (pp. 19–33). Routledge.

Racicot, K., & Mor, G. (2017). Risks associated with viral infections during pregnancy. *The Journal of Clinical Investigation*, 127(5), 1591–1599.

Rahmadiyani, R., & Widyanti, A. (2023). Prevalence of drowsy driving and modeling its intention: An Indonesian case study. *Transportation Research Interdisciplinary Perspectives,* 19, 100824. https://doi.org/10.1016/j.trip.2023.100824

Raichlen, D. A., & Alexander, G. E. (2020). Why your brain needs exercise. *Scientific American*.

Raichlen, D. A., Aslan, D. H., Sayre, M. K., Bharadwaj, P. K., Ally, M., Maltagliati, S., Lai, M. H. C., Wilcox, R. R., Klimentidis, Y. C., & Alexander, G. E. (2023). Sedentary behavior and incident dementia among older adults. *JAMA: The Journal of the American Medical Association*, 330(10), 934–940. https://doi.org/10.1001/jama.2023.15231

Raifman, J., Nunn, A., Oldenburg, C. E., Montgomery, M. C., Almonte, A., Agwu, A. L., ... Chan, P. A. (2018). An evaluation of a clinical pre-exposure prophylaxis education intervention among men who have sex with men. *Health Services Research*, 53(4), 2249–2267.

Raifman, J. R., Schwartz, S. R., Sosnowy, C. D., Montgomery, M. C., Almonte, A., Bazzi, A. R., ... Chan, P. A. (2019). Brief report: Pre-exposure prophylaxis awareness and use among cisgender women at a sexually transmitted disease clinic. *Journal of Acquired Immune Deficiency Syndromes*, 80(1), 36–39.

Raine, A. (2008). From genes to brain to antisocial behavior. *Current Directions in Psychological Science*, 17, 323–328. https://doi.org/10.1111/j.1467-8721.2008.00599

Rajan, S., McKee, M., Rangarajan, S., Bangdiwala, S., Rosengren, A., Gupta, R., ... Lopez-Jaramillo, P. (2020). Association of symptoms of depression with cardiovascular disease and mortality in low-, middle-, and high-income countries. *JAMA Psychiatry*. https://doi.org/10.1001/jamapsychiatry.2020.1351

Rajbanshi, B., Guruacharya, A., Mandell, J. W., & Bloom, G. S. (2023). Localization, induction, and cellular effects of tau phosphorylated at threonine 217 1. *Alzheimer's & Dementia*. https://doi.org/10.1002/alz.12892

Ralvenius, W. T., Mungenast, A. E., Woolf, H., Huston, M. M., Gillingham, T. Z., Godin, S. K., ... Tsai, L. (2023). A novel molecular class that recruits HDAC/MECP2 complexes to PU.1 motifs reduces neuroinflammation. *Rockefeller University Press*. https://doi.org/10.1084/jem.20222105

Ramakrishnan, S., Peng, X., Qi, Q., Hu, Q., Azabdaftari, G., Pop, E., ... Woloszynska-Read, A. (2018). DNA methylation and genetic alterations contribute to aggressive prostate cancer in African American men. *Cancer Epidemiology, Biomarkers & Prevention*, 27(7). https://doi.org/10.1158/1538-7755.DISP17-B72

Ramar, K., Malhotra, R. K., Carden, K. A., Martin, J. L., Abbasi-Feinberg, F., Aurora, R. N., Trotti, L. M. (2021). Sleep is essential to health: An American Academy of Sleep Medicine position statement. *Journal of Clinical Sleep Medicine*, 17(10), 2115–2119. https://doi.org/10.5664/jcsm.9476

Ramos-Vera, C., Saintila, J., Calizaya-Milla, Y. E., Acosta Enríquez, M. E., & Serpa Barrientos, A. (2022). Relationship between satisfaction with medical care, physical health, and emotional well-being in adult men: Mediating role of communication. *Journal of Primary Care & Community Health*, 13, 21501319221114850.

Ranby, K. W. (2019). Major research designs in health psychology. In T. E. Revenson & R. A. R. Gurung (Eds.), *Handbook of health psychology* (pp. 3–14). Routledge.

Raque-Bogdan, T. L., Lent, R. W., & Lamphere, B. (2019). Test of a social cognitive model of well-being among breast cancer survivors. *Journal of Health Psychology*, 24, 661–670.

Rasmussen, M. L. H., Poulsen, G. J., Videbech, P., Wohlfahrt,J.,&Melbye,M.(2023).Endocrinediseasehistoryandtheriskof postpartum depression. *The British Journal of Psychiatry*, 222(3), 119–124.

Ratcliff, C., & Novy, D. (2018). Treating cancer patients with persistent pain. In D. C. Turk & R. J. Gatchel (Eds.), *Psychological approaches to pain management: A practitioner's handbook* (3rd ed., pp. 485–514). The Guilford Press.

Ratzan, S. C., Bloom, B. R., El-Mohandes, A., Fielding, J., Gostin, L. O., Hodge, J. G., ... Omer, S. B. (2019). The Salzburg statement on vaccination acceptance. *Journal of Health Communication*, 24(5), 581–583.

Rawl, S. M., Skinner, C. S., Perkins, S. M., Springston, J., Wang, H. L., Russell, K. M., ... Champion, V. L. (2012). Computer-delivered tailored intervention improves colon cancer screening knowledge and health beliefs of African Americans. *Health Education Research*, 27(5), 868–885.

Ray, C. T., Gatchell, R. J., Hulla, R., & Stowell, A. W. (2018). Occupational musculoskeletal pain and disability. In D. C. Turk & R. J. Gatchel (Eds.), *Psychological approaches to pain management: A practitioner's handbook* (3rd ed., pp. 357–376). The Guilford Press.

Raymond, J. (2013, September 13). You will look better with sleep, but you have to wear your mask: Study. *NBC News*. http://www.today.com/health/you-will-look-better-sleep-you-have-wear-your-mask-8C11150914

Raymond, L. W., Morton, S. L., & Yanni, A. (2019). Workplace wellness programs and health outcomes. *Journal of the American Medical Association*, 322, 892–893.

Readdean, K. C., Heuer, A. J., Hoban, M. T., & Parrott, J. S. (2019). Integrated primary care behavioral health services in college health: Results from a national survey of health center administrators. *Journal of American College Health*. https://doi.org/10.1080/07448481.2019.1681432

Reardon, S. (2023). Alzheimer's drug donanemab: What promising trial means for treatments. *Nature*. https://doi.org/10.1038/d41586-023-01537-5

Rector, N. A., & Beck, A. T. (2001). Cognitive behavioral therapy for schizophrenia: An empirical review. *The Journal of Nervous and Mental Disease*, 189(5), 278–287.

Rector, N. A., Stolar, N., & Grant, P. (2011). *Schizophrenia: Cognitive theory, research, and therapy*. Guilford Press.

Reed, S., & Meggs, J. (2017). Examining the effect of prenatal testosterone and aggression on sporting choice and sporting longevity. *Personality and Individual Differences*, 116, 11–15.

Rehm, J., & Probst, C. (2018). What about drinking is associated with shorter life in poorer people? *PLoS Medicine*, 15(1), e1002477.

Reinisch, J. M., Mortensen, E. L., & Sanders, S. A. (2017). Prenatal exposure to progesterone affects sexual orientation in humans. *Archives of Sexual Behavior*, 46(5), 1239–1249.

Reiter, J. T., Dobmeyer, A. C., & Hunter, C. L. (2018). The Primary Care Behavioral Health (PCBH) Model: An overview and operational definition. *Journal of Clinical Psychology in Medical Settings*, 25(2), 109–126.

Remien, R. H., Stirratt, M. J., Nguyen, N., Robbins, R. N., Pala, A. N., & Mellins, C. A. (2019). Mental health and HIV/AIDS: The need for an integrated response. *AIDS (London, England)*, 33(9), 1411–1420.

Renner, M. J., & Mackin, R. S. (1998). A life stress instrument for classroom use. *Teaching of Psychology*, 25, 46–48.

Reno, J. E., O'Leary, S., Garrett, K., Pyrzanowski, J., Lockhart, S., Campagna, E., ... Dempsey, A. F. (2018). Improving provider communication about HPV vaccines for vaccine-hesitant parents through the use of motivational interviewing. *Journal of Health Communication*, 23(4), 313–320.

Rentería, E., Jha, P., Forman, D., & Soerjomataram, I. (2016). The impact of cigarette smoking on life expectancy between 1980 and 2010: A global perspective. *Tobacco Control*, 25(5), 551–557.

Reusch, J. E. B., & Manson, J. E. (2017). Management of Type 2 diabetes in 2017: Getting to goal. *Journal of the American Medical Association*, 317, 1015–1016.

Reyes-Gibby, C. C., Aday, L. A., Todd, K. H., Cleeland, C. S., & Anderson, K. O. (2007). Pain in aging community-dwelling adults in the United States: Non-Hispanic whites, non-Hispanic blacks, and Hispanics. *Journal of Pain*, 8, 75–84.

Rey, L. F., Wiglesworth, A., Prairie Chicken, M. L., Fetter, A. K., Azarani, M., Riegelman, A., . . . Gone, J. P. (2023). A systematic review of research methodologies in American Indian and Alaska Native suicide research from 2010 to 2020. *Cultural Diversity and Ethnic Minority Psychology*, 29(3), 358–371. https://doi.org/10.1037/cdp0000531

Rezaie-Keikhaie, K., Arbabshastan, M. E., Rafiemanesh, H., Amirshahi, M., Ostadkelayeh, S. M., & Arbabisarjou, A. (2020). Systematic review and meta-analysis of the prevalence of the maternity blues in the postpartum period. *Journal of Obstetric, Gynecologic, and Neonatal Nursing: JOGNN*, 49(2), 127–136. https://doi.org/10.1016/j.jogn.2020.01.001

Rhodes, R. E., & Dickau, L. (2012). Experimental evidence for the intention–behavior relationship in the physical activity domain: A meta-analysis. *Health Psychology*, 31(6), 724–727.

Rhodes, R. E., Saelens, B. E., & Sauvage-Mar, C. (2018). Understanding physical activity through interactions between the built environment and social cognition: A systematic review. *Sports Medicine*, 48(8), 1893–1912. https://doi.org/10.1007/s40279-018-0934-0

Rice, E. L., & Klein, W. M. P. (2019). Interactions among perceived norms and attitudes about health-related behaviors in U.S. adolescents. *Health Psychology*, 38(3), 268–275.

Richard, A., Rohrmann, S., Vandeleur, C. L., Schmid, M., Barth, J., & Eichholzer, M. (2017). Loneliness is adversely associated with physical and mental health and lifestyle factors: Results from a Swiss national survey. *PLoS One*, 12(7). https://doi.org/10.1371/journal.pone.0181442

Richman, L. S., Pascoe, E. A., & Lattanner, M. (2018). Interpersonal discrimination and physical health. In B. Major, J. F. Dovido, & B. G. Link (Eds.), *Handbook of stigma, discrimination, and health*. Oxford University Press.

Rigotti, N. A. (2020). Randomized trials of e-cigarettes for smoking cessation. *JAMA*, 324(18), 1835. https://doi.org/10.1001/jama.2020.18967

Rigotti, N. A., Kruse, G. R., Livingstone-Banks, J., & Hartmann-Boyce, J. (2022). Treatment of tobacco smoking. *JAMA*, 327(6), 566–577. doi: 10.1001/jama.2022.0395

Rios, R., & Zautra, A. J. (2011). Socioeconomic disparities in pain: The role of economic hardship and daily financial worry. *Health Psychology*, 30, 58–66.

Roberts, B. W., & Yoon, H. J. (2022). Personality psychology. *Annual Review of Psychology*, 73, 489–516.

Roberts, L. (2017, April 6–8). Unusual alcohol consumption methods and risky drinking. *Proceedings of the National Conference of Undergraduate Research 2017*. University of Memphis.

Robertson, K., Forbes, S., & Thyne, M. (2020). Perpetration of alcohol-related aggression by male and female college students: An examination of overt and relational aggression. *Journal of Interpersonal Violence*, 35(5–6), 1454–1475.

Robins, L. N., Helzer, J. E., & Davis, D. H. (1975). Narcotic use in southeast Asia and afterwards. An interview study of 898 Vietnam returnees. *Archives of General Psychiatry*, 32(8), 955–961.

Robinson, A. M. (2018). Let's talk about stress: History of stress research. *Review of General Psychology*, 22(3), 334–342.

Robinson, L. M., & Vail, S. R. (2012). An integrative review of adolescent smoking cessation using the transtheoretical model of change. *Journal of Pediatric Health Care*, 26(5), 336–345.

Robinson, L., Prichard, I., Nikolaidis, A., Drummond, C., Drummond, M., & Tiggemann, M. (2017). Idealised media images: The effect of fitspiration imagery on body satisfaction and exercise behaviour. *Body Image*, 22, 65–71. https://doi.org/10.1016/j.bodyim.2017.06.001

Robinson, P. J., & Reiter, J. T. (2016). *Behavioral consultation and primary care: A guide to integrating services* (2nd ed.). Springer.

Rochefort, C., Hoerger, M., Turiano, N. A., & Duberstein, P. (2019). Big Five personality and health in adults with and without cancer. *Journal of Health Psychology*, 24, 1494–1504.

Rockett, D. (2018, July 9). "If I lived on the North Side": Neighborhood may matter more than race in breast cancer survival rates. *Chicago Tribune*.

Rodgers, R. F., Berry, R., & Franko, D. L. (2018). Eating disorders in ethnic minorities: An update. *Current Psychiatry Reports*, 20(10), 90. https://doi.org/10.1007/s11920-018-0938-3

Rodrigues, D. L., Lopes, D., Pereira, M., Prada, M., & Garrido, M. V. (2018). Motivations for sexual behavior and intentions to use condoms: Development of the Regulatory Focus in Sexuality Scale. *Archives of Sexual Behavior*, 48(2), 557–575.

Rodriguez, F. (2018b). Lifestyle factors affect survival in heart disease patients: More evidence. *New England Journal of Medicine Journal Watch*. https://www.jwatch.org/na47829/2018/11/01/lifestyle-factors-affect-survival-heart-disease-patients

Rodriguez, N., Flores, R. T., London, E. F., Bingham Mira, C., Myers, H. F., Arroyo, D., & Rangel, A. (2019). A test of the main-effects, stress-buffering, stress-exacerbation, and joint-effects models among Mexican-origin adults. *Journal of Latinx Psychology*, 7(3), 212–229.

Rodriguez, S. A., Mullen, P. D., Lopez, D. M., Savas, L. S., & Fernández, M. E. (2020). Factors associated with adolescent HPV vaccination in the U.S.: A systematic review of reviews and multilevel framework to inform intervention development. *Preventive Medicine*, 131(105968), 105968. https://doi.org/10.1016/j.ypmed.2019.105968

Rodziewicz, T. L., & Hipskind, J. E. (2020). *Medical error prevention*. StatPearls Publishing. https://www.ncbi.nlm.nih.gov/books/NBK499956/

Roesch, P. T., Saiyed, N. S., Laflamme, E., De Maio, F. G., & Benjamins,M. R. (2023). Life expectancy gaps among Black and white personsand contributing causes of death in 3 large US cities, 2018–2019. *JAMA Network Open*, 6(3), e233146–e233146.

Rogers, M. M., McKinney, C., & Asberg, K. (2018). Substance use predicted by parental maltreatment, gender, and five-factor personality. *Personality and Individual Differences*, 128, 39–43.

Romero, S. (2020, April 20). Checkpoints, curfews, airlifts: Virus rips through Navajo Nation. *New York Times*. https://www.nytimes.com/2020/04/09/us/coronavirus-navajo-nation.html

Romundstad, S., Svebak, S., Holen, A., & Holmen, J. (2016). A 15-year follow-up study of sense of humor and causes of mortality: The Nord-Trøndelag Health Study. *Psychosomatic Medicine*, 78(3), 345–353.

Roozbahani, T., Nourian, M., Saatchi, K., & Moslemi, A. (2017). Effect of progressive muscle relaxation on anxiety in pre-university students: A randomized controlled clinical trial. *Advances in Nursing & Midwifery*, 27(1), 32–37.

Roque, C. G., Chung, K. M., McCurdy, E. P., Jagannathan, R., Randolph, L. K., Herline-Killian, K., ... Hengst, U. (2023). CREB3L2-ATF4 heterodimerization defines a transcriptional hub of Alzheimer's disease gene expression linked to neuropathology. *Science Advances*, 9(9). https://doi.org/10.1126/sciadv.add2671

Rosenkranz, M. A., Davidson, R. J., Maccoon, D. G., Sheridan, J. F., Kalin, N. H., & Lutz, A. (2013). A comparison of mindfulness-based stress reduction and an active control in modulation of neurogenic inflammation. *Brain, Behavior, and Immunity*, 27(1), 174–184. https://doi.org/10.1016/j.bbi.2012.10.013

Rosignoli, C., Ornello, R., Onofri, A., Caponnetto, V., Grazzi, L., Raggi, A., ... Sacco, S. (2022). Applying a biopsychosocial model to migraine: Rationale and clinical implications. *Journal of Headache and Pain*, 23(1). https://doi.org/10.1186/s10194-022-01471-3

Rosky, C. (2016). Same-sex marriage litigation and children's right to be queer. *GLQ: A Journal of Lesbian and Gay Studies*, 22(4), 541–568. https://doi.org/10.1215/10642684-3603090

Ross, K. M., Oltman, S., Baer, R., Altman, M., Flowers, E., Feuer, S., ... Jelliffe-Pawlowski, L. (2021). Socioeconomic status, diabetes, and gestation length in Native American and White women. *Health Psychology*, 40(6), 380–387. https://doi.org/10.1037/hea0001072

Rothman, E. F. (2017, December 21). In J. Whalen. The mentality of sexual assault and harassment, a Q&A. *The Wall Street Journal*.

Rotter, J. B. (1990). Internal versus external control of reinforcement: A case history of a variable. *American Psychologist*, 45, 489–493.

Rottman, B. M., Marcum, A. A., Thorpe, C. T., & Gellad, W. F. (2017). Medication adherence as a learning process: insights from cognitive psychology. *Health Psychology Review*, 11, 17–32. https://doi.org/10.1080/17437199.2016.1240624

Rowe, C. A., Sirois, F. M., Toussaint, L., Kohls, N., Nöfer, E., Offenbächer, M., ... Hirsch, J. K. (2019). Health beliefs, attitudes, and health-related quality of life in persons with fibromyalgia: Mediating role of treatment adherence. *Psychology, Health & Medicine*, 24, 962–977.

Roy, B., Ghosh, S., Sathain, B., & Banerjee, I. (2018). Genetic basis of obesity: A review. *Journal of Biomedical Sciences*, 3(2), 24–28.

Roy-Byrne, P. (2018, September 17). Chronic pain is a risk factor for suicide. *NEJM Journal Watch Psychiatry*. https://www.jwatch.org/na47486/2018/09/17/chronic-pain-risk-factor-suicide

Rozanski, A., Bavishi, C., Kubzansky, L. D., & Cohen, R. (2019). Association of optimism with cardiovascular events and all-cause mortality: A systematic review and meta-analysis. *JAMA Network Open*, 2(9), e1912200. https://doi.org/10.1001/jamanetworkopen.2019.12200

Rozenkrantz, L., Kube, T., Bernstein, M. H., & Gabrieli, J. D. E. (2022). How beliefs about coronavirus disease (COVID) influence COVID-like symptoms? – A longitudinal study. *Health Psychology*, 41(8), 519–526. https://doi.org/10.1037/hea0001219

Rozgonjuk, D., Levine, J. G., Hall, B. J., & Elhai, J. D. (2018). The association between problematic smartphone use, depression and anxiety symptom severity, and objectively measured smartphone use over one week. *Computers in Human Behavior*, 87, 10–17. https://doi.org/10.1016/j.chb.2018.05.019

Rubinstein, M. L., Delucchi, K., Benowitz, N. L., & Ramo, D. E. (2018). Adolescent exposure to toxic volatile organic chemicals from e-cigarettes. *Pediatrics*, 141(4). http://pediatrics.aappublications.org/content/141/4/e20173557

Rubinstein, S., & Caballero, B. (2000). Is Miss America an undernourished role model? *JAMA: Journal of the American Medical Association*, 283(12), 1569. https://doi.org/10.1001/jama.283.12.1569

Ruiz, J. M., & Brondolo, E. (2016). Introduction to the special issue Disparities in cardiovascular health: Examining the contributions of social and behavioral factors. *Health Psychology*, 35, 309–312.

Rumbold, J. L., & Aoun, S. M. (2019). Funerals, memorials and bereavement care. *Bereavement Care*, 38(2–3), 62–67.

Runarsdottir, V., Hansdottir, I., Tyrfingsson, T., Einarsson, M., Dugosh, K., Royer-Malvestuto, C., ... Woody, G. E. (2017). Extended-release injectable naltrexone (XR-NTX) with intensive psychosocial therapy for amphetamine-dependent persons seeking treatment: A placebo-controlled trial. *Journal of Addiction Medicine*, 11(3), 197–204.

Ruppar, T. M., Cooper, P. S., Mehr, D. R., Delgado, J. M., & Dunbar-Jacob, J. M. (2016). Medication adherence interventions improve heart failure mortality and readmission rates: Systematic review and meta-analysis of controlled trials. *Journal of the American Heart Association*, 5(6), e002606.

Ruvalcaba, Y., Rodriguez, A. L., Eaton, A. A., Stephens, D. P., & Madhivanan, P. (2022). The effectiveness of American college sexual assault interventions in highly masculine settings: A systematic review and meta-analysis. *Aggression and Violent Behavior*. https://doi.org/10.1016/j.avb.2022.101760

Ryan, K. M. (2019). Rape mythology and victim blaming as a social construct. In W. T. O'Donohue & P. A. Schewe (Eds.), *Handbook of sexual assault and sexual assault prevention* (pp. 151–174). Springer.

Sackett, P. R., & Walmsley, P. T. (2014). Which personality attributes are most important in the workplace? *Perspectives on Psychological Science*, 9, 538–551.

Sadora, J., Vilsmark, E. S., Bashara, A., Burton, D., Paschali, M., Pester, B., ... Lazaridou, A. (2023). Electromyography-biofeedback for chronic low back pain: A qualitative cohort study. *Complementary Therapies in Medicine*, 73, 102922–102922. https://doi.org/10.1016/j.ctim.2023.102922

Saglam, H. Y., & Örsal, Ö. (2020). Effect of exercise on premenstrual symptoms: A systematic review. *Complementary Therapies in Medicine*, 48, 102272. https://doi.org/10.1016/j.ctim.2019.102272

Sahler, O. J. Z., & Carr, J. E. (2009). Coping strategies. In W. B. Carey, A. C. Crocker, & H. M. Feldman (Eds.), *Developmental-behavioral pediatrics* (4th ed., pp. 491–496). https://doi.org/10.1016/B978-1-4160-3370-7.00050-X

Saini, G., Ogden, A., McCullough, L. E., Torres, M., Rida, P., & Aneja, R. (2019). Disadvantaged neighborhoods and racial disparity in breast cancer outcomes: The biological link. *Cancer Causes & Control*, 30, 677–686.

Saint-Maurice, P. F., Coughlan, D., Kelly, S. P., Keadle, S. K., Cook, M. B., Carlson, S. A., ... Matthews, C. E. (2019). Association of leisure-time physical activity across the adult life course with all-cause and cause-specific mortality. *JAMA Network Open*, 2, e190355. https://doi.org/10.1001/jamanetworkopen.2019.0355

Salamon, K. S., & Cullinan, C. C. (2019). The integrated prevention model of pain—Chronic pain prevention in the primary care setting. *Clinical Practice in Pediatric Psychology*, 7, 183–191.

Sala, M., Roos, C. R., Brewer, J. A., & Garrison, K. A. (2021). Awareness, affect, and craving during smoking cessation: An experience sampling study. *Health Psychology*, 40(9), 578–586. https://doi.org/10.1037/hea0001105

Salas, E., Kishino, N., Dersh, J., & Gatchel, R. J. (2018). Psychological disorders and chronic pain: Are there cause-and-effect relationships? In D. C. Turk & R. J. Gatchel (Eds.), *Psychological approaches to pain management: A practitioner's handbook* (3rd ed., pp. 25–50). The Guilford Press.

Salas-Wright, C. P., Kagotho, N., & Vaughn M. G. (2014). Mood, anxiety, and personality disorders among first and second-generation immigrants to the United States. *Psychiatry Research*, S0165–1781(14)00742–2. https://doi.org/10.1016/j.psychres.2014.08.045

Samtani, S. (2017). Assessing maladaptive repetitive thought in clinical disorders: A critical review of existing measures. *Clinical Psychology Review*, 53, 14–28.

Samuelson, K. W., Bartel, A., Valadez, R., & Jordan, J. T. (2017). PTSD symptoms and perception of cognitive problems: The roles of posttraumatic cognitions and trauma coping self-efficacy. *Psychological Trauma: Theory, Research, Practice, and Policy*, 9(5), 537–544.

Sancar, F. (2019). For "broken heart" syndrome, brain may hold the key. *Journal of the American Medical Association*, 321, 2270–2271.

Sanders, C., Donovan, J. L., & Dieppe, P. A. (2004). Unmet need for joint replacement: A qualitative investigation of barriers to treatment among individuals with severe pain and disability of the hip and knee. *Rheumatology*, 43, 353–357.

Sanders, L. (2006). Heart ache. *The New York Times Magazine*. https://www.nytimes.com/2006/06/18/magazine/18wwln_diagnosis.html

Sanders, L., Fortin, A. H., & Schiff, G. D. (2020). Connecting with patients—The missing links. *Journal of the American Medical Association*, 323, 33–34.

Sanders, S. H. (2018). Operant and related conditioning with chronic pain: Back to basics. In D. C. Turk & R. J. Gatchel (Eds.), *Psychological approaches to pain management: A practitioner's handbook* (3rd ed., pp. 96–114). The Guilford Press.

Sandvik, A. M., Bartone, P. T., Hystad, S. W., Phillips, T. M., Thayer, J. F., & Johnsen, B. H. (2013). Psychological hardiness predicts neuroimmunological responses to stress. *Psychology, Health & Medicine*, 18(6), 705–713.

Santos, G., Ikeda, J., Coffin, P. O., Walker, J., Matheson, T., Ali, A., ... Batki, S. (2022). Targeted oral naltrexone for mild to moderate alcohol use disorder among sexual and gender minority men: A randomized trial. *American Journal of Psychiatry*, 179(12), 915–926. https://doi.org/10.1176/appi.ajp.20220335

Santos, S., & Miller, C. (2020). The neural effects of antidepressant medication on adults with major depressive disorder: A meta-analysis. *Biological Psychiatry*, 87(9), S345.

Sarwer, D. B., & Grilo, C. M. (2020). Obesity: Psychological and behavioral aspects of a modern epidemic. *American Psychologist*, 75(2), 135–138.

Satin, J. R., Linden, W., & Phillips, M. J. (2009). Depression as a predictor of disease progression and mortality in cancer patients: A meta-analysis. *Cancer*, 115(22), 5349–5361.

Saunders, E. (2022). Flexible buprenorphine/naloxone treatment models: safe and effective in reducing opioid use among persons with prescription opioid use disorder. *American Journal of Psychiatry*. https://ajp.psychiatryonline.org/doi/10.1176/appi.ajp.20220687

Savage, J. E., Jansen, P. R., Stringer, S., Watanabe, K., Bryois, J., De Leeuw, C. A., ... Grasby, K. L. (2018). Genome-wide association meta-analysis in 269,867 individuals identifies new genetic and functional links to intelligence. *Nature Genetics*, 50(7), 912–919.

Savic, I., Garcia-Falgueras, A., & Swaab, D. F. (2010). Sexual differentiation of the human brain in relation to gender identity and sexual orientation. *Progress in Brain Research*, 186, 41–62. https://doi.org/10.1016/B978-0-444-53630-3.00004-X

Savin-Williams, R. C. (2019). Developmental trajectories and milestones of sexual-minority youth. In S. Lamb & J. Gilbert (Eds.), *The Cambridge handbook of sexual development: Childhood and adolescence* (pp. 156–179). Cambridge University Press.

Savin-Williams, R. C. (2022). Sexual and romantic spectrums: Mostly straights and mostly gays/lesbians. *Current Opinion in Psychology*. https://doi.org/10.1016/j.copsyc.2022.101503

Schafer, S. M., Colloca, L., & Wager, T. D. (2015). Conditioned placebo analgesia persists when subjects know they are receiving a placebo. *Pain*, 16, 412–420. https://doi.org/10.1016/j.jpain.2014.12.008

Scheier, M. F., Matthews, K. A., Owens, J. F., Schulz, R., Bridges, M. W., Magovern, G. J., & Carver, C. S. (1999). Optimism and rehospitalization after coronary artery bypass graft surgery. *Archives of Internal Medicine*, 159(8), 829–835. https://doi.org/10.1001/archinte.159.8.829

Schmack, K., Bosc, M., Ott, T., Sturgill, J. F., & Kepecs, A. (2021). Striatal dopamine mediates hallucination-like perception in mice. *Science*, 372(6537), eabf4740. https://doi.org/10.1126/science.abf4740

Schmitt, A., Bendig, E., Baumeister, H., Hermanns, N., & Kulzer, B. (2021). Associations of depression and diabetes distress with self-management behavior and glycemic control. *Health Psychology*, 40(2), 113–124. https://doi.org/10.1037/hea0001037

Schmitz, K. H., Campbell, A. M., Stuiver, M. M., Pinto, B. M., Schwartz, A. L., Morris, G. S., ... Matthews, C. E. (2019). Exercise is medicine in oncology: Engaging clinicians to help patients move through cancer. *CA: A Cancer Journal for Clinicians*, 69, 468–484.

Schneider, K. L., Coons, M. J., McFadden, H. G., Pellegrini, C. A., DeMott, A., Siddique, J., ... Spring, B. (2016). Mechanisms of change in diet and activity in the Make Better Choices 1 trial. *Health Psychology*, 35(7), 723–732. https://doi.org/10.1037/hea0000333

Schneider, R. H., Fields, J. Z., & Salerno, J. W. (2018). Editorial commentary on AHA scientific statement on meditation and cardiovascular risk reduction. *Journal of the American Society of Hypertension*, 12(12), e57–e58. https://doi.org/10.1016/j.jash.2018.11.005

Schoenfeld, T. J., Rada, P., Pieruzzini, P. R., Hsueh, B., & Gould, E. (2013). Physical exercise prevents stress-induced activation of granule neurons and enhances local inhibitory mechanisms in the dentate gyrus. *Journal of Neuroscience*, 33, 7770. https://doi.org/10.1523/JNEUROSCI.5352-12.2013

Schönfeld, P., Brailovskaia, J., Bieda, A., Zhang, X. C., & Margraf, J. (2016). The effects of daily stress on positive and negative mental health: Mediation through self-efficacy. *International Journal of Clinical and Health Psychology*, 16(1), 1–10.

Schrager, S., Larson, M., Carlson, J., Ledford, K., & Ehrenthal, D. B. (2020). Beyond birth control: Noncontraceptive benefits of hormonal methods and their key role in the general medical care of women. *Journal of Women's Health*. https://doi.org/10.1089/jwh.2019.7731

Schreiber, K. (2016). What does body positivity actually mean? *Psychology Today*.

Schreitmüller, J., & Loerbroks, A. (2020). The role of self-efficacy and locus of control in asthma-related needs and outcomes: A cross-sectional study. *Journal of Asthma*, 57(2), 196–204.

Schulenberg, J. E., Johnston, L. D., O'Malley, P. M., Bachman, J. G., Miech, R. A., & Patrick, M. E. (2019). *Monitoring the future national survey results on drug use, 1975–2018: Volume II, College students and adults ages 19–60*. Institute for Social Research, The University of Michigan.

Schultebraucks, K., Choi, K. W., Galatzer-Levy, I. R., & Bonanno, G. A. (2021). Discriminating heterogeneous trajectories of resilience and depression after major life stressors using polygenic scores. *JAMA Psychiatry*, 78(7), 744. https://doi.org/10.1001/jamapsychiatry.2021.0228

Schultz, L. T., & Heimberg, R. G. (2008). Attentional focus in social anxiety disorder: Potential for interactive processes. *Clinical Psychology Review*, 28, 1206–1221.

Schulz, K. F., Altman, D. G., Moher, D., & Fergusson, D. (2010). CONSORT 2010 changes and testing blindness in RCTs. *The Lancet*, 375, 1144–1146. https://doi.org/10.1016/S0140-6736(10)60413-8

Schutte, A. E., Kruger, R., Gafane-Matemane, L. F., Breet, Y., Strauss-Kruger, M., & Cruickshank, J. K. (2020). Ethnicity and arterial stiffness. *Arteriosclerosis, Thrombosis, and Vascular Biology*, 40(5), 1044–1054. https://doi.org/10.1161/ATVBAHA.120.313133

Schutte, R., Smith, L., & Wannamethee, G. (2022). Alcohol – The myth of cardiovascular protection. *Clinical Nutrition*, 41(2), 348–355. https://doi.org/10.1016/j.clnu.2021.12.009

Schütze, R., Rees, C., Slater, H., Smith, A., & O'Sullivan, P. (2017). "I call it stinkin' thinkin'": A qualitative analysis of metacognition in people with chronic low back pain and elevated catastrophizing. *British Journal of Health Psychology*, 22, 463–480.

Schwartz, J., King, C. C., & Yen, M. Y. (2020). Protecting healthcare workers during the coronavirus disease 2019 (COVID-19)

outbreak: Lessons from Taiwan's severe acute respiratory syndrome response. *Clinical Infectious Diseases*, 71(15), 858–860. https://doi.org/10.1093/cid/ciaa255

Schwarz, J., Gibson, S., & Lewis-Arévalo, C. (2017). Sexual assault on college campuses: Substance use, victim status awareness, and barriers to reporting. *Building Healthy Academic Communities Journal*, 1(2), 45–60.

Schwenk, T. L. (2017). Suboptimal diet is associated with excess mortality from cardiometabolic diseases. *NEJM Journal Watch*. http://www.jwatch.org/na43631/2017/03/16/suboptimal-diet-associated-with-excess-mortality

Schwenk, T. L. (2019). Mind-body therapies for patients who use opioids for pain. *NEJM Journal Watch Psychiatry*. https://www.jwatch.org/na50276/2019/11/21/mind-body-therapies-patients-who-use-opioids-pain?query=etoc_jwpsych&jwd=000100400036&jspc=

Schwenk, T. L., & Brett, A. S. (2019). Aspirin for primary prevention: A new meta-analysis. *NEJM Journal Watch*. https://www.jwatch.org/na48372/2019/02/06/aspirin-primary-prevention-new-meta-analysis

Schwingshackl, L., Knüppel, S., Michels, N., Schwedhelm, C., Hoffmann, G., Iqbal, K., ... Devleesschauwer, B. (2019). Intake of 12 food groups and disability-adjusted life years from coronary heart disease, stroke, type 2 diabetes, and colorectal cancer in 16 European countries. *European Journal of Epidemiology*, 34(8), 765–775. https://doi.org/10.1007/s10654-019-00523-4

Scott, K. M., de Jonge, P., Stein, D. J., & Kessler, R. C. (2018). *Mental disorders around the world: Facts and figures from the WHO World Mental Health Surveys* (1st ed.). Cambridge University Press.

Scott, W., & McCracken, L. M. (2019). Chronic pain management. In C. D. Llewellyn, S. Ayers, C. McManus, S. Newman, K. J. Petrie, T. A. Revenson, & J. Weinman (Eds.), *Cambridge handbook of psychology, health and medicine* (3rd ed., pp. 246–250). Cambridge University Press.

Sears, K. (2016, October 12). Seattle's virtual road to transcendence. Seattle Weekly. Retrived from http://www.seattleweekly.com/arts/seattles-virtual-road-to-transcendence/ (December 5, 2018).

Seaton, E. K., & Zeiders, K. H. (2021). Daily racial discrimination experiences, ethnic–racial identity, and diurnal cortisol patterns among Black adults. *Cultural Diversity and Ethnic Minority Psychology*, 27(1), 145–155. https://doi.org/10.1037/cdp0000367

Secor-Turner, M., Randall, B. A., Christensen, K., Jacobson, A., & Loyola Meléndez, M. (2017). Implementing community-based comprehensive sexuality education with high-risk youth in a conservative environment: Lessons learned. *Sex Education*, 17(5), 544–554.

Seekis, V., Bradley, G. L., & Duffy, A. L. (2020). Appearance-related social networking sites and body image in young women: Testing an objectification-social comparison model. *Psychology of Women Quarterly*. https://doi.org/10.1177/0361684320920826

Seekis, V., Bradley, G. L., & Duffy, A. L. (2021). Social networking sites and men's drive for muscularity: Testing a revised objectification model. *Psychology of Men & Masculinities*, 22(1), 189–200. https://doi.org/10.1037/men0000265

SEER Cancer Statistics Review. (2020). https://seer.cancer.gov/

Séguin Leclair, C., Lebel, S., & Westmaas, J. L. (2019). The relationship between fear of cancer recurrence and health behaviors: A nationwide longitudinal study of cancer survivors. *Health Psychology*, 38, 596–605.

Seid, M. A., Abdela, O. A., & Zeleke, E. G. (2019). Adherence to self-care recommendations and associated factors among adult heart failure patients. From the patients' point of view. *PLoS One*, 14. https://doi.org/10.1371/journal.pone.0211768

Seitz, H. H., Schapira, M. M., Gibson, L. A., Skubisz, C., Mello, S., Armstrong, K., ... Cappella, J. N. (2018). Explaining the effects of a decision intervention on mammography intentions: The roles of worry, fear and perceived susceptibility to breast cancer. *Psychology & Health*, 33(5), 682–700.

Sekar, A., Bialas, A. R., de Rivera, H., Davis, A., Hammond, T. R., Kamitaki, N., ... McCarroll, S.A. (2016). Schizophrenia risk from complex variation of complement component. *Nature*, 530, 177–183. https://doi.org/10.1038/nature16549

Seligman, M. E. P., & Maier, S. F. (1967). Failure to escape traumatic shock. *Journal of Experimental Psychology*, 74, 1–9.

Selye, H. (1946). The general adaptation syndrome and the diseases of adaptation. *The Journal of Clinical Endocrinology*, 6(2), 117–230.

Selye, H. (1956). What is stress. *Metabolism*, 5(5), 525–530.

Semaan, S., Dewland, T. A., Tison, G. H., Nah, G., Vittinghoff, E., Pletcher, M. J., ... Marcus, G. M. (2020). Physical activity and atrial fibrillation: Data from wearable fitness trackers. *Heart Rhythm*, 17(5), 842–846. https://doi.org/10.1016/j.hrthm.2020.02.013

Serbulea, V., Upchurch, C. M., Schappe, M. S., Voigt, P., DeWeese, D. E., Desai, B. N., ... Leitinger, N. (2018). Macrophage phenotype and bioenergetics are controlled by oxidized phospholipids identified in lean and obese adipose tissue. *Proceedings of the National Academy of Sciences*, 201800544. https://doi.org/10.1073/pnas.1800544115

Serpas, D. G., & Ignacio, D. A. (2022) COVID-19 fear mediates the relationship between perceived risk and preventive behaviors: The moderating role of perceived effectiveness. *Psychology & Health*, 37(12), 1457–1470. Doi:10.1080/08870446.2021.1980566

Serpentini, M. Y., & Errol, J. P. (2019). The role of coping in the relationship between stressful life events and quality of life in persons with cancer. *Psychology & Health*. https://doi.org/10.1080/08870446.2018.1545905

Serrano-Villar, M., & Calzada, E. J. (2016). Ethnic identity: Evidence of protective effects for young, Latino children. *Journal of Applied Developmental Psychology*, 42, 21–30.

Shahan, T. A. (2020). Relapse: An introduction. *Journal of the Experimental Analysis of Behavior*, 113(1), 8–14. https://doi.org/10.1002/jeab.578

Shakhnoza, I., & Asalya, A. (2022). Prevention of coronary heart disease. *The American Journal of Medical Sciences and Pharmaceutical Research*, 04(04), 19–21. https://doi.org/10.37547/tajmspr/volume04issue04-05

Shams, Y., Feldt, K., & Stålberg, M. (2015). A missed penalty kick triggered coronary death in the husband and broken heart syndrome in the wife. *The American Journal of Cardiology*, 116(10), 1639–1642. https://doi.org/10.1016/j.amjcard.2015.08.033

Shanahan, M. J., Hill, P. L., Roberts, B. W., Eccles, J., & Friedman, H. S. (2014). Conscientiousness, health, and aging: The life course of personality model. *Developmental Psychology*, 50, 1407–1425.

Sharafi, S. E., Garmaroudi, G., Ghafouri, M., Bafghi, S. A., Ghafouri, M., Tabesh, M. R., & Alizadeh, Z. (2020). Prevalence of anxiety and depression in patients with overweight and obesity. *Obesity Medicine*, 17. https://doi.org/10.1016/j.obmed.2019.100169

Sharpe, L., Jones, E., Ashton-James, C. E., Nicholas, M. K., & Refshauge, K. (2020). Necessary components of psychological treatment in pain management programs: A Delphi study. *European Journal of Pain*. https://doi.org/10.1002/ejp.1561

Sheeran, P., Abraham, C., Jones, K., Villegas, M. E., Avishai, A., Symes, Y. R., ... Mayer, D. K. (2019). Promoting physical activity among cancer survivors: Meta-analysis and meta-CART analysis of randomized controlled trials. *Health Psychology*, 38, 467–482.

Shehu, J., Mokgwathi, M., Faros, A., & Moruisi, M. (2016). Obesogenic slurs: How pervasive fat-shaming undermines the battle against juvenile obesity. *African Journal for Physical Activity and Health Sciences*, 22(41), 952–964.

Sheveland, A. C., Luchman, J. N., Mendelson, J., Xie, J., Bleiberg, M. A., Eby, D. W., ... Walton, B. R. (2020). Psychological constructs related to seat belt use: A nationally representative survey study. *Accident; Analysis and Prevention,* 148(105715), 105715. https://doi.org/10.1016/j.aap.2020.105715

Shield, K. D., Soerjomataram, I., & Rehm, J. (2016). Alcohol use and breast cancer: A critical review. *Alcoholism: Clinical and Experimental Research*, 40(6), 1166–1181.

Shields, G. S., Spahr, C. M., & Slavich, G. M. (2020). Psychosocial interventions and immune system function: A systematic review and meta-analysis of randomized clinical trials. *JAMA Psychiatry,* 77(10), 1031–1043. https://doi.org/10.1001/jamapsychiatry.2020.0431

Shiloh, S., Peleg, S., & Nudelman, G. (2021). Adherence to COVID-19 protective behaviors: A matter of cognition or emotion? *Health Psychology,* 40(7), 419–427. https://doi.org/10.1037/hea0001081

Shneidman, E. S. (2008). *A commonsense book of death: Reflections at ninety of a lifelong thanatologist*. Rowman & Littlefield.

Shor, E., Roelfs, D. J., Curreli, M., Clemow, L., Burg, M. M., & Schwartz, J. E. (2012). Widowhood and mortality: A meta-analysis and meta-regression. *Demography*, 49, 575–606.

Shuman, E. K., & Malani, P. N. (2018). Infectious diseases mortality in the United States: Ongoing investment needed for continued progress. *JAMA,* 319(12), 1205–1206

Shungu, N., & Sterba, K. R. (2021). Barriers and facilitators to informed decision-making about prostate cancer screening among Black men. *Journal of the American Board of Family Medicine,* 34(5), 925–936. https://doi.org/10.3122/jabfm.2021.05.210149

Sialvera, T. E., Papadopoulou, A., Efstathiou, S. P., Trautwein, E. A., Ras, R. T., Kollia, N., ... Koutsouri, A. (2018). Structured advice provided by a dietitian increases adherence of consumers to diet and lifestyle changes and lowers blood low-density lipoprotein (LDL)-cholesterol: The Increasing Adherence of Consumers to Diet & Lifestyle Changes to Lower (LDL) Cholesterol (ACT) randomised controlled trial. *Journal of Human Nutrition and Dietetics*, 31(2), 197–208.

Simon, L., Steinmetz, L., Feige, B., Benz, F., Spiegelhalder, K., & Baumeister, H. (2023). Comparative efficacy of onsite, digital, and other settings for cognitive behavioral therapy for insomnia: a systematic review and network meta-analysis. *Scientific Reports*, 13(1), 1929. https://doi.org/10.1038/s41598-023-28853-0

Sinclair, J., McCann, M., Sheldon, E., Gordon, I., Brierley-Jones, L., & Copson, E. (2019). The acceptability of addressing alcohol consumption as a modifiable risk factor for breast cancer: A mixed method study within breast screening services and symptomatic breast clinics. *BMJ Open*, 9(6). https://doi.org/10.1136/bmjopen-2018-027371

Singer, N. (2019, September 26). Nodding off to a cartoon therapist. *New York Times*, pp. B1, B6.

Singh, A., Khess, C. R. J., Mathew, K. J., Ali, A., & Gujar, N. M. (2020). Loneliness, social anxiety, social support, and internet addiction among postgraduate college students. *Open Journal of Psychiatry & Allied Sciences*, 11(1), 10–13.

Sirri, L., Fava, G. A., & Sonino, N. (2013). The unifying concept of illness behavior. *Psychotherapy and Psychosomatics*, 82, 74–81.

Sjøberg, K. A., Frøsig, C., Kjøbsted, R., Sylow, L., Kleinert, M., Betik, A. C., ... Richter, E. A. (2017). Exercise increases human skeletal muscle insulin sensitivity via coordinated increases in microvascular perfusion and molecular signaling. *Diabetes*, 66(6), 1501–1510.

Skin Cancer Foundation. (2019, April). Melanoma warning signs. https://www.skincancer.org/skin-cancer-information/melanoma/melanoma-warning-signs-and-images/

Skinner, C. S., Tiro, J., & Champion, V. L. (2015). The health belief model. In K. Glanz, B. K. Rimer, & K. Viswanath (Eds.), *Health behavior: Theory, research, and practice* (5th ed.). Jossey-Bass.

Skrzynski, C. J., & Creswell, K. G. (2020). Associations between solitary drinking and increased alcohol consumption, alcohol problems, and drinking to cope motives in adolescents and young adults: A systematic review and meta-analysis. *Addiction,* 115(11), 1989–2007. https://doi.org/10.1111/add.15055

Slawek, D., Syed, M., Cunningham, C. O., Zhang, C., Ross, J. D. C., Herman, M., ... Starrels, J. L. (2022). Pain catastrophizing and mental health phenotypes in adults with refractory chronic pain: A latent class analysis. *Journal of Psychiatric Research,* 145, 102–110. https://doi.org/10.1016/j.jpsychires.2021.12.001

Smart, S. E., Kępińska, A. P., Murray, R. M., & MacCabe, J. H. (2019). Predictors of treatment resistant schizophrenia: A systematic review of prospective observational studies. *Psychological Medicine*. https://doi.org/10.1017/S0033291719002083

Smith, A. R., Hames, J. L., & Joiner, T. E., Jr. (2013). Status update: Maladaptive Facebook usage predicts increases in body dissatisfaction and bulimic symptoms. *Journal of Affective Disorders*, 149, 235–240.

Smith, A., & Smith, H. (2017). Perceptions of risk factors for road traffic accidents. *Advances in Social Sciences Research Journal*, 4(1), 140–146.

Smith, B. P., & Madak-Erdogan, Z. (2018). Urban neighborhood and residential factors associated with breast cancer in African American women: A systematic review. *Hormones and Cancer*, 9, 71–81.

Smith, D. M., Donnelly, P. J., Howe, J., Mumford, T., Campbell, A., Ruddock, A., ... Wearden, A. (2018). A qualitative interview study of people living with well-controlled Type 1 diabetes. *Psychology & Health*, 33, 872–887.

Smoller, J. W. (2020). Anxiety genetics goes genomic. *American Journal of Psychiatry,* 177(3), 190–194. https://doi.org/10.1176/appi.ajp.2020.20010038

Soccorso, C. N., Picano, J. J., Moncata, S. J., & Miller, C. D. (2019). Psychological hardiness predicts successful selection in a law enforcement special operations assessment and selection course. *International Journal of Selection and Assessment*, 27(3), 291–295.

Soliani, R. D., da Silva, L. B., Lopes, A. V. B., & Santiago, F. (2024). A look at the relationship between fatigue and self-employed truck Drivers. In P. M. Arezes, R. B. Melo, P. Carneiro, et al. (Eds). Occupational and Environmental Safety and Health V (pp. 3–13). Springer Nature Switzerland.

Song, H., Fang, A., Arnberg, F. K., Mataix-Cols, D., Fernández de la Cruz, L., Almqvist, C., ... Valdimarsdóttir, U. A. (2019). Stress related disorders and risk of cardiovascular disease: Population based, sibling controlled cohort study. *British Medical Journal*, 365.

Sontate, K. V., Kamaluddin, R., Mohamed, N., Mohamed, R. M. P., Shaikh, M. F., Kamal, H., ... Kumar, J. (2021). Alcohol, aggression, and violence: From public health to neuroscience. *Frontiers in Psychology,* 12. https://doi.org/10.3389/fpsyg.2021.699726

Soth, A. (2020, September 5). Opinion. *The New York Times.*

Soto, C. J. (2019). How replicable are links between personality traits and consequential life outcomes? The Life Outcomes of Personality Replication Project. *Psychological Science*, 30(5), 711–727.

South, S. C., Jarnecke, A. M., & Vize, C. E. (2018). Sex differences in the Big Five model personality traits: A behavior genetics exploration. *Journal of Research in Personality*, 74, 158–165.

Speck, L., Brace, N., & Byrne, M. (2020). Psychosocial health. In J. Jones, J. Buckley, G. Furze, & G. Sheppard (Eds.), *Cardiovascular prevention and rehabilitation in practice* (pp. 193–225). Wiley.

Spitzer, E. G., Crosby, E. S., & Witte, T. K. (2023). Looking through a filtered lens: Negative social comparison on social media and suicidal ideation among young adults. *Psychology of Popular Media,* 12(1), 69–76. https://doi.org/10.1037/ppm0000380

Sprenger, C., Eippert, F., Finsterbusch, J., Bingel, U., Rose, M., & Büchel, C. (2012). Attention modulates spinal cord responses to pain. *Current Biology*, 22, 1019–1022. https://doi.org/10.1016/j.cub.2012.04.006

Spring, B., Champion, K. E., Acabchuk, R., & Hennessy, E. A. (2021). Self-regulatory behaviour change techniques in interventions to promote healthy eating, physical activity, or weight loss: A meta-review. *Health Psychology Review*, 15(4), 508–539. https://doi.org/10.1080/17437199.2020.1721310

Spring, B., Stump, T., Penedo, F., Pfammatter, A. F., & Robinson, J. K. (2019). Toward a health-promoting system for cancer survivors: Patient and provider multiple behavior change. *Health Psychology*, 38(9), 840–850.

Stanford, F. C., Tauqeer, Z., & Kyle, T. K. (2018). Media and its influence on obesity. *Current Obesity Reports*, 7(2), 186–192.

Stanghelle, B., Bentzen, H., Giangregorio, L., Pripp, A. H., Skelton, D., & Bergland, A. (2020). Effects of a resistance and balance exercise programme on physical fitness, health-related quality of life and fear of falling in older women with osteoporosis and vertebral fracture: A randomized controlled trial. *Osteoporosis International*, 31, 1069–1078.

Stanton, A. L., Wiley, J. F., Krull, J. L., Crespi, C. M., & Weihs, K. L. (2018). Cancer-related coping processes as predictors of depressive symptoms, trajectories, and episodes. *Journal of Consulting and Clinical Psychology*, 86, 820–830.

Stanton, A. L., Williamson, T. J., & Harris, L. N. (2019). Cancer. In T. E. Revenson & R. A. R. Gurung (Eds.), *Handbook of health psychology* (pp. 369–380). Routledge.

Starcevic, V., & Aboujaoude, E. (2017). Internet addiction: Reappraisal of an increasingly inadequate concept. *CNS Spectrums*, 22(1), 7–13.

Statista. (2019). Number of murder victims in the United States in 2018, by weapon. https://www.statista.com/statistics/195325/murder-victims-in-the-us-by-weapon-used/

Statista. (2020). Number of mHealth apps available in the Apple App Store from first quarter 2015 to first quarter 2020. https://www.statista.com/statistics/779910/health-apps-available-ios-worldwide/

Stefana, A., Dakanalis, A., Mura, M., Colmegna, F., & Clerici, M. (2022). *Instagram use and mental well-being. Journal of Nervous & Mental Disease*, 210(12), 960–965. https://doi.org/10.1097/nmd.0000000000001577

Stefanopoulou, E., Hirsch, C. R., Hayes, S., Adlam, A., & Coker, S. (2014). Are attentional control resources reduced by worry in generalized anxiety disorder? *Journal of Abnormal Psychology*, 123, 330–335.

Steinberg, D., Levine, E., Askew, S., Foley, P., & Bennett, G. (2013). Daily text messaging for weight control among racial and ethnic minority women: Randomized controlled pilot study. *Journal of Medical Internet Research*, 15, e244.

Stein, M. B., & Craske, M. G. (2017). Treating anxiety in 2017: Optimizing care to improve outcomes. *Journal of the American Medical Association*, 318, 235–236.

Stein, M. B., & Stein, D. J. (2008). Social anxiety disorder. *The Lancet*, 371, 1115–1125.

Stein, S. J., & Bartone, P. T. (2020). *Hardiness: Making stress work for you to achieve your life goals*. Wiley.

Steptoe, A., & Kivimaki, M. (2013). Stress and cardiovascular disease: An update on current knowledge. *Annual Review of Public Health*, 34, 337–354.

Stern, A. M., Yang, Y., Jin, S., Yamashita, K., Meunier, A. L., Liu, W., Cai, Y., ... Selkoe, D. J. (2023). Abundant Aβ fibrils in ultracentrifugal supernatants of aqueous extracts from Alzheimer's disease brains. *Neuron*. https://doi.org/10.1016/j.neuron.2023.04.007

Sterpenich, V., van Schie, M. K. M., Catsiyannis, M., Ramyead, A., Perrig, S., Yang, H.-D., ... Schwartz, S. (2021). Reward biases spontaneous neural reactivation during sleep. *Nature Communications*, 12(1). https://doi.org/10.1038/s41467-021-24357-5

Stetler, C. A., & Guinn, V. (2020). Cumulative cortisol exposure increases during the academic term: Links to performance-related and social evaluative stressors. *Psychoneuroendocrinology*, 114.

Stice, E., Desjardins, C. D., Rohde, P., & Shaw, H. (2021). Sequencing of symptom emergence in anorexia nervosa, bulimia nervosa, binge eating disorder, and purging disorder and relations of prodromal symptoms to future onset of these disorders. *Journal of Abnormal Psychology*, 130(4), 377–387. https://doi.org/10.1037/abn0000666

Stix, G. (2022, January). Pandemic year one saw a dramatic global rise in anxiety and depression. *Scientific American Mind*, 33(1), 14–15

Stolberg, S. G. (2001, May 10). Blacks found on short end of heart attack procedure. *New York Times*, p. A20.

Stoll, L. C., Lilley, T. G., & Pinter, K. (2017). Gender-blind sexism and rape myth acceptance. *Violence Against Women*, 23(1), 28–45.

Stolzenberg-Solomon, R. Z., Adams, K., Leitzmann, M., Schairer, C., Michaud, D. S., Hollenbeck, A., ... Silverman, D. T. (2008). Physical activity, and pancreatic cancer in the National Institutes of Health-AARP Diet and Health Cohort. *American Journal of Epidemiology*, 167, 586–597.

Stowe, R. P., Pierson, D. L., & Mehta, S. K. (2020). Stress, spaceflight, and latent herpes virus reactivation. In A. Chouker (Ed.), *Stress challenges and immunity in space* (pp. 357–372). Springer.

Strauss, C., Bibby-Jones, A., Jones, F., Byford, S., Heslin, M., Parry, G., ... Cavanagh, K. (2023). Clinical effectiveness and cost-effectiveness of supported mindfulness-based cognitive therapy self-help compared with supported cognitive behavioral therapy self-help for adults experiencing depression. *JAMA Psychiatry*, 80(5), 415. https://doi.org/10.1001/jamapsychiatry.2023.0222

Strickhouser, J. E., Zell, E., & Krizan, Z. (2017). Does personality predict health and well-being? A metasynthesis. *Health Psychology*, 36(8), 797–810. https://doi.org/10.1037/hea0000475

Strickler, G. K., Kreiner, P. W., Halpin, J. F., Doyle, E., & Paulozzi, L. J. (2020). Opioid prescribing behaviors—Prescription behavior surveillance system, 11 states, 2010–2016. *MMWR Surveillance Summaries*, 69(No. SS-1), 1–14.

Strike, P. C., Magid, K., Whitehead, D. L., Brydon, L., Bhattacharyya, M. R., & Steptoe, A. (2006). Pathophysiological processes underlying emotional triggering of acute cardiac events. *Proceedings of the National Academy of Sciences*, 103(11), 4322–4327. https://doi.org/10.1073/pnas.0507097103

Stringhini, S., Carmeli, C., Jokela, M., Avendaño, M., Muennig, P., Guida, F., ... LIFEPATH consortium. (2017). Socioeconomic status and the 25 × 25 risk factors as determinants of premature mortality: A multicohort study and meta-analysis of 1·7 million men and women. *Lancet*, 389, 1229–1237.

Stubberud, A., Omland, P. M., Tronvik, E., Olsen, A., Sand, T., & Linde, M. (2018). Wireless surface electromyography and skin temperature sensors for biofeedback treatment of headache: Validation study with stationary control equipment. *JMIR Biomedical Engineering*, 3(1). https://doi.org/10.2196/biomedeng.9062

Studd, J., & Nappi, R. E. (2012). Reproductive depression. *Gynecological Endocrinology*, 28(Suppl. 1), 42–45. https://doi.org/10.3109/09513590.2012.651932

Sturgeon, J. A., & Darnell, B. D. (2018). Facilitating patient resilience: Mindfulness-based stress reduction, acceptance, and positive social and emotional interventions. In D. C. Turk & R. J. Gatchel (Eds.), *Psychological approaches to pain management: A practitioner's handbook* (3rd ed., pp. 250–263). The Guilford Press.

Sublette, V. A., Smith, S. K., George, J., McCaffery, K., & Douglas, M. W. (2018). Listening to both sides: A qualitative comparison between patients with hepatitis C and their healthcare professionals' perceptions of the facilitators and barriers to hepatitis C treatment adherence and completion. *Journal of Health Psychology*, 23, 1720–1731.

Suh, H., Hill, T. D., & Koenig, H. G. (2019). Religious attendance and biological risk: A national longitudinal study of older adults. *Journal of Religion and Health*, 58, 1188–1202.

Sullivan, C., & Kashubeck-West, S. (2015). The interplay of international students' acculturative stress, social support, and acculturation modes. *Journal of International Students*, 5(1), 1–11.

Sullivan, M. J. L., Bishop, S. R., & Pivik, J. (1995). The Pain Catastrophizing Scale: Development and validation. *Psychological Assessment*, 7(4), 524–532.

Sullivan, P. W., Ghushchyan, V., Kavati, A., Navaratnam, P., Friedman, H. S., & Ortiz, B. (2019a). Trends in asthma control, treatment, health care utilization, and expenditures among children in the United States by place of residence: 2003–2014. *Journal of Allergy and Clinical Immunology Practice*, 7, 1835–1842.

Sun, G., Acheampong, R. A., Lin, H., & Pun, V. C. (2015). Understanding walking behavior among university students using theory of planned behavior. *International Journal of Environmental Research and Public Health*, 12, 13794–13806.

Sun, L. H. (2018, September 17). The health dangers don't stop with a hurricane's churning. They can get worse. *The Washington Post*.

Suran, M. (2022). Racial disparities in dementia diagnoses. *JAMA: The Journal of the American Medical Association*, 327(8), 709. https://doi.org/10.1001/jama.2022.0979

Süss, H., & Ehlert, U. (2020). Psychological resilience during the perimenopause. *Maturitas*, 131, 48–56. https://doi.org/10.1016/j.maturitas.2019.10.015

Swain, G. R. (2016–2017, Fall/Winter). How does economic and social disadvantage affect health? Institute for Research on Poverty.

Sweenie, R., Basch, M., Ding, K., Pinto, S., Chardon, M. L., Janicke, D. M., ... Fedele, D. A. (2020). Subjective social status in adolescents with asthma: Psychosocial and physical health outcomes. *Health Psychology*, 39, 172–178.

Swindells, S., Andrade-Villanueva, J., Richmond, G. J., Rizzardini, G., Baumgarten, A., Masia, M., ... Ki, Y. (2020). Long-acting cabotegravir and rilpivirine for maintenance of HIV-1 suppression. *The New England Journal of Medicine*, 382, 1112–1123.

Szabo, S., Tache, Y., & Somogyi, A. (2012). The legacy of Hans Selye and the origins of stress research: A retrospective 75 years after his landmark brief "letter" to the editor of Nature. *Stress*, 15(5), 472–478.

Szuhany, K. L., & Simon, N. M. (2022). Anxiety disorders. *JAMA*, 328(24), 2431. https://doi.org/10.1001/jama.2022.22744

Tabrizi, R., Saneei, P., Lankarani, K. B., Akbari, M., Kolahdooz, F., Esmaillzadeh, A., ... Asemi, Z. (2018). The effects of caffeine intake on weight loss: A systematic review and dose–response meta-analysis of randomized controlled trials. *Critical Reviews in Food Science and Nutrition*. https://doi.org/10.1080/10408398.2018.1507996

Tait, R. C., & Chibnall, J. T. (2014). Racial/ethnic disparities in the assessment and treatment of pain: Psychosocial perspectives. *American Psychologist*, 69, 131–141.

Takashima, Y., & Mandyam, C. D. (2018). The role of hippocampal adult neurogenesis in methamphetamine addiction. *Brain Plasticity*, 3(2), 157–168.

Taksler, G. B., Pfoh, E. R., Stange, K. C., & Rothberg, M. B. (2018). Association between number of preventive care guidelines and preventive care utilization by patients. *American Journal of Preventive Medicine*, 55(1), 1–10.

Talati, Z., Egnell, M., Hercberg, S., Julia, C., & Pettigrew, S. (2019). Food choice under five front-of-package nutrition label conditions: An experimental study across 12 countries. *American Journal of Public Health*, 109(12), 1770–1775.

Talwar, A., Tsang, C. A., Price, S. F., Walker, W. L., Schmit, K. M., & Langer, A. J. (2019). Tuberculosis—United States, 2018. *Morbidity and Mortality Weekly Report*, 68, 257–262.

Taquet, M., Luciano, S., Geddes, J. R., & Harrison, P. J. (2021). Bidirectional associations between COVID-19 and psychiatric disorder: Retrospective cohort studies of 62 354 COVID-19 cases in the USA. *The Lancet Psychiatry*, 8(2), 130–140. https://doi.org/10.1016/s2215-0366(20)30462-4

Tatangelo, G. L., & Ricciardelli, L. A. (2017). Children's body image and social comparisons with peers and the media. *Journal of Health Psychology*, 22(6), 776–787.

Taubes, G. (2012). Unraveling the obesity-cancer connection. *Science*, 335, 28–32. https://doi.org/10.1126/science.335.6064.28

Taylor, M. K., Pietrobon, R., Taverniers, J., Leon, M. R., & Fern, B. F. (2013). Relationships of hardiness to physical and mental health status in military men: A test of mediated effects. *Journal of Behavioral Medicine*, 36, 1–9.

Taylor, S. E. (2006). Tend and befriend: Biobehavioral bases of affiliation under stress. *Current Directions in Psychological Science*, 15(6), 273–277.

Taylor, S. E. (2011). Tend and befriend theory. In P. A. M. Van Lange, A. W. Kruglanski, & E. T. Higgins (Eds.), *Handbook of theories of social psychology* (Vol. 1, pp. 32–49). Sage.

Tchobaniouk, L. V., McAllister, E. E., Bishop, D. L., Carpentier, R. M., Heins, K. R., Haight, R. J., & Bishop, J. R. (2019). Once-monthly subcutaneously administered risperidone in the treatment of schizophrenia: Patient considerations. *Patient Preference and Adherence*, 13, 2233–2241.

Teleki, S., Zsidó, A. N., Komócsi, A., Lénárd, L., Kiss, E. C., & Tiringer, I. (2019). The role of social support in the dietary behavior of coronary heart patients: An application of the health action process approach. *Psychology, Health & Medicine*, 24, 714–724.

Teplin, L. A., McClelland, G. M., Abram, K. M., & Weiner, D. A. (2005). Crime victimization in adults with severe mental illness: Comparison with the National Crime Victimization Survey. *Archives of General Psychiatry*, 62, 911–921.

Terracciano, A., Bilgel, M., Aschwanden, D., Luchetti, M., Stephan, Y., Moghekar, A. R., ... Resnick, S. M. (2021). Personality associations with amyloid and tau: Results from the Baltimore longitudinal study of aging and meta-analysis. *Biological Psychiatry*. https://doi.org/10.1016/j.biopsych.2021.08.021

Terry, P. C., Karageorghis, C. I., Curran, M. L., Martin, O. V., & Parsons-Smith, R. L. (2020). Effects of music in exercise and sport: A meta-analytic review. *Psychological Bulletin*, 146(2), 91–117.

Tessier, A., Dupuy, M., Baylé, F. J., Herse, C., Lange, A. C., Vrijens, B., ... Misdrahi, D. (2020). Brief interventions for improving adherence in schizophrenia: A pilot study using electronic medication event monitoring. *Psychiatry Research*, 285, 112–118.

The EUGenMed, Cardiovascular Clinical Study Group, Regitz-Zagrosek, V., Oertelt-Prigione, S., Prescott, E., Franconi, F., Gerdts, E., Foryst-Ludwig, A., ... Stangl, V. (2016). Gender in cardiovascular diseases: Impact on clinical manifestations, management, and outcomes. *European Heart Journal*, 37, 24–34.

Thibeault, M. A., Stein, G. L., & Nelson-Gray, R. O. (2018). Ethnic identity in context of ethnic discrimination: When does gender and other-group orientation increase risk for depressive symptoms for immigrant-origin young adults? *Cultural Diversity and Ethnic Minority Psychology*, 24, 196–208. http://dx.doi.org/10.1037/cdp0000174

Thieme, H., Morkisch, N., Rietz, C., Dohle, C., & Borgetto, B. (2016). The efficacy of movement representation techniques for treatment of limb pain—A systematic review and meta-analysis. *The Journal of Pain*, 17, 167–180.

Thirumurthy, H., Asch, D. A., & Volpp, K. G. (2019). The uncertain effect of financial incentives to improve health behaviors. *Journal of the American Medical Association*, 321, 1451–1452.

Thøgersen-Ntoumani, C., Shepherd, S. O., Ntoumanis, N., Wagenmakers, A. J., & Shaw, C. S. (2016). Intrinsic motivation in two exercise interventions: Associations with fitness and body composition. *Health Psychology*, 35(2), 195–198.

Thomas, K. L., Shah, B. R., Elliot-Bynum, S., Thomas, K. D., Damon, K., Allen LaPointe, N. M., ... Anderson, M. (2014). Check it, change it: A community-based, multifaceted intervention to improve blood pressure control. *Circulation: Cardiovascular Quality and Outcomes*, 7(6), 828–834. https://doi.org/10.1161/CIRCOUTCOMES.114.001039

Thomas, L., Orme, E., & Kerrigan, F. (2020). Student loneliness: The role of social media through life transitions. *Computers & Education*, 146. https://doi.org/10.1016/j.compedu.2019.103754

Thompson, A., & Tapp, S. N. (2022). Criminal victimization, *2021*. Bureau of Justice Statistics, U.S. Department of Justice. https://bjs.ojp.gov/content/pub/pdf/cv21.pdf

Thompson-Brenner, H. (2013). Good news about psychotherapy for eating disorders: Comment on Warren, Schafer, Crowley, and Olivardia. *Psychotherapy*, 50, 565–567.

Thurston, G. D., & Newman, J. D. (2018). Walking to a pathway for cardiovascular effects of air pollution. *The Lancet*, 391(10118), 291–292. https://doi.org/10.1016/S0140-6736(17)33078-7

Thyme, S. B., Pieper, L. M., Li, E. H., Pandey, S., Wang, Y., Morris, N. S., ... Schier, A. F. (2019). Phenotypic landscape of schizophrenia-associated genes defines candidates and their shared functions. *Cell*, 177(2), 478–491.e20. https://doi.org/10.1016/j.cell.2019.01.048

Tian, X. (2023). The impact of feminized stigma on male socialization. *Journal of Education, Humanities and Social Sciences,* 8, 1693–1698.

Tiggemann, M., & Zaccardo, M. (2018). "Strong is the new skinny": A content analysis of #fitspiration images on Instagram. *Journal of Health Psychology*, 23(8), 1003–1011.

Tinnermann, A., Geuter, S., Sprenger, C., Finsterbusch, J., & Büchel, C. (2017). Interactions between brain and spinal cord mediate value effects in nocebo hyperalgesia. *Science*, 358, 105–108.

Titova, O. E., Baron, J. A., Michaëlsson, K., & Larsson, S. C. (2022). Anger frequency and risk of cardiovascular morbidity and mortality. *European Heart Journal Open,* 2(4). https://doi.org/10.1093/ehjopen/oeac050

Tobias, D. K., Chen, M., Manson, J. E., Ludwig, D. S., Willett, W., & Hu, F. B. (2015). Effect of low-fat diet interventions versus other diet interventions on long-term weight change in adults: A systematic review and meta-analysis. *The Lancet Diabetes & Endocrinology*, 3(12), 968–979.

Toker, A. (2019). NCER gene. *Science*, 366, 685–686.

Tolami, H. F., Sharafshah, A., Tolami, L. F., & Keshavarz, P. (2019). Haplotype-based association and in silico studies of oprm1 gene variants with susceptibility to opioid dependence among addicted Iranians undergoing methadone treatment. *Journal of Molecular Neuroscience*, 1–10. https://doi.org/10.1007/s12031-019-01443-4

Tollosa, D. N., Tavener, M., Hure, A., & James, E. L. (2019). Adherence to multiple health behaviours in cancer survivors: A systematic review and meta-analysis. *Journal of Cancer Survivorship*, 13(3), 327–343.

Tomasi, D., Gates, S., & Reyns, E. (2019). Positive patient response to a structured exercise program delivered in inpatient psychiatry. *Global Advances in Health and Medicine.* https://journals.sagepub.com/doi/10.1177/2164956119848657

Tomiyama, A. J. (2014). Weight stigma is stressful. A review of evidence for the cyclic obesity/weight-based stigma model. *Appetite*, 82, 8–15. https://doi.org/10.1016/j.appet.2014.06.108. Epub 2014 Jul 2.

Tomiyama, A. J. (2019). Stress and obesity. *Annual Review of Psychology*, 70, 703–718.

Tran, S. T., Grotkowski, K., Miller, S. A., Reed, B. W., Koven, M. L., Buscemi, J., . . . Greenley, R. N. (2021). Hassles predict physical health complaints in undergraduate students: a dynamic structural equation model analysis of daily diary data. *Psychology & Health*, 36(7), 828–846. https://doi.org/10.1080/08870446.2020.1800010

Treat, T. A., Church, E. K., & Viken, R. J. (2017). Effects of gender, rape-supportive attitudes, and explicit instruction on perceptions of women's momentary sexual interest. *Psychonomic Bulletin & Review*, 24(3), 979–986.

Troxel, W. M., Rodriguez, A., Seelam, R., Tucker, J. S., Shih, R. A., & D'Amico, E. J. (2019). Associations of longitudinal sleep trajectories with risky sexual behavior during late adolescence. *Health Psychology*, 38(8), 716–726.

Trubetskoy, B., Pardiñas, A. F., Qi, T., Panagiotaropoulou, G., Awasthi, S., Bigdeli, T. B., ... Gershon, E. S. (2022). Mapping genomic loci implicates genes and synaptic biology in schizophrenia. *Nature,* 604(7906). https://doi.org/10.1038/s41586-022-04434-5

Trunko, M. E., Schwartz, T. A., Berner, L. A., Cusack, A., Nakamura, T., Bailer, U. F., ... Kaye, W. H. (2017). A pilot open series of lamotrigine in DBT-treated eating disorders characterized by significant affective dysregulation and poor impulse control. *Borderline Personality Disorder and Emotion Dysregulation*, 4(1), 21,

Tseng, Y.-F., Wang, K.-L., Lin, C.-Y., Lin, Y.-T., Pan, H.-C., & Chang, C.-J. (2018). Predictors of smoking cessation in Taiwan: Using the theory of planned behavior. *Psychology, Health & Medicine*, 23(3), 270–276.

Tsipa, A., O'Connor, D. B., Branley-Bell, D., Day, F., Hall, L., Sykes-Muskett, B., ... Conner, M. (2020). Promoting colorectal cancer screening: a systematic review and meta-analysis of randomized controlled trials of interventions to increase uptake. *Health Psychology Review,* 15(3), 371–394. https://doi.org/10.1080/17437199.2020.1760726

Tucker, K. L., Sheppard, J. P., Stevens, R., Bosworth, H. B., Bove, A., Bray, E. P., ... McManus, R. J. (2017). Self-monitoring of blood pressure in hypertension: A systematic review and individual patient data meta-analysis. *PLoS Medicine*, 14(9). https://doi.org/10.1371/journal.pmed.1002389

Tully, J., Montgomery, C., Maier, L. J., & Sumnall, H. R. (2020). Estimated prevalence, effects and potential risks of substances used for cognitive enhancement. In K. van de Ven, K. J. D. Mulrooney, & J. McVeigh (Eds.), *Human enhancement drugs*. Routledge.

Tuman, M., & Moyer, A. (2019). Health intentions and behaviors of health app owners: A cross-sectional study. *Psychology, Health & Medicine*, 24, 819–826.

Turanovic, J. J., Pratt, T. C., & Piquero, A. R. (2017). Exposure to fetal testosterone, aggression, and violent behavior: A meta-analysis of the 2D:4D digit ratio. *Aggression and Violent Behavior*, 33, 51–61.

Turk, D. C. (2018a). A cognitive and behavioral perspective on the treatment of individuals experiencing chronic pain. In D. C. Turk & R. J. Gatchel (Eds.), *Psychological approaches to pain management: A practitioner's handbook* (3rd ed., pp. 115–137). The Guilford Press.

Turk, D. C. (2018). A cognitive and behavioral perspective on the treatment of individuals experience experiencing chronic pain. In D. C. Turk & R. J. Gatchel (Eds.), *Psychological approaches to pain management: A practitioner's handbook* (3rd ed., pp. 115–137). New York: The Guilford Press.

Turk, D. C. (2018b). Treatment of patients with fibromyalgia. In D. C. Turk & R. J. Gatchel (Eds.), *Psychological approaches to pain management: A practitioner's handbook* (3rd ed., pp. 398–424). The Guilford Press.

Turk, D. C., & Gatchel, R. J. (Eds.). (2018). *Psychological approaches to pain management: A practitioner's handbook* (3rd ed.). The Guilford Press.

Turk, D. C., & Murphy, T. B. (2019). Pain. In C. D. Llewellyn, S. Ayers, C. McManus, S. Newman, K. J. Petrie, T. A. Revenson, & J. Weinman (Eds.), *Cambridge handbook of psychology, health and medicine* (3rd ed., pp. 84–88). Cambridge University Press.

Turner, J. A., Mancl, L., & Aaron, L. A. (2006). Short and long-term efficacy of brief cognitive-behavioral therapy for patients with chronic temporomandibular disorder pain: A randomized, controlled trial. *Pain*, 121, 181–194.

Turner, L., Galante, J., Vainre, M., Stochl, J., Dufour, G., & Jones, P. (2020). Immune dysregulation among students exposed to exam stress and its mitigation by mindfulness training: Findings from an exploratory randomised trial. *Scientific Reports*. https://doi.org/10.17863/CAM.49516

Turnwald, B. P., Bertoldo, J. D., Perry, M. A., Policastro, P., Timmons, M., Bosso, C., ... Gardner, C. D. (2019). Increasing vegetable intake by emphasizing tasty and enjoyable attributes: A randomized controlled multisite intervention for taste-focused labeling. *Psychological Science*, 30(11), 1603–1615.

Tutek, J., Gunn, H. E., & Lichstein, K. L. (2020). Worry and rumination have distinct associations with nighttime versus daytime sleep symptomology. *Behavioral Sleep Medicine*, 1–16.

Twenge, J. M., Joiner, T. E., Martin, G., & Rogers, M. L. (2018a). Digital media may explain a substantial portion of the rise in depressive symptoms among adolescent girls: Response to Daly. *Clinical Psychological Science*, 6, 296–297. https://doi.org/10.1177/2167702618759321

Twenge, J. M., Joiner, T. E., Rogers, M. L., & Martin, G. N. (2018b). Increases in depressive symptoms, suicide-related outcomes, and suicide rates among U.S. adolescents after 2010 and links to increased new media screen time. *Clinical Psychological Science*, 6, 3–17. https://doi.org/10.1177/2167702617723376

Ullrich, M., Weber, M., Post, A. M., Popp, S., Grein, J., Zechner, M., ... Schuh, K. (2017). OCD-like behavior is caused by dysfunction of thalamo-amygdala circuits and upregulated TrkB/ERK-MAPK signaling as a result of SPRED2 deficiency. *Molecular Psychiatry*, 23, 444–458.

United Health Foundation. (2019). 2019 annual report. America's Health Rankings. https://www.americashealthrankings.org/learn/reports/2019-annual-report

U.S. Bureau of Justice Statistics. (2022). Criminal offenses. U.S. Department of National Center for Education Statistics.

U.S. Department of Health and Human Services. (2001). National Household Survey on Drug Abuse: Highlights 2000.

U.S. Department of Health and Human Services (USDHHS). (2018). *Physical activity guidelines for Americans* (2nd ed.). U.S. Department of Health and Human Services.

U.S. Department of Health and Human Services (USDHHS). (2020). About ending the HIV epidemic: Plan for America. https://www.hiv.gov/federal-response/ending-the-hiv-epidemic/overview

U.S. Department of Justice (2019). Facts and statistics. https://www.justice.gov

U.S. Department of Justice. (2023). Facts and statistics. https://www.justice.gov/hatecrimes/hate-crime-statistics

U.S. Preventive Services Task Force. (2017). Behavioral counseling to promote a healthful diet and physical activity for cardiovascular disease prevention in adults without cardiovascular risk factors: US Preventive Services Task Force Recommendation Statement. *Journal of the American Medical Association*, 318, 167–174.

U.S. Preventive Services Task Force. (2020). Recommendation: Healthy diet and physical activity for cardiovascular disease prevention in adults with cardiovascular risk factors: Behavioral counseling interventions. *United States Preventive Services Taskforce*.

U.S. Preventive Services Taskforce (USPSTF). (2021). Tobacco smoking cessation in adults, including pregnant persons: Interventions. https://uspreventiveservicestaskforce.org/uspstf/recommendation/tobacco-use-in-adults-and-pregnant-women-counseling-and-interventions

U.S. Surgeon General. (2010). How tobacco causes disease: The biology and behavioral basis for smoking-attributable disease: A report of the Surgeon General. https://www.ncbi.nlm.nih.gov/pubmed/21452462

Vahratian, A., Black, L. I., & Schoenborn, C. A. (2018). Percentage of adults aged ≥ 18 years who currently use e-cigarettes, by sex and age group. *National Health Interview Survey*, (xi) 2016.

Valgardson, B. A., & Schwartz, J. A. (2019). An examination of within- and between-family influences on the intergenerational transmission of violence and maltreatment. *Journal of Contemporary Criminal Justice*, 35(1), 87–102.

Vander Wal, J. S., Maraldo, T. M., Vercellone, A. C., & Gagne, D. A. (2015). Education, progressive muscle relaxation therapy, and exercise for the treatment of night eating syndrome. A pilot study. *Appetite*, 89, 136–144.

Van Dijk, H., Köke, A., Elbers, S., Mollema, J., Smeets, R. J. E. M., & Wittink, H. (2023). Physiotherapists using the biopsychosocial model for chronic pain: barriers and facilitators—A scoping review. *International Journal of Environmental Research and Public Health*, 20(2), 1634. https://doi.org/10.3390/ijerph20021634

Van Dorn, A., Cooney, R. E., & Sabin, M. L. (2020). COVID-19 exacerbating inequalities in the US. *The Lancet*. https://www.thelancet.com/journals/lancet/article/PIIS0140-6736(20)30893-X/fulltext

van Drongelen, A., Boot, C. R. L., Hlobil, H., Smid, T., & van der Beek, A. J. (2016). Process evaluation of a tailored mobile health intervention aiming to reduce fatigue in airline pilots. *BMC Public Health*, 16, 894.

Van Dyke, M., Greer, S., Odom, E., Greer, S., Odom, E., Schieb, L., ... Casper, M. (2018). Heart disease death rates among Blacks and Whites Aged ≥35 Years—United States, 1968–2015. *MMWR Surveillance Summaries*, 67(No. SS-5), 1–11.

VanFrank, B., & Presley-Cantrell, L. (2021). A comprehensive approach to increase adult tobacco cessation. *JAMA: The Journal of the American Medical Association*, 325(3), 232–233. https://doi.org/10.1001/jama.2020.23608

Van Meter, A. R., & Youngstrom, E. A. (2015). A tale of two diatheses: Temperament, BIS, and BAS as risk factors for mood disorder. *Journal of Affective Disorders*, 180, 170–178.

Van Tongeren, D. R., Aten, J. D., Davis, E. B., Davis, D. E., & Hook, J. N. (2020). Religion, spirituality, and meaning in the wake of disasters. In S. Schulenberg (Ed.), *Positive psychological approaches to disaster* (pp. 27–44). Springer.

van Tuijl, L. A., Basten, M., Pan, K.-Y., Vermeulen, R., Portengen, L., de Graeff, A., . . . Ranchor, A. V. (2023). Depression, anxiety, and the risk of cancer: An individual participant data meta-analysis. *Cancer*, 129(20), 3287–3299. https://doi.org/10.1002/cncr.34853

Vargas, P. A. (2020). Spreading the word: Comorbidity of asthma and depression is not just the product of a vulnerable personality. *The Journal of Allergy and Clinical Immunology: In Practice*, 8(1), 208–209.

Vasan, R. S. (2018). High blood pressure in young adulthood and risk of premature cardiovascular disease: Calibrating treatment benefits to potential harm. *Journal of the American Medical Association*, 320, 1760–1763.

Vasey, M. W., Vilensky, M. R., Heath, J. H., Harbaugh, C. N., Buffington, A. G., & Fazio, R. H. (2012). It was as big as my head, I swear! *Journal of Anxiety Disorders*, 26, 20. https://doi.org/10.1016/j.janxdis.2011.08.009

Vavani, B., Kraaij, V., Spinhoven, P., Amone-P'Olak, K., & Garnefski, N. (2020). Intervention targets for people living with HIV and depressive symptoms in Botswana. *African Journal of AIDS Research*, 19(1), 80–88.

Vedel, A. (2014). The Big Five and tertiary academic performance: A systematic review and meta-analysis. *Personality and Individual Differences*, 71, 66–76. https://doi.org/10.1016/j.paid.2014.07.011

Velasquez, M. M., von Sternberg, K., Dodrill, C. L., Kan, L. Y., & Parsons, J. T. (2005). The transtheoretical model as a framework for developing substance abuse interventions. *Journal of Addictions Nursing*, 16(1–2), 31–40. https://doi.org/10.1080/10884600590917174

Verduyn, P., Gugushvili, N., & Kross, E. (2021). The impact of social network sites on mental health: Distinguishing active from passive use. *World Psychiatry: Official Journal of the World Psychiatric Association (WPA)*, 20(1), 133–134. https://doi.org/10.1002/wps.20820

Villa-Alcazar, M., Aboitiz, J., Bengoechea, C., Martinez-Romera, I., Martinez-Naranjo, C., & Lopez-Ibor, B. (2019). Coping with incongruence: Mirror therapy to manage the phantom limb phenomenon in pediatric amputee patients. *Journal of Pain and Symptom Management*, 57(1), e1–e3.

Violanti, J. M., Ma, C. C., Mnatsakanova, A., Fekedulegn, D., Hartley, T. A., Gu, J. K., & Andrew, M. E. (2018). Associations between police work stressors and posttraumatic stress disorder symptoms: Examining the moderating effects of coping. *Journal of Police and Criminal Psychology*, 33(3), 271–282.

Vishkin, A. (2020). Variation and consistency in the links between religion and emotion regulation. *Current Opinion in Psychology*, 40, 6–9. https://doi.org/10.1016/j.copsyc.2020.08.005

Voelker, R. (2012). Asthma forecast: Why heat, humidity trigger symptoms. *JAMA*, 08(1). https://doi.org/10.1001/jama.2012.7533

Voelker, R. (2020). New migraine drug gains approval. *Journal of the American Medical Association*, 323, 408. https://doi.org/10.1001/jama.2020.0081

Vogel, M. E., Kanzler, K. E., Aikens, J. E., & Goodie, J. L. (2017). Integration of behavioral health and primary care: Current knowledge and future directions. *Journal of Behavioral Medicine*, 40(1), 69–84.

Vogel, R. A. (2019). Alcohol, heart disease, and mortality: A review. *Reviews in Cardiovascular Medicine*, 3(1), 7–13.

Volk, J. E., Marcus, J. L., Phengrasamy, T., Blechinger, D., Nguyen, D. P., Follansbee, S., & Hare, C. B. (2015). No new HIV infections with increasing use of HIV preexposure prophylaxis in a clinical practice setting. *Clinical Infectious Diseases*, 61(10), 1601–1603. https://doi.org/10.1093/cid/civ778

Vollmann, M., Engelhardt, G., & Salewski, C. (2021). Effects of a brief multimodal online intervention on the intention to conduct sun protective behaviours through targeting illness representations about skin cancer: A randomized controlled trial. *Psychology & Health*, 36, 3, 253–270. https://doi.org/10.1080/08870446.2020.1775831

Voorhees, S. E., Lawless, C., Ezmigna, D., & Fedele, D. A. (2020). Pediatric asthma. In A. C. Modi & K. A. Driscoll (Eds.), *Adherence and self-management in pediatric populations* (pp. 25–46). Academic Press.

Voss Jr., R. P., Corser, R., McCormick, M., & Jasper, J. D. (2018). Influencing health decision-making: A study of colour and message framing. *Psychology & Health*, 33, 941–954.

Vulczak, A., Souza, A. D. O., Ferrari, G. D., Azzolini, A. E. C. S., Pereira-da-Silva, G., & Alberici, L. C. (2020). Moderate exercise modulates tumor metabolism of triple-negative breast cancer. *Cells*, 9(3), 628.

Wachholtz, A. B., Malone, C. D., & Pargament, K. I. (2017). Effect of different meditation types on migraine headache medication use. *Behavioral Medicine*, 43(1), 1–8.

Wadden, T. A., Tronieri, J. S., & Butryn, M. L. (2020). Lifestyle modification approaches for the treatment of obesity in adults. *American Psychologist*, 75(2), 235–251.

Wahto, R., & Swift, J. K. (2016). Labels, gender-role conflict, stigma, and attitudes toward seeking psychological help in men. *American Journal of Men's Health*, 10(3), 181–191.

Waitzfelder, B., Stewart, C., Coleman, K. J., Rossom, R., Ahmedani, B. K., Beck, A., ... Simon, G. E. (2018). Treatment initiation for new episodes of depression in primary care settings. *Journal of General Internal Medicine*, 33(8), 1283–1291. https://link.springer.com/article/10.1007%2Fs11606-017-4297-2#citeas

Waldron, E. M., Burnett-Zeigler, I., Wee, V., Ng, Y. W., Koenig, L. J., Pederson, A. B., ... Miller, E. S. (2021). Mental health in women living with HIV: The unique and unmet needs. *Journal of the International Association of Providers of AIDS Care*, 20, 2325958220985665. https://doi.org/10.1177/2325958220985665

Walsh, C. (2020, April 14). COVID-19 targets communities of color. *The Harvard Gazette*. https://news.harvard.edu/gazette/story/2020/04/health-care-disparities-in-the-age-of-coronavirus/

Walsh, M. F., Cadoo, K., Salo-Mullen, E. E., Dubard-Gault, M., Stadler, Z. K., & Offit, K. (2020). Genetic factors: Hereditary cancer predisposition syndromes. In J. E. Niederhuber, J. O. Armitage, J. H. Doroshow, M. B. Kastan, & J. E. Tepper (Eds.), *Abeloff's clinical oncology* (6th ed., pp. 180–208). Elsevier. https://doi.org/10.1016/B978-0-323-47674-4.00013-X

Walters, A. (2020, January 3). Survey uncovers incorrect thinking about leading cause of death in women. WKBN.com. Youngstown, OH.

Wang, C., Lê-Scherban, F., Taylor, J., Salmoirago-Blotcher, E., Allison, M., Gefen, D., ... Michael, Y. L. (2021). Associations of job strain, stressful life events, and social strain with coronary heart disease in the women's health initiative observational study. *Journal of the American Heart Association*, 10(5). https://doi.org/10.1161/jaha.120.017780

Wang, D., Lu, Y., Han, Y., Zhang, X., Dong, S., Zhang, H., ... Wang, J. Z. (2023). The influence of etiology and stimulation target on the outcome of deep brain stimulation for chronic neuropathic pain: A systematic review and meta-analysis. *Neuromodulation: Technology at the Neural Interface*. https://doi.org/10.1016/j.neurom.2022.12.002

Wang, J. H.-Y., Gomez, S. L., Brown, R. L., Davis, K., Allen, L., Huang, E., ... Schwartz, M. D. (2019). Factors associated with Chinese American and White cancer survivors' physical and psychological functioning. *Health Psychology*, 38, 455–465.

Wang, J., Mann, F., Lloyd-Evans, B., Ma, R., & Johnson, S. (2018). Associations between loneliness and perceived social support and outcomes of mental health problems: A systematic review. *BMC Psychiatry*, 18(1), 156. https://doi.org/10.1186/s12888-018-1736-5

Wang, X., Liu, F., Li, J., Yang, X., Chen, J., Cao, J., ... Zhao, L. (2020). Tea consumption and the risk of atherosclerotic cardiovascular disease and all-cause mortality: The China-PAR project. *European Journal of Preventive Cardiology*. https://doi.org/10.1177/2047487319894685

Wang, X., Zhang, J., Feng, K., Yang, Y., Qi, W., Martinez-Vazquez, P., ... Wang, T. (2020). The effect of hypothermia during cardiopulmonary bypass on three electro-encephalographic indices assessing analgesia and hypnosis during anesthesia: Consciousness index, nociception index, and bispectral index. *Perfusion*, 35(2), 154–162.

Wansink, B., & van Ittersum, K. (2013). Portion size me: Plate-size induced consumption norms and win–win solutions for reducing food intake and waste. *Journal of Experimental Psychology: Applied*, 19, 320–332.

Wan, X., Schonfeld, P. M., & Li, Q. (2016). What factors determine metro passengers' risky riding behavior? An approach based on an extended theory of planned behavior. *Transportation Research Part F*, 42, 125–139.

Wapner, J. (2022, March 28). Cancer patients are at high risk of depression and suicide, studies find. *New York Times*. https://www.nytimes.com/2022/03/28/health/cancer-patients-depression-suicide.html?searchResultPosition=

Ward, E. M., Sherman, R. L., Henley, S. J., Jemal, A., Siegel, D. A., Feuer, E. J., ... Cronin, K. A. (2019). Annual report to the nation on the status of cancer, featuring cancer in men and women age 20–49 years. *Journal of the National Cancer Institute*, 111(12), 1279–1297. https://doi.org/10.1093/jnci/djz106

Ward, Z. J., Bleich, S. N., Cradock, A. L., Barrett, J. L., Giles, C. M., Flax, C., ... Gortmacher, S. L. (2019). Projected U.S. state-level prevalence of adult obesity and severe obesity. *New England Journal of Medicine*, 381, 2440–2450.

Washington Post. (2015, June 12). One in 5 college women say they were violated. http://www.washingtonpost.com/sf/local/2015/06/12/1-in-5-women-say-they-were-violated/

Wasielewska, M., & Bethke, K. (2019). Genetic view on intelligence and its heredity. *Journal of Education, Health and Sport*, 9(8), 481–487.

Wasserman, A. M., Crockett, L. J., Temmen, C. D., & Carlo, G. (2021). Bicultural stress and internalizing symptoms among U.S. Latinx youth: The moderating role of peer and parent support. *Cultural Diversity & Ethnic Minority Psychology*, 27(4), 769–780. https://doi.org/10.1037/cdp0000474

Watson, D., Suls, J., & Haig, J. (2002). Global self-esteem in relation to structural models of personality and affectivity. *Journal of Personality and Social Psychology*, 83, 185–197.

Watson, K. D. (2018). Women are not equally included in all cardiovascular clinical trials. *NEJM Journal Watch*. https://www.jwatch.org/na46669/2018/05/07/women-are-not-equally-included-all-cardiovascular-clinical

Watson, K. E. (2019b). The role of U.S. outcomes in acute myocardial infarction have improved in the last 20 years. *NEJM Journal Watch*. https://www.jwatch.org/na48885/2019/04/10/us-outcomes-acute-myocardial-infarction-have-improved-last

Watson, R. J., Peter, T., McKay, T., Edkins, T., & Saewyc, E. (2018b). Evidence of changing patterns in mental health and depressive symptoms for sexual minority adolescents. *Journal of Gay & Lesbian Mental Health*, 22(2), 120–138.

Waugh, M., Calderone, J., Brown Levey, S., Lyon, C., Thomas, M., DeGruy, F., & Shore, J. H. (2019). Using telepsychiatry to enrich existing integrated primary care. *Telemedicine and E-Health*, 25(8), 762–768.

Weaver, J. (2012, March 1). Twitter reveals people are happiest in the morning.

Weber, S. R., Pargament, K. I., Kunik, M. E., Lomax, J. W., & Stanley, M. A. (2012). Psychological distress among religious nonbelievers: A systematic review. *Journal of Religion and Health*, 51(1), 72–86.

Webster, R. K., Brooks, S. K., Smith, L. E., Woodland, L., Wessely, S., & Rubin, G. J. (2020). How to improve adherence with quarantine: Rapid review of the evidence. *Public Health*. https://doi.org/10.1016/j.puhe.2020.03.007

Wechsler, M. E., Szefler, S. J., Ortega, V. E., Pongracic, J. A., Chinchilli, V., Lima, J. J., ... Beigelman, A., for the NHLBI AsthmaNet. (2019). Step-up therapy in black children and adults with poorly controlled asthma. *New England Journal of Medicine*, 381, 1227–1239.

Wechsler, T. F., Kümpers, F., & Mühlberger, A. (2020). Inferiority or even superiority of virtual reality exposure therapy in phobias?—A systematic review and quantitative meta-analysis on randomized controlled trials comparing the efficacy of virtual therapy exposure to gold standard in vivo exposure in agoraphobia, specific phobia, and social phobia. In F. Pallavicini & S. Boucard (Eds.), *Assessing the therapeutic uses and effectiveness of virtual reality, augmented reality and video games for emotion regulation and stress management*. Frontiers in Psychology Research Topics.

Weidenauer, A., Bauer, M., Sauerzopf, U., Bartova, L., Meyer, B. M., Rabl, U., ... Willeit, M. (2020). On the relationship of first-episode psychosis to the amphetamine-sensitized state: A dopamine D2/3 receptor agonist radioligand study. *Translational Psychiatry*, 10, 2. https://doi.org/10.1038/s41398-019-0681-5

Weinberg, R. (2018). Theories and models of behavior change applied to exercise: Research and practice. In S. Razon & M. L. Sachs (Eds.), *Applied exercise psychology: The challenging journey from motivation to adherence* (pp. 37–48). Routledge.

Weir, K. (2016, March). Positive feedback. *Monitor on Psychology*, 47(3), 50–55.

Weitzer, J., Papantoniou, K., Lázaro-Sebastià, C., Seidel, S., Klösch, G., & Schernhammer, E. (2020). The contribution of dispositional optimism to understanding insomnia symptomatology: Findings from a cross-sectional population study in Austria. *Journal of Sleep Research*. https://doi.org/10.1111/jsr.13132

Wei, W. (2017, November 23). This 20,000-calorie burger is the craziest thing we've ever eaten. *Business Insider*. https://www.businessinsider.com/heart-attack-grill-burger-las-vegas-2015-1

Wenger, N. K. (2020). Adverse cardiovascular outcomes for women—Biology, bias, or both? *JAMA Cardiology*, 5(3), 27–28.

Wennerberg, E., Lhuillier, C., Rybstein, M. D., Dannenberg, K., Rudqvist, N. P., Koelwyn, G. J., ... Demaria, S. (2020). Exercise reduces immune suppression and breast cancer progression in a preclinical model. *Oncotarget*, 11(4), 452–461.

Whelton, P. K., & Carey, R. M. (2017). The 2017 clinical practice guideline for high blood pressure. *Journal of the American Medical Association*, 318, 2073–2074.

White, A. M., Castle, I. J. P., Hingson, R. W., & Powell, P. A. (2020). Using death certificates to explore changes in alcohol-related mortality in the United States, 1999 to 2017. *Alcoholism: Clinical and Experimental Research*. https://doi.org/10.1111/acer.14239

Whiting, D., Gulati, G., Geddes, J. R., & Fazel, S. (2022). Association of schizophrenia spectrum disorders and violence perpetration in adults and adolescents from 15 countries. *JAMA Psychiatry*, 79(2), 120. https://doi.org/10.1001/jamapsychiatry.2021.3721

Whiting, D., Lichtenstein, P., & Fazel, S. (2021). Violence and mental disorders: a structured review of associations by individual diagnoses, risk factors, and risk assessment. *The Lancet. Psychiatry*, 8(2), 150–161. https://doi.org/10.1016/S2215-0366(20)30262-5

Wilkinson, S. T., Ballard, E. D., Bloch, M. H., Mathew, S. J., Murrough, J. W., Feder, A., ... Sanacora, G. (2018). The effect of a single dose of intravenous ketamine on suicidal ideation: A systematic review and individual participant data meta-analysis. *American Journal of Psychiatry*, 175, 150–158. https://doi.org/10.1176/appi.ajp.2017.17040472

Willems, S. J., Castells, M. C., & Baptist, A. P. (2022). The magnification of health disparities during the Covid-19 pandemic. *The*

Journal of Allergy and Clinical Immunology: In Practice, 10(4), 903–908. https://doi.org/10.1016/j.jaip.2022.01.032

Williams, D. R., Priest, N., & Anderson, N. B. (2016). Understanding associations among race, socioeconomic status, and health: Patterns and prospects. *Health Psychology*, 35, 407–411.

Williams, J. E., Paton, C. C., Siegler, I. C., Eigenbrodt, M. L., Nieto, F. J., & Tyroler, H. A. (2000). Anger proneness predicts coronary heart disease risk: Prospective analysis from the Atherosclerosis Risk in Communities (ARIC) Study. *Circulation*, 101, 2034–2039.

Williams, M. T. (2020). Microaggressions: Clarification, evidence, and impact. *Perspectives on Psychological Science*, 15(1), 3–26.

Wilmot, M. P., & Ones, D. S. (2021). Occupational characteristics moderate personality–performance relations in major occupational groups. *Journal of Vocational Behavior,* 131, 103655. https://doi.org/10.1016/j.jvb.2021.103655

Wilsnack, R. W., Wilsnack, S. C., Gmel, G., & Kantor, L. W. (2018). Gender differences in binge drinking: Prevalence, predictors, and consequences. *Alcohol Research: Current Reviews*, 39(1), 57–76.

Wilson, L. C., & Newins, A. R. (2023). The role of gender, sexual assault history, and sexism in endorsement of rape myths among college students. *Violence Against Women.* 10778012231166406.

Wilson, T. E., Hennessy, E. A., Falzon, L., Boyd, R., Kronish, I. M., & Birk, J. L. (2019). Effectiveness of interventions targeting self-regulation to improve adherence to chronic disease medications: A meta-review of meta-analyses. *Health Psychology Review*, 19, 1–41.

Wilson, T. E., Hennessy, E. A., Falzon, L., Boyd, R., Kronish, I. M., & Birk, J. L. (2020). Effectiveness of interventions targeting self-regulation to improve adherence to chronic disease medications: A meta-review of meta-analyses. *Health Psychology Review*, 14, 66–85.

Wilt, J., & Revelle, W. (2018). The Big Five, everyday contexts and activities, and affective experience. *Personality and Individual Differences*, 136, 140–147. https://doi.org/10.1016/j.paid.2017.12.032

Winerip, M. (1998, January 4). Binge nights. *New York Times, Education Life*, Section 4A, pp. 28–31, 42.

Winerman, L. (2016). Snapshots of some of the latest peer-reviewed research within psychology and related fields. *Monitor on Psychology*, 47(10), 9.

Winerman, L. (2018). Making campuses safer. *Monitor on Psychology*, 49(9), 54. https://www.apa.org/monitor/2018/10/campuses-safer.aspx

Wippold, G. M., Frary, S. G., Garcia, K. A., & Wilson, D. K. (2023). Implementing barbershop-based health-promotion interventions for Black men: A systematic scoping review. *Health Psychology,* 42(7), 435–447. https://doi.org/10.1037/hea0001294

Wirga, M., DeBernardi, M., Wirga, A., Wirga, M. L., Banout, M., & Fuller, O. G. (2020). Maultsby's rational behavior therapy: Background, description, practical applications, and recent developments. *Journal of Rational-Emotive & Cognitive-Behavior Therapy*. https://doi.org/10.1007/s10942-020-00341-8

Wise, R. A., & Robble, M. A. (2020). Dopamine and addiction. *Annual Review of Psychology*, 71, 79–106.

Wittfeld, K., Jochem, C., Dörr, M., Schminke, U., Gläser, S., Bahls, M., ... Bülow, R. (2020, January). Cardiorespiratory fitness and gray matter volume in the temporal, frontal, and cerebellar regions in the general population. *Mayo Clinic Proceedings*, 95(1), 44–56.

Wittig, R. M., Crockford, C., Weltring, A., Langergraber, K. E., Deschner, T., & Zuberbühler, K. (2016). Social support reduces stress hormone levels in wild chimpanzees across stressful events and everyday affiliations. *Nature Communications*, 7. https://doi.org/10.1038/ncomms13361

Wittstein, I. S., Thiemann, D. R., Lima, J. A. C., Baughman, K. J., Schulman, S. P., Gerstenblith, G., ... Champion, H. C. (2005). Neurohumoral features of myocardial stunning due to sudden emotional stress. *New England Journal of Medicine*, 352, 539–548.

Wong, N. C. (2016). "Vaccinations are safe and effective": Inoculating positive HPV vaccine attitudes against antivaccination attack messages. *Communication Reports*, 29(3), 127–138.

Wong, P. P., & Tomer, A. (2011). Beyond terror and denial: The positive psychology of death acceptance. *Death Studies*, 35, 99–106.

Won, J., Alfini, A. J., Weiss, L. R., Michelson, C. S., Callow, D. D., Ranadive, S. M., ... Smith, J. C. (2019). Semantic memory activation after acute exercise in healthy older adults. *Journal of the International Neuropsychological Society*, 25(6), 557–568.

World Bank. (2023). Mortality rate, infant (per 1,000 live births). World Bank Open Data. https://data.worldbank.org

World Health Organization (WHO). (2003). Adherence to long-term therapies—Evidence for action. https://apps.who.int/medicinedocs/en/d/Js4883e/

World Health Organization (WHO). (2018a). HIV/AIDS. http://www.who.int/news-room/fact-sheets/detail/hiv-aids

World Health Organization (WHO). (2018). *Top ten causes of death, 2016*. Retrieved from https://www.who.int/en/news-room/fact-sheets/detail/the-top-10-causes-of-death

World Health Organization (WHO). (2020a). World immunization week. https://www.who.int/hiv/data/en/

World Health Organization (WHO). (2020b). Summary of the global HIV epidemic.

World Health Organization (WHO). (2023). Tuberculosis. https://www.who.int/news-room/fact-sheets/detail/tuberculosis

World Heart Federation. (2024). Cardiovascular health for everyone. https://world-heart-federation.org/

Wright, P. J., Tokunaga, R. S., Kraus, A., & Klann, E. (2017). Pornography consumption and satisfaction: A meta-analysis. *Human Communication Research*, 43, 315–343.

Wu, H., Ren, Q. Y., Tang, X., Zhang, H., Zhao, C. J., Yang, J. G., ... Zheng, J. (2020). Research progress of tea functional components in the prevention and treatment of lung cancer. *Food Therapy and Health Care*, 2(1), 12–23.

Wyatt, R. (2013). Pain and ethnicity. *AMA Journal of Ethics, Virtual Mentor*, 5, 449–454.

Xiang, B., Ming Wong, H. M., Perfecto, A. P., & McGrath, C. P. J. (2021) The application of theory-guided oral health interventions in adolescents: A systematic review and meta-analysis of randomized controlled trials. *Psychology & Health,* 36(7), 879–894.

Xiang, P., Geng, L., Zhou, K., & Cheng, X. (2017). Adverse effects and theoretical frameworks of air pollution: An environmental psychology perspective. *Advances in Psychological Science*, 25(4), 691–700.

Xia, N., & Li, H. (2018). Loneliness, social isolation, and cardiovascular health. *Antioxidants & Redox Signaling*, 28(9), 837–851.

Xu, J., Murphy, S., Kochanek, K., & Arias, E. (2022). *Mortality in the United States, 2021.* National Center for Health Statistics (U.S.).

Xu, J. Q., Murphy, S. L., Kochanek, K. D., & Arias, E. (2020a). Mortality in the United States, 2018. NCHS Data Brief, no. 355. National Center for Health Statistics.

Xu, X. Y., Zhao, C. N., Cao, S. Y., Tang, G. Y., Gan, R. Y., & Li, H. B. (2020b). Effects and mechanisms of tea for the prevention and management of cancers: An updated review. *Critical Reviews in Food Science and Nutrition*, 60(10), 1693–1705.

Yahr, E. (2018, June 5). Miss America eliminates swimsuit competition and won't judge contestants on physical appearance. https://www.washingtonpost.com/news/arts-and-entertainment/wp/2018/06/05/miss-america-eliminates-swimsuit-competition-and-wont-judge-contestants-on-physical-appearance/

Yamani Ardakani, B., Tirgari, B., & Roudi Rashtabadi, O. (2020). Body image and its relationship with coping strategies: The views of

Iranian breast cancer women following surgery. *European Journal of Cancer Care*, 29(1). https://doi.org/10.1111/ecc.13191

Yan, B. W., Arias, E., Geller, A. C., Miller, D. R., Kochanek, K. D., & Koh, H. K. (2023). Widening gender gap in life expectancy in the US, 2010–2021. *JAMA Internal Medicine.* https://doi.org/10.1001/jamainternmed.2023.6041

Yancy, C. W. (2020). COVID-19 and African Americans. *Journal of the American Medical Association.* https://doi.org/10.1001/jama.2020.6548

Yang, S., & Park, S. (2017). A sociocultural approach to children's perceptions of death and loss. *OMEGA-Journal of Death and Dying*, 76(1), 53–77. https://doi.org/10.1177/0030222817693138

Yang, Y. T., & Curlin, F. A. (2016). Why physicians should oppose assisted suicide. *Journal of the American Medical Association*, 315(3), 247–248. https://doi.org/10.1001/jama.2015.16194

Yanovski, S. Z., & Yanovski, J. A. (2021). Progress in pharmacotherapy for obesity. *JAMA,* 326(2), 129. https://doi.org/10.1001/jama.2021.9486

Yano, Y., Reis, J. P., & Colangelo, L. A. (2018). Association of blood pressure classification in young adults using the 2017 American College of Cardiology/American Heart Association blood pressure guideline with cardiovascular events later in life. *Journal of the American Medical Association*, 320, 1774–1782.

Yardley, L., Bradbury, K., Nadarzynski, T., & Hunter, C. (2019). Digital health psychology. In T. E. Revenson & R. A. R. Gurung (Eds.), *Handbook of health psychology* (pp. 519–525). Routledge.

Yeam, C. T., Chia, S., Tan, H. C. C., Kwan, Y. H., Fong, W., & Seng, J. J. B. (2018). A systematic review of factors affecting medication adherence among patients with osteoporosis. *Osteoporosis International*, 29(12), 2623–2637. https://doi.org/10.1007/s00198-018-4759-3

Yeary, K. H. C. K., Moore, P., Turner, J., Dawson, L., Heo, S., & Greene, P. (2018). Feasibility test of a community-relevant intervention designed to promote African American participation in translational, breast cancer disparities research: Know about Health Options for Women (Know HOW). *Journal of Cancer Education*, 33(1), 29–36.

Yi, Y., Liang, H., Jing, H., Jian, Z., Guang, Y., Jun, Z., ... Jian, L. (2020). Green tea consumption and esophageal cancer risk: A meta-analysis. *Nutrition and Cancer*, 72(3), 513–521.

Yodchai, K., Dunning, T., Savage, S., & Hutchinson, A. M. (2017). The role of religion and spirituality in coping with kidney disease and haemodialysis in Thailand. *Scandinavian Journal of Caring Sciences*, 31(2), 359–367. https://doi.org/10.1111/scs.12355

Yong, R. J., Mullins, P. M., & Bhattacharyya, N. (2021). Prevalence of chronic pain among adults in the United States. *Pain*, 163(2), e328–e332. https://doi.org/10.1097/j.pain.0000000000002291

Yoo, S. G. K., Chung, G. S., Bahendeka, S. K., Sibai, A. M., Damasceno, A., Farzadfar, F., ... Flood, D. (2023). Aspirin for secondary prevention of cardiovascular disease in 51 low-, middle-, and high-income countries. *JAMA: The Journal of the American Medical Association,* 330(8), 715. https://doi.org/10.1001/jama.2023.12905

Young, D. R., Hong, B. D., Lo, T., Inzhakova, G., Cohen, D. A., & Sidell, M. A. (2021). The longitudinal associations of physical activity, time spent outdoors in nature and symptoms of depression and anxiety during COVID-19 quarantine and social distancing in the United States. *Preventive Medicine*, 106863. https://doi.org/10.1016/j.ypmed.2021.106863

Young, K. (2014, October 1). Acupuncture shows little benefit in chronic knee pain. *NEJM Journal Watch.* http://www.jwatch.org/fw109356/2014/10/01/acupuncture-shows-little-benefit-chronic-knee-pain?query=pfw

Yu, H., Yang, T., Gao, P., Wei, X., Zhang, H., Xiong, S., ... Zhao, Y. (2016). Caffeine intake antagonizes salt sensitive hypertension through improvement of renal sodium handling. *Scientific Reports*, 6.

Yusef, S., Hawken, S., Ounpuu, S., Bautista, L., Franzosi, M. G., Commerford, P., ... INTERHEART Study Investigators. (2005). Obesity and the risk of myocardial infarction in 27,000 participants from 52 countries: A case–control study. *The Lancet*, 366, 1640–1649.

Yusuf, S., Joseph, P., Rangarajan, S., Islam, S., Mente, A., Hystad, P., Brauer, M., ... Dagenais, G. (2019). Modifiable risk factors, cardiovascular disease, and mortality in 155,722 individuals from 21 high-income, middle-income, and low-income countries (PURE): A prospective cohort study. *Lancet*, 395(10226), 795–808.

Zacher Kjeldsen, M.-M., Bricca, A., Liu, X., Frokjaer, V. G., Madsen, K. B., & Munk-Olsen, T. (2022). Family history of psychiatric disorders as a risk factor for maternal postpartum depression. *JAMA Psychiatry,* 79(10), 1004. https://doi.org/10.1001/jamapsychiatry.2022.2400

Zaitsu, M., Takeuchi, T., Kobayashi, Y., & Kawachi, I. (2020). Light to moderate amount of lifetime alcohol consumption and risk of cancer in Japan. *Cancer*, 2019. https://doi.org/10.1002/cncr.32590

Zander-Schellenberg, T., Collins, I. M., Miché, M., Guttmann, C., Lieb, R., & Wahl, K. (2020). Does laughing have a stress-buffering effect in daily life? An intensive longitudinal study. *PLoS One,* 15(7), e0235851.

Zehra, A., Burns, J., Liu, C. K., Manza, P., Wiers, C. E., Volkow, N. D., & Wang, G. J. (2019). Cannabis addiction and the brain: A review. *FOCUS, A Journal of the American Psychiatric Association*, 17(2), 169–182.

Zehra, S., Doyle, F., Barry, M., Walsh, S., & Kell, M. R. (2020). Health-related quality of life following breast reconstruction compared to total mastectomy and breast-conserving surgery among breast cancer survivors: A systematic review and meta-analysis. *Breast Cancer.* https://doi.org/10.1007/s12282-020-01076-1

Zeidman, A., Benedict, C., Zion, S. R., Fisher, S., Tolby, L., Kurian, A. W., ... Palesh, O. (2022). Association of illness mindsets with health-related quality of life in cancer survivors. *Health Psychology,* 41(6), 389–395. https://doi.org/10.1037/hea0001186

Zemore, S. E. (2017). Implications for future research on drivers of change and alternatives to Alcoholics Anonymous. *Addiction*, 112(6), 940–942.

Zengin, N., Oren, B., & Akinci, A. C. (2018). Perceived benefits and barriers of hypertensive individuals in salt-restricted diet. *International Journal of Caring Sciences*, 11(1), 488–501.

Zernike, K. (2018, April 2). "I can't stop": Schools struggle with vaping explosion. *New York Times.* https://nyti.ms/2H2goLp

Zhang, J., Fang, L., Wu, Y. W., & Wieczorek, W. F. (2013). Depression, anxiety, and suicidal ideation among Chinese Americans: A study of immigration-related factors. *Journal of Nervous and Mental Disease,* 201, 17–22. https://doi.org/10.1097/NMD.0b013e31827ab2e2

Zhang, J. G. (2020, February 28). Corona beer still struggling with confused consumers amid coronavirus fears. *Eater.* https://www.eater.com/2020/2/28/21157594/coronavirus-covid-19-corona-beer-confusion-continues

Zhang, X., Lan, T., Wang, T., Xue, W., Tong, X., Ma, T., ... Lu, Q. (2019). Considering genetic heterogeneity in the association analysis finds genes associated with nicotine dependence. *Frontiers in Genetics*, 10, 448. https://doi.org/10.3389/fgene.2019.00448

Zhao, Y.-J., Zhang, L., Feng, Y., Sha, S., Lam, M. I., Wang, Y.-Y., ... Xiang, Y.-T. (2023). Prevalence of depression and its association with quality of life among guardians of hospitalized psychiatric patients during the COVID-19 pandemic: A network perspective. *Frontiers in Psychiatry,* 14, 1139742. https://doi.org/10.3389/fpsyt.2023.1139742

Zhao, Y., Zhang, Q., Shah, C., Li, Q., Sweeney, J. A., Li, F., & Gong, Q. (2022). Cortical thickness abnormalities at different stages of the illness course in schizophrenia. *JAMA Psychiatry,* 79(6), 560. https://doi.org/10.1001/jamapsychiatry.2022.0799

Zheng, Y., Li, Y., Satija, A., Pan, A., Sotos-Prieto, M., Rimm, E., ... Hu, F. B. (2019). Association of changes in red meat consumption with total and cause specific mortality among US women and men: Two prospective cohort studies. *British Medical Journal*, 365.

Zhou, E. S., Michaud, A. L., & Recklitis, C. J. (2020). Developing efficient and effective behavioral treatment for insomnia in cancer survivors: Results of a stepped care trial. *Cancer*, 126(1), 165–173.

Zhou, E. S., Ritterband, L. M., Bethea, T. N., Robles, Y. P., Heeren, T. C., & Rosenberg, L. (2022). Effect of culturally tailored, internet-delivered cognitive behavioral therapy for insomnia in Black women. *JAMA Psychiatry,* 79(6), 538. https://doi.org/10.1001/jamapsychiatry.2022.0653

Zieman, M. (2021–2022). *Managing contraception for your pocket. Bridging the Gap Foundation.*

Zimmer, C. (2020, March 24). The virosphere is bigger than you can imagine. *New York Times*, p. D3.

Zimmer, M., Kumar, P., Vitak, J., Liao, Y., & Chamberlain Kritikos, K. (2020). "There's nothing really they can do with this information": Unpacking how users manage privacy boundaries for personal fitness information. *Information, Communication & Society*, 23(7), 1020–1037. https://doi.org/10.1080/1369118X.2018.1543442

Zink, M., & Englisch, S. (2016). Schizophrenia treatment: An obstacle course. *The Lancet Psychiatry*, 3(4), 310–312.

Zorn, J., Abdoun, O., Bouet, R., & Lutz, A. (2020). Mindfulness meditation is related to sensory-affective uncoupling of pain in trained novice and expert practitioners. *European Journal of Pain*. https://doi.org/10.1002/ejp.1576

Zucker, K. J. (2005a). Gender identity disorder in children and adolescents. *Annual Review of Clinical Psychology*, 1, 467–492.

Zucker, K. J. (2005b). Gender identity disorder in girls. In D. J. Bell, S. L. Foster, & E. J. Mash (Eds.), *Handbook of behavioral and emotional problems in girls (Issues in clinical child psychology)* (pp. 285–319). Kluwer Academic/Plenum Publishers.

Zullig, L. L., & Bosworth, H. (2017). Engaging patients to optimize medication adherence. *NEJM Catalyst*. https://catalyst.nejm.org/doi/full/10.1056/CAT.17.0489

Zulman, D. M., Haverfield, M. C., Shaw, J. G., Cati, G., Brown-Johnson, G., Schwartz, R., Tierney, A. A., ... Verghese, A. (2020). Practices to foster physician presence and connection with patients in the clinical encounter. *Journal of the American Medical Association*, 323, 70–81.

Zunhammer, M., Spisák, T., Wager, T. D., & Bingel, U. (2021). Meta-analysis of neural systems underlying placebo analgesia from individual participant fMRI data. *Nature Communications,* 12(1). https://doi.org/10.1038/s41467-021-21179-3

Index